Postgraduate
MEDICINE

Postgraduate MEDICINE

Volume 2

Editor-in-Chief

Gurpreet S Wander MD DM FACC FAMS

Professor and Head of Cardiology
Hero DMC Heart Institute
Dayanand Medical College and Hospital
Ludhiana, Punjab, India

Section Editors

PK Deb	Cardiology
SK Sharma	Clinical Medicine
Surinder K Jindal	Pulmonary Medicine
Ajay Kumar	Gastroenterology
Vivekanand Jha	Nephrology
Rohini Handa	Rheumatology
Jyotirmoy Pal	General Medicine
Gagandeep Singh	Neurology
Dhruva Chaudhry	Critical Care
Sanjay K Bhadada	Endocrinology
Bibhuti Saha	Infectious Diseases

Associate Editors

Rajesh Mahajan

NK Singh

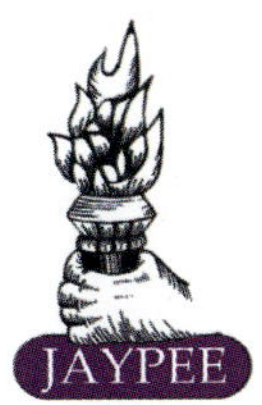

JAYPEE BROTHERS MEDICAL PUBLISHERS

The Health Sciences Publisher

New Delhi | London

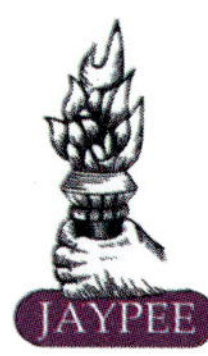

Jaypee Brothers Medical Publishers (P) Ltd

Headquarters
EMCA House
23/23-B, Ansari Road, Daryaganj
New Delhi 110 002, India
Landline: +91-11-23272143, +91-11-23272703
+91-11-23282021, +91-11-23245672
E-mail: jaypee@jaypeebrothers.com

Corporate Office
Jaypee Brothers Medical Publishers (P) Ltd.
4838/24, Ansari Road, Daryaganj
New Delhi 110 002, India
Phone: +91-11-43574357
Fax: +91-11-43574314
E-mail: jaypee@jaypeebrothers.com

Overseas Office
JP Medical Ltd.
83, Victoria Street, London
SW1H 0HW (UK)
Phone: +44-20 3170 8910
Fax: +44(0)20 3008 6180
E-mail: info@jpmedpub.com

Website: www.jaypeebrothers.com
Website: www.jaypeedigital.com

Postgraduate Medicine / *Gurpreet S Wander*

First Edition: **2022**

ISBN: 978-93-90595-46-4

Printed at: Sanat Printers

DEDICATED TO

Dr Harjit Singh

(1926–2018)

Professor and HOD Medicine
Government Medical College
Patiala, Punjab, India

"My father who taught me the value of hard work and integrity"

Dr BK Sharma

(1937–2021)

Professor and HOD Medicine
Postgraduate Institute of Medical Education and Research
Chandigarh, India

"My teacher in MD medicine from whom I learned bedside manners"

Dr SB Khurana

(1938–2011)

Professor and HOD Medicine
Dayanand Medical College Hospital
Ludhiana, Punjab, India

"Who taught me that practice of clinical medicine needs common sense and simple thinking"

Dr Siddharth N Shah

(1946–2021)

Past President API
Mumbai, Maharashtra, India

"From whom I learned how to work with others in a team with mutual respect"

Smt Raman Vij

(1957–2021)

W/o Sh Jitender Pal Vij and M/o Mr Ankit Vij
New Delhi, India

"Who was the driving force and inspiration for the Jaypee Brothers Medical Publishers (P) Ltd"

CONTRIBUTORS

VOLUME 2 (SECTION 5–8)

Section 5: Cardiology (Section Editor: PK Deb)

Abhishek Goyal MD DM
Associate Professor, Department of Cardiology, Hero DMC Heart Institute
Dayanand Medical College and Hospital
Ludhiana, Punjab, India

Ajay Bahl DM FRCP
Professor of Cardiology
Postgraduate Institute of Medical Education and Research
Chandigarh, India

Ajit S Mullasari MD DM DNB FRCP
Director and Head, Cardiology
Institute of Cardiovascular Diseases (ICVD), The Madras Medical Mission
Chennai, Tamil Nadu, India

Anita Saxena MD DM
Dean (Academics)
Chief, Cardio-Thoracic Centre
Professor and Head, Department of Cardiology, All India Institute of Medical Sciences, New Delhi, India

Ankita A Kulkarni MD
Senior Resident
Department of Cardiology
Seth GS Medical College and KEM Hospital
Mumbai, Maharashtra, India

Anunay Gupta MD DM
Assistant Professor
Department of Cardiology
Vardhman Mahavir Medical College and Safdarjung Hospital
New Delhi, India

Artur Lopes MD
Consultant Cardiologist, Cardiology Service, Hospital São Bernardo, Setúbal, Portugal

Arun Pulikkottil Jose MBBS MD
Senior Program Manager
Centre for Chronic Conditions and Injuries
Public Health Foundation of India
New Delhi, India

Aseem Basha MD
Senior Resident
Department of Cardiology
All India Institute of Medical Sciences
New Delhi, India

Ashutosh Yadav MD DM
Assistant Professor
Department of Cardiology
Vardhman Mahavir Medical College and Safdarjung Hospital
New Delhi, India

Balaji Arvind MD DM
Assistant Professor
Department of Cardiology
All India Institute of Medical Sciences
New Delhi, India

Bhupinder Singh MD DM
Associate Professor of Cardiology
Hero DMC Heart Institute
Dayanand Medical College and Hospital, Ludhiana, Punjab, India

Bishav Mohan MD DM
Professor of cardiology
Hero DMC Heart Institute
Dayanand Medical College and Hospital
Ludhiana, Punjab, India

Boban Thomas MD FRCPI
Consultant Cardiologist and Physician
Cardiology Division
Department of Medicine
University Hospital Kerry
Tralee, Republic of Ireland

Chitra Narasimhan MD DM
Associate Professor in Clinical Pediatric Cardiology, Sri Jayadeva Institute of Cardiovascular Sciences and Research
Bengaluru, Karnataka, India

CN Manjunath MD DM
Professor of Cardiology
Director, Sri Jayadeva Institute of Cardiovascular Sciences and Research
Bengaluru, Karnataka, India

Debabrata Roy MD DM FACC FSCI
Academic Coordinator and Senior Consultant Interventional Cardiologist
Rabindranath Tagore International Institute of Cardiac Sciences
Kolkata, West Bengal, India

Dorairaj Prabhakaran MD DM FRCP
Director, Centre for Control of Chronic Conditions (CCCC)
Professor, Epidemiology
Vice President - Research and Policy
Public Health Foundation of India (PHFI)
New Delhi, India

George Joseph MD DM
Professor, Department of Cardiology
Christian Medical College and Hospital
Vellore, Tamil Nadu, India

Gurpreet S Wander MD DM FACC FAMS
Professor and Head of Cardiology
Hero DMC Heart Institute
Dayanand Medical College and Hospital
Ludhiana, Punjab, India

Gurbhej Singh MD DM
Assistant Professor of Cardiology
Hero DMC Heart Institute
Dayanand Medical College and Hospital, Ludhiana, Punjab, India

Gurleen Kaur MBBS
Resident in Cardiology
Hero DMC Heart Institute
Dayanand Medical College and Hospital, Ludhiana, Punjab, India

Harikrishnan S MD DM
Professor
Department of Cardiology
Sree Chitra Tirunal institute for Medical Sciences and Technology
Thiruvananthapuram, Kerala, India

IB Vijayalakshmi MD DM DSc FAMS
Professor of Pediatric Cardiology
Super Specialty Hospital
Professor Emeritus
Bengaluru Medical College and Research Institute
Bengaluru, Karnataka, India

Jagat Narula MD PhD MACC
Professor of Cardiology
Icahn School of Medicine
Mount Sinai Health
New York, USA

Jasvinder Singh MD
DM Senior Resident
Department of Cardiology
Dayanand Medical College and Hospital
Ludhiana, Punjab, India

Jyotsna Maddury MD DM FACC
Professor of Cardiology
Nizam's Institute of Medical Sciences
Chief Editor of IJCDW
Secretary of WINCARS
Hyderabad, Telangana, India

Mandava Satya Sahitya MD
Fellow-Cardiology
Postgraduate Institute of Medical Education and Research
Chandigarh, India

Manish Bansal MD DNB FACC
Director Clinical and Preventive Cardiology, Medanta – The Medicity
Gurugram, Haryana, India

M Chenniappan MD DM
Senior Cardiologist, Ramakrishna Medical Centre and Apollo Speciality Hospital, Trichy
Adjunct Professor, The Tamil Nadu Dr MGR Medical University
Chennai, Tamil Nadu, India

Mohanan Padinhare MD DM
Director and HOD of Cardiology, Westfort Hi-Tech Hospital
Thrissur, Kerala, India

Navanil Biswas MD
Fellow In Cardiology
Rabindranath Tagore International Institute of Cardiac Sciences
Kolkata, West Bengal, India

Naved Aslam MD DM
Professor of Cardiology
Hero DMC Heart Institute
Dayanand Medical College and Hospital
Ludhiana, Punjab, India

Navjyot Kaur MD Med MRCP (UK) DNB
Fellow-Cardiology
Postgraduate Institute of Medical Education and Research
Chandigarh, India

Nazneen Ali MBBS MHA
Program Coordinator
Centre for Chronic Disease Control
New Delhi, India

Nirmal Ghati MD DM
Assistant Professor
Department of Cardiology
All India Institute of Medical Sciences
New Delhi, India

Nitish Naik MD DM
Professor of Cardiology
All India Institute of Medical Sciences
New Delhi, India

NN Khanna MD DM FRCP FACC
Senior Consultant Interventional Cardiology and Vascular Interventions
Department of Cardiology, Indraprastha Apollo Hospital, New Delhi, India

Prabhavathi MD DM
Professor of Cardiology
Sri Jayadeva Institute of Cardiovascular Sciences and Research
Bengaluru, Karnataka, India

Prafulla G Kerkar DM FACC FESC
Professor and Head of Cardiology
Seth GS Medical College and KEM Hospital, Mumbai, Maharashtra, India

Priya Chudgar DNB Radiodiagnosis FSCMR
Consultant Radiologist, Jupiter Hospital
Mumbai, Maharashtra, India

Rajeev Gupta MD PhD
Chair, Preventive Cardiology and Internal Medicine, Eternal Heart Care Centre and Research Institute
Jaipur, Rajasthan, India

Rajesh G Nair MD DM
Professor of Cardiology
Government Medical College
Kozhikode, Kerala, India

Rajesh Matta DM
Assistant Professor
Department of Cardiology
Seth GS Medical College and KEM Hospital
Mumbai, Maharashtra, India

Rajesh Vijayvergiya MD DM FACC
Professor of Cardiology
Advanced Cardiac Centre
Postgraduate Institute of Medical Education and Research
Chandigarh, India

Salil Jaura MD
DM Senior Resident
Dayanand Medical College and Hospital
Ludhiana, Punjab, India

Sandeep Bansal MD DM
Consultant, Professor and Head
Department of Cardiology
Vardhman Mahavir Medical College and Safdarjung Hospital
New Delhi, India

Sandeep Seth MD DM
Professor Cardiology
All India Institute of Medical Sciences
New Delhi, India

Sandhya Kamath MD
Former Dean, LTMG Hospital (Sion Hospital)
Former Dean, Seth GS Medical College and KEM Hospital
Mumbai, Maharashtra, India

Sanjay G MD DM
Additional Professor
Department of Cardiology
Sree Chitra Tirunal institute for Medical Sciences and Technology
Thiruvananthapuram, Kerala, India

Saurabh Dhumale MD
Fellow in Cardiology
Rabindranath Tagore International Institute of Cardiac Sciences
Kolkata, West Bengal, India

Shibba Takkar Chhabra MD DM
Professor of Cardiology
Hero DMC Heart Institute
Dayanand Medical College and Hospital, Ludhiana, Punjab, India

Smit Shrivastava MD DM FACC
Head, Department of Cardiology
Advanced Cardiac Institute
Pt J N M Medical College and Dr BRAM Hospital
Raipur, Chhattisgarh, India

Srinivasan Narayanan MD DNB FNB
Senior Consultant Cardiologist
Institute of Cardiovascular Diseases
The Madras Medical Mission Hospital
Chennai, Tamil Nadu, India

SS Kothari MD DM
Professor
Department of Cardiology
All India Institute of Medical Sciences
New Delhi, India

Sushant Mishra MD
Jr Consultant
Department of Cardiology
Indraprastha Apollo Hospital
New Delhi, India

Swati Singh MD
Jr Consultant
Department of Cardiology
Indraprastha Apollo Hospital
New Delhi, India

Thomas Alexander MD DM FACC
Senior Interventional Cardiologist
Head of Division of Cardiology
Kovai Medical Center and Hospital
Coimbatore, Tamil Nadu, India

Tiny Nair MD DM
Head of Cardiology
PRS Hospital
Thiruvananthapuram, Kerala, India

Ulhas Pandurangi MD DM
Chief, Department of Cardiac Electrophysiology and Pacing
Institute of Cardiovascular Diseases
The Madras Medical Mission Hospital
Chennai, Tamil Nadu, India

YP Munjal MD MAMS FRCP
Medical Director and Honorary Senior Consultant
Diabetes and Life Style Disease Center
Banarsidas Chandiwala Institute of Medical Sciences, New Delhi, India

Section 6: Endocrinology (Section Editor: Sanjay K Bhadada)

Aashima Dabas MD DM
Assistant Professor
Department of Pediatrics
Maulana Azad Medical College
New Delhi, India

Amit Agarwal MD DM
Professor and Head
Department of Endocrine Surgery
Sanjay Gandhi Postgraduate Institute of Medical Sciences
Lucknow, Uttar Pradesh, India

Anshita Aggarwal DM
Assistant Professor
Department of Endocrinology
Atal Bihari Vajpayee Institute of Medical Sciences and Dr RML Hospital
New Delhi, India

Ashu Rastogi MD DM
Associate Professor of Endocrinology
Postgraduate Institute of Medical Education and Research
Chandigarh, India

Avinash Patil MD DM
Assistant Professor
Department of Endocrinology
Sri Venkateswara Institute of Medical Sciences
Tirupati, Andhra Pradesh, India

Chirag Kamal Ahuja MD DM
Associate Professor
Department of Radiodiagnosis and Imaging, Postgratuate Institute of Medical Education and Research
Chandigarh, India

Kirti Gupta MD
Professor
Department of Histopathology
Postgraduate Institute of Medical Education and Research
Chandigarh, India

Liza Das MD DM
Research Scientist
Department of Endocrinology
Postgraduate Institute of Medical Education and Research
Chandigarh, India

Madhukar Mittal MD DM
Additional Professor
Department of Endocrinology
All India Institute of Medical Sciences
New Delhi, India

Manisha Sahay MD MAMS FICP
Professor and Head
Department of Nephrology
Osmania Medical College
Hyderabad, Telangana, India

Manjul Tripathi MS MCh
Associate Professor
Department of Neurosurgery
Postgraduate Institute of Medical Education and Research
Chandigarh, India

MK Garg MD DM
Professor and Head of Medicine and Endocrinology
All India Institute of Medical Sciences
New Delhi, India

Partha Pratim Chakraborty MD DM
Clinical Tutor, Department of Endocrinology and Metabolism,
Medical College Kolkata
Kolkata, West Bengal, India

Pinaki Dutta MD DM
Professor of Endocrinology
Postgraduate Institute of Medical Education and Research
Chandigarh, India

Rajat Gupta MD DM
Senior Consultant Endocrinology
Alchemist Hospital
Panchkula, Haryana, India

Rajesh Khadgawat MD DM FRCP
Professor of Endocrinology and Metabolism
All India Institute of Medical Sciences
New Delhi, India

Rakesh K Sahay MD DNB DM
Professor and Head
Department of Endocrinology
Osmania Medical College
Hyderabad, Telangana, India

Rama Walia MD DM
Associate Professor
Endocrinology and Metabolism
Postgraduate Institute of Medical Education and Research
Chandigarh, India

Ravinder Goswami MD DM
Professor
Department of Endocrinology
All India Institute of Medical Sciences
New Delhi, India

Rekha Ramot PhD
Research Scientist
Department of Endocrinology and Metabolism
All India Institute of Medical Sciences
New Delhi, India

Rekha Singh MD DM
Associate Professor
Department of Endocrinology
All India Institute of Medical Sciences
Bhopal, India

Rimesh Pal MD DM
Assistant Professor
Department of Endocrinology
Postgraduate Institute of Medical Education and Research
Chandigarh, India

Roma Pradhan MD DM
Assistant Professor and Head
Department of Endocrine Surgery
DR RML Institute of Medical Sciences
Lucknow, Uttar Pradesh, India

Sanjay K Bhadada MD DM FAMS
Professor and Head
Department of Endocrinology
Postgraduate Institute of Medical Education and Research
Chandigarh, India

Soham Mukherjee MD DM
Assistant Professor, Department of Endocrinology, Postgraduate Institute of Medical Education and Research
Chandigarh, India

Sri Venkata Madhu DM
Professor and Head
Department of Endocrinology
University College of Medical Sciences
University of Delhi, New Delhi, India

Subhankar Chowdhury MD DM
Professor and Head, Department of Endocrinology and Metabolism
Institute of Postgraduate Medical Education and Research/SSKM Hospital, Kolkata, West Bengal, India

Suneel Mattoo Mch
Resident of Endocrine Surgery
Sanjay Gandhi Postgraduate Institute of Medical Sciences
Lucknow, Uttar Pradesh, India

Suresh Vaikkakara MD DM FRCP
Professor of Endocrinology
Sri Venkateswara Institute of Medical Sciences, Tirupati, Andhra Pradesh, India

Surya K Singh MD DM
Professor of Endocrinology and Metabolism, Banaras Hindu University
Varanasi, Uttar Pradesh, India

Sushil Gupta MD DM
Professor of Endocrinology
Sanjay Gandhi Postgraduate Institute of Medical Sciences
Lucknow, Uttar Pradesh, India

Vahid Bharmal MD DM
Senior Resident
Department of Endocrinology and Metabolism, Institute of Medical Sciences, Banaras Hindu University
Varanasi, Uttar Pradesh, India

Section 7: Gastroenterology (Section Editor: Ajay Kumar)

Abhideep Chaudhary MBBS MS
Senior Director and HOD
Department of HPB and Liver Transplantation, BLK Super Speciality Hospital, New Delhi, India

Ajay Duseja MD DM FAMS
Professor and Unit Head
Department of Hepatology
Postgraduate Institute of Medical Education and Research
Chandigarh, India

Ajay Kumar MD DM
Chairman
BLK Liver and Digestive Diseases Institute, New Delhi, India

Ajit Sood MD DM
Professor and Head
Department of Gastroenterology
Dayanand Medical College and Hospital
Ludhiana, Punjab, India

Akash Roy MD DM
Senior Resident, Department of Hepatology, Postgraduate Institute of Medical Education and Research
Chandigarh, India

Amit Kumar Dutta MD DM
Professor of Gastroenterology
Christian Medical College and Hospital
Vellore, Tamil Nadu, India

Amrish Sahney DM
Senior Consultant
Institute of Digestive and Liver Diseases
BLK Hospital, New Delhi, India

Anil Kumar Mannava MD DNB
Consultant Hepatologist
Yashoda Hospitals
Hyderabad, Telangana, India

Anoop Saraya MBBS MD DM
Professor and Head, Department of Gastroenterology and Human Nutrition Unit, All India Institute of Medical Sciences, New Delhi, India

Anshuman Elhence MD DM
Advanced GI Fellow
Department of Gastroenterology
All India Institute of Medical Sciences
New Delhi, India

Anupam Kumar Singh MD DM
Assistant Professor, Department of Gastroenterology, Postgraduate Institute of Medical Education and Research, Chandigarh, India

Anuraag Jena MD DM
Senior Resident
Department of Gastroenterology
Postgraduate Institute of Medical Education and Research
Chandigarh, India

Archita Makharia MBBS MD
Junior Resident
Department of Medicine
Mahatma Gandhi Hospital
Jodhpur, Rajasthan, India

Arka De MD DM
Assistant Professor
Department of Hepatology
Postgraduate Institute of Medical Education and Research
Chandigarh, India

Arshdeep Singh MD DM
Assistant Professor
Department of Gastroenterology
Dayanand Medical College and Hospital
Ludhiana, Punjab, India

Ashish Chauhan MD DM
Assistant Professor
Department of Gastroenterology
Indira Gandhi Medical College
Shimla, India

Bimal Kumar Sahu MD DM
Consultant Gastroenterology and Hepatobiliary Sciences
Fortis Hospital, Shalimar Bagh
New Delhi, India

Dharmesh Kapoor MD DM MRCP
Consultant Hepatologist
Yashoda Hospitals
Hyderabad, Telangana, India

D Nageshwar Reddy MD DM DSc FAMS FRCP FASGE FACG AGAF FJGES
Chairman and Chief
Department of Gastroenterology
Asian Institute of Gastroenterology
Hyderabad, Telangana, India

Gaurav Sood MBBS MS DNB
Senior Consultant
Department of HPB and Liver Transplantation
BLK Super Speciality Hospital
New Delhi, India

Govind K Makharia MD DM
Professor of Gastroenterology and Human Nutrition
All India Institute of Medical Sciences
New Delhi, India

Harshad Devarbhavi MD DNB DM
Head, Department of Gastroenterology and Hepatology
St. John's Medical College Hospital
Bangaluru Karnataka, India

Kaushal Madan MBBS MD DNB DM
Director and Head
Gastroenterology and Hepatology
Max Smart Super Speciality Hospital
New Delhi, India

Mahesh K Goenka MD DM FACG
Director and Head
Department of Gastroenterology
Apollo Gleneagles Hospital
Kolkata, West Bengal, India

Mallikarjun Patil MD DM
Professor of Gastroenterology
Department of Gastroenterology and Hepatology
St John's Medical College Hospital
Bengaluru, Karnataka, India

Manav Wadhawan MD DM
Director, Institute of Liver and Digestive Diseases
Head, Hepatology and Liver Transplant, BLK Super Speciality Hospital, New Delhi, India

Mohan Ramchandani MD DM
Director of Interventional Endoscopy
AIG Hospitals
Hyderabad, Telangana, India

Neha Berry MD DM
Consultant
Institute of Digestive and Liver Diseases
BLK Hospital
New Delhi, India

Pankaj Puri MD DNB DM FRCP
Director Gastroenterology and Hepatology, Fortis Escorts Liver and Digestive Diseases Institute
New Delhi, India

Pradev Inavolu MD DM
Consultant Gastroenterologist
AIG Hospitals
Hyderabad, Telangana, India

Pramod Kumar Garg MD
Professor of Gastroenterology
All India Institute of Medical Sciences
New Delhi, India

Rakesh Kochhar MD DM
Professor
Department of Gastroenterology
Postgraduate Institute of Medical Education and Research
Chandigarh, India

Rupjyoti Talukdar MD FICP
Director, Pancreas Clinic
Asian Institute of Gastroenterology
Head, Pancreas Research Group
Asian Healthcare Foundation
Hyderabad, Telangana, India

Sanjay Khanna MD DNB
Associate Director
Institute of Digestive and Liver Diseases, BLK Super Speciality Hospital
New Delhi, India

Saurabh Kedia MBBS MD DM
Assistant Professor
Department of Gastroenterology
All India Institute of Medical Sciences
New Delhi, India

Shalimar MD DM
Additional Professor
Department of Gastroenterology
All India Institute of Medical Sciences
New Delhi, India

Shekhar Singh Jadaun MD DM
Gastroenterologist Hepatologist
Max Super Speciality Hospital Saket
New Delhi, India

Shivanand Gamanogatti MD
Professor in Radio Diagnosis
Department of Radiology
All India Institute of Medical Sciences
New Delhi, India

Shivaraj Afzalpurkar MBBS MD
Registrar of Gastroenterology
Apollo Gleneagles Hospital
Kolkata, West Bengal, India

Shobna Bhatia MD DM
Director Motility, Department of Gastroenterology and Hepatobillary Sciences, Sir HN Reliance Hospital, Former prof of Gastroenterology, KEM Hospital, Mumbai, Maharashtra, India

Soumya Jagannath Mahapatra MD DM
Assistant Professor
Department of Gastroenterology
All India Institute of Medical Sciences
New Delhi, India

Srikant Mohta DM
Senior Resident
Department of Gastroenterology and Human Nutrition Unit
All India Institute of Medical Sciences
New Delhi, India

Subrat K Acharya MD DM
Executive Director
Department of Gastroenterology
Fortis Escorts Liver and Digestive Diseases Institute, New Delhi, India

Sudheer K Vuyyuru MD DM
Fellow in Inflammatory Bowel Diseases
Department of Gastroenterology
All India Institute of Medical Sciences
New Delhi, India

Sunil Taneja MD DM
Associate Professor, Department of Hepatology, Postgraduate Institute of Medical Education and Research
Chandigarh, India

Uday C Ghoshal MD DM FRCP
Professor of Gastroenterology
Sanjay Gandhi Postgraduate Institute of Medical Sciences
Lucknow, Uttar Pradesh, India

Usha Goenka MBBS MD
Director and Head
Department of Radiology
Apollo Gleneagles Hospital
Kolkata, West Bengal, India

Vandana Midha MD
Professor of Medicine
Dayanand Medical College and Hospital
Ludhiana, Punjab, India

Vineet Ahuja MBBS MD DM
Professor of Gastroenterology
All India Institute of Medical Sciences
New Delhi, India

Section 8: Hematology and Oncology

Afaq Ahmad Khan MD DNB
Assistant Professor of Clinical Hematology, Sher-i-Kashmir Institute of Medical Sciences
Srinagar, Jammu and Kashmir, India

Davinder Paul MD DM
Assistant Professor of Medical Oncology
Dayanand Medical College and Hospital, Ludhiana, Punjab, India

Hari Krishan Dhawan MD
Associate Professor
Department of Transfusion Medicine
Postgraduate Institute of Medical Education and Research
Chandigarh, India

Manjinder Singh MBBS MD
Consultant Radiation Oncology
Dayanand Medical College and Hospital
Ludhiana, Punjab, India

Nabhajit Mallik MD DM
Assistant Professor
Department of Hematology
Postgraduate Institute of Medical Education and Research
Chandigarh, India

Pankaj Malhotra MD FRCP
Professor
Clinical Hematology
Department of Internal Medicine
Postgraduate Institute of Medical Education and Research
Chandigarh, India

Pooja Prasad MD DM
Assistant Professor
Department of Hematology
VMMC and Safdarjung Hospital
New Delhi, India

Prashant Sharma MD DNB DM
Additional Professor
Department of Hematology
Postgraduate Institute of Medical Education and Research
Chandigarh, India

Preethi Jeyaraman MD DM
Associate Consultant
Department of Hematology and Bone Marrow Transplant
Max Super Speciality Hospital
Saket, New Delhi, India

Pulkit Rastogi MD DM
Assistant Professor
Department of Histopathology
Postgraduate Institute of Medical Education and Research
Chandigarh, India

Ratti Ram Sharma MD
Professor and Head Department of Transfusion Medicine, Postgraduate Institute of Medical Education and Research, Chandigarh, India

Reena Das MD DNB
Professor and Head
Department of Hematology
Postgraduate Institute of Medical Education and Research
Chandigarh, India

Subhadeep Bose MD DM MRCP
Consultant
Department of Medical Oncology
The Royal Wolverhampton
United Kingdom

Suchet Sachdev MD
Associate Professor
Department of Transfusion Medicine
Postgraduate Institute of Medical Education and Research
Chandigarh, India

Sujith Kumar Mullapally MD DNB DM (Medical Oncology)
Consultant
Division of Medical Oncology
Apollo Proton Cancer Centre
Chennai, Tamil Nadu, India

Tushar Sehgal MD DM
Assistant Professor of Laboratory Medicine (Hematology)
All India Institute of Medical Sciences
New Delhi, India

Vijayalakshmi Aravindan Arun MD
Senior Resident
Clinical Hematology
Department of Internal Medicine
Postgraduate Institute of Medical Education and Research
Chandigarh, India

CONTENTS

VOLUME 1

SECTION 1: CLINICAL MEDICINE

SECTION 2: GENERAL MEDICINE

GENERAL TOPICS

GERIATRICS

SECTION 3: INFECTIOUS DISEASES

BASIC CONSIDERATIONS

BACTERIAL INFECTIONS

VIRAL INFECTIONS

CORONAVIRUS INFECTION

OTHER INFECTIONS

SECTION 4: CRITICAL CARE

VOLUME 2

SECTION 5: CARDIOLOGY

SECTION 7: GASTROENTEROLOGY

VOLUME 3

SECTION 9: NEPHROLOGY

SECTION 10: NEUROLOGY

SECTION 11: PULMONARY MEDICINE AND TUBERCULOSIS

SECTION 12: RHEUMATOLOGY

Free Online Resources

1. **E-version of the book chapters:** Kindly refer to the back side of the front cover to redeem the scratch code on http://www.emedicine360.com **and access the E-version.** All the chapters in the printed version can be accessed online.

2. **MCQs:** Each chapter in the printed book is followed by 5–10 MCQ's. These MCQ's have 4–5 options and one correct answer. They are from the contents of the chapter. You are advised to solve these after reading the whole chapter.

   In order to access MCQs in the E-version, kindly click the link given at the end of each chapter on www.emedicine360.com.

3. **E-Chapters:** Free elaborated E-version of the following 6 chapters is available on http://www.emedicine360.com
   - e-15 (CH-15): Chest X-ray Evaluation and Some Spotters
   - e-23 (CH-23): Electronic Health Records, Artificial Intelligence, and Big Data—Role in Medicine
   - e-38 (CH-38): Prevention and Management of Infection in Transplant Recipients
   - e-48 (CH-48): Other Virus Infections—Chikungunya, Hantavirus, Nipah Virus, and Zika Virus
   - e-88 (CH-88): Noninvasive Cardiac Imaging
   - e-118 (CH-118): Endocrine Tumors and Malignancies

4. **Videos:** Some of the chapters have videos. These videos can be accessed online in respective chapters.
   - ch-28: Falls in Elderly
   - ch-89: Cardiac Catheterization and Coronary Angiography
   - ch-185: Seizures and Epilepsy
   - ch-193: Movement Disorders: The Clinical Vignette

CHAPTER 85

Clinical Evaluation of Cardiac Patients

Prabhavathi, Bhupinder Singh

ABSTRACT

Due to huge advancement of modern technology, the diagnosis of the patient these days is largely based on investigations. Although it is necessary to adopt modern scientific advances, it is also advisable to retain the time-honored and valuable basic bed-side clinical cardiology skills. This chapter emphasizes on the clinical approach to the patient with cardiovascular disorders and is divided under two sections: History taking and clinical examination. Skillful use of "low technology" (including the cardiac history and physical examination) leads to intelligent and cost-effective use of "high technology".

"It is much more important to know what sort of a patient has a disease than what sort of disease a patient has"

—William Osler

INTRODUCTION

In present times, investigations help in the easy and fast diagnosis of cardiovascular disorders. During the 70s and 80s, diagnoses were largely based on bed-side clinical skills. Even in the present era of advanced technologies, the bed-side clinical evaluation guides clinicians to make diagnostic algorithm to reach at the final diagnosis.

A vast majority of the cardiovascular disease can still be diagnosed based on the "five fingers" approach by Dr W Proctor Harvey which included meticulous clinical history, physical examination, electrocardiogram (ECG), chest roentgenogram, and appropriate laboratory investigation. When appropriately performed, the bed-side clinical cardiovascular examination is an accurate and cost-effective method to find the structural abnormalities and their severity, and thereby planning the additional investigations needed.

Clinical assessment of the patient has two integral components: History taking and clinical examination (**Fig. 1**). Accurate history taking plays a crucial role in the assessment of patients and clinical examination follows history taking.

CLINICAL HISTORY

When a patient with confirmed or probable cardiac disease visits a physician, the clinical history taking is the first and foremost step in the assessment. The symptoms associated with cardiac illness are mentioned in the **Figure 1**.

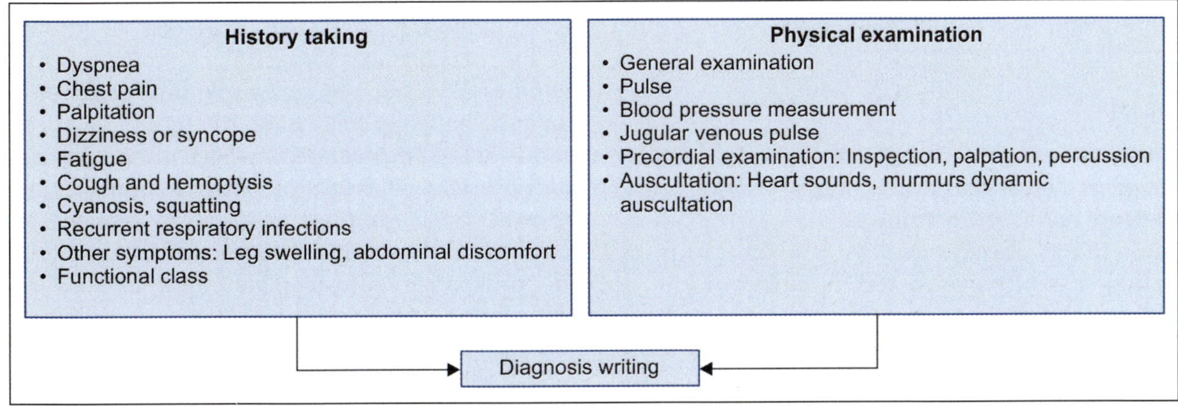

FIGURE 1: Stepwise evaluation of a cardiac patient.

BOX 1	Cardiac causes of dyspnea.
• Left heart failure	
• Acquired valvular heart disease	
• Coronary artery disease (CAD)	
• Hypertensive heart disease	
• Cardiomyopathy	
• Congenital heart disease	

DYSPNEA

Dyspnea is often referred to as "difficult, labored, and uncomfortable breathing", "awareness of respiratory distress", or uncomfortable sensation of breathing". Exertional dyspnea can be of cardiac or noncardiac origin. Therefore, it is considered less specific for cardiac ailment unless it is associated with other corroborative evidence on history and physical examination. Cardiac causes of dyspnea are tabulated in **Box 1**.

If the dyspnea is associated with orthopnea or paroxysmal nocturnal dyspnea (PND), the likelihood of underlying cardiac illness is on the left side and should lead the physician to search for various causes of pulmonary venous hypertension such as mitral stenosis (MS) and left ventricular failure (LVF).

Orthopnea: It is defined as the type of postural dyspnea that occurs when the patient is in recumbent posture and is relieved in sitting. It usually occurs after 1–2 minutes of acquiring the recumbent posture. It occurs due to increased venous return to the failing heart while in recumbent posture that causes rise in left atrial and pulmonary capillary pressure; and additionally due to elevation of diaphragm (while in supine) compromising the vital capacity of the lung.

Paroxysmal nocturnal dyspnea: It is defined as development of distressing dyspnea at night that wakes the patient from sleep. It is relieved by sitting upright and the patient often feels to get air at an open window. It usually occurs 3–4 hours after sleep and takes about half an hour to get relief. The mechanisms described for PND include: (1) Redistribution of fluid from the interstitial space to intravascular space causing the increased blood volume, (2) decreased sympathetic drive during sleep, (3) respiratory depression at night due to high vagal tone, and (4) other mechanisms like nocturnal arrhythmias.

CHEST PAIN

Chest pain is one of the cardinal symptoms of cardiology. It could be of cardiac or noncardiac origin. Various causes of chest pain are described in **Table 1**.

TABLE 1 Causes of chest pain.		
Cardiovascular	**Noncardiac**	**Sudden onset chest pain**
• Coronary artery disease (CAD) • Aortic dissection • Acute pericarditis • Pulmonary embolism (PE) • Aortic aneurysm (local compression) • Left ventricular outflow tract obstruction (LVOTO)	• Pleuritis • Costochondritis (Tietze syndrome) • Gastroesophageal disease • Herpes zoster • Esophageal rupture • Esophageal spasm	• Acute myocardial infarction (AMI) • Pneumothorax • Aortic dissection • PE • Esophageal rupture

Angina is felt as chest heaviness, pressure, burning, or squeezing. It is often retrosternal with radiation to or isolated discomfort in neck, jaw, shoulders, or arms (frequently left). It is precipitated by exertion, emotion, after eating heavy meals, or exposure to cold etc., and relieved by rest or taking sublingual nitrates. Chest pain can be classified as typical angina, atypical angina, and nonangina chest pain (**Table 2**). *Levine test* is relief of angina by carotid massage. If angina occurs only during first significant activity of the day, it is referred to as *"warm-up angina or first effort angina"*; due to no preconditioning. In patients with known obstructive coronary artery disease (CAD), if gastroesophageal reflux precipitates typical angina it is called as *"linked angina"*.

TABLE 2	Clinical classification of chest pain.
Typical angina	If patient meets three of the following features: i. Retrosternal chest pain ii. Provoked by exertion or emotional stress iii. Relieved by taking rest and/or sublingual nitroglycerine
Atypical angina	Meets two of the above features
Nonanginal chest pain	Meets one or none of the above features

The typical pattern of chest pain in common conditions is described in **Flowchart 1**.

PALPITATION

Abnormal awareness of one's own heartbeat is defined as palpitation. It can be felt as "missed" or "dropped" beats by the patients having atrial or ventricular premature ectopics (APCs or VPCs). Palpitations occur either due to sudden change in heart rate, rhythm, force of contraction, or due to volume overloading of ventricles. Its exacerbation with exertion or excessive caffeine should be highlighted as well. Fast irregular palpitation typically occurs in atrial fibrillation (AF). Rapid regular palpitation occurs in paroxysmal supraventricular tachycardia (SVT) or ventricular tachycardia (VT). Certain cardiac conditions having volume overloading of left ventricle (LV) such as mitral regurgitation (MR), aortic regurgitation (AR) cause palpitations that increase on exertion (exertional palpitations).

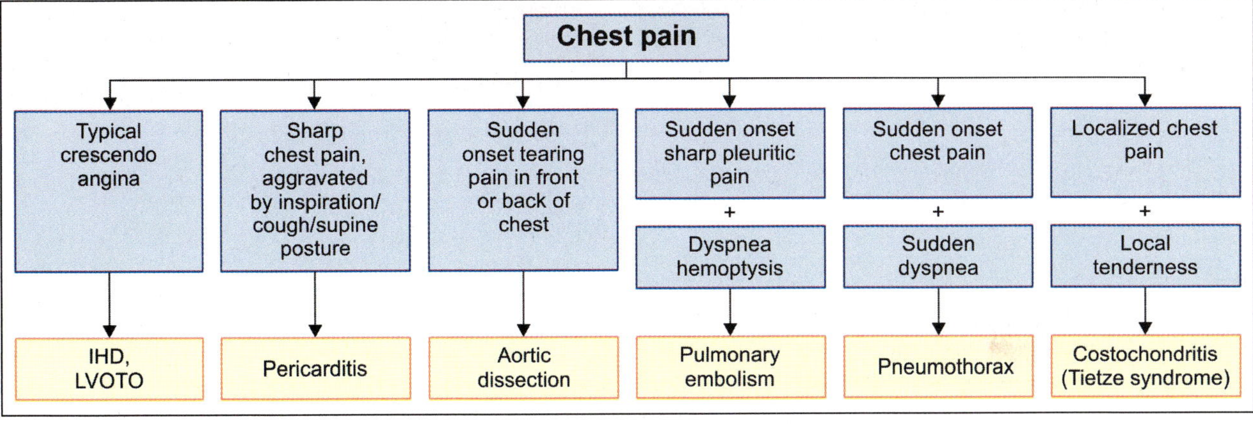

(IHD: ischemic heart disease; LVOTO: left ventricular outflow tract obstruction)

FLOWCHART 1: **Evaluation of chest pain according to its character and associations.**

BOX 2	Causes of syncope.
Cardiac causes of syncope	
Arrhythmic causes	
• Complete heart block (CHB)	
• Sick sinus syndrome (SSS)	
• Ventricular tachycardia (VT)	
Mechanical causes	
• Left ventricular outflow tract obstruction (LVOTO)	
• Left atria (LA) tumor or thrombus	
• Pulmonary embolism	
• Cyanotic spell	
• Pulmonary stenosis (PS)	
• Pulmonary hypertension (PHT)	
Non cardiac causes of syncope	
Hypovolemia	
Reflex mediated	
• Vasovagal	
• Situational	
Orthostatic hypotension	
Drug induced	
Neurological	
• Transient ischemic attack	
• Migraine	
• Seizure	
• Subclavian steal	

DIZZINESS AND SYNCOPE

Syncope is defined as the transient loss of consciousness due to cerebral hypoperfusion with rapid recovery. The causes of syncope are mentioned in **Box 2**.

"Stokes-Adams attack" is the self-limiting episode of syncope primarily described with atrioventricular blocks, but also seen with VT/fibrillation.

TABLE 3 **Various patterns of cyanosis and special subtypes of central cyanosis.**

Types of cyanosis	Site of cyanosis	Causes
Peripheral cyanosis	Only at peripheries such as fingers, toes, and lips	Heart failure and cold exposure
Central cyanosis	Both mucosa (mouth mucosa) and periphery	Cyanotic congenital heart diseases (CHDs), Eisenmenger syndrome, chronic obstructive pulmonary disease (COPD), and hemoglobinopathies
Special subtypes of central cyanosis		
Differential cyanosis	Lower limb cyanosis more than upper limb	Patent ductus arteriosus (PDA) with Eisenmenger syndrome, and interrupted aortic arch with PDA
Reverse differential cyanosis	Upper limb cyanosis more than lower limb	Transposition of great arteries with severe pulmonary arterial hypertension (PAH) with PDA, or transposition of the great arteries (TGA) with interrupted aortic arch and PDA

FATIGUE

Exertional fatigue is an important symptom of cardiac disorders with low cardiac output state such as heart failure, MR, and some of the right-sided cardiac disorders such as tricuspid valve (TV) disease, right ventricular (RV) dysfunction, pulmonary stenosis (PS), and pulmonary hypertension (PHT).

COUGH AND HEMOPTYSIS

Cough and hemoptysis can be important symptoms in conditions such as pulmonary edema, pulmonary embolism (PE) (due to peripheral wedge infarcts), and MS. Cough due to heart disease most often is dry and nonproductive. It is noted in the recumbent position and nocturnally.

BOX 3 Mechanism of lower respiratory tract infection (LRTI) in cardiac shunt lesions.

- Plethoric lung fields creating the nidus for infection
- Decreased mucociliary clearance
- Decreased immunity due to malnutrition and hypercatabolic state
- Atelectasis

TABLE 4 Other symptoms some time present in cardiac disorders.

Symptom	Causes
Fever with chills and night sweats	Infective endocarditis (IE; in predisposed heart valves)
Low grade fever	PE, AMI, and pericarditis
Right hypochondrial pain and epigastric fullness	Right-sided heart diseases such as TV disease, right heart failure
Gastrointestinal bleeding	Colonic angiodysplasia in aortic stenosis (Heyde syndrome) and anticoagulation-induced coagulopathy
TIA or stroke or limb ischemia	Thromboembolism in patients with AF or thrombosed prosthetic valves, severe LV dysfunction with cavity clot

CYANOSIS AND SQUATTING

Cyanosis is defined as the bluish discoloration of skin and mucous membrane that occurs due to increased concentration of deoxygenated hemoglobin level (at least >5 g/dL). Various causes and its patterns are described in **Table 3**.

RECURRENT RESPIRATORY INFECTIONS

Recurrent lower respiratory tract infection (LRTI) refers to two or more hospitalizations in 6 months or three hospitalizations for RTI in any time frame. It is usually seen in significant cardiac shunt lesions [atrial septa defect (ASD)/ventricular septal defect (VSD)/patent ductus arteriosus (PDA)] or congenital mitral valve (MV) diseases. The reasons for recurrent LRTI are described in **Box 3**.

OTHER SYMPTOMS

Various other symptoms giving indirect clues to the underlying cardiac illness are described in **Table 4**.

FUNCTIONAL CLASS

The functional class of a patient with underlying cardiac illness can be assessed by using New York Heart Association (NYHA) classification (**Table 5**).

The NYHA is a subjective classification of the functional class of cardiac patients. It helps in providing the prognostic information and assesses the treatment response at follow-up.

TABLE 5 New York Heart Association (NYHA) classification for dyspnea, palpitation, fatigue, and angina.

Class I	No symptoms with ordinary physical activity
Class II	Symptoms with ordinary activity, slight limitation of physical activity
Class III	Symptoms with less than ordinary activity. Marked limitation of activity
Class IV	Symptoms with any physical activity or even at rest

CLINICAL EXAMINATION

Clinical examination in a cardiovascular patient should not be limited to auscultation alone due to scarcity of time as most of the clues come from a stepwise physical examination. The components of examination are tabulated in **Figure 1**.

GENERAL PHYSICAL EXAMINATION

General appearance: Examination should be conducted in a warm, private, and quite area. Daylight or adequate artificial light is preferred. At initial step, quick assessment of the patient's illness and the level of distress are made. Start observing the patient from head to toe for relevant findings (**Table 6**).

Dysmorphic features should also be taken into account in order to look for syndromic associations. Some of the syndromes with typical dysmorphic features have been tabulated in **Table 7**.

Pulse: It is defined as the waveform felt by the fingers, produced by the ejection of blood into the arterial system, which traverses the arterial tree at a rate much faster than that of blood column. Therefore, it is the direct reflection of the physiological or pathological hemodynamic alterations produced by heart and blood vessels. Commonly felt pulses are radial, femoral, dorsalis pedis, popliteal, carotid, and brachial. Various abnormalities in arterial pulse are described in **Table 8**.

Pulse deficit (apex-pulse deficit) is the number of heart beats which are not conducted to the periphery. A deficit of >10 beats per minute is usually seen in AF while <10 beats per minutes indicates ventricular premature complexes (VPCs) or atrial premature complexes (APCs).

Character of the arterial pulse gives clues to the underlying cardiac illnesses. Normal arterial waveform and some of the typical characters of the pulse are described in **Figure 2**.

Hyperkinetic pulse is a high amplitude pulse with a rapid rise (large volume and wide pulse pressure). It is seen in anemia, fever, beriberi, and other high output states. *Collapsing pulse* is seen in AR, PDA, and ruptured sinus of Valsalva (RSOV). The rapid upstroke (due to large stroke volume) followed by the rapid downstroke (due to rapid run-off into the LV across the regurgitating aortic valve and decreased peripheral resistance) gives

TABLE 6 Some clinical signs on general physical examination.

Signs	Site	Interpretation/Associated cardiac conditions
Pallor	Lower palpebral conjunctiva, tongue, nails, and palmar crease	Anemia
Icterus	Sclera, mucosa, and skin	Jaundice
Cyanosis	Refer to symptom section	
Mitral facies	Cyanotic or dusky pink discoloration on bilateral upper cheeks	Severe MS with PH
Systemic embolism	Cold and bluish discoloration of limbs	MS
Xanthoma/Xanthelasma	On medial side of eyelids	Dyslipidemia
Earlobe crease	Diagonal crease on the ear lobule (Frank's sign)	Association with CAD
Lymphadenopathy	Cervical/axillary/groin	Infective pathology
Clubbing	Nails of hands or toes	Cyanotic CHD
Splinter hemorrhages	Under the nail bed	Infective endocarditis
Osler nodes	Painful erythematous lesions of the hands and feet	
Janeway lesion	Nontender, small, erythematous, or hemorrhagic macular lesion on palm and sole	
Polyarthritis	Migratory involvement (tender and swollen) of large joints	Acute rheumatic fever
Erythema marginatum	Skin rash on trunk and limbs	
Subcutaneous nodules	Painful nodules on the extensor surfaces of joints and bony prominences	

(CAD: coronary artery disease; CHD: congenital heart disease; MS: mitral stenosis; PH: pulmonary hypertension)

TABLE 7 Dysmorphic features characterizing syndromes having cardiac lesions.

Syndrome	Dysmorphic features	Cardiovascular lesions
Marfan syndrome	Tall, thin individual with a wide-arm span, long spider-like fingers, hyperextensible joints, high-arched palate, and dislocated lenses	Myxomatous mitral valve (MV) disease, aortic aneurysm, and dissection
William syndrome	Elfin face (short philtrum, short/flat nose bridge, and wide set eyes), small retrusive jaws, short stature, over friendly, and music lover	Supravalvular aortic stenosis (AS) and peripheral pulmonary stenosis (PPS)
Down's syndrome	Broad flat face, slanting eyes, epicanthic eye fold, flat back of head, big wrinkled tongue, dental anomalies, short/broad hands	Primum atrial septal defect (ASD), ventricular septal defect (VSD), atrioventricular canal defect, tetralogy of Fallot (TOF)
Noonan syndrome	Webbed neck, maloccluded teeth, short stature, typical chest deformity, and low set nipples	Hypertrophic obstructive cardiomyopathy (HOCM), PS, and ASD
Ellis-Van Creveld syndrome	Polydactyly, teeth abnormalities, and dystrophic nails	Common atrium
Turner syndrome	Short stature and infertility	Coarctation of aorta, bicuspid aortic valve (BAV), and AS
Alagille syndrome	Prominent forehead, deep set eyes, bulbous nose tip, pointed chin	PS, TOF, and PPS
Holt–Oram syndrome	Atriodigital dysplasia and aplasia/hypoplasia of digitals or radius	ASD
Congenital rubella syndrome	Microcephaly, cataract, and purpura	Patent ductus arteriosus (PDA) and pulmonary stenosis (PS)

TABLE 8	The abnormalities of pulse.	
Rate	Bradyarrhythmias	Sinus bradycardia, atrioventricular (AV) blocks, sick sinus syndrome (SSS), and drug induced
	Tachyarrhythmias	Sinus tachycardia, heart failure, and drug induced
Rhythm	Regular	Normal sinus rhythm
	Regularly irregular	Atrial tachycardia with fixed AV block, ventricular bigeminy or trigeminy
	Irregularly irregular	Atrial fibrillation, frequent atrial premature complexes (APCs) and ventricular premature complexes (VPCs), and atrial tachycardia with variable AV block
Volume	Low (pulse pressure <30 mm Hg)	Heart failure and cardiogenic shock
	High (pulse pressure >60 mm Hg)	Anemia, fever, beriberi, thyrotoxicosis, and aortic regurgitation (AR)
Character	Discussed elsewhere in the text	
Radio-femoral or radio-radial delay	Delay between radial and femoral pulse	Coarctation of aorta and aortoarteritis
Vessel wall	Palpable or nonpalpable	Calcified wall due to atherosclerosis will be palpable

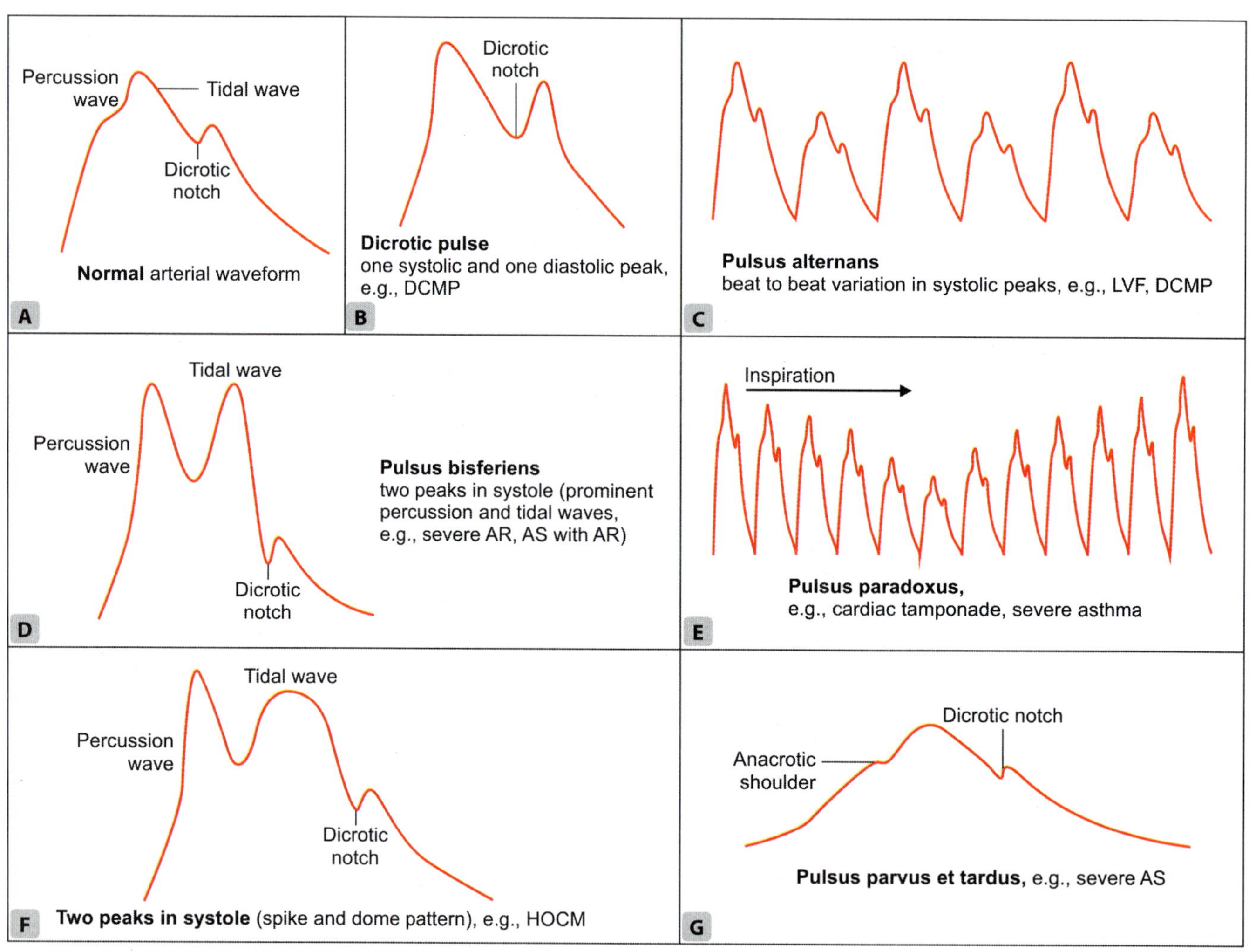

(AR: aortic regurgitation; AS: aortic stenosis; DCMP: dilated cardiomyopathy; HOCM: hypertrophic obstructive cardiomyopathy; LVF: left ventricular failure)

FIGURES 2 A to G: Graphic demonstration of characters of arterial pulse.

it a collapsing character; also known as Corrigan's or water hammer pulse. In *bisferiens pulse,* the first systolic peak occurs due to rapid ejection of large stroke volume (percussion wave) followed by another exaggerated reflected wave (tidal wave) from the peripheral high resistance circulation.

Anacrotic or pulsus parvus et tardus pulse is defined as low amplitude (parvus) and slow rising pulse (tardus): Occurs in fixed left ventricular outflow tract (LVOT) obstruction. *Pulsus bigeminus* is felt as coupled pulses of different strength due to occurrence of VPC followed by compensatory pause seen in digitalis toxicity. In *pulsus paradoxus,* there is exaggerated inspiratory fall in systolic blood pressure (SBP) of >10 mm Hg during quit breathing: Seen in cardiac tamponade and acute severe asthma. Reverse pulsus paradoxus is seen in hypertrophic obstructive cardiomyopathy (HOCM) and intermittent positive pressure ventilation.

Blood pressure: *Measurement technique*: Patient should be sitting or lying comfortably for at least 10 minutes prior to measurement. Patient should avoid smoking, caffeine, exercise, or tea half an hour prior to measurement. The appropriate cuff size should be applied at least 1 inch above the cubital fossa. The required bladder length and breadth should be 75–100% and 37–50% of the mid-arm circumference of the patient. Inflate the cuff 20–30 mm Hg above the palpatory equivalent of SBP and deflate the cuff 2 mm Hg/second listen for Korotkoff sounds (**Table 9**).

Blood pressure (BP) should be measured in all the limbs to look for disparity of BP. A BP disparity of >10 mm Hg between both upper limbs and >20 mm Hg between upper and lower limbs is considered significant. Measuring the lower limb BP can identify coarctation of aorta or other aortoiliac occlusive diseases.

Hill sign refers to the BP difference of >20 mm Hg between the upper and lower limbs. It was described to demonstrate the severity of AR. According to Hill sign, AR can be categorized as mild (20–40 mm Hg), moderate (40–60 mm Hg), or severe (>60 mm Hg).

Auscultatory gap is a silence that sometimes occurs after the first appearance of Korotkoff sounds and the second reappearance of sounds. It overestimates diastolic BP (DBP) and underestimates SBP. It usually occurs if there is venous congestion or reduced velocity of arterial flow to the extremities.

Jugular venous pulse: It is the direct reflection of right heart hemodynamics. It is seen in right internal jugular vein (IJV) as it is in straight line with superior vena cava (compared to left vein) and it does not contain valves (compared to external jugular vein). It is defined as the top oscillating level of blood column in the right IJV.

Method of measurement: Jugular venous pulse (JVP) is measured with patient sitting or reclining at an angle of 45° (or 30° if JVP is low). The neck is slightly turned to the left of the patient in order to visualize the oscillating column of the blood. A light source is put from the right shoulder towards the mid sternum at approximately 45° angle to the sagittal plane. A measuring scale is kept horizontally from the top oscillating level of IJV blood column towards the sternal angle. Another scale is kept vertically from sternal angle so that it intersects the horizontally placed scale. The vertical distance between sternal angle and the point of intersection of two scales is the JVP. This is then added to obligatory 5 cm [this is the vertical height of sternal angle from mid-right atrium (RA)] to get the mean RA pressure in cm of water. Upper limit of normal JVP is 4 cm of water and it corresponds to 6 mm Hg. Various types of abnormal JVPs are described in the **Figure 3**. The "a" wave and hence "x" descent is absent in AF.

Abdominojugular reflux or hepatojugular reflux (AJR/HJR): After making the patient position steady, firm pressure is applied at periumbilical area for 10–30 seconds while the patient is breathing quietly. Normally, jugular venous pressure rises by <3 cm of water and that too transiently while the abdominal pressure is maintained. On the contrary, in patient with raised right or left heart failure, the jugular venous pressure remains elevated for >15 seconds. A positive AJR is observed in RV systolic and/or diastolic dysfunction, TV disease, or chronic constrictive pericarditis (CCP).

Kussmaul's sign is defined as the paradoxical increase in the jugular venous pressure during inspiration. Normally, there is inspiratory decrease in the JVP. Kussmaul's sign is seen in CCP, restrictive cardiomyopathy (RCMP), RV failure, and RV infarction. It occurs due to inability of the right heart to accommodate the inspiratory increase in venous return.

TABLE 9	Korotkoff sounds.
Phase I	It is the first clear, tapping sound (represents systolic BP)
Phase II	Tapping sound is replaced by murmur
Phase III	Murmur becomes louder
Phase IV	Muffling of sound (represents diastolic BP in AR, pregnancy, and arteriovenous fistula)
Phase V	Disappearance of sounds (represents diastolic BP)

PRECORDIAL EXAMINATION

INSPECTION

Inspection should start with the chest inspection from the side or foot end of the patient. Salient points are tabulated in **Table 10**.

PALPATION

The pulsations of the heart and blood vessels are felt by the fingertips or area of the hand just proximal to that. The palpable sounds are described in the **Figure 4**.

Thrills are the vibratory sensations that are palpable manifestation of loud and harsh murmurs having low-to-medium frequencies. It is best appreciated with the flat of the hand or the fingers. Thrill can be systolic [aortic stenosis (AS), MR, and PS] or diastolic (MS).

Carotid shudder is the vibration felt on the carotid at the peak systole in AS.

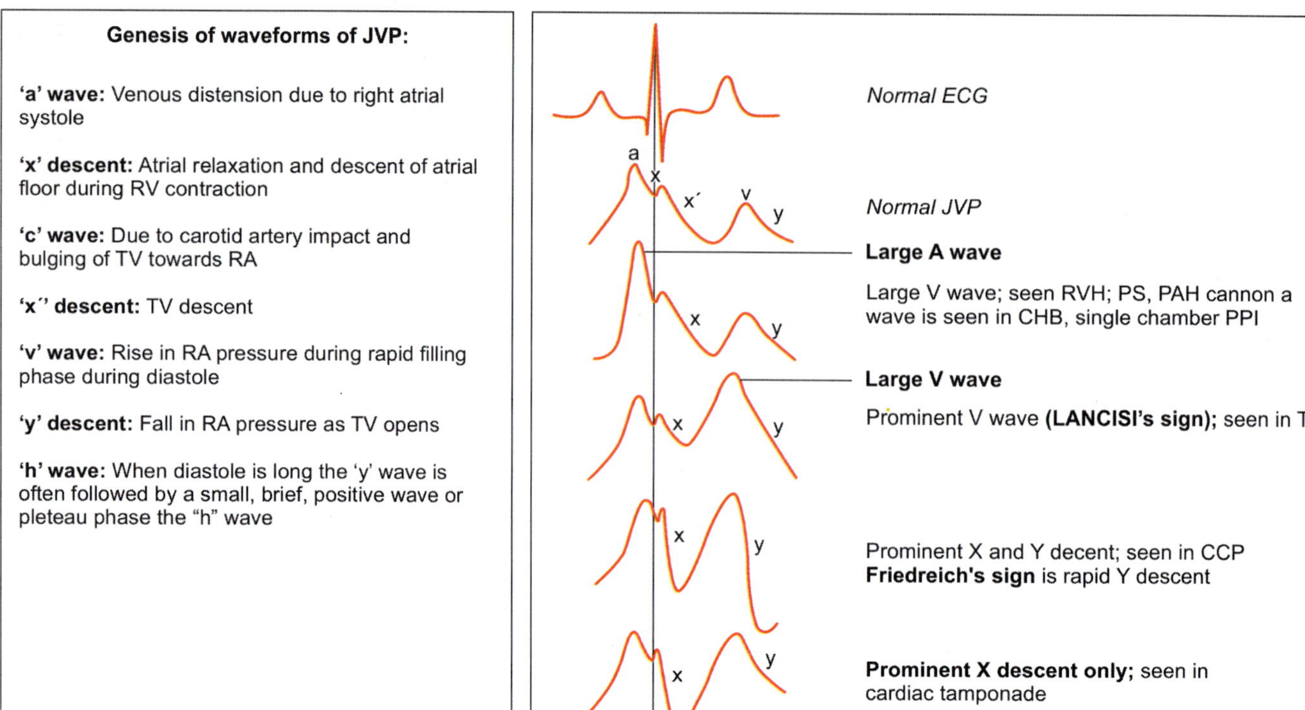

FIGURE 3: Normal waveform of JVP and its abnormalities.

TABLE 10	Various chest abnormalities on inspection.	
Shape	Pectus excavatum (cobbler's chest), pectus carinatum, kyphosis, scoliosis, and shield chest	Turner/Noonan syndrome, cor pulmonale, ankylosing spondylitis, Marfan syndrome, and other connective tissue disorders
Respiration	Rate and pattern	Tachypnea and Cheyne–Stokes breathing
Scar marks	Midline (coronary artery bypass grafting, valve replacements, and open mitral valvotomy), left thoracotomy (PDA ligation and closed mitral valvotomy), and right thoracotomy (ASD)	
Dilated veins	Venus channels on the anterior chest wall	Superior vena cava (filling from below) or inferior vena cava (filling from above) obstruction
Suprasternal pulsations	Abnormal pulsation seen in suprasternal notch	AR, aortic aneurysm, PDA, coarctation of aorta, and hyperdynamic states
Left parasternal pulsation	Right ventricular origin	RVH and MR
Apical pulsation	Left ventricular origin	LVH
Left 2nd ICS	Pulmonary artery	Pulmonary hypertension and idiopathic dilatation of main pulmonary artery

AUSCULTATION

The bell and diaphragm of the stethoscope allow the appreciation of various type of normal/abnormal sound or prolonged vibration (murmur) of varying frequency. **Table 11** and **Figure 5** describe various sounds and murmurs.

HEART SOUNDS

First heart sound (S1): The heart sound coincident with closure of the atrioventricular valves produced by vibration of the entire cardiohemic apparatus at the onset of ventricular systole. It has two components: M1 (mitral) and T1 (tricuspid). The characters and abnormalities of S1 are tabulated in **Box 4** and **Table 12**, respectively.

Normally M1 and T1 are 20–30 ms apart. Split S1 is heard in Ebstein's anomaly (sail sound), tricuspid stenosis (TS), and ASD. The first heart sounds is important in MS and MR. The mechanism of the difference in intensity and its variations in MS and MR are shown in **Box 5**.

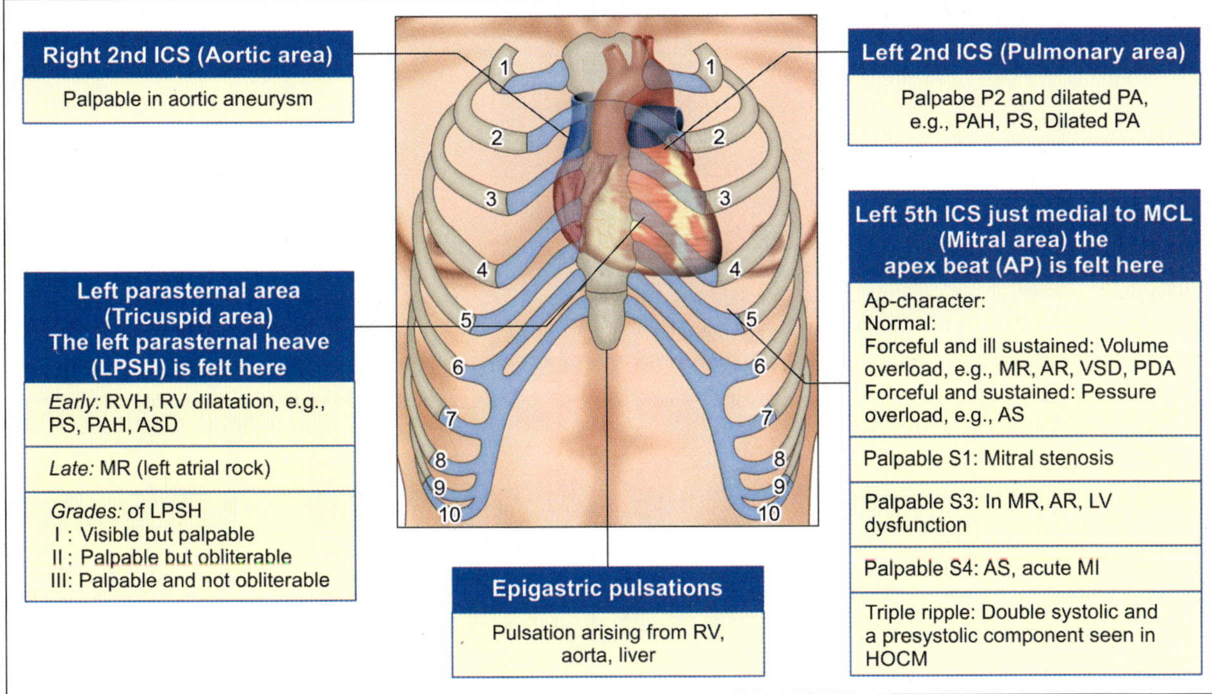

(AP: apex phonocardiogram; ICS: intercostal space; MCL: midclavicular line)

FIGURE 4: Palpatory findings on clinical cardiac examination.

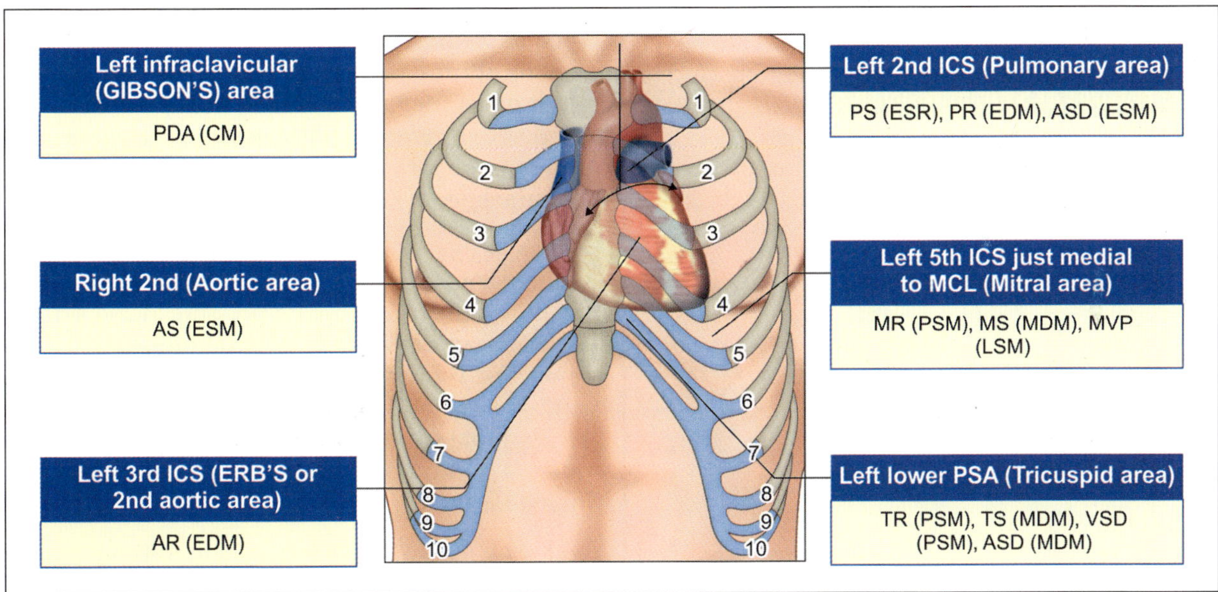

(CM: continuous murmur; LSM: late systolic murmur)

FIGURE 5: Cardiac murmurs according to the area of examination.

TABLE 11 Classifying auscultatory findings according to their frequencies.

	Low frequency	High frequency	Mixed frequency
Heart sounds	S3 and S4	S1 and S2	
Murmurs	Mid-diastolic (MS)	Early diastolic (AR and PR) and pansystolic (MR)	Ejection systolic (AS)
Added sounds	-	Pericardial knocks, opening snap, systolic clicks, and tumor plops	-

(AR: aortic regurgitation; AS: aortic stenosis; PR: pulmonary regurgitation; MR: mitral regurgitation; MS: mitral stenosis)

TABLE 12 Causes of abnormal S1.

Accentuated S1	Attenuated S1	Variable intensity of S1
• Exercise • MS/LA myxoma • Tricuspid stenosis/RA myxoma • Ebstein's anomaly (sail sound) • Hyperkinetic states • Sinus tachycardia (short PR interval) • Thin chest wall • Holosystolic MVP • AV groove calcification in CP (external MS)	• Sinus bradycardia • Prolonged PR interval (>200 ms) • LV dysfunction • Severe MR • Acute severe AR • Acute MI • Calcific MV • Emphysematous chest • Large pericardial effusion	• AF • CHB • VT with AV dissociation • Wenckebach phenomenon (bruit de canon) • Pulsus alternans (auscultatory alternans) • LA myxoma (postural)

(AF: atrial fibrillation; AR: aortic regurgitation; AV: atrioventricular; CHB: complete heart block; CP: constrictive pericarditis; LA: left atrial; LV: left ventricular; MI: myocardial infarction; MR: mitral regurgitation; MS: mitral stenosis; MV: mitral valve; MVP: mitral valve prolapse; RA: right atrial; VT: ventricular tachycardia)

BOX 4 Features of normal S1.

- Occurs 50–60 ms after electrical onset of ventricular systole
- Frequency 100–120 Hz
- Coincides with carotid upstroke
- M1-T1 separated by 20–30 ms
- M1 coincides with downstroke of LA "c" wave and T1 with RA "c" wave
- Best heard with diaphragm at apex
- T1 is usually localized to right LSB

(LA: left atrial; LSB: left sternal border RA: right atrial)

BOX 5 Features of S1 in mitral valve diseases.

Mitral stenosis

Mechanism of loud S1 in MS

- MV wide open at end diastole due to ↑ LA pressure
- Delayed closure of MV–M1 and T1 fuse
- MV closes during the high pressure of the ventricular dP/dt curve
- Thickened but pliable leaflets

When S1 can be soft in pressure of MS

- Heavily calcified valve
- Associated significant MR
- Associated severe AR
- LV dysfunction
- Prolonged PR interval (rheumatic carditis)

Mitral regurgitation

Mechanism of soft S1 in MR

- Loss of isovolumetric systole
- Fibrosis of leaflets
- Destruction of leaflets (endocarditis)
- LV dysfunction (secondary MR)
- Carditis (prolonged PR interval)

Causes of loud/normal S1 in MR

- Associated significant MS
- MVP

(AR: aortic regurgitation; LA: left atrial; MR: mitral regurgitation; MS: mitral stenosis; MV: mitral valve; MVP: mitral valve prolapse)

BOX 6 Feature of normal S2.

- Frequency 120–150 Hz
- Two components, the A2 and P2 coincide with the respective arterial dicrotic incisura
- Correlates with the downstroke of the carotid pulse
- During expiration, A2-P2 are separated by an interval of <30 ms
- Physiological split on inspiration
- Normal P2 is softer than A2 and localized to the base

Second heart sound (S2): The heart sound produced due to abrupt closure of the semilunar valves at the onset of ventricular diastole. This is produced by sudden deceleration of retrograde flow of blood column in the aorta and pulmonary artery (PA). The characters and various abnormalities of S2 are tabulated in **Boxes 6** and **7**.

Hangout interval: It is the time interval for which the pulmonary valve (PV) remains open even after the RV pressure equalizes to the PA pressure at end systole or it is the time gap between the arterial pressure curve and the respective ventricular pressure curve (PA to RV or aorta to LV) at the level of incisura. Hangout interval is <15 ms on aortic side and 40–85 ms on pulmonary side. Hangout interval is more on right side due to highly compliant pulmonary bed.

Wide and fixed S2 split: It occurs in ASD, total anomalous pulmonary venous connection (TAPVC), partial anomalous pulmonary venous connection (PAPVC), massive PE with RV failure, and severe pulmonary arterial hypertension (PAH) with RV failure.

- RV or LV stroke volume remains unchanged with inspiration
- There is a similar degree of alteration in LV/RV filling with inspiration
- Failure of the RV to augment its stroke volume during inspiration
- RV systole is substantially prolonged [e.g., right bundle branch block (RBBB) with RV failure]

In ASD, the split is wide due to maximal increase in pulmonary capacitance (hangout interval), so that no further increase occurs during inspiration and it is fixed

BOX 7	Causes of abnormal S2.
Single S2	
• Single semilunar valve (truncus arteriosus and absent PV)	
• Atresia of semilunar valve (pulmonary or aortic atresia)	
• Equal LV/RV ejection time (VSD Eisenmenger)	
• Inaudible P2 (d-TGA and dysplastic PV)	
• Masking A2 (extremely loud P2)	
Wide split S2	
Delay in P2	
• Delayed electrical activation of RV (right bundle branch block and LV pacing)	
• Prolonged RV mechanical systole (acute massive PTE and PAH with RV failure)	
• Increased pulmonary hangout interval (normotensive ASD, postoperative ASD, idiopathic PA dilatation, and early A2)	
• Shortened LV mechanical systole (MR and VSD)	
• Early electrical activation of LV (type A Wolff–Parkinson–White syndrome)	
• Other causes (straight back syndrome)	
Wide fixed split S2	
• ASD	
• Total or partial anomalous pulmonary venous connection (TAPVC or PAPVC)	
• Massive PE with RV failure	
• Severe PAH with RV failure	

(d-TGA: dextro-transposition of the great arteries; PTE: pulmonary thromboembolism)

since the phasic changes in systemic venous return with respiration are associated with reciprocal changes in the volume of L→R shunting.

Narrow split of S2: It occurs in PAH without RV failure.

Reversed S2 split: In this case, S2 split is heard in expiration and it narrows down or becomes single during inspiration. It occurs either due to delayed A2 (left bundle branch block, LVOT obstruction, PDA, and poststenotic dilatation of aorta) or due to early P2 [type-B Wolff–Parkinson–White (WPW) syndrome].

Intensity of S2 is determined by pressure beyond the valve, flow across the valve, size of the vessel beyond the valve, stenosis or regurgitation of the valve, and the chest wall transmission. The abnormalities in intensity of the two components of S2 are shown in **Table 13**.

Second heart sound (S2) is given lot of importance in congenital heart disease. It is best heard in left 2nd intercostal space. It can have various abnormalities in second heart sounds. The various types of S2 in acyanotic and cyanotic congenital heart diseases are described in **Box 8**.

TABLE 13 Causes of abnormal intensity of second heart sound (S2).

A2 component of S2	P2 component of S2
Loud A2 • Aortic root dilatation, e.g., syphilitic AR (bruit de tambour), ascending aortic aneurysm • Coarctation of aorta • Systemic hypertension • Relatively anterior placement of aorta, e.g., d-TGA and tetralogy of Fallot (TOF)	Loud P2 • Increased flow into MPA, e.g., hyperkinetic PH, ASD, and TAPVC • Dilatation of pulmonary trunk, e.g., ASD and IDPA • Increased pressure in pulmonary artery, e.g., PAH, and peripheral PS • Straight back syndrome
Soft A2 • Aortic stenosis (valvar/ supravalvular) • Masking of A2 by loud P2	Soft P2 • Pulmonic stenosis • TOF (low pressure in PA) • Dysplastic PV • Normotensive PR

(d-TGA: dextro-transposition of the great arteries; IDPA: idiopathic dilatation of pulmonary artery; TAPVC: total anomalous pulmonary venous connection; TGA: transposition of great arteries)

Third heart sound (S3): It is also known as ventricular/ protodiastolic gallop and is produced during rapid filling phase; therefore it correlates with "y" descent on JVP. S3 is produced during excessive rapid inflow of blood into a ventricle with normal/increased compliance or normal filling of a ventricle with decreased compliance. S3 indicates ventricular dilatation and systolic dysfunction with left ventricular end-diastolic pressure (LVEDP) > 25 mm Hg and cardiac index <2.0 L/min/m^2. There is increased velocity of MV inflow and short isovolumetric relaxation time (IVRT) which on Doppler is seen as tall E wave. The features of normal S3, LV S3, and RV S3 are shown in **Box 9** and the causes of S3 are shown in **Box 10**.

Fourth heart sound (S4): It is also known as atrial gallop or presystolic gallop. It occurs when artia contracts forcibly against a noncompliant ventricle, therefore it correlates with "a" wave in JVP. Unlike S3, the S4 is usually pathological when heard. It may be heard normally in some elderly. Some useful diagnostic points of the presence of S4 in various diseases are as follows. The presence of S4 in AS indicates a severe AS. It is present in all cases of HOCM. The presence of S4 rules out significant MS in multivalvular disease. The features, hemodynamic correlates and causes S4 are shown in **Box 11**.

ADDED SOUNDS

Opening snap: Opening snap (OS) is the sound generated due to the sudden early diastolic buckling of mitral or tricuspid leaflet due to elevated left or right atrial pressure. Its causes include MS and TS. In MS, OS is best heard between

BOX 8	Importance of second heart sound in congenital heart disease.
Acyanotic CHD	
• Wide fixed split in ASD	
• Wide variable split in large VSD	
• Loud A2 in a patient with VSD may indicate associated coarctation, PDA, BAV, AR, or TGA	
• Normal or paradoxical split in PDA	
Cyanosis with normal S2	
• Normally split S2 in a cyanotic patient is extremely rare and may indicate rare causes of cyanosis such as:	
◦ Pulmonary AV fistula	
◦ Persistent LSVC → LA	
◦ Abnormal IVC → LA connection	
◦ Methemoglobinemia	
Cyanosis with wide-fixed S2	
• TAPVC	
• Common atrium	
• ASD Eisenmenger	
• Ebstein's anomaly (RBBB)	
• ASD with preferential streaming	
• Absent coronary sinus with left SVC → LA connection (Raghib syndrome)	
• Severe PS or PPH with R → L shunt across PFO and RV failure	
Cyanosis with single loud P2	
• TOF and related conditions	
• Pulmonary atresia	
• d-TGA and L-TGA	
• Single ventricle	
• Truncus arteriosus	
• Tricuspid atresia	
• VSD Eisenmenger	
S2 in Eisenmenger syndrome	
• *ASD*: Narrow and fixed split	
• *VSD*: Single loud	
• *PDA*: Narrow physiological split	
• *TAPVC, common atrium*: Narrow and fixed	
• *TGA*, single ventricle: Single loud S2	

(AV: atrioventricular; BAV: bicuspid aortic valve; d-TGA: dextro-transposition of the great arteries; LA: left atrial; LSVC: left superior vena cava; L-TGA: levo-transposition of the great arteries; PPH: postpartum hemorrhage; TAPVC: total anomalous pulmonary venous connection)

BOX 9	The features of third heart sound (S3).
Features of normal S3	
• Low pitch sound	
• Best heard with bell	
• Localized sound	
• Normal S2–S3 gap is 120–160 ms	
• Early S3 is usually pathological	
LV-S3	
• At apex	
• Let lateral position	
• Increase with isometric handgrip a/w left heart failure	
RV-S3	
• At LSB	
• Better in inspiration	
• Increase with leg raising a/w rapid "y" descent in JVP	

(JVP: jugular venous pulse; LSB: left sternal border)

BOX 10	The causes of S3.
• Physiological, e.g., pregnancy and children	
• LV or RV failure	
• Acute MI	
• Dilated cardiomyopathy	
• AR	
• MR/TR	
• Left to right shunts	
• Ebstein's anomaly	

mitral and tricuspid area and A2-OS gap in inversely related to the severity of MS.

Ejection click: It can be of either vascular (due to dilated aorta or PA) or valvular (as in valvular AS or PS) origin. Pulmonary ejection click (EC) is the only right-sided event that accentuates during expiration.

Mid-systolic clicks: These are heard in mitral valve prolapse (MVP), tricuspid valve prolapse (TVP), and interatrial septal aneurysm.

Pericardial knock: It occurs due to abrupt halt to the early diastolic filling in CCP.

Tumor plop: It is a diastolic sound heard in RA or LA myxomas which are mobile and have a long pedicle.

Prosthetic sound: In mitral prosthesis, the opening sound corresponds to OS and closing sound to S1. In aortic prosthesis, the opening sound corresponds to EC and closing sound to S2.

HEART MURMURS

A murmur is defined as relatively prolonged series of audible vibrations characterized by the timing in cardiac cycle, intensity (loudness), frequency (pitch), quality, configuration, duration, and direction of radiation. According to Levine and Freeman grading, systolic murmurs have VI grades and diastolic have IV grades. Grade I being very soft to grade IV having thrill and up to grade VI being heard even with stethoscope slightly away from chest wall. The characters and causes of various murmurs are described in **Box 12**.

Dynamic auscultation: It refers to the change in hemodynamics of the heart by physiological or pharmacological maneuvers, and their effects on cardiac sounds and murmurs. These maneuvers are respiration, Valsalva, postural changes, and isometric exercise.

Respiration: All the events arising from the right side of the heart except the pulmonary EC get accentuated with deep inspiration (Carvallo's sign). AR murmur is better heard in deep expiration and leaning forward. Aortic EC is not affected by respiration except when it is associated with TOF with pulmonary atresia. S2 split is better appreciable in inspiration.

Valsalva maneuver: During phase II, the S3 and S4 are attenuated and S2 split narrows. All the murmurs get

BOX 11	Features, hemodynamic correlates, and causes of S4.
Features of S4	
• Low pitch sound	
• LV S4 usually localized to apex, while RV S4 widely heard	
• "Tennessee" sound	
• LV S4 accentuated by isometric handgrip	
• RV S4 accentuated by inspiration and passive leg raising	
Hemodynamic correlates of S4	
• Indicates nondilated and noncompliant ventricle	
• Diastolic dysfunction	
• LVEDP > 15 mm Hg	
• Sinus rhythm	
• Prominent "a" wave with E/A reversal on Doppler	
Causes of S4	
• In elderly	
• Systemic or pulmonary hypertension	
• AS/PS	
• HOCM	
• RCMP	
• AMI	
• Acute MR/AR	

(LVEDP: left ventricular end-diastolic pressure; RCMP: restrictive cardiomyopathy)

BOX 12	Characteristics and causes of various cardiac murmurs according to timing in the cardiac cycle.
Systolic	
Ejection (mid) systolic	
• Crescendo-decrescendo; begins after S1 and ends perceptibly before S2	
• Innocent and physiological	
• Outflow tract obstruction: AS, PS, and HOCM	
• Accelerated flow: ASD (pulmonary flow), pregnancy, and fever thyrotoxicosis	
Early systolic	
• Decrescendo; begins with S1, diminishes in and ends well before S2	
• Heard in acute severe MR, low pressure TR, and tiny muscular VSD	
Late systolic	
• Begins in mid to late systole and reaches up to S2	
• Heard in MVP	
Holosystolic	
• Begins with S1 and occupies all of systole till S2 on its side of origin	
• Heard in MR, high pressure TR, and restrictive VSD	
Diastolic	
Early-diastolic	
• Decrescendo; starts with A2/P2 and ends variably into diastole	
• Chronic AR (long, pure, high frequency, loud, and blowing type)	
• Hypertensive	
• In pulmonary regurgitation the EDM is called as Graham Steell murmur	
Mid-diastolic	
• Start well after S2	
• Heard in MS, TS, and in PR without PAH	
• Other examples are Austin flint murmur of AR, Rytand murmur in CHB and Carey coombs murmur of ARF and flow murmurs due to left-to-right shunt	
Continuous	
• Begins in systole and continues without interruption through S2 into variable part of diastole	
• Heard in aortopulmonary connections such as PDA, AP window, and aortopulmonary collaterals	
• Also heard in arteriovenous connections and RSOV. May be heard in Lautenbacher syndrome also	
• Differentiate murmurs due to flow disturbance in arteries and venous hum from a continuous murmur	

(AP: apex phonocardiogram; ARF: acute rheumatic fever; RSOV: ruptured sinus of Valsalva)

diminished except for MVP (clicks comes early with increased duration and intensity of murmur) and HOCM (accentuated murmur). In ASD, MS or heart failure, Valsalva maneuver produces a square wave sign in which all the phases are negated and thereby their auscultatory equivalents are also abolished.

Postural changes: Rapid lying from standing posture leads to increased venous return. Therefore, most of the murmurs get accentuated and S2 gets widened in all phases of respiration. But as the LV cavity size increases, the murmur of HOCM is attenuated while the click and murmur of MVP becomes longer. The opposite occurs from lying to standing posture. In patients in whom there is relatively wide splitting of S2 during exhalation—a finding that may be confused with fixed splitting—the width of the splitting is reduced, so that a normal pattern emerges during the respiratory cycle (from lying to standing).

Rapid attaining of squatting posture from standing leads to increased venous return and increased vascular resistance. This increases most of the cardiac murmurs and sounds. Due to increased vascular resistance the murmur of AR, RVOT murmur in TOF, and VSD murmur increase in intensity. While that of HOCM decreases in intensity and click and murmur of MVP is delayed.

Isometric exercise: Bilateral handgrip for 20–30 seconds causes transient but significant increase in systemic vascular resistance, heart rate, BP, and cardiac output. Therefore, (1) S3 and S4 of left side increases, (2) AS murmur diminishes, (3) MR, AR, and VSD murmur accentuates, (4) HOCM murmur diminishes, and (5) click and murmur of MVP is delayed.

DIAGNOSIS WRITING

The most important part of clinical evaluation is to interpret the history in lieu of the examination finding to reach at few differential diagnoses. The components of diagnosis writing include:

- Etiology
- Structural diagnosis and severity
- Pulmonary venous hypertension status
- PA hypertension status
- Cardiac rhythm
- Heart failure
- Functional class—NYHA class
- Peripheral signs of infective endocarditis or other stigmata
- Additional/other systemic findings

CONCLUSION

Good history taking and clinical examination is an important clinical skill. Despite numerous technologies, these skills remain crucial for accurate diagnosis. Intelligent use of traditional cardiac clinical medicine can narrow down the differential diagnosis and thereby help in choosing the relevant investigations and quick management. In addition, good clinical skills are a foundation for successful doctor-patient relationship.

RECOMMENDED READINGS

1. Harvey WP. Heart sounds and murmurs. Circulation. 1964;30:262-71.
2. Wright GW, Branscomb BV. Origin of the sensations of dyspnea. Trans Am Clin Climatol Assoc. 1966; 1954:66.
3. Wasserman K, Cassaburi R. Dyspnea: physiological and pathophysiological mechanisms. Annu Rev Med. 1988;39:503-15.
4. Mahler DA, Harver A, Lentine T, Scott JA, Beck K, Schwartzstein RM. Descriptors of breathlessness in cardiorespiratory diseases. Am J Respir Crit Care Med. 1996;154:1357-63.
5. Schwartzstein RM, Thibault GE. Approach to the patient with dyspnea. In: Goldman L, Braunwald E (Eds). Primary Cardiology. Philadelphia: Saunders; 1998. pp. 98-111.
6. Schmitt BP, Kushner MS, Weiner SL. The diagnostic usefulness of the history of the patient with dyspnea. J Gen Intern Med. 1986;1:386-93.
7. Mulrow CD, Lucey CR, Farnett LE. Discriminating causes of dyspnea through clinical examination. J Gen Intern Med. 1993;8:383-92.
8. Behrman RE, Kliegman RM, Jenson HB. Congenital heart disease. In: Kliegman RM, Stanton B, St Geme J, Schor NF, Behrman RE (Eds). Nelson Textbook of Pediatrics, 19th edition. Philadelphia: Saunders; 2000. pp. 1549-605.
9. Park KM. Pediatric Cardiology for Practitioners, 5th edition. Amsterdam, Netherlands: Elsevier Health Sciences; 2007. pp. 119-326.
10. Subramanyam L. Recurrent respiratory tract infection—an approach. Indian J Pract Pediatr. 2012;14(3): 245-57.
11. Muntner P, Shimbo D, Carey RM, Charleston JB, Gaillard T, Misra S, et al. Measurement of Blood Pressure in Humans: A Scientific Statement From the American Heart Association. Hypertension. 2019;73(5): e35-66.

CHAPTER

86 Epidemiology of Cardiovascular Diseases

Nazneen Ali, Arun Pulikkottil Jose, Dorairaj Prabhakaran

ABSTRACT

Cardiovascular diseases (CVDs) are a major cause of disability and premature deaths throughout the world. A large portion of these deaths occur in low and middle-income countries (LMICs). CVD has been found to be the leading cause of morbidity and mortality in India. In addition to the disease burden, CVD also contributes substantially to the healthcare costs. The epidemiological trends in India have been found to vary across different regions and have been escalating over the years. This has been influenced by both population level changes and inherent biological risks. CVD develops as a result of various risk factors that are broadly classified as modifiable and nonmodifiable risk factors. These risk factors coexist and interact in different ways. It is important to understand the dynamics of these risk factors in a population while designing and constituting preventive strategies. CVD prevention can be planned and implemented through a coordinated set of actions, at the population level or targeted at an individual, to eliminate or minimize their impact.

"Every human is the author of his own health and disease"

—Gautama Buddha

BACKGROUND

Cardiovascular diseases remain an underreported yet long-term threat to population health. Most deaths globally today are attributed to noncommunicable diseases (NCDs) (41 million), and a significant proportion of this is a result of CVD. The CVDs are a group of heart and blood vessels disorders, including coronary heart disease (CHD), cerebrovascular disease, peripheral arterial disease, rheumatic heart disease, congenital heart disease, deep vein thrombosis, and pulmonary embolism. Overall, there were 18.6 million deaths due to CVD in 2019, with over three-quarters of these deaths taking place in LMICs. However, today even in high-income countries, the age-standardized death rate of CVD has begun to rise in some locations where it was previously declining.

There has been a high-level political commitment to improve CVD outcomes by 2025. However, most countries globally are off track to meet the proposed targets. The total economic loss due to CVD in LMICs was estimated to be $3.7 trillion between 2011 and 2015, which alarmingly represents approximately half the NCD economic burden and 2% of gross domestic product (GDP) across LMICs. The existing challenges of health systems in LMICs that include insufficient health spending, poor care delivery systems, increased focus on curative care rather than prevention and poor governance, amongst many other factors—have contributed to significant economic burden. Catastrophic health spending (annual out-of-pocket health expenditures ≥40% of the total, nonfood household expenditures) and distress financing (financial activities, such as borrowing money from relatives/friends, taking loans from banks/other lenders, or selling assets/property, that were directly related to the patient's most recent hospitalization) were seen across all income strata and were the highest for India compared with three other LMICs.

EPIDEMIOLOGY

According to the State-Level Disease Burden study by the Global Burden of Disease (GBD) study group, 27.4% of mortality in India is due to CVD. The atherosclerotic vascular disease that comprises coronary artery disease, peripheral vascular disease, and associated complications is the major contributor to CVD, ischemic heart disease (IHD) and stroke are together responsible for approximately a quarter (23.61%) of all deaths and one-fifth of the years of life lost in India. Rheumatic heart disease also continues to be a problem in several parts of India, and its estimated prevalence is in the range of 1.5–2 per 1,000 individuals (2–2.5 million cases in absolute numbers). Apart from these major causes, the contribution of atrial fibrillation and flutter to the overall CVD burden in India appears to be small, according to the GBD study. Besides, the proportional mortality and morbidity burden attributed to other CVD such as aortic aneurysms, peripheral vascular disease, and endocarditis are also relatively small.

TRENDS IN CVD EPIDEMIOLOGY

The epidemiological trends of CVDs vary across regions. In addition to this, there is variability in CVD morbidity and mortality between states of the same country. The global burden disease data from 2019 reveals wide differences in DALYs within countries [DALYs: Disability Adjusted

Life Years or DALYs for a disease or health condition are calculated as the sum of the Years of Life Lost (YLL) due to premature mortality in the population and the Years Lost due to Disability (YLD) for people living with the health condition or its consequences. One DALY can be thought of as one lost year of "healthy" life].

IHD DALYs in India ranged from 506.6 per 100,000 [95% uncertainty interval (UI) 379.6–819.0 per 100,000] in Mizoram to 5,413.2 per 100,000 (95% UI 4,316.9–6,389.9 per 100,000) in Punjab, a 165.8% difference within the country. In other countries like the United States and Mexico, the regional difference of DALYs within countries was comparatively lower (99.6% and 88.9%, respectively). Additionally, there exist differences amongst sex where total CVD DALYs were higher in men than women before age 80–84 years, with a reversal in the pattern after. The sex differences in DALYs are most striking between ages 30 and 60 years (men greater) and age >80 years (women greater).

In India, the age-adjusted CVD mortality rates are higher in men than women (349/100,000 in men and 265/100,000 in women). However, these rates are 2- to 3-fold greater than in the United States, where rates are 170/100,000 in men and 108/100,000 in women. The CVD prevalence increased in India from 25.7 million (95% UI 25.1–26.0) in 1990 to 54.5 million (53.7–55.3) in 2016. In 2016, the prevalence was highest in Kerala and Tamil Nadu, followed by Andhra Pradesh, Himachal Pradesh, Maharashtra, Goa, and West Bengal.

FACTORS THAT INFLUENCE CVD BURDEN

The escalating CVD burden in India is similar to other LMICs, but also has special features. The high propensity for CVD among Indians can be attributed to two reasons. These include several population-level changes and inherent biological risk, particularly for diabetes and lipid patterns. The *population-level factors* include the following:

- The epidemiological transition
- Ageing of the population and related demographic shifts
- Rapid and unplanned urbanization and consequent downstream effects
- Changing lifestyles resulting from economic growth

The biological risks include the following:

- Ethnicity
- Genetic factors
- Fetal programing and early-life influences (the time from conception through the first 2 years)

EPIDEMIOLOGICAL TRANSITION

The epidemiological transition theory describes the changing population patterns in terms of mortality and the leading causes of death. The most evident example is the change in disease pattern in a country, away from communicable to NCDs due to improved healthcare and disease prevention. Epidemiological transition is divided into five stages: (1) *Age of pestilence and famines*, marked by malnutrition, infectious diseases, and high infant and childhood mortality with low mortality from CVD (<10%); (2) *Age of receding pandemics*, when better public health systems lead to decreased mortality from communicable diseases and the emergence of CVD (10–35% mortality); (3) *Age of degenerative and human-made diseases* is characterized by mortality from CVD surpassing mortality from communicable diseases (35–65% of all deaths); (4) *Age of delayed degenerative diseases*, when cancer and CVDs are predominant causes of deaths and CVD leads to >40% of all deaths, but there is a declining trend in death rates; and (5) *Age of inactivity and obesity*, when declining physical activity leads to epidemics of diabetes, hypertension, and lipid abnormalities, with increasing CVD deaths rates.

In a socioeconomically diverse country like India, there is evidence of all these stages of transition. The proof for this coexistence is evident from the heterogeneity in disease patterns, the urban-rural differences in CVD and risk factors, and the reversal of socioeconomic gradient for CVD (with poor and less educated becoming the predominant victims of CVD) observed in some states such as Kerala. Further, this epidemiological transition has been enhanced by the demographic shift that India is undergoing. With improving living conditions and an increased life expectancy, India has an ageing population with an increasing proportion of it becoming vulnerable to CVD every year. Based on projections, the population above 60 years is expected to rise to 19% by 2050. In addition to this, certain characteristic features of CVD epidemiology in Indians, such as an earlier age of onset as seen for acute myocardial infarction (AMI) in the INTERHEART study and the younger age of escalation of risk factors in Indians as observed by Gupta et al., have further played a role in the increase in CVD burden.

India is expected to make the greatest contribution to the global population growth of any country until at least 2050. It is projected that over half of the population will be urban by 2050. The rise in living standards and sociocultural transitions increases the susceptivity of Indians to CVD. Unhealthy dietary habits and an increasingly sedentary lifestyle may have directly influenced the increase in CVD burden and its risk factors such as hypertension, diabetes mellitus, and dyslipidemia. Smoking, a behavioral risk factor for CVD, was found to be more prevalent in people living in rural areas. Besides, the increasing level of air pollution in most large cities in India may play a role in the current high burden of CVD. A substantial 38% of the disease burden due to air pollution in India is from CVD and diabetes. Although the prevalence of CVD and its risk factors are higher in urban areas and well known, several studies have reported an increase in its prevalence in rural areas, too. This is alarming because over two-thirds of the Indian population still live in rural areas, and an increased risk in this section of the society indicates a rampant epidemic.

Throughout the industrialized world, the age-adjusted mortality rates of CVDs have decreased over the years. However, India has not experienced a decline in age-adjusted CVD event rates and continues to undergo an epidemiological transition from predominantly infectious diseases to NCDs. Addressing this significant burden of CVD in a highly populated, diverse, and rapidly developing country requires an understanding of the complex dynamics of CVD risk factors and their interactions.

RISK FACTORS IN CARDIOVASCULAR DISEASE

The development of CVD is influenced by risk factors such as tobacco use, an unhealthy diet, physical inactivity, obesity (which can result from a combination of an unhealthy diet, physical inactivity, and other factors), hypertension, dyslipidemia, and diabetes mellitus. Continuous exposure to these risk factors leads to further progression of atherosclerosis, resulting in clinical manifestations of these diseases, including angina pectoris, myocardial infarction, heart failure, and stroke. These risk factors may be classified as modifiable and nonmodifiable (**Table 1**).

A robust understanding of India's risk factors trends is essential for effective health system and policy action to improve population health. According to the India State-Level Disease Burden initiative of the GBD study, in the year 2016, the leading overlapping risk factors in terms of percentage DALYs due to CVD [%, (95% CI)] were dietary risks [56.4% (48.5–63.9)], high systolic blood pressure (BP) [54.6% (49.0–59.8)], air pollution [31.1% (29.0–33.4)], high total cholesterol [29.4% (24.3–34.8)], tobacco use [18.9% (16.6–21.3)], high fasting plasma glucose [16.7% (11.4–23.5)], and increased body mass index (BMI) [14.7% (8.3–22.0)]. The prevalence of major CVD risk factors, including high systolic BP, high fasting plasma glucose, high total cholesterol, high BMI, and exposure to ambient air pollution, increased in all states of the country.

PREVENTION OF CARDIOVASCULAR DISEASE

The word risk is commonly referred to as the percentage probability (relative frequency) of an adverse event. In CVD, the role of individual risk factors is often influenced by the presence or absence of other coexisting factors. Instead of looking at each risk factor individually, it is essential to understand the coexistence and interplay between them.

TABLE 1 Major risk factors for cardiovascular disease.

Modifiable		Nonmodifiable
Behavioral	**Biological**	
• Tobacco • Diet • Physical inactivity • Alcohol • Stress	• Hypertension • Diabetes • Dyslipidemia • Central obesity	• Family history • Age • Gender • Ethnicity • Menopause
Socioenvironmental determinants (may or may not be modifiable): Socioeconomic status, community characteristics (e.g., presence/absence of social capital), work conditions, and environmental health		

PRINCIPLES OF PREVENTION

It will be helpful to keep the following four principles in mind while designing and constituting preventive strategies.

Principle of continuous risk: Contrary to common belief, risk factors for CVD do not operate across defined cut-offs but a continuous spectrum. The risk of cardiovascular events increases in a graded and continuous fashion even within the normal range of a risk factor. For example, although two individuals with systolic BP readings of 120 mm Hg or 130 mm Hg are both within the normal range, the former has considerably lower risk as compared to the latter. Reduction in BP and lipid levels have shown to reduce cardiovascular risk irrespective of diagnostic cut-offs. This underscores the need to lower risk factor levels within the recommended range.

Principle of population-wide risk: A graphical representation of risk factors in a population produces a distribution curve, with the relative risk of events increasing as you move to the right side of the curve. It is important to note that although the relative risk increases with the increasing value of the risk factor, the absolute number of individuals (depicted by the area under the curve) decreases. In other words, most individuals fall in the midrange of the risk factor and therefore contribute to the highest burden of disease (absolute risk). For example, even though the relative risk for CHD is higher for individuals with a systolic BP of 180 mm Hg as compared with 140 mm Hg, the number of events would be higher in the latter group due to the larger number of individuals in this BP range. It is important to keep this principle in mind while designing population-level interventions that would have a greater impact if targeted for individuals in the midrange of a risk factor rather than those with extreme values.

Principle of multiplicative risk: While many risk factors exist for CVD, evidence shows that they act multiplicatively and exaggerate the damage caused by each risk factor alone. For this reason, to reduce risk, it is important to focus on all risk factors involved rather than looking into a single risk factor alone. A CVD event can occur even with minor elevations of multiple risk factors compared to elevations of a single risk factor. In practice, when the Framingham risk score is used to calculate and compare two individuals of the same gender age and risk factor profile, the individual with multiple risk factors will often score more than someone with only one single risk factor that may be alarming.

Figure 1 explains the multiple risk factor attribution to the absolute risk for individuals with CVD. In this figure, as the number of risk factors increase, the CVD risk increases in a linear fashion.

Principle of absolute risk: Absolute risk is the probability of an individual developing an adverse event over a given time period. In the context of CVD, a large number of events occur in people with moderate elevations of multiple risk factors that operate continuously rather than a significant elevation of one risk factor alone. Essentially, this principle is a mix of both the multiplicative and continuous risk as mentioned above.

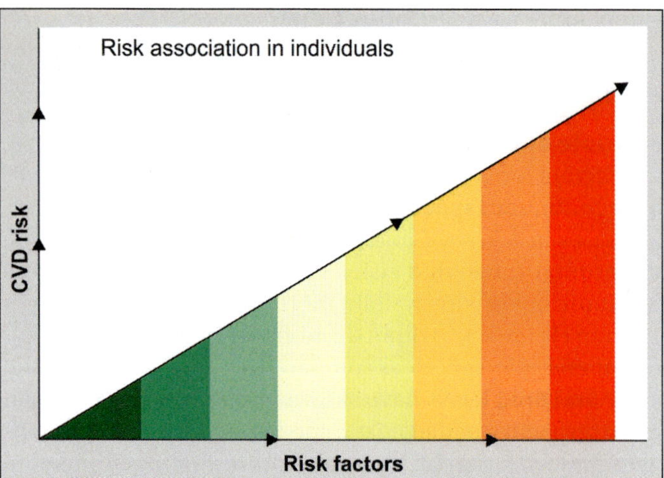

FIGURE 1: A diagrammatic representation of the multiple risk factor profile attribution to the total risk.

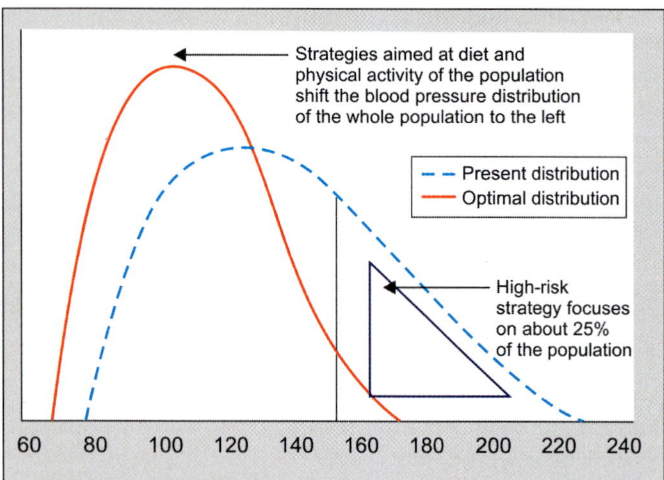

FIGURE 2: Present and optimal distribution of systolic blood pressure in adults. A combination of population and high-risk blood pressure control strategies is necessary to achieve optimal blood pressure distribution.

Source: Integrated management of cardiovascular risk, WHO.

PUBLIC HEALTH INTERVENTIONS

Cardiovascular disease prevention is defined as a coordinated set of actions, at the population level or targeted at an individual, to eliminate or minimize the impact of CVDs and their related disabilities. Prevention strategies in CVD can be planned and implemented through two different approaches as described here.

Population-wide approach: This approach intends to bring down the risk factor levels across the board in a population through collaborative efforts in the community. As mentioned above, CVD events will continue to occur in people with low- and moderate-risk levels, who are the majority in any population. Therefore, population-wide efforts will result in much greater gains and shift the overall distribution curve to the left (**Fig. 2**), primarily since risk associated with most CVD risk factors occurs continuously. This approach was found to reduce absolute and relative socioeconomic health inequalities and cost saving. For example, population-wide reduction in salt intake will decrease the population mean BP levels, shift the population BP distribution to the left, and reduce the prevalence of hypertension.

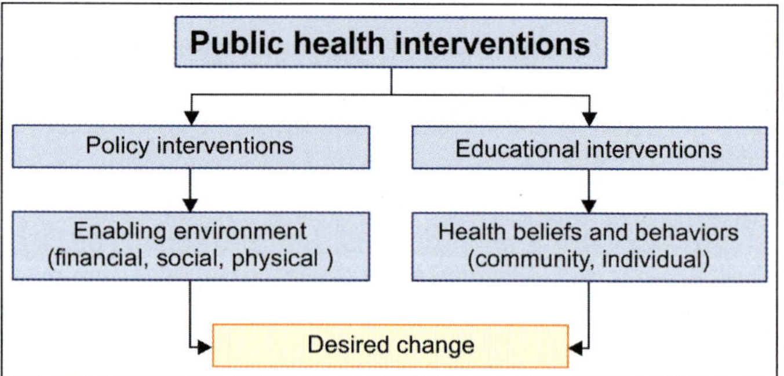

FLOWCHART 1: Public health interventions needed for health promotion.

High-risk approach: Population-wide public health strategies alone will not have an immediate impact on cardiovascular morbidity and mortality and will only have a modest absolute impact on the disease burden. The high-risk approach aims at identifying persons with markedly elevated risk factors or a prior cardiovascular event and at the highest risk. The high-risk approach is often pharmacological, but it has been found that the projected risk and anticipated benefit leads to better motivation in both patients and healthcare providers. However, given the larger risk reduction in individuals, it can save an equal proportion of lives as the population-wide approach in a cost-effective manner.

A combination of population-wide strategies and strategies targeted at high-risk individuals is necessary to reduce the CVD burden. The extent to which one approach should be emphasized over the other depends on the prevalence of the disease, cost-effectiveness, availability of resources, and public health priorities of the community.

Public health interventions in CVD prevention can be categorized as policy and educational interventions (**Flowchart 1**). They both differ in that policy interventions and focus more on creating a conducive environment. Educational interventions include promotive strategies aimed at behavior change at both the individual and community level.

Efforts to lower the burden of CVD will require early prevention of the development of risk factors (primordial prevention) rather than relying only on the treatment of existing risk factors (primary prevention). Implementation of effective public health policy has had considerable success in various countries. Major policy measures that have been implemented in the past include tobacco control, reduction of salt in processed foods, increasing fruit and vegetable intake, reduction of high fat intake, ban on trans fats, and taxes on sugar-sweetened beverages. Patients should also be empowered and have the knowledge and support to make informed decisions and to demand robust prevention efforts from healthcare groups and society.

LIFE-COURSE APPROACH IN PREVENTING CVDS

A life course approach in epidemiology investigates the biological, behavioral, and social pathways that link physical and social exposures and experiences during gestation, childhood, adolescence and adult life, and across generations, to later-life health and disease risk. The interval between exposure, disease onset, and clinical recognition in CVDs suggests that exposures early in life are involved in initiating disease processes before the appearance of clinical manifestations. Therefore, risk factors must be addressed throughout the life course. For interventions to have a lasting effect on the risk factor prevalence and the health of societies, it is also essential to change or modify the environment in which these diseases develop. Reversing the status quo will require a multifaceted public health policy approach.

RECOMMENDED READINGS

1. World Health Organization. WHO | Non Communicable Diseases Fact Sheet. WHO; 2016.
2. Roth GA, Mensah GA, Johnson CO, Addolorato G, Ammirati E, Baddour LM, et al. Global Burden of Cardiovascular Diseases and Risk Factors, 1990–2019: Update From the GBD 2019 Study. J Am Coll Cardiol. 2020;76(25):2982-3021.
3. Bowry ADK, Lewey J, Dugani SB, Choudhry NK. The Burden of Cardiovascular Disease in Low- and Middle-Income Countries: Epidemiology and Management. Can J Cardiol. 2015;31(9):1151-9.
4. Reddy KS. Measuring mortality from non-communicable diseases: broadening the band. Lancet Glob Health. 2020;8(4):e456-7.
5. Yusuf S, Wood D, Ralston J, Reddy KS. The World Heart Federation's vision for worldwide cardiovascular disease prevention. Lancet. 2015;386(9991):399-402.
6. Dandona L, Dandona R, Kumar GA, Shukla DK, Paul VK, Balakrishnan K, et al. Nations within a nation: variations in epidemiological transition across the states of India, 1990–2016 in the Global Burden of Disease Study. Lancet. 2017;390(10111):2437-60.
7. Prabhakaran D, Jeemon P, Roy A. Cardiovascular Diseases in India: Current Epidemiology and Future Directions. Circulation. 2016;133(16):1605-20.
8. Kumar RK, Tandon R. Rheumatic fever & rheumatic heart disease: The last 50 years. Indian J Med Res. 2013;137(4):643-58.
9. Gupta R, Mohan I, Narula J. Trends in Coronary Heart Disease Epidemiology in India. Ann Glob Heal. 2016;82(2):307-15.
10. Prabhakaran D, Jeemon P, Sharma M, Roth GA, Johnson C, Harikrishnan S, et al. The changing patterns of cardiovascular diseases and their risk factors in the states of India: the Global Burden of Disease Study 1990–2016. Lancet Glob Heal. 2018;6(12):e1339-51.
11. Prabhakaran D, Kumar RK, Naik N. Cardiovascular disease risk factors. In: Prabhakaran D, Kumar RK, Naik N (Eds). Tandons Textbook of Cardiology, volume 1. Wolters Kluwer; 2019. p. 1602.
12. Santosa A, Wall S, Fottrel E, Högberg U, Byass P. The development and experience of epidemiological transition theory over four decades: A systematic review. Glob Health Action. 2014;7(SUPP.1):1-16.
13. Rashid S, Khandaker N. Risk factors for early myocardial infarction in South Asians. J Am Med Assoc. 2007;297(17):1880-1.
14. Gupta R, Misra A, Vikram NK, Kondal D, Gupta SS, Agrawal A, et al. Younger age of escalation of cardiovascular risk factors in Asian Indian subjects. BMC Cardiovasc Disord. 2009;9:28.
15. Geldsetzer P, Manne-Goehler J, Theilmann M, Davies JI, Awasthi A, Danaei G, et al. Geographic and sociodemographic variation of cardiovascular disease risk in India: A cross-sectional study of 797,540 adults. PLoS Med. 2018;15(6):1-23.
16. Jose AP, Shridhar K, Prabhakaran D. Diet, nutrition and cardiovascular disease: The role of social determinants. Proc Indian Natl Sci Acad. 2018;84(4):945-53.
17. Balakrishnan K, Dey S, Gupta T, Dhaliwal RS, Brauer M, Cohen AJ, et al. The impact of air pollution on deaths, disease burden, and life expectancy across the states of India: the Global Burden of Disease Study 2017. Lancet Planet Heal. 2019;3(1):e26-39.
18. Prabhakaran D, Roy A, Praveen PA, Ramakrishnan L, Gupta R, Amarchand R, et al. 20-Year Trend of CVD Risk Factors: Urban and Rural National Capital Region of India. Glob Heart. 2017;12(3):209-17.
19. Berry JD, Dyer A, Cai X, Garside DB, Ning H, Thomas A, et al. Lifetime Risks of Cardiovascular Disease. N Engl J Med. 2012;366(4):321-9.
20. Piepoli MF, Hoes AW, Agewall S, Albus C, Brotons C, Catapano AL, et al. 2016 European Guidelines on cardiovascular disease prevention in clinical practice. Eur Heart J. 2016;37(29):2315-81.

CHAPTER 87 Electrocardiogram

M Chenniappan

ABSTRACT

The electrocardiogram (ECG) continues to remain as a crucial investigation in cardiology even after a century of its discovery in spite of so much of sophisticated investigations today. It not only gives the diagnosis but also gives other crucial information such as prognosis, management plan, and result of the treatment in many cardiac diseases. But it should be realized that the ECG gives also almost so much information in many noncardiac situations. This chapter on ECG gives a fundamental knowledge to understand the genesis of wave forms and its application in day to day reading of ECG.

"We are the survivors from the moment of diagnosis"

—Peter Jennings

BASICS

HISTORY

William Einthoven invented the ECG in 1902. He was then working in the University of Leiden in Netherlands and invented a practical method of recording the electrical activity of the heart, using a string galvanometer. He assigned the letters starting beyond the middle of the alphabet "O", to the series of deflections "P", "Q", "R", "S", and "T" which we still use today.

He won the Nobel Prize for his invention in 1924. The ECG recorded in 1902 looks better than some of the recordings with modern machines today (**Fig. 1**). For over 100 years, this investigation has contributed to diagnosis and management of numerous cardiac disorders and has not been replaced.

WHAT IS ELECTROCARDIOGRAM

Electrocardiogram is a graphic recording of the electrical properties of the heart.

From the ECG we can identify:
- Origin of impulse, its frequency
- Speed and the pathway that it is taking
- Where and how the impulse is traveling
- How the tissue is responding to the impulse

To know about the mechanical properties of the heart, we need the echocardiogram.

The echo gives us details of:
- Atrial and ventricular contraction and relaxation
- How the valves function
- About blood flow direction and velocities

Sometimes the ECG may be abnormal, and echo will be normal, and vice versa. To tell a person that his heart is normal, he should have a normal ECG and normal echo.

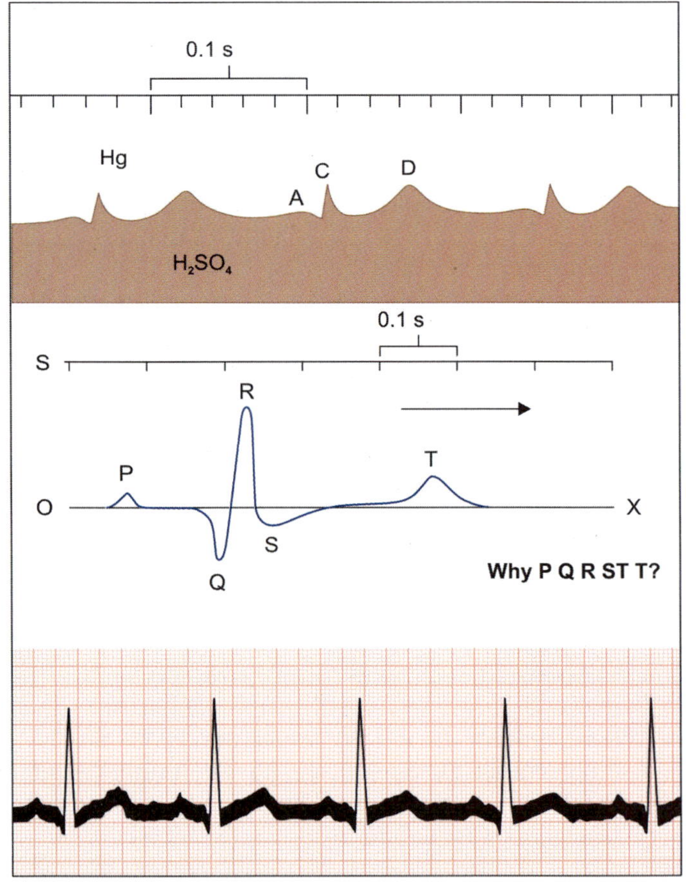

FIGURE 1: **First human electrocardiogram.**

PACEMAKERS OF THE HEART

Electrical activity is spontaneously generated in some cells and propagated in an orderly way through a conduction

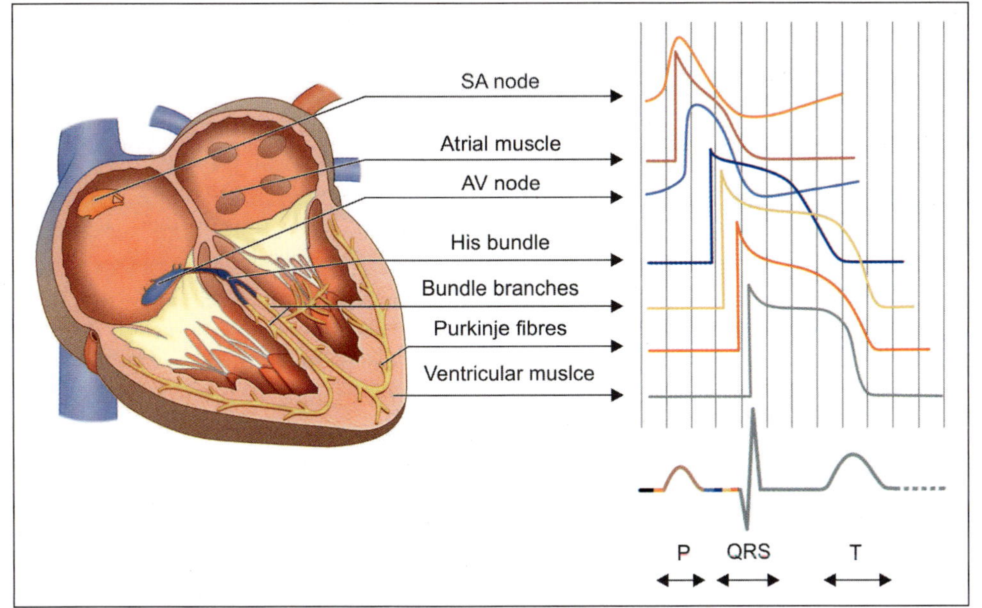

(AV: atrioventricular; SA: sinoatrial)

FIGURE 2: Active potentials of various parts of the heart.

system to other cells. This is depicted in **Figure 2** for the sinoatrial (SA) node and the atrioventricular (AV) node.

Primary pacemaker: The fastest spontaneous impulse generator in the heart is the primary pacemaker. It is the SA node which is located at the junction of the superior vena cava (SVC) and right atrium. This has the steepest spontaneous diastolic depolarization curve.

Secondary pacemaker: When the primary pacemaker fails, other pacemakers which are called secondary pacemakers take over to prevent cardiac stand still, by producing an escape rhythm. These are AV junction, His bundle, and ventricles, in whom the rate is much slower.

- Sinus rate: 60–100 beats/min
- AV junction: 40–60 beats/min
- Ventricle: 30–40 beats/min

The impulse generated from SA node travels toward the AV node by two ways (**Fig. 3**):

1. Interatrial pathways:
   - Wenckebach
   - Thorel
   - Bachman
2. Through atrial muscle

Atrioventricular node (Fig. 3): Atrioventricular node has two important roles to play:

1. To act as a speed breaker and delay the impulse conduction from atria to ventricles
2. To protect the ventricles from rapid atrial activity

The AV node delays the electrical impulse arriving from the atrium without losing its amplitude or power and conducts to His bundle (**Fig. 3**).

Delay allows atrial contraction to be completed just before ventricular systole, thereby stretching the ventricular myocardial fibers to the maximum physiological limit. Thereby it improves the force of contraction by Frank-Starling's law, (maximum end diastolic fiber length), giving the booster pump effect.

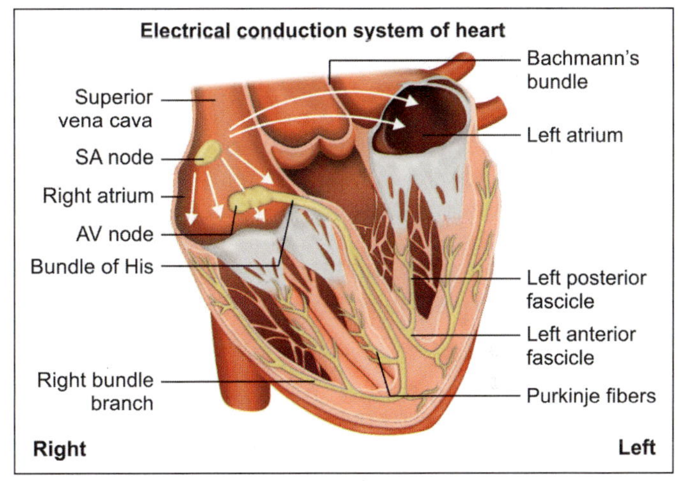

(AV: atrioventricular; SA: sinoatrial)

FIGURE 3: Conduction system of heart.

In conditions like atrial fibrillation (AF) where this "atrial boost" is lost and the efficiency of the ventricle is reduced by up to 30%.

The AV node also protects the ventricle from high atrial rates as in AF where impulses can arrive at up to 300/s but only about 120–130 impulses are conducted to the ventricle.

His bundle: From the AV node the "His Bundle" which is common bundle enters the ventricle and divides into right bundle branch block (RBBB) and left bundle branch block (LBBB) to the right ventricular (RV) and left ventricle (LV), respectively.

Bundle branches (Fig. 3): Left bundle branch (LBB) divides into left anterior fascicle and left posterior fascicle. LV being the most powerful chamber, gets two fascicles for electrical supply and two blood vessels left anterior descending (LAD) and left circumflex (LCX).

Purkinje fibers: The fascicles further divide to become the special Purkinje fibers which travel from endocardium to epicardium and supply the individual 300 billion cardiac myocytes. This arrangement allows the entire cardiac muscle to be depolarized within 0.08 seconds and the heart muscle contracts in unison.

The bundle of the His, bundle branches, fascicles, and Purkinje fibers are called the specialized conduction system of the heart.

Conduction velocities: The atrial muscle and ventricle muscle conducts electrical impulses at a rate of 0.5 m/s.

His Bundle, LBB and right bundle branch (RBB), and the fascicles conduct at a rate of 2 m/s (four times faster than ventricular muscle).

Purkinje fibers conduct at a rate of 4 m/s (eight times faster than muscle).

At the AV node the electrical impulse is conducted at only 0.05 m/s (10 times slower than muscle).

For the electrical impulse to travel from SA node to:
- AV node it takes 30 msec
- AV nodal delay 130 msec
- AV node to ventricular muscle 30 msec

Total AV conduction time is roughly the PR interval which is <200 msec (**Fig. 4**).

RESPONSE OF CARDIAC MUSCLE TO ELECTRICAL STIMULATION

- Depolarization
- Repolarization
- The resting membrane potential

The resting cardiac myocyte is in the polarized state, the interior being negative, and outside being positive (to remember, the reason for outside positivity, positively charged Na^+, and calcium are kept outside the cell, whereas less positive ions are inside the cell). The membrane is not easily permeable to sodium (**Fig. 5**).

Depolarization: The electrical impulse arriving to the cell membrane, changes the membrane permeability to sodium and it enters the cell rapidly followed by calcium.

This immediately reverses the polarity of the cell. Now when the cell is depolarized, the inside is positive and outside is negative.

Repolarization: Restoration of the electronegativity inside the cell is called repolarization.

This is done by the ion which is easily permeable from inside to outside. Potassium leaves the cell (which is also positively charged to restore electronegativity inside).

Electrocardiogram is a surface recording of the depolarization and repolarization of the entire cardiac muscle.

We can infer from the surface ECG whether the cells are depolarizing and repolarizing normally.

Depolarization starts from the endocardial surface and moves toward the epicardial surface. This produces the positive deflection in the ECG.

This is followed by repolarization:
- Repolarization being an opposite electrical event, should produce a negative wave form in the ECG. The repolarization is recorded as the "T" wave. The "T" wave also is positive because repolarization occurs from epicardium to endocardium (in the reverse direction) (**Fig. 6**).
- If the QRS is positive and "T" wave is negative, it is inferred that the repolarization is also occurring in the same direction from endocardium to epicardium which is abnormal (**Fig. 7**).

GENESIS OF THE WAVEFORMS

"P" atrial depolarization: The first wave form in the ECG is the "p" wave. The sinus node activity is not recorded in the ECG. We infer from the "p" wave characteristics, the activity of the sinus node.

PR segment: Atrioventricular nodal delay: PR segment represents AV node delay.

When there is no cardiac muscle depolarization or repolarization, lines are produced. When there is electrical activity in the muscle the waves are produced, which is the period where ionic movements occur. Therefore, lines in the

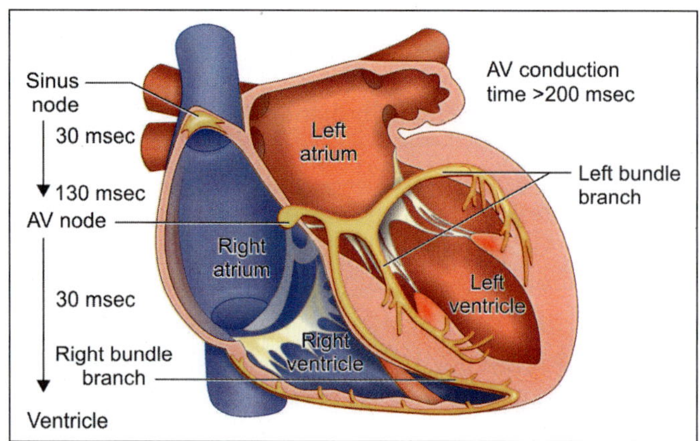

FIGURE 4: Conduction times—atrioventricular (AV) conduction is about 200 msec.

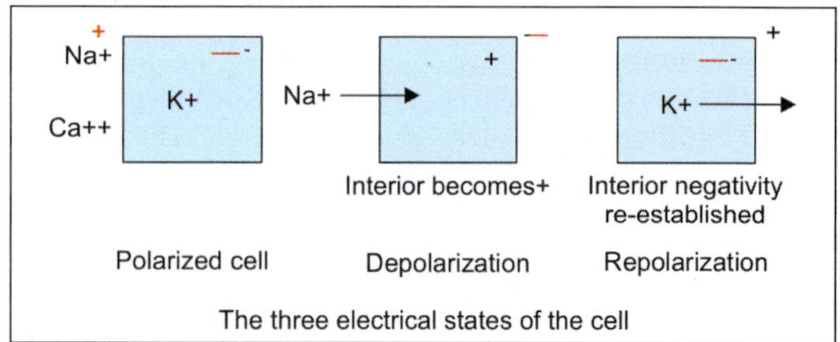

FIGURE 5: Depolarization and repolarization.

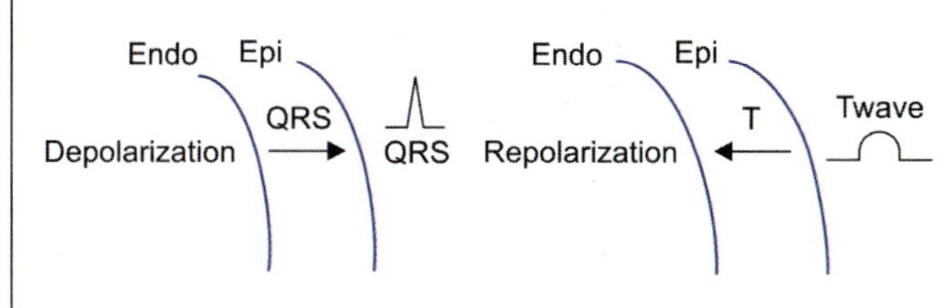

FIGURE 6: Depolarization and Repolarization producing QRS complex and T wave.

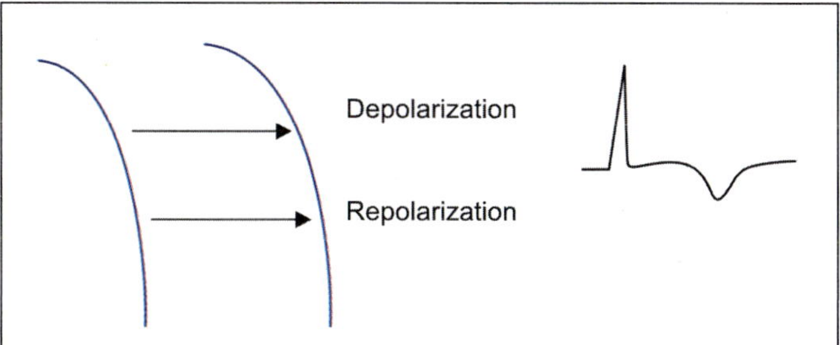

FIGURE 7: Abnormal direction of repolarization.

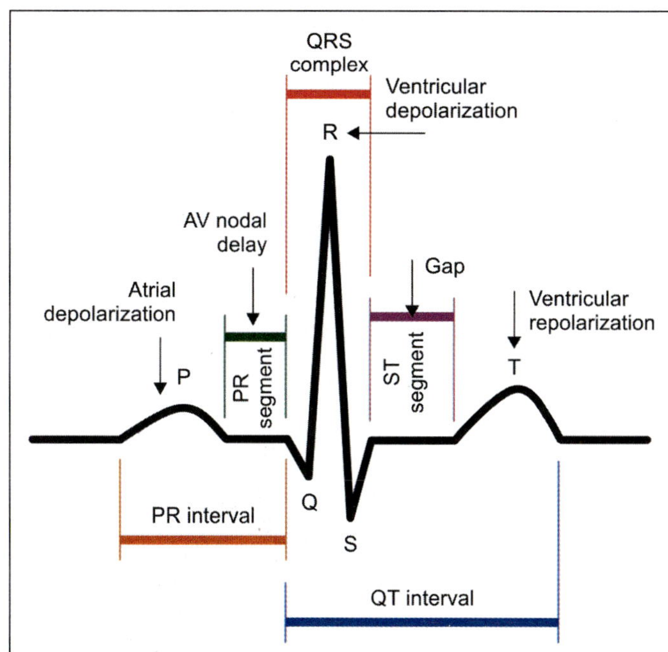

(AV: atrioventricular)

FIGURE 8: All waves, lines, and intervals.

ECG represent "no ionic movement" and waves represent "ionic movements".

QRS complex: Ventricular depolarization: The electrical impulse reaches the ventricles after AV nodal delay the ventricles are depolarized from endocardium to epicardium and QRS complex is produced.

ST segment: The segment between ventricular depolarization and repolarization represents the time when cells have been depolarized and repolarization is yet to begin.

"T" wave: Ventricular repolarization: Repolarization occurs in the reverse sequence, epicardium to endocardium and therefore, this wave is also upright, as the QRS complex.

"T" and "P" segment: End of "T" wave to beginning of "P" wave where repolarization is completed, and the cells are ready to receive the next impulse from sinus node to produce next "P" wave.

PR interval: It includes the "P" wave and PR segment. Therefore, it represents the total AV conduction time, i.e., from the origin of impulse in the sinus node to the ventricular myocardium.

PR segment: It represents AV nodal delay (**Fig. 8**).

Therefore, there are:
- Three waves—"P", "QRS", "T", and,
- Three segments or isoelectric lines—PR, ST, and TP segments (**Fig. 9**).

The Relationship between action potential and related changes in the ECG are shown in **Table 1**.

Ionic currents and waves (Fig. 10):
- QRS complex → Rapid sodium influx (upstroke of action potential)
- ST segment → Calcium influx (plateau of action potential)
- T wave → Potassium efflux (downslope of action potential)

Inference: Disorders of sodium current affects QRS complex; Na channel blockers such as type Ic antiarrhythmic drugs and tricyclic antidepressants prolong QRS complex.

Disorders of calcium affect ST segment; hypocalcemia produces long ST segment and hypercalcemia produces short ST segment.

Disorders of potassium affect T wave; hypokalemia produces low voltage T wave and hyperkalemia produces tall T wave.

Electromechanical coupling: Electrical impulse reaching the cardiac muscle changes the ionic permeability of the membrane sodium and calcium enters the cell.

Calcium stimulates sarcoplasmic reticulum to release free calcium.

This in turn removes the inhibitor Troponin "I" and stimulates acting myosin sliding to produce a contraction.

When the calcium is actively pumped back into the sarcoplasmic reticulum the myosin head relaxes the process is reversed.

VECTORS

Cardiac vector is defined as the net amplitude and direction of the resultant cardiac impulse. When the cardiac myocytes are depolarized from endocardium to epicardium the resulting wave front travels in all directions, but the net, or predominant amplitude and direction of the wave front is toward the area of maximum muscle mass toward the LV in normal heart which is directed toward

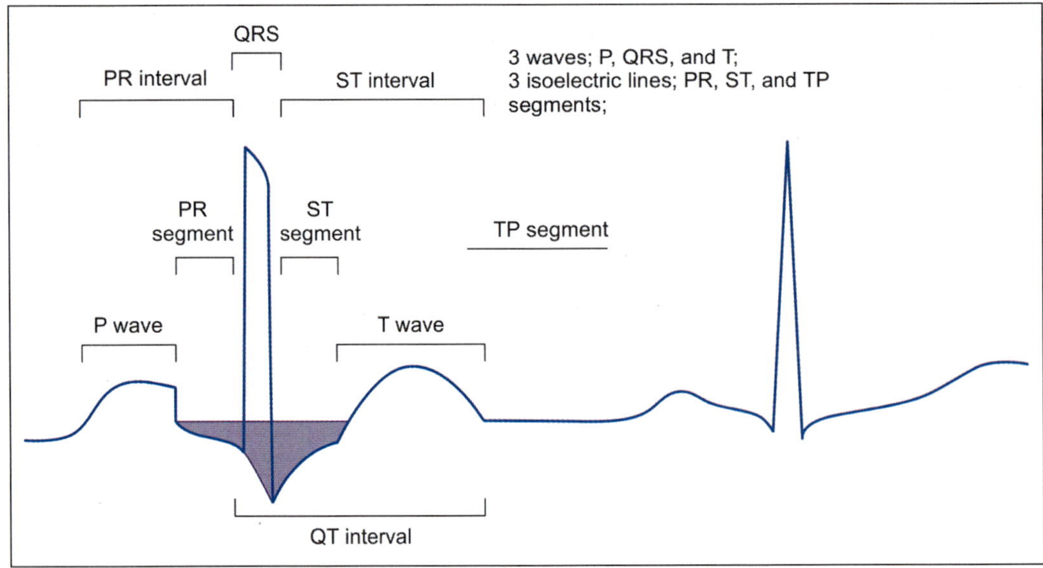

FIGURE 9: Waves and intervals.

TABLE 1 Changes in action potential at cellular level and corroborative changes in the electrocardiogram (ECG).

Action potential	ECG
Intracellular electrode recording	ECG: Recording from the surface
Single cell recording	Entire cardiac muscle
Resting membrane potential –90 mV	Isoelectric base line
Depolarization—rapid Na^+ influx	QRS complex
Plateau phase: Calcium entry into cell to maintain intracellular positivity	Represented by ST segment (absent in pace making cells)
Repolarization: Potassium leaves the cell to restore intracellular negativity	• T wave • Remains positive because of change in direction (epicardium to endocardium)

Note: Plateau phase is absent in pace making cells.

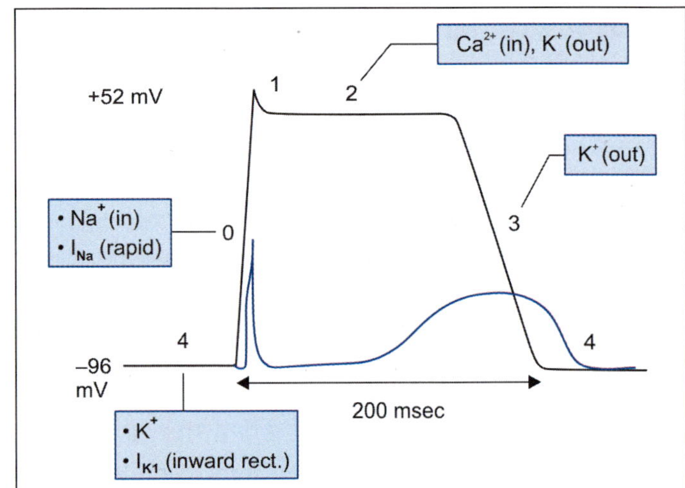

FIGURE 10: Relationship between action potential and electrocardiogram.

inferior and left direction. Therefore, the vector travels in this direction.

Direction of the vectors assessment:

- *Positive deflection in a particular lead*: When the wave of depolarization, or the vector is traveling toward that lead.
- *Negative deflection in a particular lead*: When the wave of depolarization or the vector is traveling away from that lead.
- *Equiphasic deflection in a particular lead*: When the wave of depolarization or the vector is traveling perpendicular to that lead (**Fig. 11**).

A river, which has tributaries and distributaries traveling in various directions, and yet takes one overall direction to the destination, can be likened to the vector.

Note: Depending on the various angles the vector makes with recording lead, the amplitude of the wave will change so the lead to which the vector is traveling directly will record maximum positivity.

Because of this principle in normal ECG, as the net ventricular depolarization is traveling from right to left (toward LV), the right-sided lead V_1 shows predominantly negative complex (impulse going away from V_1), and left-sided chest leads like V_5 and V_6 show positive QRS complexes (impulse coming toward them).

NAMING THE WAVES

Diagram:

"q"—first negative wave of QRS complex
"r"—first positive wave
"s"—second negative wave which follows "r" wave
"r'": "r dash"—a second r wave following s wave is usually seen in bundle branch blocks and some abnormal conduction disturbances widening QRS complexes.

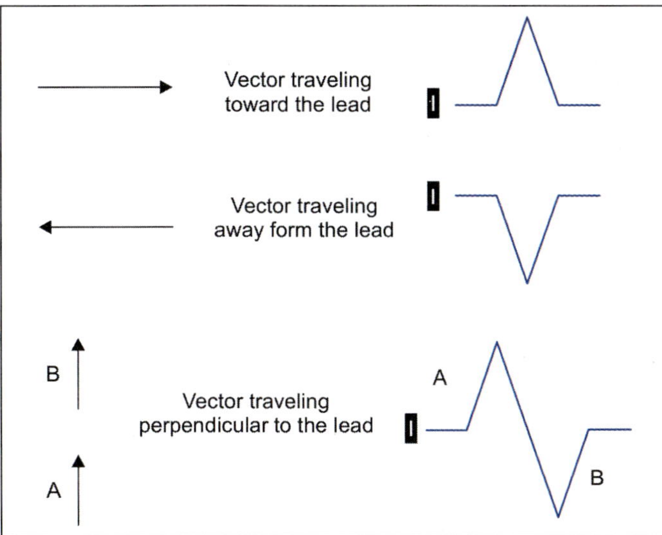

FIGURE 11: Vectors and direction assessment graphic showing the relationship between positive electrodes, depolarization wave fronts (or mean electrical vectors), and complexes displayed on the electrocardiogram (ECG).

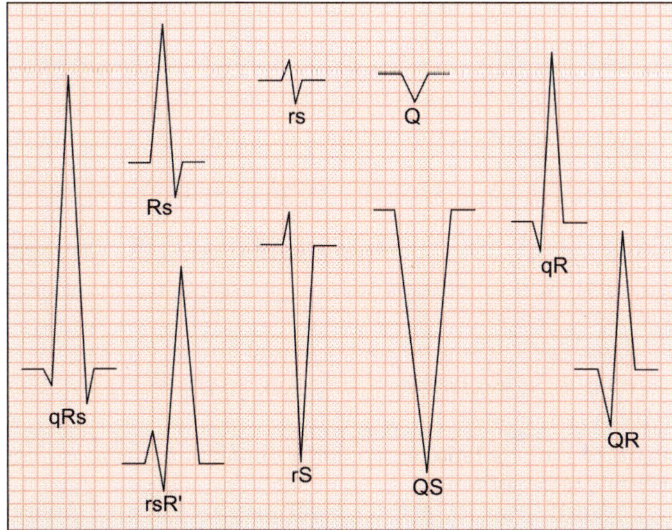

FIGURE 12: Wave nomenclature.

Small letters denote small amplitude waves and capital letters denote taller waves as shown in the diagram (**Fig. 12**).

LEAD SYSTEMS

CONCEPT

While the electrical activity that we measure at the surface of the body results from the sum of all the action potentials traveling through the heart, we should remember that an ECG does not measure an action potential. ECG records the total electrical activity generated by the heart, and so the ECG curve contains multiple waves, whereas an action potential is recorded as a single wave of depolarization and repolarization. The electrical activity generated by the heart is carried to the surface of the body in all directions, because the body is full of fluid and makes an excellent conductor! So, while we could place electrodes directly on the heart (as is sometimes done), we do not need to! We can place electrodes just about anywhere on the surface of the body, where we do not get too much interference from the skeletal system (bone is not a good electrical conductor), and still measure electrical activity emanating from the heart!

Difference between an electrode and a lead:

Electrode: An electrode is simply a measuring instrument for electrical activity. An electrode generally consists of a small metallic plate or disk that is attached to the body by means of an adhesive, or by stretchy bands (physical object).

Lead: A lead is not the same thing as an electrode. A lead is an imaginary line along which electrical activity is being measured. Some leads are created by simultaneously recording electrical activity with a positive and a negative electrode, at different locations on the body (bipolar). In this case, you can think of the lead as measuring the sum of electrical activity passing through an imaginary line between the two electrodes. In other cases, we record from one electrode at a time and you can think of the lead as being an imaginary line running from the center of the heart to the point on the body at which the recording electrode is attached (unipolar).

CLASSIFICATION OF LEADS

Limb leads: There are six limb leads which are further divided as unipolar and bipolar leads.

Bipolar leads: They simultaneously record the electrical activity of two different areas of the heart using a positive electrode and a negative electrode (**Fig. 13**). A bipolar lead gives us the potential difference of electrical activity between these two areas of the heart where the two electrodes are placed.

Lead I records the potential difference of electrical activity between left upper limb (LUL) and right upper limb (RUL). In other words, lead I records the signals coming from RUL (negative pole) to the LUL (positive pole) (**Fig. 13**). Lead I is horizontal lead and represents the lateral surface of the heart (**Table 2**).

Lead II records the signals coming from the RUL (negative pole) to the left foot (positive pole), and thus records inferior and leftward directed vector (**Fig. 13** and **Table 2**).

Lead III records signals coming from the LUL (negative pole) to left foot (positive pole) and records inferior, and rightward directed vector (**Fig. 13** and **Table 2**).

Unipolar leads: There are three unipolar limb leads—lead augmented vector right (aVR), lead augmented vector left (aVL), and lead augmented vector foot (aVF). These leads record the electrical activity of a particular area only. For example, lead aVR gives information of the right arm only (i.e., electrical signals coming toward the right arm). As mentioned earlier, a lead is an imaginary line along which

TABLE 2 Bipolar lead system.

Lead	Positive electrode	Negative electrode	Vector
Lead I	Left upper limb	Right upper limb	Horizontal, R → L
Lead II	Left foot	Right upper limb	Inferior, R → L
Lead III	Left foot	Left upper limb	Inferior, L → R

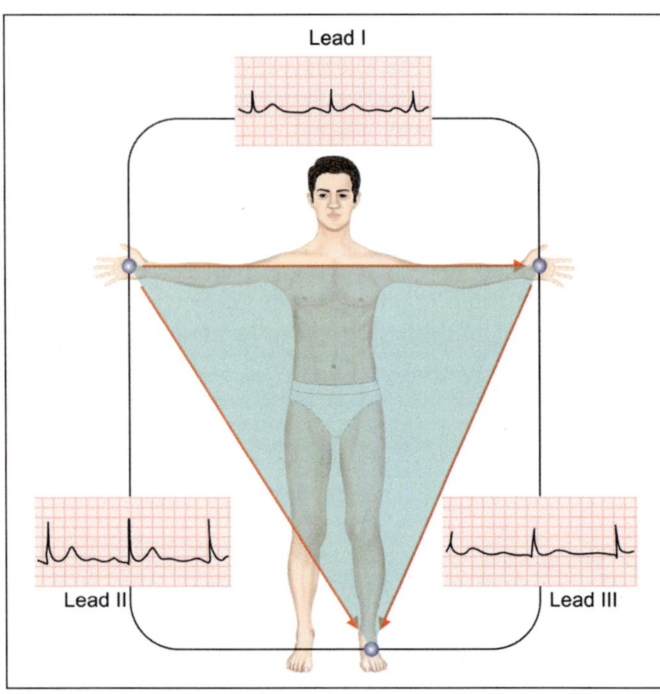

FIGURE 13: Bipolar leads record electrical activity of two different areas using a negative electrode and a positive electrode.

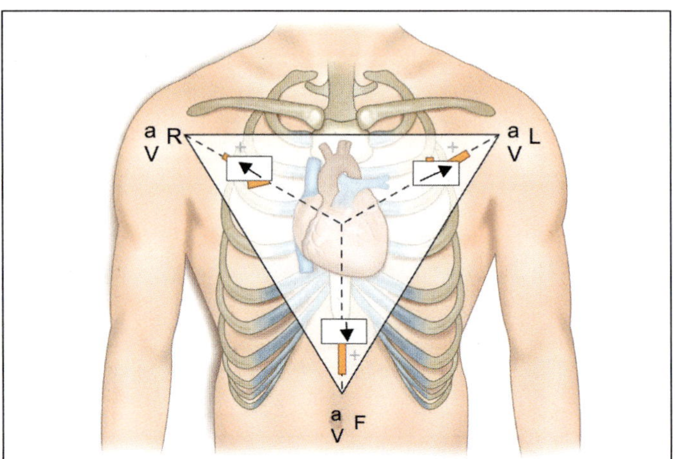

FIGURE 14: Unipolar leads, where the positive pole is the limb of interest, and the negative pole is the central terminal.

electrical activity is being measured. For unipolar leads, this imaginary line is from the center of the heart to that particular electrode (**Fig. 14**).

For example, for lead aVR, the imaginary line is from the center of the heart to the right arm, wherein the center of the heart (central terminal) serves as the negative electrode and the right arm serves as the positive electrode. This central terminal labeled as Wilson's central terminal is the negative electrodes coming from all three limbs. In other words, the negative pole of all the unipolar limb leads is connected to the central terminal. Wilson's central terminal is produced by averaging the measurements from the electrodes of right arm, left arm, and left foot to give an average potential across the body.

*Augmented leads (**Table 3**)*: The unipolar limb leads of right arm, left arm, and left foot record electrical activity of that particular area only. Since they are all located far away from the heart, the complexes recorded will be small; hence there is a need to augment these complexes. The augmentation is done by disconnecting the limb of interest from the central terminal, which serves as the negative pole. For example, in recording aVR, we disconnect the right arm lead from the negative pole, so the negative pole will be connected to the LUL and left lower limb only. Since we are not subtracting anything from the RUL, the positivity will be enhanced, and the resulting complexes will be larger (augmented).

Lead aVR gives us information about the impulses coming from the center of the heart to the RUL, i.e., high right superior surface of the heart.

Lead I aVL gives us information of the high left lateral surface of the heart.

Lead II, lead III, and lead aVF give us the information from the inferior surface of the heart.

Chest leads: Chest leads are placed over the chest and pickup electrical signals directly beneath them. They are unipolar leads giving us information from that particular area. Since the chest leads are in close proximity to the heart, the complexes are large, and there is no need for augmentation which means there is no disconnection of any electrode from the negative pole.

The chest electrodes should be placed correctly to record the ECG correctly (**Fig. 15**). The correct chest electrode placements are as follows:

- V_1: Fourth right intercostal space close to the sternum
- V_2: Fourth left intercostal space close to the sternum
- V_3: Between V_2 and V_4
- V_4: Fifth left intercostal space in the midclavicular line
- V_5: Fifth left intercostal space in the anterior axillary line
- V_6: Fifth left intercostal space in the mid axillary line

TABLE 3 Unipolar lead system.

Lead	Positive electrode	Negative electrode	Augmented
aVR	Right upper limb	Central terminal	Disconnect negative pole from RUL
aVL	Left upper limb	Central terminal	Disconnect negative pole from LUL
aVF	Left foot	Central terminal	Disconnect negative pole from left foot

(aVF: augmented vector foot; aVL: augmented vector left; aVR: augmented vector right; LUL: left upper limb; RUL: right upper limb)

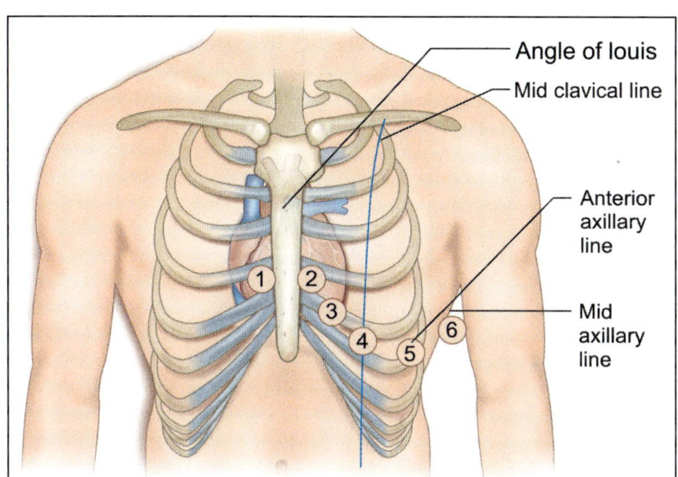

FIGURE 15: Chest leads and their positions.

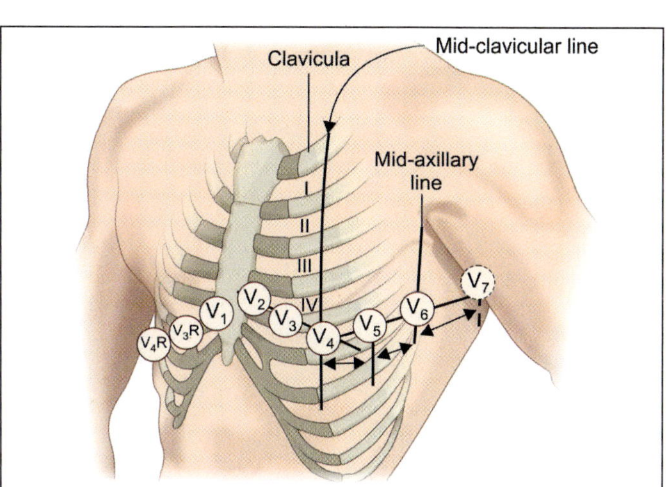

FIGURE 16: Additional leads.

Additional leads: There are certain situations where we may require additional electrodes in addition to these 12 leads (**Fig. 16**).

*Right-sided leads (**Fig. 16**)*: We record right-sided leads in three important situations: (1) dextrocardia, (2) congenital heart diseases, and (3) inferior wall myocardial infarction to diagnose RV myocardial infarction.

Additional posterior leads (V_7, V_8, and V_9): V_7 is placed in the posterior axillary line. V_8 is placed in the midscapular line, and V_9 is placed on paraspinal line. These leads are recorded whenever we have a very large LV which is away from the area of V_5, V_6, and also for recording posterior surface.

Lead aVR: It is a special lead, but often not seen while reading a routine ECG. It gives us valuable information regarding atrial depolarization (P wave), ventricular depolarization (QRS), and ventricular repolarization (T wave). In a normal ECG, P wave, QRS complex, and T wave are inverted in lead aVR as all these waves are going away from this lead. If P wave and/or QRS is upright in lead aVR, we can infer that atrial/ventricular depolarization direction is grossly abnormal.

Leads and surfaces of the heart: The leads give us valuable information of the surface.

It is important to correlate the leads to the surface of the heart for which they represent (**Table 4**).

*Leads and coronary artery disease (**Fig. 17**)*: The surfaces of the heart and thus the ECG leads represent areas of coronary artery perfusion. So, identifying changes in the ECG leads will help us in localizing the coronary artery disease. **Figure 17** will help us in converting ECG leads into coronary artery perfusion territories (**Table 5**).

*Naming of individual leads (**Fig. 18**)*: Leads are named based on the direction toward which that particular lead travels. For example, lead I is a horizontal lead with the direction of the vector going horizontally from right to left.

HOW TO LOOK

Looking at the leads in the following sequence will help to relate the leads to the corresponding cardiac surface and the relevant coronary artery (**Fig. 19**).

First look at lead I, AVL, and then V_5, V_6 (lateral surface and LCX territory).

Then look at lead II, aVF, and lead III [inferior surface and right coronary artery (RCA) territory].

Look at aVR next to confirm the normal sequence of depolarization and repolarization—all waves are negative.

Then look at V_1 (right ventricle and proximal RCA).

Finally look at V_2, V_3, and V_4 (anterior wall, anterior septum, and LAD territory).

Looking at the ECG in the above sequence will guide us in visualizing the particular surface as well as the corresponding coronary artery which supplies it.

ELECTRICAL AXIS AND AXIS DEVIATION

INTRODUCTION

We have just learnt about the leads and their positions with respect to the heart. How the QRS complexes are inscribed in the limb leads is determined by the electrical axis.

TABLE 4	Leads and corresponding surface of the heart.
Leads	**Corresponding surface**
Lead I, lead aVL	High lateral
V_5 and V_6	Anterolateral
Lead II, aVF, and Lead III	Inferior
V_1	Right ventricle
V_2, V_3, and V_4	Anterior wall and anterior IVS
Reciprocal changes in V_1 and V_2	Posterior wall

TABLE 5	Leads and coronary artery localization.
ECG leads	**Coronary artery territory**
Lead I and aVL	LCX
V_5 and V_6	LCX
Lead II, aVF, and lead III	RCA
V_1	Proximal RCA
V_2, V_3, and V_4	LAD

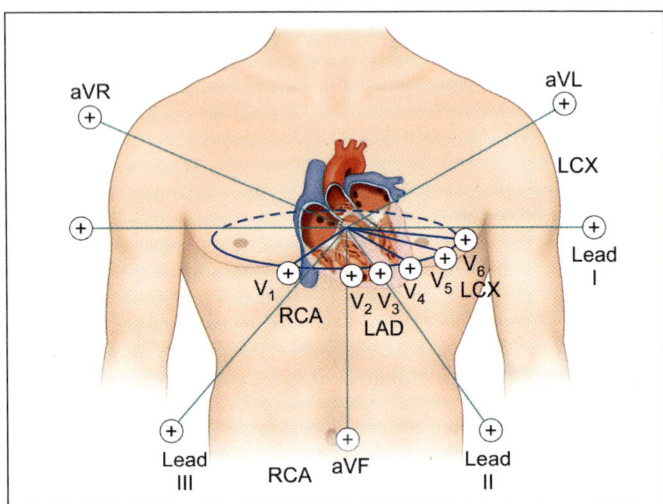

FIGURE 17: Leads and coronary artery territories.

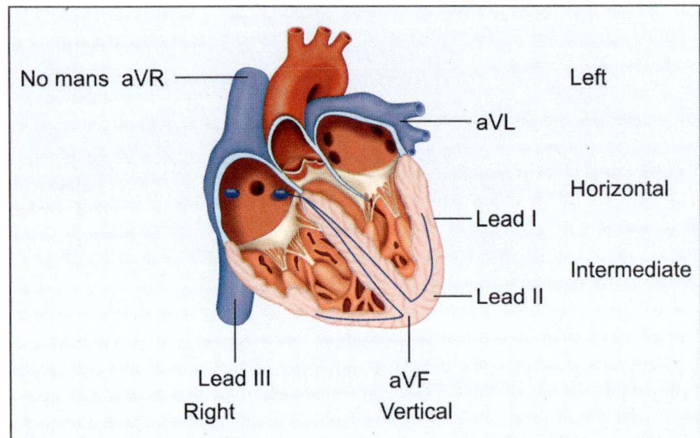

FIGURE 18: Naming of the leads based on the direction of the vector.

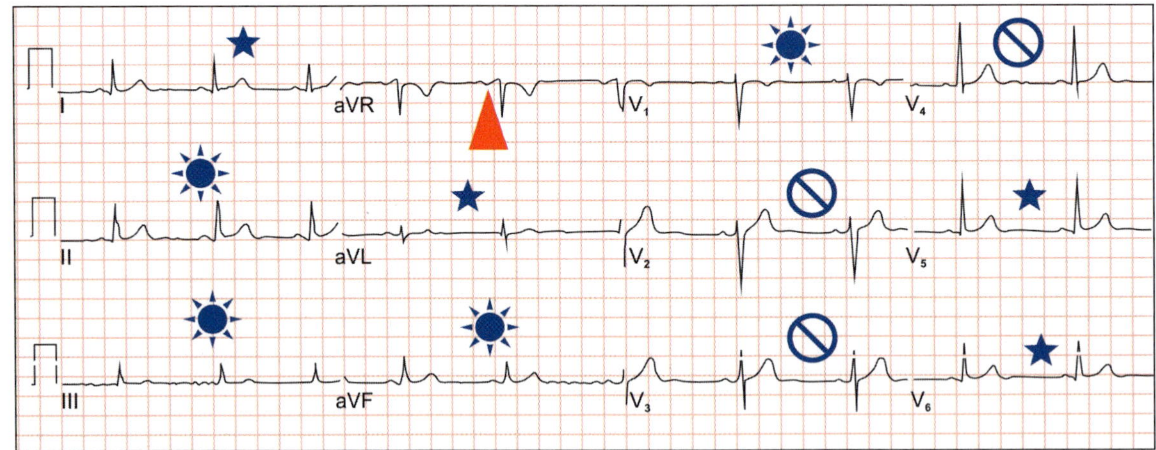

FIGURE 19: Sequence of reading an electrocardiogram.

The electrical axis of the heart is the determination of the net vector of the heart which is defined as the net direction and amplitude of the resultant cardiac impulse as described before.

Where and what to look for axis determination? As we are interested to know about the net ventricular depolarization direction in frontal plane, concentrate on QRS complexes in limb leads.

The importance of electrical axis calculation:
- To know the ultimate direction of the cardiac activity
- To know the position of the heart (horizontal heart or vertical heart, or intermediate heart)
- To diagnose the fascicular blocks, left anterior, and left posterior fascicular blocks
- To diagnose advanced conduction disturbances such as bifascicular/trifascicular blocks

METHODS OF ANALYSIS

There are various, elaborate, and complex methods of calculating the QRS axis, but learning those methods takes time and many students turn away from ECG learning because of the difficulty.

We will use a simpler but nevertheless a reasonable and practical method of calculating the axis. To recollect as discussed in the first section.

Positive deflection is recorded: When the wave of depolarization, or the vector is traveling toward that lead.

Negative deflection is recorded: When the wave of depolarization, or the vector is traveling away from that lead.

Equiphasic deflection is recorded: When the wave of depolarization or the vector is traveling perpendicular to that lead.

Simple method:

Simple rules to be followed:
- For calculation of axis always look at limb leads
- Remember the position of the leads
- Remember relationship of the leads to various surfaces of heart (**Fig. 20**)
  - Lead I is a horizontal lead.
  - Lead II is an intermediate lead.
  - Lead aVF is a vertical lead.
  - Lead III is a right-sided lead.
  - Lead aVL is a left-sided lead.
  - Lead aVR is no man's land.

If you remember this, the calculation of the axis will be easy.

How to determine the electrical heart axis:

Step 1:
Determine which of these six limb leads has the tallest QRS complex.

Look at leads I, II, and aVF.

If any one of these leads has the tallest QRS complex, the axis is normal, because the normal axis lies between leads I and aVF, and lead II lies between them (**Figs. 21** and **22**).

After diagnosing the normal axis look at the lead aVR. This is the opposite lead. It should show a negative QRS complex as in normal heart ventricular depolarization (QRS) should be away from this lead.

Step 2:
If lead I, II, or aVF does not show the tallest QRS complex, look at lead III and lead aVL.

Step 3:
If lead III shows the tallest positive QRS complex and aVL is negative, it means the impulses are moving away from the left side and going toward the right side leads. This is right axis (**Figs. 23** and **24**).

In the above ECG, note that:
- Lead I, II, or aVF does not have the tallest QRS.
- Look at lead III and aVL.
- Lead III records the tallest QRS and aVL is negative.
- Therefore, the axis is deviated to the right.

Step 4:
If lead III records a predominantly negative QRS and lead aVL records the tallest positive QRS complex, it indicates that the vector is directed to the left side and therefore, it is a left axis deviation (**Figs. 25** and **26**).

In the above ECG, note that:
- Lead I, II, or aVF does not have the tallest QRS.
- Look at lead III and aVL.
- Lead aVL records the tallest QRS and lead III is negative.
- Therefore, the axis is deviated to the left.

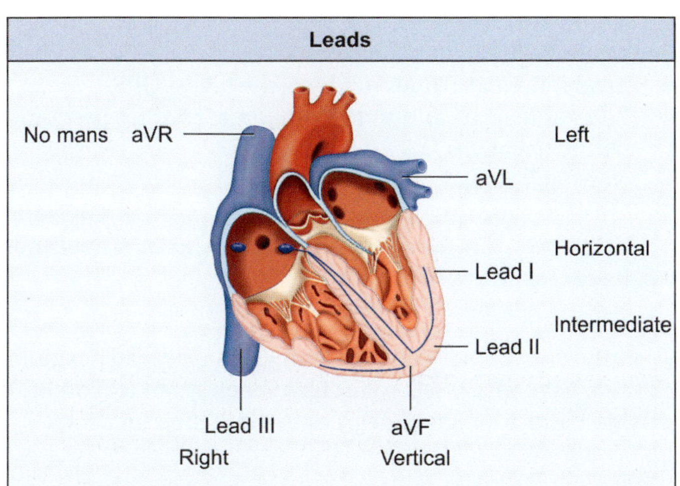

FIGURE 20: Relationship of individual limb leads to various surfaces of heart.

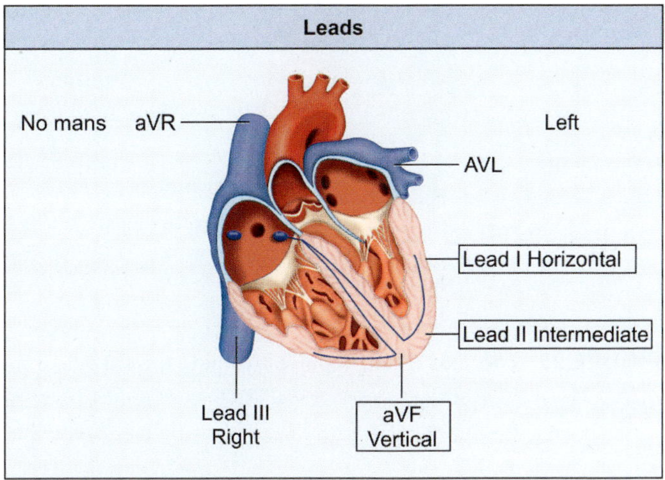

FIGURE 21: Normal axis.

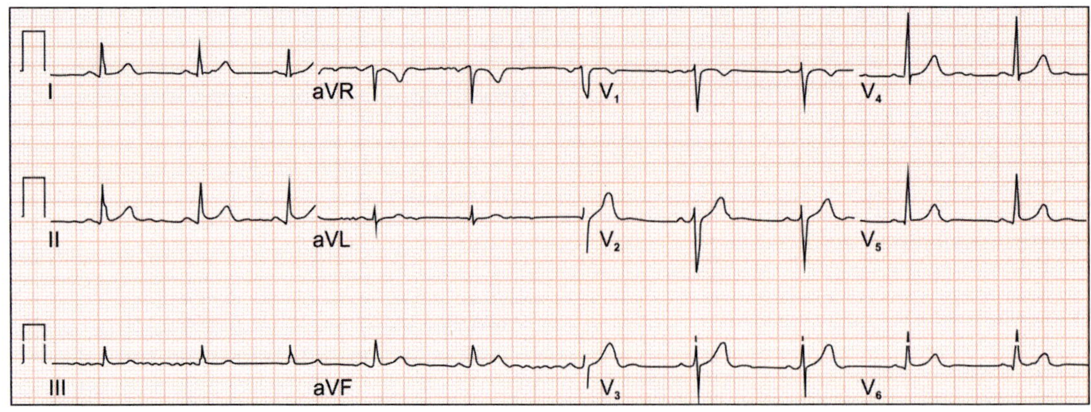

FIGURE 22: Look at leads I, II, and aVF. Lead II records the tallest QRS. aVR is negative and therefore, the axis is normal.

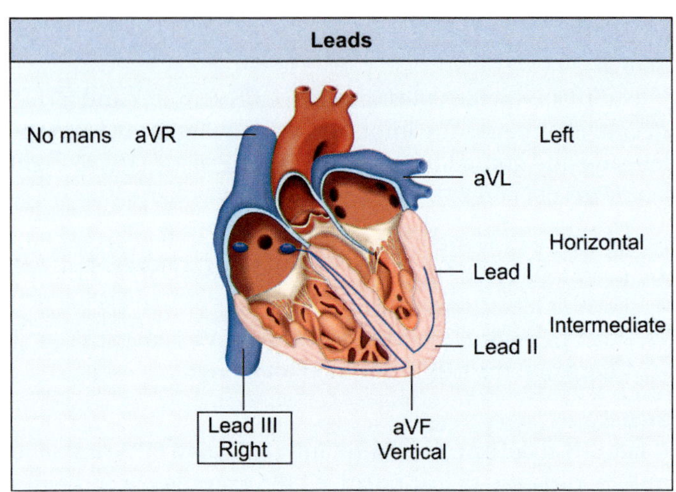

FIGURE 23: Right axis where impulse is coming toward Lead III.

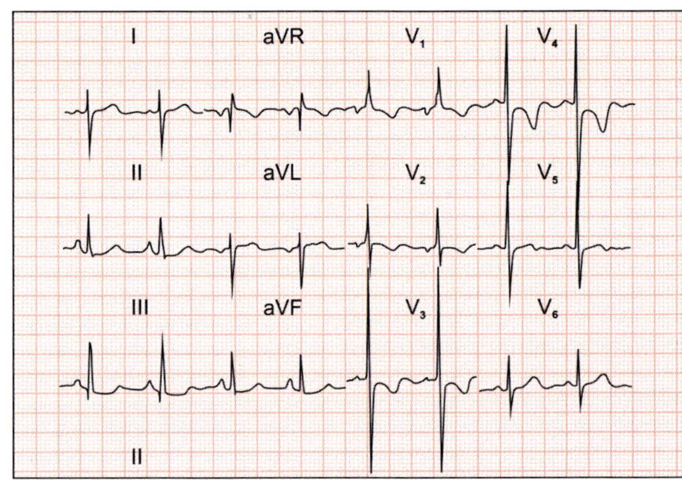

FIGURE 24: Electrocardiogram showing right axis.

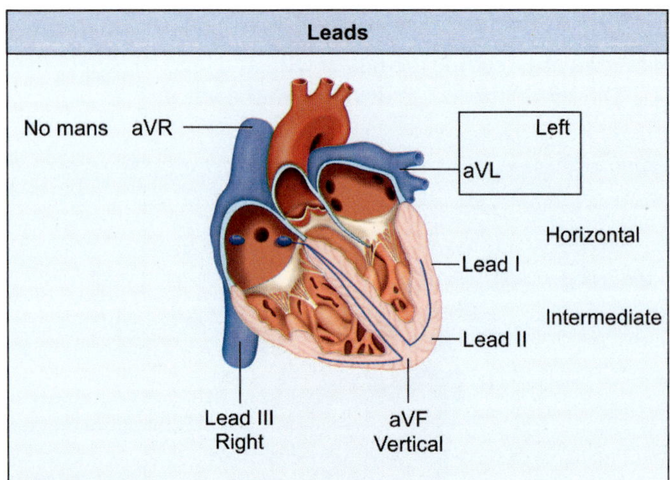

FIGURE 25: Left axis where impulse is coming toward aVL.

Step 5:
If none of the above leads (I, II, III, aVL, and aVF), records the tallest positive QRS, look at lead aVR.

If aVR is positive, then the axis is called indeterminate axis (**Figs. 27** and **28**).

In the above ECG, note that:

- Lead I, II, or aVF does not have the tallest QRS.
- Look at lead III and aVL. Both are recording predominantly negative QRS.
- Now look at lead aVR.
- This is recording a predominantly positive QRS and therefore, this is an indeterminate axis, sometimes known as North-West axis.

The next step:
Identification of the exact axis in degrees: The lead positions that we have discussed so far have been given a geometric position and is assigned degrees to mark their locations.

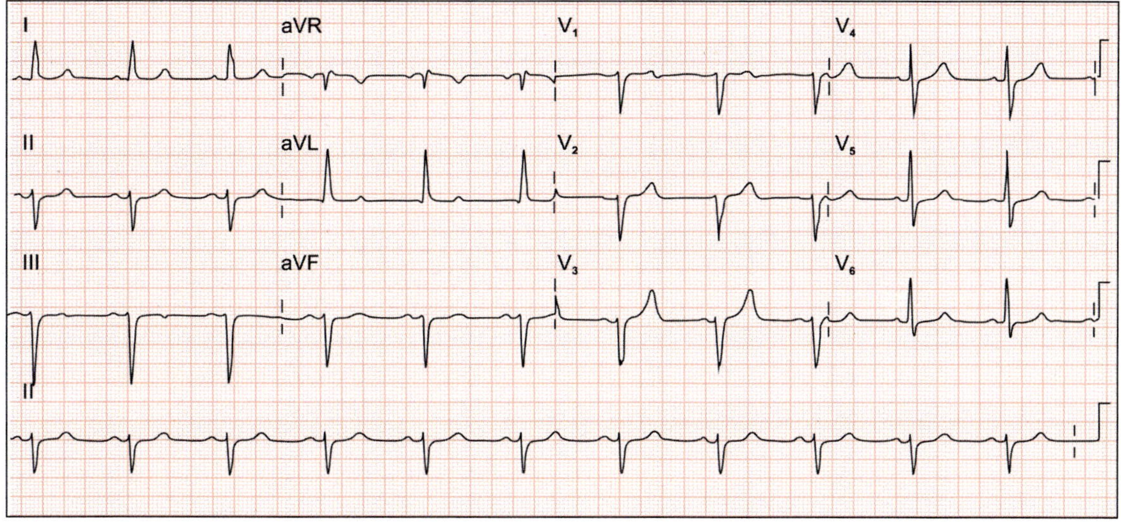

FIGURE 26: Electrocardiogram showing left axis.

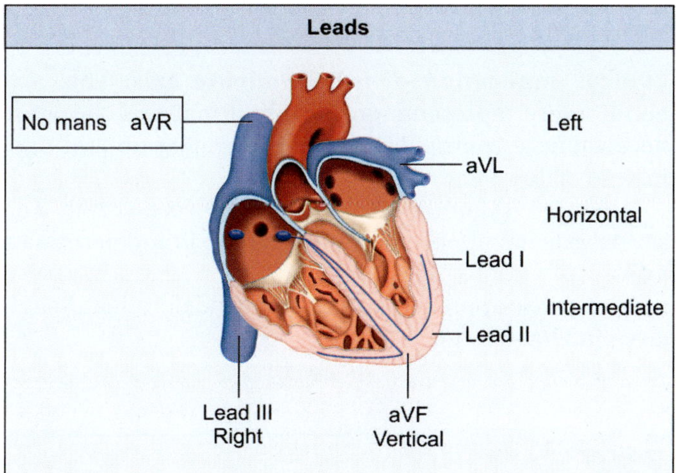

FIGURE 27: Indeterminate axis where impulse going toward aVR.

The axis diagram is divided into two halves as shown in the **Figure 29**.

Totally we have six limb leads:

- Three leads in the lower half (II, aVF, and III)
- Two leads in the upper half (aVL and aVR)
- Lower half will have positive degrees and upper half will have negative degrees as shown in the **Figure 29**.
- Lead I which lies in the horizontal plane is the starting point and is assigned "0°".
- Lead II is at +60°
- aVF at +90°
- Lead III at +120°
- aVL at –30°
- and aVR at –150° as shown in the **Figure 29**.

Now that we have moved to the next level, we have to assign degrees to the leads. For example, if you identify that lead, I is recording the tallest positive QRS you are no longer satisfied by saying that the axis is normal. You can now say that the axis is 0 degree.

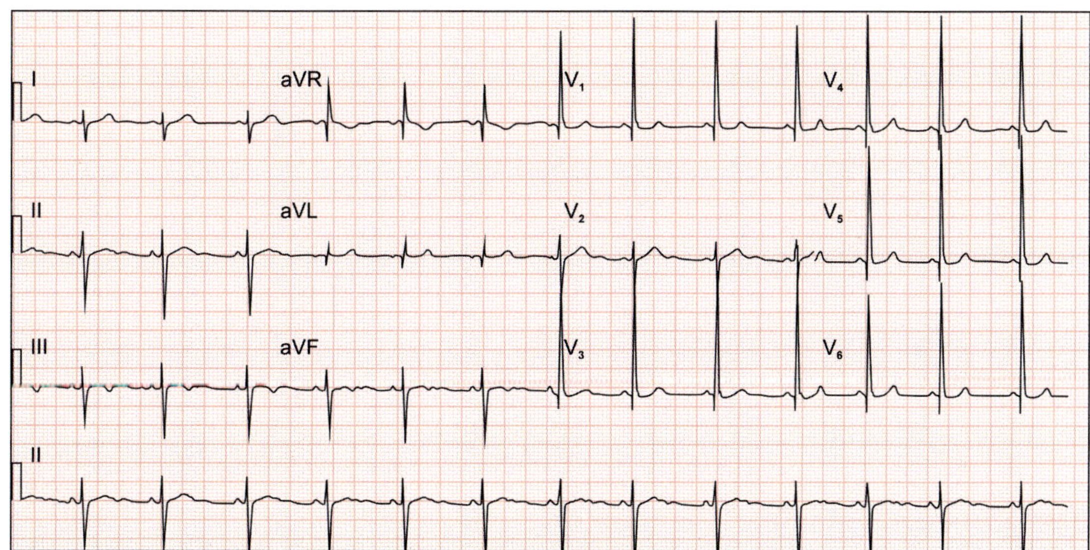

FIGURE 28: Electrocardiogram showing indeterminate axis.

Lead I, tallest positive QRS → (1) normal axis, (2) 0°,
Lead II, tallest positive QRS → (1) normal axis, (2) 60°,
aVF, tallest positive QRS → (1) normal axis, (2) 90°,
Lead III, tallest positive QRS → (1) right axis, (2) 120°,
aVL, tallest positive QRS → (1) left axis, (2) –30°, (3) left anterior fascicular block (LAFB) and left ventricular hypertrophy (LVH).

aVR has tallest positive QRS → (1) indeterminate axis, (2) –150°.

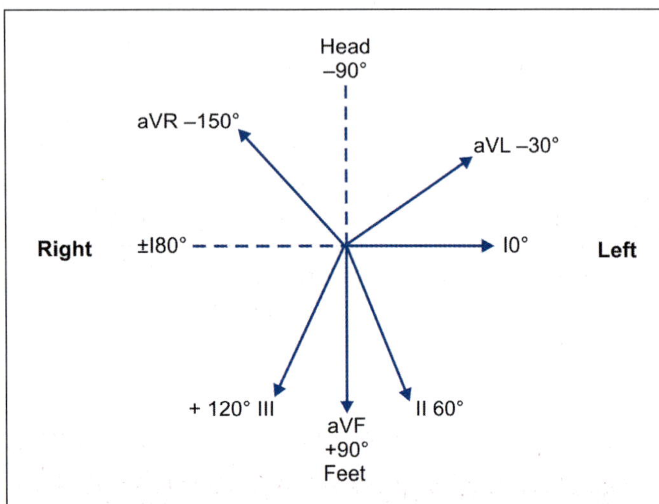

FIGURE 29: Numbers for the leads.

Clinical implications of normal axis:

Normal axis: Horizontal, vertical, or intermediate position

Horizontal heart: Ascites, pregnancy, and obesity

Vertical heart: Chronic obstructive pulmonary disease (COPD)—emphysema

Intermediate: Normal

Clinical implications of right axis deviation: Right ventricular hypertrophy (RVH) is the most common cause.

Pulmonary hypertension, pulmonary stenosis, and pulmonary thromboembolism are the conditions which can cause RVH and right axis.

Left posterior fascicular block can cause right axis which should be diagnosed only after ruling out RVH.

Clinical implications of left axis: Left anterior fascicular block is the most common cause.

Left ventricular hypertrophy due to hypertension, aortic stenosis, and hypertrophic cardiomyopathy can also have left axis.

Clinical implication of indeterminate axis: This axis abnormality represents grossly abnormal axis deviation because here ventricular vector is traveling up and right instead of down and left.

Complex cyanotic hear diseases, severe COPD, and severe skeletal abnormalities can result in indeterminate axis.

A stepwise approach to diagnosing indeterminate axis is given in **Flowchart 1**.

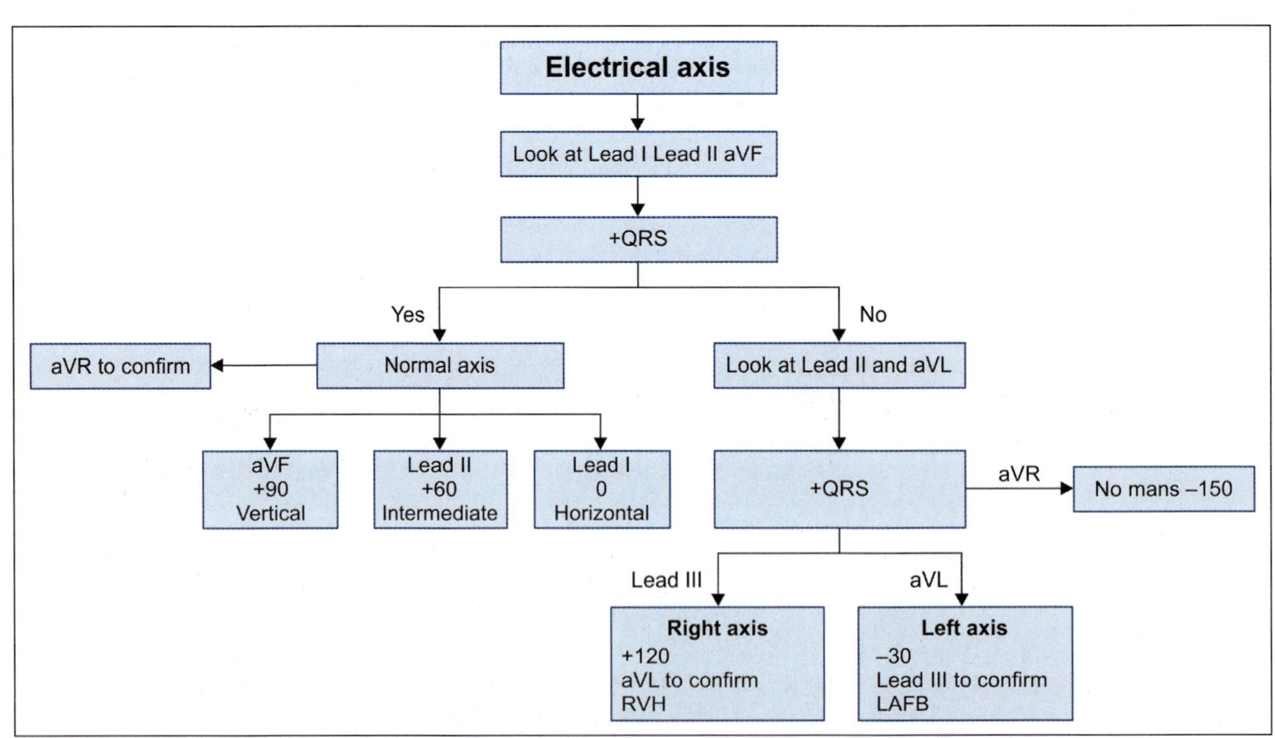

FLOWCHART 1: Stepwise approach for indeterminate axis.

MEASUREMENT OF WAVES AND INTERVALS

The measurement of waves and intervals, and their significance is shown in **Table 6**.

ELECTROCARDIOGRAM EXAMPLES

- The ECG in **Figure 30** shows a normal ECG. Note that all complexes are negative in aVR, normal axis and net QRS vector is traveling toward left in chest leads (QRS predominantly negative in V_1 and positive in V_5 and V_6).
- The ECG in **Figure 31** shows left ventricular hypertrophy. Note that the S in V_1 + R in V_5 is >35 mm.
- The ECG in **Figure 32** shows RVH. There is a tall R in V_1 of >7 mm and right axis deviation.
- The ECG in **Figure 33** shows RBBB with wide QRS having delayed terminal slurred positivity on right-sided leads (V_1).
- The ECG in **Figure 34** shows LBBB with wide QRS having delayed terminal slurred positivity on left side (V_5 and V_6).
- The ECG in **Figure 35** shows ST elevation in anterior and lateral leads—due to acute extensive anterior wall infarction.
- The ECG in **Figure 36** shows ST elevation acute coronary syndrome-ST elevated myocardial infarction (ACS-STEMI)-inferior wall infarction. There is ST elevation in lead II, III, aVF with reciprocal ST depression in lead I, aVL. (Right coronary artery occlusion related inferior wall infarction)
- The ECG in **Figure 37** shows AF fulfilling three criteria of AF: (1) Absent well-formed coordinated P waves, (2) Irregular R-R interval and (3) presence of fibrillary waves.

CONCLUSION

Basic fundamentals of ECG genesis, lead systems, and axis calculation are discussed in a simple way. This chapter on ECG at best can eliminate the fear of seeing the ECG as it explains and tries to make you understand certain essential elements of ECG interpretation. But further knowledge in ECG can be obtained only by seeing and interpreting a lot of ECGs. So, this is not the end, but the beginning of exciting journey in the interpretation of ECG.

TABLE 6 Mechanism of various waves, intervals, their normal, abnormal values, and the clinical significance.

Wave/ Segment	Cause	Normal values	Abnormal values, findings	Clinical conditions
P	Atrial depolarization	2.5 small squares, horizontally, vertically	• >2.5 vertically • >2.5 horizontally	• Tall P: Right Atrial • Enlargement • Wide P: Left atrial enlargement
PR	Atrio ventricular conduction time	0.12-0.21 s	• <0.12 short PR • >0.12 long PR	• Short PR: Pre excitation • Long PR: I degree AVB
QRS	Ventricular depolarization	Amplitude • S in V_1 + R in V_5 and V_6 35 mm • R/S ratio > 1, R in V_1 >7 mm in V_1 Width <0.08 s	• LVH • RVH • >0.08 s wide QRS	• Hypertension/AS • Pulmonary stenosis/PHT • Pulmonary thrombus • Bundle branch block
ST	Segment between depolarization and repolarization	Isoelectric ST	• ST elevation • ST depression	• ST elevation ACS • Non ST elevation ACS
T	Ventricular depolarization	20-40% of preceding QRS	• <20% low Volt. T • >40% Tall T	• Hypokalemia, Non specific T • Hyperkalemia, acute ischemia
QT interval	Ventricular depolarization, ST interval, and ventricular repolarization	0.36–0.46 s (to be corrected for HR-QTc)	• Long QTc >0.46 s • Short QTc <0.36 s	• Congenital, drugs, electrolytes; • Digoxin, hypocalcemia
U wave	After T wave goes with T wave in direction and amplitude	• Prominent u • Inverted u	• U taller than T • U in opposite direction to T	• Hypokalemia • Ischemia

***Note*: The above values are applicable only when ECG is recorded at 1 mV standardization and 25 mm/s speed.**

(ACS: acute coronary syndrome; AVB: atrioventricular block; LVH: left ventricular hypertrophy; RVH: right ventricular hypertrophy)

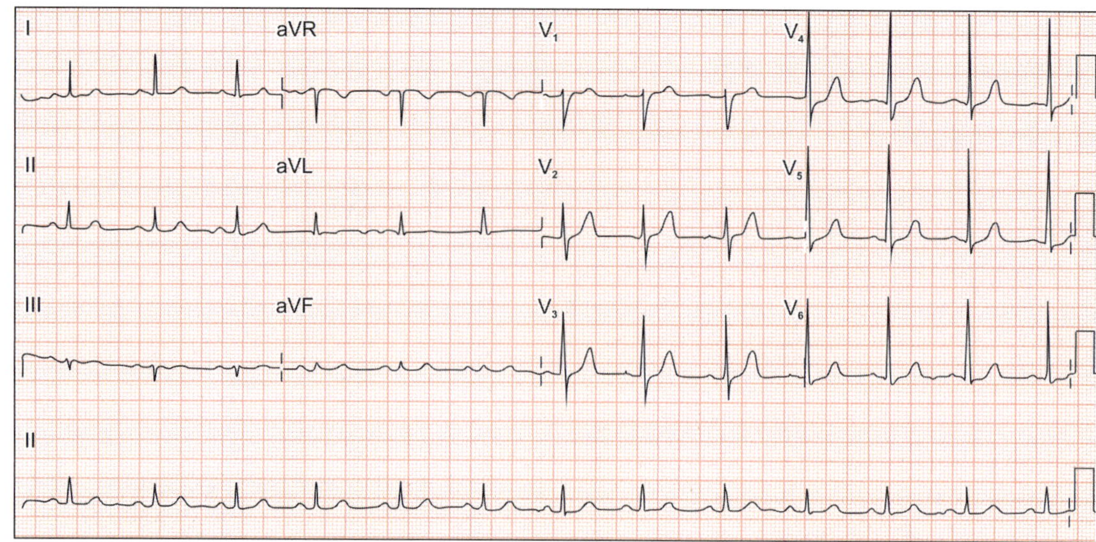

FIGURE 30: Normal ECG.

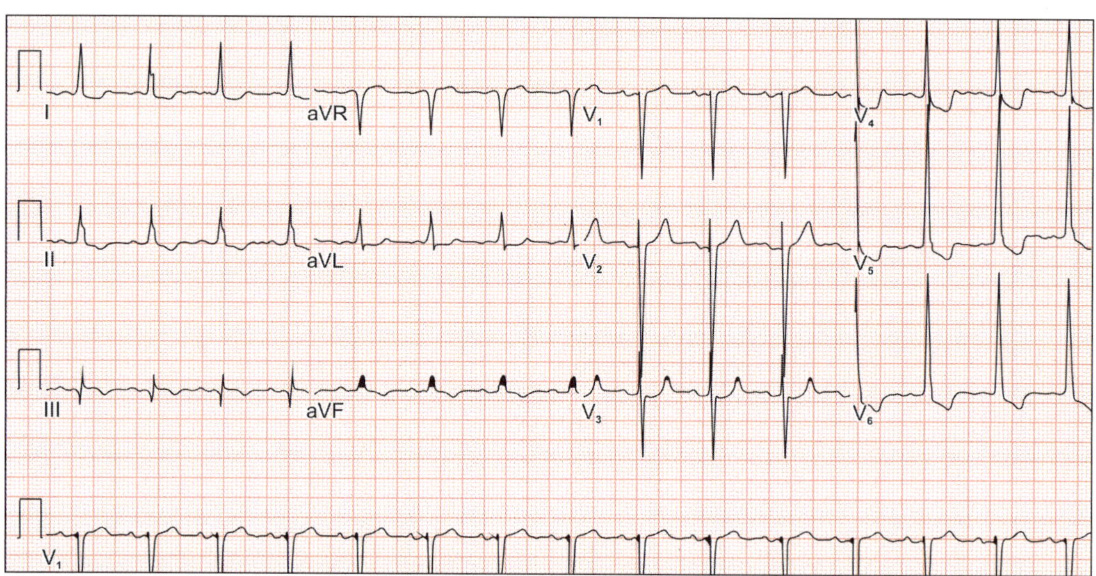

FIGURE 31: ECG showing left ventricular hypertrophy (LVH).

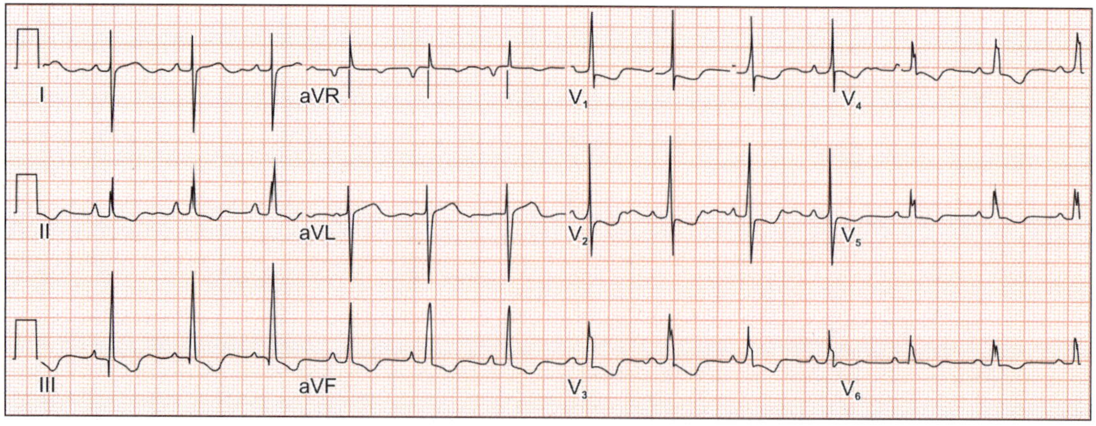

FIGURE 32: ECG showing right ventricular hypertrophy (RVH).

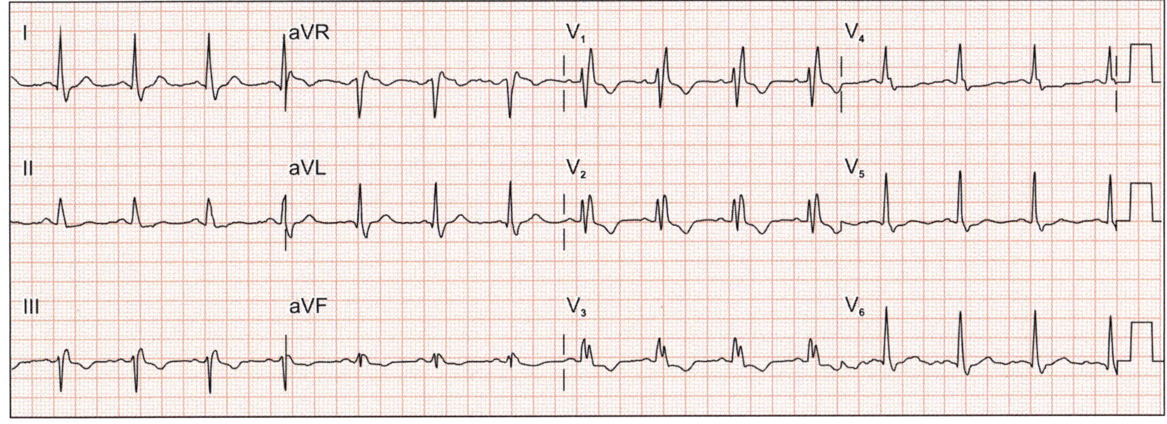

FIGURE 33: ECG showing right bundle branch block (RBBB).

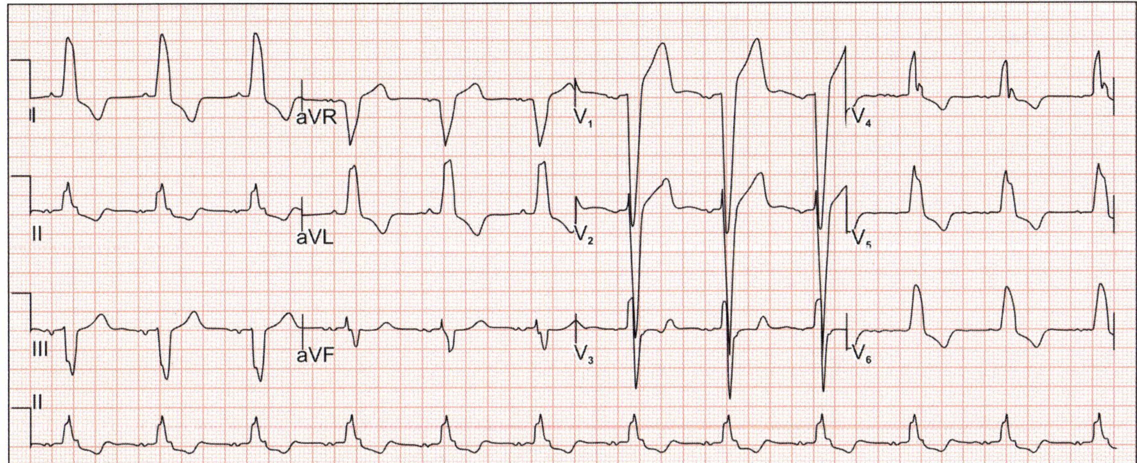

FIGURE 34: ECG showing left bundle branch block (LBBB).

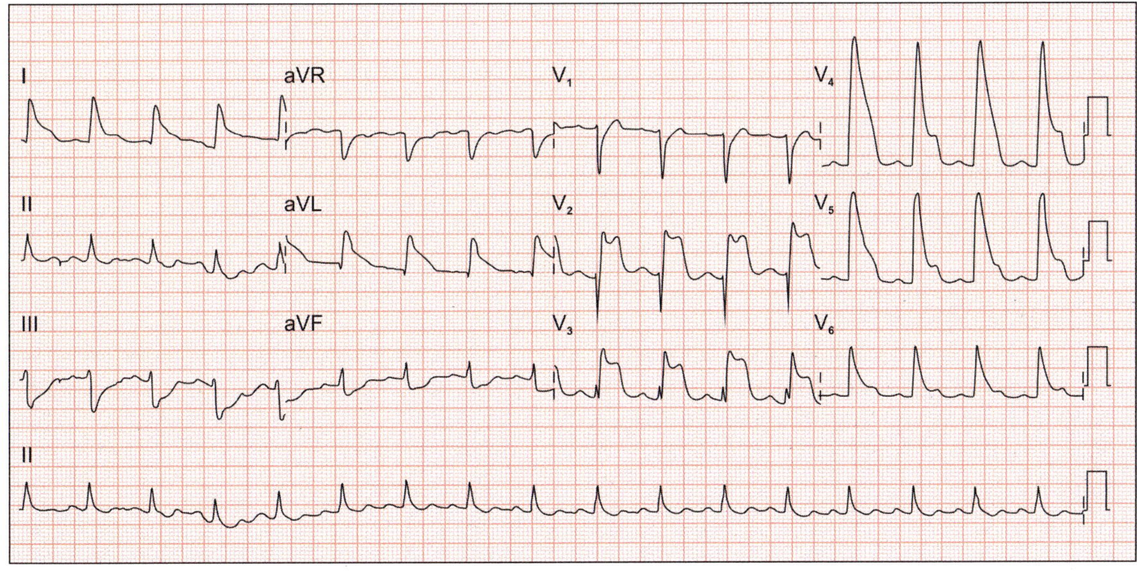

FIGURE 35: ECG showing anterior wall infarction.

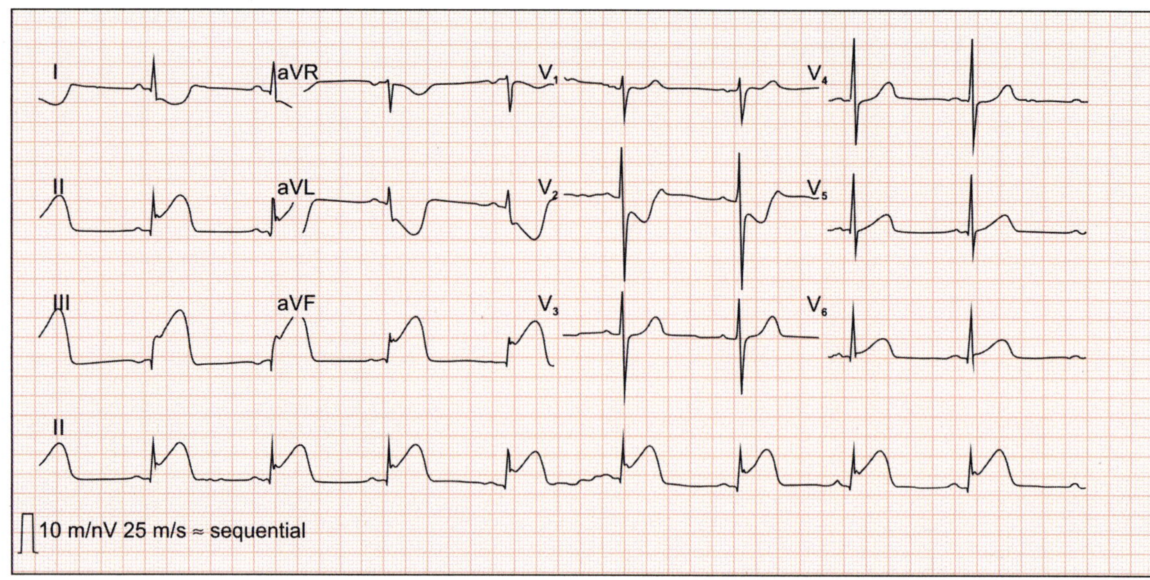

FIGURE 36: ECG showing Inferior wall STEMI.

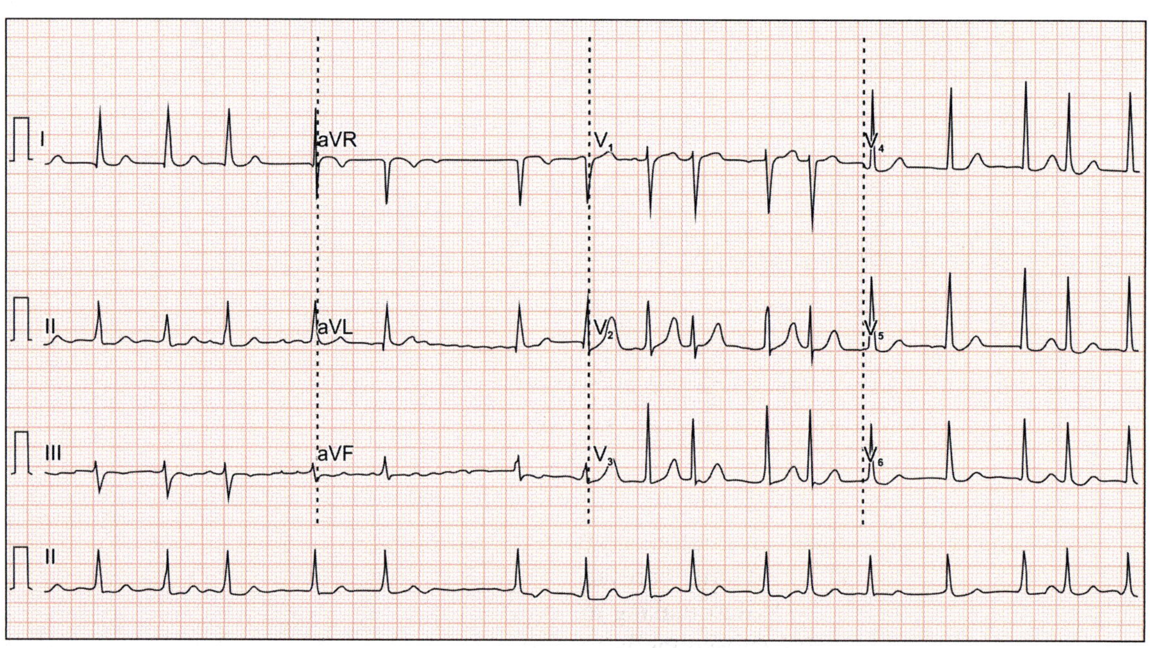

FIGURE 37: ECG showing AF.

RECOMMENDED READINGS

1. Narasimhan C, Francis J, LeoSchamroth. An introduction to electrocardiography, 8th edition.
2. Vaz M, Raj T. Guyton and Hall Textbook of medical physiology: 1st edition A South Asian edition. 2013.
3. ECG clinical interpretation: A to Z by diagnosis. (2015).
4. Garcia TB. 12_Lead ECG The Art of Interpretation. Jones and Bartlett Learning Burlington, MA. 2015.
5. Malcolm TS. The only EKG book you'll ever need. Lipincott Williams and Wilkins. Philadelphia, PA. 2012.
6. Walraven G. Basic arrhythmias seventh edition. Pearson Education Upper Saddle River, NJ. 2011.

CHAPTER

88

Noninvasive Cardiac Imaging

Manish Bansal, Priya Chudgar, Jagat Narula

ABSTRACT

Noninvasive imaging plays a pivotal role in the evaluation and management of the patients with various cardiac disorders. Chest X-ray is the basic investigation and is almost a part of clinical examination. It is discussed elsewhere in the book. Echocardiography (cardiac ultrasound) has greatly evolved and is currently the most commonly used cardiac imaging modality. Echocardiography includes M-mode, two-dimensional (2D), three-dimensional (3D) echo, Doppler for blood flow and tissue velocity measurement, strain imaging, contrast echo and stress echo. Its advantages are ease of performance, rapidity of diagnosis, low cost, safety and the ability to repeat.

Myocardial perfusion imaging (MPI), earlier with single-photon emission computed tomography (SPECT) and now also with positron emission tomography (PET) scan, is used mainly for detection of myocardial ischemia and viability in coronary artery disease (CAD). Cardiac computed tomography (CT) is used primarily for the assessment of coronary atherosclerosis and coronary anatomy. It is fast becoming an alternative to invasive coronary angiography (ICA) for excluding obstructive CAD in low-risk patients. CT-derived information about coronary atherosclerosis is also very useful for risk assessment and management of the patients requiring primary prevention of atherosclerotic cardiovascular disease. Cardiac magnetic resonance imaging (MRI) has now emerged as one of the most informative cardiac imaging modalities. It has the greatest utility for evaluation of heart muscle diseases and for quantification of cardiac chamber sizes and function.

The technical considerations of each of the four noninvasive cardiac imaging modalities are given in greater detail in the E-chapter. Salient features of these have been kept in the printed chapter. The reader is referred to E-chapter for greater details.

"Medical science has proven time and again that when the resources are provided, great progress in the treatment, cure, and prevention of disease can occur"

—Michael J Fox

INTRODUCTION

Imaging plays a pivotal role in the evaluation and management of the patients with various cardiac disorders. From initial diagnosis and decision making to guiding therapeutic interventions, and subsequently to postprocedure evaluation and long-term follow-up, some form of imaging is integral at every step. Echocardiography, nuclear scanning, cardiac CT, and cardiac magnetic resonance (CMR) are the four main noninvasive cardiac imaging techniques used in clinical practice (**Table 1**). This chapter provides an overview of the technical aspects and the clinical applications of these modalities.

ECHOCARDIOGRAPHY

Echocardiography is the most versatile of all the noninvasive cardiac imaging modalities. It is the only technique that can delineate cardiac anatomy and function simultaneously, in real-time and at the patients' bedside. This unique capability, combined with the low cost, wide availability, and ease of use and safety renders echocardiography the most used cardiac imaging modality.

TECHNICAL CONSIDERATIONS

Echocardiography is an ultrasound-based technique which uses ultrasound waves for imaging cardiac structures. In *M-mode,* the imaging is done along a single scan line. In *2D echocardiography,* the ultrasound beam is swept from one end of the image sector to the other end. *3D echocardiography* is a more recent development. It uses matrix array technology that acquires a pyramidal dataset instead of one scan line at a time. The addition of *Doppler imaging* to grayscale imaging has revolutionized echocardiography. Two primary Doppler modes exist—(1) pulsed wave (PW) and (2) continuous wave (CW). In the PW Doppler, a single piezoelectric crystal is used; this allows recording velocities from a specific site. CW Doppler is used when high velocities need to be measured.

Color Doppler is a variant of PW Doppler. Conventionally, the blood flow toward the transducer is displayed in red color and that away from the transducer is displayed in blue color. Tissue Doppler is another form of PW Doppler, which is used for measuring myocardial velocities instead of blood flow.

TABLE 1 Relative advantages and limitations of various noninvasive cardiac imaging modalities.

Echocardiography	Nuclear imaging	Computed tomography	Magnetic resonance imaging
Advantages:	*Advantages*:	*Advantages*:	*Advantages*:
• Widely available, low cost, portable • No radiation exposure, no iodinated contrast • Highest temporal resolution, excellent spatial resolution • Only modality to permit real-time, cine imaging • Least challenges due to tachycardia, arrhythmia, respiratory motion • Permits comprehensive assessment of cardiac structure and function • Excellent for hemodynamic assessment • Can be easily combined with any form of stressor • Ideal for intraprocedure imaging during surgical or percutaneous structural heart disease interventions	• Excellent modality for assessment of myocardial perfusion • Myocardial PET scan considered "gold standard" for viability assessment • Only modality to evaluate myocardial metabolism • Only modality to evaluate myocardial molecular processes • Can demonstrate active myocardial inflammation • Quantification of RV volumes and function feasible • No requirement for iodinated contrast	• Excellent modality for assessment of coronary anatomy • Excellent modality for recognition of obstructive coronary artery disease • Strong prognostic value of CT-detected nonobstructive coronary atherosclerosis and calcium score • Assessment of plaque morphology and hemodynamic significance is feasible • Excellent modality for the assessment of aortic and other vascular pathologies • Preferred modality for pre-procedural planning before TAVI	• Multifaceted, permits comprehensive assessment of cardiac structure and function • Tissue characterization feasible • Most accurate modality for quantifying cardiac chamber volumes • Excellent for assessment of myocardial fibrosis, necrosis, and edema • Excellent for evaluation of myocardial infiltrative diseases • No radiation exposure • May be performed safely even in patients with renal dysfunction
Disadvantages/limitations:	*Disadvantages/limitations*:	*Disadvantages/limitations*:	*Disadvantages/limitations*:
• Suboptimal image quality in nearly 20–30% patients • Imaging is mostly two-dimensional (3D overcomes this but has technical challenges) • Involves geometric assumptions for quantifying cardiac chamber volumes • Observer variability • Difficult to quantify myocardial perfusion • Less sensitive (although more specific) for detecting perfusion abnormalities • Tissue characterization generally not feasible	• Limited spatial resolution (at least for SPECT) • Poor temporal resolution • Virtually no diagnostic utility beyond assessment of myocardial perfusion, metabolism, and inflammation • Expensive	• Radiation exposure • Need for iodinated contrast • Predominantly an anatomic imaging modality • Coronary imaging requires good heart rate control and stable cardiac rhythm • Expensive	• Not suitable in patients with magnetically-susceptible metallic implants • Long acquisition time, claustrophobic environment • Requires good heart rate control, stable cardiac rhythm, and repeated breath-holds • Poor temporal resolution • Not yet suitable for coronary imaging • Expensive • Limited availability

(CT: computed tomography; RV: right ventricular; SPECT: single-photon emission computed tomography; TAVI: transcatheter aortic valve implantation)

Strain imaging is a relatively new development. Strain refers to the percentage change in the length of a myocardial segment during a given phase of the cardiac cycle. Speckle tracking echocardiography is the main modality used for myocardial strain imaging.

Contrast echocardiography utilizes specially designed ultrasound contrast agents. The left ventricular (LV) cavity opacification is the most important application of contrast echocardiography.

Echocardiography when performed by placing the transducer on the patient's chest wall is known as transthoracic echocardiography. It can also be performed using an endoscope which is passed into the patient's esophagus and stomach. This is known as transesophageal echocardiography (TEE). Stress echocardiography is yet another form of echocardiography in which imaging is combined with exercise or a pharmacological stressor.

CLINICAL APPLICATIONS

Left ventricular systolic function assessment: Assessment of LV systolic function is one of the most important objectives of echocardiography performed for any clinical

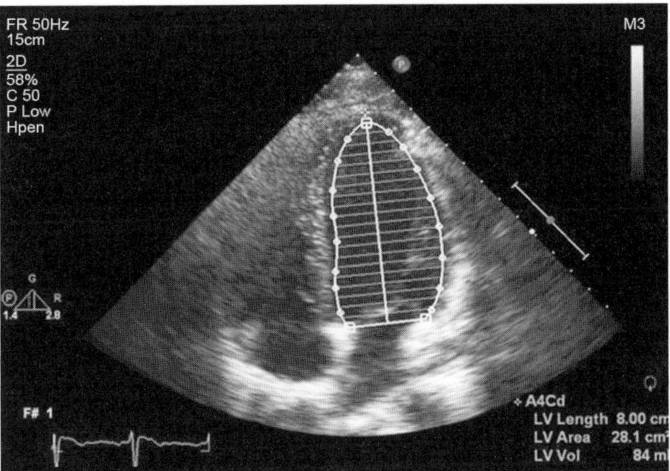

FIGURE 1: Modified Simpson's method for estimation of left ventricular volumes and ejection fraction. The left ventricular cavity border is manually traced; the automated software then divides the cavity into a stack of multiple discs and calculates the total cavity volume by adding the volume of each individual disk. This process is performed in both apical four-chamber and two-chamber views to obtain left ventricular volume.

indication. LV ejection fraction (LVEF) is the parameter used for quantifying LV systolic function. Modified biplane Simpson's method, also known as the disk summation method, is the recommended method for estimation of LVEF by 2D echocardiography (**Fig. 1**). When available, 3D echocardiography provides more accurate and reproducible measurement of LVEF as compared to 2D echocardiography, because it does not involve any geometric assumptions about the LV shape.

Although LVEF remains the most useful measure of LV systolic function in clinical practice, it is not sensitive enough to detect early myocardial dysfunction, which can be recognized using global longitudinal strain (GLS). Such subclinical LV systolic dysfunction has strong prognostic value independent of LVEF and is helpful in clinical decision-making in many conditions, such as the patients receiving cardiotoxic cancer therapies, those with valve diseases etc. It is also helpful in the differential diagnosis of various cardiomyopathies and the evaluation of heart failure with preserved LVEF.

The LV systolic dysfunction may be global or regional. This distinction has enormous clinical significance because global LV dysfunction generally indicates nonischemic etiology whereas regional dysfunction is virtually diagnostic of CAD. However, exceptions are not uncommon.

Cardiac chamber sizes: Measurement of cardiac chamber dimensions is performed routinely in every echocardiography study. Enlargement of various chamber sizes is usually reflective of the hemodynamic burden imposed on those chambers and is helpful in assessing the severity of the underlying cardiac disorder. Valvular heart disease is a classic example. In contrast, in case of cardiomyopathies, atrial fibrillation, ischemic LV systolic dysfunction etc., cardiac chamber enlargement occurs due to primary myocardial dysfunction, rather than any hemodynamic stress.

Valve lesions: Echocardiography is the most useful imaging modality for the evaluation of valve lesions (**Figs. 2 A** to **F**). Due to its high spatial and temporal resolution, it provides comprehensive information about valve structure and function that is unmatched by any other imaging modality. Furthermore, TEE often adds significant incremental value to transthoracic imaging and is frequently used for the evaluation of valve lesions, especially the mitral valve lesions.

The assessment of the valve lesions is performed by a combination of grayscale imaging and Doppler. Grayscale imaging delineates the underlying anatomic defect, helps in identifying the etiology, and provides an idea about the severity of the valve lesion. The Doppler assessment complements this information by providing hemodynamic data that reflect the severity of the valvular dysfunction. Valve gradients and area are the primary measurements used for determining severity of the stenotic lesions, whereas the regurgitant lesions are assessed using vena contracta size, jet area, effective regurgitant orifice area, regurgitation volume etc. Enlargement of the upstream and downstream cardiac chambers serves as an important corroborative evidence and is considered an essential criterion for diagnosing severe valvular regurgitation.

In addition to the above, echocardiography also provides a lot of other relevant information that is required for planning the management strategy, such as annulus size, morphological suitability of the valve for percutaneous intervention or repair, presence or absence of intracardiac thrombus, and other associated valve lesions.

Intracardiac hemodynamics: Echocardiography is an excellent modality for the assessment of intracardiac hemodynamics (**Figs. 3 A** and **B**). A variety of hemodynamic measurements can be obtained using echocardiography. Of these, pulmonary artery systolic pressure (measured using tricuspid regurgitation jet), central venous pressure (assessed using the inferior vena cava size and collapsibility), and the LV filling pressure (estimated using a combination of parameters such as mitral inflow and annular velocities) are the most useful and routinely measured.

Cardiomyopathies: Echocardiography permits a comprehensive assessment of cardiomyopathies (**Figs. 4 A** to **D**). Dilated cardiomyopathy usually presents with global LV dysfunction and dilatation, in the absence of any apparent cause for such dysfunction. Hypertrophic cardiomyopathy (HCM) most commonly presents with asymmetrical septal hypertrophy with or without LV outflow obstruction. Systolic anterior motion of the mitral leaflets or chordae is the main mechanism of LV outflow tract obstruction. Varying degree of mitral regurgitation, structural abnormalities of mitral valve apparatus, LV diastolic dysfunction, right ventricular (RV) hypertrophy etc., are also present. There are several other patterns of LV hypertrophy that can be seen, especially apical hypertrophy and midventricular hypertrophy.

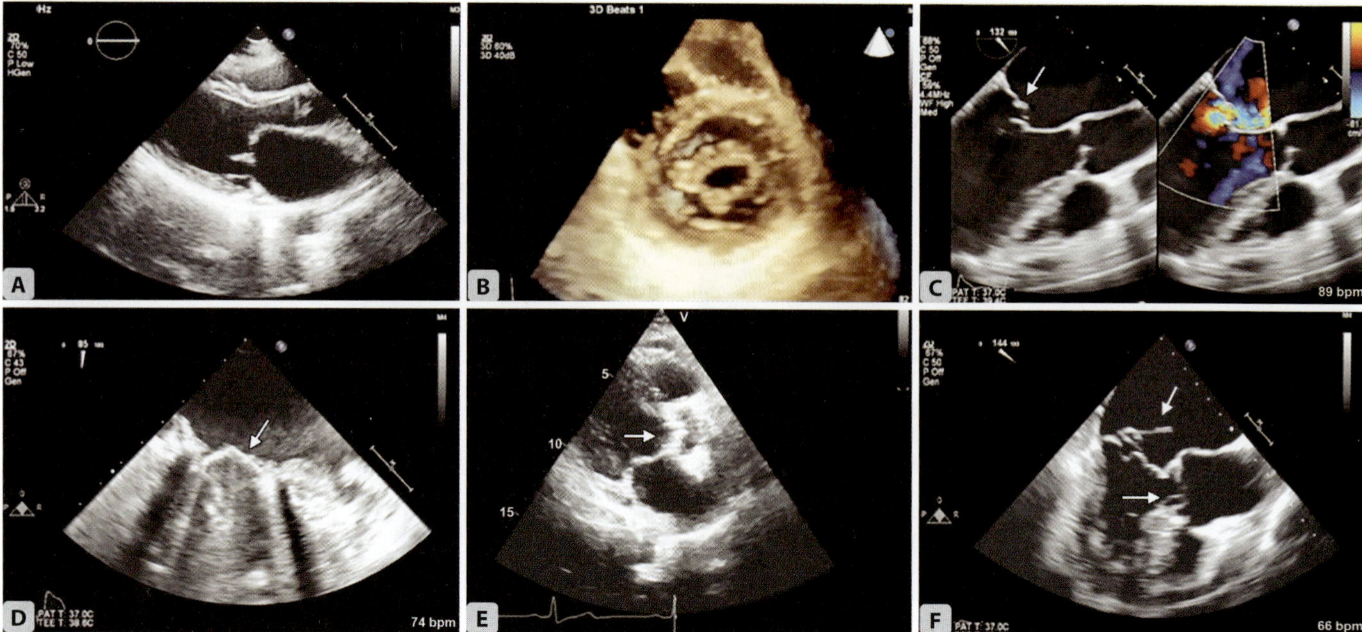

FIGURES 2 A to F: Some common valve diseases. **(A and B)** A patient with rheumatic mitral stenosis. There is doming of anterior mitral valve leaflet with restricted opening. Three-dimensional echocardiography shows the typical fish-mouth appearance of the mitral orifice. **(C)** The posterior mitral leaflet has become flail (arrow) due to chordal rupture, resulting in eccentric severe mitral regurgitation. **(D)** A bileaflet prosthetic mitral valve, one disk of which has become stuck (arrow) due to thrombosis. **(E)** Degenerative severe aortic stenosis with markedly thickened aortic leaflets (arrow) and reduced opening. **(F)** A patient with infective endocarditis of both mitral and aortic valves. Flagellar structures suggestive of vegetations can be seen attached to the valve leaflets (arrows).

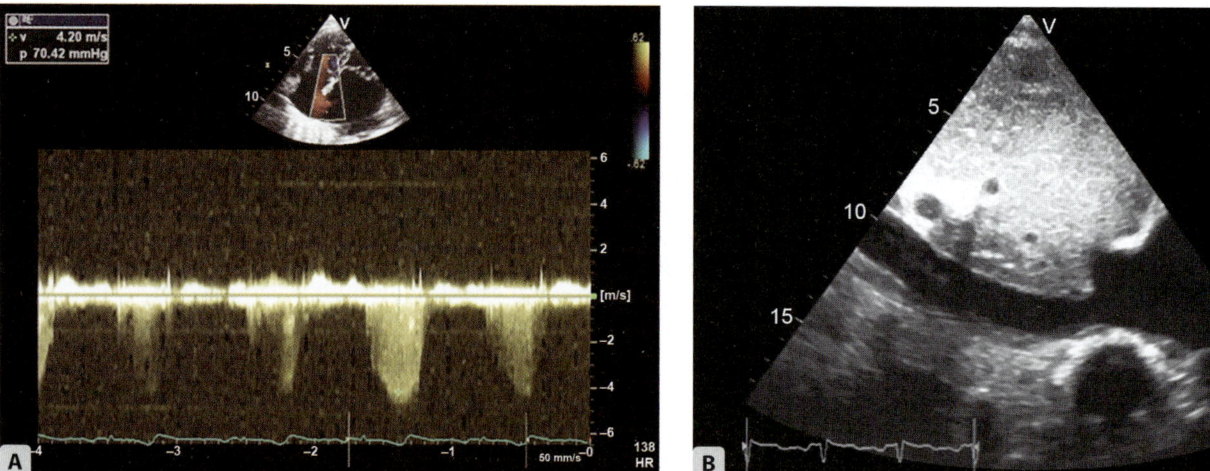

FIGURES 3 A & B: Hemodynamic assessment by echocardiography. **(A)** Estimation of right ventricular systolic pressure from tricuspid regurgitation jet. **(B)** The right atrial pressure is estimated by looking at inferior vena cava size and collapsibility with inspiration.

Restrictive cardiopathy is generally characterized by normal sized ventricles with or without increased wall thickness, atrial enlargement, and markedly increased filling pressures. LV systolic dysfunction and even dilatation may occur in late stages. In case of endomyocardial fibrosis, LV and/or RV apical obliteration is common and occurs due to thrombus formation and subsequent fibrosis.

Left ventricular noncompaction, arrhythmogenic LV or RV cardiomyopathy, Takotsubo cardiomyopathy etc., are other cardiomyopathies that are common. Cardiac involvement can also occur in several systemic diseases and may present with distinct phenotypes. Anderson–Fabry disease, Friedreich's ataxia, Duchenne muscular dystrophy etc., are some examples.

Congenital heart diseases: Echocardiography is the most useful modality for the assessment of congenital cardiac lesions. The underlying anatomic defect can be easily recognized, and its hemodynamic consequences ascertained. Cardiac catheterization and CT may be needed for further evaluation, especially for delineating the vascular connections.

Other disorders: Echocardiography is very helpful for diagnosing pericardial diseases, diseases of ascending aorta

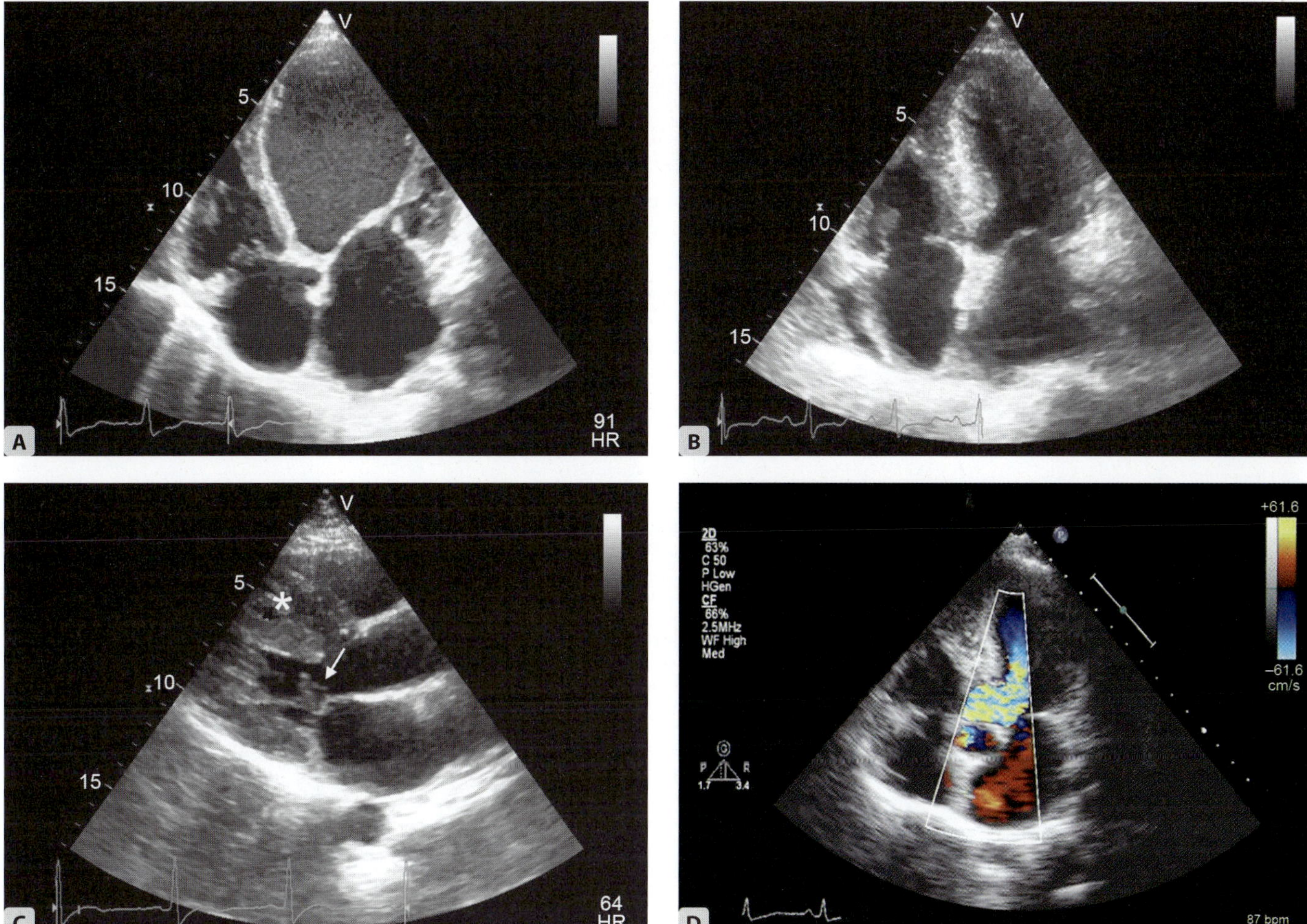

FIGURES 4 A to D: Illustrative examples of cardiomyopathies. **(A)** Dilated cardiomyopathy. **(B)** Cardiac amyloidosis resulting in restrictive cardiomyopathy. The ventricular walls are significantly thickened. The size of the ventricles is normal but both atria are enlarged. **(C and D)** Hypertrophic cardiomyopathy with markedly thickened interventricular septum (asterisk), systolic anterior motion of mitral leaflets (arrow) and flow turbulence in the left ventricular outflow tract.

(e.g., aortic dissection), intracardiac masses, right heart pathologies etc. (**Figs. 5** to **7**). Transthoracic echocardiography has a sensitivity of 77–80% and TEE ≈ 98% for diagnosing ascending aortic dissection. However, CT is invariably required to delineate the full extent of dissection and the status of branch vessels. In case of intracardiac masses, echocardiography provides valuable initial information which may be diagnostic for many conditions such as intracardiac thrombus, left atrial (LA) myxoma, and vegetations. For other lesions, CMR is often needed because of its ability to permit tissue characterization.

Guiding structural heart disease interventions: Portability and real-time imaging render echocardiography, especially TEE, an ideal imaging modality for guiding structural heart disease interventions in the cardiac catheterization laboratory. Device closure of atrial and ventricular septal defects, paravalvular leak closure, LA appendage closure, MitraClip implantation, tricuspid valve interventions etc., are all performed under TEE guidance. TEE is also routinely used in the operating room for evaluation of the immediate postoperative outcomes in patients undergoing valve surgeries.

NUCLEAR IMAGING

Nuclear scanning remains the most useful modality for imaging myocardial perfusion and metabolism. It uses a gamma camera that detects photons emitted from myocardium after injection of a suitable radiotracer. Processing of this signal allows assessment of myocardial perfusion, metabolism, inflammation, and other molecular processes.

TECHNICAL CONSIDERATIONS

There are two main forms of nuclear cardiac imaging—(1) SPECT and (2) PET.

Single-photon emission computed tomography myocardial imaging uses radiotracers that emit photons. Two main radionuclides have been in use for SPECT MPI—201-thallium (^{201}Tl) and 99m-technetium (^{99m}Tc). The use of ^{201}Tl has now been banned.

Positron emission tomography cardiac imaging uses tracers that emit positrons, instead of photons. PET yields high-quality images with excellent spatial resolution which is far superior to that obtained with SPECT. Also, PET allows absolute quantification of myocardial perfusion and

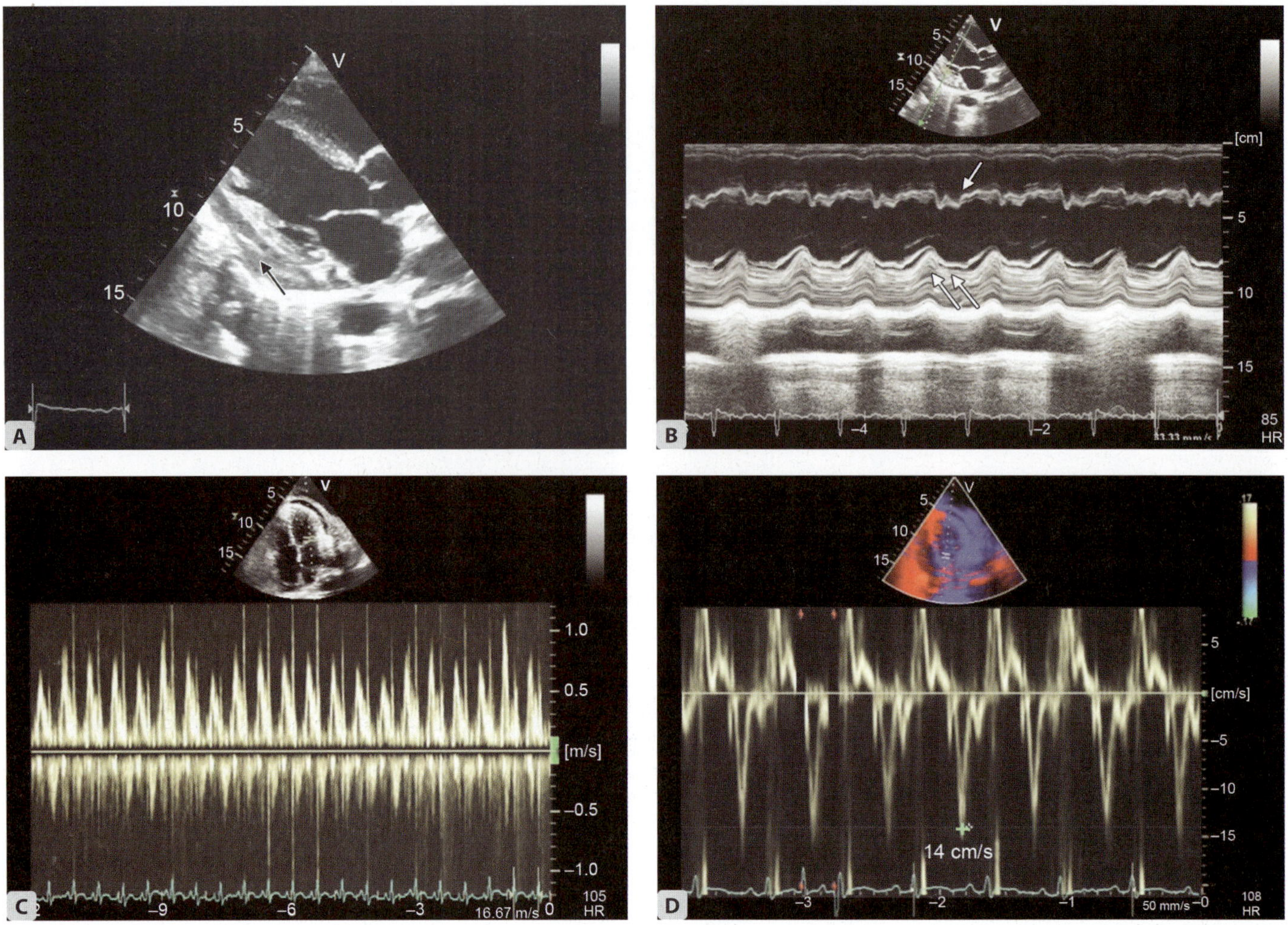

FIGURES 5 A to D: An example of constrictive pericarditis. **(A)** Markedly thickened pericardium posterior to the left ventricle (arrow). **(B)** Typical septal shudder (arrow) and dip-and-plateau motion of the posterior wall (double arrows). **(C)** Mitral inflow pattern shows increased inflow velocity with significant respiratory variation. **(D)** Exaggerated mitral annular early diastolic velocity despite increased left ventricular filling pressure.

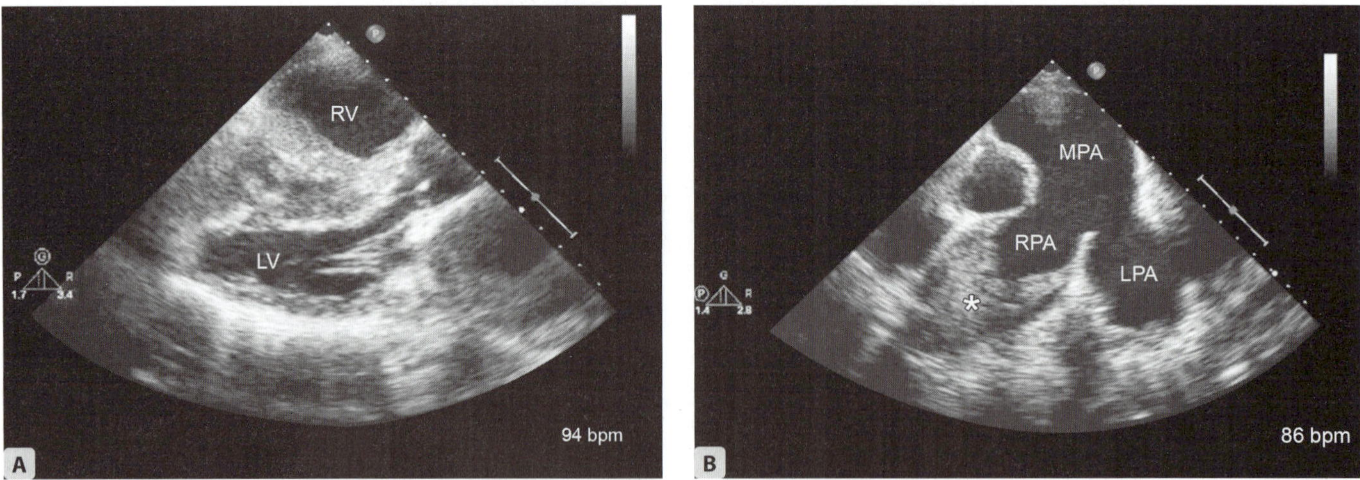

(LPA: left pulmonary artery; LV: left ventricle; MPA: main pulmonary artery; RV: right ventricle; RPA: right pulmonary artery)

FIGURES 6 A to D: *Continued...*

Continued...

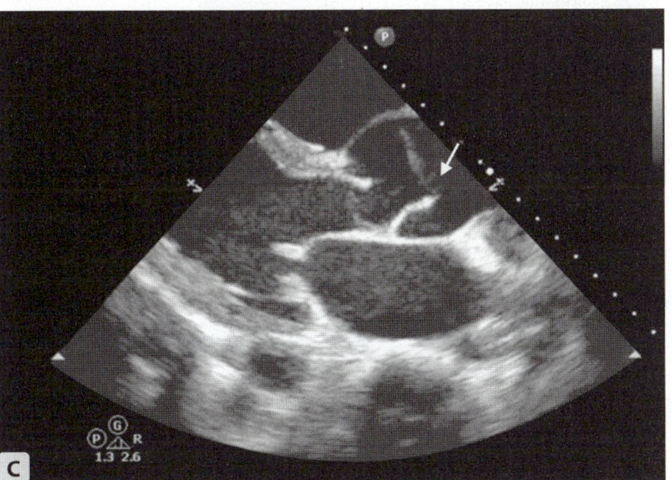

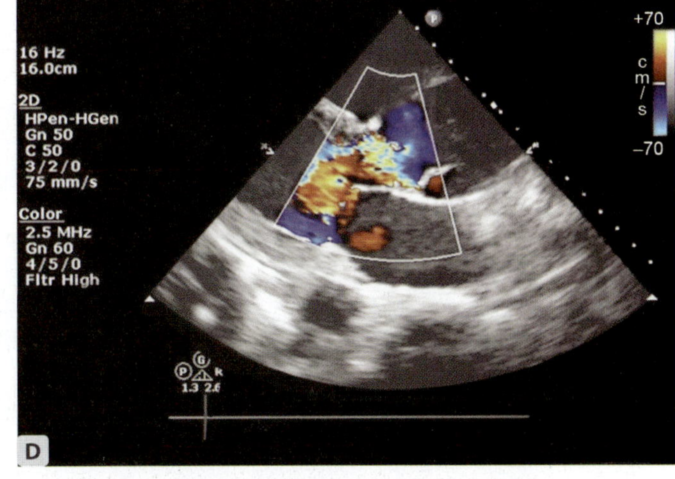

FIGURES 6 A to D: **(A and B)** A patient with massive acute pulmonary embolism. **(A)** The right ventricle is enlarged, and the interventricular septum is pushed toward the left ventricle; **(B)** pulmonary arteries are grossly dilated and the right pulmonary artery is completely occluded with a thrombus (asterisk). **(C and D)** An example of aortic dissection with a dissection flap seen just distal to the aortic valve (arrow). There is significant aortic regurgitation also.

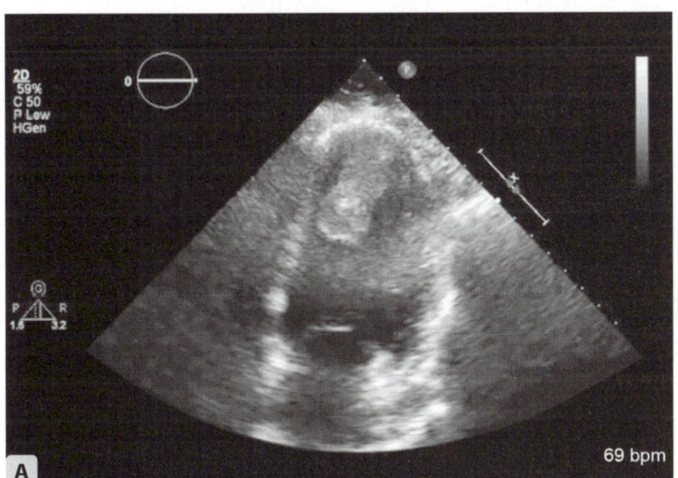

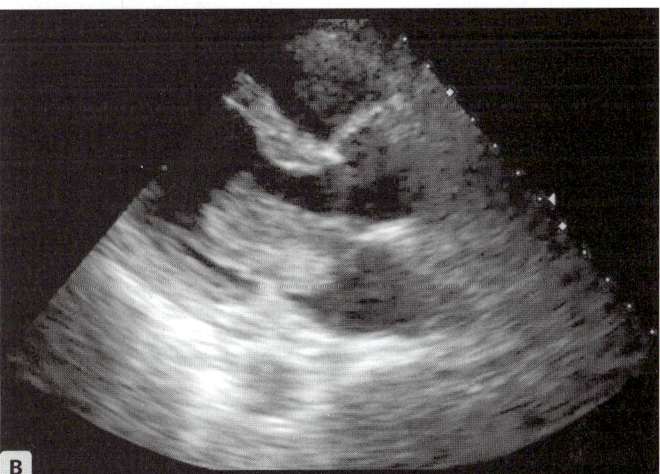

FIGURES 7 A & B: **(A)** Large thrombus at left ventricular apex in a patient with anterior wall myocardial infarction. **(B)** A left atrial myxoma which is prolapsing through the mitral orifice during diastole.

metabolism, compared with SPECT which only provides semiquantitative information. Unlike SPECT imaging, the PET scanning uses radioisotopes that can be incorporated into molecules required for normal tissue functioning.

CLINICAL APPLICATIONS

Detection of myocardial ischemia: Myocardial ischemia and viability assessment have been the two main applications of nuclear myocardial imaging. For detection of myocardial ischemia, the imaging is combined with some form of stressor which may either be exercise or a pharmacological agent such as dobutamine, adenosine, dipyridamole, or regadenoson. SPECT imaging permits use of both forms of stressors but when performing PET, only pharmacological stressors can be used due to the ultrashort half-life of PET perfusion tracers.

For ischemia detection, the radioisotope is first injected at rest and then after stress. Images are obtained after each injection and compared with each other for any stress-induced perfusion defect (**Figs. 8 A** and **B**). In some cases, the sequence is reversed. Exercise induces perfusion abnormalities by causing preferential increase in myocardial blood flow in areas supplied by the nonstenosed coronary arteries. The increase in myocardial blood flow is triggered by an increase in the myocardial oxygen demand. Dobutamine also acts by the same mechanism. In contrast, vasodilator agents such as adenosine, dipyridamole, or regadenoson cause direct vasodilatation of resistance coronary arterioles and produce flow heterogeneity between stenotic and nonstenotic segments. The increase in myocardial blood flow is maximum with the vasodilator agents (four to five times that of flow at rest) and is relatively

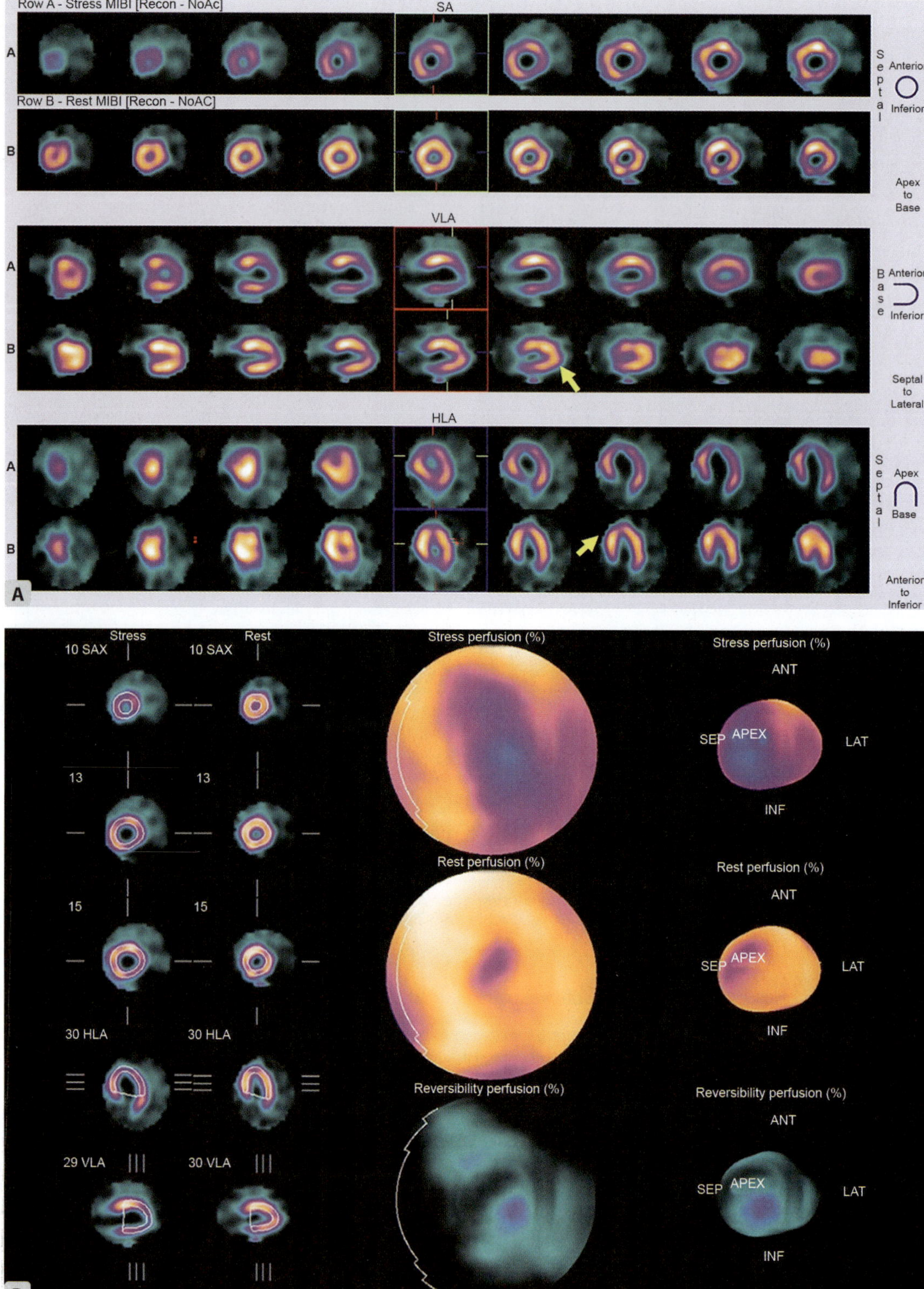

FIGURES 8 A & B: Dobutamine stress myocardial perfusion scintigraphy using 99m-technetium sestamibi. (A) Multiple images in three different orthogonal planes (SA- short-axis, VLA- vertical long-axis, and HLA- horizontal long-axis) are shown. For each stack, the upper panel shows stress images and the lower panel shows rest images. There is a large reversible stress-induced perfusion defect involving anteroapical and adjacent septal and inferior wall (arrows). **(B)** Color-coded polar map shows the same large reversible perfusion defect involving anteroapical-inferior regions.

less with dobutamine or exercise (two to three times of resting flow). However, exercise allows reproduction of the patient's symptoms and their correlation with the imaging findings. It also provides prognostically useful information such as exercise capacity and blood pressure response. Therefore, in patients who can exercise, exercise stress MPI is preferred. In those who are unable to exercise, vasodilator agents are generally preferred over dobutamine. The latter is useful mainly for the patients with contraindication to adenosine such as those with obstructive airway disease. However, at most of the centers in India, dobutamine is used more often, primarily because of the greater familiarity with this agent.

Previous studies have reported varying sensitivity and specificity of nuclear imaging for detection of obstructive CAD. In a pooled analysis, the sensitivity of SPECT imaging was 87% and specificity 73%. Notably, most of this data was derived using nongated imaging and therefore, the diagnostic accuracy may be better now with the use of electrocardiography (ECG)-gated imaging. Additionally, although the main objective of performing stress MPI is to detect obstructive CAD, the perfusion abnormalities on SPECT imaging provide prognostic information that is independent of the presence or absence of obstructive CAD on coronary angiography.

Assessment of myocardial viability: Assessment of myocardial viability by SPECT imaging has traditionally been performed using ^{201}Tl. After initial injection, ^{201}Tl is preferentially taken up by the viable, well-perfused myocytes. However, within 15–20 minutes, redistribution begins. Images taken at 4 hours after initial injection show refilling of areas that are viable but underperfused, suggestive of myocardial hibernation. When refilling is inadequate at 4 hours, additional images may be taken at 24 hours. Approximately, 40–50% "severe fixed defects" on early redistribution imaging improve on delayed redistribution. In patients in whom stress imaging is combined with viability testing, initial images are taken after stress. In such cases, reinjection of a smaller dose of tracer may be required prior to late redistribution imaging to improve the image quality.

Unlike ^{201}Tl, ^{99m}Tc does not undergo redistribution. However, ^{99m}Tc can also be used for viability assessment. The dysfunctional segments showing ^{99m}Tc uptake that is 50–60% or more of the maximal uptake, particularly after administration of sublingual nitroglycerine, are considered viable.

Positron emission tomography imaging is considered the current "gold standard" for assessment of myocardial viability. For this, simultaneous assessment of myocardial perfusion and metabolism is performed using ^{82}Rb-RbCl and ^{18}F-labeled 2-fluoro-2-deoxyglucose (^{18}F-FDG), respectively. The presence of preserved or enhanced metabolism but reduced perfusion (a mismatched defect) is suggestive of hibernation whereas a matched defect with reduced perfusion and metabolism both indicates scar tissue (**Fig. 9**). At centers where ^{82}Rb-RbCl is not available, SPECT perfusion imaging is combined with ^{18}F-FDG

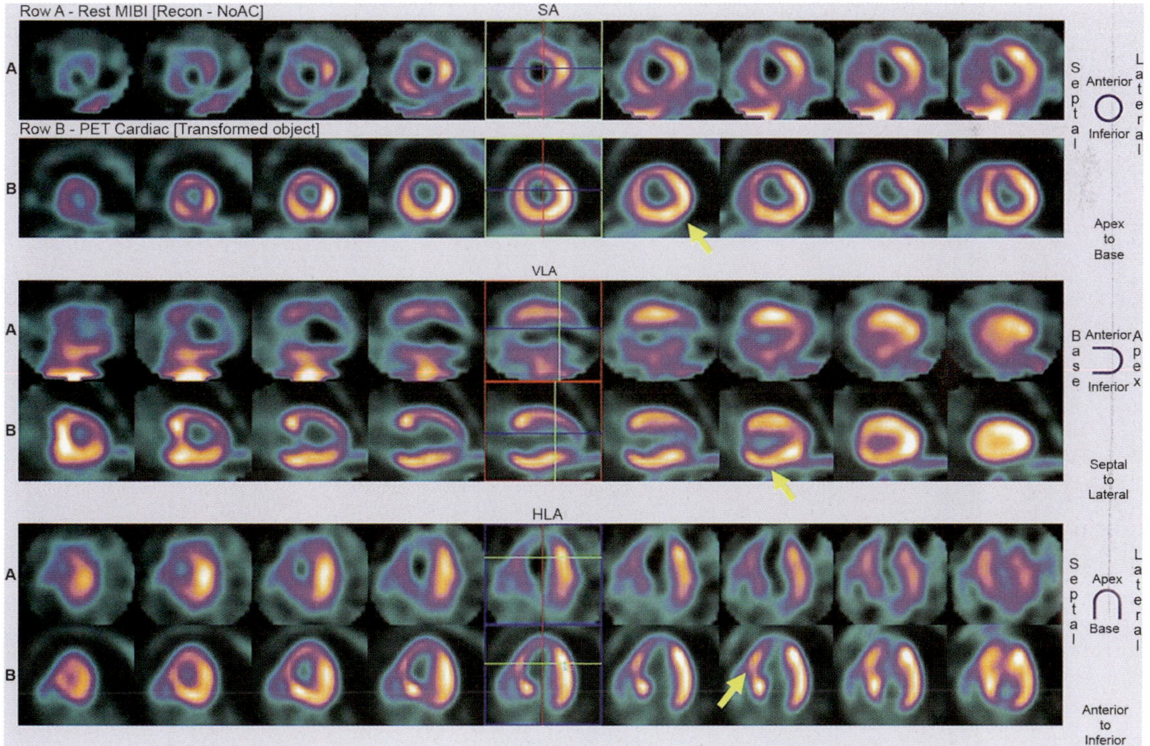

FIGURE 9: **^{18}F-fluoro-deoxyglucose myocardial positron emission tomography** for assessment of myocardial viability. Multiple images in three different orthogonal planes (SA—short-axis, VLA—vertical long-axis, and HLA—horizontal long-axis) are shown. For each stack, the upper panel shows perfusion images (obtained using 99m-technetium sestamibi at rest) and the lower panel shows metabolism images. There is reduced perfusion in the anteroapical, septal, and inferior/inferolateral walls but the metabolism is preserved (arrows) suggestive of myocardial hibernation.

imaging for viability assessment. A pooled analysis was performed of 37 studies comparing different modalities of viability assessment. Myocardial functional recovery after revascularization, although not an ideal reference, was used as the criterion for myocardial viability. ^{18}F-FDG PET had 88% sensitivity and 73% specificity, whereas ^{201}Tl rest-redistribution imaging had 90% sensitivity and 54% specificity.

Assessment of left and right ventricular volumes and function: The gated SPECT-imaging used currently for perfusion imaging can also be used for estimation of LV volumes and global and regional LV systolic function. However, radionuclide ventriculography (RVG) has been the traditional nuclear imaging technique used for the assessment of ventricular volumes and function. Unlike perfusion imaging, RVG employs blood pool labeling with radioisotopes followed by ECG-gated imaging to quantify the volume of blood present within the cardiac chambers during different phases of cardiac cycle. There are two main types of RVG-equilibrium RVG, popularly known as multigated acquisition (MUGA) scan and the first pass RVG. Equilibrium RVG is used mainly for studying the LV function. In this technique, ^{99m}Tc-labeling is applied to albumin or red blood cells and ECG-gated scanning is performed from multiple projections. Counts obtained over several hundred cardiac cycles are summated to calculate LV blood volume throughout the cardiac cycle. The volumetric data is then analyzed to derive information about LV systolic and diastolic function.

The first pass RVG is used mainly for the assessment of RV systolic function. The most used tracer for this purpose is ^{99m}Tc-labeled diethylenetriaminepentaacetic acid. It is injected rapidly into a peripheral vein and scanning is performed over the next few cardiac cycles to track the passage of the tracer as it passes through the different cardiac chambers. The temporal sequence of the tracer flow provides separation between the RV and LV counts and allows accurate assessment of the RV systolic function.

Inflammatory and infiltrative cardiac diseases: Cardiac PET scanning has emerged as a valuable technique for assessment of various inflammatory and infiltrative disorders affecting the heart.

Gallium-67 scintigraphy has been used in past as a marker of myocardial inflammation to diagnose cardiac sarcoidosis. However, it has now been superseded by ^{18}F-FDG PET, which provides much better image quality and higher sensitivity. In a patient with suspected cardiac sarcoidosis, the presence of ^{18}F-FDG myocardial uptake indicates active inflammation and is helpful in guiding treatment (e.g., steroid therapy) and monitoring response to treatment (**Fig. 10**). However, proper patient preparation is critical for achieving optimum diagnostic accuracy.

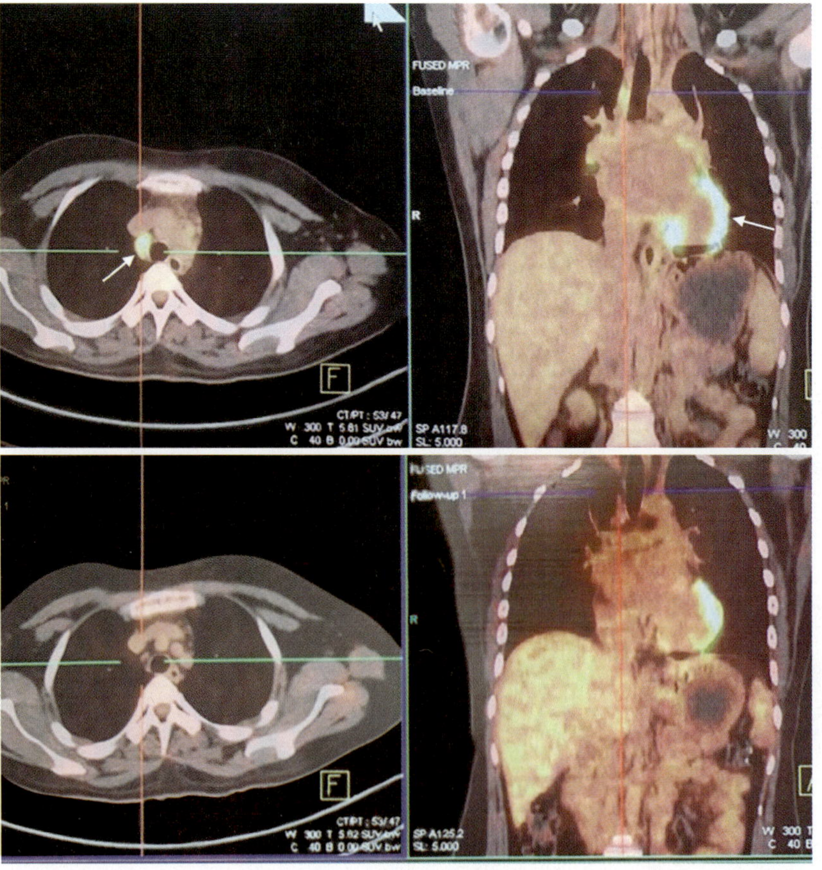

FIGURE 10: ^{18}F-fluoro-deoxyglucose positron emission tomography in a patient with sarcoidosis. Upper panel—multifocal myocardial hypermetabolism and extracardiac disease in the form of active mediastinal nodes (arrows) can be appreciated. Lower panel—significant resolution in the inflammatory activity in a follow-up scan performed after 6 weeks of treatment.

Physiological glucose uptake by normal myocardium needs to be suppressed by high-fat, high-protein, and low-carbohydrate diet combined with fasting prior to the test.

Recent studies have revealed relatively high prevalence of transthyretin (TTR) amyloidosis, especially in elderly patients presenting with low-gradient aortic stenosis. ^{99m}Tc-pyrophosphate is the most useful modality for diagnosing this condition with a sensitivity of 99% and specificity of 86%. Although, mild uptake of ^{99m}Tc-pyrophosphate can also occur in light-chain amyloidosis, it can be easily differentiated with the help of serum or urine light-chain analysis.

CARDIAC COMPUTED TOMOGRAPHY

TECHNICAL CONSIDERATIONS

Computed tomography involves X-rays for imaging the heart. At present, 256-, 512-, and 640-slice CT scanners are being commonly used for imaging in clinical practice. For cardiac imaging, heart rate control is an important requirement to minimize motion artifacts. Currently, cardiac CT scan can be performed with as small as 3 mSv radiation exposure.

Estimation of coronary artery calcium score (CACS) is performed using the Agatston method (**Fig. 11**). Several recent studies using invasive *fractional flow reserve (FFR)* have clearly demonstrated the value of functional significance of a coronary lesion. To provide a noninvasive alternative to invasive FFR, CT-FFR has been developed and is being used commonly now.

Plaque morphology and coronary calcium score: Different tissues have different attenuation density on CT. This property can be used for characterizing coronary plaque morphology especially for diagnosing vulnerable plaques.

CLINICAL APPLICATIONS

Detection of obstructive coronary artery disease: Detection of obstructive CAD by CT coronary angiography (CTCA) is perhaps the most common application of cardiac CT at present (**Fig. 12**). Several studies have evaluated diagnostic accuracy of CTCA for this purpose. These studies have shown that CTCA currently has sensitivity and specificity both above 90% for detecting obstructive CAD on ICA, both on per-patient and per-vessel basis. CTCA has also been compared with functional stress testing in a few studies. A recent large study showed that CTCA had the highest diagnostic accuracy for detecting significant CAD defined as >70% luminal stenosis on ICA, with a sensitivity and specificity of 91% and 92%, respectively. In comparison, stress MPI had a sensitivity and specificity of 74% and 73%, respectively, whereas the same for stress echocardiography were 49% and 92%. An added advantage of CTCA over functional assessment is its ability to show nonobstructive CAD and coronary calcification both of which have considerable prognostic and therapeutic significance (**Fig. 13**). CTCA can also demonstrate high-risk features such as low-attenuation plaque (suggestive of higher lipid content) and positive remodeling which may have incremental value in predicting coronary event risk.

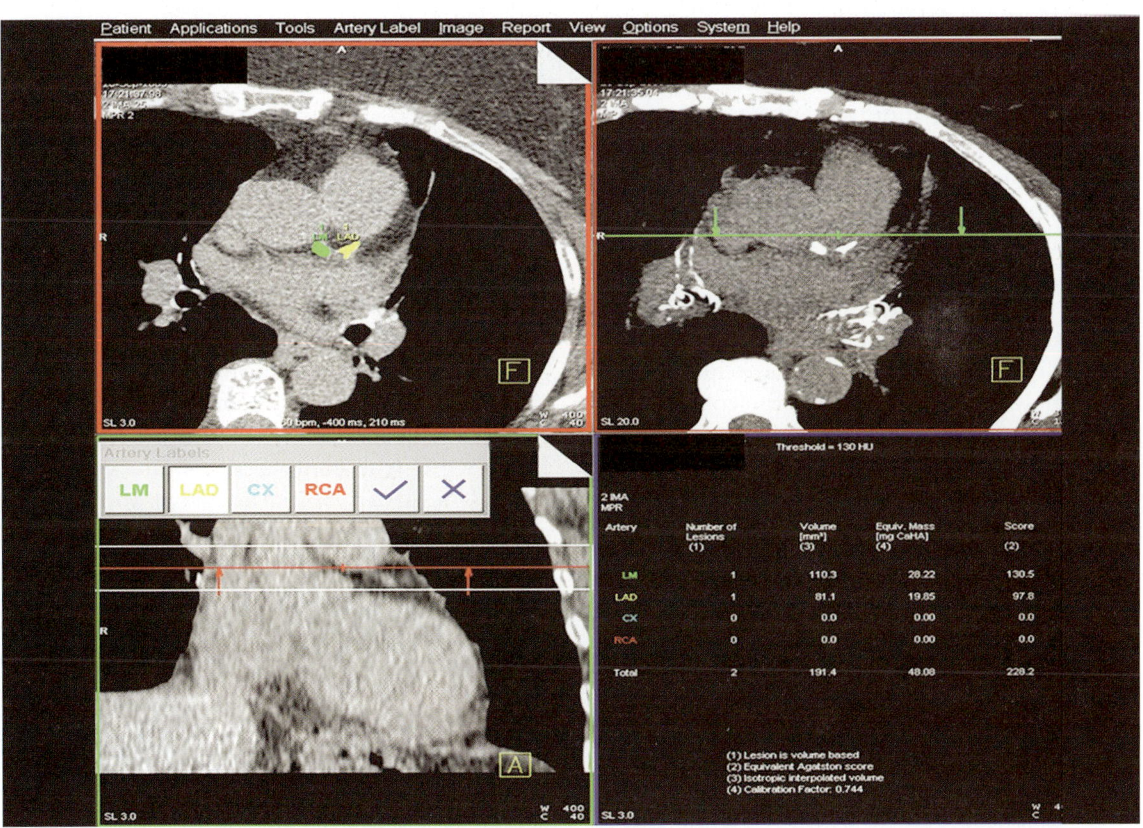

FIGURE 11: Estimation of coronary artery calcium score. Presence of calcium in each vessel is quantified and total score can be obtained, which is considered a reproducible measure of coronary atherosclerotic burden.

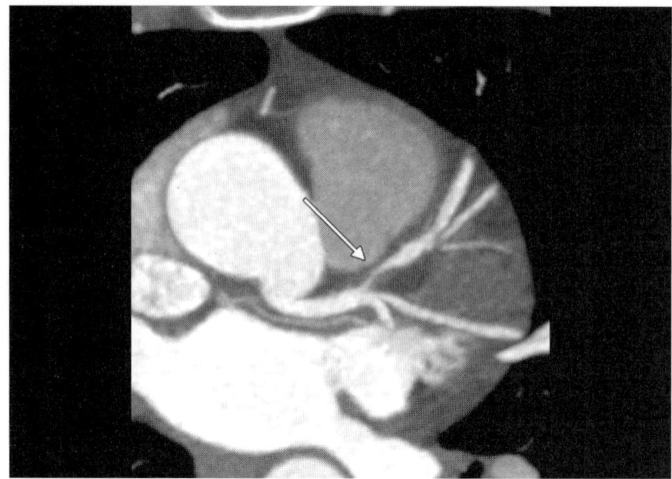

FIGURE 12: Contrast-enhanced axial image of computed tomographic coronary angiography reveals concentric low-density plaque in the proximal left anterior descending artery causing significant stenosis.

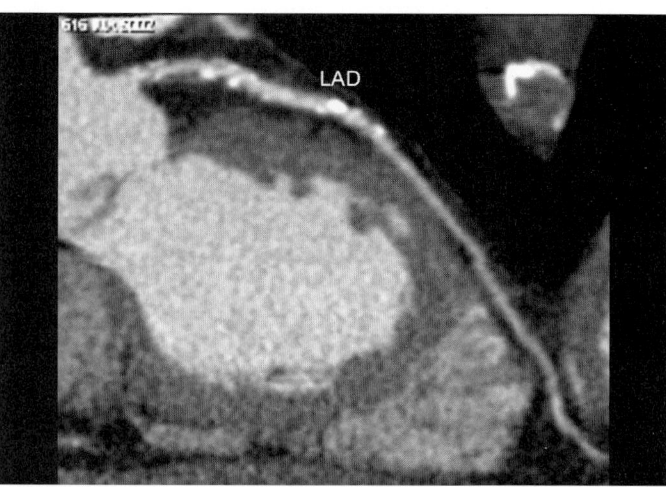

FIGURE 13: Curved multiplanar reconstruction image of left anterior descending (LAD) coronary artery reveals calcific and low-density plaques in proximal and midsegments. No evidence of significant obstructive lesion is, however, seen.

Given the high diagnostic accuracy of CTCA for diagnosing obstructive CAD, it has been used for guiding decision-making in various clinical settings. *In patients presenting to emergency room with chest pain,* ruling out an acute coronary event is an immediate priority. In such patents, if there are no high-risk ECG changes and the initial troponin is not elevated, several different options are available for further evaluation, including serial troponin assay, stress testing, CTCA, or ICA. CTCA has been consistently shown to have high negative predictive value for ruling out underlying CAD in this setting. Extremely low event rates are reported in patients discharged from emergency room based on normal CTCA findings. CTCA thus may reduce emergency room stay duration, improve workflow efficiency, and may lead to potential cost-savings. However, there have been concerns that CTCA-based approach may result in higher rates of ICA and coronary revascularization. Although the initial ICA and revascularization rates may be higher with CTCA, this gets balanced out by lower rates during subsequent follow-up. As a result, the overall major adverse cardiac event (MACE) rates during long-term follow-up are not different between CTCA-guided management and the conventional functional assessment-based management.

In patients presenting with acute chest pain, CT has the advantage of being able to exclude the three most dreaded possibilities, namely (1) acute coronary syndrome, (2) acute pulmonary embolism, and (3) aortic dissection. However, the routine use of this "triple rule out" is not recommended due to overall low incidence of these pathologies and the issues related to image quality, contrast use, and radiation exposure.

The role of CTCA in the *evaluation of patients with stable chest pain syndromes* has been assessed in a few large studies. In the Prospective Multicenter Imaging Study for Evaluation of Chest Pain (PROMISE) trial, 10,003 symptomatic patients were randomly assigned to undergo CTCA or functional testing. A greater number of patients in the CTCA group underwent ICA within 90 days after randomization (12.2% vs. 8.1%). However, after a median follow-up of 25 months, there was no difference between the two arms in the rates of primary endpoint, which was a composite of death, MI, hospitalization for unstable angina, or major procedural complication.

In contrast, the use of CTCA significantly improved clinical outcomes in the SCOT-HEART (Scottish Computed Tomography of the Heart) trial. It was an open-label trial in which 4,146 patients with stable chest pain were randomly assigned to standard care plus CTCA or to standard care alone. The 5-year rate of the primary endpoint, a composite of death from coronary heart disease or nonfatal MI, was significantly lower in the CTCA group (2.3% vs. 3.9%, hazard ratio 0.59, $p = 0.004$). Although more patients in the CTCA group underwent ICA and coronary revascularization during the initial few months, the overall rates at 5 years were not different. The reduction in the primary endpoint with CTCA was believed to be due to greater use of preventive therapies in these patients, driven by demonstration of nonobstructive plaques during CT coronary imaging.

More recently, the International Study of Comparative Health Effectiveness with Medical and Invasive Approaches (ISCHEMIA) trial compared a strategy of initial medical management with initial invasive approach in patients with stable chest pain with moderate or severe ischemia on functional testing. CTCA was performed in most of the patients to rule out left main coronary disease and nonobstructive CAD. Over a median follow-up duration of 3.2 years, there was no difference in the primary outcome (a composite of death from cardiovascular causes, MI, or hospitalization for unstable angina, heart failure, or resuscitated cardiac arrest) between the two groups. Although this trial did not compare CTCA with other diagnostic strategies, it did show that in patients with stable CAD in whom left main CAD was ruled out by CTCA, initial medical management could be an effective treatment option, despite the presence of moderate or severe ischemia on stress testing.

An important finding from the previous prospective studies has been the prognostic significance of nonobstructive disease detected by CTCA (**Fig. 13**). It has been seen that the presence of nonobstructive CAD on CTCA is associated with high risk of cardiovascular mortality or MI during follow-up, in a manner analogous to obstructive CAD. The risk increases with increasing number of coronary artery involvement. Conversely, a normal CTCA is associated with an extremely low risk of events during the next few years and has been suggested to confer a warranty for at least 5 years.

Computed tomography coronary angiography is also an excellent modality for recognition of coronary anomalies and the assessment of coronary bypass grafts (**Figs. 14** and **15**). For evaluation of coronary in-stent restenosis, it has traditionally been limited by the blooming artifacts caused by the metallic stents. However, the current generation coronary stents are more conducive to CT imaging, resulting in high diagnostic accuracy of CTCA for detection of significant in-stent restenosis (sensitivity 82–91% and specificity 91–93%) (**Fig. 16**).

Coronary artery calcium score: Normally, there is no calcium in the coronary arteries. Calcification occurs as a part of atherosclerotic process or much less commonly due to dystrophic calcification seen in conditions such as chronic kidney disease and hyperparathyroidism. Thus, the presence of any calcium in the coronary arteries, for all practical purposes, can be considered an evidence of ongoing atherosclerosis. This is the rationale for using CACS as a marker of coronary atherosclerosis. Autopsy studies have shown that CACS has an excellent correlation with the total coronary atherosclerotic burden, although the site of maximum luminal stenosis may not correlate.

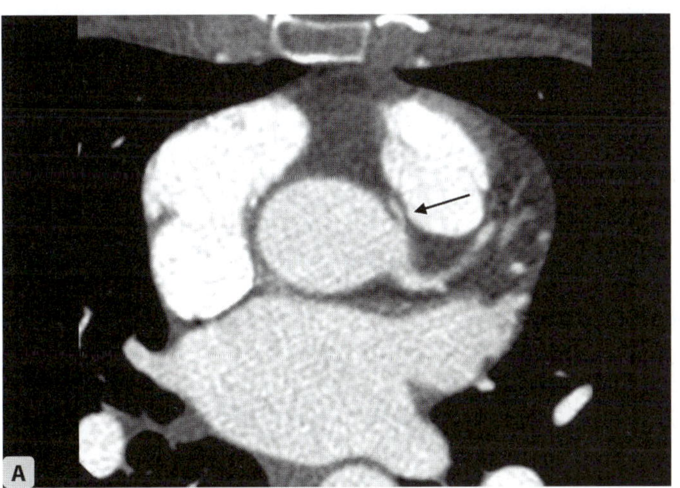

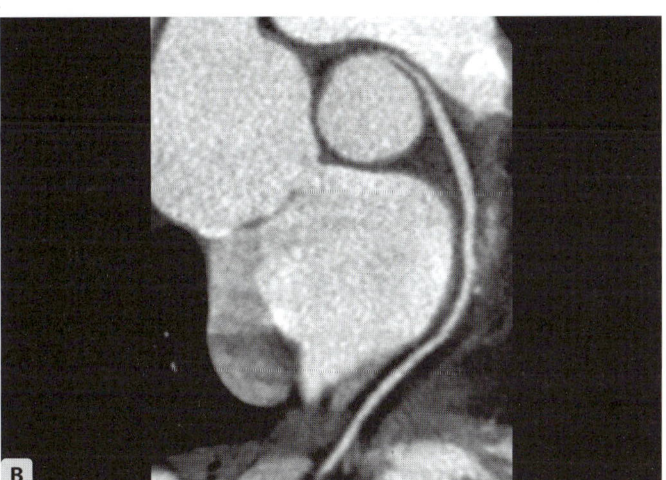

FIGURES 14 A & B: Computed tomographic coronary angiogram shows anomalous origin of right coronary artery from the left coronary sinus. It then courses between aorta and main pulmonary artery. This anomaly is dangerous and is known as malignant right coronary artery.

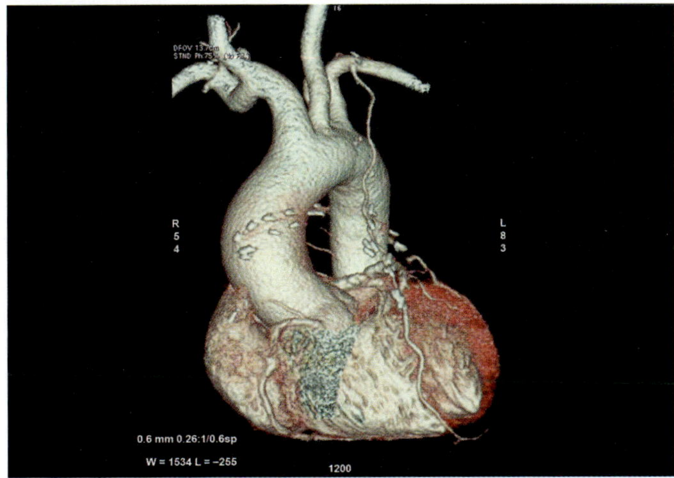

FIGURE 15: Volume-rendered image of the heart performed to evaluate bypass grafts.

Note: Only staples are visualized over aorta, suggestive of graft occlusion.

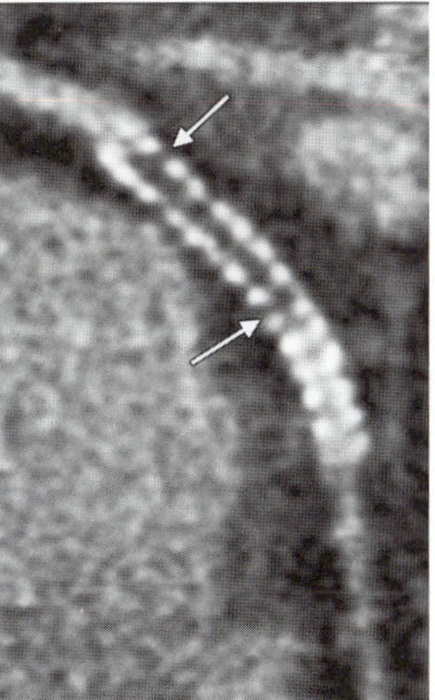

FIGURE 16: High resolution image of coronary stent shows occlusion of the stent suggestive of in-stent restenosis.

Numerous large-scale multicentric studies have shown that CACS is an excellent predictor of incident cardiovascular events and this predictive accuracy is incremental to any of the conventional risk factors and risk algorithms. In asymptomatic individuals, a CACS value of zero is associated with an extremely low risk of atherosclerotic vascular events during follow-up. The risk increases with increasing CACS, with values >100 generally associated with event rates comparable to those observed in the secondary prevention setting.

Due to its strong correlation with the MACE rates, CACS has been proposed as a useful tool for guiding preventive therapies. Several retrospective studies have consistently shown that the use of CACS in the primary prevention setting may lead to a more appropriate patient selection for statin therapy, as compared to the current strategy of using clinical risk algorithms. Among those with estimated 10-year atherosclerotic vascular disease risk of 5–20%, the addition of CACS results in significant reclassification of individuals into "statin eligible" and "statin ineligible" groups that match better with the observed event rates. However, CACS does not provide any incremental benefit in individuals who are already at high risk (estimated 10-year risk >20%). CACS >100 may also help in identifying patients who might benefit from low-dose aspirin therapy even in the absence of documented obstructive atherosclerotic vascular disease. Finally, CACS estimation may also favorably influence physician and patient behavior and may lead to greater adoption of preventive therapies and a healthier lifestyle.

Aortic diseases: Computed tomography is currently the most useful noninvasive modality for the assessment of aortic diseases. It is highly accurate for measuring aortic dimensions (**Fig. 17**). In patients with aortic aneurysms, CT permits comprehensive delineation of the aneurysm anatomy and its relationship with the adjacent structures. For aortic dissection, contrast-enhanced CT scan has a sensitivity and specificity of 98–100%. CT scan is also an excellent modality for the evaluation of other aortic pathologies such as aortic intramural hematoma, aortoarteritis, and aortic arch anomalies.

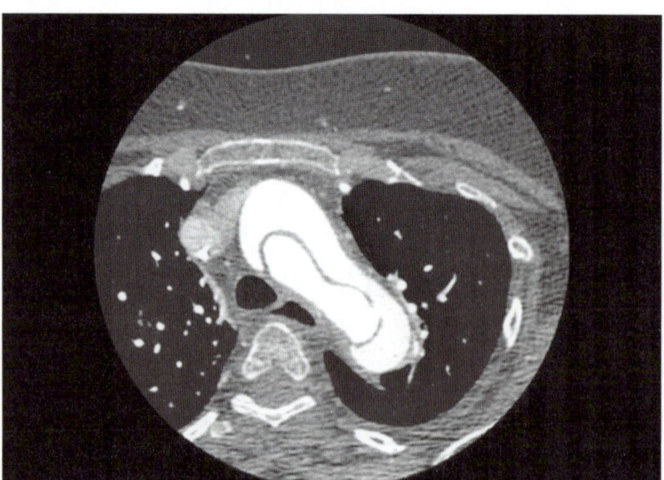

FIGURE 17: Contrast-enhanced axial image of aorta reveals presence of intimal dissecting flap in the arch of aorta.

Valvular heart diseases: Nearly, one-third of all patients with severe aortic stenosis defined as aortic valve area < 1 cm^2 have valve gradients below the threshold for severity (i.e., mean gradient ≥40 mm Hg). This is known as "low-gradient severe aortic stenosis" and often presents a major diagnostic and therapeutic dilemma. In such patients, the presence of dense aortic valve calcification on CT (aortic valve calcium score >2,000 in men and >1,200 in women) favors the diagnosis of severe aortic stenosis.

Structural heart disease interventions: Computed tomography is the most useful modality for preprocedure planning in patients undergoing percutaneous aortic valve replacement [transcatheter aortic valve replacement (TAVR)] (**Fig. 18**). It permits accurate assessment of the aortic annulus and aortic root size, extent and distribution of annular calcification, coronary ostial height in relation to the valve leaflet tips, extent of atherosclerotic involvement of the aorta, and finally the size of the peripheral vessels being used for vascular access. Apart from TAVR, CT is also being increasingly used for preprocedural planning for other structural heart disease interventions such as LA appendage occlusion, mitral valve-in-valve or valve-in-ring implantation, and tricuspid valve interventions.

Congenital heart disease: In patients with congenital heart diseases, CT is used routinely for delineating cardiac anatomy when echocardiography is not sufficiently informative (**Fig. 19**). CT is especially useful for evaluating vascular structures such as great vessels, systemic and pulmonary veins, anomalous vascular channels, and collaterals (**Fig. 20**).

Other uses: Cardiac CT is also useful in the assessment of many other cardiac diseases such as pericardial effusion, constrictive pericarditis, cardiac tumors, and cardiomyopathies. Cardiac CT can also provide cardiac chamber volumes and function and may complement echocardiography. However, for most of these indications, CMR is preferred over cardiac CT.

CARDIAC MAGNETIC RESONANCE IMAGING

TECHNICAL CONSIDERATIONS

Cardiac magnetic resonance utilizes the magnetic field produced by the hydrogen nuclei to generate images of various tissues. The CMR scanner uses a strong magnetic field (B_0) which is oriented in the patient's head-to-foot direction (z-axis). Once the protons are aligned to the z-axis, a brief radiofrequency (RF) pulse is delivered at Larmor frequency to flip them completely or partially from z-axis to x-y plane. The time taken by the magnetic vector in the z-axis to recover to 63% of its original value is known as T1-relaxation time whereas the time taken by the magnetic vector in the x-y plane to decay to 37% of its original value (in other words, decay by 63%) is known as T2- or T2*-relaxation time.

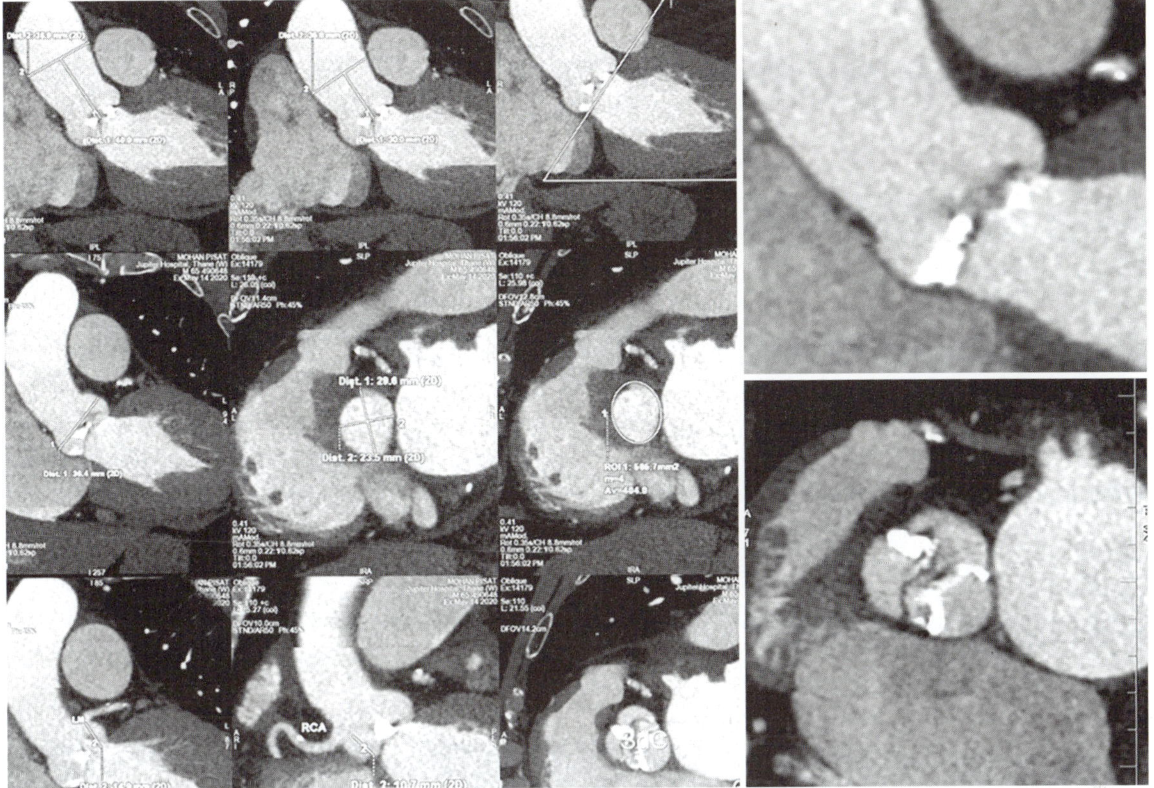

FIGURE 18: Contrast-enhanced computed tomographic angiogram with double oblique reconstructions provides different views and measurements required for planning of transcatheter aortic valve implantation.

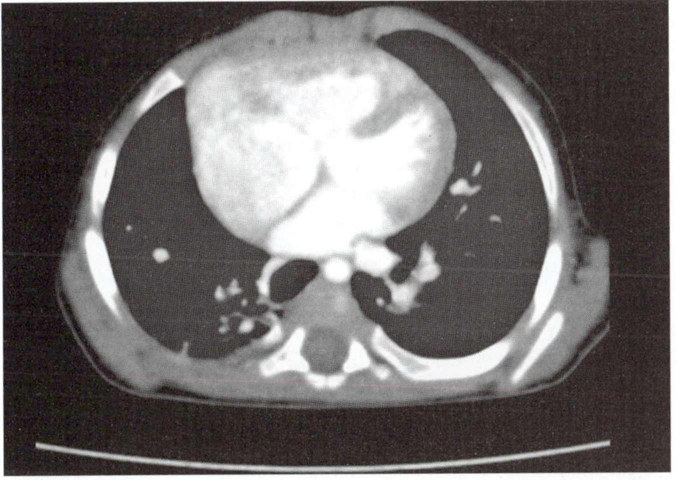

FIGURE 19: Contrast-enhanced computed tomography showing a defect in the ventricular septum. Also note, dilated right-sided heart chambers.

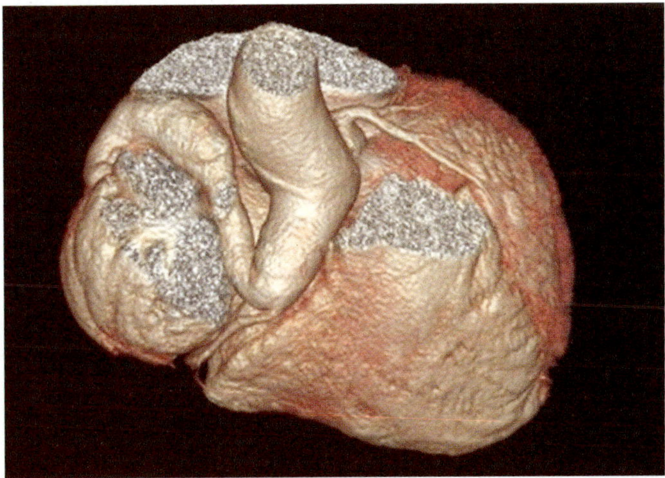

FIGURE 20: Volume-rendered image of the heart showing dilated tortuous vessel arising from aorta and ending in right atrial chamber. This is a coronary-cameral fistula.

The CMR signal strength depends mainly on two factors—(1) the availability, at the beginning of each imaging sequence, of protons in z-axis that can be flipped to x-y plane, and (2) the strength of the magnetic vector in the x-y plane. T1-wieghting uses a short repetition time. Since fat has shorter T1-relaxation time than muscle, it produces brighter signal because of its rapid recovery. Myocardium produces intermediate density signal whereas water produces the weakest signal (appears black). T2-weighting uses long repetition time. Water produces brighter signal as compared to fat or muscle.

Gadolinium-based contrast agents are used for performing contrast-enhanced CMR studies. They are injected intravenously. The interpretation of CMR grayscale images is typically a qualitative process. However, there are specific imaging sequences that allow measurement.

Unlike CT, CMR does not use any ionizing radiation; hence, there are no radiation-safety issues. There are also no major renal safety issues with the currently available gadolinium-based contrast agents. The most important limitation with CMR (other than the presence of metallic implants) is its slow acquisition time and the claustrophobic environment.

CLINICAL APPLICATIONS

Cardiomyopathies: Because of the ability of CMR to permit tissue characterization with excellent spatial resolution (2–3 mm), cardiomyopathies and myocardial disorders represent the most useful application for CMR in clinical practice. Distinct morphological patterns seen in various specific cardiomyopathies can be recognized by CMR, allowing a noninvasive diagnosis of these conditions.

Nonischemic dilated cardiomyopathy is characterized by LV dilatation and dysfunction, accompanied by varying degree of secondary mitral regurgitation, all of which can be accurately quantified by CMR. Late gadolinium enhancement (LGE) may be present in one-third of all cases, typically in midmyocardial layers. This LGE pattern is useful for distinguishing it from ischemic LV systolic dysfunction in which there is subendocardial or transmural LGE that follows coronary vascular distribution. However, in about 13–16% of the patients with nonischemic cardiomyopathy, there may be subendocardial or transmural scar on LGE. This may indicate prior MI with spontaneous recanalization of the coronary artery. The presence and extent of LGE are also predictive of arrhythmic as well as overall mortality risk in these patients. CMR may also assess LV dyssynchrony, provide information about scar location and extent, and delineate coronary venous anatomy, all of which may help in guiding lead placement if cardiac resynchronization therapy is contemplated.

In HCM, CMR permits excellent visualization of the location and extent of LV hypertrophy, site of intracavity flow obstruction, papillary muscle abnormalities, LA enlargement, and RV hypertrophy (**Fig. 21**). CMR is the best modality for diagnosing apical hypertrophy and apical aneurysms which are common in patients with midventricular or apical variants of HCM. LGE in HCM is seen mostly in the hypertrophied segments, at the site of insertion of RV wall into the ventricular septum and in aneurysmal segments. As with any other cardiomyopathy, the presence of LGE in HCM is associated with increased arrhythmic risk.

Cardiac magnetic resonance is an excellent modality for the diagnosis of cardiac amyloidosis, which is characterized by increased LV and RV wall thickness, biatrial enlargement, thickened atrial septum, dilated inferior vena cava etc., (**Figs. 22 A** and **B**). Characteristic LGE abnormalities are seen in cardiac amyloidosis. There is intense accumulation of gadolinium in the LV myocardium with marked extracellular volume expansion on T1-mapping. There is typically diffuse subendocardial LGE but in some patients, it may be patchy. The presence of gadolinium makes it extremely difficult to null the myocardium during T1-weighing which is also a characteristic finding in cardiac amyloidosis.

FIGURE 21: Four-chamber cine magnetic resonance image of the heart reveals asymmetric hypertrophy of the interventricular septum. This is the most common phenotypic variant of hypertrophic cardiomyopathy.

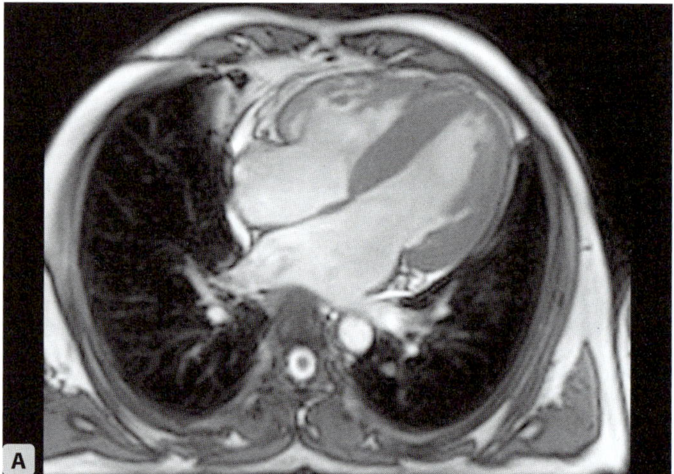

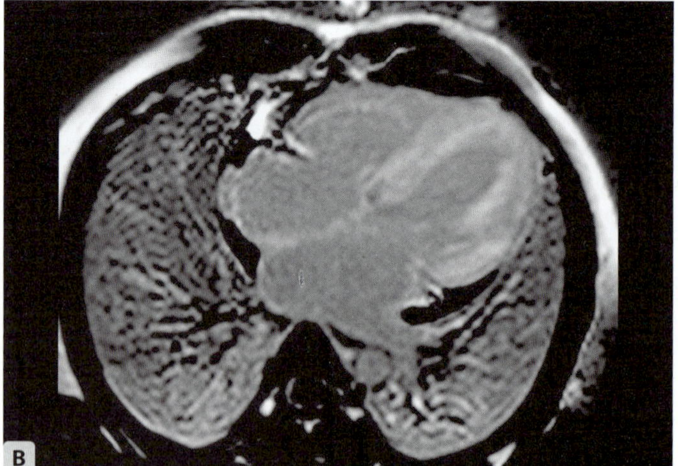

FIGURES 22 A & B: Four-chamber image in steady-state free precession **(A)** and late gadolinium enhancement **(B)** sequences reveal left ventricular wall hypertrophy. There is diffuse global subendocardial hyperenhancement with dark blood pool. These features represent cardiac amyloidosis.

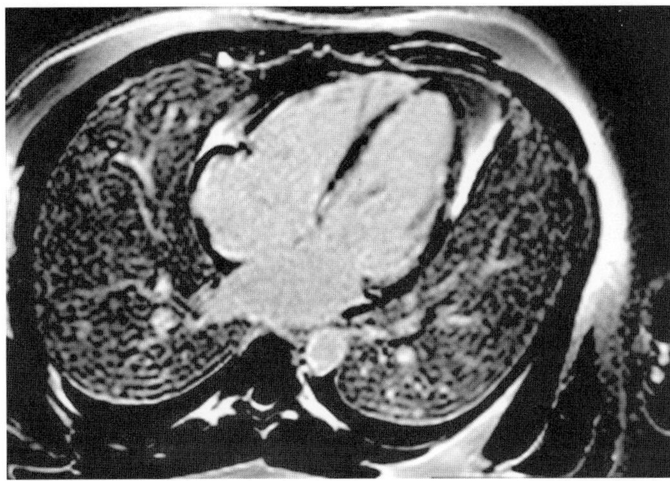

FIGURE 23: Four-chamber view of the heart with late gadolinium enhancement shows patchy midmyocardial and epicardial hyperenhancement in the classical basal septal distribution suggestive of cardiac sarcoidosis.

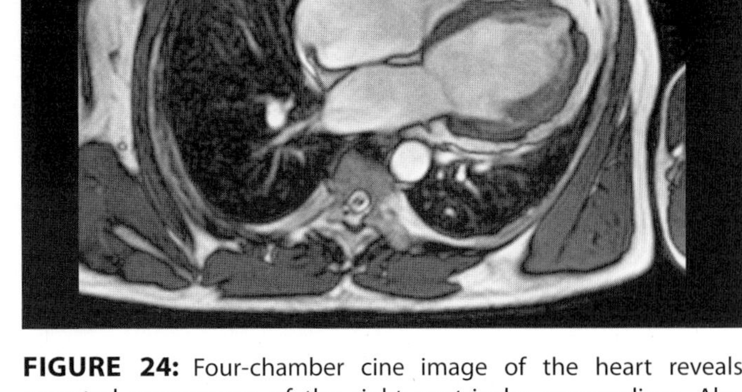

FIGURE 24: Four-chamber cine image of the heart reveals crenated appearance of the right ventricular myocardium. Also note microaneurysms involving free wall of the right ventricle.

In Anderson–Fabry disease, there is often thickening of basal inferolateral segments with increased T2 time (due to fat accumulation) compared with the normal myocardium. Sarcoidosis often shows patchy LGE involving basal inferolateral segments of LV, ventricular septum, and RV and right atrial walls (**Fig. 23**). The presence of LGE is associated with the risk of ventricular tachyarrhythmia in these patients. In patients with thalassemia undergoing repeated blood transfusions, marked shortening of T2* time (<20 ms) is highly suggestive of iron deposition in the myocardium and indicates the need for iron chelation therapy. Timely institution of chelation therapy based on CMR findings has been able to significantly improve survival in children with thalassemia. CMR can also be used for monitoring response to chelation therapy by serially measuring T2* times. In arrhythmogenic RV cardiomyopathy, there may be aneurysmal dilatation, thinning, and/or fatty infiltration of the RV free wall (**Fig. 24**). Noncompaction cardiomyopathy is characterized by typical spongy appearance of the myocardium with trabeculations and recesses. Specific criteria have been laid down for diagnosing noncompaction by CMR.

Coronary artery disease: Cardiac magnetic resonance is useful in the assessment of almost entire spectrum of CAD. In patients with acute MI, regional wall motion abnormalities can be detected by cine imaging whereas perfusion imaging will demonstrate perfusion defects. With its high spatial resolution (usually <3 mm), CMR can identify even small regions of subendocardial perfusion defects. Additionally, T2-weighted images can demonstrate myocardial edema whereas LGE shows the areas of irreversible injury. During acute MI, the extent of myocardial edema detected by T2-weighting is usually much greater than the areas of irreversible myocardial injury identified by LGE after reperfusion. This represents the area of salvaged myocardium. CMR also helps in differentiating an acute coronary event with other conditions that can have similar clinical presentations. In acute myocarditis, myocardial edema can be detected by T2-weighted imaging, myocardial hyperemia, and capillary leak by early gadolinium enhancement (EGE), and irreversible myocardial injury by LGE. LGE is typically seen in the subepicardial or midmyocardial layers and in a patchy distribution which does not correspond to any coronary vascular territory. The combined use of all these three features achieves the best diagnostic accuracy for recognition of acute myocarditis. In patients with Takotsubo cardiomyopathy, which has a clinical presentation very similar to an acute coronary event, CMR shows typical regional myocardial dysfunction with no or minimal subendocardial LGE. Patchy, intermediate intensity LGE without the loss of wall thickness and T2-weighted evidence of myocardial edema may also be seen.

In patients recovering from an acute MI, CMR can demonstrate areas of "no-reflow" and microvascular obstruction as well as intramyocardial hemorrhage. Late after an acute MI, the extent of LGE serves as an excellent predictor of reversibility of myocardial dysfunction, LV remodeling and clinical outcomes (**Figs. 25** and **26**). The transmural extent of scar by LGE is a reliable predictor of improvement in myocardial contractile function after coronary revascularization. A transmural thickness of >50% of LGE is accepted as a threshold of irreversibility. The number of segments with transmural LGE is a strong predictor of LV remodeling, development of heart failure, need for cardiac transplantation, risk of ventricular tachyarrhythmias, and sudden cardiac death and overall cardiac mortality. LGE involving >5% of the LV mass has been reported to be a risk marker in both ischemic and nonischemic cardiomyopathies.

In patients with stable CAD, CMR can permit detection of obstructive diseases by showing reversible perfusion defects and regional contractile dysfunction during pharmacological stress imaging using adenosine, dipyridamole, or dobutamine.

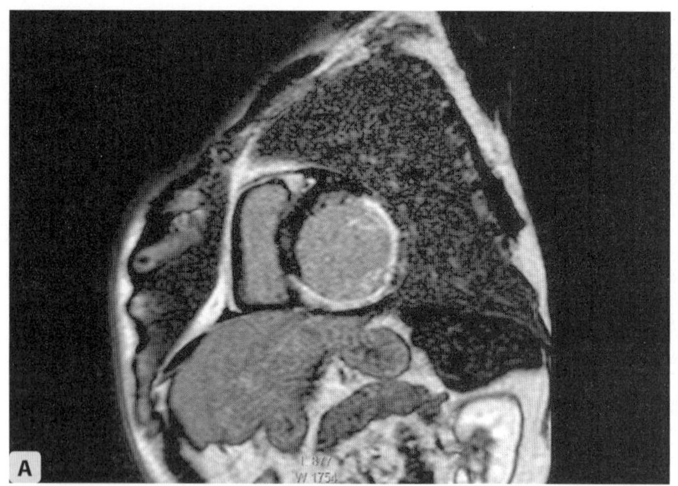

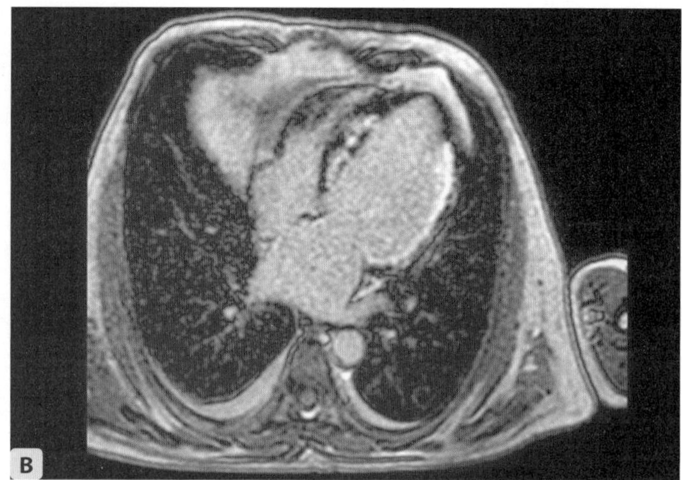

FIGURES 25 A & B: Late gadolinium-enhanced images obtained in short-axis and four-chamber views reveal presence of delayed hyperenhancement in the lateral wall of the left ventricle. The gadolinium enhancement is confined to the subendocardial region.

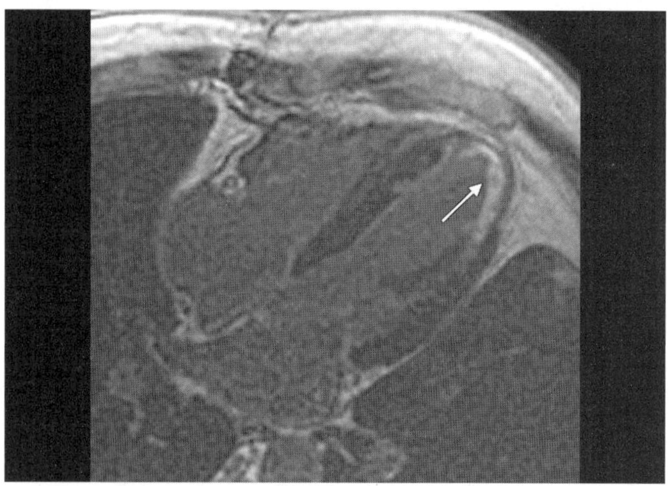

FIGURE 26: Four-chamber view showing transmural (full thickness) hyperenhancement (marked with white arrow), suggestive of scarred, nonviable myocardium.

Cardiac chamber volumes and function: The excellent delineation of tissue blood interface during CMR permits accurate quantification of cardiac chamber volumes and function (**Fig. 27**). Furthermore, unlike echocardiography, complete tomographic reconstruction with CMR allows direct quantification of chamber volumes without involving any geometric assumptions. For these reasons, CMR is considered the current gold standard for estimation of LV volumes, mass, and ejection fraction, whereas it is almost the only noninvasive modality available for estimation of RV volumes and ejection fraction. Although the advent of 3D echocardiography has now enabled the assessment of RV by echocardiography, it remains technically challenging and a much inferior alternative to CMR for this purpose. CMR is the current recommended modality for serial follow-up of the patients with congenital heart diseases who are at risk of developing RV dysfunction, such as those operated earlier for tetralogy of Fallot. CMR can also reliably estimate left or right atrial volumes.

Valve diseases: As mentioned above, CMR has better accuracy and reproducibility than echocardiography for volumetric assessment. Hence, CMR is now considered the gold standard for quantification of the severity of the regurgitant valve lesions. A combination of phase-contrast imaging and stead-state free precession (SSFP) imaging permits accurate quantification of regurgitant volumes, net stroke volume, and regurgitant fraction in patients with aortic or mitral regurgitation (**Fig 28**). Several studies have shown better correlation of clinical outcomes with CMR-derived estimates of regurgitant lesions than with the echocardiography-based measurements. However, CMR is much inferior to echocardiography for evaluation of the valve anatomy and function.

Intracardiac masses: Cardiac magnetic resonance provides excellent anatomic visualization of various intracardiac masses and in combination with tissue characterization, can provide etiological diagnosis in many of these cases (**Fig. 29**). Thrombus is the most common intracardiac mass and CMR has an excellent diagnostic accuracy for recognizing an intracardiac thrombus. EGE or LGE with long inversion time is recommended for this purpose.

Others: Cardiac magnetic resonance is an excellent modality for the assessment of various other cardiac diseases such as chronic constrictive pericarditis, certain congenital heart diseases, and evaluation of anatomic substrate for cardiac arrhythmias (**Fig. 30**). CMR is the current test of choice for differentiating constrictive pericarditis from restrictive cardiomyopathy. Pericardial thickness can be easily measured by either black-blood fast spin echo or cine imaging, and up to 3 mm is accepted as normal. Real-time cine SSFP and phase-contrast imaging can be used for assessing the hemodynamic abnormalities associated with constrictive pericarditis. Cine myocardial tagged imaging may be useful to identify perimyocardial adhesions by demonstrating lack of deformation of tag lines with the cardiac motion. LGE within the thickened pericardium suggests active inflammation or pericardial fibrosis which

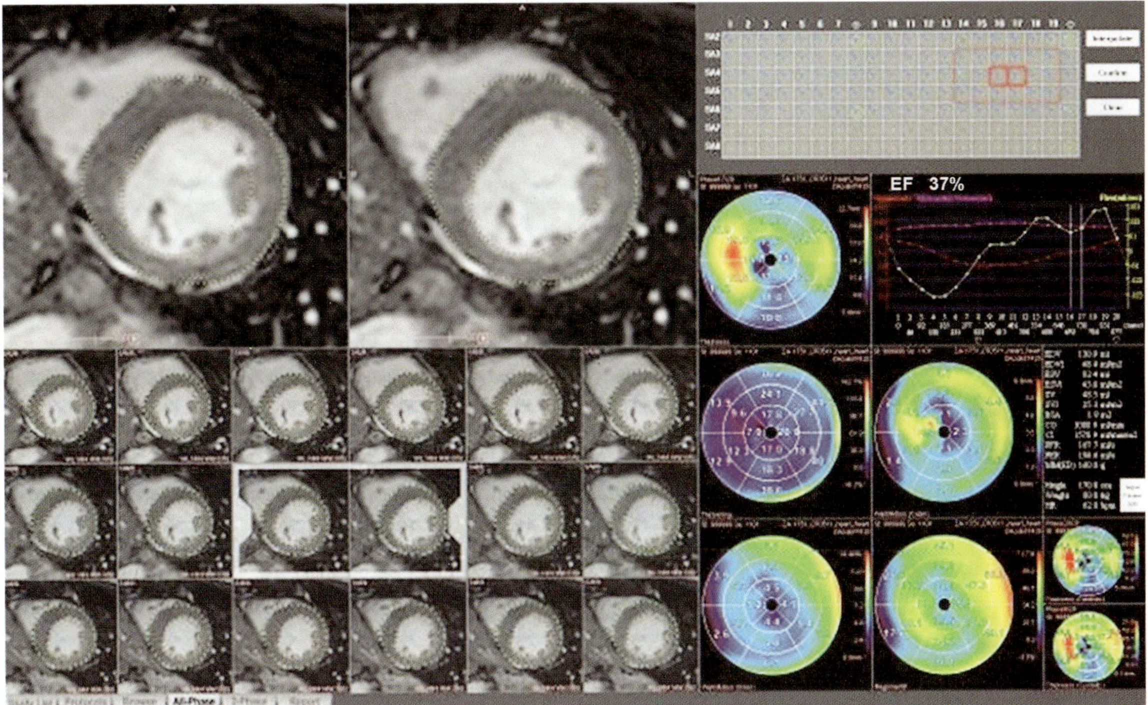

FIGURE 27: Short-axis image stack obtained using gradient echo cine images to calculate left ventricular volume and mass. Contouring of left ventricular myocardium in end systole and end diastole is performed to obtain the same.

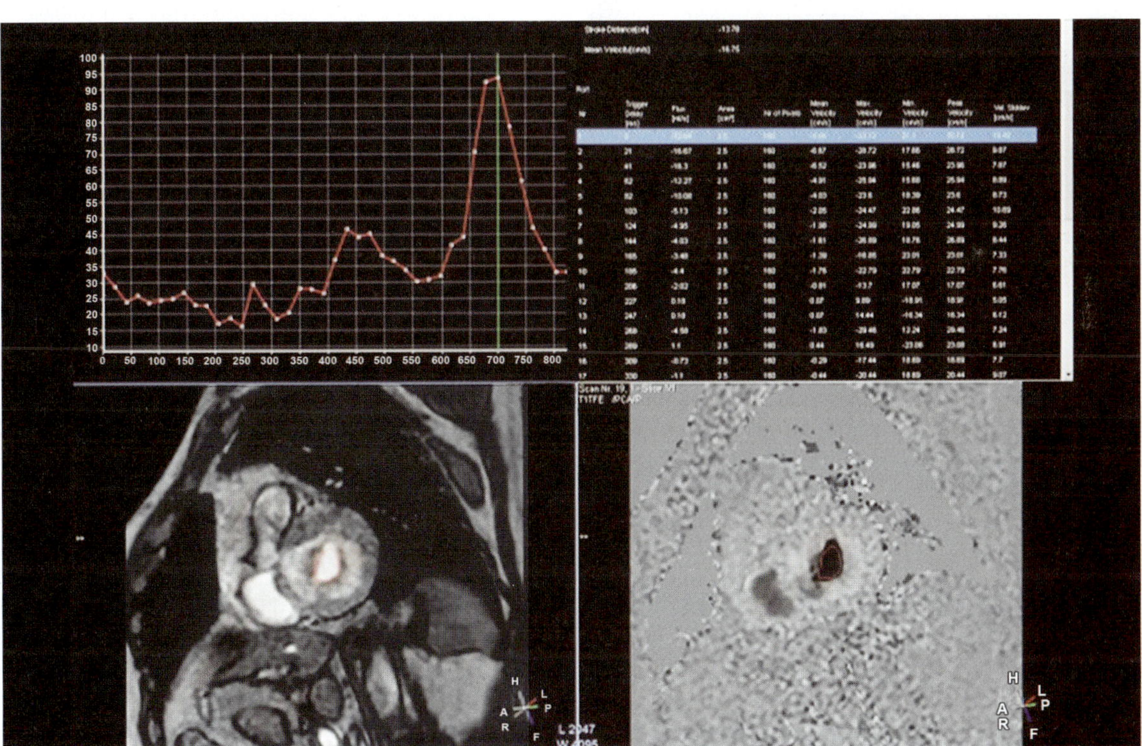

FIGURE 28: Phase contrast image of the heart consisting of phase and magnitude images can be used for quantification of flow, intracardiac shunts, and valvular abnormalities.

can be further differentiated using T2-weighted myocardial edema imaging. The presence of active inflammation has therapeutic implications as anti-inflammatory therapies may help in reversing pericarditis and may obviate the need for pericardiectomy.

ACKNOWLEDGMENTS

The authors are thankful to Drs Atul Pathak and Surbhi Pande from Medanta - The Medicity Hospital India for providing **Figures 8** to **10**.

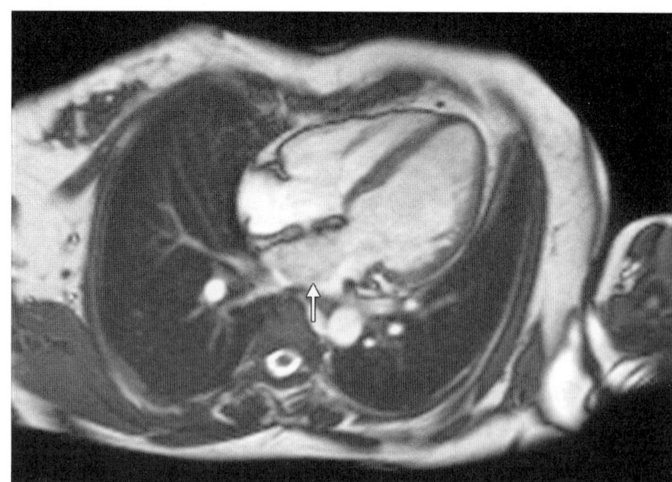

FIGURE 29: Four-chamber cine image of the heart reveals well-marginated lobular lesion (arrow) in the left atrium attached to interatrial septum suggestive of myxoma.

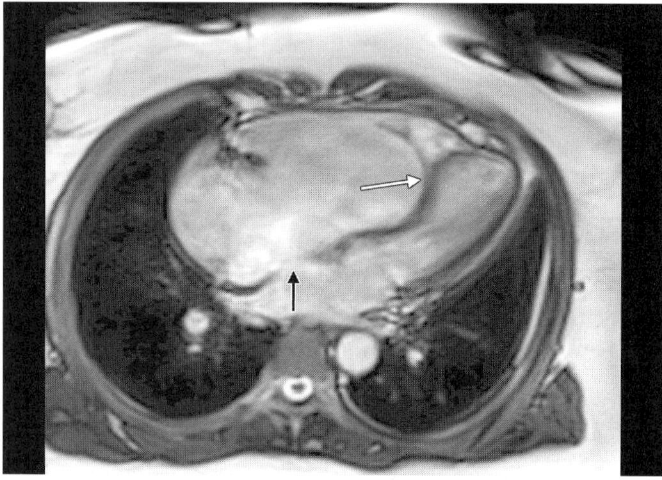

FIGURE 30: Four-chamber image of the heart in a patient with Ebstein anomaly reveals apical displacement of tricuspid valve leaflet (white arrow). This results in enlarged right atrial chamber (arterialization of right ventricle). Also note, bowing of the interventricular septum and a defect in the interatrial septum (black arrow) suggestive of ostium secundum atrial septal defect.

RECOMMENDED READINGS

1. Armstrong WF, Ryan T. Ultrasound physics and instrumentation. In: Armstrong WF, Ryan T, (Eds). Feigenbaum's Echocardiography, 7th ed. Philadelphia, PA: Lippincott, Williams and Wilkins; 2018. pp. 9-38.
2. Mitchell C, Rahko PS, Blauwet LA, Canaday B, Finstuen JA, Foster MC, et al. Guidelines for performing a comprehensive transthoracic echocardiographic examination in adults: recommendations from the American Society of Echocardiography. J Am Soc Echocardiogr. 2019;32(1):1-64.
3. Lang RM, Badano LP, Mor-Avi V, Afilalo J, Armstrong A, Ernande L, et al. Recommendations for cardiac chamber quantification by echocardiography in adults: an update from the American Society of Echocardiography and the European Association of Cardiovascular Imaging. J Am Soc Echocardiogr. 2015;28(1):1-39.
4. Nagueh SF, Smiseth OA, Appleton CP, Byrd BF 3rd, Dokainish H, Edvardsen T, et al. Recommendations for the evaluation of left ventricular diastolic function by echocardiography: an update from the American Society of Echocardiography and the European Association of Cardiovascular Imaging. J Am Soc Echocardiogr. 2016;29(4):277-314.
5. Zoghbi WA, Adams D, Bonow RO, Enriquez-Sarano M, Foster E, Grayburn PA, et al. Recommendations for noninvasive evaluation of native valvular regurgitation: a report from the American Society of Echocardiography developed in collaboration with the Society for Cardiovascular Magnetic Resonance. J Am Soc Echocardiogr. 2017;30(4):303-71.
6. Baumgartner H, Hung J, Bermejo J, Chambers JB, Evangelista A, Griffin BP, et al. Echocardiographic assessment of valve stenosis: EAE/ASE recommendations for clinical practice. J Am Soc Echocardiogr. 2009;22(1): 1-23; quiz 101-2.
7. Baumgartner H, Hung J, Bermejo J, Chambers JB, Edvardsen T, Goldstein S, et al. Recommendations on the echocardiographic assessment of aortic valve stenosis: a focused update from the European Association of Cardiovascular Imaging and the American Society of Echocardiography. J Am Soc Echocardiogr. 2017;30(4):372-92.
8. Bansal M, Sengupta PP. How to interpret an echocardiography report (for the non-imager)? Heart. 2017;103(21):1733-44.
9. Bansal M, Kasliwal RR. How do I do it? Speckle-tracking echocardiography. Indian Heart J. 2013; 65(1):117-23.
10. Collier P, Phelan D, Klein A. A test in context: myocardial strain measured by speckle-tracking echocardiography. J Am Coll Cardiol. 2017;69(8):1043-56.
11. Udelson JE, Dilsizian V, Bonow RO. Nuclear cardiology. In: Zipes DP, Libby P, Bonow R, Mann DL, Tomaselli GF, Braunwald E (Eds). Braunwald's Heart Disease: A Textbook of Cardiovascular Medicine, 11th edition. Philadelphia, PA: Elsevier; 2019. pp. 261-300.
12. Kansal M, Bansal M, Narula J, Sengupta PP. Imaging in advanced heart failure. In: Domanski MJ, Mehra MR, Pfeffer MA (Eds). Oxford Textbook of Advanced Heart Failure and Cardiac Transplantation. New York, NY: Oxford University Press; 2016. pp. 102-136.
13. Bax JJ, Wijns W, Cornel JH, Visser FC, Boersma E, Fioretti PM. Accuracy of currently available techniques for prediction of functional recovery after revascularization in patients with left ventricular dysfunction due to chronic coronary artery disease: comparison of pooled data. J Am Coll Cardiol. 1997;30(6):1451-60.

14. Narula J, Chandrashekhar Y, Ahmadi A, Abbara S, Berman DS, Blankstein R, et al. SCCT 2021 expert consensus document on coronary computed tomographic angiography: a report of the Society of Cardiovascular Computed Tomography. J Cardiovasc Comput Tomogr. 2020;S1934-5925(20)30473-1.
15. Shaw LJ, Blankstein R, Bax JJ, Ferencik M, Bittencourt MS, Min JK, et al. Society of Cardiovascular Computed Tomography / North American Society of Cardiovascular Imaging - Expert Consensus Document on Coronary CT Imaging of Atherosclerotic Plaque. J Cardiovasc Comput Tomogr. 2021;15(2):93-109.
16. Douglas PS, Hoffmann U, Patel MR, Mark DB, Al-Khalidi HR, Cavanaugh B, et al. Outcomes of anatomical versus functional testing for coronary artery disease. N Engl J Med. 2015;372(14):1291-300.
17. Newby DE, Adamson PD, Berry C, Boon NA, Dweck MR, Flather M et al. Coronary CT Angiography and 5-year risk of myocardial infarction. N Engl J Med. 2018;379(10):924-33.
18. Maron DJ, Hochman JS, Reynolds HR, Bangalore S, O'Brien SM, Boden WE, et al. Initial Invasive or Conservative Strategy for Stable Coronary Disease. N Engl J Med. 2020;382(15):1395-407.
19. Bansal M, Agarwala R, Kasliwal RR. Imaging atherosclerosis for cardiovascular risk prediction- in search of the holy grail! Indian Heart J. 2018;70(5):587-92.
20. Biglands JD, Radjenovic A, Ridgway JP. Cardiovascular magnetic resonance physics for clinicians: Part II. J Cardiovasc Magn Reson. 2012;14:66.

CHAPTER 89

Cardiac Catheterization and Coronary Angiography

Mandava Satya Sahitya, Navjyot Kaur, Rajesh Vijayvergiya

ABSTRACT

Cardiac catheterization and coronary angiography (CAG) remain the gold standard for intracardiac pressure measurements, hemodynamic assessment of various shunt and valvular lesions, and diagnosis of coronary artery disease, besides allowing the therapeutic intervention, if required. Nonetheless, due to the invasive nature, requirement of contrast and radiation, there are guidelines for the appropriate indications, the preprocedural work up, and procedural and postprocedural monitoring of patients undergoing cardiac catheterization and CAG. In this chapter, we shall discuss in brief, the technical aspects of CAG, common diagnostic catheters, and coronary angiographic views, besides the preprocedural evaluation and possible complications of the procedure. The cardiac catheterization laboratory is used for many therapeutic interventional procedures. These are mentioned in the chapters on specific disorders.

"If you take shortcuts, you get cut short"

—Gary Busey

INTRODUCTION

Cardiac catheterization refers to the invasive direct catheter-based assessment of the heart. It is useful for anatomical assessment of the heart including coronaries, hemodynamic measurement in various chambers, evaluation of regurgitant, and various shunt lesions. Cardiac catheterization has come a long way since Forssmann first performed self-right heart catheterization in 1929. André Cournand and Dickinson Richards redesigned Forssmann's catheter which allowed for a safer procedure, longer indwell times, and easy multiple collections of true mixed venous blood. Sones pioneered selective CAG, which was improved with the development of specialized catheters by Judkins and Amplatz. Till date, CAG remains the gold standard for the evaluation of coronary artery disease.

Since Gruentzig performed the first angioplasty in 1977, the number of percutaneous coronary intervention (PCI) has increased at an enormous rate, such that in 2018, nearly 438,351 PCI were performed in India itself with an annual growth rate of about 13%. There is also an increase in the number of complex PCI such as left main coronary artery (LMCA) stenting by 2.45% and intervention to previous surgical bypass grafts by 1%. Overall 4.32% of PCI were for bifurcation disease and 3.5% for chronic total occlusions (CTOs), out of which 0.29% were performed through a retrograde approach.

CARDIAC CATHETERIZATION AND CAG

INDICATIONS

- *Coronary artery disease*: CAG is indicated in patients with symptomatic coronary artery disease including acute coronary syndrome and chronic stable angina with high-risk features on noninvasive stress tests. Besides, new-onset left ventricle dysfunction or regional wall motion abnormality, ventricular arrhythmias, lesions of unclear severity or ≥50% on computed tomography CAG, and resuscitated cardiac arrest also warrant a CAG.
- *Valvular heart disease*: Cardiac catheterization helps in objective hemodynamic assessment of various valvular lesions including cardiac chamber and pulmonary artery pressures. The invasive evaluation is indicated when the symptoms are out of proportion to the severity of valvular heart disease and when there is concomitant unexplained left ventricular dysfunction. Besides, diagnostic CAG is indicated in any patient of >40 years of age, before he/she is taken up for valve surgery.
- In certain situations, cardiac catheterization is indicated to distinguish between restrictive and constrictive physiology.
- Coronary angiography is indicated in patients with left ventricular dysfunction of unknown etiology. Also in certain conditions, like cardiac amyloidosis, cardiac catheterization is done to get the tissue diagnosis.
- Cardiac catheterization remains the gold standard for diagnosing pulmonary hypertension, and also to assess the response to vasodilators.
- In congenital heart diseases, cardiac catheterization remains the cornerstone for defining the anatomy, hemodynamic measurement, and deciding the operability of intracardiac left to right shunts and for defining the major aortopulmonary collaterals.

CONTRAINDICATIONS

There are no absolute contraindications for catheterization. The relative contraindications are as follows:

- Acute gastrointestinal bleeding
- Uncontrolled hypertension
- Decompensated heart failure and pulmonary edema
- Severe hypokalemia
- Uncorrected digoxin toxicity
- International normalized ratio (INR) >1.8 or severe coagulopathy
- Previous anaphylactoid reaction to contrast media
- Acute stroke
- Acute renal failure or severe chronic nondialysis-dependent kidney disease
- Unexplained fever or untreated active infection
- Severe anemia
- Recent cerebrovascular event (<1 month)
- Pregnancy

PREPROCEDURE PREPARATION

A detailed history and examination is a must before any invasive procedure. A note of comorbidities like diabetes mellitus, chronic kidney disease, chronic liver disease, hematological diseases and infections like human immunodeficiency virus (HIV) and hepatitis B and C should be made. Any history of allergy to drugs/contrast material should be recorded. Blood investigations include complete blood counts, coagulation profile, serum electrolytes, blood urea nitrogen, and creatinine. The INR should be <1.8 for a transfemoral approach and <2.2 for a transradial approach to minimize bleeding risk.

Medications to be withheld prior to catheterization: Oral anticoagulants such as warfarin should be withheld at least 2–3 days prior to catheterization to achieve the desired INR limits. In case of an emergency, transradial instead of transfemoral catheterization is preferred to avoid local access site vascular complications secondary to high INR. The direct thrombin inhibitor such as dabigatran should be discontinued 24 hours before catheterization in those with estimated glomerular filtration rate (eGFR) of 80 mL/min or greater, 36 hours if eGFR is 50–79 L/min, and 48 hours if it is 30–49 mL/min. If PCI is likely to be performed, these timelines should be extended by a factor of two. Direct Xa inhibitors (rivaroxaban, apixaban, or edoxaban) should be discontinued 24 hours before the procedure if the eGFR is 30 mL/min or higher, otherwise at least 36 hours prior. In case PCI is a possibility, the timeline for discontinuation is at least 48 hours. Metformin is withheld on the morning of the procedure and resumed if the renal functions remain stable for the next 48 hours. Aspirin and other antiplatelets should be continued without interruption.

Hydration: The risk of contrast-induced nephropathy (CIN) should be assessed in all patients. The risk factors for CIN include diabetes, chronic kidney disease, congestive heart failure, low ejection fraction, anemia, and advanced age. The only proven strategy to reduce the risk of CIN is adequate hydration. As a general rule, the total contrast volume used during the intervention should be <3.7 times the eGFR.

Fasting: The patient should be fasting for 6 hours before catheterization, so that emergency intubation and general anesthesia can be safely given, without the risk of aspiration.

Consent: Written informed consent and indoor admission is must for any cardiac catheterization and PCI.

POSTPROCEDURE CARE

All patients, postprocedure, are monitored hemodynamically in a cardiac care unit. The vascular access sheaths used for diagnostic procedures are usually removed in the catheterization laboratory unless there is a need for invasive blood pressure monitoring. Local hemostasis is achieved either by manual compression or by balloon inflatable devices for transradial access. For femoral access, manual compression or suture/collagen plug-based vascular devices are used.

COMPLICATIONS

Bleeding complications: Arterial access site bleeding is the most common complication of cardiac catheterization. This includes minor oozing, ecchymosis, hematoma, retroperitoneal bleeds, arteriovenous fistula, or pseudoaneurysm formation. These complications are more common following PCI than diagnostic catheterization because of the use of anticoagulation, i.e., heparin. An activated clotting time (ACT) value of <160–180 seconds is required before removing the post PCI access sheath. Nonaccess site bleeds include pericardial bleed and the comorbidities unmasked due to anticoagulation and antiplatelet therapy (e.g., peptic ulcer disease).

Contrast-induced nephropathy: The reported incidence of CIN varies between 3.3% and 16.5% in patients undergoing cardiac catheterization. It is defined as a rise in creatinine levels by 0.5 mg/dL or by 25% from baseline and occurs 24–72 hours after exposure to contrast. The risk is higher in patients with underlying kidney disease (eGFR <60 mL/min/1.73 m^2), diabetes, elderly, females, patients on diuretics, angiotensin-converting enzyme inhibitors, and metformin. Adequate prehydration, use of iso-osmolar agents, and a lesser amount of contrast decrease the risk of this complication. The CIN Consensus Working Panel recommends that an infusion of 1.0–1.5 mL/kg/h of isotonic saline solution from 3 to 12 hours before and until 6–24 hours after the procedure is suitable to minimize CIN.

Reactions to contrast material: These are classified as allergic and nonallergic reactions.

- Allergic reactions: These range from itching to skin rash, local edema, asthma, and full-blown anaphylactoid reaction. These occur due to the activation of various components of the immune system.
- Allergic-like reactions: They present similarly as the classic allergic response but are independent of immune system activation. Allergic-like reactions revolve around a physiologic response to contrast (e.g., nausea, vomiting, vasovagal reaction, hypotension, and flushing).

Neurological complications: The risk of stroke is 0.05–0.1% after diagnostic procedures and 0.18–0.4% for patients undergoing intervention. Embolic risk is increased with increased length of procedure and volume of contrast, use of intra-aortic balloon pumps, urgent indication, and presence of diabetes mellitus, hypertension, previous stroke, renal failure, and presence of atherosclerotic plaques at ascending aorta/aortic arch.

Rare complications: The rare but potentially fatal complications of cardiac catheterization include cardiac chamber perforation/coronary artery perforation with resultant tamponade, coronary artery dissection, air embolism, pulmonary artery dissection/perforation, and cardiac arrhythmias. Death related to diagnostic cardiac catheterization is rare (<0.05%). The strongest predictors are heart failure (especially advanced stages), hypotension and shock, acute coronary syndrome, severe aortic or mitral valve disease, renal failure, and moribund state.

TECHNICAL ASPECTS AND PROCEDURE

Procedures are performed under conscious sedation and local anesthesia with 1% xylocaine.

Vascular access: The various access sites used are as follows:

- *Femoral artery*: It has been the standard vascular access for many years and is also known as the Judkins technique. The point of entry is 1–3 cm (1–2 finger breadths) below the inguinal ligament, in line with the palpable course of the common femoral artery. The inguinal crease can be misleading in obese as well as very thin individuals. Hence, in clinical practice, the optimal point of skin entry over the inferior edge of the femoral head is often identified using fluoroscopy guidance. The femoral artery technique is disadvantageous for patients unable to endure long bed rest times, those with high bleeding risk, and those with peripheral artery disease.
- *Radial artery*: Radial access is associated with a lower risk of bleeding and is more comfortable for the patient postprocedurally. Adequate dual blood supply to the hand is tested by either the Allen or the Barbeau test. To perform the Allen test, manual compression of the radial and the ulnar artery is done during fist clenching until blanching of the hand is seen, at which point the pressure over the ulnar artery is released. Under normal conditions, normal color returns within 10 seconds, and significant reactive hyperemia is absent on the release of pressure over the radial artery. The Barbeau test is performed similarly, but with the use of pulse oximetry; it has higher accuracy and reproducibility. The radial artery has a high propensity for spasm as it is extremely vasoactive. Therefore, as soon as access is obtained, an intra-arterial spasmolytic agent such as nitroglycerin (100–200 μg) or verapamil (2.5 mg) diluted into 10 mL of saline should be administered. To prevent thromboembolic events and radial artery occlusion, weight-adjusted unfractionated heparin (UFH), 40–70 units/kg up to 5,000 units, is administered either intravenously or intra-arterially. A hydrophilic-coated sheath further reduces the likelihood of spasm and regional pain.
- *Brachial artery*: It should be used sparingly, but may be required if radial access is not available or fails. Being the end artery for the forearm, there is no alternative blood supply to the forearm, in case of closure.

Continuous electrocardiogram (ECG) and invasive blood pressure monitoring are required during the procedure. As the procedure is performed under local anesthesia, other systems such as respiration and neurologic status can also be monitored as per the requirement. Special efforts should be taken by the primary operator to use the minimal amount of contrast and limit the radiation exposure.

Under fluoroscopic guidance, a flexible J-tipped guidewire is advanced through the sheath into the arterial axis until the aortic root is reached. Maintaining the wire in place, a catheter is then advanced over the guidewire into the aortic root, which is then flushed and connected to the contrast media injection apparatus. Under fluoroscopic imaging, the tip of the catheter is engaged to the coronary ostium and angiographic images are then obtained while injecting contrast directly into the cannulated coronary artery.

Hardware and catheters used: *A diagnostic CAG catheter* has three parts: Hub, shaft, and tip (**Fig. 1**). While the hub connects the catheter to the contrast injection system; the shaft, which is usually strong and rigid, transmits the torque to the tip (**Fig. 1**). The tip can be divided into three curves: Primary, secondary, and tertiary; starting from the distal end (**Fig. 1**). The diagnostic catheters, unlike the guiding catheters used for PCI, have a thicker wall, which considerably reduces their internal lumen. The standard length for adult left-heart catheterization by both the radial and the femoral approach is 100 cm (40 inches), while 80 cm is suitable for brachial access.

The most commonly used catheters are as follows:

Judkins catheter: The catheters consist of primary, secondary, and tertiary curves. There are two types of preformed Judkins catheter: Judkins right (JR) and Judkins left (JL) (**Fig. 2**). The distance between the primary and secondary curves (termed *arm*) is variable; for example, JL4, JL5, and JL6 have 4.2 cm, 5.2 cm, and 6.2 cm long arms, respectively. JL presents a primary curve of 90° and a secondary curve of 180°. JR presents a primary curve of 90° and a secondary curve of 30°. In addition to their conventional use, JR catheters may be used for saphenous vein graft (SVG) and left internal mammary artery (IMA) graft study through femoral and left radial approach.

Amplatz catheters: Similar to Judkins, there are preformed Amplatz left (AL) and Amplatz right (AR) catheters (**Fig. 2**). AL catheter tip allows for easier coronary engagement in specific settings, such as short left main ostium, separate origin of left circumflex (LCx) and left anterior descending (LAD) arteries and right coronary artery (RCA) with anterior-high origin. AR catheter allows engagement of RCA with inferior orientation. Amplatz catheters may also be used for the study of SVGs.

Multipurpose (MP) catheters: They are used for the engagement of coronary ostia as well as the study of SVGs. MPA 1 and 2 have a 45–60° primary curve, while MPB 1 and 2 have approximately an 80° primary curve (**Fig. 2**).

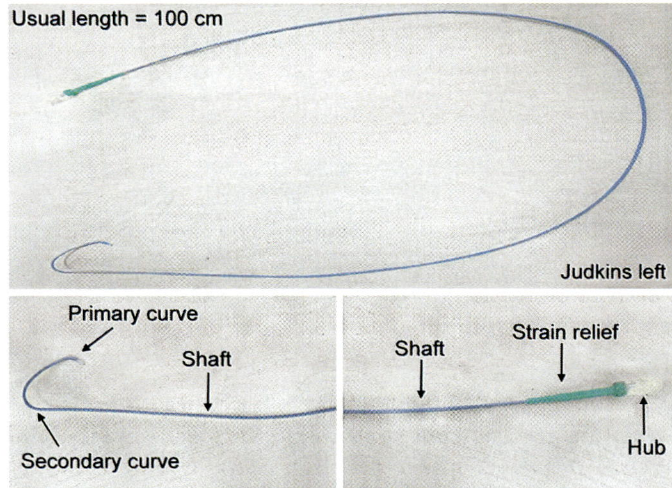

FIGURE 2: Diagnostic catheter (Judkins left) and its parts.

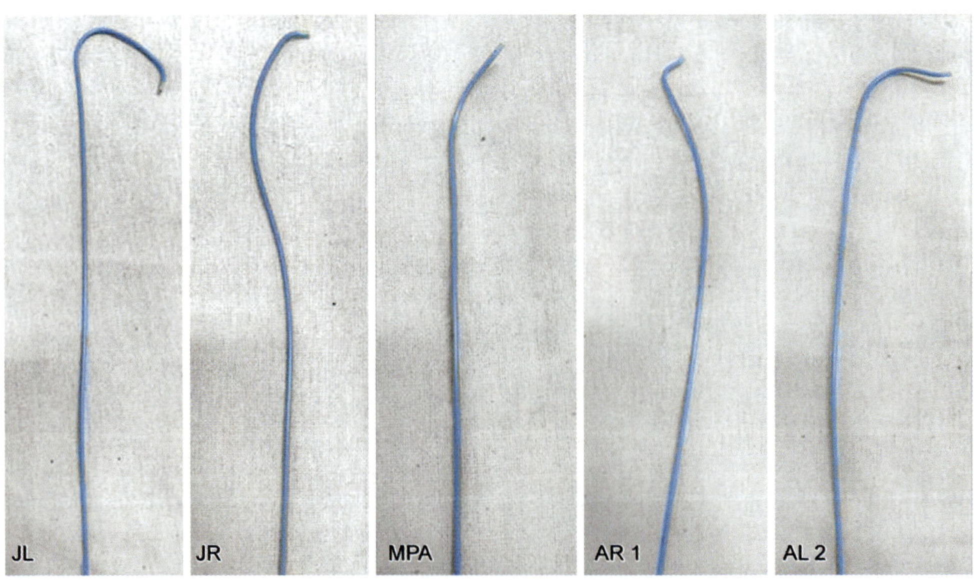

FIGURE 1: Diagnostic catheters.

IMA catheters: They have a high angulated primary curve tip (80°), to facilitate the engagement of the IMA. These catheters can also be used to engage the upward-pointing RCA.

Contrast material: The contrast agents are most commonly classified into high-osmolar (HOCA), low-osmolar (LOCA), and iso-osmolar (IOCA) contrast agents (**Table 1**).

The high osmolality and calcium-chelating proprieties of HOCAs often alter the heart rhythm and left ventricular contractibility, besides being toxic to kidneys. New-generation IOCAs with low osmolality and neutral chemical characteristics allow a significant reduction of adverse events. In large cohort studies, the incidence of all types of adverse reactions to contrast was approximately 12% with a high-osmolality agent, compared to only 3% with a low-osmolality contrast agent. For this reason, LOCAs and IOCAs are now considered the safest contrast agents to use for vascular diagnostic procedures.

Radiation safety: The radiation hazard remains an important concern with cardiac catheterization. As low as reasonably achievable (ALARA) radiation principles should be used to reduce both deterministic and stochastic effects. *Deterministic effects* are dose-related which increase in severity with increasing dose. These include cataract, hair loss, and skin injury. *Stochastic effects* are not dose-related and related to probability, though probability increases with increasing exposure. These include neoplasms and genetic defects. Even after applying this principle, the radiation dose for cardiac catheterization is in the range of 1–10 millisieverts.

Besides using personal protective gear like lead aprons, collars, glasses, gloves, and radiation dosimeters, best practices to minimize radiation exposure include minimization of fluoroscopy time, use of beam collimation, application of the least magnification possible, and optimal positioning of X-ray tube-image receiver unit with avoidance of extreme angles and rotation of the radiographic projection during long procedures. The maximum allowable whole-body radiation dose per year for those working with radiation is five roentgen-equivalents-man (rem), or a maximum of 50 rem in a lifetime.

TABLE 1 Types of contrast agents.

Contrast agent	Osmolality	Examples Ionic (I), nonionic (NI)
High-osmolar contrast agent (HOCA)	4–5 times the blood osmolality	Diatrizoate (I) Iothalamate (I)
Low-osmolar contrast agent (LOCA)	Two times the blood osmolality	Ioxaglate (I) Iodapamide (I) Iohexol (NI) Ioversol (NI) Iopromide (NI)
Iso-osmolar contrast agent (IOCA)	Same as blood osmolality	Iodixanol (I)

INTERPRETATION

Every coronary artery should be angiographically viewed in its entire length for morphological and extent of the lesion, percentage of stenosis, presence of collaterals, and downstream flow (**Figs. 3 A** to **D**). To avoid overlapping of vessels and for best angiographic delineation of vessels, some standard views are used, as in **Table 2**. **Figures 4 A** to **C** show CAG in a patient with no lesions. **Figures 5 A** to **C** show LMCA disease with triple vessel disease. LMCA disease is often called "widow maker" disease since it carries high mortality and these patients need early coronary artery bypass grafting (CABG). **Figure 6** shows angiogram in a patient with a tight proximal LAD lesion of 95%. This patient will be a candidate for percutaneous transluminal coronary angioplasty (PTCA) with stenting. **Figures 7 A** and **B** show a patient with three discrete lesions in LAD, LCx, and RCA. All three lesions are type A since they are small in length and there is no calcium. These can be amenable to multiple vessel PTCA.

Description of coronary lesion: The degree of the stenosis can be evaluated by comparing the minimum diameter of the vessel at the level of the lesion to the diameter of the adjacent segment upstream of the stenosis. This is usually underestimated as compared to estimates from post-mortem or intravascular imaging studies, as the proximal segment can be in vasospasm or there may be diffuse atherosclerosis. While commenting on stenosis severity, the diameter and length of the lesion are two main important characteristics. The moderate narrowing is defined as 50–70% and severe narrowing is defined as ≥70% stenosis. American Heart Association has classified the coronary lesions into three types (**Table 3**) depending on their morphological characteristics, probability of PCI success, and possible complications.

The complexity of coronary lesion is increased by the presence of thrombus, calcification, and by the tortuosity of the vessel. CTO, complete or almost complete blockage of a coronary artery for ≥30 days, is considered a complex lesion and contribute greatly to the SYNTAX score. Another challenging anatomy for percutaneous intervention is bifurcation lesions, which have less than optimal long-term outcomes with PCI. Coronary artery dissections may occur spontaneously or they may occur as a complication of CAG/PCI. Spontaneous coronary artery dissections are more common in premenopausal females and are usually managed conservatively. Angiographically these are divided into five types (**Table 4**).

Limitations of CAG: Apart from the possible complications listed above, the radiation hazards, and the risk of CIN, CAG is associated with few important limitations:

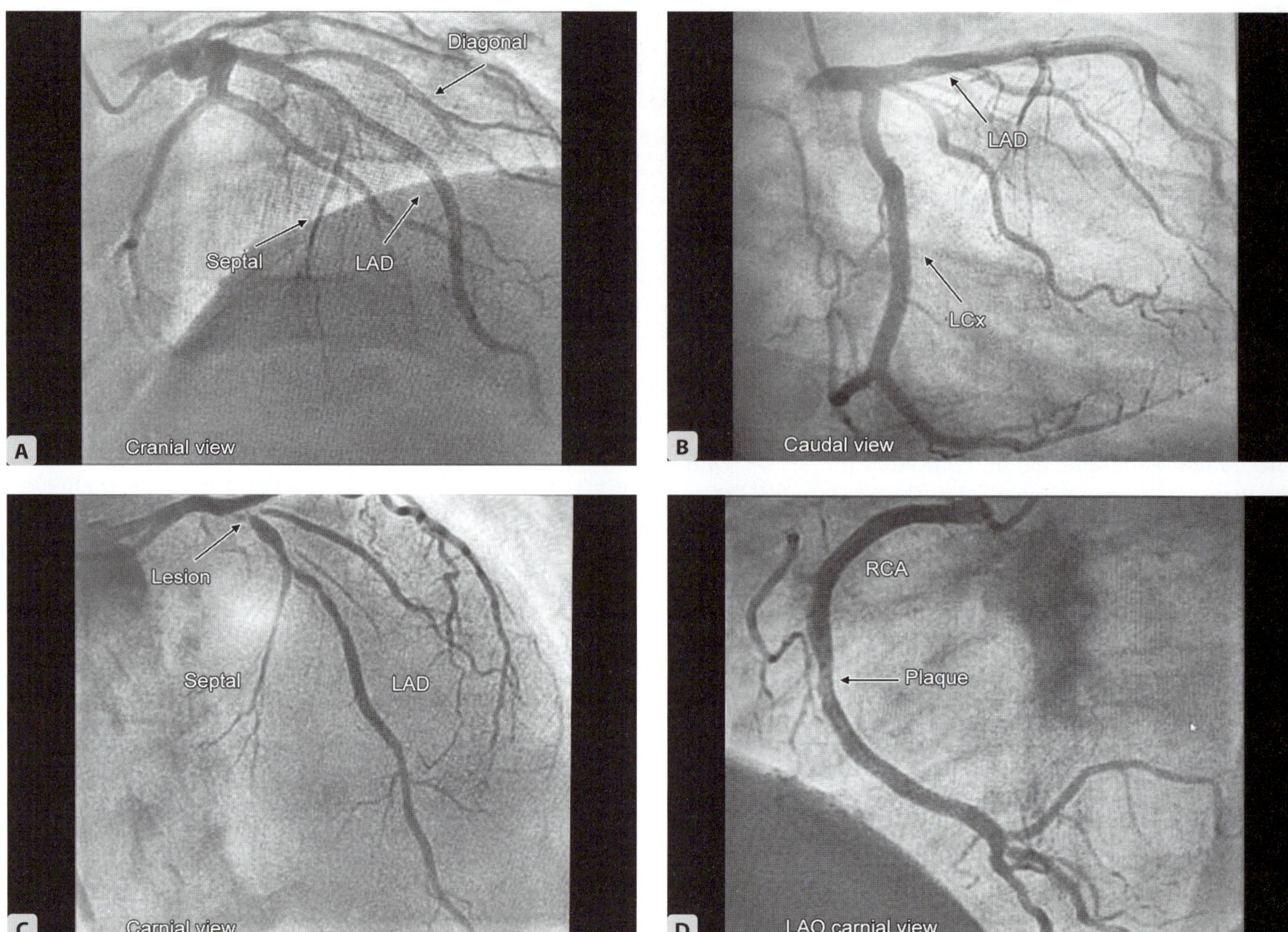

FIGURES 3 A to D: **(A)** Cranial view: Left anterior descending (LAD) and its branches; **(B)** Caudal view: Left main, LAD, and left circumflex (LCx) artery; **(C)** Cranial view: Proximal LAD and diagonal lesion (bifurcation lesion); and **(D)** Left anterior oblique (LAO) cranial view: Right coronary artery (RCA) with plaque in mid portion.

TABLE 2 Standard angiographic views for coronaries.

Right coronary artery (RCA)	
• LAO 45–60, cranial 20	• Vessel engagement projection • RCA ostium and vessel along AV sulcus
• AP, cranial 20	• RCA beyond crux; PDA and PLV branches
• RAO 30	• RV branches, PDA ostium, and septal branches
• Lateral view	• The mid-part of RCA
Left coronary artery (LCA)	
• AP caudal 20	• LM ostium, LCx, and proximal LAD
• RAO 30	• LM, proximal-mid LAD, and LCx
• LAO 45–60, caudal 20 (spider projection)	• LM and proximal segments of LAD, LCx, and ramus
• LAO 40–60, cranial 20	• Mid-distal LAD, diagonal, and septal branches, left PDA/PLV if present
• RAO 30, caudal 20	• Proximal LAD, LCx, and their branches
• RAO 30, cranial 20–30	• Mid-distal LAD, left PDA/PLV

(AP: anteroposterior; LAO: left anterior oblique; RAO: right anterior oblique; LM: left main; PDA: posterior descending artery; PLV: posterolateral ventricle)

- It does not give any information about the vessel wall and is highly insufficient for eccentric lesions and diffuse disease, where there is no "normal" vessel.
- The physiological significance of intermediate lesions cannot be ascertained with CAG alone.
- Coronary angiography is highly insufficient for the evaluation of calcified coronary lesions, which require additional intravascular imaging for better morphological characterization.
- Only optimal and multiple angiographic views can define the lesions in tortuous segments, bifurcations and in very short lesions.
- There is wide interobserver variability in CAG interpretation and it usually leads to overestimation of lesions.

Besides diagnosis of CAD diagnostic cardiac catheterization helps to diagnose significance of left to right shunts with an oximetry run. The step up in oxygen saturation helps to measure the ratio of pulmonary to systemic blood flow (QP:QS, the quantity of pulmonary and systemic blood flow). Patients with significant shunts are operable.

In valvular heart disease cardiac catheterization and measurement of intracardiac pressures help to confirm the level and extent of stenosis. The cardiac chamber

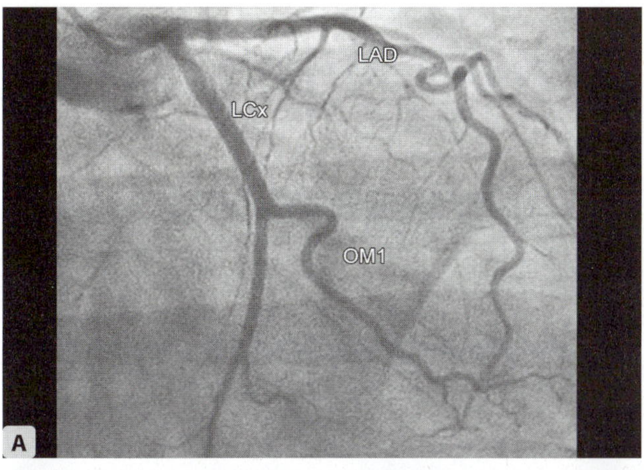

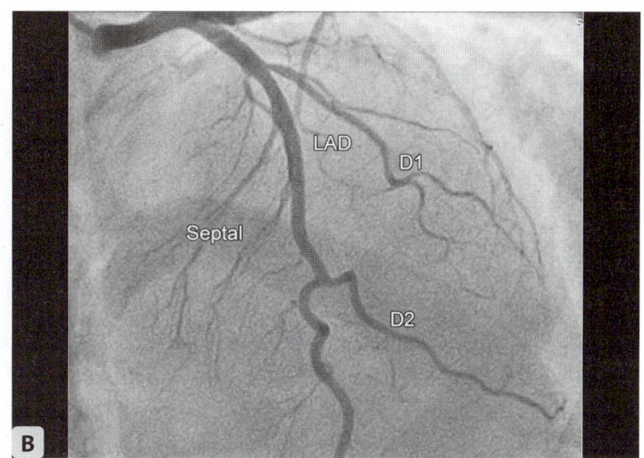

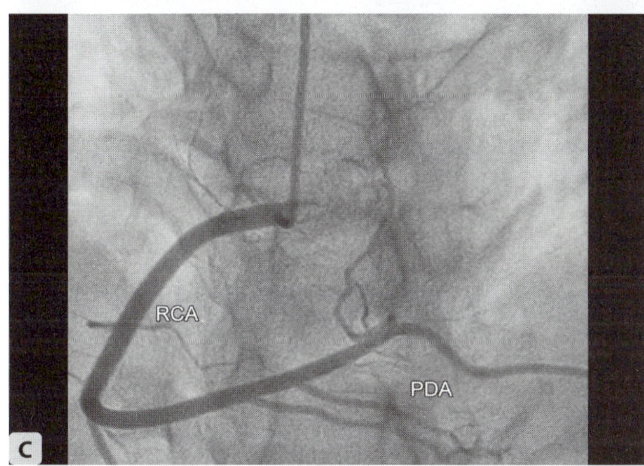

(D1: diagonal artery; OM1: obtuse marginal artery; PDA: posterior descending artery)

FIGURES 4 A to C: Normal angiogram showing no lesion in any vessel. **(A)** Caudal view of left coronary shows LCx and LAD; **(B)** Apical view shows LAD with its diagonal and septal branches; **(C)** Right coronary injection showing the RCA with the posterior descending artery.

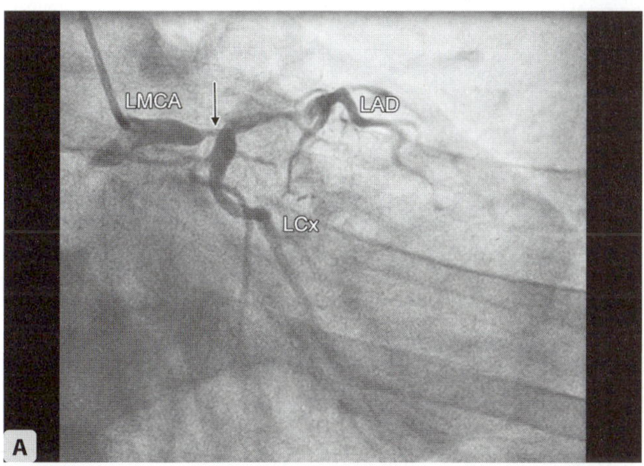

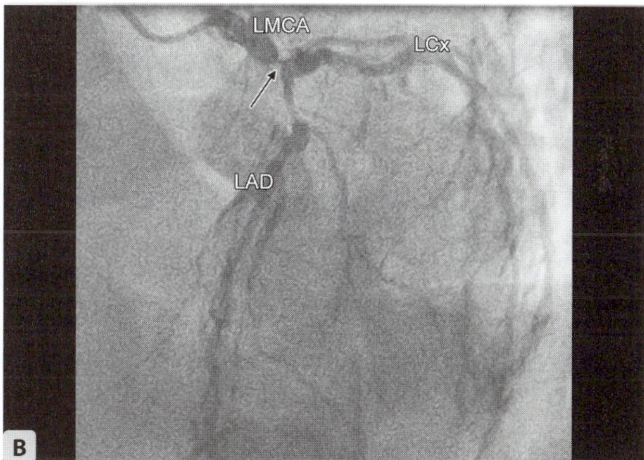

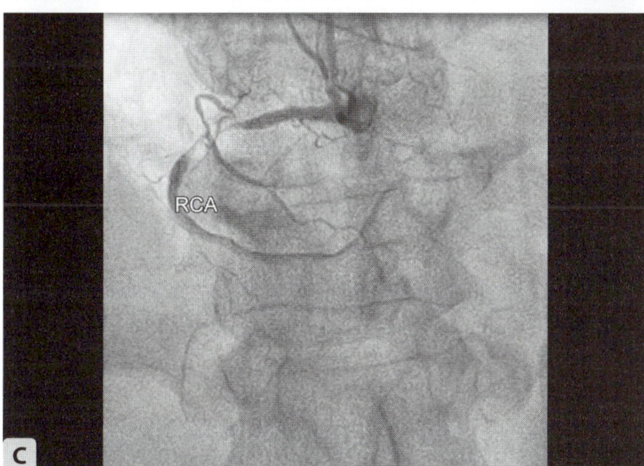

(LAO: left anterior oblique; LMCA: left main coronary artery; RAO: right anterior oblique; TVD: triple vessel disease)

FIGURES 5 A to C: Pictures of a coronary angiography in a patient with left main coronary artery disease and TVD. **(A)** RAO cordial view shows lesion indicated by arrow at the distal end of LMCA; **(B)** Apical view shows lesion in LMCA and proximal LAD also; **(C)** Right coronary injection in a LAO view shows lesion in proximal RCA. Such patients need coronary artery bypass grafting.

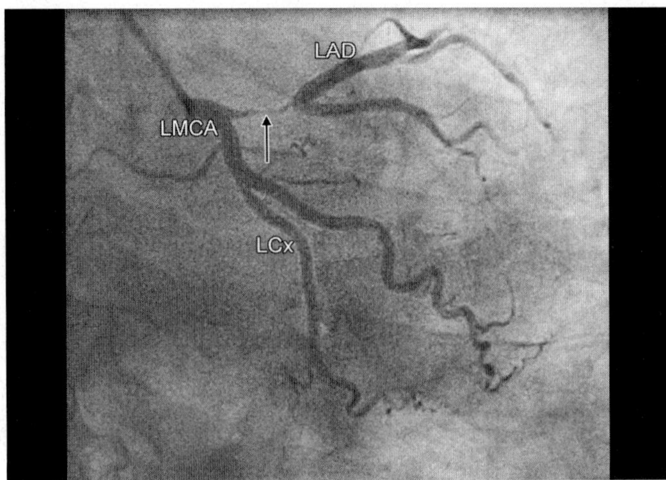

(RAO: right anterior oblique)

FIGURE 6: RAO caudal view in a patient with proximal LAD tight 95% lesion. Such patients with single vessel disease are best treated with percutaneous transluminal coronary angioplasty (PTCA) with stenting.

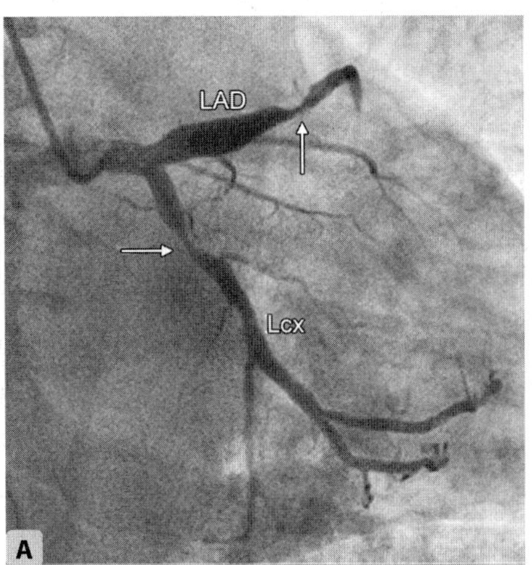

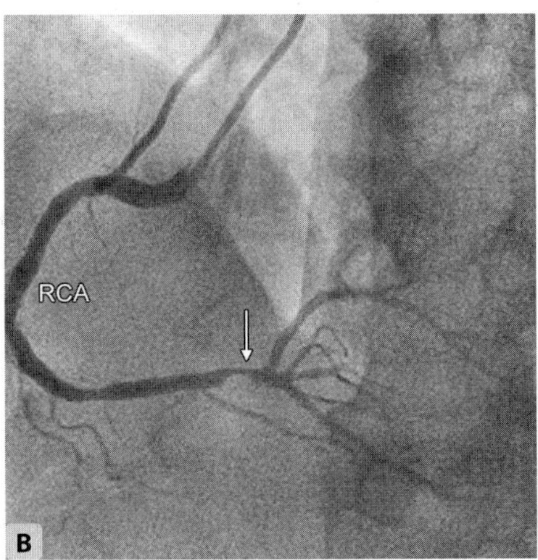

FIGURES 7 A & B: Coronary angiography in a patient with triple vessel disease (TVD) arrows shows a three lesions in the LAD, LCx, and RCA. **(A)** Left coronary injection in a right anterior oblique caudal view shows lesions in LCx and LAD; **(B)** Right coronary injection in a left anterior oblique view shows lesion at the crux (bifurcation of RCA into posterior descending and posterior left ventricular branch).

angiography (LV and aortic root) helps to look at the amount of regurgitation. This can of course be better looked at with echocardiography. With advances in echocardiography many more patients with valvular heart disease and congenital heart disease are being operated on the basis of echocardiography without a diagnostic cardiac catheterization study.

Figure 8 shows left ventricular angiogram in a patient with mitral regurgitation. This is often not required since MR can be well seen and quantified on color Doppler echocardiography. **Figure 9** shows aortic root angiogram in a patient with aortic regurgitation. This also is better seen in color Doppler echocardiography. **Figures 10** and **11** show left ventricular angiograms in two patients with ventricular septal defect (VSD). The VSD is visible and the right ventricle is getting opacified. **Figures 12 A** to **C** shows aortic angiogram with flow across patent ductus arteriosus (PDA). Device closure of the PDA is also seen in subsequent frames. Series of 7 videos are given with the e-chapter. The **Video 1** shows normal coronary angiogram. **Video 2** shows patient with left main and RCA lesion. **Video 3** shows proximal LAD 99% lesion. **Video 4** shows patent ductus arteriosus. **Video 5** shows aortic regurgitation. **Video 6** shows mitral regurgitation and **Video 7** shows left ventricle will VSD closure device in situ.

TABLE 3 American Heart Association/American College of Cardiology (AHA/ACC) classification of coronary lesions.

	Type A	Type B	Type C
Lesion characteristics	• Length <10 mm • Concentric/discrete • Smooth contour • Mild tortuosity (<45° angle) • Little or no calcification • Less than totally occluded • No major side branch involvement • No thrombus • Nonostial	• Length 10–20 mm • Eccentric • Irregular contour • Moderate tortuosity of the proximal segment • Moderate to heavy calcification • Total occlusion <3 months old • Bifurcation lesion requiring two guidewires • Presence of any thrombus • Ostial	• Length >20 mm • Diffuse • Irregular contour • Excessive tortuosity of the proximal segment • Moderate to heavy calcification • Total occlusion >3 months old and/or bridging collaterals • Inability to protect major side branch • Degenerated vein graft with friable lesions
Probability of procedural success	92%	72%	62%
Probability of complication	Low	10%	20%

TABLE 4 Classification of coronary artery dissection.

Type of dissection	Description
Type A	Minor radiolucent area in the lumen, with no persistence of contrast
Type B	Parallel track separated by radiolucent area, with no persistence of contrast
Type C	Persistent "Extraluminal contrast cap" which stays after contrast has cleared from the lumen
Type D	Spiral luminal filling defect
Type E	Persistent filling defect within the lumen
Type F	Total occlusion of a vessel without antegrade flow

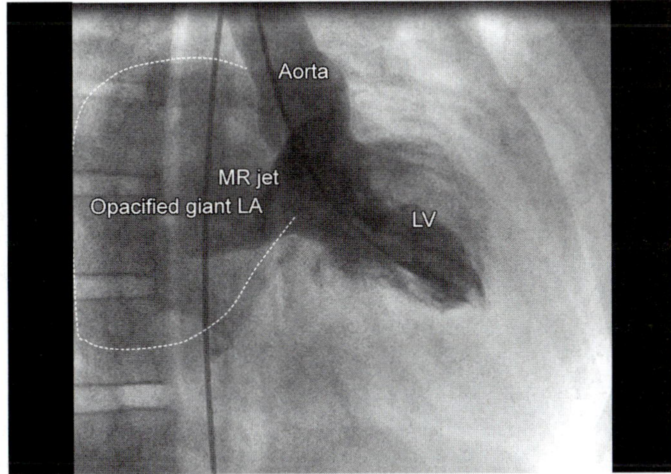

(LA: left atrium; MR: mitral regurgitation; LV: left ventricular; RAO: right anterior oblique)

FIGURE 8: Left ventricular angiogram in RAO view showing grade 4 mitral regurgitation and giant LA.

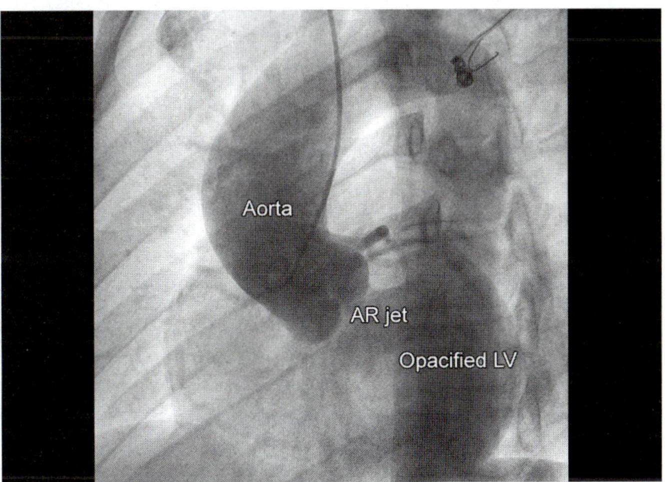

(AR: aortic regurgitation; LV: left ventricular; LAO: left anterior oblique)

FIGURE 9: Ascending aortogram in LAO view showing grade 3 aortic regurgitation.

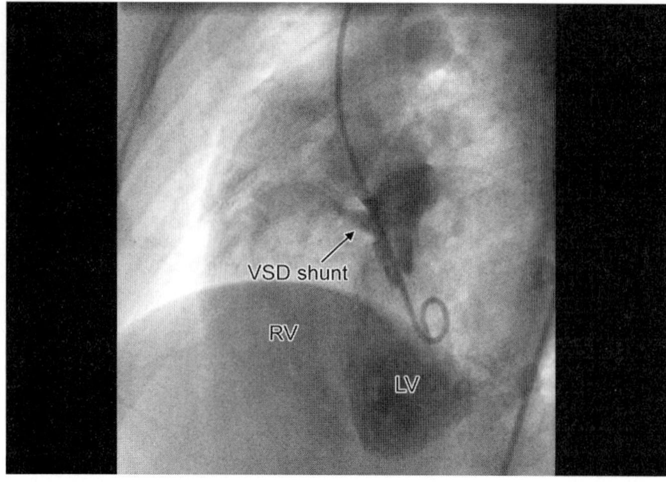

(VSD: ventricular septal defect; RV: right ventricular; LV: left ventricular; LAO: left anterior oblique)

FIGURE 10: Left ventricular angiogram in LAO view showing jet of dye flowing from LV to RV across the perimembranous ventricular septal defect. The pig tail catheter is visible in the left ventricle.

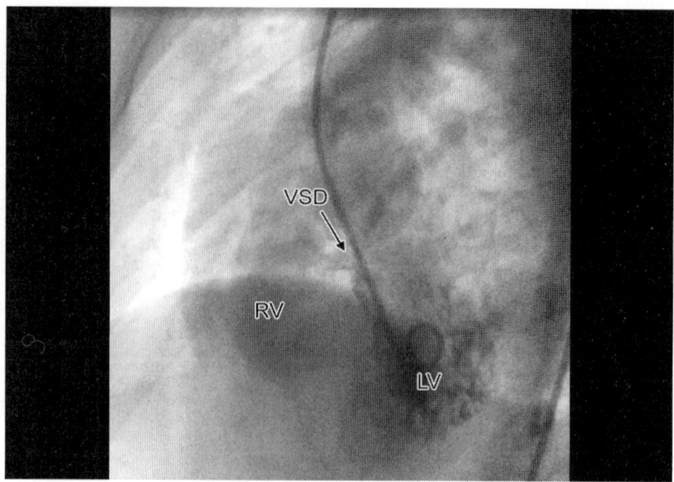

(VSD: ventricular septal defect; RV: right ventricle; LV: Left ventricle)

FIGURE 11: Left ventricular angiogram in a patient with ventricular septal defect. The pigtail catheter is seen in left ventricular.

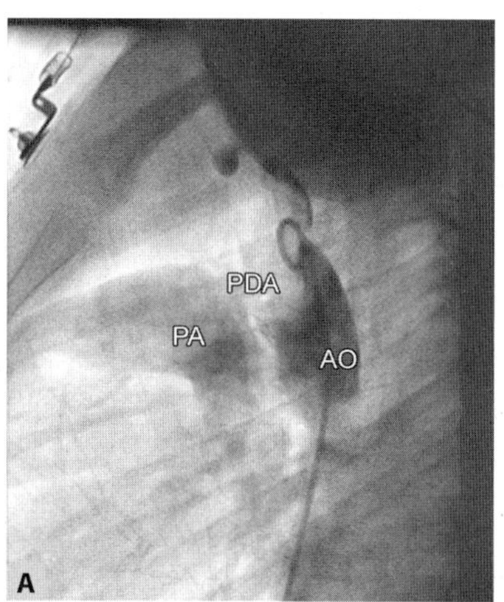

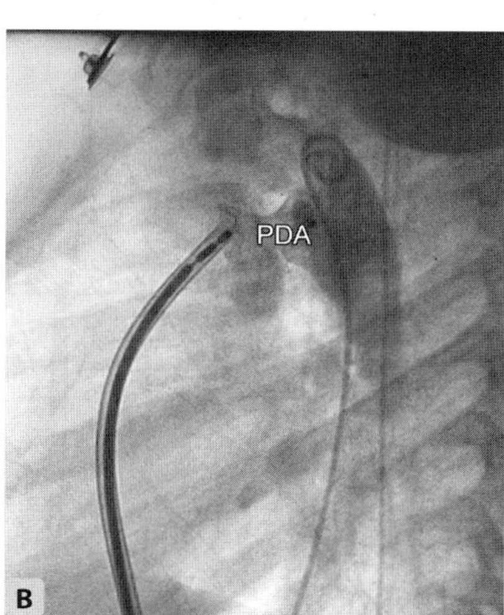

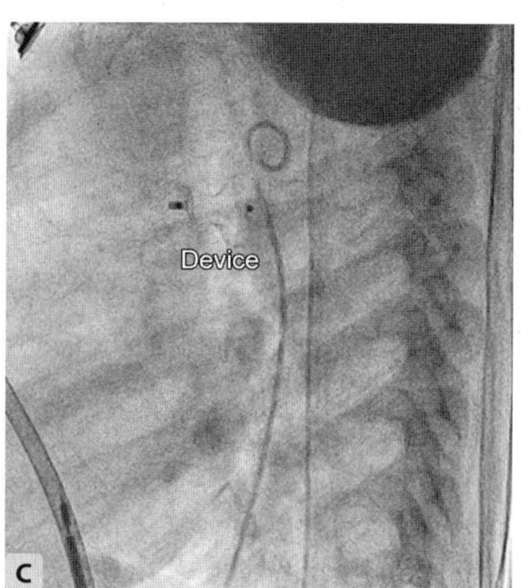

(AO: aorta; PA: pulmonary artery; PDA: patent ductus arteriosus)

FIGURES 12 A to C: Steps of device closure of PDA. **(A)** Preclosure injection shows dye flowing from aorta to pulmonary artery across PDA; **(B)** Device being positioned with the catheter across the PDA; **(C)** Post PDA device closure picture showing the device in position.

RECOMMENDED READINGS

1. Sones FM Jr. Cine-coronary arteriography. Ohio State Med J. 1962;58:1018-9.
2. Judkins MP. Selective coronary arteriography. I. A percutaneous transfemoral technic. Radiology. 1967; 89(5):815-24.
3. Amplatz K, Formanek G, Stanger P, Wilson W. Mechanics of selective coronary artery catheterization via femoral approach. Radiology. 1967;89(6):1040-7.
4. Arramraju SK, Janapati RK, Sanjeeva KE, Mandala GR. National interventional council data for the year 2018-India. Indian Heart J. 2020;72(5):351-5.
5. K Viktor. The coronary angiography – An old-timer in great shape. Cor et Vasa. 2015;57(6):e419-24.
6. Bashore TM, Balter S, Barac A, Byrne JG, Cavendish JJ, Chambers CE, et al. ACCF Task Force Members. 2012 American College of Cardiology Foundation/ Society for Cardiovascular Angiography and Interventions expert consensus document on cardiac catheterization laboratory standards update: A report of the American College of Cardiology Foundation Task Force on Expert Consensus documents developed in collaboration with the Society of Thoracic Surgeons and Society for Vascular Medicine. J Am Coll Cardiol. 2012;59:2221-305.
7. Solomon RJ, Mehran R, Natarajan MK, Doucet S, Katholi RE, Staniloae CS, et al. Contrast-induced nephropathy and long-term adverse events: cause and effect? Clin J Am Soc Nephrol. 2009;4:1162-9.

8. Arora N, Matheny ME, Sepke C, Resnic FS. A propensity analysis of the risk of vascular complications after cardiac catheterization procedures with the use of vascular closure devices. Am Heart J. 2007;153(4):606-11.
9. Wagener JF, Rao SV. A comparison of radial and femoral access for cardiac catheterization. Trends Cardiovasc Med. 2015;25:707-13.
10. McCullough PA. Acute kidney injury with iodinated contrast. Crit Care Med. 2008;36 (4 Suppl):S204-11.
11. Dickinson MC, Kam PCA. Intravascular iodinated contrast media and the anaesthetist. Anaesthesia. 2008;63:626-34.
12. Theuerle J, Yudi MB, Farouque O, Andrianopoulos N, Scott P, Ajani AE, et al. Utility of the ACC/AHA lesion classification as a predictor of procedural, 30-day and 12-month outcomes in the contemporary percutaneous coronary intervention era. Cathet Cardiovasc Intervent. 2018;92:E227-34.

CHAPTER 90

Bradyarrhythmias

Naved Aslam, Salil Jaura, Ulhas Pandurangi

ABSTRACT

Bradyarrhythmia can be broadly divided into three categories. Sinus bradycardia can be physiological and asymptomatic. This does not require any treatment. The other two set of conditions are usually pathological and need active management. These are sinus node dysfunction (sick sinus syndrome) and atrioventricular (AV) blocks. Sick sinus syndrome patients have abnormality in impulse initiation from the sinus node. They have severe sinus bradycardia, sinus pauses, and sinus arrests. Patients who present with Stokes–Adams attacks (syncope due to bradyarrhythmia) need pacemaker after we have ruled out reversible factors like drugs (beta blockers, nondihydropyridine calcium channel blockers etc.).

Atrioventricular blocks involve block in the conduction system from the AV node to the His bundle and the left and right bundle. Those patients also present with syncope and those with infra-Hisian high-grade AV blocks need permanent pacemaker after ruling out transient and reversible causes such as myocardial infarction (MI) and some drugs.

The pacemakers are devices which increase heart rate externally. These can be temporary (external or internal) or permanent (implanted subcutaneously in infraclavicular area). Significant advances have occurred in the pacemaker devices which are discussed in the chapter.

"It is better to change an opinion than to persist in a wrong one"

—Socrates

INTRODUCTION

The heart contracts in a regular, repetitive, rhythmic, and continuous fashion at a defined rate. Bradyarrhythmias are a common clinical problem and are said to occur when the heart rate falls below 60 beats per minute. This may be physiological, i.e., in athletes or pathological when it is caused by disturbances in the conduction system at the level of sinoatrial (SA) node, AV node, and His-Purkinje system. The clinical presentation and prognosis depend on level of abnormality, presence or absence of structural heart disease, and the duration. Sinus bradycardia is almost always benign and asymptomatic and requires no treatment. On the other hand, sick sinus syndrome and complete heart block usually cause severe symptoms and require early treatment.

Common symptoms caused by bradyarrhythmias are fatigue, dyspnea, lightheadedness, exercise intolerance, presyncope, or syncope. Symptoms may be transient or persistent. **Box 1** shows classification of bradyarrhythmia and **Box 2** shows common causes of bradyarrhythmia.

TYPES OF BRADYARRHYTHMIAS

SINUS NODE DISEASE

Sinus node disease is characterized by atrial rate which is inappropriate for physiological requirements. It is commonly called as sick sinus syndrome as it encompasses a variety of electrocardiographic manifestations due to abnormalities of impulse generation and/or conduction in sinus node, and conduction within the atria. The clinical spectrum varies from asymptomatic to mild symptoms to frank syncope. Other symptoms include fatigue, lightheadedness, chronotropic incompetence heart failure, and thromboembolic episodes. Primarily it is a disease of

BOX 1	Classification of bradyarrhythmias.
Sinus node dysfunction	
• Sinus bradycardia and chronotropic incompetence	
• Sick sinus syndrome	
○ Sinus pause	
○ Arrest	
○ Sinoatrial exit block	
Atrioventricular (AV) conduction abnormalities	
• First-degree heart block	
• Second-degree heart block (Mobitz type I and Mobitz type II)	
• High grade AV block	
• Third-degree (complete) heart block	

BOX 2	Common causes of bradyarrhythmias.
• Degenerative fibrosis of conduction system	
• Ischemic heart disease (IHD)	
• Infiltrative diseases	
• Postradiation fibrosis	
• Drugs	
• Hypothyroidism	
• Electrolytes (K^+ and Ca^{++})	
• Postoperative blocks after cardiac surgeries	
• Congenital	

elderly but can occur early also. The mean age is 65 years and accounts for 50% of pacemaker implantations.

Causes: Most of the cases are idiopathic but can be caused by a variety of disease as mentioned in **Table 1**.

Types of sinus node disease: Electrocardiographically sick sinus syndrome manifests with one or a combination of the following:

- Persistent sinus bradycardia
- Sinus pause or sinus arrest
- SA exit block
- Bradycardia-tachycardia syndrome

Persistent sinus bradycardia: It is defined as heart rate of <60 beats per minute. Mostly it is physiological and asymptomatic and is caused by increased vagal tone. It is mainly seen in trained athlete or as the nocturnal fall in heart rate. Other causes include raised ICT, myxedema, severe hypoxia, hypothermia, and fibro degenerative diseases.

Sinus pause or sinus arrest: On surface electrocardiogram (ECG) it manifests as, absence of expected "P" wave and the following QRS-T complexes, due to abnormality of impulse formation or conduction in the sinus node. Sinus pause of >3 seconds usually require pacemaker in symptomatic patients.

Sinoatrial exit blocks: The impulse is formed within the SA node but fails to conduct to the atria. On ECG, it manifests as absence of sinus P waves and the duration of pause is a multiple of the preceding P-P interval.

TABLE 1 Diseases/Conditions causing sinus node dysfunction.

Intrinsic (in heart)	Extrinsic
• Idiopathic degenerative disorder • Ischemic heart disease: ○ Chronic ischemia ○ Acute myocardial infarction • Hypertensive heart disease • Cardiomyopathy • Surgery for congenital heart disease • Inflammation: ○ Collagen vascular disease ○ Rheumatic fever ○ Pericarditis • Infection: ○ Viral myocarditis ○ Lyme's disease • Neuromuscular disorders: ○ Friedreich ataxia ○ X-linked muscular dystrophy • Familial disorder	• Autonomically mediated: ○ Carotid sinus hypersensitivity ○ Vasovagal syncope • Electrolyte abnormalities: ○ Hyperkalemia ○ Hypokalemia • Hypothermia • Hypothyroidism • Hypoxemia, hypercarbia, and acidosis • Sleep apnea • Drugs: ○ Beta-blockers, nondihydropyridine calcium channel blockers, digoxin, antiarrhythmic drugs, lithium, methyldopa, risperidone, and cisplatin

Bradycardia-tachycardia syndrome: Alternation of atrial flutter and fibrillation with episodes of slow heart rates (**Fig. 1**).

ATRIOVENTRICULAR CONDUCTION ABNORMALITIES

It encompasses a variety of electrocardiographic manifestations due to abnormalities in impulse conduction in AV node and the conduction system below it (bundle of His and the main bundles left and right). Normally the impulse is generated from the SA node. It depolarizes the atria and reaches the AV node where after some delay it conducts to the His-Purkinje system and thus depolarizes the ventricles (**Box 3**).

Causes: The various causes of AV conduction abnormalities intrinsic to the heart and various extensive factors are shown in **Box 3**.

Types of AV blocks:

- *First-degree AV block*: When delay at the AV node is abnormally prolonged it results in a prolonged PR interval on surface ECG (>200 ms). The P wave is normal in contour and morphology and every P wave is conducted to the ventricle resulting in a regular ventricular rate. The QRS morphology is normal (**Fig. 2**).
- *Second-degree AV block*: Second-degree AV blocks occur when some P waves are not conducted to ventricle. The nonconducted P waves may occur at regular or irregular intervals. Second-degree AV block

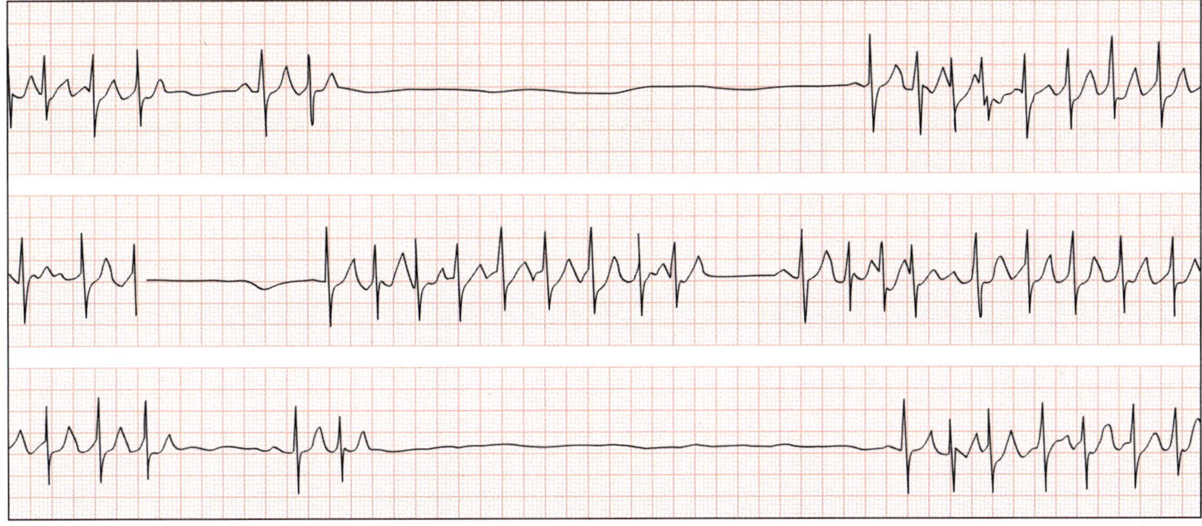

FIGURE 1: Sick sinus syndrome with bradycardia-tachycardia.

BOX 3	Causes of AV conduction abnormalities.
Intrinsic causes	
• *Degenerative*: Lev's and Lenègre disease	
• *Infectious*: Lyme carditis, bacterial endocarditis with perivalvular abscess, acute rheumatic fever, Chagas disease, and toxoplasmosis	
• *Inflammatory*: Myocarditis and rheumatologic disease, systemic sclerosis, SLE, and RA	
• *Infiltrative*: Amyloidosis, sarcoidosis, and lymphoma	
• *Ischemic*: Acute MI and chronic ischemic cardiomyopathy	
• *Neuromuscular diseases*: Myotonic dystrophy, Kearns–Sayre syndrome, and Erb's dystrophy	
• *Procedural*: Catheter ablation, cardiac surgery, especially valve surgery, TAVR and alcohol septal ablation	
• *Congenital*: AV block (associated with maternal SLE) and congenital cardiac defects (L-TGA)	
Extrinsic causes	
• *Increased vagal tone*: OSA, neurocardiogenic, and high-level athletic training	
• *Acid-base disorders*: Acidosis and hyperkalemia	
• *Poisoning/Overdose*: Mercury, cyanide, carbon monoxide, and mad honey	
• *Endocrine diseases*: Thyroid disease (both hypothyroidism and hyperthyroidism) and adrenal disease (e.g., pheochromocytoma and hypoaldosteronism)	
• *Drugs*: Beta-blockers, verapamil, diltiazem, digoxin, antiarrhythmic drugs, and nutraceuticals	

(AV: atrioventricular; L-TGA: L-looped transposition of the great arteries; MI: myocardial infarction; OSA: obstructive sleep apnea; RA: rheumatoid arthritis; TAVR: transcatheter aortic valve replacement)

is of two types. *Mobitz type I second-degree AV block* (Wenckebach) is characterized by gradual lengthening of PR interval till a P wave is not conducted (**Fig. 3**). Usually, block occurs at AV nodal level. The QRS morphology is normal. Generally, it is a benign condition, reversible, common in acute inferior wall MI, and usually does not require temporary pacemaker. It can be a normal phenomenon in well-trained athletes due to high resting vagal tone.

In *Mobitz type II second-degree AV block*, PR interval remains constant until a P wave is dropped (**Fig. 4**). It usually occurs in a 2:1 conduction ratio. The R-R interval surrounding the nonconducted P wave is twice the basic R-R interval. QRS is of bundle branch morphology. The block is usually at His-Purkinje level. It is commonly seen in acute anterior wall MI, symptomatic, commonly needs temporary, and/or permanent pacemaker and carries a bad prognosis due to large infarct resulting in pump failure.

- *Third-degree AV block*: The atria are beating at their own rate and ventricles are beating at their own rate. There are two independent pacemakers controlling the atrial rhythm and ventricular rhythm, atrial rate being higher than ventricular rate. The latent pacemaker controlling the ventricular rhythm may be in AV node, His bundle, or more distal Purkinje system, determining ventricular rate and morphology of QRS. If the block is in AV node or proximal His bundle, the ventricular escape rhythm is relatively fast and QRS morphology is a bit narrow (**Fig. 5**). If the block is in distal Purkinje system, the ventricular rate is usually <40/min and QRS morphology is wider.

The ventricular rate is relatively higher in congenital complete heart block compared to acquired complete heart block.

CLINICAL MANIFESTATION

Those with sick sinus syndrome and high-grade AV blocks can present with near syncope, blackouts, and vertigo. When syncope occurs due to bradyarrhythmias it is called as Stokes–Adams attacks. Episodes of syncope can be recurrent. When it is prolonged it can result in seizures.

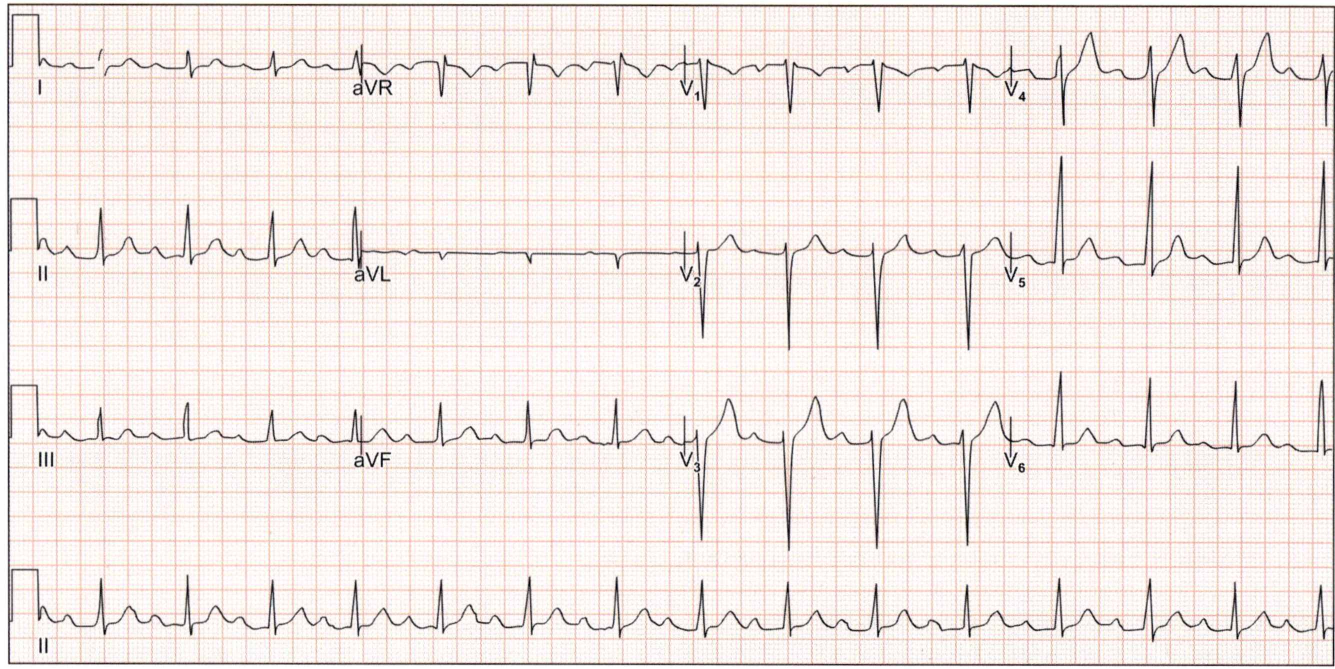

FIGURE 2: First-degree atrioventricular (AV) block.

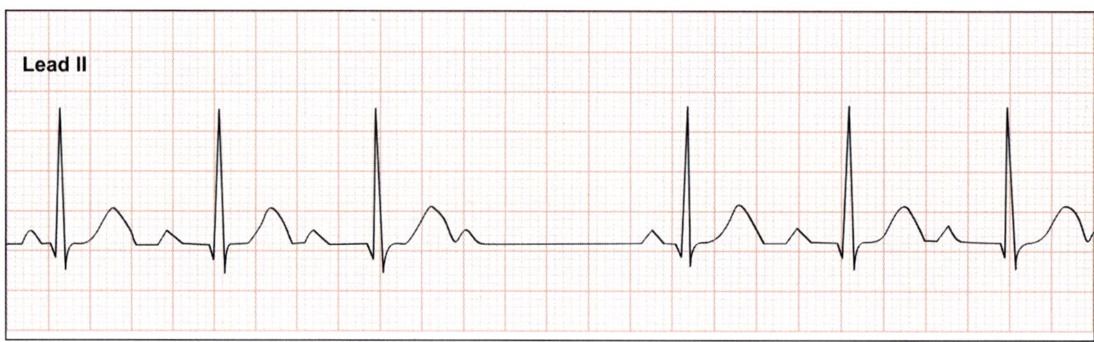

FIGURE 3: Mobitz type I atrioventricular (AV) block.

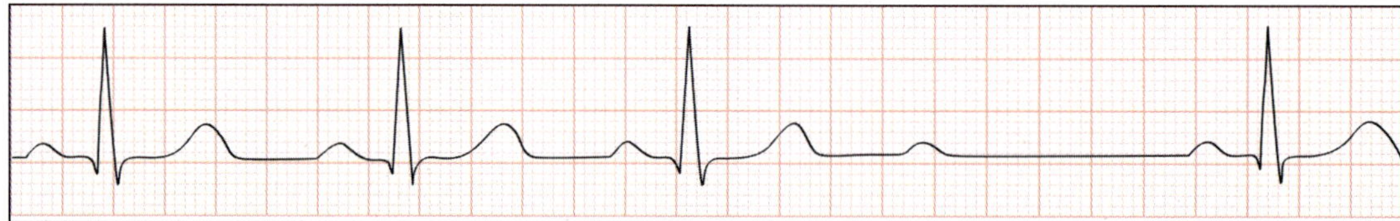

FIGURE 4: Mobitz type II atrioventricular (AV) block.

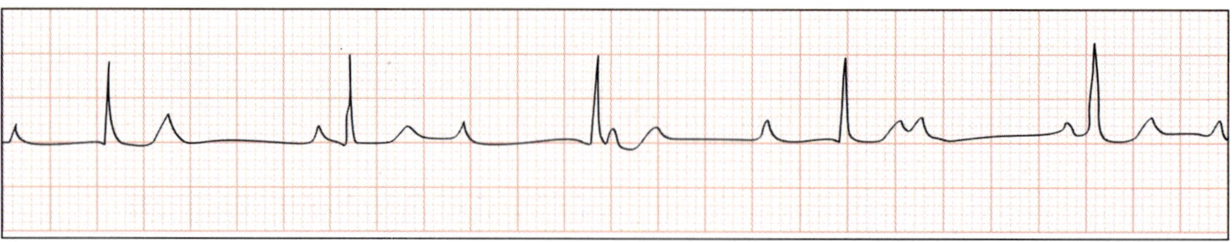

FIGURE 5: Complete heart block.

Some patients may be asymptomatic or may present with palpitation, fatigue, or exercise intolerance. Some patients with prolonged bradyarrhythmias can have heart failure, ventricular tachyarrhythmias, or altered sensorium.

DIAGNOSTIC EVALUATION

Bradyarrhythmias can be diagnosed by ECG when they are persistent. In those with intermittent blocks Holter monitoring is useful. Patients who present with syncope and we have ruled out other causes for it will need prolonged rhythm monitoring with loop recorders. The use of electrophysiological testing for bradyarrhythmias is less than for tachyarrhythmia. Each of these investigations is discussed below.

Electrocardiogram: A simple, easily available, cost-effective, noninvasive test, and can be repeated many times. "*P*" wave presence or absence, contour, and relation with QRS, and morphology of QRS are useful to establish a diagnosis. The ECG may miss the diagnosis since sick sinus syndrome and AV blocks may be transient.

Echocardiography: It is useful to assess left ventricular function, infiltrative disorders, ischemic heart disease, and congenital heart diseases. Echocardiogram is often normal in the degenerative and idiopathic varieties of sick sinus syndrome and AV block which are the most common variety.

Holter monitors: Ambulatory Holter recording is useful in patients with frequent symptoms suggestive of arrhythmias. These devices use three leads and continuously record the ECG for 24–48 hours. Prolonged monitoring may increase the diagnostic yield. The recorded events require correlation with symptoms.

Loop recorders: The loop recorders may be categorized as external loop recorders (ELRs) or implantable loop recorders (ILRs). These devices are useful in less frequent symptoms. ELR does not require electrodes and can monitor rhythm for 30 days. ILR is implanted in chest wall subcutaneously and can monitor rhythm for 3 years.

Post-event recorders: Patient is advised to place the device on chest as soon as he/she experiences the symptoms.

Electrophysiological studies: This is an invasive procedure and is recommended in patients with unexplained symptoms when noninvasive assessment is noncontributory.

MANAGEMENT

A good history is important since we need to rule out transient causes such as use of drugs and electrolyte disturbances. Ischemia and more often infarction can cause bradyarrhythmias and most of them revert in a few days. There is no definite drug therapy to increase heart rate for long period of time. Pacemaker therapy is the mainstay of treatment in symptomatic patients.

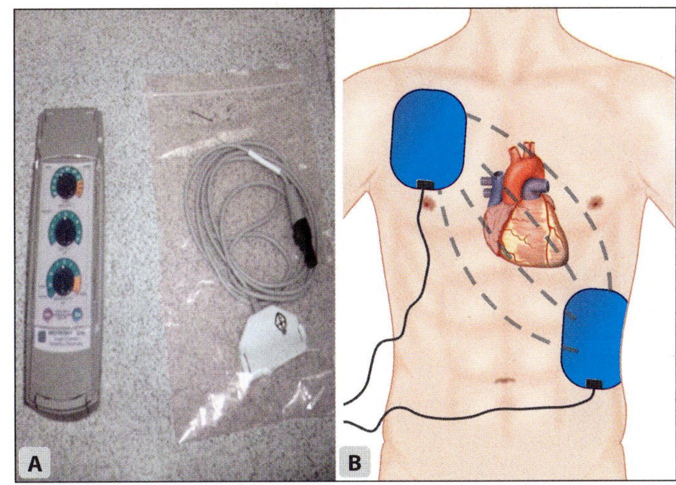

FIGURES 6 A & B: Two types of temporary pacemakers. **(A)** Pulse generator of transvenous temporary pacemaker; **(B)** Location of pads for the external temporary pacemaker.

Patients admitted in emergency with syncope and bradyarrhythmia need urgent temporary transvenous pacemaker. This is usually done under fluoroscopic guidance. The temporary pacing is done through femoral vein puncture although it can be done from the internal jugular or subclavian veins also. Temporary pacemaker can be kept for 5–8 days by which time a diagnosis is made. Patient is evaluated and if no reversible factor (drugs or ischemia) is found then patient is planned for permanent pacemaker implantation. In some patients with very marked bradycardia external temporary pacing can be done with pads on the chest wall. This causes discomfort to the patient and is done only till the patient can have a transvenous temporary pacemaker under fluoroscopy (**Fig. 6**).

The permanent pacemakers are put under local anesthesia. The pulse generator which has the battery is placed under the clavicle. The pacing lead is inserted and is made to touch the right atrium and right ventricle. It is insulated till the terminal electrode. Permanent pacemakers that were use earlier were single chamber (VVI pacemaker) with one lead placed in the right ventricle. However, these have fixed rate and the atrial kick is lost. So the VVI pacemakers were associated with low cardiac output and pacemaker syndrome. The dual chamber pacemaker (DDD pacemaker) has one lead in the right atrium and the other in the right ventricle. So the atrial contraction contributes to the ventricular filling and the DDD pacemakers have the ability to increase heart rate with activity. The five-digit numeric coding system for definition of pacemaker type is shown in **Table 2**. The appearance of various types of pacemakers on chest X-ray is shown in **Figure 7**.

Coronary artery disease (CAD) is an important cause of bradyarrhythmias although the most common cause of sick sinus syndrome and high-grade AV blocks is sclerodegenerative and they have a normal heart on echocardiography. Patients who present with bradyarrhythmias to the emergency we should rule out

TABLE 2 The international five-digit coding system for classification of pacemakers.

Position I	Position II	Position III	Position IV	Position V
Pacing chamber	Sensing chamber	Response to sensing	Rate modulation	Multisite pacing
0 = None	0 = None	0 = None	0 = None	0 = None
A = Atrium	A = Atrium	T = Triggered	R = Rate modulation	A = Atrium
V = Ventricle	V = Ventricle	I = Inhibited		V = Ventricle
D = Dual (atrium and ventricle)	D = Dual (atrium and ventricle)	D = Dual (triggered and inhibited)		D = Dual (atrium and ventricle)

VVI pacemaker is single chamber and senses and paces ventricle only. DDD pacemaker is dual chamber and senses and paces both atrium and ventricle.

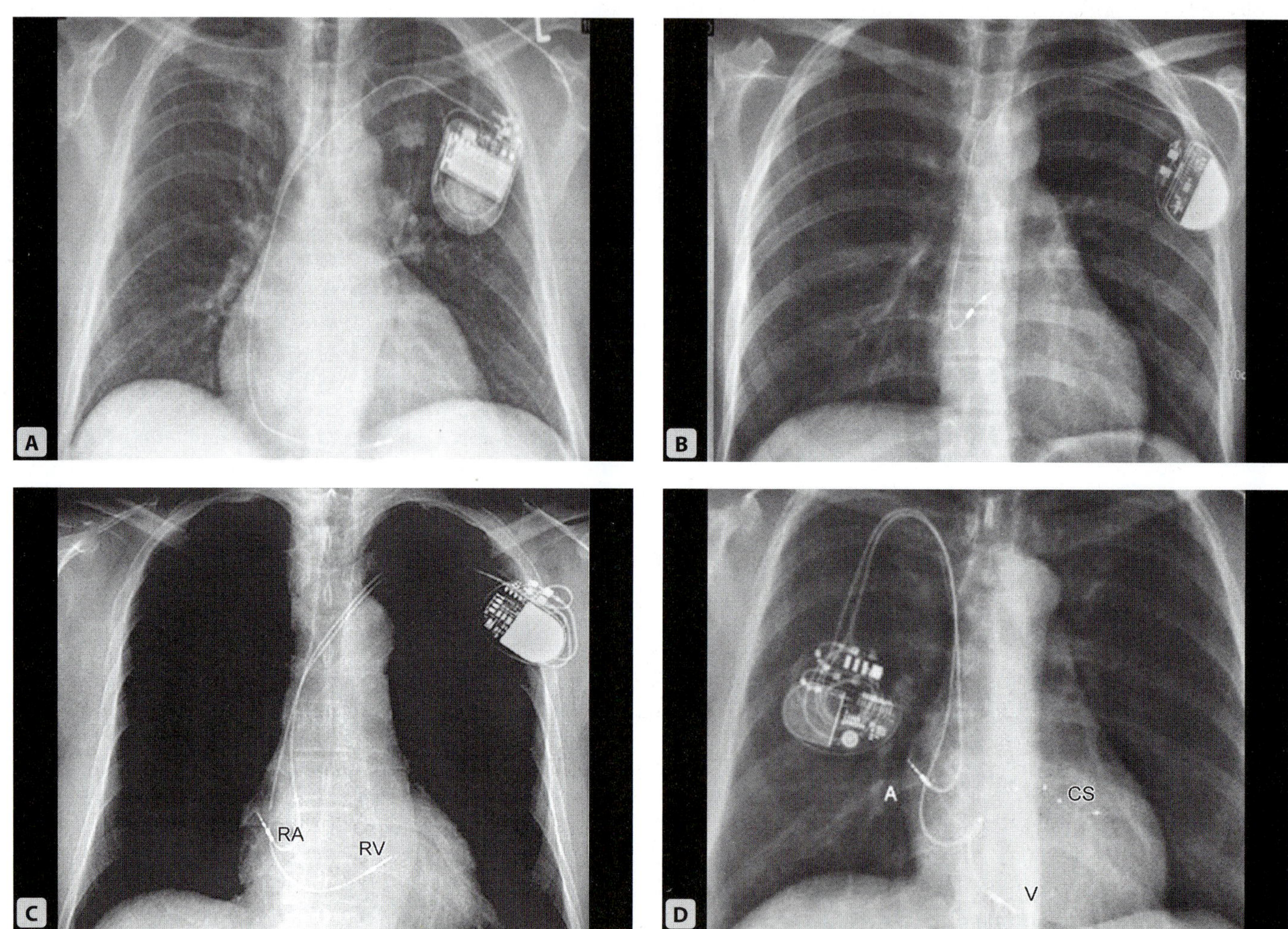

FIGURES 7 A to D: Chest X-ray from four different patients with pacemakers. **(A)** Single chamber VVI pacemaker with lead tip at right ventricular (RV) apex; **(B)** Single chamber AAI pacemaker with lead tip in right atrial (RA) appendage; **(C)** Dual chamber DDD pacemaker with two leads one at RA appendage other in RV pacing the septum; **(D)** Cardiac resynchronization therapy by triple lead pacemaker used in patients with left ventricular (LV) dysfunction and left bundle branch block (LBBB). One lead in RA, other in RV, and third pacing the left ventricle through the coronary sinus (CS).

CAD with biomarkers and echocardiography. Sick sinus syndrome and complete AV block, both can be seen in inferior wall infarctions. The differences between the complete heart block seen in inferior wall MI and that in anterior wall MI are shown in **Table 3**.

SINUS NODE DISEASE

Permanent pacemaker implantation is recommended in symptomatic patients (chronotropic insufficiency and sinus pauses >3 s). While evaluating a patient for device therapy, it is important to document symptoms concurrent with arrhythmias. Randomized trials have shown that DDD pacemakers reduce risk of atrial fibrillation (AF) or congestive heart failure (CHF) compared to VVI. VVI/VVIR should be considered in sick sinus disease with chronic AF. The risk of AF, congestive cardiac failure (CCF), embolic strokes, morbidity, and mortality is less with atrial versus ventricular pacing.

ATRIOVENTRICULAR BLOCKS

Complete AV blocks are most common indication for permanent pacemaker implantation. Pacemaker implantation is recommended in type 2 AV block as progression to complete AV block is high. The indications for permanent pacemaker implantation in sick sinus syndrome AV blocks, fascicular blocks, and patients with heart blocks due to MI are shown in **Box 4**.

TABLE 3 Differences in complete heart block in inferior wall myocardial infarction (MI) and anterior wall MI.

	Inferior wall MI	Anterior wall MI
Incidence	More common	Less common
QRS complex	Narrow	Wide
Site of block	Atrioventricular (AV) nodal	Infra-Hisian
Morality in those with block	~15%	~50%
Treatment	Almost never need permanent pacemaker	May need permanent pacemaker implantation

RECENT ADVANCES

Leadless pacemakers: This is a small device without lead. It is delivered via femoral vein into RV directly. Complications related to puncture, pocket site, and lead can be avoided. Two prospective and nonrandomized trials have shown high success rate and low rate of complications with comparable follow-up results. The leadless Micra pacemaker and as it looks on chest X-ray are shown in **Figures 8 A** and **B**.

Battery-less pacemaker: To prevent pocket infections battery-less devices are tested in animals.

Physiological pacing (his bundle pacing/left bundle branch pacing): Conduction system pacing is more physiological as it alleviates the dys-synchrony associated with RV apical pacing, thus decreasing risk of heart failure.

His bundle pacing activates the ventricle via intrinsic conduction system results in narrow QRS. In patients with heart failure, His bundle pacing is used in conjunction with cardiac resynchronization therapy (CRT) or substitution to CRT (**Fig. 9**).

BOX 4 Indications of permanent pacemaker implantation.

Patients with sinus node dysfunction

Class I

- Symptomatic bradycardia or frequent symptomatic sinus pauses
- Symptomatic chronotropic incompetence
- Symptomatic bradycardia that results from required drug therapy

Patients with atrioventricular (AV) block

Class I

- Third-degree or advanced second-degree AV block at any anatomic level associated with any one of the following conditions:
  - Symptoms (including heart failure) or ventricular arrhythmias attributable to AV block
  - Arrhythmias and other medical conditions requiring drugs that result in symptomatic bradycardia
  - Documented periods of asystole >3.0 s, any escape rate <40 beats/min, or any escape rhythm below the AV junction in awake
  - A documented period of asystole >5 s in awake and asymptomatic patients in atrial fibrillation
- Symptomatic second-degree AV block regardless of type or site of block
- Asymptomatic third-degree AV block at any anatomic site with an average awake ventricular rate >40 beats/min in patients with cardiomegaly or left ventricular dysfunction or if the site of block is below the AV node

Patients with chronic bifascicular and trifascicular block

Class I

- Advanced second-degree AV block or intermittent third-degree AV block
- Type II second-degree AV block
- Alternating bundle branch block

Patients after acute myocardial infarction

Class I

- Persistent second-degree AV block in the His-Purkinje system with alternating bundle branch block or third-degree AV block within or below the His-Purkinje system after ST-segment elevation myocardial infarction
- Transient second- or third-degree intranodal AV block and associated bundle branch block
- Persistent and symptomatic second- or third-degree AV block

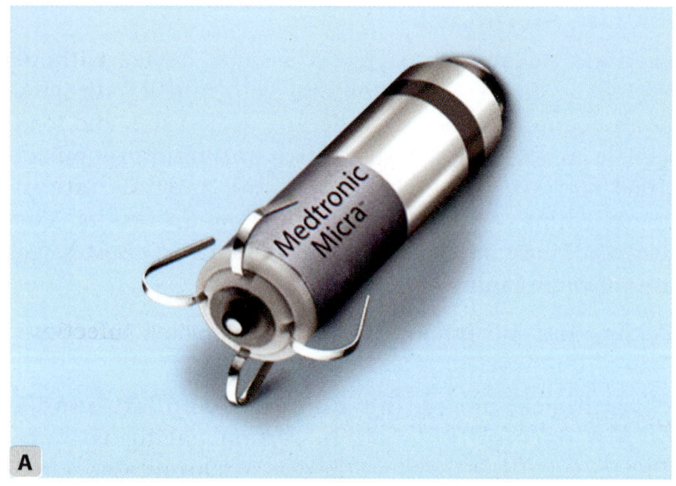

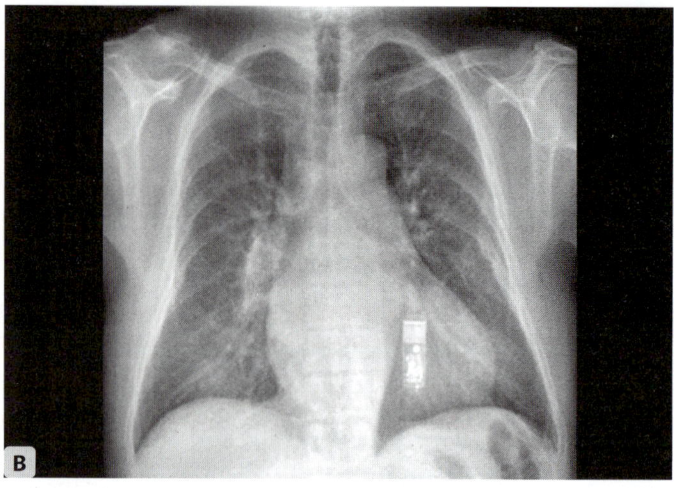

FIGURES 8 A & B: **(A)** Leadless Micra pacemaker; **(B)** The leadless pacemaker (Micra) seen at the right ventricular (RV) apex.

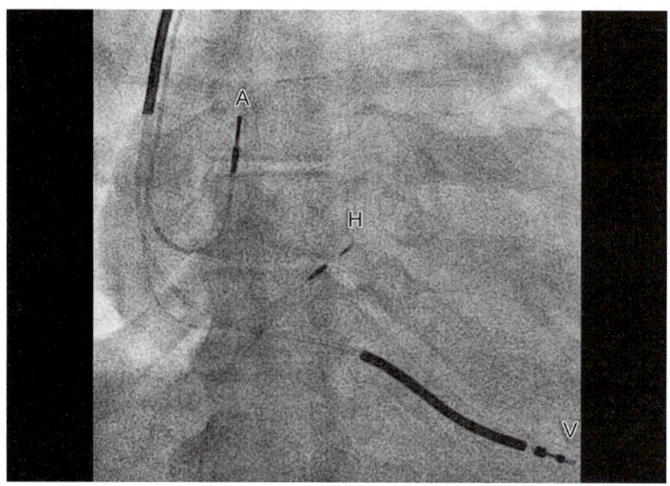

FIGURE 9: Fluoroscopic image showing His bundle pacing marked as H, the right ventricular coiled lead for defibrillation marked as V, and the atrial lead marked as A.

Left bundle branch (LBB) pacing is emerging as a good alternative to His bundle pacing with stable threshold and narrow QRS. It overcomes many technical issues of His bundle pacing. Although results are encouraging, more data is required.

RECOMMENDED READINGS

1. Zimetbaum P, Goldman A. Ambulatory arrhythmia monitoring: choosing the right device. Circulation. 2010;122:1629-36.
2. Brignole M, Vardas P, Hoffmann E, Huikuri H, Moya A, Ricci R, et al. Indications for the use of diagnostic implantable and external ECG loop recorders. Europace. 2009;11:671-87.
3. Giada F, Bertaglia E, Reimers B, Noventa D, Raviele A. Current and emerging indications for implantable cardiac monitors. Pacing Clin Electrophysiol. 2012;35: 1169-78.
4. Mangrum JM, DiMarco JP. The evaluation and management of bradycardia. N Engl J Med. 2000;342:703-9.
5. Wahls SA. Sick sinus syndrome. Am Fam Physician. 1985;31:117-24.
6. Alagona P Jr. Advances in pacing for the patient with sick sinus syndrome. Curr Opin Cardiol. 1997;12:3-11.
7. Bernstein AD, Camm AJ, Fletcher RD, Gold RD, Rickards AF, Smyth NP, et al. The NASPE/BPEG generic pacemaker code for antibradyarrhythmia and adaptive-rate pacing and antitachyarrhythmia devices. Pacing Clin Electrophysiol. 1987;10:794-9.
8. Andersen HR, Nielsen JC, Thomsen PE, Thuesen L, Mortensen PT, Vesterlund T, et al. Long-term follow-up of patients from a randomised trial of atrial versus ventricular pacing for sick-sinus syndrome. Lancet. 1997;350:1210-6.
9. Wilkoff BL, Cook JR, Epstein AE, Greene HL, Hallstrom AP, Hsia H, et al. Dual-chamber pacing or ventricular backup pacing in patients with an implantable defibrillator: the Dual Chamber and VVI Implantable Defibrillator (DAVID) Trial. JAMA. 2002;288(24):3115-23.
10. Deshmukh P, Casavant DA, Romanyshyn M, Anderson K. Permanent, direct His bundle pacing: a novel approach to cardiac pacing in patients with normal His-Purkinje activation. Circulation. 2000;101(8):869-77.
11. Kronborg MB, Mortensen PT, Poulsen SH, Gerdes JC, Jensen HK, Nielsen JC. His or para-His pacing preserves left ventricular function in atrioventricular block: a double-blind, randomized, crossover study. Europace. 2014;16(8):1189-96.
12. Vijayaraman P, Naperkowski A, Ellenbogen KA, Dandamudi G. Electrophysiologic Insights Into Site of Atrioventricular Block: Lessons From Permanent His Bundle Pacing. JACC Clin Electrophysiol. 2015;1(6): 571-81.
13. Lustgarten DL, Crespo EM, Arkhipova-Jenkins I, Lobel R, Winget J, Koehler J, et al. His bundle pacing versus biventricular pacing in cardiac resynchronization therapy patients: A crossover design comparison. Heart rhythm. 2015;12(7):1548-57.

CHAPTER 91

Tachyarrhythmias and Sudden Cardiac Death

Aseem Basha, Nirmal Ghati, Nitish Naik

ABSTRACT

Sudden cardiac death (SCD) is the most common mode of death due to cardiovascular causes. It is usually based on a ventricular fibrillation (VF). Coronary artery disease (CAD) is the most common cause of SCD, especially in those >40 years. In younger patients, hypertrophic cardiomyopathy (HCM) and primary electric disorders are the most common causes. The sudden death survivors in hospital and those who have survived SCD out-of-hospital are a high-risk subset and need to be evaluated in detail. The risk stratification of patients with various cardiac disorders can help to prevent SCD before it occurs. The various individual diseases causing SCD are discussed here.

Supraventricular tachycardias (SVTs) are common and need to be diagnosed and managed. Most of these patients present with history of repeated palpitations and frequent visits to emergency room for its termination. Unlike ventricular tachycardia (VT) and VF, these are well-tolerated hemodynamically and most of them have structurally normal heart. They are amenable to radiofrequency ablation (RFA) if they are recurrent and can be cured with this procedure. Atrioventricular (AV) nodal reentry and anomalous AV pathways can both result in SVT's.

Ventricular tachycardias usually occur in structural heart disease with significant left ventricular (LV) dysfunction usually due to CAD. Some electrical disorders can also cause VT in a structurally normal heart. The VT can be monomorphic (scar VT) or polymorphic (ischemia trigger) in morphology. The most common cause of VT is CAD. VT usually results in hypotension and is a medical emergency. It can degenerate into VF and can then be fatal. The use of implantable cardioverter-defibrillator (ICD) in patients with VT and LV dysfunction [LV ejection fraction (LVEF) <30%) helps to reduce the mortality in vulnerable patients. Various conditions that can cause VT are also discussed in the chapter.

"The problem with heart disease is, the first symptom is often fatal"

—Michael Phelps

INTRODUCTION

Sudden cardiac death is defined as natural unexpected death from cardiac causes heralded by an abrupt loss of consciousness within 1 hour of the onset of an acute change in cardiovascular status, in a person in whom preexisting heart disease may or may not have been known to be present. The time and mode of death are unexpected. For those who succumb to an unwitnessed death, a time frame of 24 hours is accepted as definition of SCD. VF is the first recorded arrhythmic abnormality in 75% of patients who sustain cardiac arrest. Sustained VT as the initial rhythm is documented rarely as it rapidly degenerates into VF. With increasing age, CAD becomes the most common cause of SCD. However, SCDs associated with nonischemic etiologies and genetic channelopathies are increasingly being recognized. Risk stratification of these patients, timely detection of vulnerable substrates, and their specific triggers and appropriate primary prevention interventions are the need of the hour in the management of these at-risk patients.

EPIDEMIOLOGY

Annual incidence of SCD in an overall adult population varies from 0.1 to 0.2% (1–2/1,000) in different studies. The incidence of SCD increases with age as the prevalence of CAD increases with age. SCD accounts for >50% of all CAD and 15–20% of all deaths. There exists an inverse relation between incidence and event rates, indicating that subgroups with high-risk indices [arrhythmic risk markers/post-myocardial infarction (MI)] have higher incidence of SCD but lower absolute number of events per annum. Low-risk groups such as the general population have maximum number of events annually despite a lower absolute risk due to the large number of cumulative events in this group. In many individuals, SCD may be the first clinical manifestation of an underlying heart disease. Patient subgroups with known high-risk markers known to be associated with increased risk of SCD constitute about 30% of population burden of SCD.

Accurate estimation of incidence and burden of *SCDs in Indian scenario* is challenging and only limited data is available from our country. SCDs contributed to 10.3% of total deaths in a study from Southern India. SCDs peaked in the age group of 50–70 years in this study in contrast to Western population (age group: 75–85 years). No obvious risk factors were evident in 56%, while history of MI was present in 33% of cases from SCD cohort. Unwitnessed cardiac arrest and SCD tend to be under reported and a proportion of patients dying from primary electrical diseases go unaccounted. However, lack of population-based data makes reliable estimation of this burden very hazardous.

AGE, SEX, RACE, AND HEREDITY

The incidence of SCD increases with age as the prevalence of CAD increases. Risk of SCD in adolescents/young adults is 1 per 100,000, while the risk is 1 per 1,000 for general population beyond 35 years of age. The risk is further increased on acquisition of modifiers such as CAD, valvular heart disease (VHD), and cardiomyopathies. Studies have demonstrated a higher risk of cardiac arrest and SCD in blacks than in whites.

Men are at higher risk of SCD than women before 65 years. Risk in perimenopausal women increases proportionately as risk of coronary events increase. Numerous primary electrical diseases of the heart exist in which an apparently "structurally normal heart" is predisposed to fatal arrhythmias and SCD. Many of these manifest with just an abnormal electrocardiogram (ECG) (prolonged or shortened QT interval, Brugada pattern, short-coupled premature ventricular beats etc.).

ETIOPATHOGENESIS

Although *CAD is the major cause* underlying a witnessed or unwitnessed cardiac arrest, there are multiple predisposing conditions comprising of a vulnerable substrate which with an appropriate trigger can result in fatal tachyarrhythmia and SCD. **Flowchart 1** enlists various conditions which can result in tachyarrhythmias and possible SCD.

VULNERABLE SUBSTRATE AND TRIGGERS

A hit by an appropriate trigger on a baseline vulnerable substrate is usually the basis for electrical instability resulting in fatal arrhythmias. Enhanced normal automaticity, abnormal automaticity, reentry, and triggered activity are the underlying mechanism of arrhythmogenesis. The vulnerable substrates include various structural and electrical diseases. Specific triggers such as stress, emotions, sleep, exercise, and dyselectrolytemia predispose to tachyarrhythmias, cardiac arrest, and SCD. **Figure 1** summarizes the pathogenesis of SCD in this context. In patients with heart with poor ventricular function, SCD may not be due to a new precipitating event but due to abrupt failure due to an additional minor worsening of already failing heart.

In witnessed cardiac arrests where there is only a brief delay between collapse and preterminal rhythm, ventricular tachyarrhythmias remains the predominant documented cardiac rhythm comprising 75–80% of initial rhythms. Rapidly, over a few minutes, the VT/VF degenerates to asystole or pulseless electrical activity. However, consequent to improvement in emergency care, population awareness, and bystander cardiopulmonary resuscitation patterns, there is a progressive decrease in prevalence of SCD presenting as VF and emergence of non-VF deaths.

RISK STRATIFICATION FOR SUDDEN CARDIAC DEATH

Risk of SCD can be assessed by various invasive and noninvasive means which can help us in assessing probability of SCD in these patients with vulnerable substrates. The following tools help us in risk stratification of these patients in addition to appropriate using of implantable cardiac defibrillators for primary or secondary prevention (**Flowchart 2**).

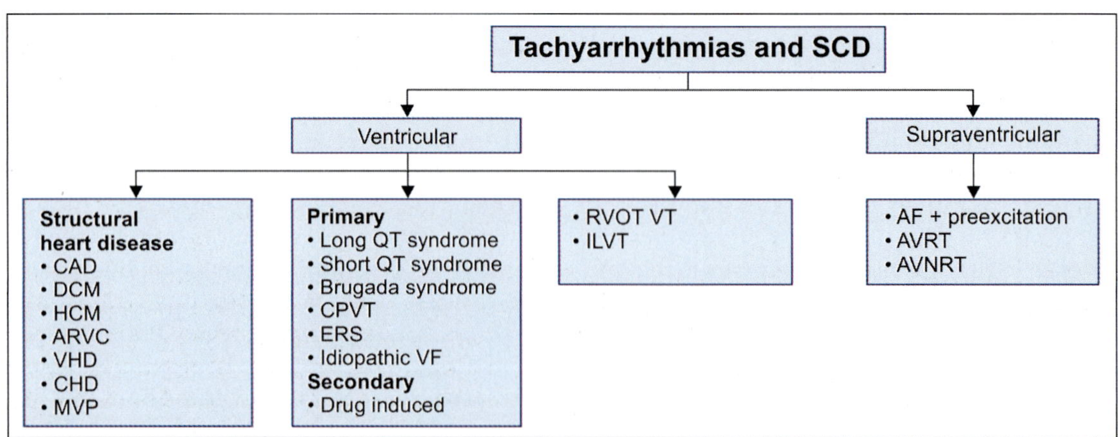

(ARVC: arrhythmogenic right ventricular cardiomyopathy; AVNRT: atrioventricular nodal reentrant tachycardia; AVRT: atrioventricular reentrant tachycardia; CPVT: catecholaminergic polymorphic ventricular tachycardia; ERS: early repolarization syndrome; ILVT: idiopathic left ventricular tachycardia; MVP: mitral valve prolapse; RVOT: right ventricular outflow tract; VHD: valvular heart disease)

FLOWCHART 1: Etiologies for tachyarrhythmias predisposing to SCD.

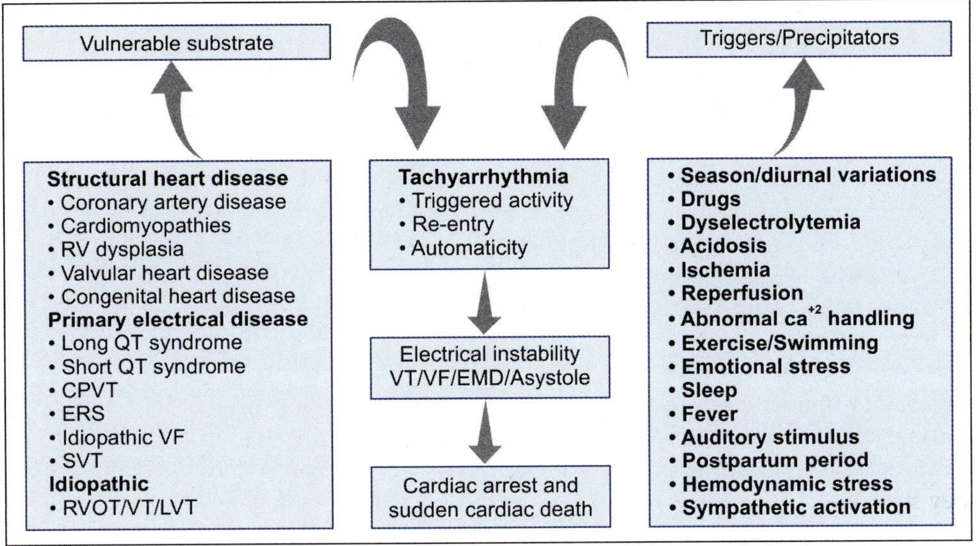

(CPVT: catecholaminergic polymorphic ventricular tachycardia; EMD: empirical mode decomposition; ERS: early repolarization syndrome; ILVT: idiopathic left ventricular tachycardia; RVOT: right ventricular outflow tract)

FIGURE 1: Pathogenesis of SCD in tachyarrhythmias.

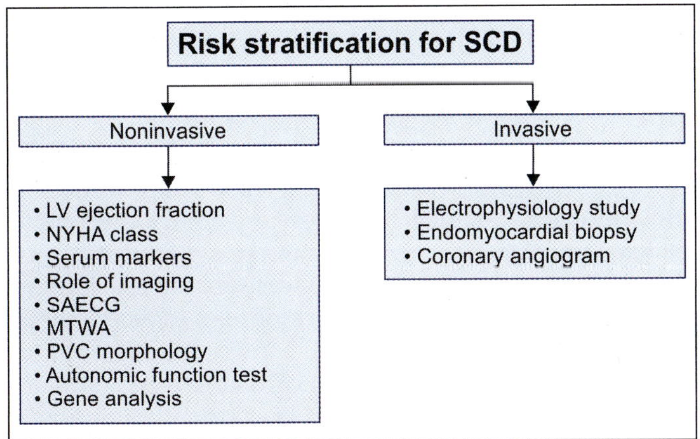

(NYHA: New York Heart Association; MTWA: microvolt T-wave alternans; SAECG: signal-averaged electrocardiogram)

FLOWCHART 2: Risk stratification for tachyarrhythmias and SCD.

PRESENTATION

The New York Heart Association (NYHA) functional class is an important determinant. The relative probability of death being sudden is higher and absolute mortality risk is lower in patients with better functional capacity.

SERUM MARKERS

Elevated levels of C-reactive protein, N-terminal pro B-type natriuretic peptide (NT-proBNP), BNP, ST2, and other markers of membrane stability such as nonesterified fatty acids, n-3 fatty acids, and trans-fatty acids have been found to be associated with increased risk of SCD.

ELECTROCARDIOGRAM

- *Signal-averaged electrocardiogram (SAECG)*: MI is associated with prolonged and fragmented myocardial activation pattern which results in low-amplitude, high-frequency electrical signals in the terminal portions of the QRS complex referred as "late potential". These potentials are typically not recorded on surface ECG. Hence, signal averaging of ECG allows noise reduction and amplification to detect these potentials. In the MUSTT (Multicenter Unsustained Tachycardia Trial) study, SAECG was strong predictor of arrhythmic death and total mortality. Prolonged and fragmented myocardial activation pattern facilitates reentry and detection of it might identify patient at risk of slow coronary flow (SCF). However, the positive predictive value is relatively low (30%) which limits its usefulness in guiding the preventive therapies.
- *Microvolt T-wave Alternans (MVTWA)*: MVTWA reflects spatiotemporal heterogeneity of repolarization of ventricles. It is the beat-to-beat alternation of the T-wave amplitude which occurs as a consequence of abnormal calcium handling. Occurrence of T-wave alternans (TWA) at lower rates has been hypothesized to demonstrate an arrhythmic risk. Regardless of etiology and LV function, MVTWA has a very high negative predictive value for predicting ventricular arrhythmias. However, at present, there is not enough clinical evidence to support the use of TWA testing in routine clinical practice to guide therapy.
- *Premature ventricular contraction (PVC) morphology and nonsustained ventricular tachycardia (NSVT)*: Short, coupled PVCs, R on T phenomenon, polymorphic PVCs, and long runs of NSVT (>10 beats per minute) are important predictors of imminent SCD and warrant timely intervention to prevent their degeneration into VT/VF which tend to be fatal.

AUTONOMIC FUNCTION TESTS

The autonomic system may have a role in the genesis of ventricular arrhythmias. Impaired heat rate variability, baroreflex sensitivity, and heart rate turbulence are associated with increased total and cardiac mortality in survivors of acute myocardial infarction (AMI). However, the role of autonomic function tests in nonischemic cardiomyopathies remains to be proven.

NONINVASIVE TOOLS

- *Echocardiography*: The LVEF is one of the most powerful predictors of all-cause deaths as well as cardiac mortality. However, it has a relatively low specificity to predict SCD from arrhythmic causes. Most of the SCD in survivors of MI occurs in those patients with LVEF >30% whereas few patients who received an ICD required appropriate defibrillation. Many patients with very low LVEF may not benefit with ICD with primary intent since they have lower individual risk of SCD to begin with.
- *Cardiac magnetic resonance imaging (MRI)*: Tissue characterization using late-gadolinium enhancement, T1 mapping, and extracellular volume fraction calculation can provide vital information on arrhythmogenic substrates that can predispose to lethal arrhythmias in various cardiomyopathies. There exists a significant association of SCD with presence and extent of late gadolinium enhancement (LGE) in HCM patients such that in patients without any of the conventional SCD risk marker and extensive LGE, ICD for primary prevention has been proposed for.
- *Metaiodobenzylguanidine (MIBG) uptake scan*: I-123 tagged MIBG scan can be used to image adrenergic receptors in the heart with single-photon emission computed tomography (SPECT). In patients with dilated cardiomyopathy (DCM), reduced MIBG uptake and increased washout rate resulting in low heart-to-mediastinum (H/M) ratio has been found to be an independent predictor of SCD.

GENETIC TESTING

Genetic testing for culprit genes is typically useful in disorders of Mendelian inheritance/single gene disorders. The utility is best depicted in long QT syndrome (LQTS) patients where there is a specific genotype-phenotype correlation which not only helps in risk stratification and genetic counseling, but also helps in guiding medical therapy and preventing SCD in patients who refuse ICD/cannot afford ICD. CAD is polygenic in nature with several genes contributing to its predisposition and each having only mild-to-moderate influence. Hence, genetic testing may not be beneficial in evaluation of CAD unless it is caused by monogenic disorders like familial hypercholesterolemia.

INVASIVE TESTING

- *Coronary angiogram*: Presence of signs of ischemia should point towards ischemic etiology and a coronary angiogram may help in identifying the culprit vessel and planning an appropriate strategy. ECG may fail to detect ischemia in up to 30% of the SCD survivors where a culprit vessel may be found. Thus, all survivors of cardiac arrest warrant an angiogram for delineation of coronary anatomy.
- *Endomyocardial biopsy*: The role of endomyocardial biopsy is in diagnosing inflammatory or infiltrative cardiomyopathies. However, with widespread availability of advanced imaging modalities such cardiac magnetic resonance (MR) and positron emission tomography-computed tomography (PET-CT) it is done less frequently now.
- *Electrophysiology study (EPS)*: Inducibility of VT during EPS had long been proposed as marker of SCD and also a substrate to be ablated. Inducibility of sustained VT during EP testing is a well-established marker for SCD in patients with CAD. However, in patients with nonischemic heart disease, its value remains controversial. Likewise, inducibility of VT in patients with Brugada syndrome has also been used as an indication of ICD.

APPROACH IN A SPECIFIC PRESENTATION

PATIENT WITH UNEXPLAINED CARDIAC ARREST

The outcomes of witnessed cardiac arrest are more favorable when compared to unwitnessed or out-of-hospital cardiac arrests (OHCAs). Survival to hospital discharge in case of OHCAs is only 7.9% despite major advances in emergency medical services and cardiopulmonary resuscitation patterns. Immediate recognition of cardiac arrest, activation of emergency response team, prompt defibrillation for shockable rhythms, effective chest compressions as per the advanced cardiac life support, and prevention of recurrence of cardiac arrest in addition to post-cardiac arrest care are corner stone for improving survival to discharge.

Approximately 50% of cardiac arrests occur in individuals without a known heart disease, but most suffer from concealed ischemic heart disease. Careful history regarding sequence of events leading to cardiac arrest, chest pain, palpitations, presyncope, syncope, dyspnea, and a likely trigger in addition to detailed family history of SCD and risk factors such as diabetes, hypertension, dyslipidemia, smoking, and drug abuse should be sought.

A standard 12-lead ECG remains the most important investigation in evaluation. Characteristic patterns might point towards primary electrical disorders. Approximately 30% of OHCAs patients still have a culprit lesion on coronary angiogram when ECG did not show any signs of ischemia or infarction. This warrants assessment of all patients who survive cardiac arrest with ECG and a coronary angiogram. A complete diagnostic work has to be performed to identify the predisposing condition utilizing various imaging modalities, provocation tests, and invasive modalities as well. A stepwise approach to a patient with unexplained cardiac arrest is shown in the **Flowchart 3**.

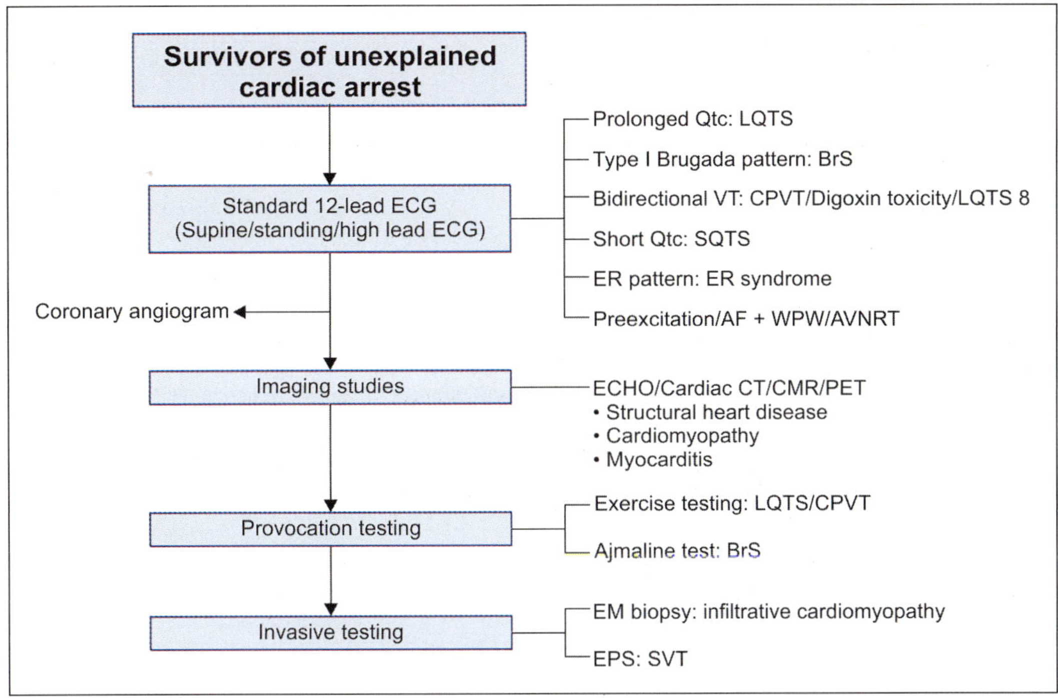

(AVNRT: atrioventricular nodal reentrant tachycardia; BrS: Brugada syndrome; CPVT: catecholaminergic polymorphic ventricular tachycardia; EM: endometrial; ER: early repolarization; LQTS: long QT syndrome; SQTS: short QT syndrome)

FLOWCHART 3: Stepwise approach to a patient with unexplained cardiac arrest.

SUDDEN CARDIAC DEATH SURVIVOR WITH DOCUMENTED TACHYARRHYTHMIA

An ECG documented tachyarrhythmia in the periarrest period is the most valuable clue to the underlying diagnosis. Reversible causes such as ischemia, infarction, drug toxicity, and dyselectrolytemia should be promptly recognized and treated. This should be followed by appropriate risk stratification and counseling with a stringent follow-up to anticipate and prevent recurrence of cardiac arrest. Nonreversible causes such as those with channelopathies, nonischemic cardiomyopathies, and scar VTs should receive an ICD for secondary prevention. One such management algorithm for patients with survivors of cardiac arrest is shown in **Flowchart 4**.

DISEASE STATES AND MANAGEMENT

CORONARY ARTERY DISEASE

Coronary artery disease is the most common substrate underlying SCD in the Western world, being responsible for 80% of SCDs and SCD accounts for up to 50% of all CAD-related deaths. CAD is a result of complex interplay between traditional risk factors, environmental factors, and polygenic influences which in conjunction with resultant atherosclerosis influence the arrhythmia expression and confers the risk of SCD.

Transient or persistent ischemia results in membrane instability with potassium efflux and calcium influx resulting in myocardial inhomogeneity. This results in a vulnerable substrate with a nidus for reentrant mechanism to come in action setting up the stage for fatal peri-MI polymorphic VT/VF, which is a characteristic arrhythmia in early stages of ischemia (**Flowchart 5** and **Figs. 2 A** and **B**). The irritable myocardium in the first few days post MI is especially vulnerable to short-coupled ventricular premature complexes (VPCs) consequent to abnormal automaticity and result in SCD due to VF. In late phases of MI when scar has formed, reentrant mechanism becomes the principal mechanism of ventricular arrhythmias.

Early intervention with a successful myocardial reperfusion strategy might influence the occurrence, recurrence, and outcomes of these fatal arrhythmias. Angiographic findings in survivors of OHCAs reveal CAD (≥1 lesion with >50% disease) in approximately 64% of patients, while only 37% had clinical or angiographic evidence of acute coronary syndrome (ACS) due to acute occlusion or ruptured plaque or thrombus.

Currently, the only strategy to reduce the risk of SCD in the peri-MI period is timely reperfusion of occluded vessels. In patients with scar VT, which is usually monomorphic in nature, drug therapy with beta-blockers and other antiarrhythmic drugs and ICD with secondary prevention intent remains the mainstay of management strategy.

CARDIOMYOPATHIES

Nonischemic dilated cardiomyopathy: Mortality in nonischemic dilated cardiomyopathy (NIDCM) is primarily because of progressive pump failure, while SCD occurs in up to 10% of these patients. SCD is usually consequent to a malignant form of PVC triggering a monomorphic or

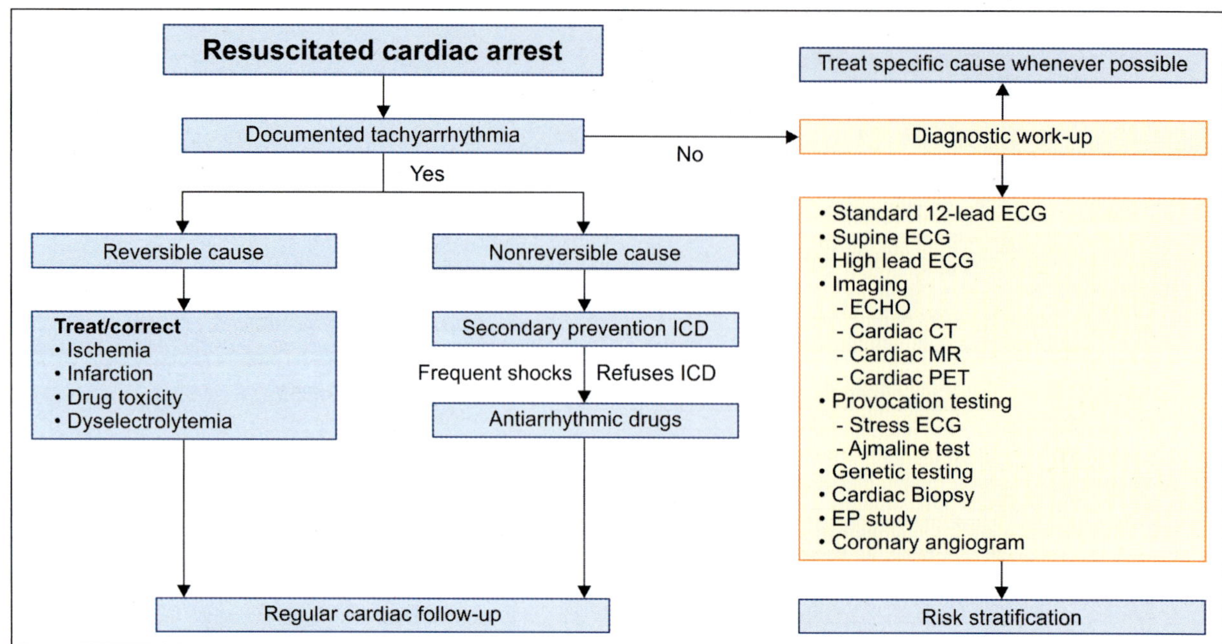

(EP: electrophysiology; ICD: implantable cardioverter-defibrillator)

FLOWCHART 4: Management algorithm in patients with survivors of cardiac arrest.

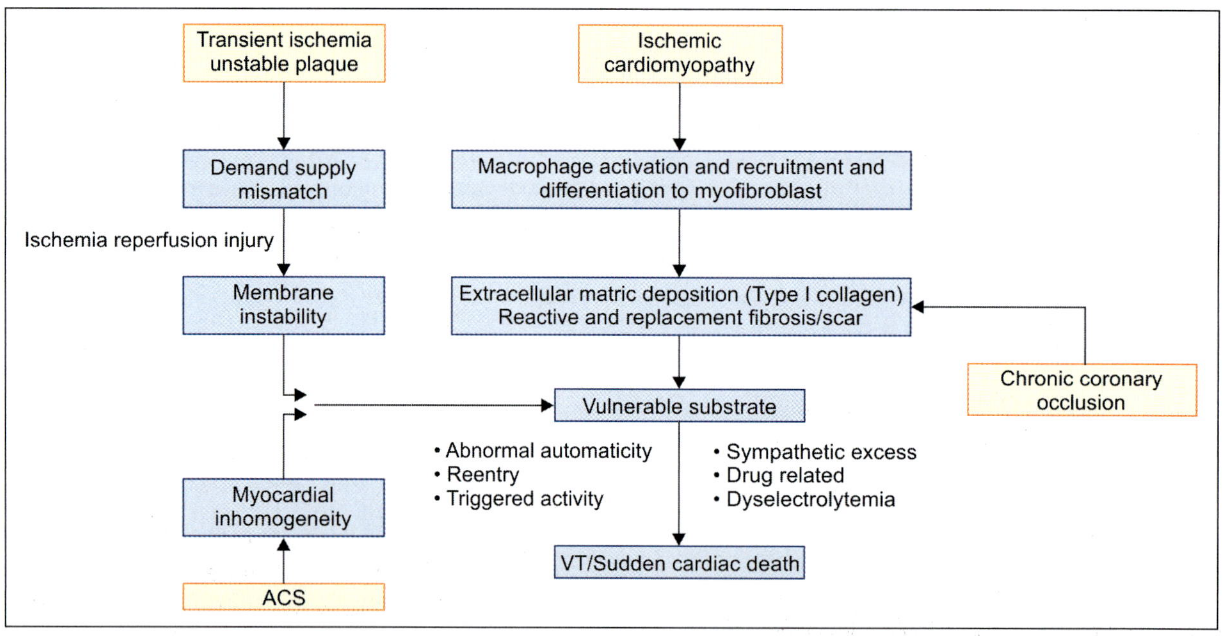

(ACS: acute coronary syndrome)

FLOWCHART 5: Pathophysiology of SCD in arrhythmias secondary to CAD.

polymorphic VT. Unexplained syncope, complex ventricular ectopy, and nonsustained VT stratify the patient into high risk and should warrant therapeutic and preventive strategies to mitigate the risk of evolution into fatal arrhythmias and SCD.

HYPERTROPHIC CARDIOMYOPATHY

Hypertrophic cardiomyopathy is one of the most common heritable genetic cardiomyopathy with a prevalence of 1 in 200–500. It is the most common cause of SCD in young athletes. SCD may be the first clinical manifestation of HCM. It has marked genotypic and phenotypic heterogeneity with sarcomeric gene mutations contributing to up to 60% of the cases. While MYBPC3 mutations are associated with later onset hypertrophy and good prognosis, TNNT2 mutations seem to cause SCD more frequently.

Management of SCD consequent to tachyarrhythmias in HCM warrants implantable cardiac defibrillator for

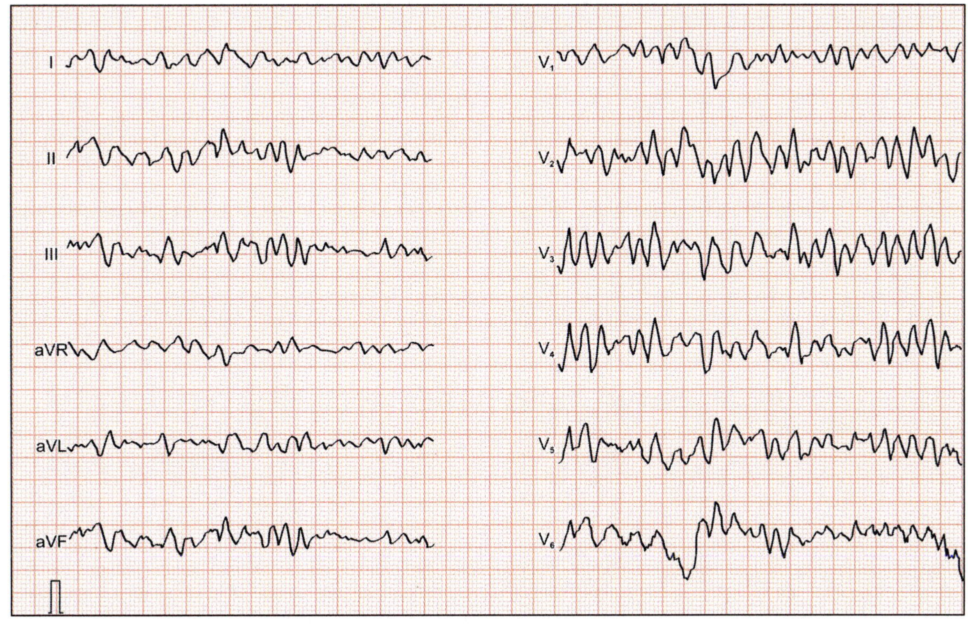

FIGURE 2 A: ECG of a patient with acute coronary syndrome showing polymorphic VT/VF.

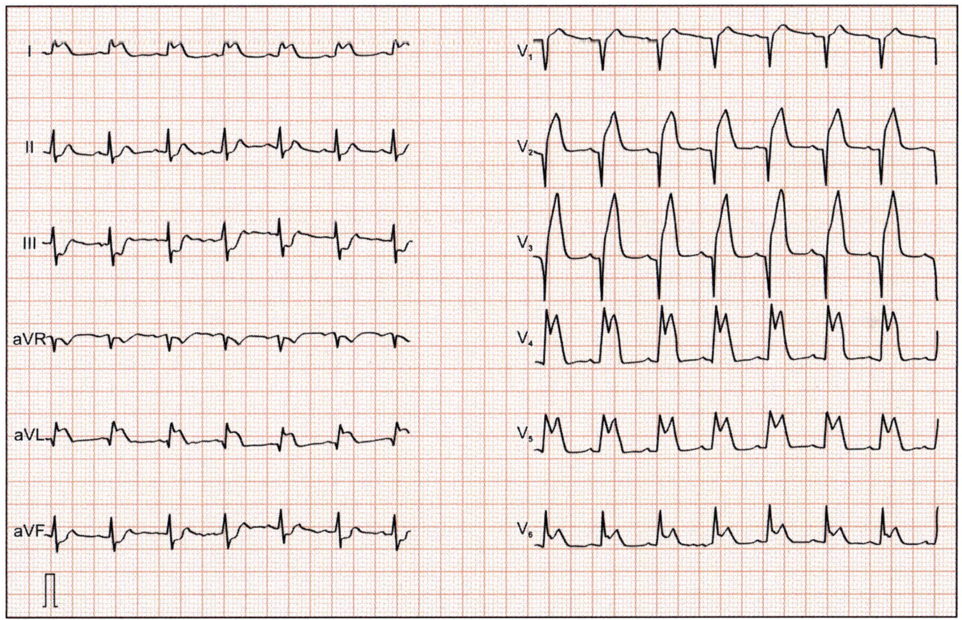

FIGURE 2 B: ECG of the same patient post direct current cardioversion showing anterolateral wall MI.

survivors of cardiac arrest. In those with 5-year HCM-SCD risk score of ≥6%, an ICD is indicated for primary prevention. A summary of established risk factors, risk modifiers, and SCD risk score is shown in **Flowchart 6**. **Figures 3 A** and **B** show a patient with apical HCM who presented with recurrent episodes of VT, while cardiac MRI revealed clot in apex of left ventricle.

Right ventricular cardiomyopathy: Arrhythmogenic right ventricular cardiomyopathy (ARVC) is a genetic cardiomyopathy involving the desmosomes, characterized by fibrofatty replacement of myocardium which may result in multiple left bundle branch morphology VTs in addition to recurrent PVCs, NSVT, and VFs predisposing to SCD. The concealed phase of ARVC that precedes the ECG changes is presumed to be associated with high burden of lethal arrhythmias and SCD.

Surface ECG usually provides a clue to the diagnosis with epsilon waves (**Fig. 4**) seen in up to 30% of cases, the presence of which may be associated with high risk of VT and SCD. However, ECG may be normal in nearly 50% of the patients.

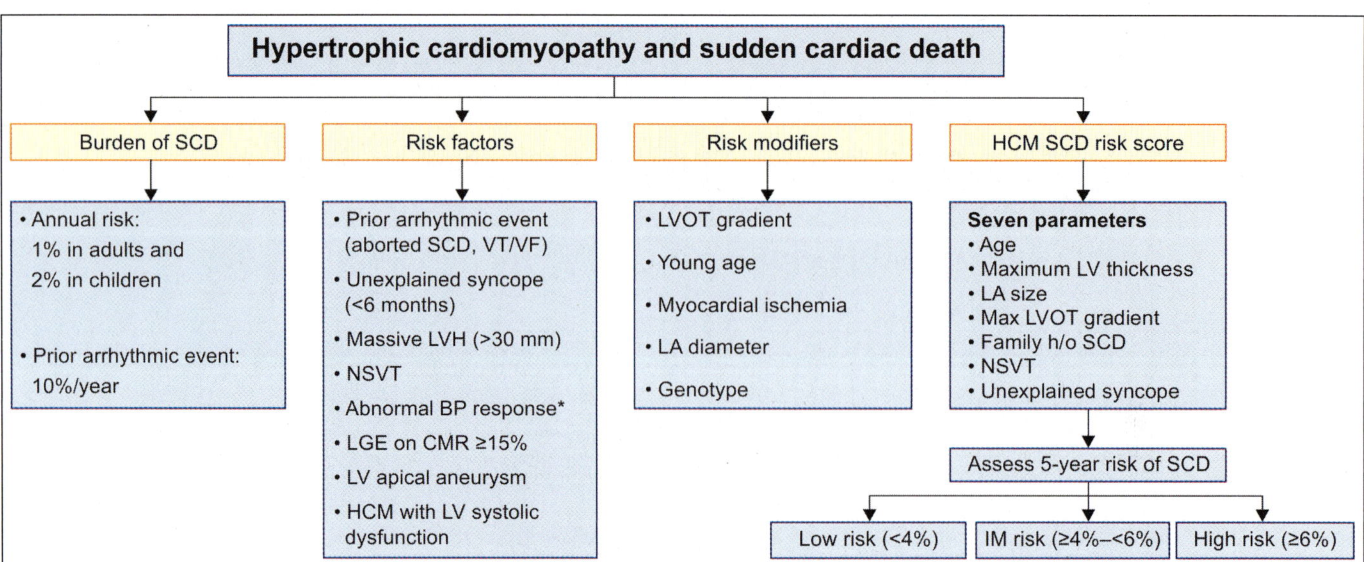

* Failure to increase by at least 20 mm Hg or a drop of at least 20 mm Hg during effort.

(LA: left atrial; LGE: late gadolinium enhancement; LV: left ventricular; LVH: left ventricular hypertrophy; LVOT: left ventricular outflow tract; NSVT: nonsustained ventricular tachycardia)

FLOWCHART 6: Hypertrophic cardiomyopathy and SCD.

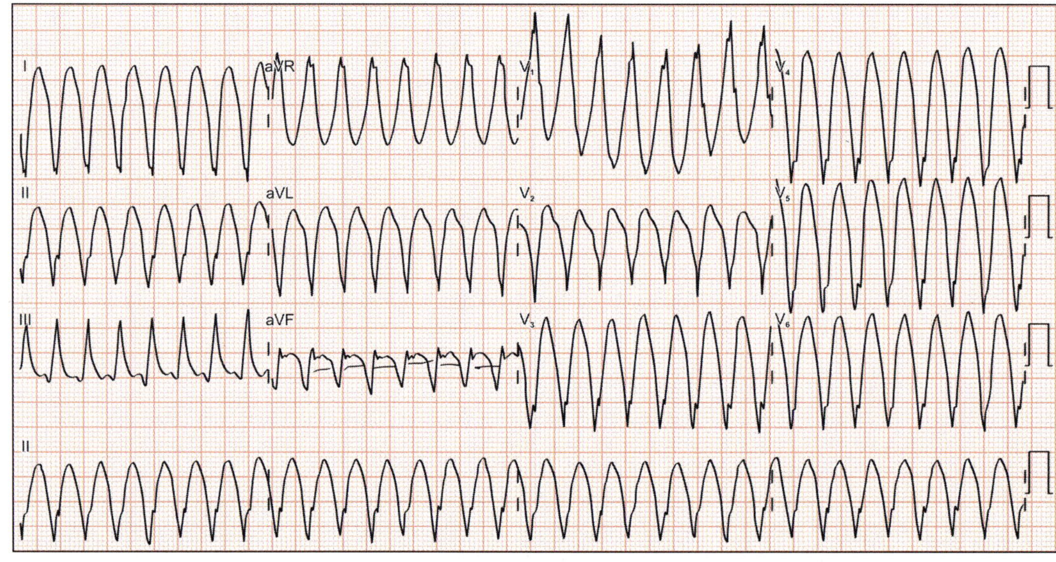

FIGURE 3 A: ECG during episodes of palpitation showing monomorphic VT in a patient with apical hypertrophic cardiomyopathy.

Young age at diagnosis, unexplained syncope, prior cardiac arrest/VT/VF, LV involvement, ventricular dysfunction, increased QRS dispersion, ARVC type 2 and type 4, and Naxos disease are considered high-risk groups. Thus, risk stratification is important, although not standardized.

Drug therapy/catheter ablation in low-risk groups and ICD in high-risk patients have been standard of care as of now. Survival benefits of up to 5 years have been shown with ICDs. Problems which are unique to ICD therapy in ARVC patients include higher defibrillation thresholds, lead sensing and pacing issues, higher rates of redo procedures, and higher complication rates.

OTHER STRUCTURAL HEART DISEASES

Valvular heart disease and congenital heart disease: Risk of tachyarrhythmias and SCD occur more frequently in patients post valve surgery or post open-heart surgery for congenital heart disease (CHD). Although less frequent than bradyarrhythmias/heart blocks, tachyarrhythmias can turn fatal warranting appropriate drug/catheter ablation/ ICD therapies whenever applicable.

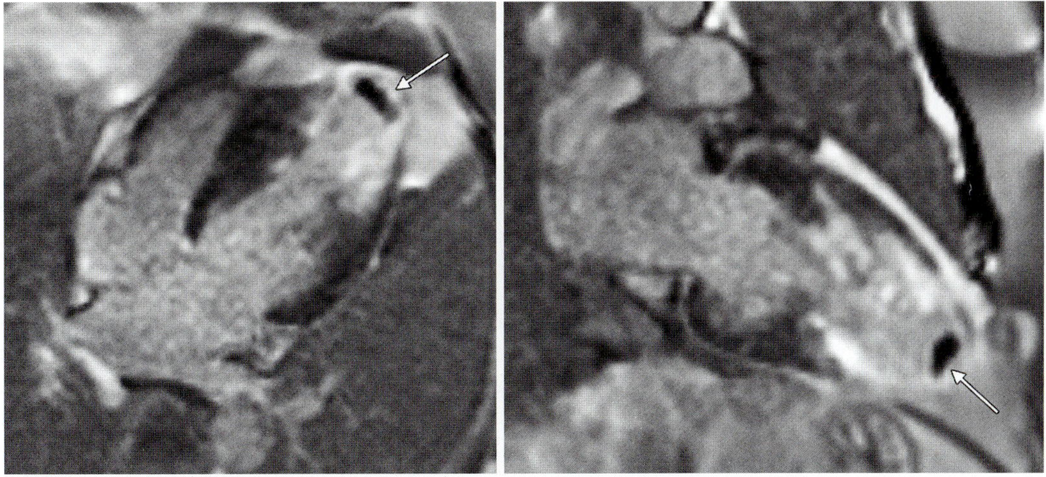

FIGURE 3 B: Late gadolinium enhancement (LGE) sequences in four-chamber and two-chamber view showing LGE in the apical segments and apex of the left ventricle with nonenhancing hypointense clot in the left ventricular (LV) apex (arrow): end systole (left) and end diastole (right).

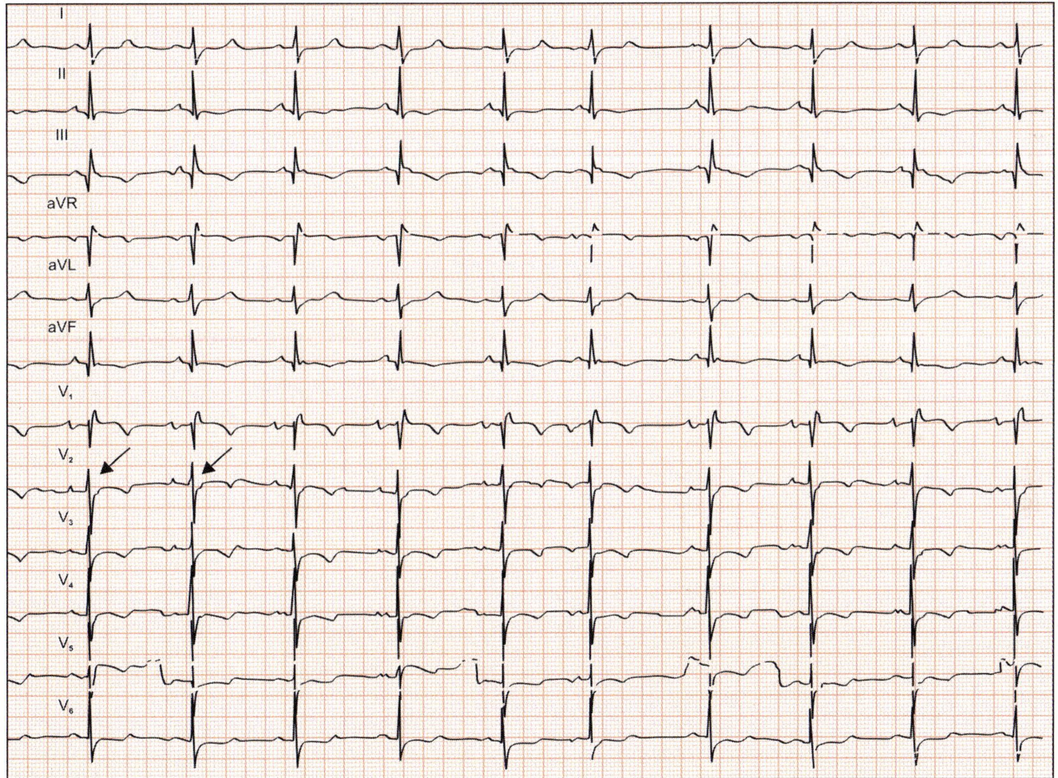

FIGURE 4: Electrocardiogram (ECG) of a 15-year-old boy showing depolarization (epsilon wave—arrow) and repolarization [inverted T in V_1–V_4 in >14 years in the presence of complete right bundle branch block (CRBBB)] changes consistent with arrhythmogenic right ventricular cardiomyopathy (ARVC).

Arrhythmic mitral valve prolapse: A subset of patient with mitral valve prolapse present with SCD and are frequently found to have a malignant phenotype. This phenotype is associated with ST segment depression, T-wave inversions on baseline ECG, mitral annular disjunction, and leaflet redundancy on echocardiography and ventricular arrhythmias of variable severity. Patients with these findings are predisposed to tachyarrhythmias and SCD.

CHANNELOPATHIES

Long QT syndrome: Long QT syndrome is a disorder of myocardial repolarization. It is an important cause of SCD due to its propensity to increase the risk of a life-threatening arrhythmia—torsades de pointes. LQTS may be either acquired or congenital. *Acquired LQTS* is mainly due to drug side effects. However, hypokalemia, hypocalcemia, hypothermia, and intracranial diseases may also increase the risk. Although up to 17 genes have been discovered to cause *congenital LQTS*, only three major genetic subtypes have been identified to result in three major subtypes—LQTS1 [35%(KCNQ1)], LQTS2 [25–35%(KCNH2)], and LQTS3 [5–10%(SCN5A)]. All these genetic mutations alter myocardial ion channel function resulting in either a decrease in repolarizing K^+ current or an increase in depolarizing Na^+ or Ca^{2+} current leading to the pathological increase in QT interval. A representative ECG of a patient with LQTS is shown in the **Figure 5**.

Although the time at presentation greatly varies, LQTS is most commonly diagnosed during the first three decades of life. The most common presentation is arrhythmogenic syncope. However, seizure or sudden cardiac arrest may occur in case of prolonged arrhythmia. SCD has been reported as initial presentation in approximately 13% patients. In Pediatric Electrophysiology Society registry, 61% of patients were symptomatic at presentation. Among them, syncope, seizures, and cardiac arrest were present in 2,610 and 9% patients, respectively.

Ventricular tachyarrhythmia is the most common arrhythmia in LQTS. However, bradycardia, AV block, and atrial tachycardias are not uncommon. The most feared arrhythmia is torsades de pointes, which, if prolonged, may cause SCD. It is a polymorphic VT with a characteristic twisting of QRS peaks around the isoelectric line. The last sinus beat preceding the arrhythmia characteristically has prolonged QT interval.

The most important diagnostic test in LQTS is 12-lead electrocardiography. The normal QTc in a healthy adult is 420 ± 20 ms. QTc interval >460 ms, >470 ms, and >480 ms are considered abnormal in prepuberty, postpubertal male, and postpubertal females, respectively. LQTS diagnostic score ("Schwartz score") and exercise test are additional diagnostic tools to identify subtle cases. Genetic testing identifies LQTS genetic variants in approximately 80% of cases and, together with characteristic symptoms, confers the definitive diagnosis.

Beta-blockers (propranolol and nadolol) are the main drugs used in case of LQTS with syncope or seizures. ICD is also recommended if there is a history of SCD survivor. If symptom recurs even after the maximum tolerated dose of beta-blocker or in case of discontinuation of beta-blockers due to side effects, cardiac sympathetic denervation is recommended.

Brugada syndrome: Brugada syndrome is caused by loss of function mutation involving sodium channel (SCN5A). It is characterized a typical ECG pattern consisting of coved-type ST-segment elevation (≥2 mm) followed by a negative T wave in the right precordial leads V_1 through V_3 (type I Brugada pattern). The mechanism of lethal arrhythmias is a phase 2 reentry, typically resulting in syncope and SCD during rest or sleep. SCD may well be the first manifestation of the disease typically occurring in third to fourth decade of life. Other triggers which can precipitate type I Brugada pattern include fever, heavy meals, alcohol consumption, or few provocation agents such as ajmaline, flecainide, procainamide, or pilsicainide. The clinical variables which predict worse outcomes include syncope, spontaneous type I ECG pattern, male gender, and inducibility of arrhythmia on electrophysiology studies.

Implantable cardioverter-defibrillator seems to be the most beneficial therapy in survivors of cardiac arrest or those patients with syncope and type I Brugada pattern. Type I ECG pattern in absence of symptoms or family history or inability to induce VT/VF on EPS stratify patients in low-risk category. They need close follow-up. The only drug which (inhibiting Ito current) is found to be effective in Brugada syndrome is quinidine, although it is just considered to be an adjunctive therapy in patients with high risk of SCD, to reduce the number of ICD shocks in these patients.

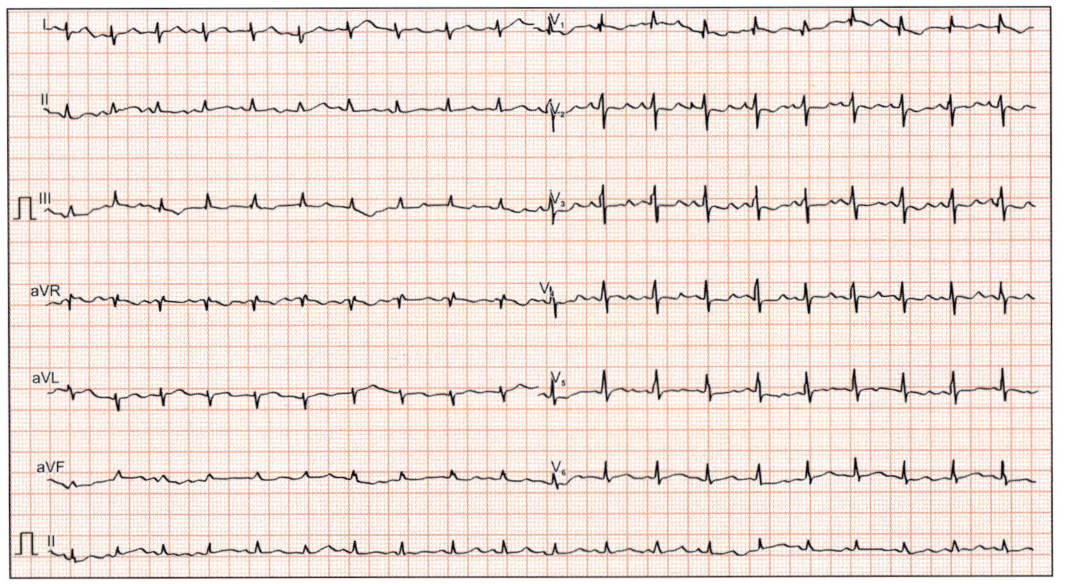

FIGURE 5: Electrocardiogram (ECG) of a patient with long QT syndrome with QTc of 520 ms.

Short QT syndrome: Short QT syndrome (SQTS) is another congenital channelopathy that has been recently recognized as a cause of SCD. It is characterized by short QT interval due to either hyperfunction of delayed rectifier potassium current or hypofunction of calcium current leading to a high risk of atrial and VF. Five subtypes of SQTS [SQTS1 (KCNH2), SQTS2 (KCNQ1), SQTS3 (KCNJ2), SQT4 (CACNA1C), and SQTS5 (CACANB2B)] have been recognized. Most of these inherit with an autosomal dominant pattern.

Short QT syndrome is considered as a highly lethal syndrome where sudden cardiac arrest is the most frequent (34%) and most common first presentation (28%). Other symptoms are syncope (24%) and atrial fibrillation (31%). Diagnosis is mainly based on 12-lead ECG. Males with QTc <330 ms and females with <340 ms should be diagnosed with SQTS even if they are asymptomatic. For symptomatic males and females, the QTc cutoffs are 360 ms and 370 ms, respectively. The role of genetic tests as a diagnostic tool for SQTS is still not established.

Because of a very high risk of fatal arrhythmia, ICD is indicated in SQTS patients if there are clinical symptoms or family history, or positive genetic tests. Quinidine is the first-line pharmacological therapy as it prolongs the QTc interval by blocking several K^+ channels and inward sodium and calcium currents. Disopyramide is another drug that has shown promising effects by increasing ventricular effective refractory period in SQTS1 patients.

Catecholaminergic polymorphic ventricular tachycardia: Catecholaminergic polymorphic ventricular tachycardia (CPVT) is a genetic channelopathy characterized by abnormal calcium handling, unremarkable resting ECG, and exercise-induced bidirectional VT or polymorphic VT and SCD. It is also reproducible by catecholamine infusion. Both autosomal dominant forms involving *RYR2* gene and autosomal recessive form involving *calsequestrin (CASQ2)* gene exist. *KCNJ2* gene involvement which is involved in Andersen–Tawil syndrome is also known to be associated with bidirectional VT (**Fig. 6**). The sequela of these mutations is inappropriate calcium leakage because of increased channel opening or increased sensitivity of calcium concentration in sarcoplasmic reticulum, which predisposes to the development of delayed afterdepolarization and triggered activity on provocation.

Beta-blockers are the drugs of choice. The other options include flecainide and verapamil. However, in patients with sustained VTs despite maximally tolerated beta-blockers, ICD remains the mainstay of therapy to prevent SCD.

Early repolarization syndrome and idiopathic polymorphic VT/VF syndromes: Early repolarization syndrome (ERS) is yet another J wave syndrome which has also been associated with increased risk of SCD. Features consistent with risk of severe arrhythmias and SCD include survivors of SCD, positive family history, transient augmentation of J waves, high amplitude (>0.2 mV) J waves, short-coupled VPCs, overlap syndromes, and J waves in inferolateral leads

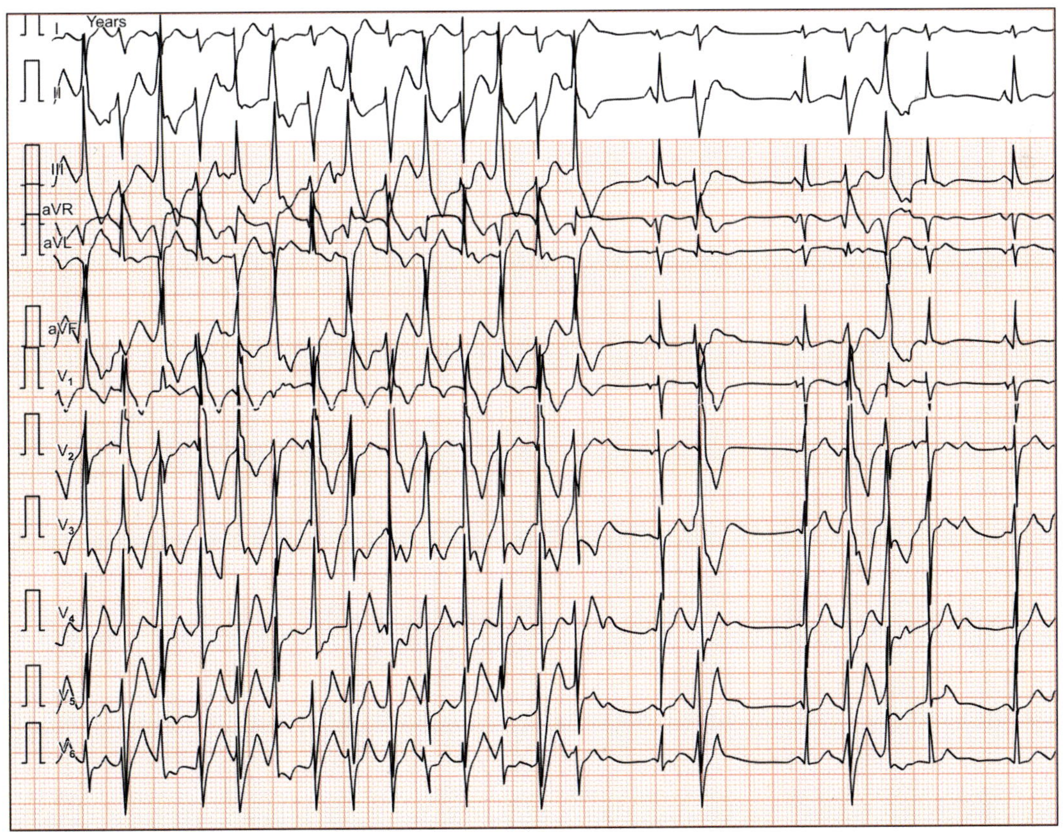

FIGURE 6: 12-lead electrocardiogram shows atrioventricular (AV) dissociation and 180° change in the QRS axis in the alternate beat (better appreciated in lead II, aVL, and aVF).

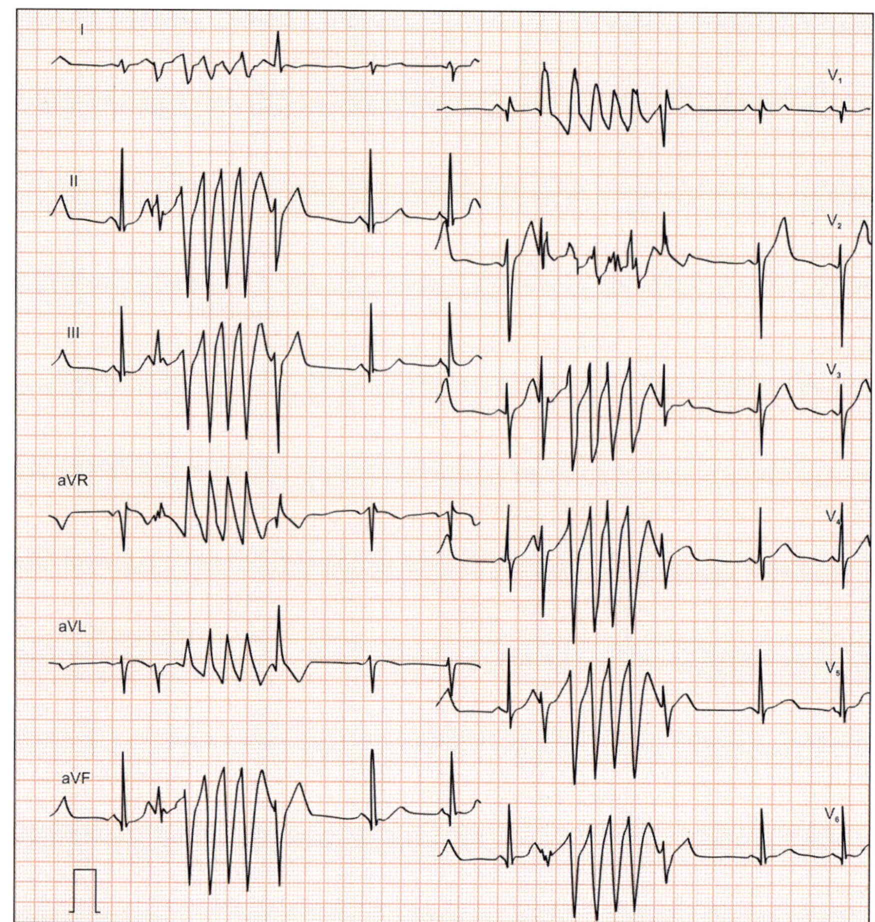

FIGURE 7: Holter trace demonstrating an early-coupled ventricular premature beat of right bundle branch block (RBBB) morphology initiating a short run of polymorphic ventricular tachycardia.

or globally. However, due to lack of consistent association between these high-risk features and SCD, there are no specific recommendations in patients with asymptomatic early repolarization (ER) pattern on ECG. Currently, ICD is indicated only in survivors of cardiac arrest or sustained ventricular arrhythmias. **Figure 7** shows Holter trace of a patient with idiopathic VF, demonstrating an early-coupled ventricular premature beat of left bundle branch block (LBBB) morphology initiating a short run of polymorphic VT.

Idiopathic ventricular tachycardias: Right ventricular outflow tract VT and idiopathic left VTs are usually well tolerated and more commonly present with tachycardia-induced cardiomyopathy rather than SCD. The risk of SCD in these arrhythmias is very low.

SUPRAVENTRICULAR TACHYCARDIAS

Supraventricular tachycardias are usually associated with low risk of SCD except in few specific subsets such as atrial fibrillation with preexcitation. SCD occurs in Wolff–Parkinson–White (WPW) in relation to rapid preexcited atrial fibrillation with fast ventricular response in up to 50% of cases. However, risk of SCD in asymptomatic WPW is to the tune of 0.15–0.39% over 3–10 years follow-up. Although, asymptomatic WPW is associated with low risk of SCD overall, there are certain markers which can increase the risk of SCD. Patients with increased risk of SCD require ablation of these accessory pathways to prevent SCD. These markers which can increase the risk of SCD include anterograde effective refractory period of accessory pathway (APERP) 240–250 ms (on isoproterenol APERP <200 ms), shortest preexcited RR interval (SPERRI) <250 ms, inducible AV reciprocating tachycardia or atrial fibrillation lasting ≥1 minute, multiple accessory pathways, Ebstein anomaly, and familial WPW syndrome.

CONCLUSION

Ventricular tachycardias/ventricular fibrillations constitute up to 75–80% of preterminal rhythm in patients sustaining cardiac arrest. Pertinent history, stepwise diagnostic approach, risk stratification, and prompt usage of implantable cardiac defibrillators to prevent recurrence of cardiac arrest and SCD are keys to improve survival rates in these patients.

RECOMMENDED READINGS

1. Deo R, Albert CM. Epidemiology and genetics of sudden cardiac death. Circulation. 2012;125(4):620-37.
2. Rao BH, Sastry BK, Chugh SS, Kalavakolanu S, Christopher J, Shangula D, et al. Contribution of sudden cardiac death to total mortality in India—a population based study. Int J Cardiol. 2012;154(2):163-7.
3. Mäkikallio TH, Barthel P, Schneider R, Bauer A, Tapanainen JM, Tulppo MP, et al. Prediction of sudden cardiac death after acute myocardial infarction: role of Holter monitoring in the modern treatment era. Eur Heart J. 2005;26(8):762-9.
4. Gräni C, Benz DC, Gupta S, Windecker S, Kwong RY. Sudden Cardiac Death in Ischemic Heart Disease: From Imaging Arrhythmogenic Substrate to Guiding Therapies. JACC Cardiovasc Imaging. 2020;13(10):2223-38.
5. Goldberger JJ, Basu A, Boineau R, Buxton AE, Cain ME, Canty JM Jr, et al. Risk stratification for sudden cardiac death: a plan for the future. Circulation. 2014;129(4):516-26.
6. Myerburg RJ, Junttila MJ. Sudden cardiac death caused by coronary heart disease. Circulation. 2012;125(8):1043-52.
7. Davies MJ, Thomas A. Thrombosis and acute coronary-artery lesions in sudden cardiac ischemic death. N Engl J Med. 1984;310(18):1137-40.
8. Elliott PM, Anastasakis A, Borger MA, Borggrefe M, Cecchi F, Charron P, et al. 2014 ESC Guidelines on diagnosis and management of hypertrophic cardiomyopathy: the Task Force for the Diagnosis and Management of Hypertrophic Cardiomyopathy of the European Society of Cardiology (ESC). Eur Heart J. 2014;35(39):2733-79.
9. Schwartz PJ, Ackerman MJ, George AL Jr, Wilde AAM. Impact of genetics on the clinical management of channelopathies. J Am Coll Cardiol. 2013;62(3):169-80.
10. Priori SG, Schwartz PJ, Napolitano C, Bloise R, Ronchetti E, Grillo M, et al. Risk stratification in the long-QT syndrome. N Engl J Med. 2003;348(19):1866-74.
11. Al-Khatib SM, Stevenson WG, Ackerman MJ, Bryant WJ, Callans DJ, Curtis AB, et al. 2017 AHA/ACC/HRS Guideline for Management of Patients With Ventricular Arrhythmias and the Prevention of Sudden Cardiac Death: A Report of the American College of Cardiology/American Heart Association Task Force on Clinical Practice Guidelines and the Heart Rhythm Society. J Am Coll Cardiol. 2018;72(14):e91-220.
12. Kusumoto FM, Bailey KR, Chaouki AS, Deshmukh AJ, Gautam S, Kim RJ, et al. Systematic review for the 2017 AHA/ACC/HRS guideline for management of patients with ventricular arrhythmias and the prevention of sudden cardiac death: A Report of the American College of Cardiology/American Heart Association Task Force on Clinical Practice Guidelines and the Heart Rhythm Society. Heart Rhythm. 2018;15(10):e253-74.
13. Viskin S. The QT interval: too long, too short or just right. Heart Rhythm. 2009;6(5):711-5.
14. Wu SH, Lin XX, Cheng YJ, Qiang CC, Zhang J. Early repolarization pattern and risk for arrhythmia death: a meta-analysis. J Am Coll Cardiol. 2013;61(6):645-50.

CHAPTER 92

Heart Failure: Pathophysiology and Diagnosis

Tiny Nair

ABSTRACT

Heart failure (HF) results from a complex interplay of altered hemodynamics, deranged neurohormonal regulations as well as biochemical, molecular, and transcriptional changes at cellular levels. Knowledge in this area is constantly evolving. An updated insight into the pathophysiology would help in better diagnosis and treatment of this complex disease. Advances in imaging and biomarkers in HF have changed the entire approach of HF diagnosis. Understanding pathophysiology would help us connect the dots, identify specific subsets who are likely to benefit from emerging therapies in HF such as the angiotensin receptor-neprilysin inhibitor (ARNI) and sodium-glucose cotransporter inhibitors (SGLT2i).

Heart failure is defined as failure of the heart to supply oxygen, commensurate to the demand of the tissues, despite adequate filling.

"There is no limit to how complicated things can get, on account of one thing always leading to another"
—EB White

INTRODUCTION

Heart failure is subdivided into heart failure with reduced ejection fraction (HFrEF) with left ventricular ejection fraction (LVEF) <40%, heart failure with preserved ejection fraction (HFpEF) LVEF >50%, and the new gray area of heart failure with midrange ejection fraction (HFmrEF) LVEF between 40 and 49%.

In both HFrEF and HFpEF there is reduction of stroke volume; in HFrEF the diastolic volume [end-diastolic volume (EDV)] is normal, with reduction of systolic volume [end-systolic volume (ESV)], while in HFpEF the diastolic volume (EDV) is reduced (inability to relaxation).

PATHOPHYSIOLOGY

The failing heart tries to compensate by activating multiple compensatory mechanisms. All the compensatory mechanisms are initially helpful and directed towards maintenance of blood pressure to preserve organ perfusion. However, as these compensatory mechanisms overshoot with progressive HF these become harmful. Blocking this overshoot in compensatory mechanisms helps to retard cell damage and improve mortality. Thus, the beta-blockers (BBs), renin-angiotensin-aldosterone system (RAAS) blockers, neprilysin inhibitors, and aldosterone antagonists all have shown mortality benefit as they block overshoot in the compensatory mechanisms.

NEUROHORMONAL ACTIVATION

The failing heart tries to compensate the reduction of stroke volume by augmentation of multiple neurohormonal support pathways in an endeavor to correct the deranged physiology. The activation of sympathetic pathway and RAAS play the predominant role, but multiple other pathways including the neprilysin pathway, endothelin (ET) system, and inflammatory pathways also contribute to this effect. Understanding them gives us a logical insight to plan treatment strategies in HF.

Most of these mechanisms are compensatory and helpful in the short term, resulting in the following benefits (**Fig. 1**):

- Increased rate and contractility of the heart
- Vasoconstriction—increased peripheral vascular resistance
- Salt and water retention (volume expansion)
- Mobilization of inflammatory mediators to trigger cardiac repair and healing

But these compensatory "life-saving" systems, in the long-term turn detrimental, starting off a downward spiral of progressive cardiac damage.

Activation of sympathetic system: Normal sympathetic and parasympathetic tone is delicately balanced in a healthy heart.

The carotid sinus receptors and the aortic arch baroreceptors act as high-pressure sensors, while cardiac and pulmonary mechanoreceptors act as low-pressure sensors (**Fig. 2**). The input from these sensors inhibits the sympathetic tone. In contrast, the peripheral chemoreceptors and muscle metabolic receptors act as excitatory signal for the sympathetic system. A normal cardiovascular system has a low sympathetic discharge and a high heart rate variability (HRV).

Activation of the sympathetic system happens very early in the failing heart. The sympathetically overdriven failing heart results in increased contractility, sinus tachycardia, and a low HRV.

The high sympathetic activity produces a higher circulating norepinephrine (NE) level. A higher NE level portends a poor survival in HF. But over time many patients of chronic HF show low NE levels, which may be evidence of "storage exhaustion". A high NE level increases the heart rate (HR), increases myocardial contractility, and increases peripheral resistance (by alpha receptor mediated vasoconstriction) in the short run. These effects over time, becomes detrimental, by increasing the energy demand by the failing heart and increase chances of major cardiac arrhythmias.

Downregulation of beta-1 receptors in the failing heart result in loss of catecholamine-induced ionotropic effect and further myocardial failure and development of major cardiac arrhythmias. Institution of beta-blocker early in HF corrects this hyperadrenergic state resulting in improvement in the long run. Since sympathetic activation occurs very early in HF, it is logical to use BBs as the first line of drugs for prevention of progression of HF as well as for preventing cardiac arrhythmias, which are the leading cause of death in HF with milder symptoms.

Recent evidence shows that, along with sympathetic activation, there is withdrawal of parasympathetic effect.

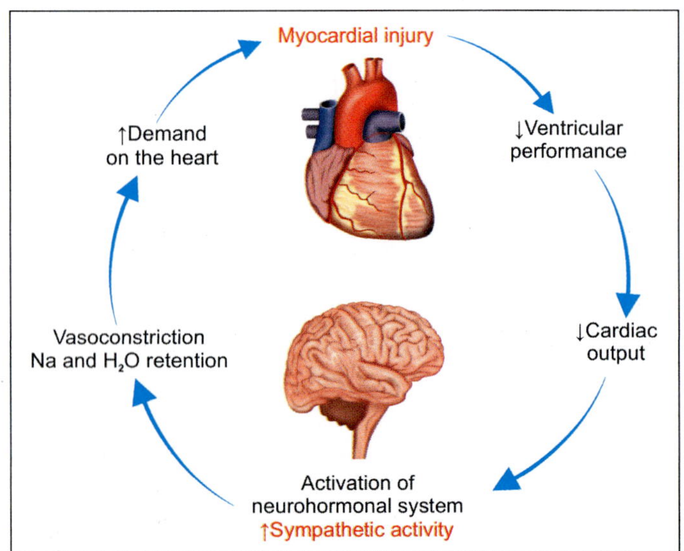

FIGURE 1: The vicious cycle of onset and progression of heart failure by the neurohormonal activation.

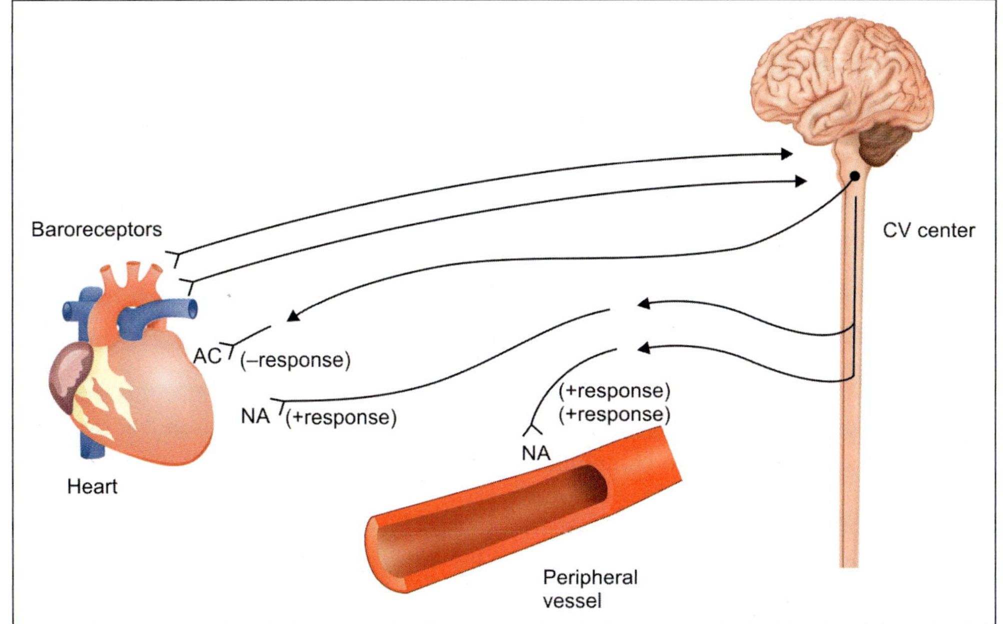

(CV: cardiovascular)

FIGURE 2: Role of baroreceptors in the heart and the great vessels in reflex sympathetic activation.

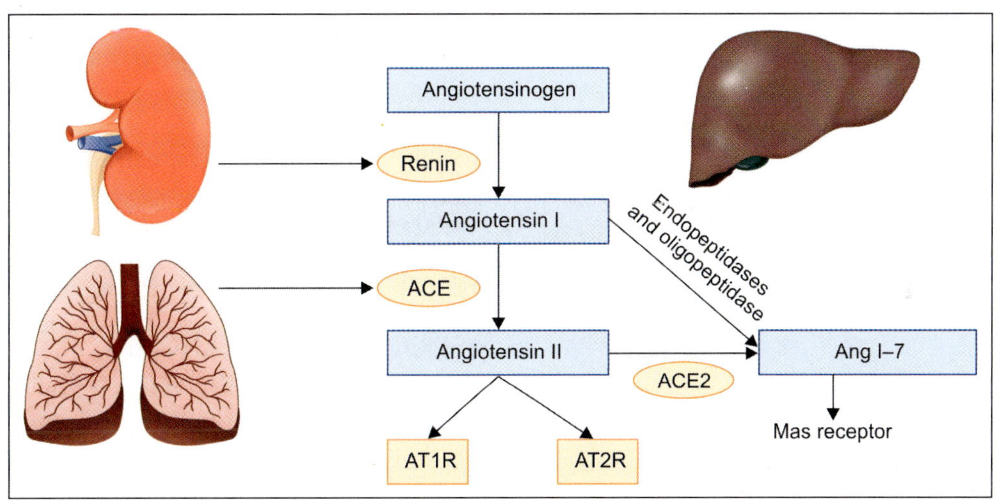

FIGURE 3: The renin–angiotensin system showing the source of angiotensinogen, renin, and angiotensin-converting enzymes (ACEs) and the sites of action of angiotensin II.

This withdrawal of parasympathetic activity has been shown to result in reduction of vascular nitric oxide (NO) which is a potent vasodilator, augmentation of inflammation as well as adverse cardiac remodeling.

Activation of renin–angiotensin–aldosterone system: The kidney produces renin that cleaves the angiotensinogen to angiotensin I (decapeptide) and then to angiotensin II (octapeptide) by angiotensin-converting enzyme (ACE). In HF, renal hypoperfusion as well as increased filtered sodium load to macula densa trigger off secretion of renin, consequently producing more angiotensin II. Angiotensin II through AT1 receptors causes vasoconstriction, cell growth, sympathetic stimulation, and stimulates aldosterone production, which in turn retains sodium. Stimulation of AT2 receptors causes vasodilation and other beneficial effects including inhibition of cell growth, sodium loss, and release of vasodilators like bradykinin. Angiotensin is also converted to Ang 1–7 which is a vasodilator, acting through the Mas receptors (**Fig. 3**).

The short-term effects of activation of RAAS are beneficial, but it quickly becomes maladaptive and detrimental. Also, stimulation of sympathetic system pours out excess of NE. Suppression of RAAS by ACE inhibitors or angiotensin receptor blockers or ARNI has been clearly shown to suppress RAAS axis and result in improved outcome.

Reduction of blood pressure, cardiac output, and effective blood volume leads to renal hypoperfusion. Renal hypoperfusion causes release of sympathetic hyperactivity as well as activation of RAAS. Both cause salt and water retention as well as peripheral vasoconstriction. The peripheral vasoconstriction is mediated by NE and angiotensin II. Other vasoconstrictors are thromboxane A2, ET, and arginine vasopressin (AVP).

PEPTIDES IN HEART FAILURE

Arginine vasopressin: Arginine vasopressin is a peptide hormone secreted from the pituitary gland in response to increased plasma osmolality.

Arginine vasopressin increases water reabsorption from collecting ducts to normalize the osmolality. In chronic HF, AVP production is triggered initially in response to altered osmolality, but subsequently, even after osmolality is corrected, there continues to be increased production of AVP. This increase in AVP in a state of "normo-osmolality" results in hyponatremia, which is commonly seen in chronic HF. AVP acts through a series of receptors called vasopressin receptors with subtypes of V_{1a}, V_{1b}, and V_2 (**Fig. 4**).

Natriuretic peptides: Natriuretic peptides are a family of small molecules secreted by the atria or ventricle of the heart, that have autocrine, endocrine, and paracrine functions. The existence of such peptides was suspected long back when diuresis was noted following conversion of atrial tachyarrhythmias to sinus rhythm.

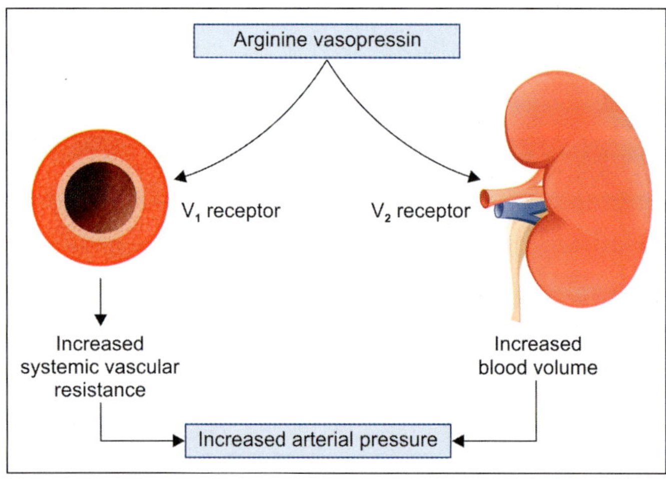

FIGURE 4: Arginine vasopressin system with V_1 and V_2 receptors and their site of action.

Atrial natriuretic peptide (ANP) was discovered in 1984. It is secreted from the atrial muscles where it is stored as granules (pro-ANP). Pro-ANP is stripped up into an "omega"-shaped ANP with 28-amino acid and a linear N-terminal (NT) pro-ANP with 98-amino acid.

B-type natriuretic peptide (BNP) was discovered in 1988. It is secreted from the ventricular myocardium in response to stretch. Stored pro-BNP is further cleaved out into NT pro-BNP with 75-amino acid and BNP with 36-amino acid.

Subsequently in 1990 a third natriuretic peptide (NP), C-type natriuretic peptide (CNP) was isolated from the pig brain. The structures of three NP receptors; the ANP, BNP, and CNP have significant similarity as shown in **Figure 5**.

There are three kinds of receptors for NPs, natriuretic receptor A (NPR-A), B (NPR-B), and C (NPR-C). NPR-B is biologically least active. The main effects are carried out by A and C. NPR-A acts as a stimulatory receptor which regulates most of actions of both ANP and BNP. In contrast, the NPR-C is associated with destruction of the ANP and BNP.

It is now understood that the receptor system C (NPR-C) is not the only system that regulate the destruction and neutralization of NPs. One other mechanism by which NPs are neutralized and inactivated is by "endopeptidase system" called neprilysin. There is great interest in this after the clinical studies have shown that its modulation by ARNIs can result in mortality reduction in HFrEF.

The "NPR-C" receptors are in adipose tissue and kidney while neprilysin is seen in high concentrations in vascular endothelium, cardiomyocytes, and fibroblasts. Both NPR-C and neprilysin play an important role in the body by controlling the degradation of NPs.

HEMODYNAMIC CHANGES

Hemodynamic changes depend on the inciting event (acute/chronic), etiology (ischemia, inflammation, and toxic), and the hemodynamic burden (volume overload/pressure overload). Acute events tend to preserve the ventricular size with rapid increase in pressures while in chronic HF, the pressures are compensated by volume expansion.

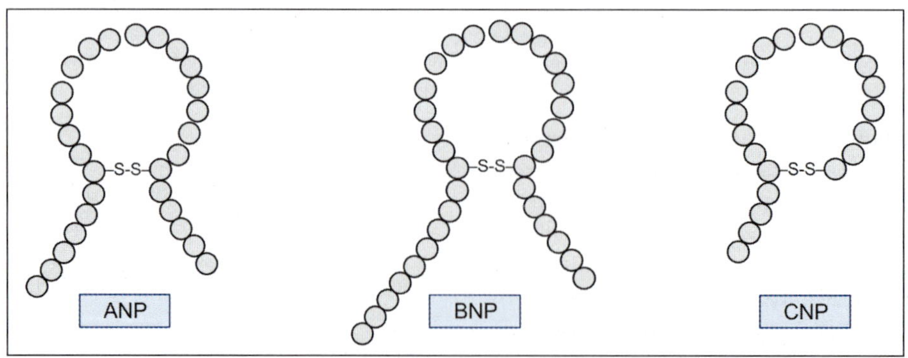

(ANP: atrial natriuretic peptide; BNP: B-type natriuretic peptide; CNP: C-type natriuretic peptide)

FIGURE 5: The structural similarity of the three natriuretic peptide receptors, the ANP, BNP and CNP.

BOX 1	Effects of increased wall stress.
	• Stretch activates relatively suppressed genes. It causes neurohormonal activation and causes a proinflammatory condition by activation of tumor necrosis factor (TNF) and interleukin-6 (IL-6)
	• It sends signals to activate mediators of hypertrophy
	• It results in subendocardial hypoperfusion resulting in myocardial ischemia
	• It causes abnormal traction on the papillary muscle and results in functional mitral regurgitation

Preload and afterload: *Preload* is the initial stretching of the cardiac myocytes (CMs) before contraction. It depends on venous filling of ventricle. Increase in preload increases the stroke volume by "Frank–Starling mechanism" which states that to a certain level, stretching of the myocytes improves its contractility. The curve plateaus beyond a certain level and then there is no increase in stroke volume with further increase in preload.

Afterload is the force or load against which the heart has to contract. It depends on the peripheral vascular resistance. It is proportional to the mean arterial pressure. According to the "Laplace law", the wall stress on the heart muscle is directly related to the pressure in the ventricle multiplied by the volume and is inversely related to the wall thickness. So, as afterload (pressure) or left ventricular (LV) volume increases the wall stress increases. The increase in thickness of ventricle helps to reduce the wall stress (helpful compensatory mechanism). The increase in wall stress activates some processes which are detrimental for the failing heart. These are as shows in **Box 1**.

Concentric versus eccentric hypertrophy: A pressure overload typically increases the sarcomeres in parallel, thereby thickening the myocardium (concentric hypertrophy) as well as increasing the myocardial cross-sectional area. This is typically seen in aortic stenosis and systemic hypertension. The mechanism involves activation of "calcium calmodulin-dependent protein kinase II" dependent signaling.

Volume overload, in contrast increases the sarcomere length in series, resulting in elongation of the ventricle (eccentric hypertrophy). In contrast to the concentric hypertrophy, this is driven by "protein kinase B" activation (**Fig. 6**).

The change in geometry with pressure and volume overload results in significant functional alterations in the left ventricle. The typical prolate ellipse geometry of the LV helps in propelling blood efficiently as the base of the LV contract inward, narrowing the neck while the rest pushes the blood out acting like a piston, fitting well inside a cylinder. In early HF, the shape of LV changes to a spherical shape resulting is some degree of hemodynamic inefficiency. Subsequently the ventricle dilates in size. Damage to a particular segment resulting in thinning and loss of function coupled with the shape and/or size change result in increase in wall stress as well as increased afterload.

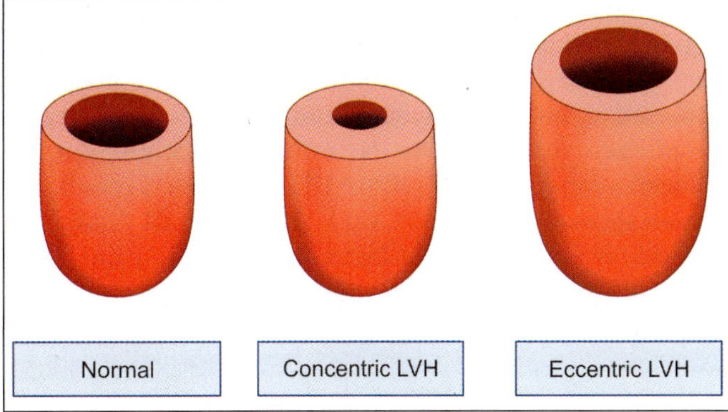

FIGURE 6: Shape of normal left ventricle in comparison with that in concentric left ventricular hypertrophy (LVH) as seen in aortic stenosis and hypertension and eccentric LVH as seen in volume overload (aortic regurgitation and mitral regurgitation).

CHANGES AT CELLULAR LEVEL

Cardiac myocyte: The hallmark of cardiac failure is damage and or destruction of myocytes, anatomically, pathologically, or functionally. The damage can occur by three different pathological processes:

1. *Necrosis*: When the myocyte damage is substantial, the cell dies. This can result from ischemia [as in myocardial infarction (MI)], inflammation (myocarditis), or with toxic damage (cytotoxic anticancer drugs). The cells tend to swell up and get destroyed. It releases danger-associated molecular patterns (DAMPs), which in turn causes features of inflammation with mobilization of inflammatory cells (neutrophils). This eventually results in a scar replacing the myocyte, which causes a loss of function of that area and increases the chance of arrhythmias.
2. *Apoptosis*: Apoptosis or programmed cell death is body's defense of selectively killing cells without setting up the intense inflammation, so typical of necrosis. Here the cell shrinks (rather than swell) and destroys the intracellular organelles into a dense apoptotic body. The tissue architecture is undisturbed and there is no scar. The process is powered by the *caspase pathway*, which is triggered by the alteration in mitochondria and is driven by hypoxia, reduced nutrition, and oxidative stress. It releases apoptotic protein which through cytochrome C damages the endoplasmic reticulum (ER). The damaged ER pours out calcium into the cytosol to trigger and start-off the process of apoptosis.
3. *Autophagy*: In cases where the damage is limited and localized, the myocyte tries to sacrifice part of its cellular organelle, proteins, and lipids. It packs it into an *autophagosome* and bundles it to be trashed. The tissue architecture is undisturbed and there is no inflammatory tissue response. In dilated cardiomyopathy, there is increase in autophagy.

Extracellular matrix: Extracellular matrix (ECM) consists of a foundation of basement membrane, over which a scaffold of collagen and glycosaminoglycan scaffold stack myocytes and matricellular proteins. Unlike older view, it is now believed that ECM is as dynamic as the CM. A specific protein called osteopontin (OPN) communicates and cross talks between CM and ECM. The turnover of collagen is increased in the failing myocardium as is shown by markers of collagen turnover like N-terminal peptide type III collagen propeptide (PIIINP). PIIINP has been correlated to mortality of HF. In the RALES (Randomized Aldactone Evaluation Study) trial, aldosterone inhibition has been shown to reduce PIIINP levels as well as improve outcomes. This is the connecting link between aldosterone and ECM turnover.

The increase in an enzyme like matrix metalloproteinase (MMP) and its modulator tissue inhibitor of MMP (TIMP) in HF alters the ECM turnover and is considered a future molecular target of therapy for HF management.

Excitation–contraction coupling (connecting link): The electrical impulse producing the action potential needs to translate to a coordinated muscular contraction. Such a healthy relationship is the excitation–contraction coupling. In HF, it can go wrong in multiple areas and understanding the complex interaction can lead to better therapeutic approaches in the treatment of HF.

The phase 0 of action potential results from rapid influx of sodium into the cell, after which the sodium channels shut off. In the failing heart, this does not happen, and sodium continues to seep into the cell as late sodium current (sodium leak). This slow sodium poisoning results in multiple adverse consequences:

- Prolonged action potential duration
- Increased early after depolarization
- Cellular acidosis
- Altered sodium calcium exchange (NCX)

All these factors tend to produce an abnormal cellular milieu, conducive for production of an arrhythmic substrate even in the absence of a scar, quite early in the development of HF. The anti-ischemic drug ranolazine acts by inhibiting this sodium flux.

Heart rate and calcium flux: In the cardiac cell, the sarcolemma lets the calcium in, by opening of the calcium channel. This increase in cytosolic calcium triggers large flux of "calcium-mediated calcium release" from the sarcoplasmic reticulum (SR) supplying the calcium, essential for interaction between actin and myosin, causing the cardiac contraction.

During diastole, calcium is rapidly removed both by the SR [by sarcoendoplasmic reticulum calcium transport ATPase (SERCA)] and sarcolemma (by NCX). Failure of these mechanisms results in suboptimal myocyte function and consequent HF.

DIAGNOSIS OF HEART FAILURE

CLINICAL SIGNS AND SYMPTOMS

The left HF is characterized by important symptoms of exertional dyspnea, orthopnea, and paroxysmal nocturnal dyspnea (PND). Nocturnal postural cough can occur. Orthopnea and PND are unique to dyspnea due to left HF. The right HF is characterized by signs of raised jugular venous pressure (JVP), tender hepatomegaly, and pedal edema. In some patients, pleural effusion (right sided more often) and ascites can also occur. Palpitations are a common symptom in conditions with volume overload and arrhythmias.

The three common and important clinical symptoms and signs of HF are orthopnea (82%), hepatojugular reflux (80%), and S3 gallop (64%). These might be missed unless there is a high index of suspicion. It is important to distinguish a cardiac from a respiratory cause of dyspnea. Orthopnea, PND, palpitations, and syncope point towards cardiac cause. Productive cough, fever, and audible wheeze go in favor of a respiratory cause. Less common sign and symptoms are ascites and gross hepatomegaly. In a cohort of 200 patients of HF, ascites, chest rales, and hepatomegaly were found in 16%, 14%, and 12% cases, with a positive predictive value (PPV) of 80% in each of these. "Bendopnea" is an unusual form of dyspnea which occurs on bending down (tying the shoelace). It tends to point to a diagnosis of HFpEF.

DIAGNOSTIC WORKUP

The diagnostic workup includes all the following.

Basic investigations: This includes blood biochemistry such as sugar profile, renal functions, and liver functions. Cardiorenal syndrome is common and hence renal function test (RFT) and estimated glomerular filtration rate (eGFR) should be calculated.

In special circumstances we need to do thyroid function tests and other specific tests like serum free light chain (kappa and lambda) to rule out amyloidosis (AL) may be required. Screening for hemochromatosis, obstructive sleep apnea (OSA), immunodeficiency states, and collagen vascular disease is done sometimes depending on clinical presentation.

Genetic testing is required in selected cases such as in arrhythmogenic right ventricular dysplasia (ARVD), familial hypertrophic cardiomyopathy (HCM), and familial dilated cardiomyopathy.

Electrocardiogram: Electrocardiogram (ECG) is often abnormal in HF. Bundle branch blocks are common. Presence of left bundle branch block (LBBB) indicates ventricular desynchrony. Ischemic heart disease (IHD) is the most common cause of HF and the ECG will show its features. Some patients will have arrhythmias [atrial fibrillation (AF) and ventricular premature complexes (VPCs)]. Holter monitoring is done for suspected or detected arrhythmias or for diseases with higher arrhythmic risk (HCM).

Chest X-ray: Cardiomegaly and increased computed tomography (CT) ratio is common. Presence of upper lobar veins and Kerley B lines indicate pulmonary venous hypertension. Prominent main and right pulmonary artery indicates pulmonary arterial hypertension.

Biomarkers: *BNP and NT-proBNP* are released from the damaged myocyte and is a sensitive marker of myocardial dysfunction. Its value is more to rule out HF in a patient who is symptomatic (orthopneic). A valve of BNP of >35 pg/mL and NT-proBNP of >125 pg/mL is considered abnormal in the HF.

In the PRIDE study, patients presenting with orthopnea, single value of elevated NT-proBNP indicated worse prognosis at 1 year. ADHERE registry showed that admission BNP value was a predictor of in hospital mortality regardless of LV ejection fraction. OPTIMIZE registry showed that compared to admission BNP, discharge BNP was a better long-term prognostic marker.

High-sensitive troponin: Introduction of "high-sensitive" troponin assay has changed the predictive value of troponin from a marker of MI to one of myocyte injury. It is now clear that large proportion of patients with acute decompensated heart failure (ADHF) may have elevated troponin levels, even in the absence of IHD.

In the RELAX AHF database, 90% of patients of ADHF had a troponin level above the 99 percentiles above the upper reference limit, and it indicated a poor prognosis.

Echocardiography: Two-dimensional echo and Doppler echo are important to make the diagnosis of HF. Ejection fraction, valve regurgitations, atrial size and ventricular thickness, and dilation all should be looked at. It is the most important investigation to make the diagnosis and find out the etiological cause.

Advanced imaging: For assessment of myocardial viability single-photon emission computed tomography (SPECT) or positron emission tomography (PET) scan can be done. Cardiac magnetic resonance imaging (MRI) is being used increasingly now in patients with muscle disease and HF. It helps to diagnose uncommon causes (sarcoidosis and AL) and to define the arrhythmic risk (HCM).

Invasive investigations: These are done only when indicated. A coronary angiogram is done in HF due to IHD. Left main disease and/or triple vessel disease with LV dysfunction are indications for myocardial revascularization. Endomyocardial biopsy may be required in patients of heart muscle disease due to infiltrative conditions.

DIAGNOSTIC CRITERIA

The *Framingham group* has grouped the clinical features of HF into major and minor criteria. As per these criteria HF can be diagnosed by the presence of two major or one major and two minor criteria. The major and minor criteria are given in **Table 1**.

The diagnostic process involves suspicion based on symptoms and physical signs. Then do an ECG and chest X-ray for further evaluation. Confirmation of the diagnosis is done with echocardiography and biomarker evaluation. For etiology further imaging or invasive investigations are done according to the pointers from the above investigations. Diagnosis of HF and its classification into HFrEF, HFmrEF, and HFpEF is important for management, which is discussed in the next chapter.

TABLE 1 Framingham group clinical criteria for diagnosis of heart failure.

Major criteria	Minor criteria
• Paroxysmal nocturnal dyspnea • Elevated JVP • Rales • Acute pulmonary edema • Hepatojugular reflux • CVP > 16 cm water • Weight loss of >4.5 kg in 5–7 days with treatment • S3 gallop • Cardiomegaly in CXR	• Nocturnal cough • Effort dyspnea • Reduced FVC • Pleural effusion • Tachycardia of >120 bpm • Hepatomegaly • Bilateral ankle edema

(CXR: chest X-ray; FVC: forced vital capacity; JVP: jugular venous pressure)

RECOMMENDED READINGS

1. Floras JS. Sympathetic nervous system activation in human heart failure: clinical implications of an updated model. J Am Coll Cardiol. 2009;54(5):375-85.
2. Sudoh T, Minamino N, Kangawa K, Matsuo H. C-type natriuretic peptide (CNP): a new member of natriuretic peptide family identified in porcine brain. Biochem Biophys Res Commun. 1990;168(2):863-70.
3. Mukoyama M, Nakao K, Hosoda K, Suga S, Saito Y, Ogawa Y, et al. Brain natriuretic peptide as a novel cardiac hormone in humans. Evidence for an exquisite dual natriuretic peptide system, atrial natriuretic peptide and brain natriuretic peptide. J Clin Invest. 1991;87(4):1402-12.
4. Korinek J, Boerrigter G, Mohammed SF, Burnett JC Jr. Insights into natriuretic peptides in heart failure: an update. Curr Heart Fail Rep. 2008;5(2):97-104.
5. Hein S, Arnon E, Kostin S, Schönburg M, Elsässer A, Polyakova V, et al. Progression from compensated hypertrophy to failure in the pressure-overloaded human heart: structural deterioration and compensatory mechanisms. Circulation. 2003;107(7):984-91.
6. Abbate A, Narula J. Role of apoptosis in adverse ventricular remodeling. Heart Fail Clin. 2012;8(1):79-86.
7. Deschamps AM, Spinale FG. Matrix modulation and heart failure: new concepts question old beliefs. Curr Opin Cardiol. 2005;20(3):211-6.
8. Kakkar R, Lee RT. Intramyocardial fibroblast myocyte communication. Circ Res. 2010;106(1):47-57.
9. Zhang W, Chancey AL, Tzeng HP, Zhou Z, Lavine KJ, Gao F, et al. The development of myocardial fibrosis in transgenic mice with targeted overexpression of tumor necrosis factor requires mast cell-fibroblast interactions. Circulation. 2011;124(19):2106-16.
10. Neubauer S. The failing heart—an engine out of fuel. N Engl J Med. 2007;356(11):1140-51.
11. Mann DL, Barger PM, Burkhoff D. Myocardial recovery and the failing heart: myth, magic, or molecular target? J Am Coll Cardiol. 2012;60(24):2465-72.

12. Small EM, Olson EN. Pervasive roles of microRNAs in cardiovascular biology. Nature. 2011;469(7330): 336-42.
13. Thum T. Facts and updates about cardiovascular non-coding RNAs in heart failure. ESC Heart Fail. 2015;2(3):108-111.
14. Ho KK, Pinsky JL, Kannel WB, Levy D. The epidemiology of heart failure: the Framingham Study. J Am Coll Cardiol. 1993;22(4 Suppl A):6A-13A.
15. Lindenfeld J, Albert NM, Boehmer JP, Collins SP, Ezekowitz JA, Givertz MM, et al. HFSA 2010 Comprehensive Heart Failure Practice Guideline. J Card Fail. 2010;16(6):e1-194.
16. Ponikowski P, Voors AA, Anker SD, Bueno H, Cleland JGF, Coats AJS, et al. ESC Scientific Document Group. 2016 ESC Guidelines for the diagnosis and treatment of acute and chronic heart failure. Eur Heart J. 2016;37(27):2129-200.

CHAPTER 93

Management of Heart Failure

Sanjay G, Harikrishnan S

ABSTRACT

Management of patients with heart failure depends on the clinical presentation of the patient and ventricular ejection fraction. Patients can present with acute heart failure to the emergency which necessitates attaining hemodynamic stability. Generally, those who get admitted with acute decompensation are sicker and have 5–8% in-hospital mortality. Readmissions are common in some of these patients, and it indicates a worse prognosis. The other mode of presentation is chronic compensated heart failure. These patients present in outpatient department (OPD) and need a long-term treatment plan. Treatment objectives include symptom relief, control of risk factors attempt to modify ventricular remodeling treatment of the underlying cause, improving the longevity of life, and rehabilitation.

Three classes of agents reduce mortality in heart failure with reduced ejection fraction (HFrEF). The renin–angiotensin–aldosterone system (RAAS) blockers [angiotensin-converting enzyme inhibitors (ACEIs) and angiotensin receptor blockers (ARBs) in angiotensin receptor-neprilysin inhibitor (ARNIs)], beta blockers (BBs), and mineralocorticoid receptor antagonists (MRAs) all reduce mortality. Besides these agents, the diuretics are used for symptom relief. Patients with heart failure with preserved ejection fraction (HFpEF) benefit from good blood pressure control and diuretics for relief of fluid overload. The three classes of agents that reduce mortality in HFrEF have not been shown to prolong life in patients with HFpEF. The HFmrEF (mr—midrange) patients behave more like the HFpEF. This chapter focuses on pharmacotherapy of heart failure in detail and mentions other therapies also which are useful.

"What we have most to fear is the failure of the heart"

—S Johnson

STAGING OF HEART FAILURE

The original staging of heart failure (HF) from A to D by American College of Cardiology Federation and American Heart Association (ACCF/AHA) which has been recently revised and incorporated into Universal Definition of Heart Failure (**Table 1**) enables stepwise implementation of a continuum of measures against HF viz., prevention of occurrence, arrest of progression, control of symptoms and pathophysiology, advanced therapies, and palliation. Stages A and B call in for preventive strategies; later stages require both definitive therapy in tandem with risk factor prevention and control. The therapeutic strategies depend on the modes of presentation also which include acute HF (when a patient presents with new-onset HF or decompensation of the patient known to have HF previously) and chronic HF (patients who are in stage C or D HF with stable symptoms). The stages of HF are described as progressive and inviolate, once a patient moves to a higher stage, regression to an earlier stage of HF is not observed.

The heart failure clinical syndrome can be with reduced ejection fraction, preserved ejection fraction, or mildly reduced ejection fraction. The diagnosis is based on symptoms of heart failure and raised B-type natriuretic peptide (BNP) levels. The three types of heart failure according to the ejection fraction and their special features are shown in **Table 2**.

TABLE 1 Stages of HF.

Stage of HF	Description	Treatment principles
A (At risk for HF)	• At high risk of HF • No structural heart disease • No symptoms/signs of HF	• Control of risk factors that contribute to cardiovascular disease (CVD) such as hypertension, diabetes, lipids, tobacco cessation etc.
B (Pre-HF)	• Structural heart disease present • No symptoms/signs of HF	• Treatment of CVD that can cause HF, like MI and valve regurgitations • Disease modifying agents β-blockers and RAAS blockers
C (HF)	• Structural/functional heart disease present • Symptoms/signs of HF present	• Agents that prolong life • Drugs for symptom relief (diuretics)
D (Advanced HF)	• Refractory HF requiring specialized interventions	• Continue treatments listed under stage A, B, and C • Advanced therapies—mechanical therapy, inotrope infusion, and heart transplantation

TABLE 2 Phenotypes of heart failure according to the ejection fraction as given by the 2016 European Society of Cardiology guidelines.

	HFpEF	HFmrEF	HFrEF
Criterion 1	Symptoms and/or signs	Symptoms and/or signs	Symptoms and/or signs
Criterion 2	LVEF ≥50%	LVEF 40–49%	LVEF <40%
Criterion 3	1. Elevated natriuretic peptides 2. At least one additional criterion: i. Structural heart disease (i.e., LVH and/or LAE) ii. Diastolic dysfunction	1. Elevated natriuretic peptides 2. At least one additional criterion: i. Structural heart disease (i.e., LVH and/or LAE) ii. Diastolic dysfunction	None

(HFpEF: heart failure with preserved ejection fraction; HFrEF: heart failure with reduced ejection fraction; HFmrEF: heart failure with midrange ejection fraction; LAE: left atrial enlargement)

From here on we are discussing the HFrEF. The preserved and midrange ejection fraction heart failure are mentioned in the end where the special features of this type of heart failure are listed.

ACUTE DECOMPENSATED HEART FAILURE

Acute HF is a condition with high mortality, with 5–8% of patients succumbing to it during hospitalization. The principles of treatment include correcting hemodynamic instability, relieving symptoms, and transitioning into long-term treatment pathways aimed at improving survival and quality of life. Patients should be quickly evaluated for high-risk features (**Box 1**) and hospitalized for emergency care.

BOX 1 High-risk clinical features in patients with acute heart failure.

- Rapid decompensation
- Evidence of systemic hypoperfusion: Shock, decreased urine output, and confusion
- Tachypnea with arterial desaturation (SaO_2 <90%)
- Arrhythmias causing hemodynamic compromise: Ventricular tachyarrhythmias, supraventricular arrhythmias with rapid ventricular rate (e.g., atrial fibrillation), and bradyarrhythmias
- Acute coronary syndrome
- Metabolic/electrolyte imbalances: Hyperkalemia, hypokalemia, and metabolic acidosis
- Associated comorbidities: Pneumonia, pulmonary embolism

MANAGEMENT OF HEMODYNAMICS

Oxygen should be supplemented in patients with acute HF displaying features of hypoxia (SpO_2 <95%) and respiratory distress. Noninvasive ventilation (NIV) should be instituted when patients continue to be hypoxic. Patients who have severe distress, hypotension, acidosis, and those who do not improve with NIV need endotracheal intubation and mechanical ventilation. Assisted ventilation helps to improve the oxygenation of the blood in presence of pulmonary edema, decrease work of breathing, and thereby decrease the LV afterload. However, O_2 should not be routinely administered in the absence of hypoxemia, because of the risk of systemic vasoconstriction induced by hyperoxia.

The immediate choice of therapeutic agents depends on the hemodynamic profile of the patient. At one end of the

TABLE 3 Inotropes and vasodilators used in HF.

Drug	Dose	Remarks
Inotropes		
Dobutamine	2.5–5 μg/kg/min	Decreases SVR
	5–20 μg/kg/min	No effect on SVR
Dopamine	Up to 5 μg/kg/min	No effect on SVR
	10–20 μg/kg/min	Increases SVR
Norepinephrine	0.2–10 μg/kg/min Maximum 20 μg/kg/min	Increases SVR, causes myocardial ischemia. Generally, first agent used in hypotension after giving fluids
Epinephrine	0.05–0.5 μg/kg/min	Used when hypotension with bradycardia
Milrinone	0.125–0.75 μg/kg/min	Needs dose modification in renal failure, used in patients on β-blockers
Levosimendan	0.05–0.2 μg/kg/min	Opens K-dependent ATP channels, causes PDE-3 inhibition. Decreases SVR
Vasodilators		
Nitroglycerine	10–20 μg/kg/min initial dose 40–400 μg/kg/min (dose range)	Headache, hypotension, tolerance on continuous infusion
Sodium nitroprusside	0.3–5 μg/kg/min	Light sensitive, isocyanate toxicity use, only when BP very high
Nesiritide	Bolus 2 μg/kg Infusion 0.01–0.03 μg/kg/min	Hypotension

Note:
1. Inotropes that decrease SVR should be avoided in patients with hypotension.
2. Concomitantly, IV dopamine or dobutamine may be administered if SBP <110 mm Hg and depressed left ventricular systolic function.
3. If SBP >120 mm Hg, IV nitroglycerine may be administered.

(ATP: adenosine triphosphate; IV: intravenous; PDE: phosphodiesterase inhibitor; SVR: systemic vascular resistance)

spectrum, patients with cardiogenic shock characterized by hypotension and low cardiac output require inotropes and mechanical circulatory support. Agents more commonly used here are norepinephrine and dopamine. Patients with hypoperfusion and venous congestion, in absence of severe hypotension, are treated with agents having combined inotrope-vasodilatory effects, (dobutamine) and diuretics are added when perfusion is maintained. Patients with acute pulmonary edema who are hypertensive, require a combination of diuretics and vasodilators. The usual doses of commonly used inotropes and vasodilators used in acute decompensated heart failure (ADHF) are shown in **Table 3**.

Inotropes: Hypotension and other features of systemic hypoperfusion occur in patients with markedly impaired cardiac contractility. Such patients require inotropes that include sympathomimetic amines (norepinephrine, epinephrine, dopamine, and dobutamine), phosphodiesterase inhibitors (milrinone), or vasopressin. Systolic arterial pressures <70 mm Hg in adult patients often necessitate potent vasoconstrictors such as norepinephrine and vasopressin. However, these increase the myocardial oxygen demand and can worsen contractility. Inotropes with vasodilatory action such as dobutamine should be used only if the filling pressures are maintained. Long-term use of inotropes increases the risk of arrhythmias and mortality.

Vasodilators: In patients without hypotension, vasodilators are useful to improve congestive symptoms and act by altering the loading conditions (preload and afterload) of the heart. Apart from decreasing the congestion, vasodilators attempt to modify the contractility in a failing ventricle. Vasodilator therapy requires intensive monitoring of cardiac hemodynamics, due to their rapid and strong effects. They should be avoided in patients with fixed cardiac output states such as obstructive valve lesions, severe pulmonary hypertension, and in pericardial diseases. The various vasodilators available include sodium nitroprusside (SNP), nitroglycerin, and nesiritide (recombinant B-natriuretic peptide). Nitroglycerine causes venous dilatation predominantly and often is preferred in patients with underlying ischemic heart disease (IHD). SNP causes balanced arterial and venous dilatation. SNP is not recommended in patients with acute coronary syndrome because of intense intramyocardial vasodilatation resulting in preferential perfusion away from the ischemic myocardium (coronary steal). Nesiritide is a synthetic analog of human BNP manufactured using recombinant DNA technology, from *Escherichia coli*. This causes both arterial and venous dilatation. Novel therapeutic agents including serelaxin—a recombinant human relaxin-2 which increases intracellular nitric oxide and upregulates endothelin type-B receptors—and soluble guanylate cyclase stimulators which increase the levels of c-GMP have been assessed in acute heart failure trials and have been shown to have modest efficacy.

MANAGEMENT OF CONGESTIVE SYMPTOMS—(DIURETIC THERAPY)

Intravenous (IV) loop diuretics (furosemide, torsemide, and bumetanide) are the cornerstones of decongestive treatment. Irrespective of left ventricular ejection fraction (LVEF), diuretics relieve symptoms and improve exercise capacity in patients with acute HF. Apart from rapid decongestion, diuretics decrease the preload and attempt to improve the contractility of a failing ventricle. For patients already on oral loop diuretics, it is recommended to initiate the IV bolus therapy with 1–2.5 times the oral dose. Furosemide causes venodilatation before its diuretic action. To avoid ototoxicity, the rate of injection of furosemide should not exceed 4 mg/min.

Once the initial dose is administered and the patient is on the path of decongestion, subsequent doses of loop diuretics should be spaced appropriately, not to exceed >4 half-lives of the agent ($T_{1/2}$ of furosemide = 1.5 h and $T_{1/2}$ of torsemide = 3.5 h). This avoids the postdiuretic sodium retention and rebound fluid accumulation. Other considerations about dosing include associated impaired glomerular filtration in HF that can decrease the amount of available drug in the loop of Henle and intestinal wall edema interfering with the absorption of the drug orally. They may be administered as infusion when the response to high-dose boluses is not adequate.

In the adult patient presenting with acute HF, up to 3–5 L of fluid removal per day may be required till euvolemia is achieved, depending on the volume load. Most patients lose at least 1 kg weight per day during the hospitalization. Daily weight chart, urine output, edema, jugular venous pressure (JVP), chest rales, and blood pressure should be done. Check the hematocrit for hemoconcentration, electrolytes, and renal functions on alternate days to detect cardiorenal syndrome early.

A third of the patients with acute HF have concomitant renal dysfunction. This necessitates aggressive volume management with intensive monitoring.

During treatment of HF, some patients exhibit features of fluid reaccumulation, despite appropriate doses of diuretics. A reduction in diuretic efficacy is often driven by renal compensatory mechanisms such as activation of renin–angiotensin–aldosterone axis and hypertrophy of distal tubular epithelial cells resulting in enhanced Na^+ reabsorption. However, the effect of other factors such as concomitant drug use [e.g., nonsteroidal anti-inflammatory drugs (NSAIDs)], excess Na^+ dietary intake in provoking acute HF and in diminishing diuretic response should not be forgotten. Diuretic resistance can be managed by:

- Increasing the dose or administering loop diuretics as infusion
- Achieving sequential nephron blockade (predosing another class of diuretic acting at a different site in nephron, e.g., aldosterone antagonists like spironolactone, thiazides, e.g., metolazone)
- Ultrafiltration
- Correcting precipitating reasons (e.g., high sodium intake)

BOX 2	Common clinical factors that precipitate acute HF episodes.
• Nonadherence to therapy	
• Use of NSAIDs and other drugs known to worsen HF	
• Excess salt intake	
• Excessive physical exertion	
• Infections	
• Systemic diseases: Renal dysfunction, anemia, thyroid diseases, and uncontrolled diabetes	
• Arrhythmias: Especially atrial fibrillation	
• Coronary ischemia	
• Diuretic resistance	
• Alcohol, tobacco, and other substance abuse	
• Rheumatic reactivation in patients with pre-existing RHD	

Aggressive diuresis occasionally causes worsening of serum creatinine, though this may not indicate adverse outcomes if the volume loss is adequate. If dilutional hyponatremia results due to ineffective diuresis, as indicated by features of continuing volume overload along with low plasma osmolality and decreasing urine sodium concentration, addition of tolvaptan (V2 receptor blocker) or acetazolamide (inhibits proximal tubular Na^+ reabsorption) to loop diuretics improves free water excretion.

MANAGEMENT OF PRECIPITATING CAUSES

During hospitalization, every effort should be made to identify and correct the factor(s) that often coexist and provoke acute HF (**Box 2**). Correction of these factors will help in improvement of ADHF faster. The common drugs that can precipitate worsening are nondihydropyridine calcium channel blockers, thiazolidinediones, class I and III antiarrhythmics (can cause ventricular arrhythmias), cilostazol, carbamazepine, tricyclic antidepressants, anthracyclines, and other chemotherapeutic agents.

To prevent recurrence of decompensation besides removing the precipitating cause and ensuring adherence to medicines that are used, we should treat the underlying cause of heart failure after stabilization. Patients with underlying IHD should undergo revascularization and medical treatment to minimize the risk of acute coronary events in future. Patients with underlying structural heart diseases such as valvular heart disease should be recommended corrective surgery or percutaneous interventions based on the diagnosis.

CHRONIC CONGESTIVE HEART FAILURE

Management of patients with HF and reduced ejection fraction; HFrEF, i.e., (EF <40%) is currently centered on comprehensive disease-modifying pharmacological agents aimed at decreasing mortality, morbidity, repeat hospitalizations, and improving quality of life. The ideal combination includes a renin angiotensin blocker (ACEIs, ARBs, or an ARNI), β-adrenoceptor blocker, and an MRA. More recently sodium-glucose cotransporter-2 inhibitors (SGLT-2i) have also been shown to reduce morality.

The drugs acting on various components of the RAAS and adrenergic nervous system are cumulatively termed as neurohormonal antagonists. Patients with acute HF after initial stabilization and those with stable chronic heart failure should be prescribed the initiating doses of these classes of medications with a structured up-titration plan. However, use of BBs is delayed in patients with persistent congestive symptoms. Likewise, use of RAAS blockers is delayed in azotemia, hypotension, and hyperkalemia. Based on these, patients can be initiated on low doses of one of these and the other added as permitted by the clinical status. The effective strategy is to prescribe low dose of ACEIs or ARBs, add BBs and step-up gradually, rather than waiting for attaining full dose of one of them to begin the other. The up titration of these drugs should be cautious, graded (once in 2 weeks, to the next higher dose) and deliberate, with periodic monitoring of symptoms, blood pressure, heart rate, clinical features of HF, renal function, and electrolyte status. The upscaling should aim for maximum tolerated dose or the guideline-recommended dose. Whenever possible, abrupt withdrawal should be avoided because of the risk of clinical deterioration. If they have been withdrawn for some reason we should restart on stabilization. All patients in stage II and III and after stabilization of stage IV should be on these three classes of agents. The list of medications that have been demonstrated to provide significant survival benefits in HFrEF trials is provided in **Table 4**.

RENIN–ANGIOTENSIN–ALDOSTERONE AXIS INHIBITORS

Activation of RAAS axis, resulting in vasoconstriction, increased sympathetic tone, and eventually remodeling is one of the key maladaptive responses in HF. RAAS inhibitors have been shown to decrease mortality and morbidity in patients with HFrEF and mild, moderate, or severe symptoms, as a class-effect.

TABLE 4 Guideline-directed medical therapy (GDMT) in HF: Initial and target doses.

Class	Starting dose	Target dose	Remarks
ARNI			
Sacubitril–Valsartan	24/26 mg BD	97/103 mg BD	Double the dose q 2–4 weeks
ACEIs			
Captopril	6.25 mg TDS	50 mg TDS	Increase every 2 weeks
Enalapril	2.5 mg BD	10–20 mg BD	
Ramipril	1.25 mg OD	10 mg OD	
Lisinopril	2.5 mg OD	20–40 mg OD	
Perindopril	2 mg OD	8–16 mg OD	
ARBs			
Candesartan	4–8 mg OD	32 mg OD	Increase every 2 weeks
Losartan	25–50 mg OD	50–150 mg OD	
Valsartan	20–40 mg BD	160 mg BD	
BBs			
Carvedilol	3.125 mg BD	25–50 mg BD	Increase every 2 weeks
Metoprolol succinate	12.5–25 mg OD	200 mg OD	
Bisoprolol	1.25 mg OD	10 mg OD	
MRAs			
Spironolactone	12.5 mg OD	50–100 mg OD	
Eplerenone	25 mg OD	50–100 mg OD	
SGLT-2i			
Dapagliflozin	10 mg OD	10 mg OD	
Empagliflozin	10 mg OD	10 mg OD	
Vasodilators combination			
Nitrate-hydralazine (H) fixed dose combination	20 mg ISDN/37.5 mg (H) TDS	40 mg/75 mg TDS	Double every 2 weeks

(ACEIs: angiotensin-converting enzyme inhibitors; ARBs: angiotensin receptor blockers; ARNI: angiotensin receptor-neprilysin inhibitor; BB: beta blocker; MRA: mineralocorticoid receptor antagonist; SGLT-2i: sodium-glucose cotransporter-2 inhibitors)

The efficacy of ACEIs and ARBs is dependent on the volume status of the patient. In hypovolemic patients they can cause hypotension. To avoid first dose hypotension patients should be euvolemic when we start these drugs. Hypotension can develop in patients with significant bilateral renal artery stenosis or patients with stenotic lesions in descending or abdominal aorta also. Both neprilysin inhibitors and ACEIs prevent breakdown of bradykinin and can cause angioedema in about 1% of the patients. About 10–15% of patients on ACEIs can manifest cough due to accumulation of bradykinin. Renal function and serum potassium should be estimated within 1–2 weeks of onset or change in dose and when found to be stable, should be periodically checked every 3 months. Comparative studies between ACEIs and ARBs such as ELITE-II and VALIANT (Valsartan in Acute Myocardial Infarction) showed that ARBs are noninferior to ACEIs in reducing mortality. We should prefer ACEIs over ARBs in patients with HFrEF, unless the patients had previous intolerance to ACEIs. RAAS inhibitors are contraindicated during pregnancy.

Apart from ACEIs, ARBs, and MRAs a new class of agents the ARNIs has been added to this group. This involves a combination of sacubitril (neprilysin inhibitor that prevents breakdown of natriuretic peptides) and valsartan, an ARBs. Neprilysin also causes breakdown of angiotensin-II and hence a neprilysin inhibitor is used in combination with ARBs. ARNI was found to be more effective than ACEIs (enalapril) in the landmark PARADIGM-HF (Prospective Comparison of ARNI with ACEI to Determine Impact on Global Mortality and Morbidity in Heart Failure) trial of patients with chronic HFrEF, with an absolute reduction of composite of cardiovascular death and hospitalization by 4.7%, and a 20% reduction in sudden cardiac death. ACEIs/ARBs/ARNI can be initiated in patients with acute HF after attaining features of hemodynamic stability. A 36-hour washout period should be allowed when switching-over from ACEs to ARNI.

Renin–angiotensin–aldosterone system axis activation also results in increased production of aldosterone. Aldosterone causes vascular and myocardial remodeling with fibrosis. MRA such as spironolactone and eplerenone improve mortality in patients with HFrEF with mild to severe symptoms. Serum creatinine and serum potassium should be monitored during therapy as with other RAAS inhibitors, with caution exercised when serum creatinine concentration exceeds 2.5 mg/dL and serum potassium levels >5 mmol/L. Spironolactone decreases testosterone production and stimulates its conversion to estradiol, resulting in gynecomastia in about 10% of patients. Antiandrogenic effects are less pronounced with eplerenone which is more expensive.

BETA-ADRENOCEPTOR BLOCKERS

Sympathetic nervous system (SNS) activation is a key feature in HF and has deleterious effects on cardiovascular system in the long run. BBs inhibit cardiac remodeling, decrease myocardial oxygen demand, and have antiarrhythmic effects. BBs inhibit renin secretion and RAAS activation. They have been found to demonstrate survival benefit in trials regardless of etiology of HFrEF. Unlike ACEIs, only some BBs have been identified to have favorable outcomes in patients with HFrEF, and the prescription should be restricted to carvedilol (including long-acting form), metoprolol succinate, or bisoprolol. While carvedilol is a nonselective BB which competitively inhibits β1, β2, and α-receptors, metoprolol succinate and bisoprolol are long-acting BBs that show high selectivity to β1 receptors. Nebivolol, a highly selective β1 antagonist, having vasodilatory properties mediated by nitric oxide, did not demonstrate significant mortality reduction in elderly stable HF patients in the SENIORS trial. BBs should be started at low doses and up titrated gradually to target doses. Some patients may experience fluid retention in the 1st week of therapy which may be treated by increasing diuretic doses. Patients may be instructed to weigh themselves daily. Sudden withdrawal of BB can result in rebound HF.

OTHER AGENTS

Nitrate-hydralazine combination: A combination of venous dilator (nitroglycerine) and arterial dilator (hydralazine) has been found to be beneficial in HFrEF. Patients especially among those of African origin, in whom ACEIs have been found to be less effective. In fact this combination of nitrates and hydralazine was the fast vasodilator to show mortality benefit in the Vasodilator-Heart Failure (V-HeFT) trial in 1986. The ACEIs and the ARBs showed greater benefit and so this combination is now used primarily in patients of HF with renal failure and reduces glomerular filtration rate (GFR) of ≤30 mL/min/1.73m^2 when the RAAS blockers cannot be used.

Sodium-glucose cotransporter-2 inhibitors: Sodium-glucose cotransporter-2 inhibitors have demonstrated reduction in cardiovascular death and hospitalization due to HF in patients irrespective of diabetic status in trials such as DAPA-HF and EMPEROR-Reduced. SGLT-2i are known to cause osmotic diuresis, natriuresis, and reduced systemic vascular resistance. These class of drugs are contraindicated in patients with type 1 diabetes mellitus due to the risk of ketoacidosis, and in patients with advanced kidney failure. Because of the diuretic effect, patients with blood pressure in lower limit of normal need close monitoring.

Ivabradine: It is a selective blocker of cardiac pacemaker if current was found to have benefits in patients with HFrEF in sinus rhythm and resting HR ≥70 beats/min. It is not effective in atrial fibrillation (AF) and should be used with caution in presence of conduction abnormalities.

Digoxin, often used in patients with HF and AF, did not confer any long-term survival benefit, though was shown to decrease hospitalizations for HF.

Diuretics, as described previously, confer symptomatic benefit without any effect on survival, barring MRA. Various classes of diuretics are available for treatment of patients with HF, though loop diuretics are the most preferred.

Correcting iron deficiency using parenteral preparations have been found to decrease mortality and improve functional capacity in patients with HF. Iron deficiency is defined as serum ferritin <100 ng/dL or ferritin 100–299 ng/dL *plus* transferrin saturation <20%. Oral preparations, with inconsistent GI absorption, have not been found to be as useful.

Vaccination for *Haemophilus influenzae* and pneumococcus should be done yearly and every 5 years, respectively. Patients of heart failure have frequent chest infections and preventive vaccination has been shown to be beneficial.

The essence of management of HFrEF is to combined therapies so as to impart maximal benefit to the patient. In those who do not response we need to add additional therapies in a stepwise manner. The treatment algorithm guide as given in the 2016 European Society of Cardiology (ESC) guidelines on heart failure is given in **Flowchart 1**. The 2017 ACC/AHA algorithm is given in **Flowchart 2** and is essentially similar to the ESC algorithm although there are some subtle differences. The Indian guidelines depict the treatment choices in a stepwise manner according to the distance from the center as shown in **Figure 1**.

NONPHARMACOLOGICAL TREATMENT

Devices are very important part of treatment of HFrEF. *Cardiac resynchronization therapy* with biventricular pacemakers helps to improve left ventricular (LV) contraction (resynchronization). These are indicated in significantly symptomatic patients with prolonged QRS duration (>120 ms) and left bundle branch block with ejection fraction of <30%. Those with prolonged PR interval and mitral regurgitation derive greater benefit. Though the primary myocardial pathology is not corrected, the adverse remodeling often improves in those who respond to the treatment (about 66%).

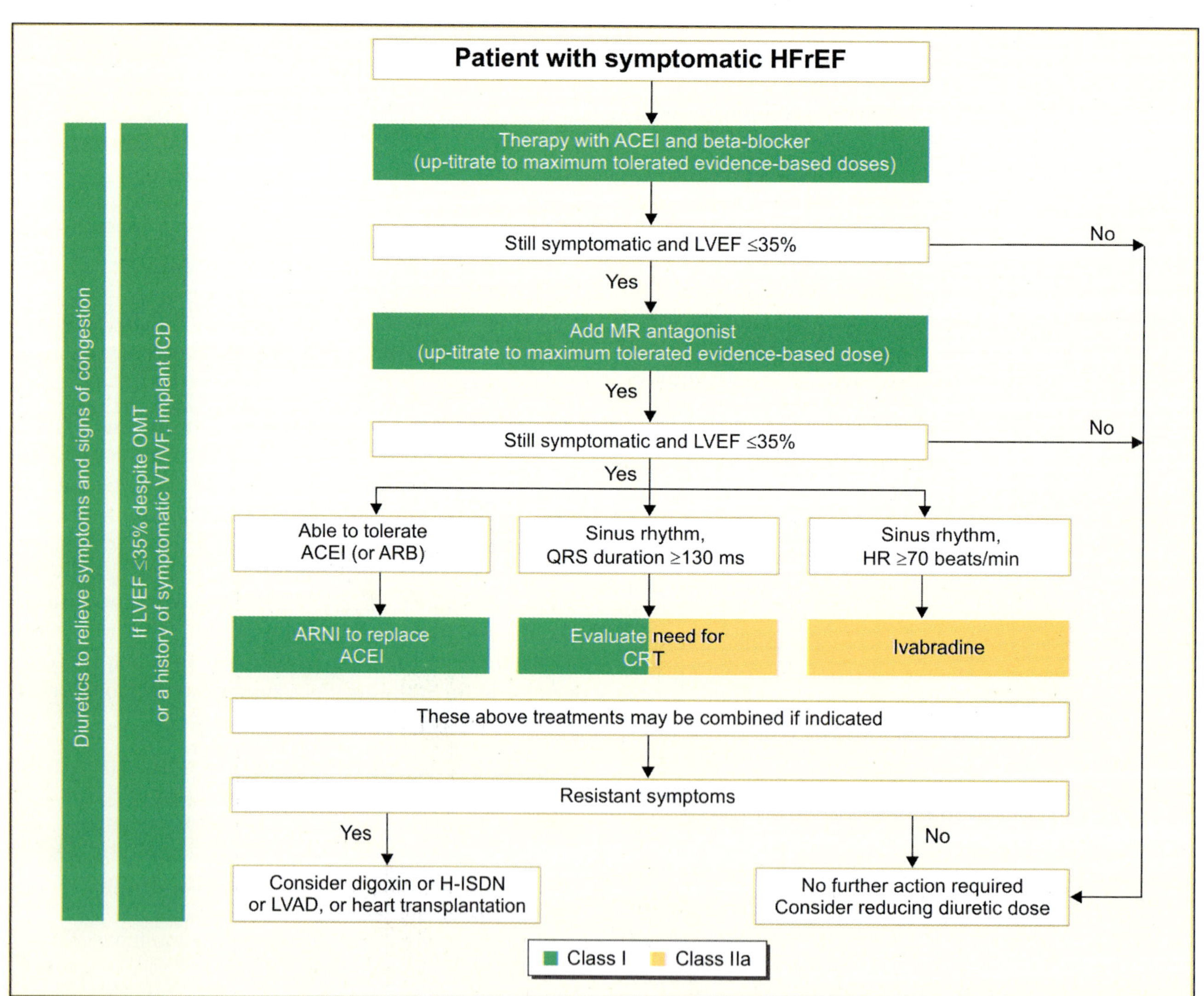

(CRT: cardiac resynchronization therapy; ESC: European Society of Cardiology; H-ISDN: hydralazine and isosorbide dinitrate; ICD: implantable cardioverter-defibrillator; LVAD: left ventricular assist device; MR: mineralocorticoid receptor; OMT: optimal medical therapy)

FLOWCHART 1: 2016 ESC guidelines for management of HFrEF.

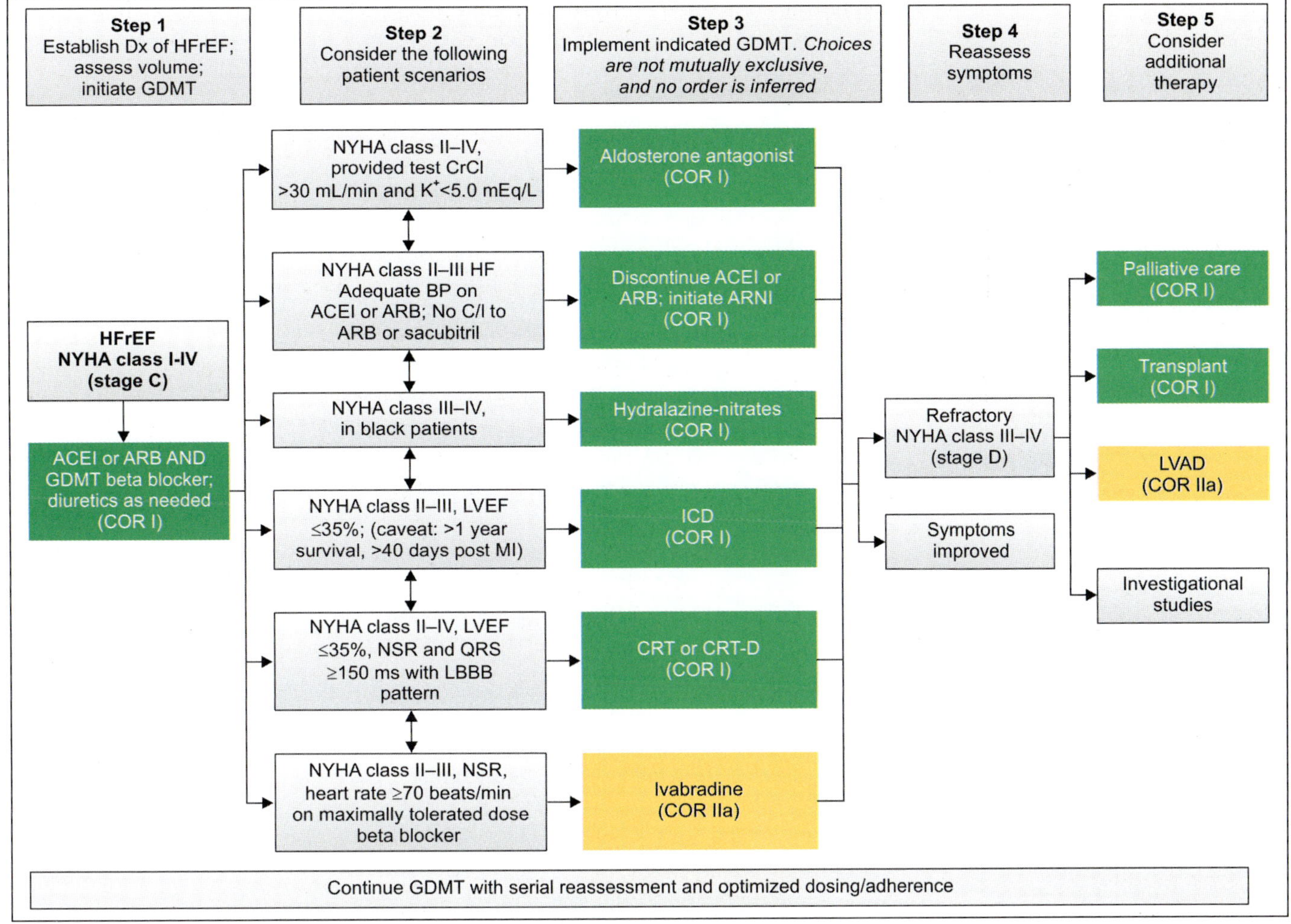

(COR: class of recommendation; CRT: cardiac resynchronization therapy; GDMT: guideline-directed medical therapy; LVAD: left ventricular assist device)

FLOWCHART 2: 2017 ACC/AHA guidelines algorithm for management of HFrEF.

In patients with ejection fraction of <30% sudden death is common. An *automatic implantable cardioverter-defibrillator (AICD)* has been shown to reduce mortality in those with documented ventricular arrhythmias and syncope (secondary prophylaxis) and even in those without documented arrhythmias (primary prophylaxis). AICDs and CRT combined devices are also available and are known as "Combo device." These are expensive but help reduce mortality significantly in those where indicated.

TREATMENT OF UNDERLYING DISEASE

It is very important. Since *coronary artery disease* (*CAD*) is the most common cause of heart failure, in some patients revascularization [surgery or percutaneous coronary intervention (PCI)] is useful especially where viable ischemia myocardium is documented. Option of surgery and PCI must be explored in patients with heart failure due to IHD.

MECHANICAL ABNORMALITY

It can be corrected in some patients. In those with secondary severe mitral regurgitation due to IHD surgery with repair or replacement has been helpful. More recently percutaneous initial clip application with mitraclip has been shown to be beneficial even in patients with dilated benefits and secondary severe mitral regurgitation in dilated cardiomyopathy.

In patients who are terminally ill with very low ejection fraction and require repeated hospitalization *LV assist devices* have been shown to be beneficial. Initially they were used as a "bride to heart transplantation." Now with their documented survival benefits the LV assist devices are used as "end therapy" also. The earlier HeartMate 2 device is less expensive. The HeartMate 3 is technically more proficient and has 2 years survival rates of 70%.

HEART TRANSPLANTATION

The heart transplantation is increasingly being done for terminally sick patients of heart failure. The 5-year survival rate is 50%. The difficulty in finding cadaveric donors, lack of public awareness, problems of declaring brain death, and developing a program are some of the obstacles in it being used more. However, many centers in

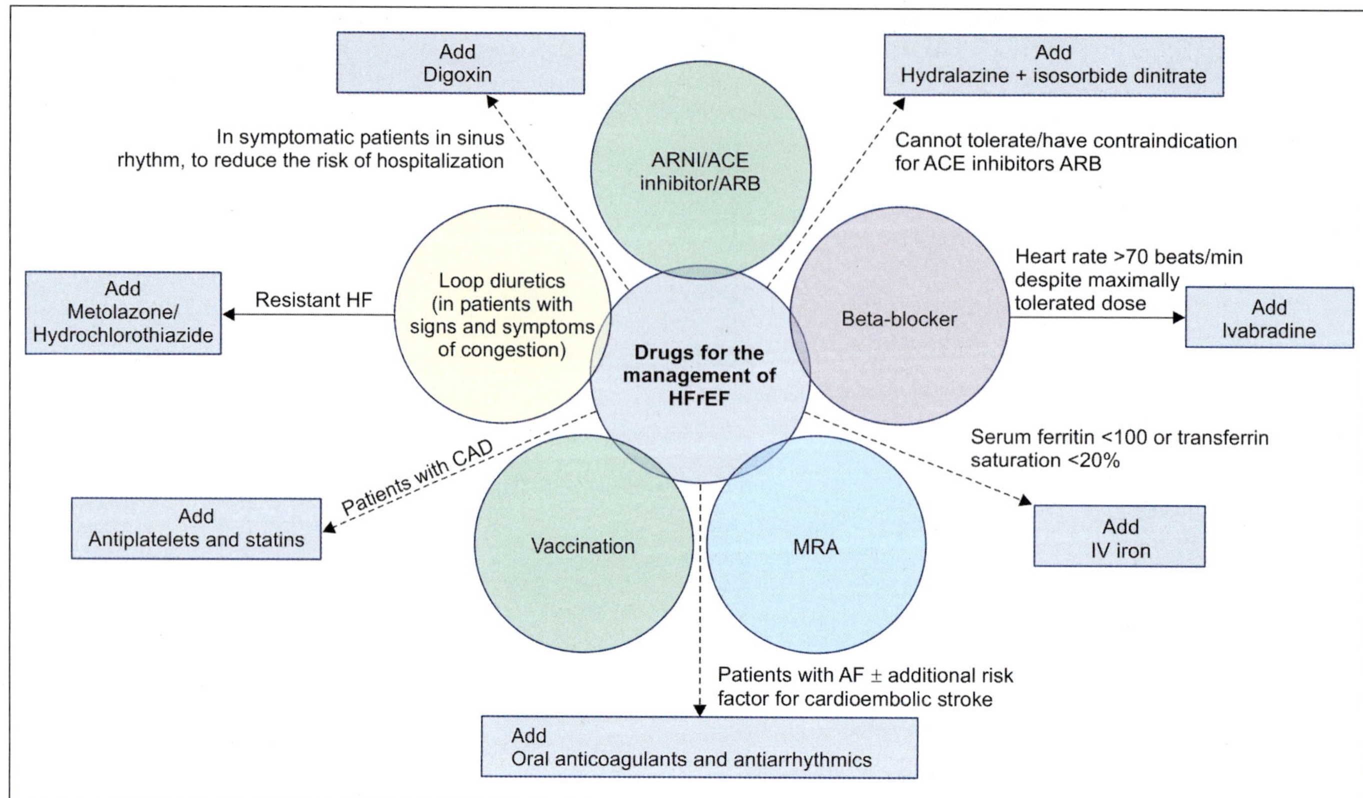

FIGURE 1: Management protocols for chronic heart failure in India consensus document published in Indian Heart Journal. 2018;70: 105-27.

India now have a heart transplant program and they have sick patients listed in the clinics for the same.

HFpEF AND HFmrEF

About half of all heart failure patients in the high-income countries are comprised of patients having LVEF ≥50% and predominant diastolic dysfunction; HFpEF. However, registry-based data from India point to lesser prevalence of HFpEF. Patients with HFpEF are often elderly, have higher prevalence of cardiovascular risk factors, and coexisting medical illnesses. Though cardiovascular mortality is lesser in HFpEF, the incidence of other causes of mortality is higher among them. Treatment is focused on alleviation of symptoms, improving risk factors, and comorbidities. No specific therapy has been found to confer mortality reduction. Good blood pressure control, rate control if AF is present, and low-dose diuretics are the main treatment. Associated diseases like anemia, obstructive sleep apnea (OSA), and respiratory problems need to be managed effectively. RAAS blockers and β-blockers do not impart any mortality benefits in HFpEF. Patients with LVEF between 41 and 49% are categorized as HFmrEF and often exhibit features of either groups.

HEART FAILURE CLINICS

The heart failure clinics help in cardiac rehabilitation and regular follow-up of these patients. Institution of disease-modifying therapy at the earliest is tantamount to improve the survival of patients with HF, especially in those with depressed LVEF. Only a fourth of eligible patients have been found to be prescribed GDMT in the Asian HF trial. We should give the ACEIs/ARBs, β-blockers, and MRAs in maximally tolerated or recommended doses to patients with chronic congestive cardiac failure (CCF). In this context, dedicated HF clinics can improve focused care of such patients which will translate into improvement of quality and length of life. Such clinics may effectively institute structured exercise training programs and help to improve the drug compliance of patients.

RECOMMENDED READINGS

1. Yancy CW, Jessup M, Bozkurt B, Butler J, Casey DE Jr, Drazner MH, et al. 2013 ACCF/AHA guideline for the management of heart failure: a report of the American College of Cardiology Foundation/American Heart Association Task Force on practice guidelines. Circulation. 2013;128(16):e240-327.

2. Bozkurt B, Coats AJS, Tsutsui H, Abdelhamid CM, Adamopoulos S, Albert N, et al. Universal definition and classification of heart failure: A report of the Heart Failure Society of America, Heart Failure Association of the European Society of Cardiology, Japanese Heart Failure Society and Writing Committee of the Universal Definition of Heart Failure: Endorsed by Canadian Heart Failure Society, Heart Failure Association of India, the Cardiac Society of Australia and New Zealand, and the Chinese Heart Failure Association. Eur J Heart Fail. 2021 Mar;23(3):352-80.
3. Farmakis D, Agostoni P, Baholli L, Bautin A, Comin-Colet J, Crespo-Leiro MG, et al. A pragmatic approach to the use of inotropes for the management of acute and advanced heart failure: An expert panel consensus. Int J Cardiol. 2019;297:83-90.
4. Hollenberg SM, Warner Stevenson L, Ahmad T, Amin VJ, Bozkurt B, Butler J, et al. 2019 ACC Expert Consensus Decision Pathway on Risk Assessment, Management, and Clinical Trajectory of Patients Hospitalized With Heart Failure: A Report of the American College of Cardiology Solution Set Oversight Committee. J Am Coll Cardiol. 2019;74(15):1966-2011.
5. Grodin JL, Stevens SR, de Las Fuentes L, Kiernan M, Birati EY, Gupta D et al. Intensification of Medication Therapy for Cardiorenal Syndrome in Acute Decompensated Heart Failure. J Card Fail. 2016;22(1): 26-32.
6. Costanzo MR. Hypertonic Saline: The Genesis of the Exodus of Fluid in Heart Failure? JACC Heart Fail. 2020;8(3):209-11.
7. Maddox TM, Januzzi JL Jr, Allen LA, Breathett K, Butler J, Davis LL, et al. 2021 Update to the 2017 ACC Expert Consensus Decision Pathway for Optimization of Heart Failure Treatment: Answers to 10 Pivotal Issues About Heart Failure With Reduced Ejection Fraction: A Report of the American College of Cardiology Solution Set Oversight Committee. J Am Coll Cardiol. 2021;77(6):772-810.
8. McMurray JJ, Packer M, Desai AS, Gong J, Lefkowitz MP, Rizkala AR, et al.; PARADIGM-HF Investigators and Committees. Angiotensin-neprilysin inhibition versus enalapril in heart failure. N Engl J Med. 2014;371(11):993-1004.
9. Harikrishnan S, Jeemon P, Ganapathi S, Agarwal A, Viswanathan S, Sreedharan M, et al. Five-year mortality and readmission rates in patients with heart failure in India: Results from the Trivandrum heart failure registry. Int J Cardiol. 2021;326:139-43.
10. Vaduganathan M, Claggett BL, Jhund PS, Cunningham JW, Pedro Ferreira J, Zannad F, et al. Estimating lifetime benefits of comprehensive disease-modifying pharmacological therapies in patients with heart failure with reduced ejection fraction: a comparative analysis of three randomised controlled trials. Lancet. 2020;396(10244):121-8.

CHAPTER

94

Acute Rheumatic Fever

IB Vijayalakshmi, Chitra Narasimhan

ABSTRACT

Acute rheumatic fever (RF) is an autoimmune disease due to a throat infection caused by group A β-hemolytic streptococci (GAS). The long-term sequela of acute RF can result in rheumatic heart disease (RHD), which can cause heart failure and premature mortality. The mainstay of diagnosis of acute RF is clinical as there is no laboratory gold standard and no treatments have been shown to reduce progression to RHD. The recently updated Jones criteria in 2015 have supplemented the major criteria with echocardiographic examination, introduction of the concept of subclinical carditis, and separation of low-, medium-, and high-risk populations among the patients. All suspected RF cases are now required to undergo Doppler echocardiography examination after the Jones criteria have been verified, even if no clinical signs of carditis are present. Primary prevention of RF consists of proper treatment of streptococcal pharyngitis. Secondary prevention of RF involves long-term administration of benzathine penicillin.

"Rheumatic fever sparks from the throat, licks the joints and bites the heart"

—Aadil C

INTRODUCTION

Acute RF and its long-term sequel, RHD, are important global health problems especially in children, adolescents, and young adults. In many developing countries including India, RHD has remained a common problem. Hence precise and early diagnosis and management of RF is very important.

EPIDEMIOLOGY

The annual incidence of RF ranges from <0.5/100,000 in developed countries to >100/100,000 in developing countries. Annually, approximately 500,000 new cases of RF occur worldwide and RHD affects ≈40 million people and claims nearly 300,000 lives each year. Most cases occur in low- and middle-income countries and among indigenous groups. RF occurs equally in boys and girls in the age group of 5–15 years and is rare in children younger than 5 years. The first episode of RF is rare beyond 30 years. Although recurrences can occur at older ages, they are rare beyond 40 years. Nearly 0.3–3% of cases of group A β-hemolytic streptococcal pharyngitis (GAS) can develop RF and nearly 60% of cases with RF in endemic communities subsequently develop RHD. The 2015 American Heart association (AHA) guidelines have risk stratified the population according to the incidence of RF. Low-risk population is where the incidence of RF in children aged 5–14 years is <2/100,000/year or an all age prevalence of RHD ≤1/1,000 population/year. Patients are assigned to the medium- and high-risk category if they are not low risk. The aim of this risk stratification is to improve the diagnostic pickup rate in high-risk endemic areas.

ETIOPATHOGENESIS

The pathogenesis of RF and RHD is a complex maze of events that are immunologically intricate, pathologically significant, and clinically devastating for the patients. The pathogenesis of RF has eluded scientists for decades. In susceptible individuals RF occurs 2–3 weeks following throat infection with GAS through an inflammatory process, characterized by rheumatologic, cardiac, and neurologic manifestations. The long-term damage to cardiac valves causes RHD which occurs as a result of a severe initial or multiple episode of RF. Chronic valvular disease can lead to heart failure and ultimately death.

The pathogenesis of RF is most likely attributable to "molecular mimicry," whereby the immune system attacks and damages body tissues. The streptococcal antigens activate both humoral and cell-mediated immune responses which produce antibodies against streptococcal components, which cross-react with human proteins in the myocardium, synovial tissue, and the basal ganglia. In carditis, activated monoclonal autoantibodies produce T-cell infiltration in the valve endothelium. Although, the genetic pattern of RF has not been fully established, it is generally accepted that an immunologic mechanism is responsible for the injury. In families prone to the disorder, it is difficult to distinguish between heredity factor and the effects of lifestyle factors such as overcrowding and poor medical care.

MANIFESTATIONS

The clinical manifestations of RF are usually a combination of fever, joint manifestations, and cardiac involvement. A smaller proportion has chorea and skin manifestations occur rarely. The diagnosis of RF is based on the Jones criteria and there is no single confirmatory clinical sign or laboratory test. The Jones criteria were first established in 1944 and since then have undergone multiple modifications, revisions, and updates, most recently in 2015. The criteria include major and minor manifestations and risk stratification has recently been applied to populations, dividing them into low risk and moderate to high risk. The words "major" and "minor" are related to their importance as a diagnostic criteria and do not refer to the severity of the process, its activity, or to prognosis.

The common presentations (the major criteria) are carditis (50–78%), arthritis (35–88%), erythema marginatum (<6%), subcutaneous nodules (<1–13%), and Sydenham's chorea (2–19%). In our prospective study of 452 cases of RF, the incidences of the major manifestations were—arthritis in 53%, carditis in 36%, chorea in 9%, subcutaneous nodules in 2.4%, and erythema marginatum in 0.4%. Polyarthralgia which has been made as major criterion in endemic areas now was a minor criterion then. It was present in 47%. Besides carditis, polyarthritis, chorea, erythema marginatum, and subcutaneous nodules, in the recent guidelines, echocardiographic evidence of carditis including "subclinical carditis" is also accepted as a major manifestation. The minor criteria are arthralgia, hyperpyrexia, high erythrocyte sedimentation rate (ESR), and/or high C-reactive protein (CRP), and prolonged PR interval.

The diagnosis of first episode of RF is made when the patient presents with two major manifestations or one major manifestation and at least two minor manifestations. In addition, evidence of preceding infection with GAS must be observed by using streptococcal serology. The exceptions to these criteria are patients who present with chorea or indolent carditis because these manifestations might only become apparent months after the causative streptococcal infection and hence additional manifestations might not be present and streptococcal serology testing might be normal. The diagnosis of subsequent episodes of RF requires either two major criteria, one major and two minor criteria or three minor criteria. **Table 1** shows the 2015 revised Jones criteria.

TABLE 1 Revised Jones criteria for diagnosis of acute rheumatic fever (2015).

Low-risk populations	Moderate- and high-risk populations
Major criteria	

• Carditis
  ◦ Clinical and/or subclinical
• Arthritis
  ◦ Polyarthritis only
• Chorea
• Erythema marginatum
• Subcutaneous nodules
	• Carditis
	  ◦ Clinical and/or subclinical
	• Arthritis
	  ◦ Monoarthritis or polyarthritis
	  ◦ Polyarthralgia
	• Chorea
	• Erythema marginatum
	• Subcutaneous nodules

Minor criteria	
• Polyarthralgia • Fever (≥38.5°C) • ESR ≥60 mm in the 1st hour and/or • CRP ≥3.0 mg/dL • Prolonged PR interval, after accounting for age variability (unless carditis is a major criterion)	• Monoarthralgia • Fever (≥38°C) • ESR ≥30 mm in the 1st hour and/or • CRP ≥3.0 mg/dL • Prolonged PR interval, after accounting for age variability (unless carditis is a major criterion)

(CRP: C-reactive protein; ESR: erythrocyte sedimentation rate)

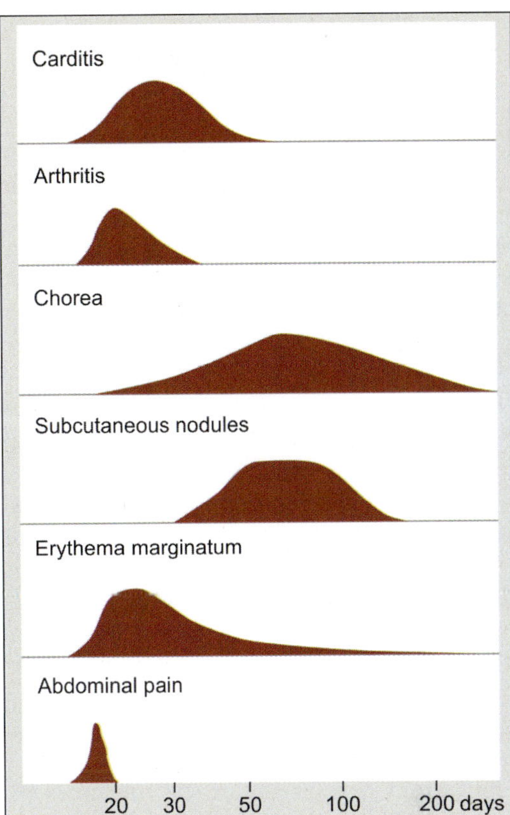

FIGURE 1: Time lag for various clinical manifestations after streptococcal infection (in days from sore throat).

The clinical manifestations usually occur 2–5 weeks after the onset of pharyngitis and the average interval was 18 days in one of the studies. The average latent period is the same for recurrent attacks as for initial episodes. Chorea and indolent carditis may occur after a long latent period of 3–6 months (**Fig. 1**).

ARTHRITIS

Rheumatic fever owes its name to its most common major manifestation which is involvement of the joints "rheumatism," even though carditis is far more serious and important manifestation. Arthritis is characteristically asymmetrical, migratory, and very painful. It usually affects the peripheral large joints (knees, ankles, elbows, and wrists) whereas, small joints and axial skeleton are rarely involved. The arthritis improves dramatically with anti-inflammatory therapy. It usually resolves spontaneously in 2–3 weeks. In 2015, Jones criteria guidelines polyarthralgia and aseptic monoarthritis, commonly seen in endemic regions, are considered as major manifestations for diagnosis in moderate-to-high risk populations and monoarthralgia is considered a minor manifestation. RF never causes permanent joint damage. A very rare exception is the so called "Jaccoud's type of deformity" of the metacarpophalangeal joints described in a patient with RF. Jaccoud first described the chronic arthritis appearing after frequent and severe attacks of RF.

The incidence and severity of cardiac involvement is lower in patients with severe polyarthritis than in those with milder joint manifestations. Carditis was observed in 26% of patients with red, hot, or swollen joints and in 40% of those with tender joints. Therefore prognosis in patients with severe arthritis is generally better than in patients with mild arthritis. Thus, the severity of the articular symptoms and signs are inversely proportional to the degree of carditis. In our study, out of 213 cases of arthralgia, echocardiographic evidence of subclinical carditis or valvulitis was present in 88 cases (41%). Polyarthritis is rarely seen simultaneously with active chorea, mainly due to disparity in the latency period following the antecedent streptococcal infection. The mechanism or the reason for migratory polyarthritis which is so characteristic of RF is not known.

CARDITIS

Carditis is a major clinical manifestation of RF. It is the most important and serious manifestation of RF as it results in life-long disability from its sequel RHD. The clinical presentation is quite variable, ranging from the asymptomatic patient with a characteristic heart murmur to the critically ill patient presenting in heart failure. The latest update recommends using echocardiography with Doppler to diagnose carditis and subclinical carditis in all patients, regardless of the risk stratification. The subclinical carditis is defined as positive findings of mitral or aortic valvulitis on an echocardiogram without heart murmurs or other clinical signs. This has now emerged as a major criterion. The diagnosis of carditis is characterized by valvulitis of the mitral valve or less commonly aortic valve causing mitral regurgitation (MR) or aortic regurgitation (AR), respectively. The clinical diagnosis of carditis is classically made in the presence of a pathological murmur(s) not previously present, enlargement of the heart, congestive heart failure (CHF), and pericardial friction rubs or signs of effusion. The RF causes a pancarditis involving all three layers of the heart. It can present with (1) heart murmur of MR, with or without the murmur of AR or TR or both due to involvement of endocardium (values), (2) pericarditis (friction rub, pericardial effusion, chest pain with ECG changes) may be present. Pericarditis does not occur without mitral valve involvement in RF. Pericardial effusion is usually of small amount and almost never causes cardiac tamponade. Pericarditis is the least common finding in RF. It is not seen as a sole manifestation and occurs in 4–11% of patients with acute rheumatic carditis. (3) Myocardial involvement can present with cardiomegaly on chest X-ray, signs of CHF, gallop rhythm, and distant heart sounds which indicate severe cardiac dysfunction.

The important and characteristic murmurs in acute carditis are: (1) apical soft high-pitched pan systolic murmur of MR with muffled S1 and S2, (2) early diastolic blowing murmur of AR in Erb's area, (3) Carey Coombs murmur, (4) pan systolic murmur in the left lower sternal border due to tricuspid regurgitation, and (5) Seagull murmur (**Table 2**). The murmurs indicative of carditis are usually present during the 1st week of the illness. They are present in about three-fourths of the patients who are eventually diagnosed as carditis. By the 2nd or 3rd week, murmurs will become manifest in 85% and <15% of patients with carditis will develop murmurs after the 4th week.

CHOREA

Sydenham's chorea (St. Vitus' dance) may be the sole manifestation of RF and commonly occurs in the absence of other manifestations. It occurs in about 15% of cases and is more common in females and adolescents. Chorea has a prolonged latent period after GAS infection, developing 1–6 months after the initial illness. By this time the other inflammatory features of RF have all resolved. Chorea is a neurological disorder characterized by rapid involuntary, quasi purposeful or purposeless movements of facial and skeletal muscles associated with generalized muscular weakness and emotional liability. The movements are neither purposeful nor repetitive but abrupt and erratic. The abnormal movements disappear during sleep. Child may initially become fretful, irritable, and inattentive to schoolwork, fidgety, or even severely disturbed. Physical incoordination manifests as clumsiness and a tendency to drop objects. Facial movements include grimaces, grins, and frowns. When the tongue is protruded it resembles a "bag of worms" and speech is jerky and staccato. Handwriting becomes illegible. When the hands are extended, the dorsum assumes a "spoon" or "dish" configuration due to flexion of the wrist and hyperextension of the metacarpophalangeal joints. When raising the hands above the head, the patient may pronate one or both hands (pronator sign). When asked to grip the examiner's hand the irregular, repetitive squeezes have been termed as "milkmaid grip." Although, the choreiform movements are usually bilateral, they may be unilateral (hemichorea). There may be "hung up" reflexes. Chorea is a self-limiting illness and the duration is quite variable, ranging from 1 week to >2 years and the manifestations may wax and wane during its course. Three quarters of the patients recover within 6 months. In our study, rheumatic chorea was found in 9% patients and nearly 70% had associated echocardiographic evidence of carditis/valvulitis.

SUBCUTANEOUS NODULES

They are small (<2 cm diameter), firm, painless, movable nodules that occur over the extensor surfaces of elbows, wrists, knees, ankles (**Fig. 2**) and occasionally over the spinous processes of the thoracic or lumbar vertebrae, suboccipital area, and Achilles tendon. They appear during the 1st weeks of the illness and last rarely for more than a month and have no long-term sequelae. They almost

TABLE 2 Various murmurs heard in rheumatic carditis.

Type of murmur	Characteristic feature of murmur
Mitral regurgitation murmur	• Mitral regurgitation is the most typical and most common form of valvulitis in RF • Pansystolic, soft blowing, high-pitched murmur best heard at the apex radiating to the axilla
Aortic regurgitation murmur	• Soft blowing early diastolic murmur in aortic or Erb's area. Better heard in sitting and bending forward • It always indicates significant carditis when it appears abruptly in RF
Carey Coombs murmur	• The murmur is best heard at the apex or just above it, by using the bell applied lightly. Patient in left lateral decubitus • No thrill or presystolic accentuation (unlike mitral stenosis) • It is due to acute edematous thickened mitral valve chordae tendinae in RF
Seagull murmur	• High-pitched raucous cooing or crying of sea gull murmur rarely heard transiently in aortic or mitral valvulitis

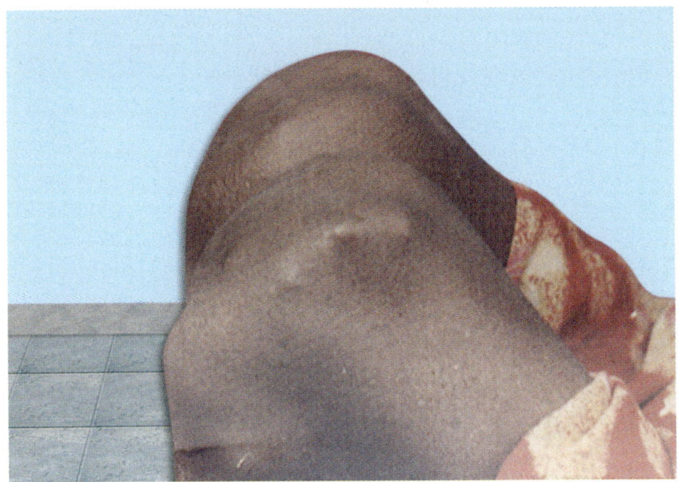

FIGURE 2: **Subcutaneous nodules** over the extensor surfaces of knees in a 12-year-old girl with rheumatic fever.

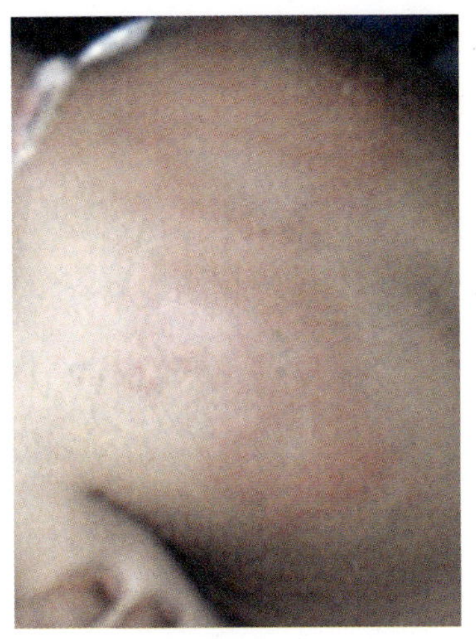

FIGURE 3: **Erythema marginatum** in a 1-year 11-month-old child with rheumatic fever.

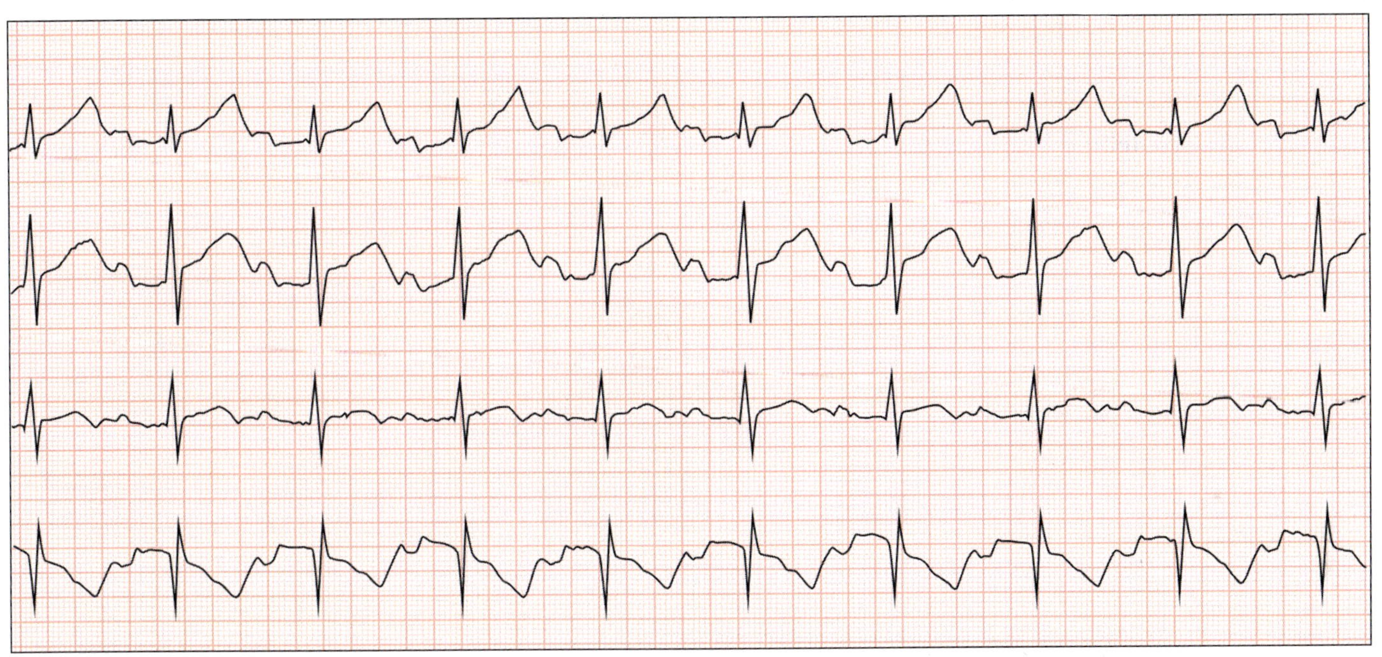

(ASO: antistreptolysin)

FIGURE 4: ECG shows prolonged P-R interval in a 14-year-old boy who presented with fever, migrating joint pains. The ASO titer was 410 units.

always appear in association with carditis. In our study, subcutaneous nodules were seen in 2.4%.

ERYTHEMA MARGINATUM

This rash may occur early in the course of the disease and may be more frequently detected with concomitant carditis. It is rare and occurs in ≤1% of the cases. This rash is an evanescent, erythematous, nonpruritic rash with pale center and rounded or serpiginous margins. It is usually found on the back and sometimes the limbs but not the face. The rash is evanescent, appearing and disappearing within hours. A warm bath or contact with hot towel characteristically accentuates it. It is difficult to detect it in dark-skinned patients. In our study, erythema marginatum was seen in 0.4% of patients. The youngest child with erythema marginatum was 1 year and 11 months (**Fig. 3**).

MINOR MANIFESTATIONS

The minor manifestations of RF include fever, arthralgia, elevated acute phase reactants, and prolonged PR interval on ECG (**Fig. 4**). Polyarthralgia is considered as a major manifestation only in moderate- to high-risk populations whereas in low-risk population it is considered a minor criterion. Monoarthralgia is considered a minor manifestation in moderate- to high-risk populations. Fever (≥38.5°C) in low-risk population and fever (≥38°C) in moderate to high-risk populations is considered as a minor manifestation. The evidence of inflammation in the form of elevated CRP of >3 mg/dL and ESR of >60 mm in the 1st hour in low-risk populations (>30 mm in high-risk populations) are considered as minor manifestations. The CRP value must be greater than upper limit of normal for the laboratory. As ESR can evolve during the course of RF, peak ESR values should be used. A prolonged PR interval (after adjustment for age) is considered a minor manifestation (in the absence of carditis). Electrocardiographic evidence of delayed AV conduction with inverted T waves may appear within 9 days after streptococcal infection and as early as 7 days before the onset of arthritis. Abdominal pain and epistaxis may occur in about 5% of patients with RF. Due to lack of specificity of these symptoms, they have not been considered a part of the Jones criteria. However, they may be of considerable clinical importance because they often appear hours or days before major manifestations of the disease and may mimic a variety of other acute abdominal conditions.

TABLE 3 Vijaya's echo score to diagnose carditis of rheumatic etiology.

S. No.	Echo feature	Score
1.	MV and AV thickness ≥4 mm	2
2.	MV regurgitation and AV/TVR	2
3.	MV prolapse	2
4.	Rheumatic nodules	2
5.	Pancarditis	2
6.	Chordal tear	2
7.	Reduced mobility of valves	2
8.	↑ echogenicity of submitral structures	2
	Total score	**16**

Echo score ≥6 is diagnostic of rheumatic carditis

INVESTIGATIONS

EVIDENCE OF PRECEDING STREPTOCOCCAL INFECTION

The evidence of prior GAS infection is needed whenever possible for diagnosis of RF. The exception to this is chorea. Any one of the following can serve as evidence of preceding GAS infection.

- Increased or rising *antistreptolysin O titer (ASO)* or other streptococcal antibodies (anti-DNASE B- ADB). A rising titer is a better evidence than a single titer result.
- A *positive throat culture* for GAS
- A positive rapid group A *streptococcal carbohydrate antigen test* in a child whose clinical presentation suggests a high pretest probability of streptococcal pharyngitis.

In the setting of RF, antistreptococcal antibodies have a high sensitivity for the documentation of streptococcal infection. Titers vary with age, season, and geography, but published normal values are available for children in the US and children in tropical settings. A positive ASO titer is generally accepted as >333 in children and >250 Todd units in adults. ASO titers can be normal in up to 20% of RF patients. The antibody response of ASO peaks at approximately 3–5 weeks following GAS pharyngitis, which usually is during the first to third week of RF, while ADB titers peak at 6–8 weeks.

ECHOCARDIOGRAPHY

The echocardiography helps in early and precise diagnosis by using Vijaya's echo criteria (**Table 3**). As per the 2015 Jones criteria all patients with suspected or confirmed RF or a new murmur should undergo echocardiography with Doppler. We look for both morphologic valvular involvement of mitral and/or aortic valves and Doppler evidence of pathologic valvular regurgitation. Serial echocardiography should be performed if carditis is not present on first examination. Also, in moderate- to high-risk populations when RF is considered likely, it should be performed even in the absence of auscultatory findings (subclinical carditis). A normal echocardiogram excludes the diagnosis of clinical carditis. The morphological and Doppler findings in rheumatic valvulitis as per the revised 2015 Jones criteria are shown in **Table 4**. Echocardiography is the key to diagnosis of pancarditis. Often small nodules are present on the tips of mitral valve which can be seen on autopsy (**Fig. 5**) as club-like nodule. On echocardiogram it gives a beaded appearance which is a characteristic feature of carditis in RF (**Figs. 6 A** and **B**).

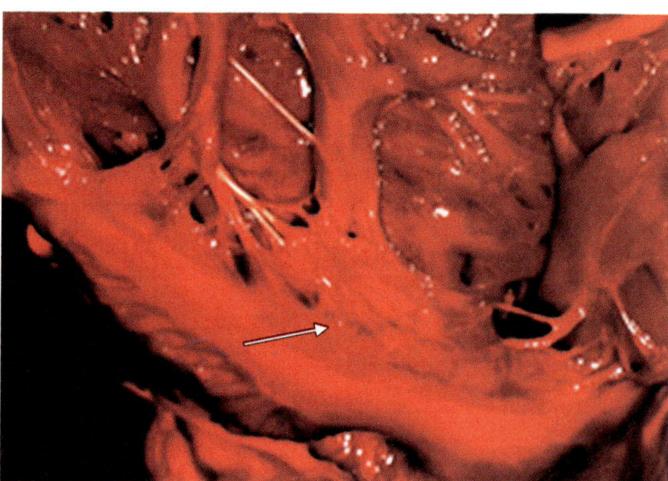

FIGURE 5: Autopsy picture of carditis shows thickened irregular nodules on the free edge of mitral valve (MV).

TREATMENT

The main goals of management of RF are:

- The management of the current infection with eradication of GAS infection
- Anti-inflammatory treatment for the symptoms of RF
- Treatment of chorea, carditis, and cardiac failure

TABLE 4 Echocardiographic features of carditis in RF by AHA guidelines.

Doppler features	Morphological features	
	Mitral valve	Aortic valve
• A regurgitant jet ≥2 cm (MR) or ≥1 cm (AR) in length in at least one view • A regurgitant jet in at least two planes • Peak velocity >3 m/s • Jet persists throughout systole (MR) or diastole (AR) in at least one envelope	• Annular dilation • Chordal elongation • Chordal rupture resulting in flail leaflet with severe MR • Anterior (or less commonly posterior) leaflet tip prolapse • Beading/nodularity of leaflet tips	• Irregular or focal leaflet thickening • Coaptation defect • Restricted leaflet motion • Leaflet prolapse

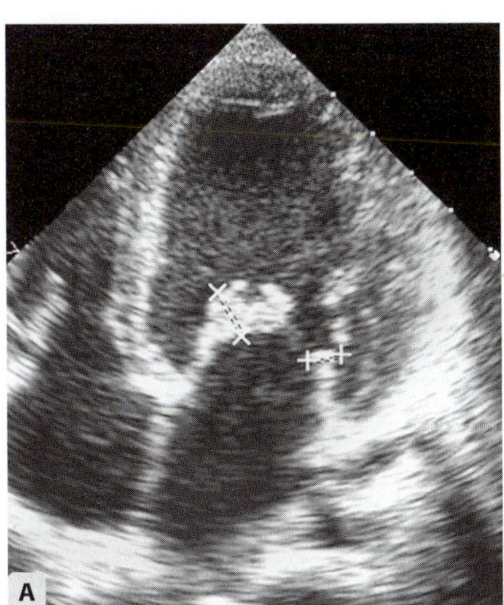

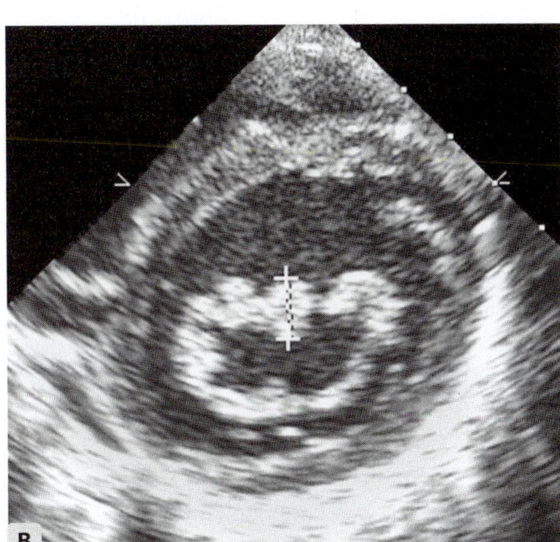

FIGURES 6 A & B: Transthoracic echocardiography in a 12-year-old girl of RF. **(A)** Apical four-chamber view showing thickened mitral valve (MV) with club-like nodule on body and tip of mitral leaflet. It does not have the chaotic motion of vegetations (distinguishing feature); **(B)** Short-axis view showing beaded appearance of MV. It is a classical feature of carditis.

- Prevention of recurring episodes of RF with long-term secondary prophylaxis and infective endocarditis prophylaxis
- Surgery for severe regurgitation

The primary prevention of RF is accomplished by proper identification and adequate antibiotic treatment of GAS tonsillopharyngitis. Diagnosis of GAS pharyngitis is best accomplished by differentiating clinical presentation of streptococcal tonsillopharyngitis from other upper respiratory tract infections (**Table 5**). The antimicrobials to be used for GAS pharyngitis are penicillin (either oral penicillin V or injectable benzathine penicillin) which is the treatment of choice, because it is cost-effective, has a narrow spectrum of activity, and has long-standing proven efficacy. GAS resistant to penicillin have not been documented. The drugs used in primary prevention are given in **Table 6**. The treatment for clinical manifestations of RF is given in **Table 7**. The antibiotics for secondary prophylaxis are shown in **Table 8**. In Indian subcontinent, as RF is endemic, penicillin prophylaxis once in 3 weeks is preferable. The duration for secondary prophylaxis is shown in **Table 9**. **Flowchart 1** shows the whole gamut of RF ending with RHD and its complications.

TABLE 5 Clinical presentation of streptococcal tonsillopharyngitis.

Common findings	Findings not suggesting of GAS infection
Symptoms	
• Sudden onset sore throat • Pain on swallowing • Fever • Headache • Abdominal pain • Nausea and vomiting	• Coryza • Hoarseness • Cough • Diarrhea
Signs	
• Tonsillopharyngeal erythema • Tonsillopharyngeal exudate • Soft palate petechiae ("doughnut" lesions) • Beefy red, swollen uvula • Anterior cervical adenitis • Scarlatiniform rash	• Conjunctivitis • Anterior stomatitis • Discrete ulcerative lesions

TABLE 6 Primary prevention of rheumatic fever (treatment of streptococcal tonsillopharyngitis).

Agent	Dose	Mode	Duration
Penicillins			
Penicillin V (phenoxymethylpenicillin)	• Children: 250 mg 2–3 times daily for ≤27 kg (60 lb) • Children >27 kg (60 lb), adolescents, and adults: 500 mg 2–3 times daily Or	Oral	10 days
Amoxicillin Or	• 50 mg/kg once daily (maximum 1 g)	Oral	10 days
Benzathine penicillin G	• 600,000 U for patients <27 kg (60 lb) • 1200,000 U for patients >27 kg (60 lb)	Intramuscular	Once
For individuals allergic to penicillin			
Narrow-spectrum cephalosporin† (cephalexin, cefadroxil)	Variable Or	Oral	10 days
Clindamycin	20 mg/kg/day divided in three doses (maximum 1.8 g/day) Or	Oral	10 days
Azithromycin	12 mg/kg once daily (maximum 500 mg) Or	Oral	5 days
Clarithromycin	15 mg/kg/day divided into bid (maximum 250 mg bid)	Oral	10 days

† To be avoided in those with immediate (type I) hypersensitivity to a penicillin.

Note: The following are not acceptable: sulfonamides, trimethoprim, tetracyclines, and fluoroquinolones.

TABLE 7 Management of rheumatic fever in patients with different clinical manifestations.

Symptom	Management
Arthritis	• *Aspirin* is the first line of therapy. The dose is 100 mg/kg/day divided into 4–5 times. In children, the dose may be increased up to 125 mg/kg/day and to 6–8 g/day in adults. After 2 weeks, the dosage can be decreased to 60–70 mg/kg/day for an additional 3–6 weeks • *Naproxen* may have equivalent efficacy with fewer side effects and is given twice daily, at a dose of 10–20 mg/kg/day
Carditis	• The *mainstays of management* are early diagnosis, severity assessment by echocardiography, management of heart failure, and other complications when present and commencement of secondary prophylaxis • In *case of mild cardiac involvement*, treatment is aspirin in a similar dose to arthritis, mentioned above • In *case of moderate to severe carditis*, oral prednisone (2 mg/kg/day, maximum 80 mg/day) is used for 2 weeks and the dose is tapered down over 2–4 weeks by decreasing the dose to 2.5–5 mg every 3 days. Aspirin at a dose of 50–75 mg/kg/day should be administered concomitantly and should continue for 12 weeks • In the *case of heart failure*, bed rest, diuretics, fluid restriction, and angiotensin-converting enzyme inhibitors are required
Chorea	• Treatment should only be considered if the movements interfere substantially with normal activities, place the person at risk of injury or are extremely distressing • Valproic acid (15–20 mg/kg/day) and carbamazepine (7–20 mg/kg/day) are now the first-line drugs and are preferred to haloperidol

TABLE 8 Antibiotics used in secondary prophylaxis of RF (AHA 2009).

Antibiotic	Route	Dose
Benzathine Penicillin G	Single IM injection every 4 weeks (3 weeks in high risk)	600,000 IU for children ≤27 kg (60 LB), 1,200,000 IU for those >27 kg
Penicillin V	Oral	250 mg twice daily
Sulfadiazine	Oral	0.5 gm once daily for patients ≤27 kg ,1.0 g once daily for patients >27 kg
For individuals allergic to penicillin and sulfadiazine		
Macrolide or azalide	Oral	Variable

TABLE 9 Duration of secondary prophylaxis of RF (AHA 2009).

Category	Duration after last attack
Rheumatic fever with carditis and residual heart disease (persistent valvular disease*)	10 years or until 40 years of age (whichever is longer), sometimes lifelong prophylaxis
Rheumatic fever with carditis but no residual heart disease (no valvular disease*)	10 years or until 21 years of age (whichever is longer)
Rheumatic fever without carditis	5 years or until 21 years of age (whichever is longer)

*Clinical or echocardiographic evidence

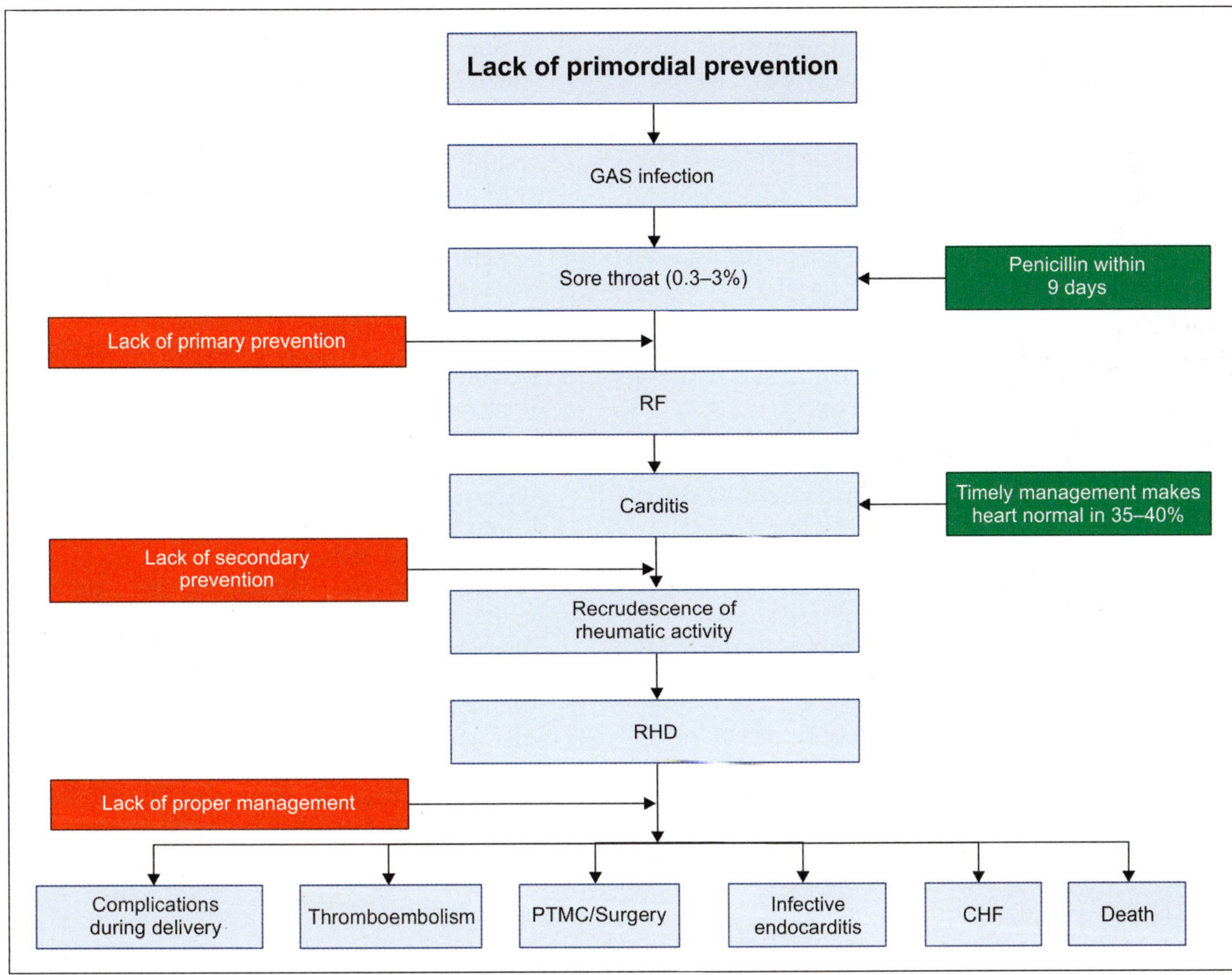

(GAS: group A β-hemolytic streptococci; PTMC: percutaneous transvenous mitral commissurotomy)

FLOWCHART 1: Rheumatic fever (RF) and its complications highlighting the levels at which prevention and management can help.

SUMMARY

Acute RF and its long-term sequel, RHD, are major health problems in children, adolescents, and young adults, as morbidity and mortality and financial burden of surgical and nonsurgical treatment are very high. Clinical profile of RF is changing. Adherence to revised new Jones criteria with echocardiography as a major criteria to detect subclinical carditis, will lead to early and precise diagnosis. Also with polyarthralgia now as a major criterion in high prevalence area it will lead to more children getting the needed secondary prophylaxis. This will avoid morbidity, mortality, and heavy expenditure on sophisticated treatment with balloon and valve repair/replacement in the future. Until vaccine is available primordial, primary, and secondary prophylaxis are essential. New Jones criteria will take the bite from RF which was known in the past as "licks the joints and bites the heart."

RECOMMENDED READINGS

1. Gewitz MH, Baltimore RS, Tani LY, Sable CA, Shulman ST, Carapetis J, et al. Revision of the Jones Criteria for the Diagnosis of Acute Rheumatic Fever in the Era of Doppler Echocardiography: A Scientific Statement From the American Heart Association. Circulation. 2015;131:1806-18.
2. Carapetis JR, Steer AC, Mulholland EK, Weber M. The global burden of group A streptococcal diseases. Lancet Infect Dis. 2005;5:685-94.
3. GBD 2017 Disease Injury Incidence Prevalence Collaborators. Global, regional, and national incidence, prevalence, and years lived with disability for 354 diseases and injuries for 195 countries and territories, 1990–2017: a systematic analysis for the Global Burden of Disease Study 2017. Lancet. 2018;392:1789-858.

4. World Health Organization. Rheumatic fever and rheumatic heart disease, 2018: Executive Board, 141st Session: resolutions and decisions, annexes, summary records. Geneva, Switzerland. [online] Available from https://www.who.int/cardiovascular_diseases/publications/trs923/en/.
5. Noonan S, Zurynski YA, Currie BJ, McDonald M, Wheaton G, Nissen M, et al. A national prospective surveillance study of acute rheumatic fever in Australian children. Pediatr Infect Dis J. 2013;32:e26.
6. Carapetis JR, McDonald M, Wilson NJ. Acute rheumatic fever. Lancet. 2005;366:155-68.
7. Bisno AL. Acute pharyngitis. N Engl J Med. 2001;344:205-11.
8. Wannamaker LW. The chain that links the heart to the throat. Circulation. 1973;48:9-18.
9. Jones TD. The diagnosis of rheumatic fever. J Am Med Assoc. 1944;126:481-4.
10. Taranta A, Stollerman GH. The relationship of Sydenham's chorea to infection with group A streptococci. Am J Med. 1956;20:170-5.
11. Bhardwaj R, Sood A. Clinical profile of acute rheumatic fever patients in a tertiary care institute in present era. J Assoc Physicians India. 2015;63:22-4.
12. Rammelkamp Jr. CH, Stolzer BL. The latent period before the onset of acute rheumatic fever. Yale J Biol Med. 1961-1962;34:386-98.
13. Jaccoud S (Ed). Lerons de clinique medicale faites a l'Hospital de la Charite, 2nd edition. Paris: Delahaye; 1869.
14. Vijayalakshmi IB, Vishnuprabhu RO, Chitra N, Rajasri R, Anuradha TV. The efficacy of echocardiographic criterions for the diagnosis of carditis in acute rheumatic fever. Cardiol. Young. 2008;18:586-92.
15. Arora R, Subramanyam G, Khalilullah M, Gupta MP. Clinical profile of rheumatic fever and rheumatic heart disease: a study of 2,500 cases. Indian Heart J. 1981;33:264-9.
16. Seckeler MD, Hoke TR. The worldwide epidemiology of acute rheumatic fever and rheumatic heart disease. Clin Epidemiol. 2011;3:67-84.
17. Rantz LA, Randall E, Rantz HH. Antistreptolysin O; a study of this antibody in health and in hemolytic *Streptococcus* respiratory disease in man. Am J Med. 1948;5:3-23.
18. Saxena A, Kumar RK, Gera RP, Radhakrishnan S, Mishra S, Ahmed Z. Consensus guidelines on pediatric acute rheumatic fever and rheumatic heart disease. Indian Pediatr. 2008;45:565-73.
19. Vijayalakshmi IB. Consensus and controversies in the management of acute rheumatic fever. In: Vijayalakshmi IB (Ed). Acute Rheumatic Fever and Chronic Rheumatic Heart Disease. New Delhi: Jaypee Brothers Medical Publishers; 2011. pp. 225-39.
20. Vijayalakshmi IB. Prevention and vaccine for rheumatic fever: How far are we? In: Vijayalakshmi IB (Ed). Acute Rheumatic Fever and Chronic Rheumatic Heart Disease. New Delhi: Jaypee Brothers Medical Publishers; 2011. pp. 265-82.

CHAPTER 95

Mitral Valve Disease

CN Manjunath, Prabhavathi

ABSTRACT

Mitral valve (MV) can be affected by many diseases. Mitral stenosis (MS) and mitral regurgitation (MR) can occur in isolation or in combination.

Most common cause of MS is rheumatic heart disease (RHD). Earliest symptom of MS is progressive exertional dyspnea due to pulmonary venous hypertension (PVH). Low-pitched rumbling diastolic murmur best heard at the apex is the hallmark of MS. Loud sound (S_1) and opening snap (OS) indicate leaflet pliability. Long diastolic murmur with presystolic accentuation and a short A2-OS interval suggest tight MS. Pulmonary hypertension (PH) is a feature of severe MS. Atrial fibrillation (AF) is the most common complication of MS and the incidence increases with increasing age. Left atrial enlargement (LAE) (P mitrale) is the earliest finding in electrocardiogram (ECG), seen in 90% of patients with significant MS. Chest X-ray may show cephalization and Kerley lines in addition to LAE. Echo features suggestive of severe MS are MV orifice area (MVOA) of <1 cm^2 and mean gradient >10 mm Hg. Balloon mitral valvotomy (BMV) is the preferred treatment in patients with symptomatic severe MS with suitable morphology.

Mitral regurgitation is classified as primary (or organic), caused by intrinsic diseases of the mitral leaflets, and secondary (or functional), caused by diseases of the left ventricle (LV) or mitral annulus. Many patients with severe MR remain completely asymptomatic for long periods. Palpitations due to LV volume overload and fatigue due to decreased cardiac output (CO) are more common features in MR. Dyspnea is a late manifestation. Systolic murmur of at least grade 3/6 is the most prominent finding in chronic severe MR. ECG and chest X-ray may show features suggestive of left atrial and LV enlargement (LVE). Echocardiography helps to identify the presence, severity, and mechanism of MR. Surgery is considered only for severe MR. Surgical options are MV repair and MV replacement (MVR). MV repair is preferred to replacement in primary MR, whenever anatomically feasible.

"A comprehension of 'the wisdom of the body and the understanding of the heart', and thereby to the mastery of disease and pain....will enable us to relieve the burden of mankind"

—Ernest Sterling

MITRAL STENOSIS

ETIOLOGY

Most common cause of MS is RHD. Rheumatic changes were present in 99% of stenotic MV excised at the time of MVR. Pure MS is seen in one-fourth of the patients with RHD and two-thirds of the cases of MS occur in female. Pathological changes seen in MS due to RHD are thickening and calcification of the valve leaflets, and commissural or chordal fusion.

Mitral valve deformity is rarely congenital. Among the acquired causes, myxoma in the left atrium (LA), severe annular calcification of MV, and radiation rarely cause MV obstruction. MS, though uncommon, can also occur as a complication of autoimmune conditions like systemic lupus erythematosus (SLE) and rheumatoid arthritis (RA), mucopolysaccharidosis, malignant carcinoid, and methysergide therapy (**Box 1**).

BOX 1	Causes of mitral stenosis.
• RHD (most common)	
• Congenital	
• Severe mitral annular calcification	
• Left atrial myxoma (mimics MS)	
• Post MV repair for MR	
• Very rarely—SLE, RA, carcinoid, radiation, mucopolysaccharidosis, and methysergide therapy	

(MR: mitral regurgitation; MS: mitral stenosis; MV: mitral valve; RA: rheumatoid arthritis; RHD: rheumatic heart disease; SLE: systemic lupus erythematosus)

PATHOPHYSIOLOGY

When the MVOA is reduced to 2 cm^2, from the normal 4–6 cm^2, a pressure gradient is generated to maintain the blood flow from LA to LV. Pressure in LA is raised, which also leads to elevated pressure in pulmonary venous circulation, pulmonary venous pressure (PVP), and pulmonary arterial (PA) pressure. As MS becomes severe, secondary vasoconstriction in the pulmonary bed causes further increase in PA pressure, and PH may become extreme. This leads to right ventricular hypertrophy (RVH), RV dysfunction, and tricuspid regurgitation (TR). Cardiac output (CO) may be normal at rest but decreases on exertion as the severity of MS increases (MVOA < 1 cm^2). Although, well-defined symptoms appear when there is marked reduction in MVOA usually to <1.0 cm^2, gradual limitation of functions and exercise limitation occurs at MVOA of 1–2 cm^2.

SYMPTOMS

Exertional dyspnea occurring as a result of PVH, is the most common symptom, and can progress to orthopnea and paroxysmal nocturnal dyspnea (PND) later. Cough and wheezing may also occur as initial symptoms. The tachycardia occurring from exercise, emotional stress, and pregnancy can trigger the dyspnea in early stages. As CO decreases, fatigue ensues. With marked increase in PH, symptoms of right heart failure (RHF) begin to appear. Hemoptysis, though uncommon, can be severe and have sudden onset. Mild hemoptysis can occur due to pulmonary infarction. Pink frothy sputum seen in pulmonary edema may be seen due to rupture of alveolar capillaries. Various causes of hemoptysis in MS are shown in **Box 2**.

BOX 2	Causes of hemoptysis in mitral stenosis.
• Pulmonary apoplexy	
• Pulmonary edema	
• Pulmonary infarction	
• Winter bronchitis	
• Pulmonary infections	

Around 15% cases of MS present with chest pain occurring due to increased pressure and ischemia in RV. MS is complicated by AF in around 40% cases. AF is rare in juvenile MS. Systemic embolism occurs in 20% of patients, with 60–75% occurring to the brain. Infective endocarditis (IE) is very rare in isolated MS (0.17 per 1,000 patient-years). Dilated LA with increased pressure causes left recurrent laryngeal nerve to get compressed causing cardiovocal syndrome, also known as Ortner syndrome. This is characterized by hoarseness of voice.

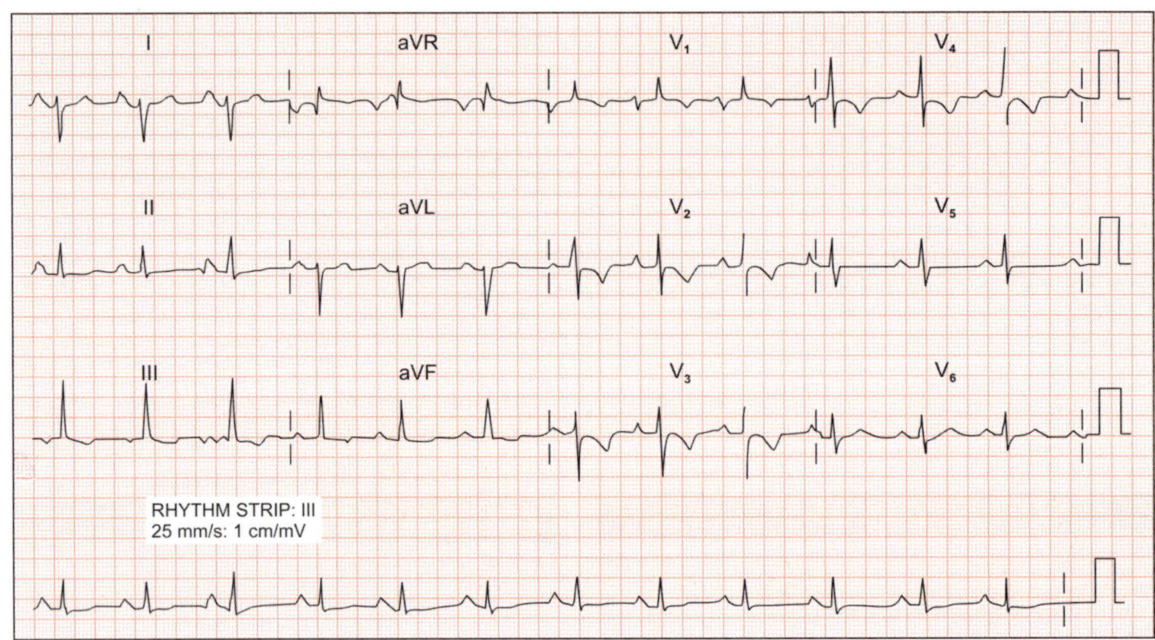

(LAE: left atrial enlargement; MS: mitral stenosis; PH: pulmonary hypertension; RAD: right axis deviation; RVH: right ventricular hypertrophy)

FIGURE 1: ECG in severe MS with PH—LAE, RVH, and RAD.

PHYSICAL SIGNS

Patients with severe chronic MS, low CO, and systemic vasoconstriction may have typical "mitral facies", characterized by pinkish purple patches on the cheeks. Arterial pulse is usually normal but in patients with a reduced stroke volume, pulse volume may be low. Pulse is irregular in patients with AF. The jugular venous pulse (JVP) may show prominent "a" wave in the presence of PH. With the onset of AF, "a" wave disappears.

In cardiovascular system (CVS), the apical impulse (AI) is usually in normal position and is "tapping" due to palpable S_1. A loud, palpable S_1 and presence of OS indicate soft and pliable anterior mitral leaflet (AML). S_1 is of variable intensity when accompanied with AF. The most distinguishing sign of MS is diastolic murmur, which is low pitched and rumbling, heard best at the apex, and accompanied with a presystolic accentuation. As the leaflets get calcified and their mobility gets restricted, the intensity of murmur decreases. Silent MS can occur in cases of very severe MS, severe PH, congestive cardiac failure (CCF), extensive calcification, and marked enlargement of RV. A less prominent murmur is heard if aortic stenosis (AS) or atrial septal defect (ASD) coexist with MS. Chronic obstructive pulmonary disease (COPD), obesity, and thick chest wall can also reduce the intensity of murmur.

In patients with PH and secondary TR, pansystolic murmur which increases on inspiration may be heard in lower left sternal border. Neck vein distention, ascites, hepatomegaly, and edema reflect RHF.

ELECTROCARDIOGRAM

Left atrial enlargement (P mitrale) is the earliest finding, seen in 90% of patients with significant MS. AF is common in adults. Tall R waves in precordial leads suggest RVH. RVH, right axis deviation (RAD), and right atrial enlargement (RAE) are seen in patients with severe PH and TR (**Fig. 1**).

CHEST X-RAY

Patients with hemodynamically significant MS invariably have evidence of LAE in the form of double density, prominent left atrial appendage (LAA), and widening of carinal angle. PA segment is enlarged due to PH. Straightening of left heart border results from prominent LAA, dilated PA, and underfilled aortic knuckle. Redistribution of blood flow to lung apices (cephalization), and Kerley lines in the lung fields reflect chronic PVH (**Box 3**) (**Fig. 2**).

ECHOCARDIOGRAPHIC FINDINGS

Box 4 and **Figures 3 A** to **D** show the echocardiographic findings of MS.

3D has better reproducibility than 2D to calculate the valve area using direct planimetry (**Figs. 3 B** and **C**). Continuous wave Doppler (CWD) can determine the mean pressure gradient across MV (**Fig. 3 D**). Echo can be helpful in evaluation of patients before BMV.

Echocardiography can assess the severity of MS from the calculated MV area by planimetry or from pressure half time. We can also assess the pliability of valve and the subvalvular apparatus. The LA cavity thrombi can be seen by transthoracic echo (**Figs. 4 A** and **C**). The clots in LA in fact form initially in the LAA as shown in **Figures 4 B** and **D** (B: Transesophageal and D: Transthoracic).

NATURAL HISTORY

Mitral stenosis has an insidious course in younger age group and accelerates in later life. The asymptomatic

BOX 3	Chest X-ray findings in mitral stenosis.
• LAE (earliest sign), prominent LAA	
• PVH: Prominent upper lobe veins	
• Kerley lines: Peribronchial cuffing	
• PAH: Dilated pulmonary arteries	
• RV enlargement, RAE	
• Calcification of MV	
• Pulmonary hemosiderosis–long-standing MS	

(LAE: left atrial enlargement; LAA: left atrial appendage; PVH: pulmonary venous hypertension; RAE: right atrial enlargement)

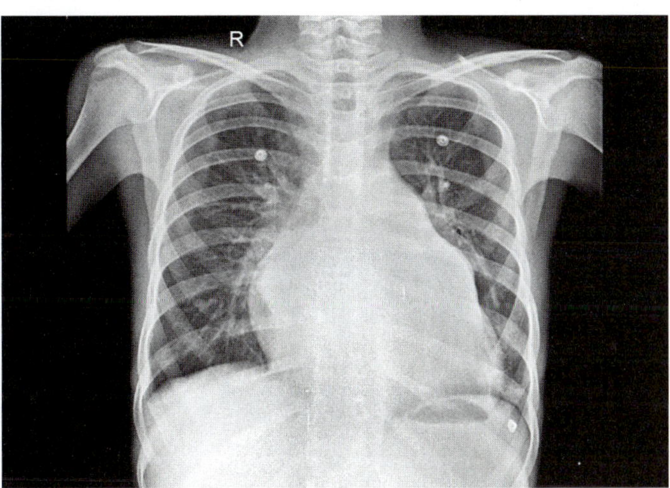

FIGURE 2: Chest X-ray in severe MS—LAE, PVH, and PAH.

period of MS can be as long as 15–20 years and progression from mild to severe disability can take 5–10 years. In India, critical MS has been reported in children as young as 6 years (Juvenile MS < 20 years). The 10-year survival rate is ≥80% which drops to the 10–15% with appearance of limiting symptoms. If untreated, death due to progressive pulmonary and systemic congestion occurs in 60–70%. The other causes of death include systemic embolism (20–30%), pulmonary embolism (10%), and infection (1–5%). 10-year survival rate is as high as 90% with timely interventions.

MANAGEMENT

- *Medical management*: Consists of the following principles**:** (A) Penicillin prophylaxis: It aims to prevent recurrence of rheumatic fever (RF); (B) Prevention and management of complications; (C) Monitoring the disease progression for timely intervention.
- BMV/PTMC (percutaneous transvenous mitral commissurotomy)
- *Surgical*: Closed mitral valvotomy (CMV), open mitral valvotomy (OMV), and MVR.

Secondary prevention of RF, preferably with long-acting benzathine penicillin should be continued at least up to the age of 40 years. Current guidelines do not recommend antibiotic prophylaxis for prevention of IE.

BOX 4	Echocardiographic findings in mitral stenosis.
• Thickening of leaflets and subvalvar apparatus	
• Restricted movement of the mitral leaflets	
• Fusion of commissures	
• Diastolic doming of AML ("hockey stick appearance")	
• MVOA decreases—"fish mouth" appearance	
• Turbulent high velocity flow with increased gradient across MV	
• "Candle flame" appearance on color flow Doppler	
• LAE, RVH, PH, and TR	
• LA thrombus (**Figs. 4 A** to **D**)	

(MVOA: mitral valve orifice area; TR: tricuspid regurgitation)

Mild cases of MS can be managed using diuretics and beta blockers. The latter reduces the increased heart rate (HR) during exertion and optimizes diastolic filling in patients with normal sinus rhythm. Treatment of coexisting anemia and infections is essential.

In case of AF accompanying MS, there is risk of development of acute pulmonary edema and shock due to LA hypertension and reduced CO. Hence, immediate normalization of HR is crucial. In chronic AF, adequate HR control is achieved with beta blocker and rate-reducing calcium channel blockers (CCBs)—verapamil and diltiazem. Digoxin may be added if optimal HR control is not achieved. A resting HR of 60–80 beats per minute and after moderate exercise, HR 100–110 beats per minute is recommended. Adequacy of rate control should be monitored not only at rest but also during activity, because in many patients, apparently adequate rate control at rest belies tachycardia with even mild activity.

Patients with MS in chronic AF are at risk of embolic stroke (at a rate of 7–15% per year). Accordingly, all such patients require anticoagulation (AC) with vitamin K antagonist (VKA) such as warfarin or acenocoumarin, with a target international normalized ratio (INR) of 2.0–3.0. After a first embolic event, the recurrence rate is increased twofold without AC. Hence, AC needs to be continued indefinitely. AC is also recommended in patients with LA thrombus. Newer oral anticoagulants are not approved for MS with indication for AC.

Balloon mitral valvotomy: For treatment of symptomatic rheumatic MS, BMV is the most preferred treatment as it has excellent hemodynamic and functional results. BMV is particularly useful when the valve leaflets are thin and mobile. Considering BMV in early course of disease can prevent AF and PH, and preserve functional status in younger age group (**Table 1**).

Indications for BMV: BMV is indicated in patients with moderate-to-severe MS in the absence of LA thrombus and moderate-to-severe MR:

- Symptomatic [New York Heart Association (NYHA) class II–IV] with valve morphology favorable for BMV (Class I)

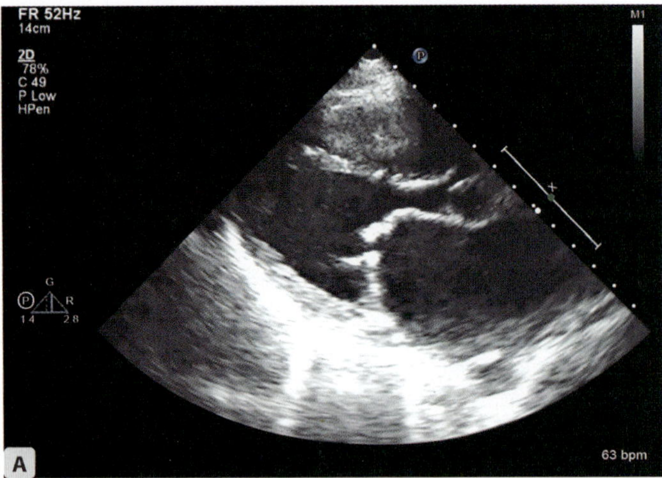

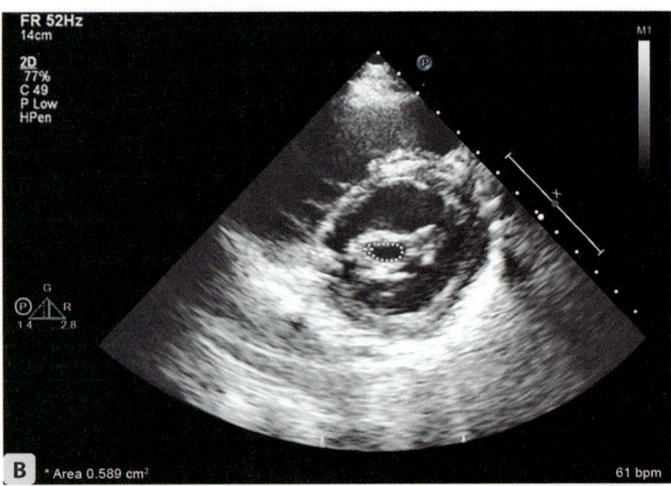

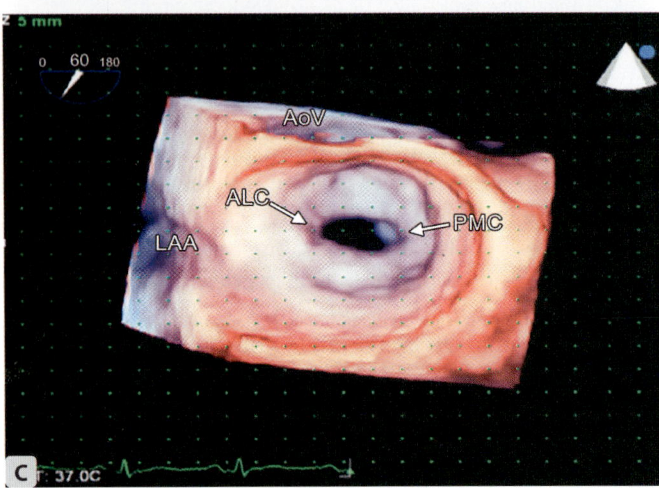

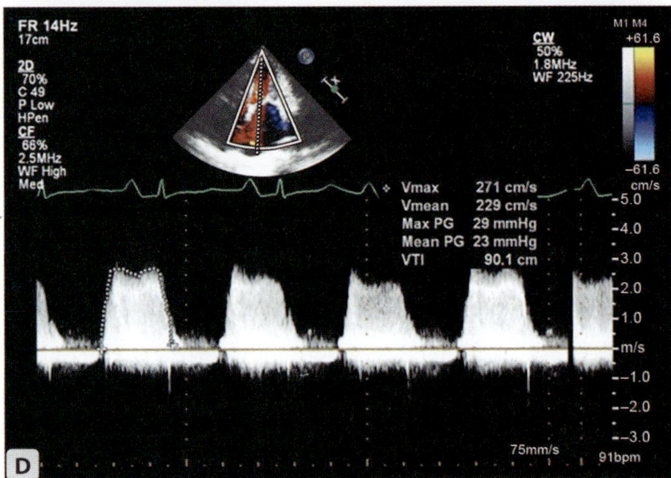

(ALC: anterolateral commissure; AoV: aortic valve; CWD: continuous wave Doppler; LAA: left atrial appendage; MVOA: mitral valve orifice area; PMC: posteromedial commissure)

FIGURES 3 A to D: **(A)** Parasternal long-axis view: Hockey stick appearance of AML. **(B)** Parasternal short-axis view: MVOA. **(C)** MVOA by 3D echo. **(D)** Assessment of severity of mitral stenosis by CWD: MV gradient (peak and mean).

- Asymptomatic patients with severe MS, MVOA < 1 cm^2 (Class IIa)
- Asymptomatic patients with PH [pulmonary arterial systolic pressure (PASP) >50 mm Hg at rest] (Class IIa)

Balloon mitral valvotomy is contraindicated in the situations mentioned in **Box 5**.

Technique: BMV is most commonly performed using transseptal technique with the help of self-positioning Accura or Inoue balloon (**Fig. 5**). Balloon is dilated and then echocardiographic and hemodynamic assessment done in the catheterization laboratory. An MVOA > 1.5 cm^2 or 50% increase in MVOA after procedure compared to preprocedure area, is considered as a successful procedure (**Figs. 6 A** and **B**).

Immediate hemodynamic results: MVOA increases from an average of 1 to 2 cm^2. Transmitral pressure gradient reduces from an average of 18 to 6 mm Hg and the PA pressure declines rapidly. MV morphology is found to be a strong predictor of successful BMV.

Complications of BMV: In general, BMV is a safe procedure with high success rate in patients with optimal valve morphology. Reported rates of complications are summarized in **Box 6**.

Balloon mitral valvotomy in special circumstances:

- *Balloon mitral valvotomy in pregnancy*: Due to raised intravascular volume and tachycardia in pregnancy, a large proportion of moderate to severe MS patients deteriorate with worsening of symptoms. A maternal mortality rate of 6.8% has been observed in the absence of any intervention, for those in NYHA classes III and IV, particularly during labor and delivery. BMV (when indicated due to worsening symptoms and MVA ≤ 1.2 cm^2) should be done in late second trimester or early third trimester when risk of radiation to the fetus is minimal. Few steps that can be taken to reduce radiation exposure are shielding the abdominal and pelvic regions, conducting procedure after 20 weeks and reducing the fluoroscopy time.
- *Balloon mitral valvotomy in juvenile MS*: Special features of MS in children are fibrotic, rubbery valve with severe subvalvular disease. Calcification and AF are rare. Significant PH is seen in majority of children. BMV appears to be safe and effective like in adults.

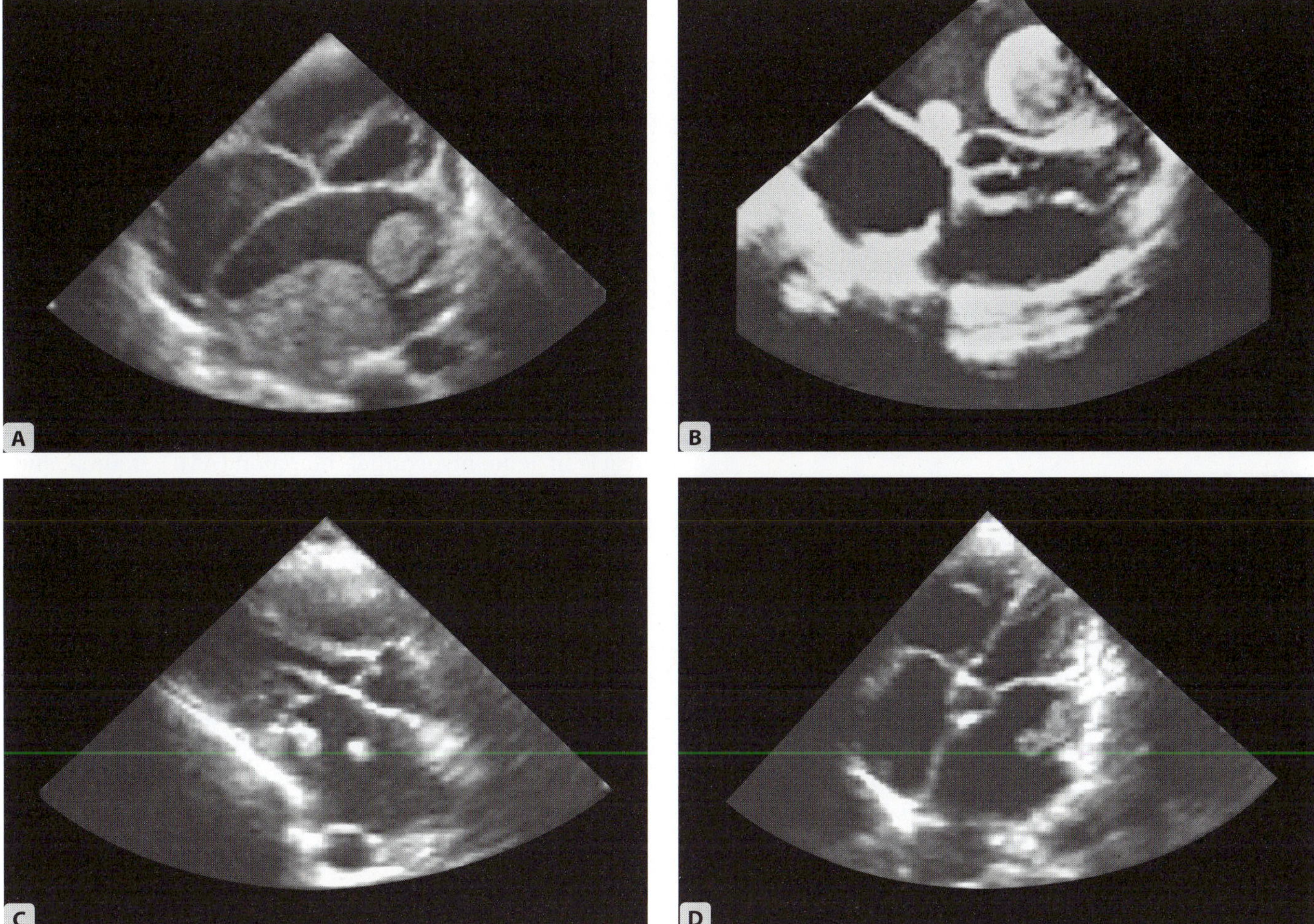

FIGURES 4 A to D: **LA and LAA clot.**

TABLE 1 Assessment of severity of mitral stenosis.

Severity	Mean gradient	MVOA	PASP
Normal	–	4–6 cm^2	
Mild MS	<5 mm Hg	1.5–2 cm^2	<30 mm Hg
Moderate MS	5–10 mm Hg	1.0–1.5 cm^2	30–50 mm Hg
Severe MS	>10 mm Hg	<1.0 cm^2	>50 mm Hg

(PASP: pulmonary arterial systolic pressure)

BOX 5 Contraindications for balloon mitral valvotomy.

- LA clot
- Grade II or more MR
- Bicommissural calcification
- Lack of expertise
- Marked subvalvular chordal adhesions

- *Balloon mitral valvotomy in mitral restenosis*: Criterion for defining mitral restenosis is return of symptoms with >50% loss of MVOA achieved after the procedure or MVOA < 1.5 cm^2 at follow up. In approximately 5 8% BMV procedures, restenosis occurs over a period of 8 years. Good results are seen with BMV in restenosis when the valve is not calcified.
- *Indications for MV surgery in patients with MS*: CMV was the procedure of choice in isolated severe MS before 1990. It is rarely done now and has been largely replaced by BMV. OMV is performed in patients with persistent LA body clot with suitable morphology. OMV is feasible and successful in >80% of patients referred for this procedure, with an operative mortality of 1%. MVR is recommended for symptomatic patients when BMV or surgical OMV is not possible because of moderate or severe MR, extensive commissural calcification, severe fibrosis, and subvalvar fusion. The operative mortality rate for MVR ranges from 3% to 8% in most centers. In patients with AF sometimes a surgical procedure called LA Maze operation or AF ablation is done along with MVR to maintain long-term sinus rhythm.

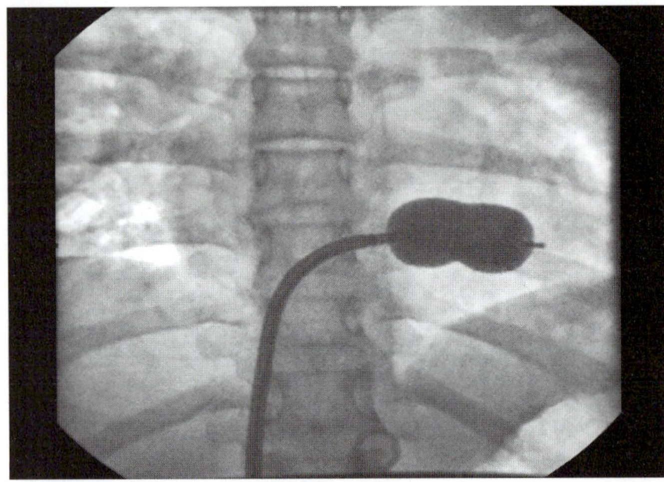

FIGURE 5: Balloon across mitral valve.

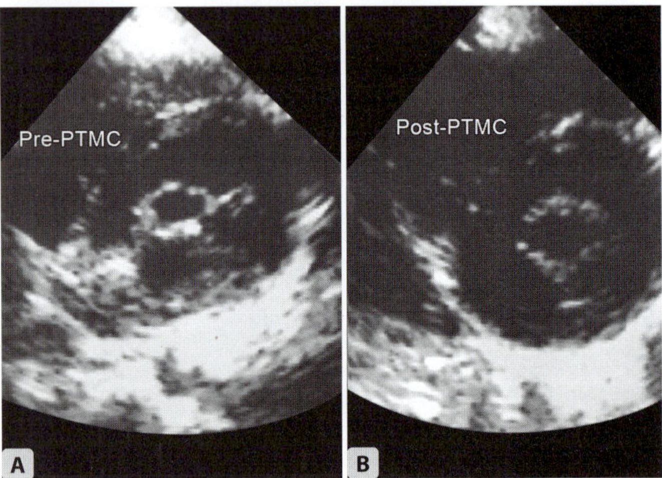

(BMV: balloon mitral valvotomy; MVOA: mitral valve orifice area; PSX: parasternal short axis)

FIGURES 6 A & B: Pre- and post-BMV—MVOA in PSX view—both commissures split.

BOX 6	Complications of balloon mitral valvotomy.
• Mortality: 0–0.5%	
• Cerebral embolism: 0.5–1%	
• Cardiac perforation and tamponade: 0.7–1%	
• Severe MR requiring emergency surgery: 2%	
• Mild to moderate MR: 15%	
• Small ASD: 20% (closes or decreases in size in most patients)	

MITRAL REGURGITATION

ETIOLOGY AND CLASSIFICATION

Mitral valve apparatus is complex. It includes anterior and posterior mitral leaflets, two commissures, annulus, chordae tendineae, two papillary muscles (anterolateral and posteromedial), and subjacent LV myocardium (**Fig. 7**). Abnormalities of any of these structures may cause MR.

Causes of MR are many and diverse. They can involve any part of the MV apparatus. For clinical purposes, MR is classified as primary (or organic) MR when it is caused by intrinsic diseases of the mitral leaflets, and secondary (or functional) MR when caused by diseases of the LV and/or mitral annulus. Chronic ischemic MR is a subset of secondary MR caused by regional ventricular dysfunction from prior MI. Primary and secondary MR are two distinctly different disease conditions, with different causes (**Table 2**) pathophysiologies, outcomes, and management considerations.

Mitral regurgitation can be acute or chronic. Important causes of acute MR are spontaneous rupture of chordae tendineae, IE with disruption of valve leaflets or chordal rupture, ischemic dysfunction or rupture of a papillary muscle in acute myocardial infarction (AMI), trauma, and malfunction of a prosthetic valve (**Box 7**). MR is usually severe in these conditions.

SYMPTOMS

The nature and severity of symptoms in patients with chronic MR depends on interrelated factors, including severity of MR; rate of its progression; level of LA, pulmonary venous, and PA pressures; presence of episodic or chronic atrial tachyarrhythmias; and presence of associated valvular, myocardial, or coronary artery disease (CAD). Many patients with severe MR remain completely asymptomatic for long periods. They may have palpitations due to volume overload of LV. Chronic weakness and fatigue due to decreased CO are more prominent features in MR. In patients with severe chronic MR who have a greatly enlarged LA and relatively mild LA hypertension (compliant LA), LA pressure does not usually rise markedly. Hence symptoms of PVH like exertional dyspnea, PND, and orthopnea occur late in the natural history of MR, only when LV decompensates. However, acute on chronic MR or new-onset AF can cause sudden increase in LA pressure and cause acute dyspnea. Development of AF affects the course adversely but not as dramatically as in MS. Right-sided HF, characterized by congestive hepatomegaly and edema, may be seen in patients with acute MR.

Vast majority of patients with myxomatous degeneration and MVP are asymptomatic and remain so throughout life. Chest discomfort may be typical of angina but is more often atypical. Discomfort may be secondary to abnormal tension on papillary muscles. In patients with MVP and severe MR, fatigue, dyspnea, and exercise limitation predominate. Patients with MVP may also develop symptomatic arrhythmias.

PHYSICAL EXAMINATION

Pulse is brisk in severe MR. Pulse volume may be normal or reduced. AF is common (less common than in MS) in patients with chronic severe MR, related to age and LA dilatation. AI is usually displaced to the left and downward and is hyperdynamic. Systolic thrill and S_3 may be palpable in thin individuals. Late systolic left parasternal pulsation due to reflux of large regurgitant jet into LA is a feature

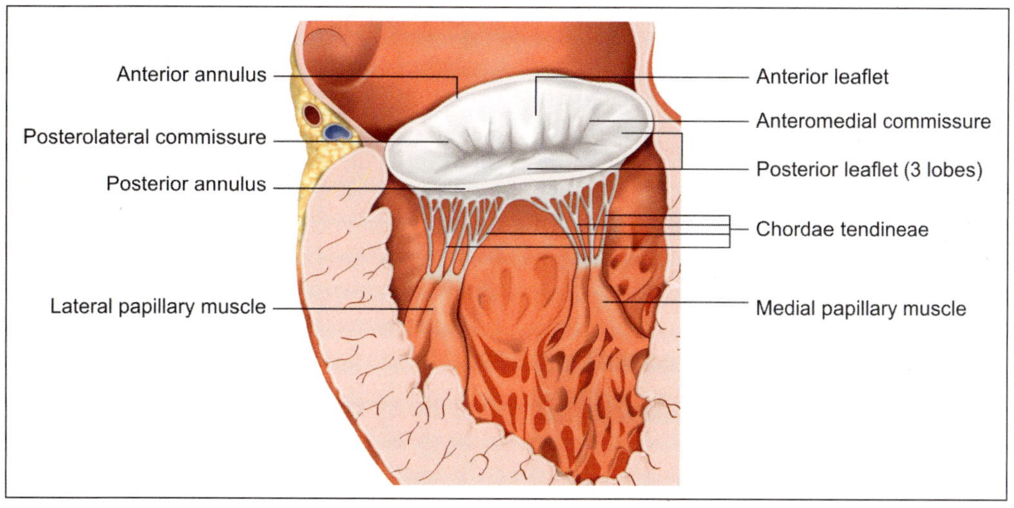

FIGURE 7: Components of mitral valve.

TABLE 2 Causes of mitral regurgitation.

Primary	Secondary
• Rheumatic heart disease (RHD) • Mitral valve prolapse (MVP) • Infective endocarditis • Congenital heart disease (CHD), cleft mitral valve • Trauma • Rare causes: Collagen vascular diseases, hypereosinophilic syndrome, and carcinoid	• Ischemic heart disease (IHD) • Dilated cardiomyopathy • Hypertrophic obstructive cardiomyopathy (HOCM) • Mitral annular calcification in elderly and in renal failure

BOX 7 Causes of acute mitral regurgitation.

- Spontaneous chordal rupture
- Rupture of papillary muscle in (acute myocardial infarction)
- Infective endocarditis
- Trauma
- Iatrogenic (after balloon mitral valvotomy)
- Malfunction of a prosthetic valve

of severe MR. This appears as a rocking movement of the precordium.

AUSCULTATION

S_1 is usually diminished in RHD MR. But S_1 can be loud in associated MS and MVP with severe MR. Wide split S_2 is common and results from earlier A2 due to shortened LV ejection time. In patients with severe PH, P2 is louder than A2. S_3 is a feature of severe MR. It results from increase in the flow across the MV during the rapid filling phase and this may be accompanied by a brief diastolic rumble.

Systolic murmur of at least grade 3/6 is the most prominent finding in chronic severe MR. In most patients with severe MR, the murmur is pansystolic, commences with the soft S_1 and continues till and may obscure the A2. The murmur of chronic MR is usually constant in intensity, blowing, high-pitched, and loudest at the apex, with frequent radiation to the left axilla (in RHD with anterior leaflet involvement). Radiation toward the sternum or aortic area may occur with abnormalities of the posterior leaflet. This is seen in patients with MVP.

The murmur shows little change, even in the presence of large beat-to-beat variations of LV stroke volume, as in AF. This finding contrasts with that in most ejection murmurs, such as in AS, which vary greatly in intensity with stroke volume. The systolic murmur of MR may be less prominent when it is caused by LV dilatation, acute MI, or paraprosthetic valvular regurgitation, or in those who have marked emphysema, obesity, or chest deformities.

Murmur of MR may also be late systolic, or early systolic. A midsystolic click preceding a mid to late systolic murmur and the response of that murmur to a number of maneuvers, helps to establish the diagnosis of MVP. Occasionally, a late systolic murmur of papillary muscle dysfunction may be noted, becoming louder or holosystolic during acute myocardial ischemia, and may disappear when ischemia is relieved. Early systolic murmurs are typical of acute MR. Clinical features suggestive of severe (chronic) MR are listed in **Box 8**.

ELECTROCARDIOGRAM

The principal ECG findings are LAE and AF. ECG evidence of LV hypertrophy occurs in about one third of patients with severe MR. Approximately 15% of patients exhibit RVH that reflects the presence of PH of sufficient severity to counterbalance the dilated LV of MR (**Figs. 8 A** and **B**).

CHEST X-RAY

Cardiomegaly with LVE and LAE is a common finding in patients with chronic severe MR. LA may be severely enlarged. Cephalization and interstitial edema with Kerley lines are seen in acute MR or with progressive LV failure. Calcification of the mitral annulus, an important cause of MR in older adults, is most prominent in the posterior third of the cardiac silhouette. The lesion is best visualized on lateral chest films (**Fig. 9**).

BOX 8	Clinical features suggestive of severe mitral regurgitation.
• Apical impulse—hyperdynamic, displaced to left	
• Late systolic left parasternal pulsations—LA pulsations	
• Wide variable split of S_2 (early A2)	
• Features of PH-loud P2	
• LV S_3/diastolic flow rumble in apex	

ECHOCARDIOGRAPHY

Echocardiography allows reliable identification of the presence, severity, and mechanism of MR (**Fig. 10**). The severity of MR can be quantitated by several approaches, including calculation of regurgitant volumes and fraction using continuity equation, proximal isovelocity surface area (PISA), or by measurement of vena contracta on color flow imaging. In practice, many clinicians rely on the simpler, albeit less quantitative, evaluation by color flow imaging in multiple views. When transthoracic imaging is suboptimal, transesophageal echo and 3D imaging provide excellent visualization of MV anatomy and allow an accurate assessment of the etiology and likelihood of surgical repair. Important echo features of severe MR are listed in **Box 9**.

NATURAL HISTORY

Numerous studies indicate that patients with chronic severe MR have a high likelihood of developing symptoms or LV dysfunction over the course of 6–10 years. However, patients at risk of death are predominantly those with

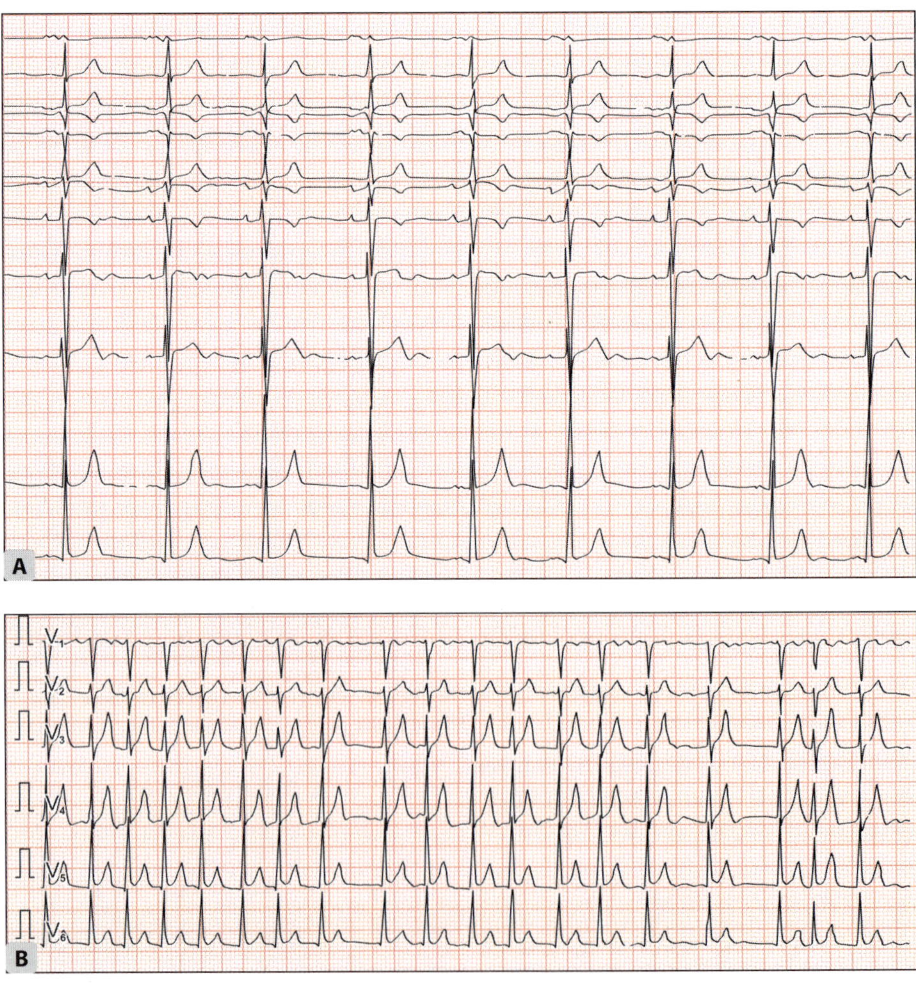

FIGURES 8 A & B: ECG in MR: (A) Sinus rhythm, left atrial enlargement, and LV volume overload; **(B)** Atrial fibrillation with LV hypertrophy (chest leads only).

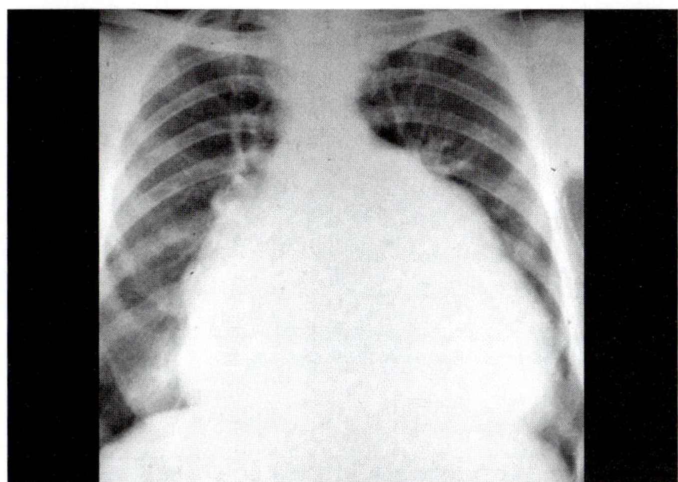

FIGURE 9: Chest X-ray in severe MR showing cardiomegaly, LVE, LAE, and PVH.

BOX 9	Echo features of severe mitral regurgitation.
• Dilated LV, LA	
• Flail leaflet, ruptured papillary muscle	
• Large color flow jet, jet area >40% of LA	
• CW Doppler of MR jet—dense, full envelop	
• Systolic flow reversal in pulmonary veins	
• Vena contracta >7 mm	
• PISA radius >10 mm	
• Regurgitant fraction >50%	
• Regurgitant volume >60 mL	
• Regurgitant orifice >0.4 cm^2	

LV ejection fraction (EF) <60% or with NYHA class III–IV symptoms, and less so in those who are asymptomatic and have normal LV function (**Fig. 11**).

Severe MR develops slowly in patients with MVP after a long delay and is rare before the age of 50 years. It occurs in about 15% of patients over 10–15 years period. Serious complications including cardiac death, need for cardiac surgery, IE, or cerebral events were seen in 1 per 100 patient-years.

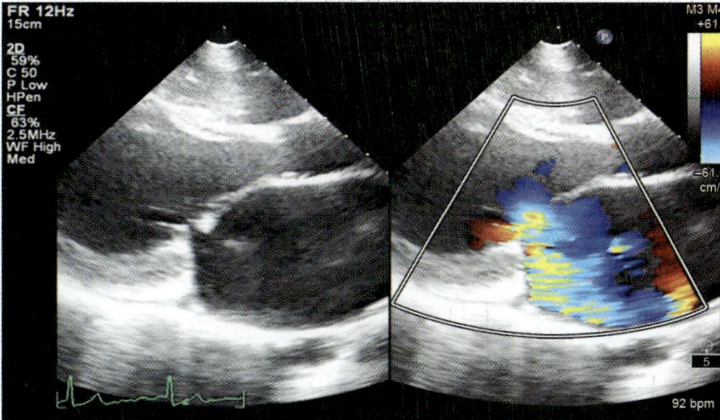

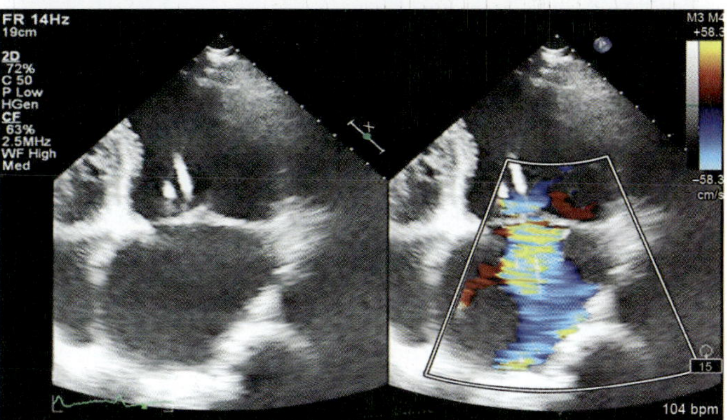

FIGURE 10: Echo showing severe mitral regurgitation.

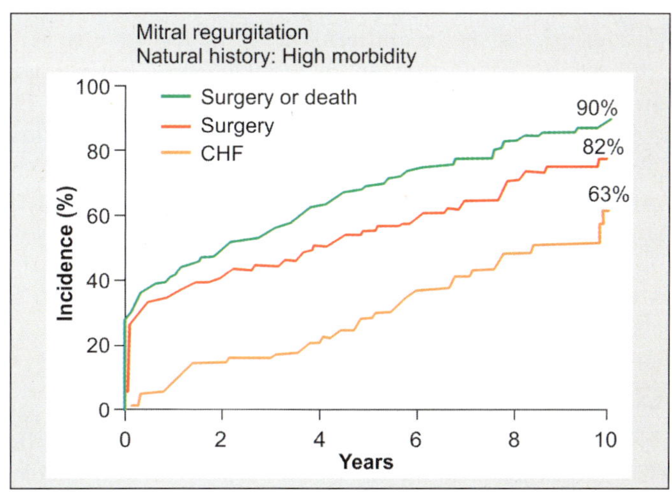

FIGURE 11: Natural history of severe mitral regurgitation.

MEDICAL TREATMENT

Secondary prophylaxis for RF should be continued indefinitely or at least up to the age of 40 years in patients with rheumatic MR. Routine antibiotic prophylaxis to prevent IE is no longer recommended for patients with MR unless there is previous history of IE. All patients with AF, paroxysmal or chronic, should receive chronic AC and appropriate measures should be taken to control the ventricular rate and restore sinus rhythm, if possible.

Role of pharmacologic therapy for MR remains uncertain. Afterload reduction therapy undoubtedly is indicated and may be lifesaving in patients with acute MR and secondary forms of chronic MR. At present, convincing data are lacking that vasodilator therapy (like ACE inhibitors) affects LV volumes or systolic function favorably in the absence of LV dysfunction or hypertension. Current guidelines do not recommend the use of these agents for chronic therapy of primary MR.

There is no specific treatment for mild to moderate MR. Monitoring disease progression to allow intervention at the optimal time point is an important aspect of medical follow-up.

BOX 10	Advantages of mitral valve repair over mitral valve replacement.
• Avoid long-term anticoagulation	
• Maintains normal LV geometry and systolic function	
• Less operative mortality (1% vs. 5%)	
• Improves long-term outcome	
• Avoids prosthetic valve-related complications	

SURGERY

Surgery is considered only for severe MR. Surgical options include MV repair and MVR, with or without chordal preservation. When annular-papillary continuity is preserved, EF remains stable after MV surgery in contrast to a decline by an average of 10% when this continuity is disrupted. MV repair is possible in >95% of patients with MR due to MVP. MV repair offers several advantages over MVR (**Box 10**). MV repair is durable with a low rate of reoperation for recurrent MR, with an event-free survival of 80–90% at 5–10 years. Hence *MV repair is preferred to replacement whenever anatomically feasible and durable especially in nonrheumatic primary MR.* Patients of RHD with severe MR and LV dilatation and /or symptoms need MVR as the valve is fibrotic and is not amendable to repair.

Indications for surgery: Surgery is indicated on an emergency basis in patients with acute severe MR. Indications for surgery in primary chronic severe MR are listed in **Box 11**. MVR is contraindicated in severe LV dysfunction [EF < 30% and/or end-systolic dimension (ESD) > 55 mm].

A transcatheter procedure of MV clip application has shown promise in patients with severe secondary MR in patients with ischemic and dilated cardiomyopathy. In future transcatheter MVR might become possible as it is also being evolved.

CONCLUSION

Mitral valve disease is a common clinical problem. Symptoms, physical findings, and basic investigations like ECG and chest X-ray help in assessing the lesion severity and need for intervention. Echo is pivotal in confirming the diagnosis, assessing the etiology and severity and choosing appropriate therapy. Medical management is aimed at prevention and treatment of complications. Periodic evaluation is necessary to optimize timing of intervention. Valve-sparing procedure is always preferred to valve replacement. BMV has shown encouraging results in the management of rheumatic MS, and hence it is preferred. For patients with MR, MV repair is preferred where the valve morphology is not too bad and it is feasible. For rheumatic MR when indicated, we have to do valve replacement usually with mechanical prosthetic valves. In some special situations like young women wanting to be pregnant and very old persons (age >70) bioprosthetic valve may have to be used.

BOX 11	Indications for surgery in primary chronic severe mitral regurgitation.
• Symptomatic patients, in the absence of severe LV dysfunction (Class I)	
• Asymptomatic patients with mild to moderate LV dysfunction, EF-30%–60%, and/or ESD ≥ 40 mm (≥2.6 cm/m^2) (Class I)	
• Asymptomatic patients with preserved LV function and new onset AF (Class IIA)	
• Asymptomatic patients with preserved LV function, and PH (PASP > 50 mm Hg at rest)	
• NYHA class III-IV symptoms and severe LV dysfunction if MV repair is highly likely	

RECOMMENDED READINGS

1. Zipes DP, Libby P, Bonow RO, Mann DL, Tomaselli GF. Braunwald's Heart Disease: A Textbook of Cardiovascular Medicine, 11th edition. Elsevier Health Sciences; 2018.
2. Fuster V, Harrington R, Narula J, Eapen Z. Hurst's the heart: Textbook of cardiology, 14th edition. McGraw-Hill Education; 2017.
3. Bonow RO, O'Gara PT, Adams DH, Badhwar V, Bavaria JE, Elmariah S, et al. 2020 focused update of the 2017 ACC expert consensus decision pathway on the management of mitral regurgitation: A report of the American College of Cardiology solution set oversight committee. J Am Coll Cardiol. 2020;75(17):2236-70.
4. Otto CM, Nishimura RA, Bonow RO, Carabello BA, Erwin JP 3rd, Gentile F, et al. 2020 ACC/AHA guideline for the management of patients with valvular heart disease: Executive summary: A report of the American College of Cardiology/American Heart Association Joint Committee on Clinical Practice Guidelines. Circulation. 2021;143(5):e35-e71.
5. Manjunath C, Srinivas Kh, Dattatreya P, Sinha N, Sarkar A, Chag M, et al. The 7th report of the non-coronary cardiac interventions registry of India. Indian Heart J. 2008;60(1):73-8.
6. Manjunath CN, Srinivasa KH, Patil CB, Venkatesh HV, Bhoopal TS, Dhanalakshmi C. Balloon mitral valvuloplasty: our experience with a modified technique of crossing the mitral valve in difficult cases. Cathet Cardiovasc Diagn. 1998;44(1):23-6.
7. Manjunath CN, Srinivasa KH, Ravindranath KS, Manohar JS, Prabhavathi B, Dattatreya PV, et al. Balloon mitral valvotomy in patients with mitral stenosis and left atrial thrombus. Catheter Cardiovasc Interv. 2009;74(4):653-61.

8. Manjunath CN, Panneerselvam A, Srinivasa KH, Prabhavathi B, Rangan K, Dhanalakshmi C, et al. Incidence and predictors of atrial septal defect after percutaneous transvenous mitral commissurotomy-a transesophageal echocardiographic study of 209 cases. Echocardiography. 2013;30(2):127-30.
9. Khandenahally Shankarappa R, Dwarakaprasad R, Karur S, Bachahally Krishnanaik G, Panneerselvam A, Cholenahally Nanjappa M. Balloon mitral valvotomy for calcific mitral stenosis. JACC Cardiovasc Interv. 2009;2(3):263-4.
10. Manjunath CN, Srinivas P, Ravindranath KS, Dhanalakshmi C. Incidence and patterns of valvular heart disease in a tertiary care high-volume cardiac center: a single center experience. Indian Heart J. 2014;66(3):320-6.
11. Manjunath CN, Srinivasa KH, Panneerselvam A, Prabhavathi B, Ravindranath KS, Rangan K, et al. Incidence and predictors of left atrial thrombus in patients with rheumatic mitral stenosis and sinus rhythm: a transesophageal echocardiographic study. Echocardiography. 2011;28(4):457-60.
12. Panneerselvam A, Ananthakrishna R, Srinivas BC, Hemanna Setty SK, Manjunath SC, Basavanna D, et al. Hemopericardium following transseptal puncture during balloon mitral valvotomy: management strategies and outcomes. J Invasive Cardiol. 2020;32(2):70-5.

CHAPTER 96

Diseases of the Aortic Valve

Prafulla G Kerkar, Rajesh Matta, Ankita A Kulkarni

ABSTRACT

Aortic valve (AV) stenosis is commonly encountered, resulting from degenerative, bicuspid, or rheumatic causes. Typical symptoms of angina, dyspnea, and syncope along with classical signs help clinically suspect aortic stenosis (AS). Echocardiography is diagnostic; however, multimodality imaging and testing help decision making regarding its severity and timing of intervention to alter its natural history. Many drugs have long been tried to retard progression of the disease, but without fruition. Much progress, however, has been made in last two decades, with a paradigm shift from surgical management in symptomatic patients historically; to current transcatheter therapies performed safely and effectively, even for low risk individuals. Long-term data for transcatheter intervention are however lacking.

Aortic regurgitation (AR) can be either acute or chronic with varying clinical presentation and management. Chronic regurgitation presents with symptoms of palpitations, dyspnea, fatigue, and classical signs on examination which have fascinated physicians since centuries. Diagnosis is generally confirmed on echocardiography and optimal timing of intervention after symptom onset prevents rapid progression of disease and deterioration of left ventricular function. Contrary to this, acute severe regurgitation is an emergency and needs surgical intervention to prevent mortality.

"The cause is hidden; The effect is visible to all"

—Ovid

INTRODUCTION

Diseases of the AV generally manifest as either AS, or AR, or as mixed AS and AR. Due to common occurrence, their diagnosis and appropriate management become mandatory for the practicing physician and cardiologist. In this chapter, we shall briefly review these AV diseases.

NORMAL AORTIC VALVE

Normal AV is tricuspid and has three symmetrical cusps which are mobile and free up to their commissures so as to achieve complete overlap upon closure. It has a cross-sectional area of 3-4 cm^2 and a mean systolic pressure gradient between the left ventricle (LV) and aorta is <5 mm Hg.

A competent and normally functioning AV guards the LV outflow tract (LVOT). It ensures forward flow during ventricular systole and prevents regurgitation of blood from aorta into LV during diastole.

AORTIC STENOSIS

It occurs due to narrowing of the AV orifice caused by failure of leaflets to open normally and is caused by cusp and/or annular abnormalities. Valvar AS is the most common cause of LVOT obstruction (LVOTO), others being subvalvar and supravalvar. Subvalvar obstruction could occur due to hypertrophic obstructive cardiomyopathy, fibrous ridge, and diffuse fibromuscular thickening of LVOT. Supravalvar LVOTO includes membranes, aortic bands, and constrictions.

EPIDEMIOLOGY

The prevalence of AS increases with age, being 1–2% in >65 years age-group and 12% at age >75 years, based on echocardiography. Indian studies have shown senile valvular degeneration to be the most common cause of acquired AS, majority presenting before 60 years of age. Another study found AS to be third most common valve abnormality (7.3%) of all valvular lesions, being more common in males across all age groups. With an aging population, the incidence of AS is expected to increase, thereby increasing the burden on Indian healthcare system. In the western world, however, valvar AS remains the most common valvular heart disease and the third most common cardiovascular disease.

ETIOLOGY

Valvar AS has three predominant causes—rheumatic, degenerative calcification of AV, and degenerative affection of congenital bicuspid AV (**Figs. 1 A** to **C**). Other causes include radiation-induced AS, alkaptonuria, and familial hyperlipidemia (**Table 1**).

BICUSPID AORTIC VALVE

Bicuspid AV caused by fusion of two AV cusps is the most common congenital cardiac abnormality, occurring

TABLE 1 Various etiologies of aortic stenosis.

Cause	Clinical presentation	Associated findings
Calcific degeneration	• Advanced age • Atherosclerotic risk factors	• Atherosclerotic coronary disease • Frailty
Congenital		
• Bicuspid AV	• Family history, younger age	• Aortic aneurysms or coarctation
• Subvalvular	• Asymptomatic with a murmur • Subaortic membrane or fibromuscular ridge	• Associated AR and other congenital defects
	• Williams syndrome	• Short stature, elfin facies
• Supravalvular	• Homozygous familial hypercho-lestrolemia	• Renal abnormalities • Impaired cognition • Tuberous xanthomas • LDL-cholesterol >500 mg/dL
Rheumatic	• History of rheumatic fever	• Affection of other valves
Autoimmune	• Lupus rash, joint pains, kidney disease	• Leaflet thickening and verrucous vegetations, antibodies positive
Metabolic	• Alkaptonuria (arth-ritis, high levels of homogentisic acid)	• Brown or blue pigment deposition
Radiation	• Hodgkin's lymphoma • Breast cancer • Mediastinal irradiation	• Premature coronary disease • Pericardial and myocardial disease • Fibrosis/calcification of other valves and annulus

(LDL: low-density lipoprotein)

Source: Adapted from Lilly LS, Braunwald E. Braunwald's Heart Disease: A Textbook of Cardiovascular Medicine. Philadelphia: Elsevier Health Sciences; 2012.

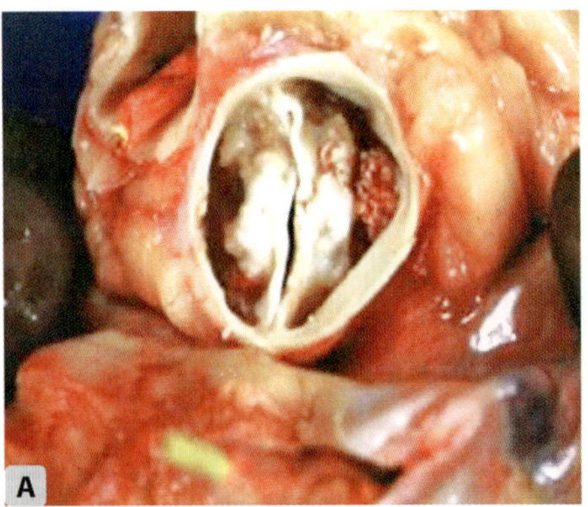

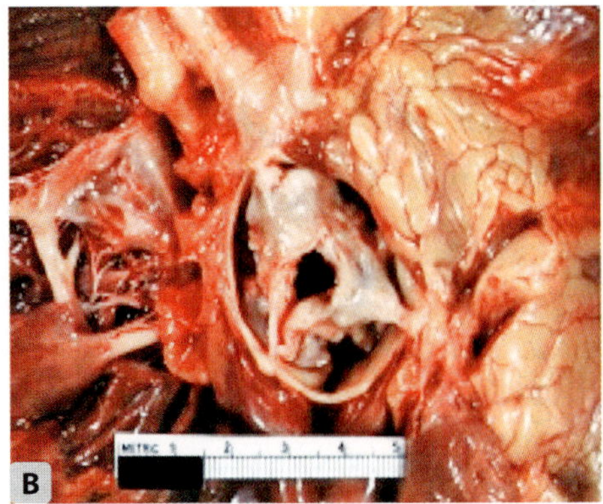

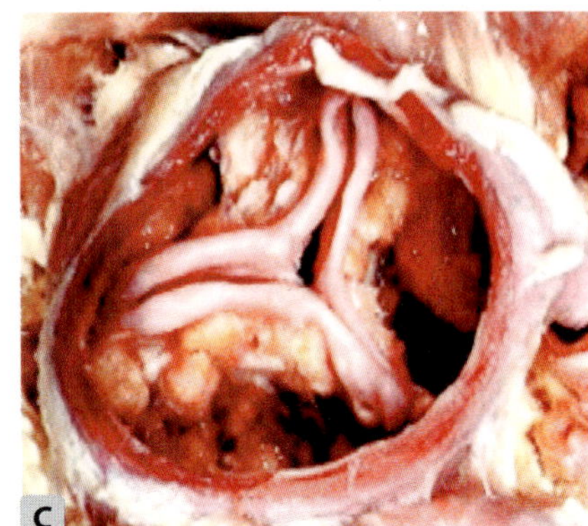

FIGURES 1 A to C: Pathologic specimen showing common etiologies of aortic stenosis (AS); **(A)** congenital bicuspid AV; **(B)** rheumatic; and **(C)** calcific degeneration.

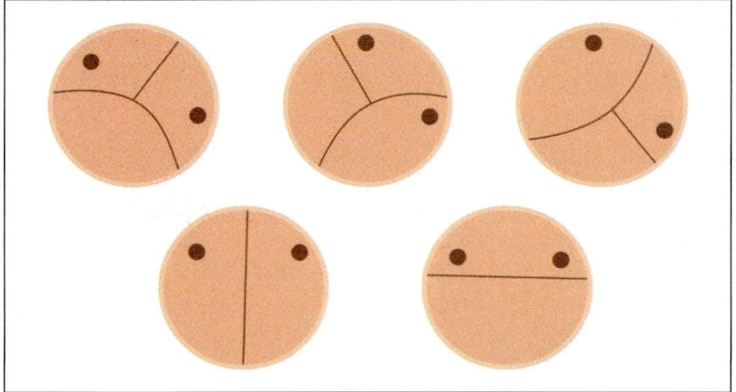

FIGURE 2: Siever's types of bicuspid aortic valve (as seen on parasternal short-axis). Top row (left to right): Type I has fusion of the right coronary cusp (RCC) and left coronary cusp (LCC); Type II has fusion of the RCC and non-coronary cusp (NCC); and Type III with fusion of LCC and NCC. Bottom row: Seiver's type zero: symmetrical bicuspid valve with no raphe (left to right). The common lateral subtype with right and left cusps and the less common anteroposterior subtype with anterior and posterior cusps.

in 1.5–2% of the population with male preponderance (M:F of 3:1).

It is classified depending on presence/absence of raphe and fusion of right, left or noncoronary cusps into Sievers types (**Fig. 2**). It can be associated with Turner syndrome, or with other anomalies such as hypoplastic left heart syndrome, coarctation of aorta, or other obstructive lesions of left heart (Shone complex).

Majority of bicuspid AV patients remain asymptomatic, but have hemodynamic disadvantages such as uneven systolic flow patterns, increased strain in systole, and high stress in raphe. Dysfunctional bicuspid AV may present as symptomatic AS (75%) or AR (15%) or both. Bicuspid AV associated with aortic dilation is seen in 40% of patients and they are at increased risk of dissection/rupture/aneurysm, independent of valve disease.

SENILE DEGENERATIVE (CALCIFIC)

Many patients with a normal tricuspid AV develop senile degeneration of valve leaflets and calcification, thus producing AS.

Calcification is not a passive process related to wear and tear; rather is an active process with risk factors similar to atherosclerosis. This process is initiated by lipid infiltration and oxidative stress with resultant cytokine release by activated inflammatory cells. Cells undergo osteogenic reprogramming promoting mineralization of the extracellular matrix and fibrocalcific remodeling of the valve.

Familial clustering suggests genetic and hereditary components to this disease. Genes including vitamin D receptor, estrogen receptor, transforming growth factor (TGF)-β, interleukin-10 (IL-10), apolipoprotein E4, and lipoprotein-associated phospholipase A2 (Lp-associated PLA2) are implicated in it.

Sclerosis of AV (AV calcification without LVOTO) is common and associated with cardiovascular mortality and morbidity. It is a precursor of calcific AS, but its progression is variable.

RHEUMATIC

Rheumatic AS remains relatively common in India. Adhesion and fusion of commissures and cusps with vascularization of leaflets of the valve ring lead to retraction and stiffening of the borders of the cusps with calcific nodules on leaflets leading to triangular/round small opening of the valve; manifesting as combined AS and AR, usually with accompanying mitral valve abnormalities.

PATHOPHYSIOLOGY

When AS leads to significant LVOTO, flow across the AV is impeded during systole. Progressive LVOTO requires elevation of left ventricular systolic pressure (LVSP) to overcome impedance to flow into aorta. A measurable gradient between LV and aorta is detected only when the AV area is reduced by 50%. Compensatory mechanisms allow adequate cardiac output (CO) in the initial stages and include elevation of LV systolic pressure and increase in LV ejection time. LV compensates by concentric hypertrophy [left ventricular hypertrophy (LVH)] to overcome pressure overload imposed by AS. Initially, LVH is adaptive because it reduces the systolic stress developed by the myocardium (Laplace law) and patient remains asymptomatic.

Progression of AS results in exhaustion of capacity for LVH, impaired contractility of LV, increased LV end-systolic volume (due to inadequate contraction) and then, the Frank–Starling effect (dilation with augmented fiber stretch) attempts to maintain CO. With exhaustion of this, pump failure ensues and symptoms develop.

Over time LVH reduces LV compliance with increase in LV end-diastolic pressure (LVEDP) and increased left atrial (LA) pressure. To facilitate adequate filling of LV, contraction of LA provides atrial kick to maintain adequate LV preload [contributes about 25% of LV stroke volume (SV)]. Hence, loss of effective atrial contraction [e.g., development of atrial fibrillation (AF), complete heart block (CHB)] causes clinical deterioration of patients with AS.

Ischemia occurs due to myocardial supply–demand mismatch. Elevated LVSP with hypertrophy increases oxygen consumption. Reduced coronary perfusion can be attributed to increased LV ejection time (prolonged systole and reduced relative time in diastole, when coronary perfusion occurs) and reduced aortic pressure distal to AS. Acutely, it precipitates angina, syncope, or arrhythmia. Over long run, it impairs LV function and causes conduction disturbance. Also, calcific AS has high incidence of associated atherosclerotic coronary artery disease (CAD).

Stages of progression of AS are described in **Table 2**. When LV dysfunction sets in, Doppler echocardiography may not show gradients across stenosed AV (as gradient depends on flow across AV which is reduced with LV dysfunction). Such a condition is termed as "Low-Flow/Low-Gradient AS".

TABLE 2	Stages of progression of aortic stenosis (AS).				
Stage	**Definition**	**Valve anatomy**	**Hemodynamics**	**Consequences**	**Symptoms**
A	**At risk**	BAV or sclerosis	$AV_{vmax} < 2$ m/s, normal leaflet motion	None	None
B	**Progressive disease**	Mild-to-moderate leaflet calcification/ fibrosis rheumatic affection	• Mild AS: V_{max} 2.0–2.9 m/s or mean AVG < 20 mm Hg • Moderate AS: V_{max} 3.0–3.9 m/s or mean AVG 20–39 mm Hg	• LV diastolic dysfunction may be present	None
C	**Asymtomatic severe AS**				
C1	Without LV dysfunction	Severe leaflet calcification or fibrosis with severely reduced leaflet opening	• $AV_{vmax} \geq 4$ m/s or mean AVG ≥ 40 mm Hg • AVA ≤ 1.0 cm^2 (indexed ≤ 0.6 cm^2/m^2) • Very severe AS V_{max} ≥ 5 m/s or mean AVG ≥ 60 mm Hg	• LV diastolic dysfunction • Mild LV hypertrophy • Normal LVEF	Exercise testing is reasonable to confirm the symptom status
C2	With LV dysfunction	Severe leaflet calcification or fibrosis with severely reduced leaflet opening	• $AV_{vmax} \geq 4$ m/s or mean AVG ≥ 40 mm Hg • AVA ≤ 1.0 cm^2 (indexed ≤ 0.6 cm^2/m^2) • Very severe AS V_{max} ≥ 5 m/s or mean AVG ≥ 60 mm Hg	• LVEF < 50%	None
D	**Symptomatic severe AS**				
D1	High-gradient AS	Severe leaflet calcification or fibrosis with severely reduced leaflet opening	• $AV_{vmax} \geq 4$ m/s or mean AVG ≥ 40 mm of Hg • AVA ≤ 1.0 cm^2 (indexed ≤ 0.6 cm^2/m^2) • Very severe AS V_{max} ≥ 5 m/s or mean AVG ≥ 60 mm Hg	• LV diastolic dysfunction • Mild LV hypertrophy • Normal LVEF • Pulmonary hypertension may be present	Exertional dyspnea, exertional angina, exertional syncope
D2	Low-flow, low-gradient with reduced LVEF	Severe leaflet calcification or fibrosis with severely reduced leaflet opening	• $AV_{vmax} < 4$ m/s or mean AVG ≤ 40 mm Hg • DSE shows: AVA ≤ 1.0 cm^2 (indexed ≤ 0.6 cm^2/m^2) • Very severe AS V_{max} ≥ 5 m/s or mean AVG ≥ 60 mm Hg	• LV diastolic dysfunction • LV hypertrophy • LVEF < 50%	HF, angina, syncope/ presyncope
D3	Low-flow, low-gradient with normal LVEF or paradoxical low-flow, low gradient	Severe leaflet calcification or fibrosis with severely reduced leaflet opening	• AVA ≤ 1.0 cm^2 (indexed ≤ 0.6) with an AV_{vmax} < 4 m/s or mean AVG < 40 mm Hg *and* SVI < 35 mL/m^2 measured when patient is normotensive (SBP < 140 mm Hg)	• Increased LV thickness; small LV chamber with low stroke volume Restricted diastolic filling • LVEF ≥ 50%	HF, angina, syncope/ presyncope

(AV: aortic valve; AVA: aortic valve area; AVG: aortic valve gradient; SVI: Stroke Volume Index)

Source: Adapted from the American College of Cardiology/the American Heart Association (ACC/AHA) guidelines for the management of patients with valvular heart disease 2020.

CLINICAL FEATURES

SYMPTOMS

Patients of bicuspid AV with severe AS present by 5th–6th decade and those with degenerative calcific AS by seventh decade. Symptoms usually occur after valve area is <1 cm^2, or the mean pressure gradient is >40 mm Hg (severe AS).

Three cardinal symptoms of AS are angina, syncope, and dyspnea. Eventually, LV failure sets in. Symptoms portend poor prognosis unless intervention is performed.

1. *Dyspnea*: Exertional dyspnea occurs due to elevated pulmonary capillary wedge pressures secondary to elevated LVEDP.
2. *Angina*: It can be attributed to (i) myocardial oxygen supply-demand mismatch, (ii) coexistent coronary artery disease (CAD), especially in older adults, and (iii) calcific embolization to coronaries, rarely.
3. *Syncope*: Sudden, transient, and spontaneously reversible loss of consciousness as a result of reduced cerebral perfusion can occur due to (i) inability to increase CO with increasing exertion in the face of a "fixed cardiac output" with peripheral vasodilation, manifesting as exertional syncope, (ii) complete AV conduction block presenting as nonexertional syncope even while patient is supine, (iii) AF which hampers the "atrial kick" essential to maintain CO, (iv) atherosclerotic CAD with ischemia and transient severe LV dysfunction/tachyarrhythmia, and (v) elevated LVSP leading to reflex peripheral vasodilation and syncope.

Uncommon presentations include: (i) bleeding from gastrointestinal tract, known as Heyde's syndrome, which is an acquired von Willebrand disease caused by shear stress across stenotic AV and associated colonic vascular dysplasia and (ii) embolism to brain, kidney, or other organ systems which may rarely be initial presentation of severe AS.

Eventually, LV failure manifesting as orthopnea, paroxysmal nocturnal dyspnea, pulmonary edema, and fatigue ensues.

SIGNS

Pulse is typically described as pulsus parvus et tardus (low volume with delayed peaking) which is specific for AS, palpated best in carotid artery, along with shudder (usually on left carotid). It may be absent if AS is not severe or associated with other valve abnormality.

Blood pressure (BP) is typically normal or elevated, but systolic decapitation may be seen in severe AS.

Jugular venous pulse (JVP) may show elevated pressure and prominent "a" wave due to Bernheim effect (LVH affecting the interventricular septum and causing it to bulge into right ventricle, reducing its compliance).

Apex is well sustained, heaving, and is displaced laterally in advanced disease. Double beating apex due to palpable S4 can be present. Palpable systolic thrill over second right intercostal space with carotid shudder is usually present.

A2 is delayed and soft if the valve is calcified. If A2 is audible, paradoxically split S2 indicates severe AS. Audible S4 might be present. S3 indicates LV dysfunction.

Ejection click (EC) may be present in young patients with pliable leaflets and is better heard at the apex. It localizes the LVOTO to valve level.

Low pitched, rough, rasping, and harsh ejection systolic murmur is heard along the right second intercostal space with radiation to carotid. Murmur begins after S1 and can follow an EC. The high-pitched components of the murmur may also be heard at the apex (Gallavardin phenomenon). It must not be confused with pansystolic murmur of mitral regurgitation. With worsening severity, the murmur peaks later in systole. With LV dysfunction, the intensity of murmur may diminish due to reduced flow.

INVESTIGATIONS

ELECTROCARDIOGRAM

It shows LVH with strain pattern (pressure overload). A deep S in V_1–V_2 and tall R in V_5–V_6 with T-wave inversion in anterolateral lead. However, LVH, LA hypertrophy, and secondary repolarization-ST and T wave abnormalities (strain pattern) may not be there in severe AS (**Fig. 3**).

CHEST X-RAY

Initially cardiac silhouette appears normal, but with progression, rounded LVH develops with poststenotic dilation of aorta. AV calcification may be appreciated. With LV dysfunction, cardiomegaly with features of pulmonary venous hypertension and pulmonary edema become apparent.

ECHOCARDIOGRAPHY

When appropriately performed, it is sufficient for the diagnosis and estimation of severity, prognosis, need for intervention, and for diagnosis of associated valvular disorders. M mode and two-dimensional (2D) echocardiography show valve thickening, calcification, and reduced movements of valve leaflets; LVH and LV dysfunction. Doppler measures gradients and estimates severity of AS by measuring flow velocity across AV. Estimation of effective orifice area with help of continuity equation can be done (**Figs. 4 A** to **D**).

Three-dimensional (3D) echocardiography can help to estimate AV area with planimetry. Transesophageal echocardiography is not routinely recommended in these patients.

Dobutamine stress echocardiography (DSE) is used to distinguish patients with severe AS with LV dysfunction (low-flow/low-gradient AS), attributable to afterload mismatch from primary myocardial dysfunction with moderate AS. **Table 3** demonstrates echocardiographic parameters used in assessment of severity and progression of AS.

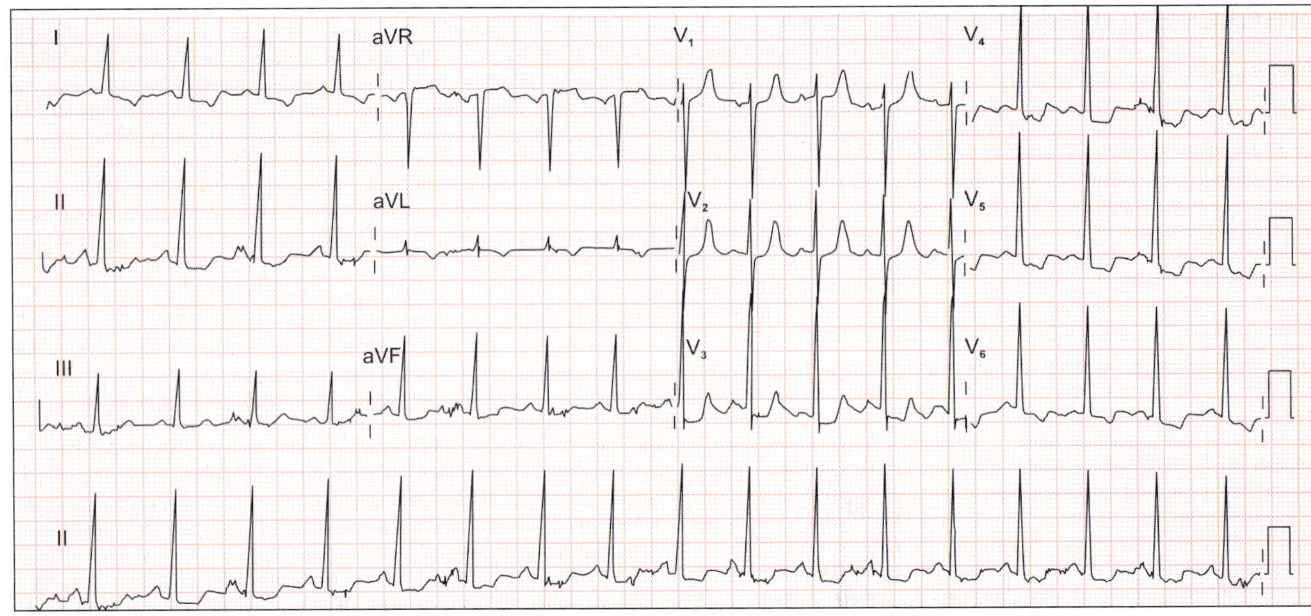

FIGURE 3: Echocardiography (ECG) showing severe left ventricular hypertrophy (LVH) with systolic overload (LV strain) in severe aortic stenosis (AS).

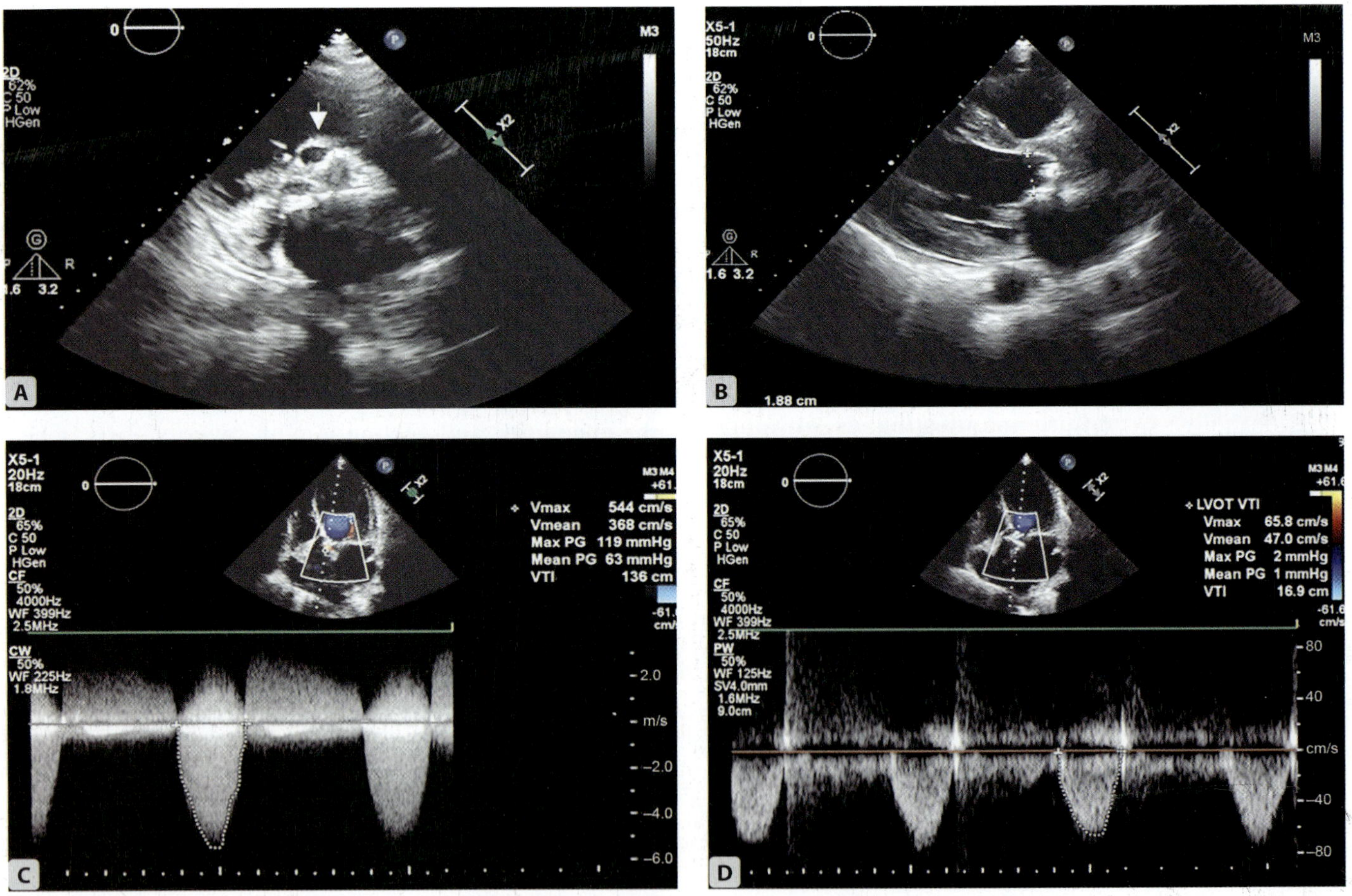

FIGURES 4 A to D: Echocardiographic tracing of aortic valve gradients: **(A)** Parasternal short axis view showing calcific degeneration of a tricuspid aortic valve (white arrow); **(B)** parasternal long axis view measuring aortic annulus diameter; **(C)** continuous-wave Doppler across aortic valve showing severe aortic stenosis (AS) gradients (dotted line); and **(D)** pulsed wave Doppler across left ventricular outflow tract (LVOT) measuring velocities across LVOT (dotted line).

TABLE 3 Etiology of acute and chronic aortic regurgitation.	
Leaflet abnormalities	**Aortic root abnormalities**
Acute aortic regurgitation	
• Acute infective endocarditis • Acute prosthetic valve dysfunction • Traumatic rupture • Post-aortic balloon valvuloplasty	• Acute aortic dissection • Perivalvular leak or dehiscence of prosthetic valve
Chronic aortic regurgitation	
• Rheumatic fever • Infective endocarditis • Trauma • Myxomatous degeneration • Whipple's disease • Crohn's disease • Drug-induced valvulopathy • Congenital aortic regurgitation • Systemic lupus erythematosus • Rheumatoid arthritis • Ankylosing spondylitis • Takayasu's arteritis	• Age-related aortic dilation • Cystic medial necrosis of the aorta (isolated bicuspid AV or Marfans syndrome) • Systemic hypertension • Annuloaortic ectasia • Reiter's syndrome • Ankylosing spondylitis • Psoriatic arthritis • Behçet's syndrome • Ehlers–Danlos syndrome • Aortitis (syphilis and giant cell arteritis) • Osteogenesis imperfecta • Relapsing polychondritis

Source: Adapted from Griffin B. Valvular Heart Disease.

CARDIAC CATHETERIZATION AND CAG

Coronary angiography is indicated in all patients above 40 years prior to valve replacement. Cardiac catheterization is recommended only in case of equivocal noninvasive evaluation or discrepancy between clinical and echocardiographic severity of AS.

OTHER DIAGNOSTIC MODALITIES

Exercise treadmill test (ETT): It is indicated in apparently asymptomatic severe AS patients to assess effort tolerance and symptom status, as patients limit their activity due to symptoms or attribute them to ageing and deconditioning. Patients who develop symptoms or exhibit a decrease in BP should be considered to have symptomatic disease.

Cardiac CT: AV calcification is a strong predictor of outcomes in patients with AS. Quantification by CT imaging is useful in patients with low-flow/low-gradient AS of unclear severity with either a normal or reduced LVEF. Agatston unit thresholds for severe AS are 1,300 in women and 2,000 in men.

CT is performed prior to transcatheter aortic valve replacement (AVR) to determine annulus area, leaflet length, annular to coronary ostial distance, and peripheral vascular anatomy. CT coronary angiography rules out CAD requiring revascularization in low-risk patients prior to AVR. Cardiac MRI or PET are not routinely recommended in these patients.

NATURAL HISTORY

There is marked individual variation in the progression of disease. Patients with mild and asymptomatic disease have long latent period and slow progression over 20 years with only 20% progressing to severe, symptomatic AS, and have clinical outcomes similar to age-matched normal population. Moderate AS requires regular follow-up and average annual rate of progression in disease severity is decrease in valve area of 0.1 cm^2, increase in velocity of 0.3 m/s, and mean pressure gradient of 7 mm Hg. Severe AS has a high rate of progression to symptoms. Asymptomatic severe AS needs periodic monitoring as symptoms can be insidious. Symptomatic severe AS has an event-free survival of only 30–50% at 2 years.

Survival after onset of symptoms of angina, syncope, and dyspnea was 5 years, 3 years, and 2 years respectively in preintervention era. Sudden death, usually from arrhythmia, occurred in 10–20%; mostly in symptomatic patients. Sudden death as the first manifestation of severe AS is uncommon (~1%/year) in asymptomatic patients.

MANAGEMENT

MEDICAL MANAGEMENT

Medical therapy has no effect on disease progression. Hypertension, hyperlipidemia, and concomitant CAD is managed according to guidelines. In heart failure (HF)/LV dysfunction, diuretics provide symptom relief and help to stabilize patients prior to intervention.

INTERVENTION

Important issues in intervention for severe AS are indication and/or timing and the modality of intervention. *Intervention is indicated* in all symptomatic patients with severe AS, asymptomatic patients with LV dysfunction or undergoing other cardiac surgery or reduced exercise capacity on exercise stress test, moderate AS patients undergoing cardiac surgery for another reason, low-flow/low-gradient AS.

The decision of transcatheter AVR (TAVR) versus surgical AVR requires a "Heart Team" approach and discussion with patients. While TAVR has been proven to be noninferior to surgical AVR even for low surgical risk subset patients (debatable); long-term durability data, and anatomic suitability of patients to undergo TAVR are its current limitations. The American College of Cardiology/the American Heart Association (ACC/AHA) 2020 guidelines for valvular heart disease recommendations are shown in **Flowchart 1**.

Transcatheter balloon aortic valvotomy alone is performed as a palliative procedure only in adolescents and young adults presenting with severe AS. This is done to delay surgery (**Figs. 5 A** and **B**).

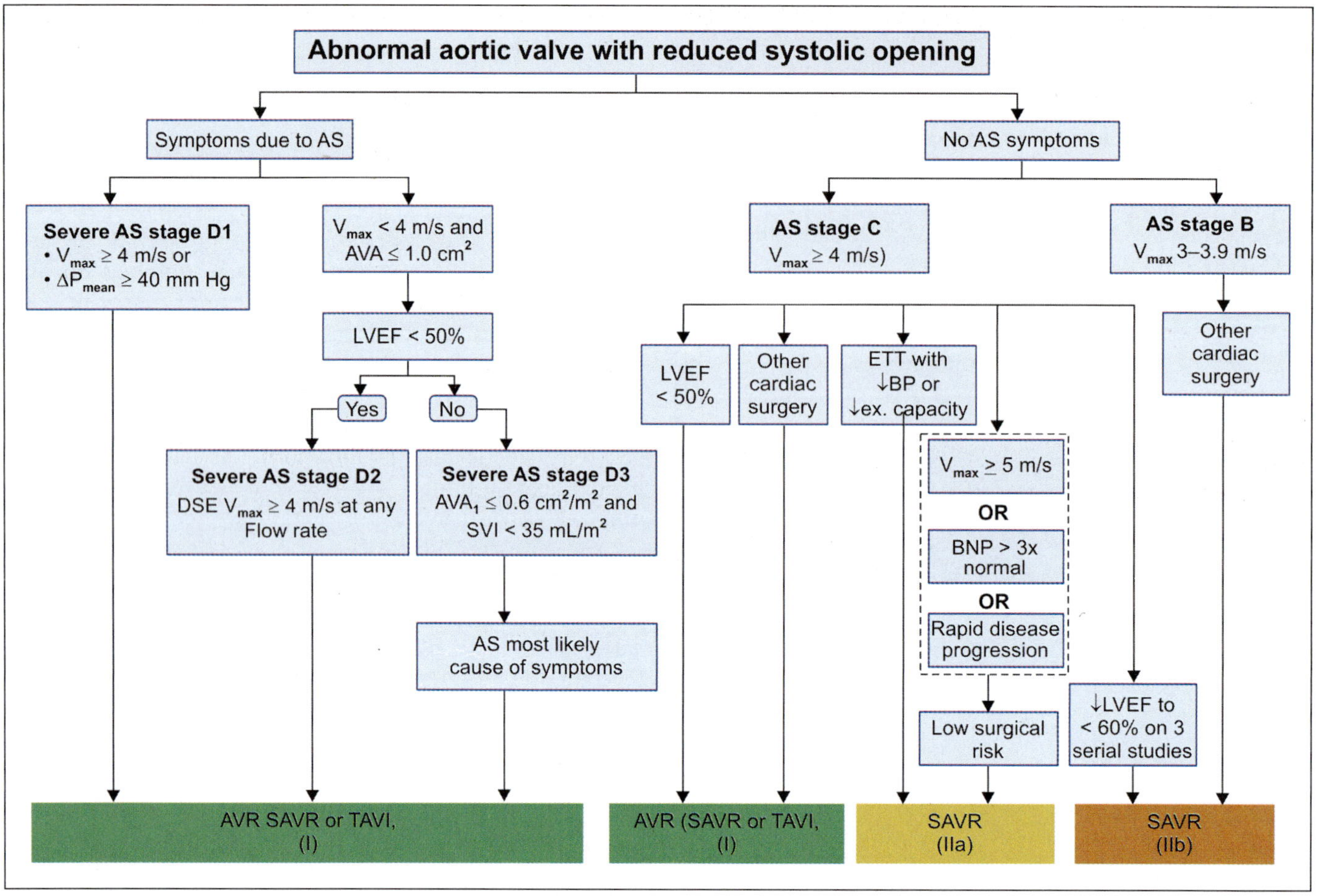

Abnormal aortic valve with reduced systolic opening

- **Symptoms due to AS**
  - **Severe AS stage D1**
    - $V_{max} \geq 4$ m/s or
    - $\Delta P_{mean} \geq 40$ mm Hg
    - → AVR SAVR or TAVI, (I)
  - $V_{max} < 4$ m/s and AVA ≤ 1.0 cm^2 → LVEF < 50%
    - Yes → **Severe AS stage D2**: DSE $V_{max} \geq 4$ m/s at any Flow rate → AVR SAVR or TAVI, (I)
    - No → **Severe AS stage D3**: $AVA_i \leq 0.6$ cm^2/m^2 and SVI < 35 mL/m^2 → AS most likely cause of symptoms → AVR SAVR or TAVI, (I)
- **No AS symptoms**
  - **AS stage C** ($V_{max} \geq 4$ m/s)
    - LVEF < 50% → AVR (SAVR or TAVI, (I)
    - Other cardiac surgery → AVR (SAVR or TAVI, (I)
    - ETT with ↓BP or ↓ex. capacity → SAVR (IIa)
    - $V_{max} \geq 5$ m/s OR BNP > 3x normal OR Rapid disease progression → Low surgical risk → SAVR (IIa)
    - ↓LVEF to < 60% on 3 serial studies → SAVR (IIb)
  - **AS stage B** (V_{max} 3–3.9 m/s)
    - Other cardiac surgery → SAVR (IIb)

[AVA: aortic valve area; AVAi: aortic valve area index; AVR: aortic valve replacement; DSE: dobutamine stress echocardiography; ΔP_{mean}: mean systolic pressure gradient between left ventricle (LV) and aorta; SAVR: surgical aortic valve replacement; SVI: Stroke Volume Index; TAVI: transcatheter aortic valve implantation; V_{max}: maximum velocity]

FLOWCHART 1: Decision pathway for recommendations for aortic valve (AV) intervention.

Source: Adapted from 2020 ACC/AHA (the American College of Cardiology/American Heart Association) guidelines for the management of patients with valvular heart disease.

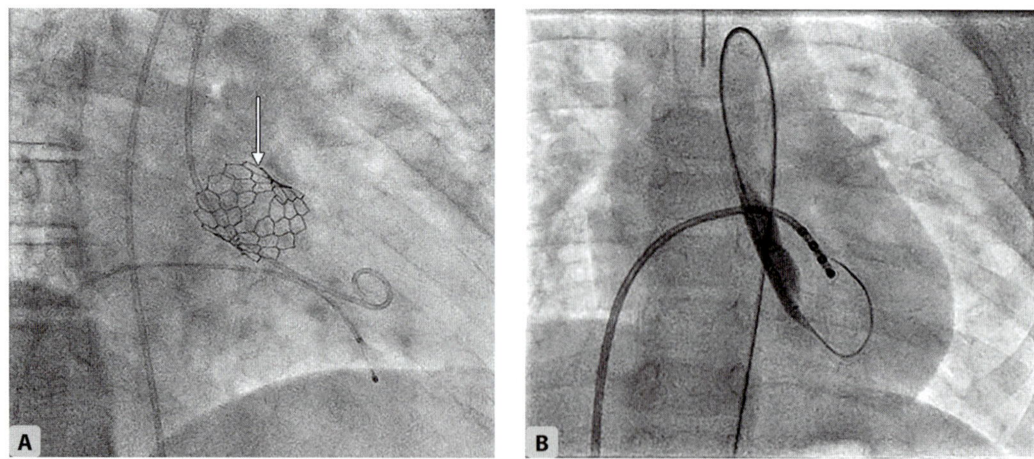

FIGURES 5 A & B: Aortic valve (AV) interventions: (A) transcatheter aortic valve replacement (white arrow shows stent-valve); and **(B)** balloon aortic valvuloplasty.

AORTIC REGURGITATION

Aortic regurgitation is backflow of blood from aorta into the LV, in diastole, due to failure of valve to close properly. Normally, the integrity of the aortic orifice in diastole is maintained by intact aortic root and firm apposition of free margins of AV cusps. AR may thus be caused by disorders affecting the valve cusps and/or aortic root.

EPIDEMIOLOGY

The prevalence of AR was estimated at 4.9% in the Framingham study with moderate and severe AR occurring in 0.5% of the study population. The incidence of significant AR increases with age, peaking at 40–60 years and is more common in men than women. In an Indian study, isolated AR had a prevalence of 5.8%, main etiology being rheumatic, followed by congenital bicuspid AV.

ETIOLOGY

Aortic regurgitation can be due to AV disease (primary/organic AR) or diseases of the aortic root (secondary/functional AR). Various etiologies of AR are listed in **Table 4**.

TABLE 4 Stages of progression of aortic regurgitation (AR).

Stage	Definition	Valve anatomy	Hemodynamics	Consequences	Symptoms
A	**At risk**	Bicuspid AV (or other congenital valve anomaly) • Aortic valve sclerosis • Diseases of the aortic sinuses or ascending aorta • History of rheumatic fever or known rheumatic heart disease • IE	AR: None or trace	None	None
B	**Progressive disease**	• Mild-to-moderate calcification of a trileaflet valve BAV (or other congenital valve anomaly) • Dilated aortic sinuses • Rheumatic valve changes • Previous IE	**Mild AR:** • Jet width < 25% of LVOT • Vena contracta < 0.3 cm • Regurgitant volume < 30 mL/beat • Regurgitant fraction < 30% • ERO < 0.10 cm^2 • Angiography grade 1 **Moderate AR:** • Jet width 25%–64% of LVOT • Vena contracta 0.3–0.6 cm • Regurgitant volume 30–59 mL/beat • Regurgitant fraction 30–49% • ERO 0.10–0.29 cm^2 • Angiography grade 2	• Normal LV systolic function • Normal LV volume or mild LV dilation	None
C	**Asymptomatic severe AR**				
C1	Without LV dysfunction	• Calcific aortic valve disease • Bicuspid valve (or other congenital abnormality) • Dilated aortic sinuses or ascending aorta • Rheumatic valve changes • IE with abnormal leaflet closure or perforation	**Severe AR:** • Jet width ≥ 65% of LVOT • Vena contracta > 0.6 cm • Holodiastolic flow reversal in the proximal abdominal aorta • Regurgitant volume ≥ 60 mL/beat • Regurgitant fraction ≥ 50% • ERO ≥ 0.3 cm^2 • Angiography grade 3 to 4 • In addition, diagnosis of chronic severe AR requires evidence of LV dilation	Normal LVEF (>55%) and mild-to-moderate LV dilation (LVESD < 50 mm)	None; exercise testing is reasonable to confirm symptom status

Continued...

Continued...

Stage	Definition	Valve anatomy	Hemodynamics	Consequences	Symptoms
C2	With LV dysfunction	• Calcific aortic valve disease • Bicuspid valve (or other congenital abnormality) • Dilated aortic sinuses or ascending aorta • Rheumatic valve changes • IE with abnormal leaflet closure or perforation	**Severe AR:** • Jet width ≥ 65% of LVOT • Vena contracta > 0.6 cm • Holodiastolic flow reversal in the proximal abdominal aorta • Regurgitant volume ≥ 60 mL/beat • Regurgitant fraction ≥ 50% • ERO ≥ 0.3 cm^2 • Angiography grade 3–4 • In addition, diagnosis of chronic severe AR requires evidence of LV dilation	Abnormal LV systolic function with depressed LVEF (≤55%) or severe LV dilation (LVESD > 50 mm or indexed LVESD > 25 mm/m^2)	None; exercise testing is reasonable to confirm symptom status
D	**Symptomatic severe AR**	• Calcific aortic valve disease • Bicuspid valve (or other congenital abnormality) • Dilated aortic sinuses or ascending aorta • Rheumatic valve changes • IE with abnormal leaflet closure or perforation	**Severe AR:** • Jet width ≥ 65% of LVOT • Vena contracta > 0.6 cm • Holodiastolic flow reversal in the proximal abdominal aorta • Regurgitant volume ≥ 60 mL/beat • Regurgitant fraction ≥ 50% • ERO ≥ 0.3 cm^2 • Angiography grade 3 to 4 • In addition, diagnosis of chronic severe AR requires evidence of LV dilation	• Symptomatic severe AR may occur with normal systolic function (LVEF > 55%), mild-to-moderate LV dysfunction (LVEF 40–55%), or severe LV dysfunction (LVEF < 40%) • Moderate to severe LV dilation is present	Exertional dyspnea or angina or more severe HF symptoms

(ERO: effective regurgitant orifice; LVESD: left ventricular end-systolic dimension; LVOT: left ventricular outflow tract)

Source: Adapted from the American College of Cardiology/the American Heart Association (ACC/AHA) guidelines for the management of patients with valvular heart disease 2020.

PRIMARY AORTIC REGURGITATION

Bicuspid AV and degenerative calcific AV leaflets are the most common valvular causes of AR in developed countries, while rheumatic disease is the leading cause in India.

Rheumatic AR: Rheumatic AV is characterized by fibrosis and thickening of leaflet edges with resultant retraction and restricted leaflet motion and consequent AR. The AV is the second most common valve after the mitral valve to have rheumatic affection. Isolated involvement of the AV is uncommon. A common rheumatic multivalvular disease is mitral stenosis and AR.

Bicuspid AV: Bicuspid AV with incomplete closure and prolapse of cusp may result in isolated AR or a combination of AR and AS. Aortopathy with bicuspid AV may result in aortic dilation which may worsen AR.

Other etiologies for valvular AR include:
- Older patients with calcific AS have associated AR.
- Infective endocarditis (leaflet perforation or vegetation interfering with coaptation)
- Traumatic rupture of ascending aorta/root with cusp prolapse
- Ventricular septal defect/subaortic membrane with cusp prolapse
- After aortic balloon valvuloplasty, TAVR, structural deterioration of bioprosthetic valve
- Associated with inflammatory disorders such as systemic lupus erythematosus, rheumatoid arthritis, and ankylosing spondylitis

SECONDARY AORTIC REGURGITATION

Dilation of ascending aorta with dilated aortic annulus and failure of leaflet apposition also causes AR, the resultant LV dilation exaggerates root dilation which further intensifies AR, resulting in a vicious cycle. Etiologies include age-related dilation, annulo-aortic ectasia, aortic cystic medial necrosis, aortitis, hypertension, inflammatory and connective tissue disorders.

PATHOPHYSIOLOGY AND HEMODYNAMICS

In AR, abnormal regurgitation of blood occurs from the aorta into the LV during diastole (regurgitant volume/

fraction). LV pumps that regurgitant volume plus blood entering from the LA. Total SV equals combined regurgitant fraction and effective forward SV.

Besides severity the pathophysiology of AR also depends on rapidity of its onset. Acute severe AR results in acute volume and consequently pressure overload of LV since the compensatory mechanisms of LV dilation and eccentric hypertrophy do not happen in a short time. Hallmark of chronic AR is the compensatory mechanism in LV and the hemodynamics.

CHRONIC AORTIC REGURGITATION

Volume overload evokes compensatory mechanisms based on Frank-Starling principle. With AR there is an increase in left ventricular end-diastolic volume (LVEDV). However, LV starts dilating with increased LV compliance, hence LVEDP does not increase. The increase in EDV translates into an increase in total SV, resulting in maintenance of normal forward SV.

Patient develops eccentric LVH by production of new sarcomeres in series. Overall preload increases enhancing total SV and ejection fraction. LV performance is normal, and patient remains asymptomatic for decades.

Increase in LV volume elevates LVSP (Laplace law), thereby increasing LV afterload. Both preload and afterload are increased in AR (compared to decreased afterload in MR); resulting in continued recruitment of preload reserve and LVH. In AR, LV mass is greatly increased resulting in extremely enlarged heart (Cor Bovinum).

Compensation cannot be maintained and afterload mismatch ensues with progressive decrease in LV systolic performance indices (including LVEF) to subnormal range. With LV decompensation, LV compliance declines, LVEDP increases, and myocardial interstitial fibrosis progresses. In advanced stages, elevated LVEDP is reflected backward in pulmonary circulation and forward CO falls, at first during exercise and then at rest. Symptoms of HF develop, particularly those secondary to pulmonary congestion.

Diastolic aortic pressure declines due to AR, coronary perfusion pressure falls thereby reducing myocardial oxygen supply. Dilated LV cavity and increased LVSP increase myocardial oxygen demand with ischemia manifesting as angina even without concomitant CAD. This ischemia may further impair LV function.

ACUTE AORTIC REGURGITATION

As mentioned earlier the severity and the rapidity of onset of AR determine its hemodynamics. Acute AR is caused by infective endocarditis, aortic dissection, and trauma. Other causes include prosthetic valve dysfunction/dehiscence, complication of balloon aortic valvuloplasty/TAVR. In acute AR, LVH/increase in LV compliance does not occur. As a result, AR causes increased LVEDV with increase in LVEDP. The suddenly elevated LVEDP is transmitted to left atrium and pulmonary circulation with resulting dyspnea and pulmonary edema. The total SV is not increased and the effective forward SV drops. To compensate for low output, sympathetic stimulation with tachycardia and peripheral vasoconstriction occurs, worsening AR. Such situation is a surgical emergency, requiring immediate intervention.

CLINICAL FEATURES

SYMPTOMS

Chronic AR remains asymptomatic for prolonged period. Dyspnea on exertion, effort intolerance, and fatigue are the common symptoms. Palpitations may be present in apparently asymptomatic patients for years. It may be exertional or on lying down due to awareness of forceful LV contraction. They develop gradually and insidiously. In late stages, they have dyspnea on minimal exertion, paroxysmal nocturnal dyspnea, and orthopnea.

Angina, though uncommon, can be due to coexisting CAD. An unusual form of nocturnal angina has been described in AR and is attributed to nocturnal bradycardia with fall in arterial diastolic pressure and coronary perfusion pressures. It is paroxysmal and associated with dyspnea and diaphoresis and generally not relieved by nitrates. Syncope is an uncommon symptom compared to AS.

In acute AR patient has sudden onset of dyspnea, orthopnea, dry cough, and weakness with rapid progression to hemodynamic collapse if untreated. Presentation gives clue to underlying etiology. Abrupt chest/back pain with acute AR is characteristic of aortic dissection. Fever and chills indicate infective endocarditis. History of blunt chest/abdominal trauma indicates disruption of AV.

SIGNS

Chronic AR: Most signs of chronic AR are related to high SV being ejected into aorta with rapid runoff as regurgitation occurs, accounting for peripheral signs (**Table 5**) that might be absent in mild AR, acute AR, LV dysfunction, and associated stenotic lesions masking the AR.

Arterial pulse is classically described as "water hammer"; an abrupt thud imparted due to rapid upstroke. It also has a collapsing nature (fades away quickly, caused by runoff into periphery). Pulse volume is large because of wide pulse pressure (steep upstroke due to rapid ejection, ill-sustained peak, and steep downslope). The bisferiens character is better felt in carotids/brachial artery in severe AR and is large volume, twice beating pulse with two peaks in systole. It is explained by Venturi forces that are created at aortic root when a large SV is ejected rapidly causing suction and thus a dip in forward flow.

Systolic pressure is elevated, diastolic pressure is abnormally low (peripheral runoff), resulting in wide pulse pressure. Korotkoff sounds persist to zero and muffling of these sounds in phase IV indicates diastolic pressure. Diastolic pressures may rise in presence of LV dysfunction.

Apex is diffuse and hyperdynamic, displaced laterally and inferiorly. S3 may be palpable. Systolic thrill at the base of the heart and over the carotid arteries indicates augmented SV. A diastolic thrill is rare. Presence of palpable carotid shudder does not necessarily signify concomitant AS.

TABLE 5	Peripheral signs of chronic severe aortic regurgitation (AR).*
Lighthouse sign	Alternate blanching and flushing of forehead with the arterial pulse
Landolfi sign	Pulsatile iris causing rhythmical alteration of pupil size
Ashrafian sign	Pulsatile pseudoproptosis, a rhythmical anterior propulsion of both eyes in systole
Becker sign	Presence of retinal arterial pulsations
Müller sign	Pulsating uvula
Morton and Mahon sign	Facial flushing and blanching
Alfred de Musset sign	Anteroposterior bobbing of the head with the arterial pulse
Bozzolo sign	Pulsatile nasal mucosa
Minervini's sign	Pulsation of tongue
Corrigan sign	Dancing of carotids caused by abrupt distention and rapid collapse of arterial pulse
Locomotor brachii	Rhythmical pulsation of a serpentine brachial artery
Mayne sign	>15 mm Hg diastolic pressure reduction with arm elevation
Quincke's pulse	Capillary pulsation (normally capillary flow is nonpulsatile) detected at the nail bed
Palmar click	Pulsating palms—palpable systolic flushing of palms
Rosenbach sign	Systolic pulsation of enlarged liver
Gerhardt sign (Sailer's sign)	Systolic pulsation of enlarged spleen
Lincoln sign	Rhythmic movement of leg crossed over the other
Hill's sign	Disproportionate elevation of lower limb blood pressures when compared to upper limb blood pressure in patients
Pistol shot sound	A sharp sound heard over the femoral artery during rapid ejection of large volume of blood into the arterial tree
Duroziez sign	The double intermittent murmur heard over femoral arteries
Sherman sign	Prominent and easily palpable dorsalis pedis in elder
Watson pulse	Waterhammer pulse

*Signs listed as found during examination from head to toe.

S1 is usually normal or soft in absence of associated mitral valve disease. S2 may be normal in intensity and splitting, A2 may be soft/inaudible in case of calcific immobile aortic leaflets or rarely may be loud in root disease(syphilis). S3 may be audible with the onset of LV dysfunction. S4 may occasionally be heard due to hypertrophy. An EC signifies dilated aortic root or bicuspid AV.

A high-pitched, soft, blowing, decrescendo early diastolic murmur is heard best in the third intercostal space along the left sternal border with diaphragm of stethoscope with patient sitting up and leaning forward and breath held in expiration. Duration of murmur correlates with the severity of AR. A short murmur suggests mild AR while a long diastolic murmur suggests severe AR. In very severe AR, the late diastolic equilibration of the aortic and LV pressures may obliterate later part of murmur. In valvular AR, murmur is usually louder along the left sternal border; whereas loud murmur along the right sternal border suggests dilation of the aortic root as cause of AR. Musical/"cooing dove"/seagull murmur usually signifies eversion/perforation of an aortic cusp (syphilis/infective endocarditis/rheumatic fever/trauma). Occasionally, murmur of AR may radiate up to the left axilla (Cole-Cecil murmur).

Harsh systolic ejection murmur may be present, caused by increased SV, often radiating to carotids. It may be more readily audible than diastolic murmur. It is higher-pitched and less rasping than the murmur of AS and often accompanied by thrill. Presence of other peripheral signs of AR differentiates it from AS.

Occasionally, a soft, low-pitched, and rumbling mid-to-late diastolic (Austin Flint) murmur is heard. It is caused by the posterior displacement of anterior leaflet of the mitral valve by the jet of AR. However, it is not associated with hemodynamically significant mitral obstruction and must be differentiated from coexisting mitral stenosis (mid diastolic murmur).

Acute AR: Classic peripheral signs of chronic AR are usually absent. The patient is gravely ill with peripheral vasoconstriction, cyanosis, and pulmonary edema. Tachycardia is a rule and hypotension may be present. The precordium is conspicuously quiet and apex undisplaced. S1 is usually soft (due to raised LVEDP with premature closure of mitral valve). S2 may be soft or even absent if cusps are damaged with resultant noncoaptation and S3 is frequently present. Patient has a short, low-pitched early diastolic murmur (raised LVEDP with rapid equilibration of aortic and LV pressures). Austin flint murmur and short ejection systolic murmur are frequently present.

INVESTIGATIONS

ELECTROCARDIOGRAM

Left ventricular hypertrophy with left axis deviation, LA enlargement may be present. Features of LV volume overload (q waves and upright T waves) are seen in moderate/early stages of severe AR (**Fig. 6**). LV pressure overload (ST depression and T wave inversion in leads I and aVL) might be present in later stages of chronic AR.

Tachycardia is usually the only manifestation in acute AR.

PR prolongation/AV block might indicate infective endocarditis with perivalvular abscess or degenerative calcific AV.

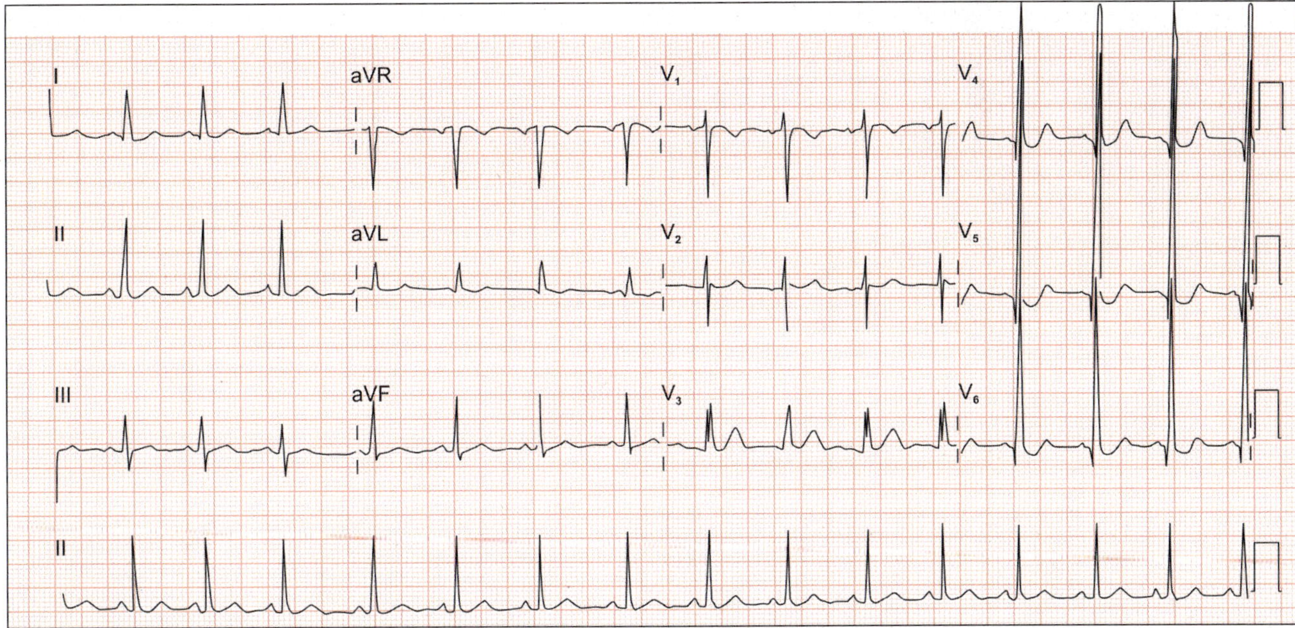

FIGURE 6: Electrocardiogram (ECG) showing volume overload in a patient with severe aortic regurgitation (AR).

CHEST X-RAY

Cardiac silhouette shows cardiomegaly, dilation of aortic root, and calcification of valve. Calcified ascending aorta may be present. Pulmonary vascular redistribution, interstitial and alveolar edema, and LA enlargement indicate LV dysfunction.

In acute AR, cardiac size is usually normal with pulmonary edema. Mediastinal widening indicates associated aortic dissection.

ECHOCARDIOGRAPHY

Transthoracic echocardiography (TTE) is indicated for assessment of the presence, cause and severity of regurgitation, LV size and systolic function, prognosis, and timing of valve intervention.

Two-dimensional echocardiography and M-mode help to identify presence of bicuspid AV, thickened cusps, prolapse of the valve, and a flail leaflet or vegetation. Aortic leaflet anatomy and motion, the size and shape of the aortic root, LV systolic and diastolic function, and LV end-systolic and end-diastolic dimensions can be evaluated. Diastolic fluttering of the anterior mitral leaflet or septum caused by impingement of regurgitant flow. Although specific it is not very sensitive in AR and is unrelated to the severity.

Doppler echocardiography is the best noninvasive method for detecting AR, manifested as a diastolic flow abnormality arising from the AV, directed toward the LV. Use of color Doppler has more advantages over continuous or pulsed wave Doppler (**Figures 7 A** to **D**). The global longitudinal strain measured on TTE is also a useful predictor of mortality in patient with chronic AR. 3D echocardiography is valuable tool, especially for evaluation of LV volumes.

Transesophageal echocardiography is rarely indicated with suboptimal TTE images.

Quantification, grading of severity of AR, and progression of AR on echocardiography involve a number of parameters as described in **Table 5**.

CARDIAC CATHETERIZATION AND CAG

Coronary angiography is indicated in patients with risk factors for CAD prior to intervention.

Diagnostic cardiac catheterization is indicated in case of discrepancy between clinical and TTE findings. Aortic root angiogram can grade severity of AR with dye injected at rapid rates.

OTHER INVESTIGATIONS

CT aortogram is indicated to assess aortic root/ascending aorta in cases of dissection prior to surgery.

Exercise stress testing is useful in assessing objective exercise capacity and symptoms in patients with AR but who report no symptoms or those with equivocal symptoms.

Recent data indicate *serum BNP or NT-proBNP* may be an early sign of LV dysfunction, and it is possible that this will be added to recommendations for surgical intervention in the future.

NATURAL HISTORY

Asymptomatic patients with moderate-to-severe AR without LV dysfunction remain so for many years. In a large follow-up study AVR was required at rate of 4% per year, with 90% remaining asymptomatic at 3 years, 81% at

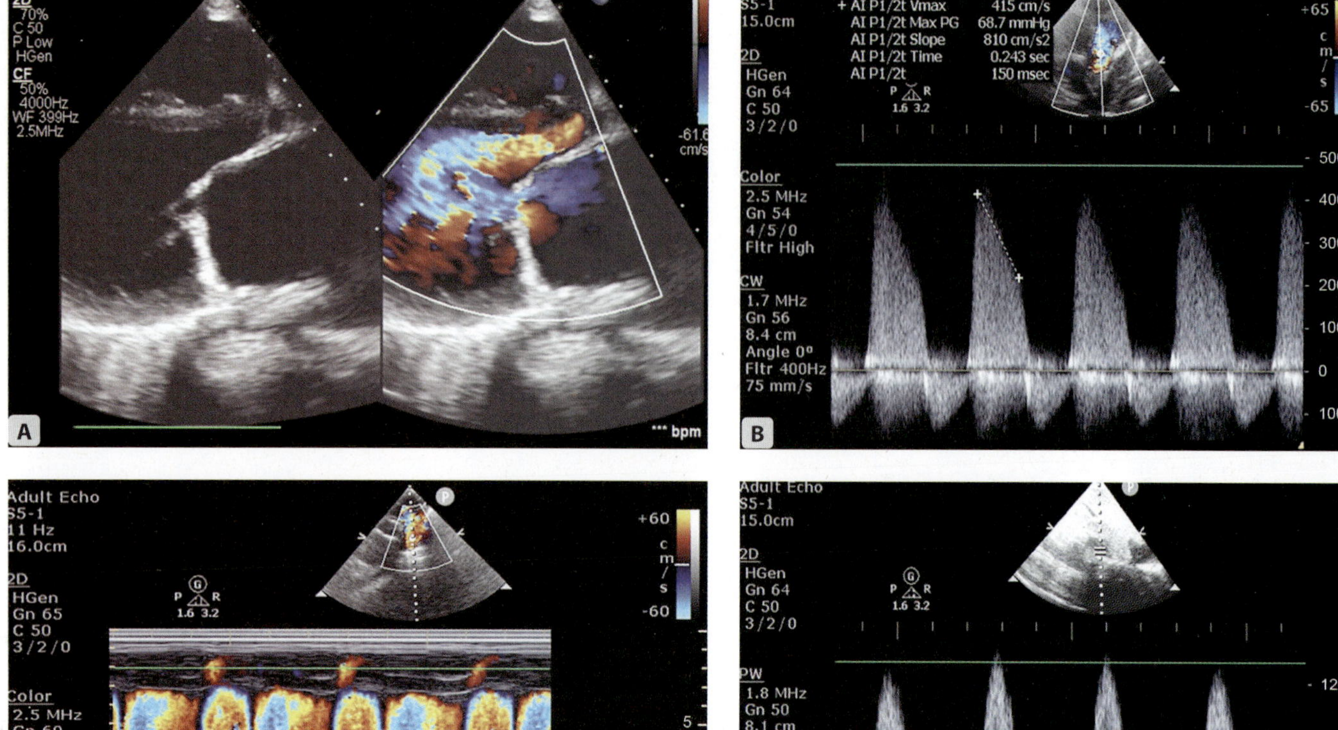

FIGURES 7 A to D: Echocardiographic tracings showing severe aortic regurgitation (AR): **(A)** color Doppler image; **(B)** continuous wave Doppler across the aortic valve with measurement of pressure half time; **(C)** M-mode with color Doppler across descending thoracic aorta showing holo-diastolic flow reversal; and **(D)** Pulsed-wave Doppler across the abdominal aorta showing holo-diastolic flow reversal.

5 years, and 75% at 7 years after diagnosis. Conservative management of moderate-to-severe AR results in a 5-year and 10-year survival rate of 75% and 50%, respectively.

Quantitative measures of AR, LV size, and LV function predict clinical outcome. Once the patient becomes symptomatic, course becomes rapidly progressive. HF, episodes of acute pulmonary edema, and sudden death may occur in symptomatic patients with LV dilation.

Early death caused by LV failure is common in patients with acute severe AR.

MANAGEMENT

CHRONIC AORTIC REGURGITATION

Medical therapy: Patients with asymptomatic chronic AR must be advised clinical and echocardiographic follow-up. Specific therapy to prevent disease progression is currently unavailable.

There is no evidence that vasodilating drugs reduce severity of AR or alter history of AR in absence of hypertension, although they are commonly used.

Management of hypertension and HF is done according to guidelines. Control of BP (goal systolic BP < 140 mm Hg) is important. Medications which reduce heart rate may paradoxically increase systolic BP due to increased SV. Since ACE inhibitors do not affect heart rate and lower BP they are commonly used.

In symptomatic patients, medical therapy helps to stabilize the patients prior to intervention and is helpful in alleviating symptoms in patients at prohibitive risk of AVR. HF management with salt restriction, diuretics, and ACE inhibitors is indicated.

Intervention: Most symptomatic patients eventually need valve replacement with a mechanical or bioprosthetic valve. The American Heart Association/The American College of Cardiology (AHA/ACC) 2020 valvular heart disease guidelines proposed management strategy for patients with chronic severe AR which is shown in **Figures 4 A** to **D**.

Briefly, indications/timing for intervention include symptomatic chronic severe AR, asymptomatic patients with LV dysfunction (LVEF <55%)/undergoing cardiac surgery for another indication/LV end systolic dimension >50 mm (or >25 mm/m^2) with preserved LV systolic function. AVR may be performed in low surgical risk patients with progressive decrease in LVEF or increase in LV end-diastolic dimension >65 mm in three successive

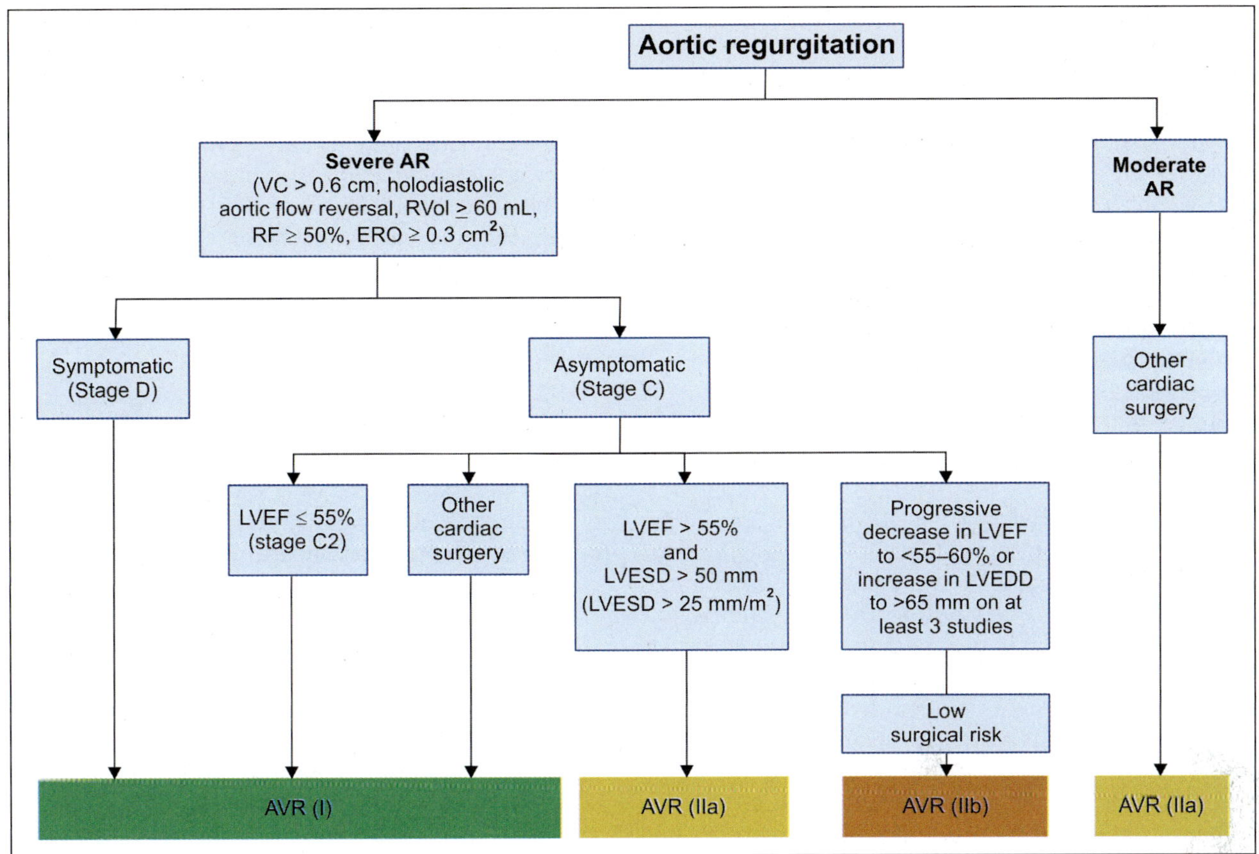

(EDD: end-diastolic dimension; ERO: effective regurgitant orifice; LVESD: left ventricular end-systolic dimension; RF: regurgitant fraction; RVol: regurgitant volume; VC: vena contracta)

FLOWCHART 2: Recommendations for aortic valve intervention in aortic regurgitation (AR).

Source: Adapted from 2020 ACC/AHA (the American College of Cardiology/American Heart Association) guidelines for the management of patients with valvular heart disease.

studies. AVR in moderate AR may be recommended if patient is undergoing another cardiac surgery.

Surgical AVR is the preferred option. Assessment of the size of aortic root and ascending aorta (>45 mm) is important to evaluate the need for concomitant aortic root replacement surgery (**Flowchart 2**).

Transcatheter aortic valve replacement for isolated chronic AR is anatomically challenging and is hence not routinely done.

ACUTE AORTIC REGURGITATION

Most guidelines recommend prompt surgical intervention for acute severe AR. While waiting for surgery, medical therapy aims to augment forward flow and achieve hemodynamic stability. Positive inotropes and/or vasodilators should be carefully chosen based on arterial pressures. The placement of an intra-aortic balloon counterpulsation (IABP) is contraindicated in severe AR.

Although β-blockers are recommended for aortic dissection, its use is not recommended in acute severe AR because it worsens AR by causing bradycardia.

Antibiotics are indicated in acute severe AR due to endocarditis. Surgical intervention may be delayed for 5–7 days of antibiotic therapy in hemodynamically stable patients.

CONCLUSION

- The high prevalence of AV disease in community makes it likely for practitioners to encounter such patients. Hence, its diagnosis, assessment of severity, and appropriate management become crucial.
- There is significant difference in the etiology and prevalence of AV disease in India as compared to the western world.
- Timely and accurate diagnosis and management can significantly alter the natural history of AV disease.
- Transcatheter aortic valve replacement has brought about a paradigm shift in management of AS.

RECOMMENDED READINGS

1. Rajamannan NM, Bonow RO, Rahimtoola SH. Calcific aortic stenosis: an update. Nature clinical practice Cardiovascular medicine. 2007;4(5):254-62.
2. d'Arcy JL, Coffey S, Loudon MA, Kennedy A, Pearson-Stuttard J, Birks J, et al. Large-scale community echocardiographic screening reveals a major burden of undiagnosed valvular heart disease in older people: the OxVALVE Population Cohort Study. Eur Heart J. 2016;37:3515-22.

3. Sahu AK, Sagar P, Khanna R, Kumar S, Tewari S, Kapoor A, et al. Etiology and distribution of isolated aortic stenosis in Indian patients–A study from a large tertiary care hospital in north India. Indian heart j. 2020;72(4):272-7.
4. Levinson GE. Valvular heart disease. In: Gordon BL (Ed). Clinical Cardiopulmonary Physiology, 3rd edition. New York: Grune and Stratton; 1969. pp. 245-58.
5. Manjunath CN, Srinivas P, Ravindranath KS, Dhanalakshmi C. Incidence and patterns of valvular heart disease in a tertiary care high-volume cardiac center: a single center experience. Indian heart j. 2014;66(3):320-6.
6. Verma S, Siu SC. Aortic Dilatation in Patients with Bicuspid Aortic Valve. N Engl J Med. 2014;370:1920-9.
7. Ridley CH, Vallabhajosyula P, Bavaria JE, Patel PA, Gutsche JT, Shah R, et al. The Sievers classification of the bicuspid aortic valve for the perioperative echocardiographer: the importance of valve phenotype for aortic valve repair in the era of the functional aortic annulus. J. Cardiothorac Vasc Anesth. 2016;30:1142-51.
8. Sabet HY, Edwards WD, Tazelaar HD, Daly RC. Congenitally bicuspid aortic valves: a surgical pathology study of 542 cases (1991 through 1996) and a literature review of 2,715 additional cases. Mayo Clin Proc. 1999; 74:14-26.
9. Lindman BR, Clavel M-A, Mathieu P, Iung B, Lancellotti P, Otto CM, et al. Calcific aortic stenosis. Nat Rev Dis Primers. 2016;2:16006.
10. Otto CM, Nishimura RA, Bonow RO, Carabello BA, Erwin JP 3rd, Gentile F, et al. 2020 ACC/AHA guideline for the management of patients with valvular heart disease: a report of the American College of Cardiology/ American Heart Association Joint Committee on Clinical Practice Guidelines. J Am Coll Cardiol. 2021;77(4):e25-197.
11. Singh JP, Evans JC, Levy D, Larson MG, Freed LA, Fuller DL, et al. Prevalence and clinical determinants of mitral, tricuspid, and aortic regurgitation (the framingham heart study). Am J Cardiol. 1999;83: 897-902.
12. Enriquez-Sarano M, Tajik AJ. Clinical practice. Aortic regurgitation. N Engl J Med. 2004;351(15):1539-46.
13. Griffin B. Valvular heart disease. In: Griffin BP, Callahan TD, Menon V, Wu WM, Cauthen CA, Dunn JM (Eds). Manual of cardiovascular medicine, Vol. 1, 4th edition. Philadelphia, PA: Lippincott Williams and Wilkins; 2013. pp. 238-355.
14. Detaint D, Messika-Zeitoun D, Maalouf J, Tribouilloy C, Mahoney DW, Tajik AJ, et al. Quantitative echocardiographic determinants of clinical outcome in asymptomatic patients with aortic regurgitation: a prospective study. JACC Cardiovasc Imaging. 2008;1: 1-11.

CHAPTER

97

Tricuspid, Pulmonary, and Multivalvular Diseases

Smit Shrivastava

ABSTRACT

The right-sided valves (tricuspid and pulmonary) are less often affected in chronic rheumatic heart disease. Also, hemodynamic implications are less than the mitral and aortic valve disease. Since right side of heart is a low-pressure circuit as the pulmonary vascular resistance (PVR) is low the valve replacement of tricuspid and pulmonary valve is rarely done. Tricuspid valve (TV) involvement when overlooked in left-sided rheumatic heart disease can result in poor surgical outcomes. The involvement of TV can be primary or secondary to pulmonary artery (PA) hypertension. The pulmonary valve stenosis is always congenital. It is amenable to balloon pulmonary valvotomy (BPV) will very good outcome.

Patients with rheumatic heart disease often have multivalvular involvement. Although, we discuss each valve disease separately, clinically we often encounter mixed valve disease. The hemodynamics of one affect the hemodynamics of the other. The relative severity of the lesions has to be the assessed clinically and then confirmed on echocardiography since it has implications on the management plan.

"We fail when we try to give simple answers to complicated problems"

—T Ramadan

INTRODUCTION

The right-sided valves possess striking anatomical and hemodynamic differences to command secernate approach. The recent interest and enthusiasm into understanding and treating tricuspid, pulmonary and multivalvular diseases have been kindled with the advent of transcatheter therapies for the left-sided valves and epidemiological evidence of worse outcomes for patients with added or residual tricuspid disease.

TRICUSPID VALVE

The TV regulates the flow from the right atrium into the right ventricle (RV) over a small gradient while electrically isolating the two chambers. The TV diseases more often are diagnosed late and are denied treatment till their surgery becomes a must. The TV diseases are predictors of morbidity and mortality.

The TV anatomy is far more complex and mobile than the mitral valve. The TV is the largest valve with flexible annulus, usually three thin and fragile leaflets, anchoring chordae tendinae and papillary muscles. The TV annulus is asymmetric and saddle shaped. The annulus can grow twice the size of neighboring mitral annulus. The shape and size alter with cardiac cycle with 20% reduction in the annular circumference with atrial systole. TV has three leaflets. The semicircular anterior leaflet is the largest, fastening to a single papillary muscle at anterior or free wall of RV, affected most by annular dilatation. The septal leaflet has papillary muscle attachment to the septum. The posterior leaflet often has multiple scallops, without clear divisions.

The TV has three relatively constant papillary muscles, one for each commissure. The anterior papillary muscle arising from the moderator band is largest. The inferior or posterior papillary muscle arises from the acute margin between the anterior and inferior walls. The medial papillary muscle (papillary muscle of the conus or the muscle of Lancisi or Luschka) marks the junction between the inflow and outflow portions of the RV.

The anatomically unique features of TV are its tendency to lack calcium deposits; the right ventricular apical approach for interventions is not favored by trabeculated and thin RV. The high compliance of the RV doubles its size before functions deterioration. The right ventricular dilatation and dysfunction change its shape from natural oval shape to a more circular one.

TRICUSPID STENOSIS

Most of the tricuspid stenosis (TS) occurs with tricuspid regurgitation (TR) of varying severity. Rheumatic TS is the most common cause. It is seen in 5% of symptomatic cases and in 15–25% at autopsy. It is more common in females. It is almost always associated with rheumatic involvement of the left-sided valves. Congenital stenosis, more common in males, occurs in 0.3% of all congenital heart diseases. The other causes are rare (**Table 1**).

CLINICAL FEATURES

The symptoms of TS are often masked by coexisting rheumatic mitral valve disease. Clinical presentation depends on the severity and duration of stenosis. Patients with significant stenosis can have low forward output symptoms of easy fatigue, weakness, and exercise intolerance. There can be masking of symptoms of left-sided lesions. The backward systemic venous congestion symptoms of neck vein dilatation, ascites, peripheral edema, and anorexia can be there. Patients with carcinoid syndrome can have diarrhea and flushing.

The physical examination is also overshadowed by the coexisting other valvular lesions; however, the suspicion for TS is raised when signs of mitral stenosis (MS) are unexpectedly ameliorated and/or the venous pressure are out of proportion to the pulmonary congestion. Patients have ascites, peripheral edema and anasarca, and tender hepatomegaly with presystolic pulsations. The elevated jugular venous pressure (JVP) demonstrating a prominent presystolic a wave with slow inappreciable y descent is seen. Kussmaul sign (absence of decrease or a rise in JVP with inspiration) may be appreciable.

In cardiovascular system (CVS), they have a widely split first heart sound. Opening snap of the pliable TV at the left lower sternal border is often drowned by preceding mitral valve opening snap. A low frequency rumbling mid-diastolic crescendo-decrescendo murmur before first heart sound is heard in the fourth intercostal space. The murmur is shorter, softer, and higher pitched than the mitral counterpart. The dynamic maneuvers that increase flow across the valve increase the murmur, like inspiration (Carvallo sign), leg

TABLE 1 The causes of tricuspid stenosis.

Cause	Features
Rheumatic heart disease	Female preponderance, 3–5% in rheumatic valve disease
Congenital tricuspid stenosis	Male preponderance, often associated with pulmonary obstruction
Right atrial tumors	Atrial myxoma is the most common
Carcinoid heart disease	Fibrotic plaques and serotonin thicken the valve in 40%
Endomyocardial fibrosis	Uncommon cause
Valvular vegetations	Large fungal, vegetations in intravenous drug abusers
Extracardiac tumors	External compression, very rare
Devices	Obstruction by pacemaker leads
Iatrogenic	Radiation drugs like fenfluramine, methysergide, and ergotamine

TABLE 2 Causes of tricuspid regurgitation.

Primary TR (25%)	Secondary TR (75%)
• **Congenital:** ◦ Ebstein anomaly, TV tethering associated with perimembranous VSD, atrioventricular canal defect, corrected transposition of great vessels, and rarely TV dysplasia • **Acquired:** ◦ Rheumatic, degenerative myxomatous prolapse, endocarditis, carcinoid, endomyocardial fibrosis, toxins, trauma, iatrogenic (pacing leads, RV biopsy, and radiation) and rarely ischemic papillary muscle dysfunction/rupture	• **Left heart disease:** ◦ LV dysfunction or valve disease especially mitral • **Right ventricular dysfunction:** ◦ RV ischemia, RV volume overload, and RV cardiomyopathy • **Pulmonary hypertension:** ◦ Chronic lung disease, pulmonary thromboembolism, and intracardiac shunts • **Right atrial abnormalities:** ◦ Atrial fibrillation • **Postoperative:** ◦ Recurrent TR, postsurgical intervention

raising, inhalation of amyl nitrate, squatting, or exercise and decreased by expiration and Valsalva.

DIAGNOSIS

Chest radiograph shows enlarged right atrium or biatrial enlargement in mitral disease and dilated azygos and superior vena cava.

Electrocardiogram is often not rewarding but for atrial fibrillation and tall peaked P waves in II, III, and aVF depicting enlarged right atrium in sinus rhythm.

Echocardiography (2D and Doppler) is diagnostic as TS is often not detected on clinical examination. The rheumatic TV has thickened, malformed, and restricted leaflets. The dilated right atrium, vena cava can be demonstrated. The echocardiographic findings of mean pressure gradient >5 mm Hg, pressure half-time ≥190 ms, valve area ≤1.0 cm^2 by the continuity equation, and associated right atrial and inferior vena cava (IVC) enlargement aid in diagnosis. The concomitant TR can alter the hemodynamics.

Three-dimensional transesophageal echocardiography (TEE) though not validated provides better qualitative data on the morphological abnormalities by enface visualization of the valve.

Cardiac catheterization for hemodynamic assessment of the severity of TS is routinely not required. A double lumen catheter can facilitate simultaneous recording of right atrial and ventricular pressures. The Fick principle can provide the valve area. A TV area of <1 cm^2 indicates severe TS.

MANAGEMENT

Patients are advised symptom limited activities with fluid and salt restriction to reduce venous congestion. The diuretics can relieve congestion in early stages but may worsen the low cardiac output symptoms. The stenosis may be relieved by percutaneous dilation, removal of pacemaker leads, or surgical valve repair or replacement (rarely).

The criteria for intervention are mean diastolic pressure gradient >5 mm Hg, TV area <2.0 cm^2. TV surgery is preferred over percutaneous interventions for greater surgical experience and accompanying TR. Percutaneous TV balloon valvotomy is reserved for isolated TS without more than mild TR that may be done concomitant with balloon mitral valvotomy.

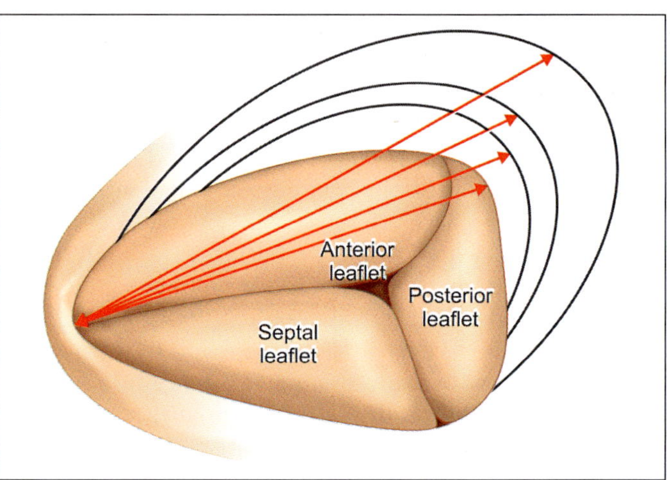

FIGURE 1: Stages of tricuspid regurgitation with progressive annular dilation.

The majority of TV surgeries are performed consequent to or as part of other cardiac surgeries and surgical mortality is about 10% for combined surgery. The magnitude of valvular and subvalvular pathology governs the choice between TV repair and replacement. The long-term mortality rates are similar; however, the in-hospital mortality rates are lower with the valve repair. The limited life expectancy and higher thrombotic risks favor bioprosthetic valves, scientific evidence is lacking. The prognosis is largely dictated by the accompanying cardiac conditions.

TRICUSPID REGURGITATION

It is of two types. Secondary TR (75%) is due to left heart and pulmonary diseases causing pulmonary hypertension. It is also sometime called as functional TR since there is no primary structural abnormality of the valve. Primary TR (25%) is due to valve involvement in a disease process (rheumatic or others). Primary TR is uncommon and generally less severe (**Table 2**).

The pathophysiology of secondary TR is better understood in three phases (**Fig. 1**):

- *First phase*: The left heart disease, atrial fibrillation, and resultant pulmonary hypertension cause right ventricular and annular dilatation without causing significant TR.

- *Second phase*: Progress to leaflet (edge-to-edge) separation causing significant TR.
- *Third phase*: Noncoaptation of anterior and posterior leaflet causing severe TR. The volume overload in moderate to severe TR causes further worsening of TR by increasing right ventricular and TV annular dilation.

CLINICAL FEATURES

The symptoms of TR are variable. The physiologic TR is asymptomatic and benign. The primary TR remains asymptomatic till the RV fails. The symptoms in secondary TR are regulated by etiology, pulmonary hypertension, and chronicity. Pulmonary hypertension can cause low output symptoms of easy fatigability, exercise intolerance, shortness of breath and weakness, rarely peripheral cyanosis, and cold skin. Severe TR can result in distended neck vein sensation, right hypochondrial discomfort, ascites, and peripheral edema. In chronic TR with right ventricular failure, there can be cachexia with ascites and peripheral edema.

The physical examination shows signs of right heart failure which are most prominent. They have ascites, peripheral edema and anasarca, and tender pulsatile hepatomegaly. The JVP shows distended pulsatile jugular veins with distinct c-v regurgitant wave (x-x' disappears) and sharp y descent, with occasional Kussmaul's sign and systolic thrill. The peripheral pulse is diminished. Atrial fibrillation is common.

On cardiac examination, precordium is hyperdynamic with thrusting right ventricular apex and right ventricular heave. In secondary TR due to pulmonary arterial hypertension (PAH), there is dullness and fullness in left second intercostal space. A loud pulmonary second heart sound (P2) will be there. Third and fourth heart sounds increasing on inspiration can be there in RV failure. Late or midsystolic clicks in TV prolapse can be there. The murmur of secondary TR is high pitched and pansystolic, in fourth intercostal space in parasternal region. Occasionally, it is loudest in subxiphoid area when severe TR is associated with pulmonary hypertension. The murmur can translocate to the apex with dilated RV. Murmur increases with inspiration (Carvallo sign), exercise, leg raising, and hepatic compression. In absence of pulmonary hypertension, the murmur is low intensity and is protosystolic.

DIAGNOSIS

Electrocardiogram shows frequent atrial fibrillation, right bundle branch block, and q in V_1 lead.

Chest radiograph may reveal marked cardiomegaly, distention of the azygos vein and pleural effusions, diaphragmatic elevation with ascites, and pulmonary arterial and venous hypertension.

Echocardiography: The assessment of degree of TR can be difficult due to dynamic changes with cardiac and respiratory cycle. The echocardiographic interrogation mandates assessment of the (1) severity of TR, (2) TV annular size, (3) mode of TV leaflet coaptation, and (4) the extent of TV leaflet tethering. Echocardiography assessment of TR severity according to the American Society of Echocardiography guidelines is shown in **Table 3**. The three-dimensional echocardiography can reveal TV tenting area that correlates with surgical outcomes.

Cardiac catheterization is reserved for those with inadequate noninvasive interrogation to measure PA pressures and PVR, thermodilution or Fick cardiac output can be measured.

MANAGEMENT

The chief determinants for TR management are the severity of heart failure and of TR, and the associated abnormalities. In isolated severe TR, physical activity is not limited. Patients with severe secondary TR need restriction

TABLE 3 Echocardiographic features for severity of tricuspid regurgitation.

Echocardiographic features	Mild TR	Moderate TR	Severe TR
Qualitative			
Interventricular septal motion	Normal	Typically normal	Paradoxical/volume overload
Color flow TR jet	Small RA penetration or not holosystolic	Moderate RA penetration or late systolic	Deep RA penetration and holosystolic
Flow convergence zone	Not visible, transient, or small	Intermediate in size and duration	Large throughout systole
CW signal TR jet	Faint/parabolic or partial contour	Dense, variable contour	Dense, triangular with early peaking contour (peak <2 m/s in very severe TR)
IVC diameter	Normal	2.1–2.5 cm	>2.5 cm
Semi-quantitative			
Color flow jet area (cm^2)	<5	5–10	>10
Vena contracta (cm)	<0.3	<0.6	>0.7
PISA radius (cm)	≤5	0.6–0.9	>0.9
Hepatic vein flow	Systolic dominance	Systolic attenuation	Systolic flow reversal
RV and RA size	Usually normal	Normal/mild dilation	Dilated

(PISA: proximal isovelocity surface area)

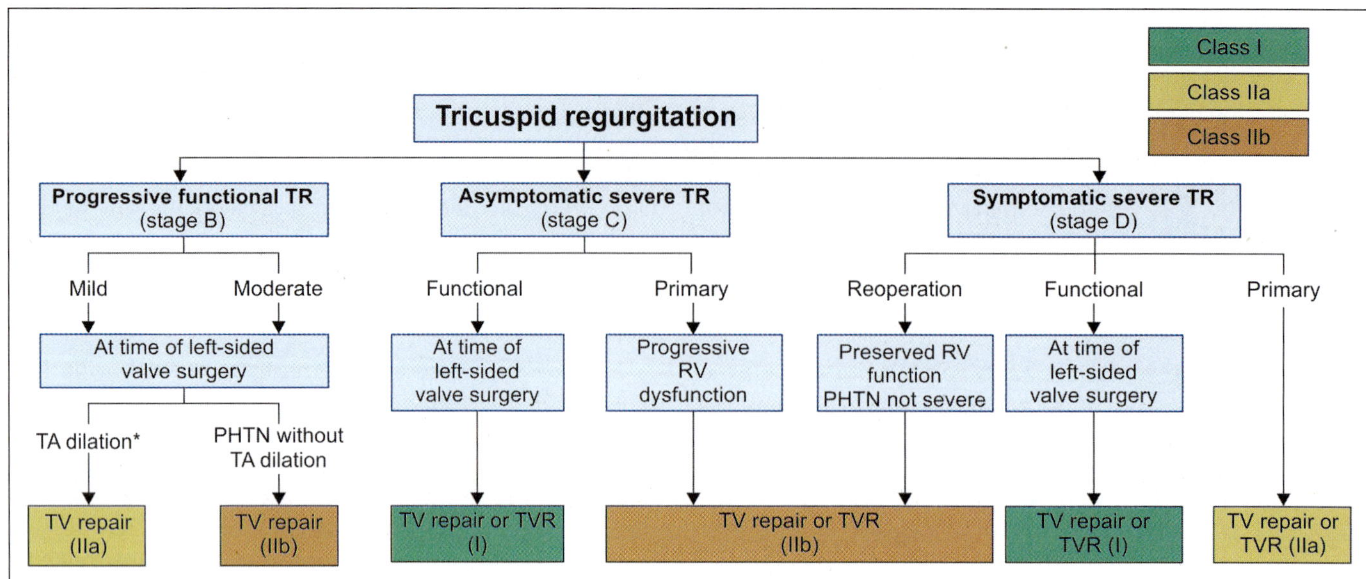

Notes: I: Indicates there is consensus of its benefit, IIa: Indicates it is usually done, IIb: Indicates generally not done.

FLOWCHART 1: Indications of surgery in tricuspid regurgitation (TR).

of activity since they have severe PAH. We should restrict fluid and sodium to manage volume status. Make cautious use of diuretics and fluid restriction to reduce systemic congestion.

Criteria for intervention: The TV surgery involves repair in most cases. Since it is a low-pressure area, replacement of TV is rarely done, since it is associated with valve thrombosis. Whenever replaced a bioprosthetic valve is used instead of a metallic valve. It may be required sometime in TR due to infective endocarditis. The indications for intervention (mostly repair) as per 2014 American Heart Association/ American College of Cardiology (AHA/ACC) valvular heart disease (VHD) guidelines are shown in **Flowchart 1**.

Class I: TV surgery is recommended for patients with severe TR undergoing left-sided valve surgery. Class IIa: TV repair can be beneficial for patients with mild, moderate, or greater functional TR at the time of left-sided valve surgery with either tricuspid annular dilation or prior evidence of right heart failure. TV surgery can be beneficial for patients with symptoms due to severe primary TR that are unresponsive to medical therapy. Class I indicates there is consensus of its benefit. Class IIa indicates that it is usually done.

Some basic principles and features of TVs are: No surgery is indicated in the absence of pulmonary hypertension as TR is well tolerated. Even total vulvectomy is well tolerated as dilation of RV-RA occurs after years. TV repair is favored over valve replacement. For repair ringed or flexible band annuloplasty, DeVega (purse-string) annuloplasty, edge-to-edge (Alfieri-type) repairs, and posterior annular bicuspidization can be done.

PULMONARY VALVE

The pulmonary valve is located anterolateral to the aortic valve. It separates the RV from the PA. It is situated apart from the other three cardiac valves. The PV complex is formed by PV leaflets and commissures, the infundibular RV and PA wall. The three semilunar leaflets are attached by convex edges partly to the infundibular wall of the RV and partly to the origin of the pulmonary trunk without the proper supporting circular annulus. It has three leaflets, the anterior, right, and left cusps.

PULMONARY VALVE STENOSIS

Pulmonic valve stenosis (PS) is caused by a congenital or genetic disorder in 95% of cases. Pulmonic stenosis can occur at three locations (**Figs. 2 A** to **C**): (1) Valvular (90%), (2) subvalvular, and (3) in frequently supravalvular. Noonan syndrome has additional narrowing of the pulmonic annulus and outflow tract. Pulmonary valve is rarely affected by rheumatic heart disease.

The PS is caused by fusion of leaflets along the commissural lines from periphery toward central orifice. It can be of various types:

Acommissural: Prominent systolic doming of the valve cusps with an eccentric orifice

Unicommissural: A single asymmetric commissure, especially in those presenting very early

Bicuspid: Fused commissures, most commonly the valvular PS is of this type.

Dysplastic: Severely thickened and deformed valve cusps

PREVALENCE

Congenital pulmonary stenosis occurs in 8–12% of all congenital heart disease. Pulmonary stenosis is the second most common congenital cardiac malformation. The isolated PS occurs in 80% of the cases, the rest occur in combination with other cardiac lesions like tetralogy

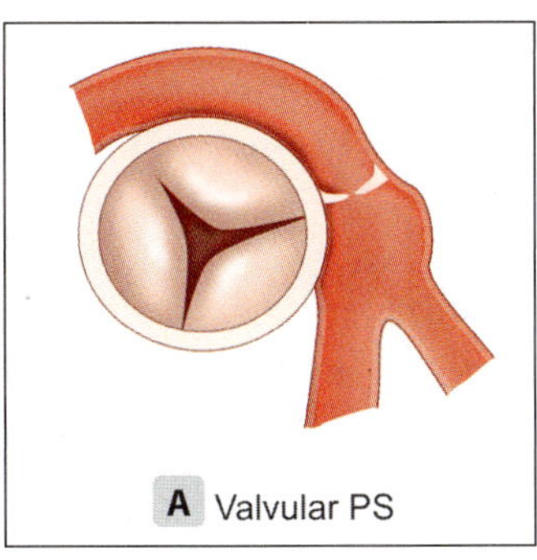

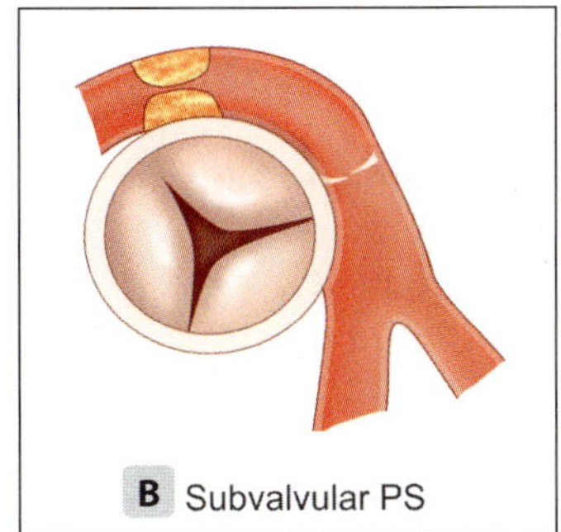

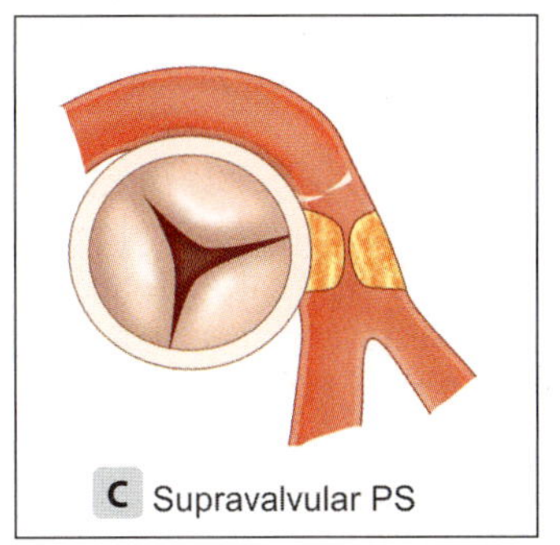

FIGURES 2 A to C: Types of pulmonic valve stenosis (PS); **(A)** Valvular PS, **(B)** Subvalvular PS, and **(C)** Supravalvular PS.

of Fallot and other Fallot-like physiologies. There is some female and family preponderance.

Mild PS is mostly asymptomatic and nonprogressive in unoperated adults. Moderate PS is usually asymptomatic too; however, the stenosis may progress during adulthood due to subvalvular hypertrophy. Most of the patients with severe PS require intervention (60% in the first 10 years after diagnosis). As a result of the increased pressure in the RV, right ventricular hypertrophy including muscular hypertrophy of the infundibulum develops. A valvular stenosis causes poststenotic dilatation of the PA due to the turbulent blood flow.

Pulmonic valve stenosis may be often associated with other cardiac anomalies like patent foramen ovale or atrial septal defect (ASD), ventricular septal defect (VSD), patent ductus arteriosus (PDA), tetralogy of Fallot, and single ventricle. Supravalvular PS can occur in combination with other syndromal diseases like Williams-Beuren syndrome [supravalvular PS, with a supravalvular aortic stenosis (AS)], Noonan syndrome (valvular or supravalvular PS with dysplastic pulmonary valve), and rubella embryopathy.

CLINICAL FEATURES

Mild-to-moderate PS patients are usually asymptomatic. Those with severe PS can develop symptoms like exertional dyspnea, fatigue, or chest pain. In late stages, they can have features of right heart failure.

On physical examination, the JVP is usually normal with prominence of the "A" wave. On cardiac palpation, they have a prominent right ventricular systolic impulse (left parasternal heave). There is a thrill in the second left intercostal space which does not radiate to the carotid arteries. On auscultation, the second heart sound has prolonged split as the severity delays the pulmonary component. The splitting becomes fixed with conduction abnormalities or right ventricular failure. The pulmonary component of the second heart sound is soft. A right-sided fourth heart sound may be there in those with decreased RV compliance. A high-pitched ejection click increasing upon inspiration is heard. It becomes inaudible in severe valvular PS as it gets buried in first heart sound. An ejection-type systolic murmur (grade 2–5 of 6), best audible at the upper left sternal border is heard. It is transmitted to the back and becomes louder and longer with increasing severity.

TABLE 4 Physical signs and severity of pulmonary stenosis.

Sign	Mild PS	Moderate PS	Severe PS
Cyanosis	–	–	+ with atrial shunt
JVP	Normal	Normal	"A" wave
Thrill	–	+/–	++
RV heave	–	+/–	++
Ejection click	+	Expiratory	Buried in S1
Murmur	Ejection mid systole	Long ejection systolic	Long ejection systolic beyond A2
Second heart sound	Normal	Wide variable	Absent P2

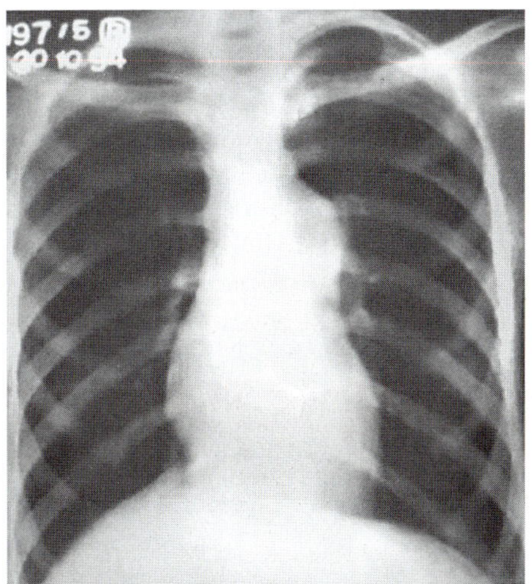

FIGURE 3: Chest radiograph of valvular pulmonary stenosis patient showing poststenotic dilatation of the pulmonary artery.

The severity of PS can be assessed from clinical features as shown in **Table 4**.

DIAGNOSIS

Electrocardiogram—it is normal in mild PS. There is right ventricular hypertrophy or conduction delay in moderate to severe cases.

Chest radiograph—no cardiomegaly without heart failure, poststenotic PA dilation may be seen, oligemic lung in severe PS (**Fig. 3**)

Echocardiography—the 2014 ACC/AHA guidelines concluded that echocardiography [generally transthoracic echocardiography (TTE)] is the preferred test for evaluating the severity of pulmonic stenosis. It shows the domed and thickened pulmonary valve leaflets with poststenotic dilated main pulmonary trunk. The instantaneous pressure gradient estimated by Doppler echo is slightly greater than the peak-to-peak systolic pressure gradient obtained by cardiac catheterization. The severity of PS on echocardiography is based on peak velocity across the pulmonary valve. It is graded as mild, moderate, and severe as shown here.

- Mild PS—peak velocity <3 m/s, peak gradient <36 mm Hg
- Moderate PS—peak velocity 3–4 m/s, peak gradient 36–64 mm Hg
- Severe PS—peak velocity >4 m/s, peak gradient >64 mm Hg

Cardiac catheterization—diagnostic cardiac catheterization is rarely required. Usually, it is performed during BPV.

MANAGEMENT

Balloon pulmonary valvuloplasty with oversized balloon is the intervention of choice when transvalvular pressure gradient is >60 mm Hg (severe PS). The procedure has high success rate and is very rewarding. Those with mild-to-moderate PS can be left alone. Patients with unfavorable valve morphology like in Noonan syndrome need surgical valvotomy. These patients have a dysplastic valve which cannot be opened with balloon valvuloplasty.

PULMONARY REGURGITATION

Pulmonary regurgitation can be present in three different situations: (1) An isolated PR (usually mild, no hemodynamic significance and no symptoms); (2) Idiopathic dilatation of PA (IDPA) may be associated with PR. These patients are also usually asymptomatic, have dilatation of PA on chest X-ray with normal lung fields; and (3) Secondary to severe PA hypertension. This is usually seen as part of Eisenmenger syndrome when severe irreversible PAH develops in some patients of left-to-right shunts.

CLINICAL FEATURES

Isolated PR and IDPA in absence of any other cardiac lesion are usually of no hemodynamic significance and do not cause any symptoms. Patients with PR due to severe PAH will of course be symptomatic since they have fixed cardiac output due to PAH. This can also be a part of idiopathic PAH (primary pulmonary hypertension). Even though patients with left-sided valvular disease (mostly MS) can develop severe PAH, they usually do not have secondary PR as is seen in PAH related to Eisenmenger syndrome.

On clinical examination, the murmur of pulmonary regurgitation with PAH will be high pitched, decrescendo, and heard in the left second intercostal space (Graham–Steell murmur). The murmur of PR in IDPA is low pitched, short, and nonsignificant. The clinical findings of PR in the three situations are shown in **Table 5**.

DIAGNOSIS

Electrocardiogram—normal in isolated PR and in IDPA. In severe PAH-related PR, there will be features of RV hypertrophy.

Chest radiograph—enlarged PA. In PAH-related PR, main and level one branches of right PA (RPA) and left PA (LPA) will be dilated with oligemic lung fields. In IDPA, lung fields will be normal with mild dilatation of main PA (MPA).

Echocardiography—deformed PV in primary PR. Dilated PA in IDPA. In PR due to PAH, there will be all the features of PA hypertension.

MANAGEMENT

Pulmonary regurgitation itself does not require any treatment. Patients with isolated PR and IDPA are left alone. In PR due to PAH, the treatment of basic disease and PA hypertension is done.

TABLE 5 Signs of pulmonary regurgitation (PR) as per etiology.

Sign	Isolated PR	Secondary PR with PA dilation (IDPA)	Secondary PR due to PAH
Pulse	Normal	Normal	Low volume
JVP	Normal	Normal	Prominent "a" wave
Left parasternal heave	Absent	Absent	Present, prominent
Second heart sound	• Not palpable normal intensity • S2 widely split	• Normally heard • P2 loud in dilated PA	• Palpable and very loud P2 • Split closely
Ejection click	Absent	Present	Loud up to apex
RV fourth heart sound	Absent	Absent	Common
Early diastolic murmur (EDM)	Short, low-pitched, mid diastolic murmur	Short and faint EDM Decrescendo murmur	Long, high-pitched, decrescendo early diastolic murmur (Graham–Steell murmur)
TR murmur	Absent	Absent	Usual

(IDPA: idiopathic dilatation of pulmonary artery)

MULTIVALVULAR DISEASES

Multiple VHD (MVHD) is the combination of stenotic or regurgitant lesions occurring on ≥2 cardiac valves. Mixed VHD is the combination of stenotic and regurgitant lesions on the same valve. Multiple valve disease is a common condition, more so in rheumatic and degenerative heart disease. The less common causes are infective endocarditis, radiation induced, drug-induced, carcinoid, and systemic inflammatory diseases. Downstream valvular lesions may induce secondary mitral regurgitation (MR) and TR and rarely PR. The congenital causes include connective tissue diseases—Marfan syndrome, Ehlers-Danlos syndrome, trisomy 18, 13 and 15, ochronosis (alkaptonuria), and Shone's syndrome.

PREVALENCE

In the Euro Heart Survey, multiple VHD was seen in 20% of the patients. In the American Society of Thoracic Surgeons Database of 290,000 surgical patients between 2003 and 2007, 11% had double valve procedures (replacement or repair), most often aortic and mitral, and triple valve surgery had been performed in 1% of cases. The most frequent associations were AS + aortic regurgitation (AR), AS + MR and AR + MR. In India, MVHD has been seen in more than a third (36.8%) of all cases (**Fig. 4**).

In an echocardiographic record study from a single center in India, the combination of MS and MR (MS + MR) was the most common followed by the combination of MS and AR (MS + AR) and the least common lesion combination was that of MS and AS (MS + AS). MVHD was observed slightly more often in females. The lesion combinations involving MS were more common in females and those with AS were more common in males. In rheumatic heart disease, the combinations were in the following order of involvement: MS + MR (46.6%) > MS + AR (26.5%) > MR + AR (23.3%) > MS + AS (2.4%) > MR + AS (0.9%) > AS + AR (0.3%) (**Fig. 5**). The Euro Heart Survey of 5,001 patients from 92 centers in 25 European countries had most common lesions as AS and MR, mostly of degenerative etiology. The natural history of MVHD depends on the complex interplay of pathophysiological factors including the severity of individual valve lesions, loading conditions, and ventricular compensation for these loading conditions.

Hemodynamically, significant disease involving the mitral, aortic, and TVs is uncommon. Patients with trivalvular disease may present in advanced heart failure with marked cardiomegaly, and surgical correction of all three valvular lesions may be necessary. However, the operative and postoperative complications are high.

CLINICAL FEATURES

The hemodynamic derangements associated with the more proximal valve disease can conceal the clinical features of the more distal valve lesion. Downstream valvular lesions may induce secondary MR and TR and rarely PR. Finally, symptoms of heart failure may prevail over individual lesions.

Multiple or mixed valve disease may develop symptoms at a relatively earlier stage than the single valve disease patients in the natural history of their disease. The symptoms can be predominantly either of low output state or downstream congestion or a combination depending upon the summed hemodynamics. Symptoms related to right heart failure (abdominal fullness/bloating, edema) are late manifestations of advanced disease.

The manner in which the hemodynamic effects of one valve affect the other valve disease, its pathophysiological relationship and effect on clinical findings and management plan are shown in **Table 6**.

DIAGNOSIS

Electrocardiogram indicative of right-sided cardiac abnormalities with left-sided valve lesions should alert PA

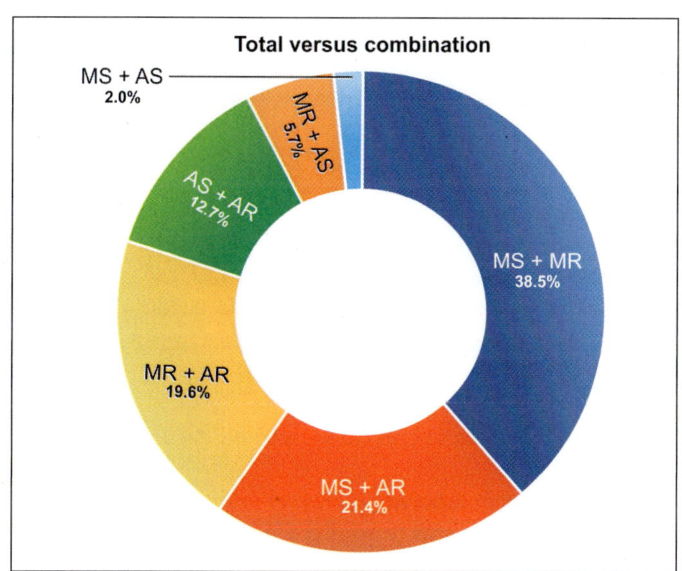

FIGURE 4: Multiple valve heart disease in India.

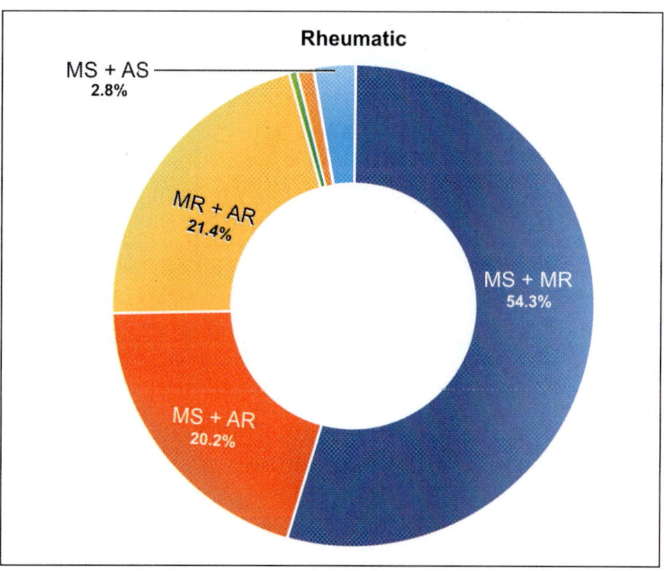

FIGURE 5: Multiple rheumatic valve heart disease in India.

TABLE 6 Pathophysiology, clinical features, and management principles of multivalvular disease.

Combination	Characteristics and pathophysiology	Findings and treatment
MS + MR	• In patients with dominant MS, the size of LV may be normal • MR backflow can increase transmitral gradient	• Most frequently, the systolic murmur typical of MR is prominent and may mask the soft rumble typical of MS. The first heart sound may be increased in intensity • Percutaneous valvuloplasty is contraindicated, hence mitral valve replacement is done
MS + AR	• MS reduces LV volume overload and can mask AR • Impaired LV filling from left atrium is compensated by reverse blood flow through aortic valve	• Typical signs of MS and diastolic murmur along left sternal border, loud S1 and opening snap may be clue to MS • Percutaneous balloon mitral valvuloplasty considered before aortic valve replacement
MR + AR	• AR frequently dominant. AR leads to LV dilation and secondary MR • In such cases, it is difficult to distinguish primary from secondary MR due to LV enlargement	• Apical systolic murmur caused by MR and diastolic murmur caused by AR • Simultaneous aortic valve and mitral valve replacement when both are hemodynamically significant
MS + AS	MS restricts blood inflow to LV and aggravates the drop of cardiac output caused by AS, underestimation of both stenotic lesions	• Typical signs of MS and murmur caused by AS (less prominent than in isolated AS) • Atrial fibrillation is clue to MS • Simultaneous replacement of both valves • Percutaneous balloon mitral valvuloplasty in patients with significant AS may result in pulmonary edema
MR + AS	AS leads to LV hypertrophy and secondary MR; impaired aortic valve outflow can further aggravate MR	• Ejection AS murmur radiating to carotid arteries and murmur caused by MR radiating to axilla • Handgrip reduces AS and increases MR murmur. Postventricular premature contractions the AS murmur increases and MR does not change • Simultaneous aortic valve replacement and mitral repair or replacement • MR may be reduced after aortic valve replacement (or TAVI) without specific mitral valve intervention
AS + AR	• Common causes are congenital (most commonly a bicuspid aortic valve), degenerative, rheumatic disease, or prior balloon valvuloplasty for AS in childhood • AR increases severity of AS	• The coexisting AR causes a louder systolic murmur by increasing transvalvular flow across the stenotic valve • Prominent conduction to neck vessels clue to AS • Aortic valve replacement
MR + TR	• MR most commonly the dominant lesion • Chronic MR causes pulmonary hypertension, leading to RV dilation and secondary TR	• At times relief of MR alone may result in decrease in TR • Apical systolic murmur caused by MR and lower sternal border murmur of TR • Mitral repair or replacement with TV repair or annuloplasty
MS + TR	MS leads to pulmonary hypertension and secondary regurgitation of anatomically normal TV; in some patients TV also affected by rheumatic fever	• Typical signs of MS and holosystolic murmur (more prominent during inspiration) caused by TR • Hemodynamically significant TR may improve following mitral valve valvuloplasty (or surgery) without specific surgical treatment of the TV • Mitral valve replacement (or mitral valvuloplasty) and tricuspid annuloplasty

hypertension and/or right-sided valve disease. The presence of atrial fibrillation in patients with aortic valve disease may be a clue to mitral valve disease.

Chest radiograph can suggest cardiac chamber enlargement, valve and/or annular calcification, and any abnormalities in the pulmonary vasculature. Patients with multivalvular disease can have marked cardiomegaly (CT ratio >70%).

Transthoracic echocardiography is the most commonly used and most helpful modality for the identification and characterization of multiple and/or mixed VHD. TEE may be required for more accurate assessment of valve anatomy and infective endocarditis. Echocardiography will permit establishing the etiopathogenesis, mechanisms, severity, progression, and hemodynamic interactions of each valvular lesion. It is a critical determinant of timing, indication, and likelihood of success for surgery or transcatheter intervention.

Cardiac catheterization of right and left heart hemodynamics may be required to characterize more completely the individual contributions of each valvular heart lesion. It is recommended when there is a discrepancy between the clinical and noninvasive findings in a symptomatic patient. Patients of VHD if they have to go for open heart surgery (repair or replacement) and are >40 years, should have a coronary angiogram before surgery since 6–8% of them can have asymptomatic coronary artery disease (CAD).

MANAGEMENT

Patients of multiple valve heart disease who have to undergo surgery need a detailed assessment of the other valve disease. In case of moderate to severe affection of the other valve, they will also need to be replaced. Mild lesions of the other valves can be left alone. Double valve replacement carries greater mortality than single valve replacement. However, it still has to be done along with one valve surgery since patient will have immediate postoperative complications in case the other valve has significant involvement. Also, a moderate lesion in the other valve can progress in the next few weeks and so it is better to deal with it in the same operation. Some patients with severe MS and mild-to-moderate AR can have balloon mitral valvotomy and then kept on follow-up for AR. Each patient's management needs to be individualized.

RECOMMENDED READINGS

1. Nath J, Foster E, Heidenreich PA. Impact of tricuspid regurgitation on long-term survival. J Am Coll Cardiol. 2004;43(3):405-9.
2. Colombo T, Russo C, Ciliberto GR, Lanfranconi M, Bruschi G, Agati S, et al. Tricuspid regurgitation secondary to mitral valve disease: tricuspid annulus function as guide to tricuspid valve repair. Cardiovasc Surg. 2001;9(4):369-77.
3. Acar C, Périer P, Fontaliran F, Deloche A, Carpentier A. Anatomical study of the tricuspid valve and its variations. Surg Radiol Anat. 1990;12(3):229-30.
4. Dreyfus GD, Martin RP, Chan KM, Dulguerov F, Alexandrescu C. Functional tricuspid regurgitation: a need to revise our understanding. J Am Coll Cardiol. 2015;65(21):2331-6.
5. Nishimura RA, Otto CM, Bonow RO, Carabello BA, Erwin JP 3rd, Fleisher LA, et al. 2017 AHA/ACC Focused Update of the 2014 AHA/ACC Guideline for the Management of Patients With Valvular Heart Disease: A Report of the American College of Cardiology/American Heart Association Task Force on Clinical Practice Guidelines. Circulation. 2017;135(25):e1159-95.
6. Baumgartner H, Falk V, Bax JJ, De Bonis M, Hamm C, Holm PJ, et al. ESC Scientific Document Group. 2017 ESC/EACTS Guidelines for the management of valvular heart disease. Eur Heart J. 2017;38(36):2739-91
7. Vassileva CM, Shabosky J, Boley T, Markwell S, Hazelrigg S. Tricuspid valve surgery: the past 10 years from the Nationwide Inpatient Sample (NIS) database. J Thorac Cardiovasc Surg. 2012;143(5):1043-9.
8. Shrivastava S, Singh A. Percutaneous Tricuspid Valvular Interventions: Emerging Origin. In: Arulrhaj S (Ed). Medicine Update 2020 (2 Volumes) and Progress in Medicine 2020. New Delhi: Jaypee Brothers Medical Publishers Pvt. Limited; 2019. pp. 114-8.
9. Topilsky Y, Nkomo VT, Vatury O, Michelena HI, Letourneau T, Suri RM, et al. Clinical outcome of isolated tricuspid regurgitation. JACC Cardiovasc Imaging. 2014;7(12):1185-94.
10. Singh JP, Evans JC, Levy D, Larson MG, Freed LA, Fuller DL, et al. Prevalence and clinical determinants of mitral, tricuspid, and aortic regurgitation (the Framingham Heart Study). Am J Cardiol. 1999;83(6):897-902.
11. Zoghbi WA, Adams D, Bonow RO, Enriquez-Sarano M, Foster E, Grayburn PA, et al. Recommendations for noninvasive evaluation of native valvular regurgitation: A report from the American society of echocardiography developed in collaboration with the society for cardiovascular magnetic resonance. J Am Soc Echocardiogr. 2017;30(4):303-71.
12. Ton-Nu TT, Levine RA, Handschumacher MD, Dorer DJ, Yosefy C, Fan D, et al. Geometric determinants of functional tricuspid regurgitation: insights from 3-dimensional echocardiography. Circulation. 2006; 114(2):143-9.
13. Lancellotti P, Moura L, Pierard LA, Agricola E, Popescu BA, Tribouilloy C, et al. European Association of Echocardiography. European Association of Echocardiography recommendations for the assessment of valvular regurgitation. Part 2: Mitral and tricuspid regurgitation (native valve disease). Eur J Echocardiogr. 2010;11(4):307-32.
14. Iung B, Baron G, Butchart EG, Delahaye F, Gohlke-Bärwolf C, Levang OW, et al. A prospective survey of patients with valvular heart disease in Europe: The Euro Heart Survey on Valvular Heart Disease. Eur Heart J. 2003;24(13):1231-43.
15. Andell P, Li X, Martinsson A, Andersson C, Stagmo M, Zöller B, et al. Epidemiology of valvular heart disease in a Swedish nationwide hospital-based register study. Heart. 2017;103(21):1696-1703.
16. Manjunath CN, Srinivas P, Ravindranath KS, Dhanalakshmi C. Incidence and patterns of valvular heart disease in a tertiary care high-volume cardiac center: A single center experience. Indian Heart J. 2014;66(3):320-6.

CHAPTER 98 Congenital Heart Disease in the Adults

Balaji Arvind, Anita Saxena

ABSTRACT

Adults with congenital heart disease (CHD) comprise a heterogenous population. They may either be diagnosed with CHD for the first time during adulthood or present for follow-up after having had some form of intervention during childhood. With improvement in cardiac care, more patients born with CHD are surviving into adulthood. It is important that the physician is aware of the modified and unmodified natural history of the most common CHDs at least, so that they could be actively involved in the care of these patients. Though few of these patients require specialized care by a cardiologist, adequate care may be provided by the physician in a majority of these patients, especially those with simple CHDs and those with completely repaired CHDs without any significant residual lesions. The physician should be competent enough to provide the general measures and basic medical therapy in these patients and decide whenever it is appropriate to seek cardiologists' opinion. This knowledge also would help the physician in efficiently managing concomitant illnesses that are seen in adults with CHD.

"Don't be pushed by the fears in your mind. Be led by the dreams in your heart"

—Roy T Bennett

INTRODUCTION

- Congenital heart diseases are the most common malformations constituting almost a quarter of all birth defects. CHDs are of variable severity with few lesions requiring early intervention in infancy or childhood, whereas some lesions may be well tolerated until adulthood.
- Adult CHD encompasses patients with both native and operated (repaired or palliated) CHDs. The aim of this chapter is to provide a concise overview regarding the most common and important issues encountered by the physician during management of an adult with CHD.

Magnitude of the problem: Steadily increasing numbers of adults with CHD

- Globally, the number of adults with CHD is steadily increasing due to advancements in cardiac surgical/interventional techniques and perioperative care. Data from west estimates that greater than 90% of individuals born with CHD are able to survive into adulthood. This has resulted in the number of adults with CHD outnumbering children with CHD.
- The Indian scenario is completely different wherein it is estimated that only a quarter of children born with serious CHD receive optimal care, although these numbers have steadily improved over the years.
- An unpublished internal audit of adults with CHD presenting to our institute showed that the percentage of patients with operated CHDs has increased from 13.9 to 33% between 2012 and 2019.

What constitutes adult CHD?

- Adult CHD includes patients born with CHDs and present in their adulthood either after an intervention (surgical or transcatheter, corrective or palliative) or as native CHD without been intervened previously. They may belong to any of the categories as shown in **Figure 1**.
- A study from Europe showed that the most common CHD encountered in adults is atrial septal defect (ASD) followed by ventricular septal defect (VSD), whereas the most common cyanotic CHD is tetralogy of Fallot (TOF). Similarly, in a study from India, it was reported that ASD is the most common lesion diagnosed among adults with native CHD presenting to a tertiary care center for evaluation.
- Some native CHDs known to have survival into adulthood are shown in **Figure 2**.
- Some of these lesions may not require any intervention, e.g., small VSD, mild aortic stenosis/aortic regurgitation (AS/AR) or mild pulmonary stenosis (PS). Some may need intervention, e.g., ASD, PDA, TOF, and severe valvular lesions. Unfortunately, a small number of patients present with an inoperable condition known as Eisenmenger Syndrome (ES) which occurs due to irreversible changes in pulmonary vasculature secondary to an unattended large left-to-right shunt, such as a large VSD. It is important for the physician to recognize these different subsets of patients and promptly refer to a cardiologist whenever in doubt.

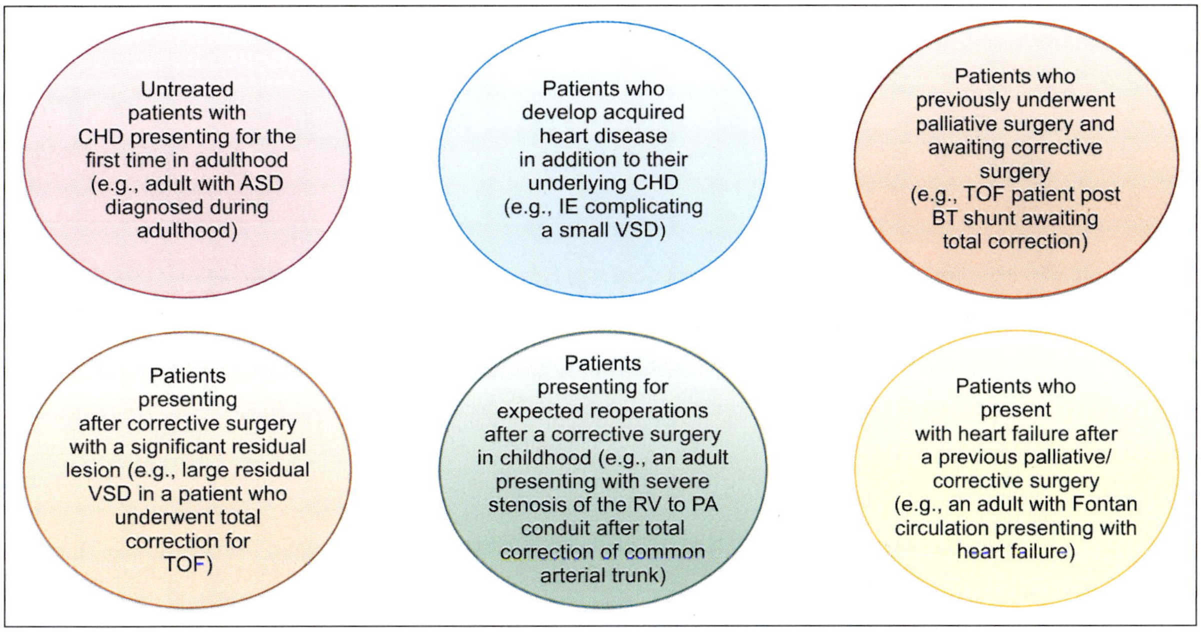

(BT: Blalock–Taussig; TOF: tetralogy of Fallot)

FIGURE 1: Categories into which adults with CHD may be grouped.

Acyanotic CHD	Cyanotic CHD	Miscellaneous
• Atrial septal defect (ASD) • Ventricular septal defect (VSD) • Patent ductus arteriosus • Coarctation of aorta **Congenital valvular defects** • Bicuspid aortic valve (Normal/stenostic/ regurgitant) • Mitral valve prolapse • Pulmonary stenosis (PS) • Pulmonary regurgitation	• Tetralogy of fallot (TOF) • TOF-like physiologies including SV with PS • Eisenmenger syndrome (secondary to VSD, PDA, or ASD)	• CC-TGA • Ebsteins anomaly • Coronary arteriovenous fistula • Sinus of Valsalva aneurysm (ruptured or unruptured) • Pulmonary arteriovenous malformations

(CC-TGA: congenitally corrected transposition of great arteries; SV: single ventricle)

FIGURE 2: Native CHDs known to have survival into adulthood.

NATIVE CONGENITAL HEART DISEASES IN ADULTS

ACYANOTIC CONGENITAL HEART DISEASES

Atrial septal defects (ostium secundum type):

- Atrial septal defects are the most common defects to remain asymptomatic till adulthood. They cause left-to-right shunt at the atrial level resulting in volume overload of the right atrium and right ventricle (**Fig. 3**).
- The magnitude of shunt increases with age, due to progressive reduction of left ventricular compliance (due to hypertension, ischemic heart disease etc.); hence, majority of patients become symptomatic beyond the third or fourth decade of life.
- Pulmonary artery hypertension (PAH) is rare (<5%) and majority remain operable. However, the benefits of closure are maximum if done before 25 years of age.
- Device closure has become the preferred mode of closure whenever feasible.
- In the presence of associated conditions such as PAH, left ventricular (LV) dysfunction, atrial flutter, or atrial fibrillation, detailed evaluation at a cardiac facility is required before decision-making.

Ventricular septal defects:

- Ventricular septal defect (VSD) results in left-to-right shunt at the ventricular level and results in volume overload of left heart (**Fig. 3**). Magnitude of shunt is mainly determined by the size of the defect.

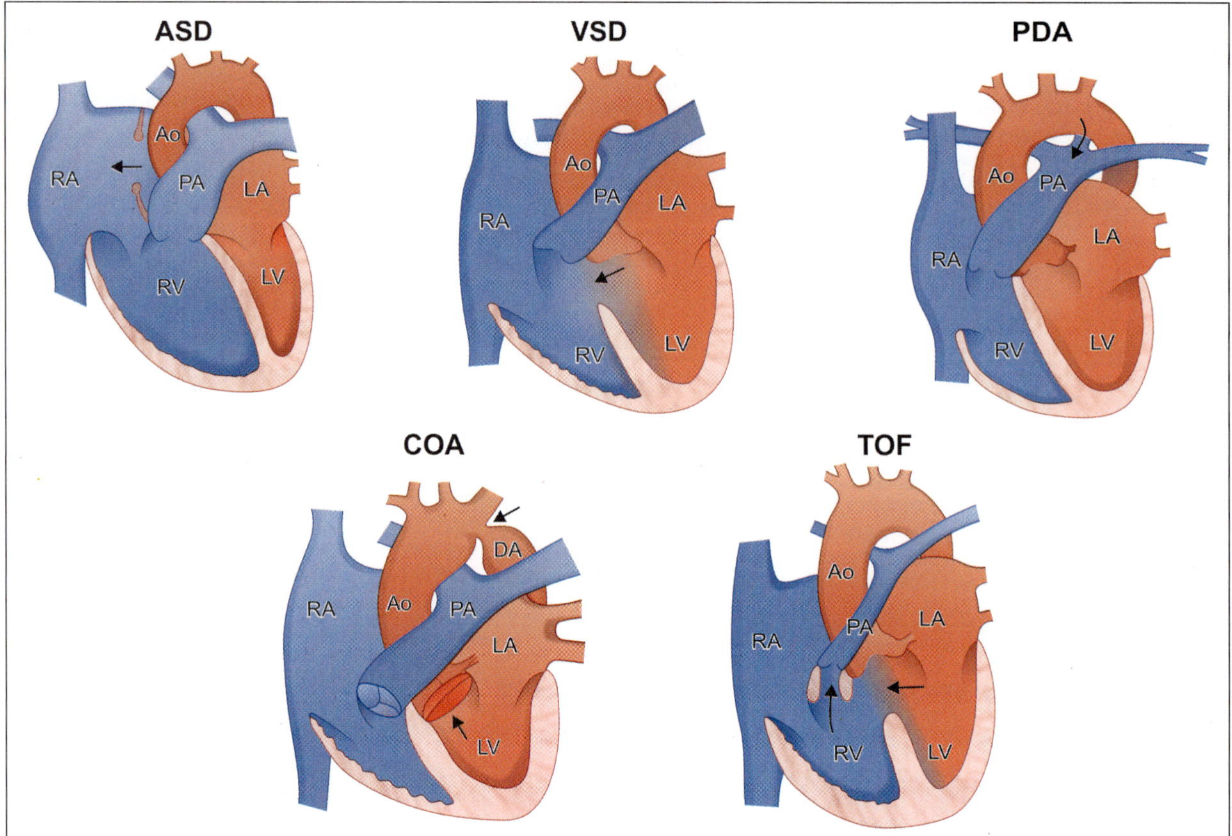

(COA: coarctation of aorta; TOF: tetralogy of Fallot)

FIGURE 3: **Schematic representation of hemodynamics in some of the most common CHDs.**

- Large defects are invariably associated with severe PAH, since there is direct transmission of the systemic LV pressures to the pulmonary artery (PA) through the nonrestrictive defect.
- When these patients are young (first 2 years of life) the pulmonary vascular resistance (PVR) is low, which allows large left-to-right shunt across the defect: "Hyperkinetic" or "flow-related" PAH.
- If untreated, these patients develop pulmonary vascular occlusive disease leading to rise in PVR. As a result, the magnitude of shunt decreases and may even reverse (right to left). Beyond a stage, the pulmonary vascular changes become irreversible: "Irreversible" PAH or "fixed" PAH.
- Native VSDs in adults are either small defects that have not resulted in PAH or large defects that are almost always associated with irreversible PAH and right-to-left shunt across VSD: ES.
- Ventricular septal defects, especially in the outlet part or the perimembranous part of septum can result in prolapse of aortic cusps leading to AR, thereby necessitating surgical closure even if the defect is small.
- Small VSDs need not be closed unless associated with AR or are complicated by infective endocarditis (IE).
- All adults with large VSD need detailed evaluation including a cardiac catheterization to test for operability before decision making.

Atrioventricular septal defects:

- Atrioventricular septal defect (AVSD) results due to faulty development of endocardial cushion during embryogenesis.
- Atrioventricular septal defect is characterized by common atrioventricular (AV) junction. It encompasses a spectrum of defects ranging from septum primum atrial septal defect (also known as partial AVSD), where there is no VSD component, to complete AVSD, characterized by presence of septum primum ASD and a inlet VSD.
- Complete AVSD is uncommon in adults; however, partial AVSD is not unusual. The clinical presentation in partial AVSD is similar to that of a secundum ASD and that of complete AVSD depends on the size of the VSD component (similar to the natural history of VSD).
- The presentation may be altered by the presence of incompetent AV valves, which is a frequent finding in patients with AVSD.

Patent ductus arteriosus:

- Patent ductus arteriosus (PDA) is abnormal persistence of the communication between left pulmonary artery and descending aorta (**Fig. 3**). Ductus arteriosus plays a crucial role in fetal circulation.
- PDA, like VSD, is known to result in early development of irreversible PAH and should be evaluated cautiously when encountered in adults.

- Large PDA in adults are almost always associated with irreversible severe PAH. A cardiac catheterization study with or without a temporary balloon occlusion of PDA may be required before deciding status of operability.
- Moderate-sized PDA may still be considered operable if it demonstrates features of left-to-right shunt and LV volume overload.
- Small PDA may be incidentally picked up in an adult. A small PDA that is not producing a murmur may even be left untreated since they are unlikely to result in PAH.
- All PDAs considered operable should be closed, device closure is a preferred option over surgical ligation.

Coarctation of aorta:

- Coarctation of Aorta (COA) is characterized by narrowing of the aorta usually at the region where the ductus arteriosus joins the aorta (**Fig. 3**).
- The commonest presentation of COA in adults is hypertension that is picked up incidentally: So, rule out COA in all young hypertensives.
- A systolic blood pressure gradient of >20 mm Hg between upper and lower limb suggests significant COA (requires confirmation by invasive measurement).
- Intervention is indicated in patients with hypertension and an invasive pressure gradient of >20 mm Hg (Class 1).
- Interventions may be considered in patients without hypertension (with significant gradient) and in patients who have >50% narrowing of aorta (despite no significant gradient) (Class IIa).
- In adults with COA, transcatheter interventions (stent or balloon aortoplasty) are preferred over surgery in view of lower rates of complication.
- These patients are at increased risk of developing intracranial hemorrhage (from berry aneurysms), IE, premature coronary artery disease, and aortic rupture or dissection (especially in patients with Turner syndrome).

CYANOTIC CONGENITAL HEART DISEASES

Tetralogy of fallot:

- Tetralogy of Fallot is the most common cyanotic CHD seen in adults.
- Tetralogy of Fallot is characterized by a large non-restrictive VSD with aortic override (<50%) and severe PS (**Fig. 3**). Hence, these patients do not have PAH. Pulmonary atresia is the most severe form where there is lack of continuity between the RV outflow and main pulmonary artery.
- With increasing severity of obstruction, less blood traverses the RV outflow: Shorter murmur and greater cyanosis (because of more right-to-left shunt across VSD).
- Cyanosis is noticed from early childhood. Nevertheless, it is not uncommon for TOF patients to present for the first time in adulthood, especially in developing countries.
- Corrective surgery (VSD closure and relief of RV outflow obstruction) may be performed in adult patients with favorable anatomy. However, the perioperative risks of adverse events are higher in adults compared to that in young children.
- In patients whose anatomy would not permit a corrective surgery, a variety of palliative systemic arterial to pulmonary shunts can be performed to augment pulmonary blood flow and alleviate cyanosis.
- There are few lesions other than the "classic" TOF that are characterized by a nonrestrictive interventricular communication and severe PS. These lesions are labeled as "TOF-like physiologies" [e.g., double outlet right ventricle (with large VSD and severe PS), transposition of great arteries (TGA) (with large VSD and severe PS)]. Though the hemodynamics of these lesions are similar to that of "classic" TOF, the presentation and management are highly variable and are beyond the scope of discussion here.

Eisenmenger syndrome:

- Eisenmenger syndrome occurs in patients with increased pulmonary blood flow situations who are left untreated for long. Such lesions initially result in "hyperkinetic" PAH, however, with time, the PVR rises, PAH becomes "fixed" and "irreversible" leading to fall in pulmonary blood flow and cyanosis ensues.
- Eisenmenger syndrome is considered the end stage of shunt-related PAH when the patients are deemed "inoperable."
- Eisenmenger syndrome develops earlier in cyanotic CHDs (e.g., TGA, Truncus arteriosus, and Single ventricles without PS) compared to acyanotic CHD.
- Eisenmenger syndrome develops earlier in post-tricuspid shunt lesions [e.g., VSD, PDA, aortopulmonary (AP) window] compared to pre-tricuspid shunt lesions (e.g., ASD).
- Markers of poor survival in patients with ES include presence of syncope, arterial saturation < 85%, and right heart failure.
- Conditions such as pregnancy, hypovolemia, strenuous exercise, high altitude, and iron deficiency increase the risk of adverse events in these patients and should be avoided. Medical therapy for patients with ES is discussed below.

Tetralogy of fallot versus eisenmenger syndrome: Clues to differentiation:

- The differentiation of these two conditions is extremely important because TOF (or TOF-like physiologies) is not associated with PAH and may remain amenable for surgical intervention whereas ES is associated with severe PAH, thereby precluding corrective surgery. Some clues that help differentiate these two conditions are shown in **Table 1**.

ADULTS WITH CHD POST INTERVENTION

- The number of adult patients with postoperative or posttranscatheter intervention CHD is steadily increasing. It is important for the physician to be aware of specific issues that are sought out in an adult with postoperative CHD (**Table 2**).

TABLE 1 Points to differentiate TOF physiology and Eisenmenger physiology in an adult patient with cyanotic CHD.

Features	TOF physiology	Eisenmenger physiology
Growth and weight gain	Normal or only mildly affected	Severe failure to thrive present from infancy
Heart failure in infancy and early childhood	Absent	Present
Onset of cyanosis	Early (usually in the first decade), but can be variable	Late
Degree of cyanosis	Variable (usually deep)	Usually mild
History of squatting	Present	Absent
Syncope	Uncommon	Common
Hemoptysis	Uncommon	Common
Chest pain/Angina	Rare	Common
Prominent "a" wave in JVP	In older patients	Common
Left parasternal heave	Grade 1 (Mild)	• Present in ASD • Grade 1 (mild) in VSD, PDA
Cardiomegaly	Absent	Absent (present in ASD)
Systolic thrill	May be present	Absent
Second heart sound	Single	Single (VSD), narrow (PDA), wide (ASD)
Pulmonary component of S2	Absent or attenuated	Loud and palpable
Ejection click	Present (Aortic)	Present (Pulmonary)
Ejection systolic murmur	Yes	Not more than grade 2
Early diastolic murmur	Of AR may be heard rarely	Of PR may be heard in PDA

- Few cardiac surgeries require placement of a conduit to establish continuity between RV and pulmonary arteries (e.g., in VSD with pulmonary atresia, truncus arteriosus). These patients are at a definitive risk for conduit dysfunction (stenosis or incompetence) and related complications (ventricular dysfunction).

GENERAL ISSUES IN ADULTS WITH CHD

- Congenital heart diseases may be considered a "lifelong chronic" condition. Irrespective of the severity of cardiac lesion, these patients encounter multiple challenges, both cardiac and noncardiac. Important ones are discussed in further detail in **Table 3**.

HEART FAILURE

- Heart failure is an important cause of mortality in this patient population.
- Some cardiac lesions are at higher risk of developing ventricular dysfunction. (e.g., single ventricle and right ventricle as systemic ventricle)
- Any adult CHD patients with ventricular dysfunction should be carefully evaluated for reversible etiologies and promptly corrected if found (**Box 1**).
- No separate guidelines exist for medical therapy of heart failure in this population. They are managed based on general heart failure guidelines.
  a. Diuretics alleviate symptoms.
  b. Beta blockers, angiotensin-converting enzyme (ACE) inhibitors, and angiotensin II receptor blockers (ARB) are usually prescribed, despite no definitive evidence demonstrating clinical benefit in this population.
  c. For patients with end-stage heart failure, heart transplantation may be a therapeutic option.

PULMONARY HYPERTENSION

- Pulmonary artery hypertension in CHD is an important concern and has prognostic implications.
- Pulmonary artery hypertension is defined as a mean pulmonary artery pressure >20 mm Hg and a PVR ≥3 wood units. They can be further classified as precapillary, postcapillary, or combined types of PAH.
- Prevalence of CHD-associated PAH increases with biological age and age at defect closure.
- Congenital heart disease-associated PAH may be grouped into four broad categories as shown in **Table 4**.
- Cardiac catheterization is required in all patients with CHD-associated PAH for prognostication and risk assessment.
- *General measures*: Avoid excessive physical stress and supplemental oxygen (if PaO_2 is <60 mm Hg).
- All patients with CHD–PAH should be strongly counseled against pregnancy.

TABLE 2 Important issues to be sought out in adults with specific CHDs who have undergone some form of intervention in the past.

Congenital heart disease (CHD)	Interventions performed	Important issues to be sought out when these patients are seen in adulthood
Acyanotic CHD		
ASD, VSD, PDA	Corrective: Surgical or transcatheter	• Residual defects • Ventricular dysfunction • Persistence or recurrence of pulmonary hypertension • Arrhythmias, AV blocks • AV valve regurgitation (AVSD)
AVSD	Corrective surgery	LV outflow tract obstruction (AVSD)
COA	Surgical repair	Hypertension
	Balloon dilation	Recoarctation
	Stenting	Intracranial aneurysms
		Aortic aneurysms, dissection
Cyanotic CHD		
Tetralogy of Fallot	Total correction (A conduit may have been used If the RV outflow had been atretic)	• Pulmonary regurgitation (and resultant RV enlargement) • Residual obstruction (RV outflow, branch PA stenosis etc.) • RV dysfunction • Residual VSD • Arrhythmias: Monomorphic VT, supraventricular arrhythmias • Risk of sudden cardiac death
	Palliative shunt between systemic arterial and pulmonary artery (e.g., modified Blalock–Taussig shunt, Potts shunt, central shunt)	• Blocked shunt • Hemoptysis (from aortopulmonary collaterals) • Problems due to persistent intracardiac right to left shunting • Effects of chronic cyanosis (see text given below)

(AVSD: atrioventricular septal defect; COA: coarctation of aorta; VT: ventricular tachycardia)

TABLE 3 Significant problems encountered by adults with congenital heart disease (CHD).

Cardiac	Noncardiac
• Mortality, morbidity, and quality of life • Postoperative residual lesions, sequelae • Need for reintervention (surgical, transcatheter) • Arrhythmia • Heart failure • Pulmonary hypertension • Sudden cardiac death • Infective endocarditis • Aortopathy, aortic dilatation, and aortic dissection • Acquired cardiovascular diseases (ischemic heart disease, obesity, diabetes mellitus etc.)	• Perioperative risks during noncardiac surgery • Cyanosis and its multisystem effects • Pregnancy, reproductive issues, risks of inheritance • Exercise, competitive sports participation • Air travel • Employment issues • Psychosocial considerations • Renal and hepatic diseases • Transition of care issues

BOX 1 Reversible etiologies contributing to heart failure symptoms in patients with adult CHD.

- Anemia
- Arrhythmia: Atrial tachycardia, atrial flutter, bradyarrhythmia, and complete heart block
- Metabolic and nutritional causes: Hypocalcemia, vitamin D deficiency, and hypothyroidism
- Infective endocarditis
- Hypertension
- Coexisting ischemic heart disease
- Presence of significant postoperative residual lesion, e.g., severe pulmonary regurgitation or severe stenosis of RV outflow or branch pulmonary arteries in a patient with TOF post complete correction
- Chronic hypoxia/cyanosis

TABLE 4 Categories of CHD associated PAH.

Category	Mechanism	Closure of defect indicated	Role of pulmonary vasodilators
Hyperkinetic PAH	Due to large left-to-right shunt causing increased pulmonary flow	Yes	No
Eisenmenger syndrome	Irreversible PAH due to pulmonary vascular changes secondary to unoperated long standing large shunt lesions	No	Yes
PAH with small/coincidental defects	• Similar to primary/idiopathic PAH • PAH is not attributed to the defect	No	Yes
PAH after complete correction	PAH that persists or progresses even after closure of defect	NA	Yes

(CHD: congenital heart disease; PAH: pulmonary artery hypertension)

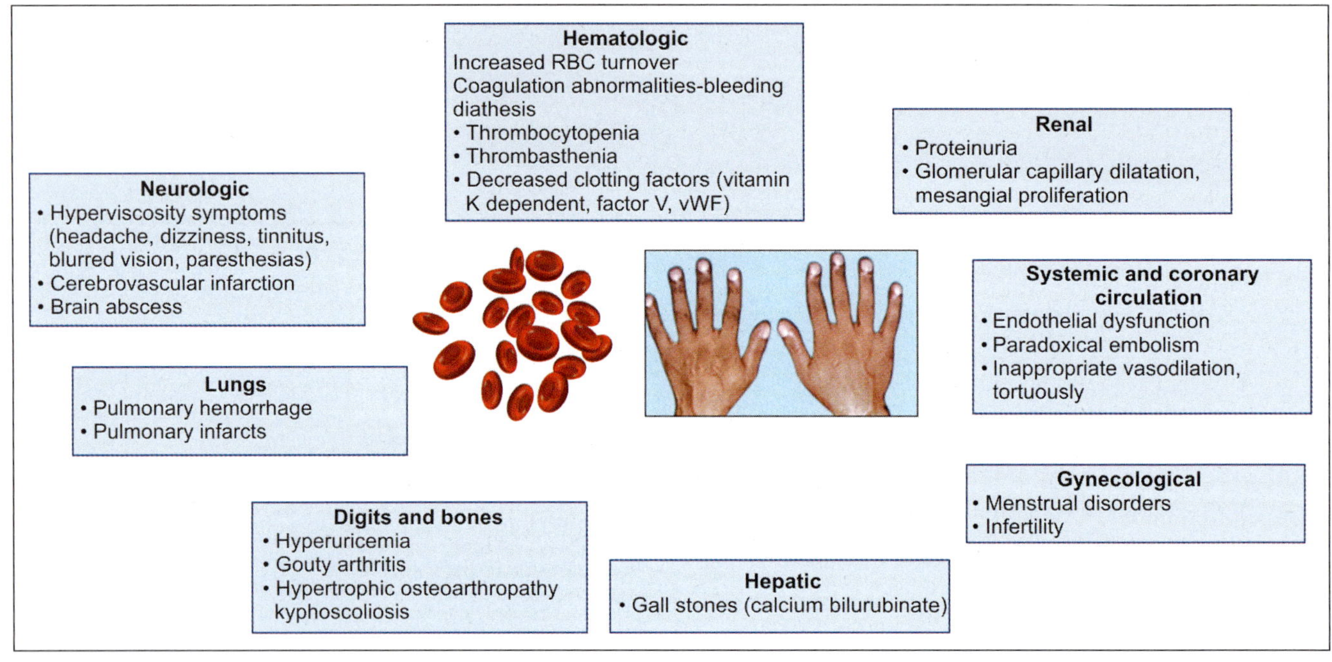

(vWF: von Willebrand factor)

FIGURE 4: The multisystem effects of chronic cyanosis and related secondary erythrocytosis.

- Pulmonary artery hypertension-directed medical therapy, Bosentan, an endothelin receptor antagonist (ERA), has shown beneficial effect on exercise capacity and quality of life in symptomatic ES patients. Phosphodiesterase type 5 (PDE-5) inhibitors such as sildenafil and tadalafil have also shown favorable hemodynamic and functional response in these patients; however, none of the therapies has been proven to provide mortality benefit.
- Patients at low or intermediate risk of events may be initiated on a sequential combination therapy. High-risk patient should be started on upfront combination therapy with a PDE-5 inhibitor and an ERA.

CYANOSIS

- A significant proportion of adult CHD patients are cyanotic.
- Mortality is significantly higher in patients with cyanosis, especially those with PAH.
- Cyanosis induces adaptive mechanisms to improve tissue oxygen delivery, most important of which is secondary erythrocytosis. Chronic hypoxia may lead to unregulated secondary erythrocytosis leading to excessive rise in hematocrit which affects multiple organ systems (**Fig. 4**).
- Iron deficiency is associated with adverse outcomes in these patients. Iron deficiency exacerbates microcytosis and is a strong predictor of cerebrovascular events.
- Therapeutic phlebotomy to relieve hyperviscosity symptoms is reserved for patients with hematocrit levels >65% only after ruling out dehydration and iron deficiency. Inappropriate phlebotomies may in fact be detrimental since it aggravates iron deficiency.
- A higher hemoglobin (of at least 14 g/dL) is targeted in cyanotic patients. Blood transfusion may be required even in the presence of iron replete anemia and should not be based on conventional indications. Iron should be supplemented in these patients if iron deficiency is detected.

- Precautions during ordering investigations in patients with cyanosis:
  - Diagnosis of anemia should not be made solely based on hemoglobin levels.
  - A complete assessment including measurement of mean corpuscular volume (MCV), serum ferritin, iron, transferrin levels, and transferrin saturation help in reliable assessment of iron status.
  - Folate levels and B12 levels may be required in the presence of elevated or normal MCV and low serum ferritin.
  - High hematocrit causes proportionate decrease in plasma volume in these patients. This results in a falsely high prothrombin time if vacutainers using standard doses of anticoagulants are used. The amount of anticoagulant (sodium citrate) should be adjusted for each patient as per the hematocrit to avoid erroneus results.
  - High hematocrit also results in spurious hypoglycemia and spurious hyperkalemia, especially when the analysis is delayed.
- Hemoptysis is a common problem in these patients. The most common source of bleeding is the bronchial arteries.
  - Chest radiograph should be screened for evidence of infection. Computed tomography angiography is the most useful test for evaluating the etiology and sources of bleed. There is no role for bronchoscopy.
  - *Management*: Good hydration should be maintained. Blood transfusion is done if required. Discontinue antiplatelets or anticoagulants. Cough suppressants may be beneficial. Antifibrinolytic agents (ethacrynic acid) are used commonly, though its benefits are not proven.
  - Selective bronchial artery embolization may be required in refractory cases.
- *Hyperuricemia* is commonly encountered in cyanotic patients with polycythemia. They are usually asymptomatic and require no treatment. Occasional patient may experience acute gouty arthritis: Colchicine and anti-inflammatory agents help provide symptomatic benefit. Allopurinol may be considered to avoid recurrences.
- General prophylactic measures to be followed in these patients to avoid complications are listed in **Box 2**.

PREGNANCY

- Few cardiac lesions are associated with high risk of maternal adverse events during pregnancy. The overall risk of maternal mortality in this patient population is 0–1%. The World Health Organization (WHO) has classified CHDs into various risk categories (**see Chapter 101, Fig. 2**).
- Cyanosis poses significant risk to the fetus with only a 12% chance of live birth at maternal oxygen saturation <85%.
- All women with CHD should be evaluated and counseled by a multidisciplinary team comprised of cardiologist, obstetrician, and anesthetist prior to planning pregnancy.

BOX 2 Prophylactic measures and risk-reduction strategies to avoid complications in patients with cyanosis.

- Pregnancy (Patients with Eisenmenger syndrome and patients with arterial saturation <90% should be counseled strongly against pregnancy)
- Avoid dehydration
- Use of air filter in intravenous lines to prevent air embolism
- Prompt treatment of iron deficiency and anemia—avoid inappropriate phlebotomies
- Infectious disease prevention: Routine administration of influenza and pneumococcal vaccines
- Prompt antibiotic therapy of upper respiratory tract infections
- Drugs to avoid:
  - Inappropriate anticoagulation
  - Estrogen-containing contraceptives
  - Agents that impair renal function
- Lifestyle modifications:
  - Avoid acute exposure to heat (hot showers and hot tub) or extreme cold
  - Avoid strenuous exercise
  - Avoid cigarette smoking, recreational drug use, and excess alcohol intake
  - Use of barrier contraceptive
- Regular consultation with the primary treating cardiologist every 6–12 monthly or before administration of any new drug or procedure
  - Infective endocarditis prophylaxis in all patients

- Pregnancy is not recommended in patients with severe PAH and severe systemic ventricular dysfunction. Other patients belonging to the WHO risk class IV are also counseled against pregnancy.
- The *teratogenic effects of cardioactive medications* should be considered. ACE inhibitors (Enalapril and Ramipril), ARB (Losartan), aldosterone antagonists (spironolactone), and Bosentan are the common cardiovascular drugs that are contraindicated during pregnancy.
- Patients with *prosthetic mechanical valves* are on lifelong anticoagulation with vitamin K antagonists such as Warfarin. Embryopathy is known to occur with warfarin, especially, if administered at high doses (>5 mg/day). Hence, warfarin should be substituted with heparin during the first trimester.
- The timing and mode of delivery should be decided together by the obstetrician and the cardiologist. Those belonging to the WHO risk category III and IV should be cared for at a tertiary care facility.
- *Contraception*: Barrier contraceptives are most preferred. Estrogen containing oral contraceptives are best avoided especially in patients with high risk of thrombosis such as those with cyanosis, Fontan physiology, mechanical valves and those with PAH.

NONCARDIAC SURGERY

- Adults with CHD are at an increased risk of perioperative adverse events, especially those with cyanosis. Patients with residual cardiac abnormalities such as ventricular dysfunction, severe PAH, history of malignant arrhythmia, need for anticoagulation, presence of cyanosis or heart failure, and those with Fontan physiology constitute the subsets with highest risk.
- Risk also depends on the nature of surgery being planned. Surgeries of respiratory and gastrointestinal system including the hepatobiliary system are associated with substantial risk.
- A comprehensive evaluation involving the cardiologist, cardiac anesthetist, and the surgeon with respect to the functional capacity and risk quantification of every adult CHD patient is essential before any noncardiac surgery for formulating the most appropriate perioperative plan.
- Perioperative considerations to be addressed: Presurgical hydration, precautions to avoid air embolism, need of arterial and central venous catheters, IE prophylaxis, strategies for antiplatelets or anticoagulation, preference of inotropic agents etc.
- In patients with ES hypotension and conditions that worsen PVR (hypothermia, metabolic acidosis, and hypercarbia) should be avoided since they are poorly tolerated.
- In the postoperative period, aggressive control of fever, bleed, and pain is important. Early ambulation is advised to avoid deep vein thrombosis.
- It is preferable that elective noncardiac surgeries in patients with elevated risk take place in tertiary care centers with facilities for managing patients with CHD.

INFECTIVE ENDOCARDITIS PROPHYLAXIS

- Adults with CHD constitute a high-risk group for IE with the magnitude of risk varying depending on the underlying lesion. Patients at highest risk of IE and undergoing a high-risk procedure should receive prophylactic antibiotics.
- Those at highest risk include those with cyanotic CHD, surgically or percutaneously repaired CHD (till 6 months after procedure in the absence of any residual lesion, lifelong in the presence of residual lesion) presence of prosthetic materials (valves, prosthetic ring used during valve repair etc.), and those with prior history of IE.
- Procedures which are considered to be at high risk for IE: Dental procedures that involve manipulation of gingival tissue, periapical region of teeth or perforation of oral mucosa, procedures on respiratory tract or infected skin or musculoskeletal system.
- *Drugs recommended* for IE prophylaxis: Oral amoxycillin 2 g or oral Clindamycin 600 mg (in those allergic to penicillin) to be administered 30–60 minutes before the procedure.
- Nonspecific measures, such as maintenance of good oral and cutaneous hygiene, and strict asepsis during any invasive procedure should be applied in all CHD patients.

ACQUIRED CARDIOVASCULAR DISEASES

- The number of patients with CHD who survive to advanced ages up to and beyond fifth decade of life is increasing in the western world.
- These patients have a greater prevalence of cardiovascular comorbidities such as hypertension, diabetes mellitus, and renal disease than those in general population. Also, the adverse impact of these risk factors may be amplified in adults with CHD due the underlying abnormalities in myocardial substrate and cardiovascular physiologies.
- Primary prevention measures for risk factors of coronary artery disease are recommended for all adults with CHD. The American Heart Association (AHA) has issued scientific statement for managing older adults with CHD.

CONCLUSION

Adults with CHD constitute a heterogeneous group of patients. Though a few require specialized care by a cardiologist, adequate care may be provided by a physician in a majority of these patients, especially those with simple CHDs and those with completely repaired CHDs without significant residual lesions. The physician should be competent enough to provide general measures and basic medical therapy in these patients and decide whenever it is appropriate for referral to a cardiologist. It is important for the physician to have basic knowledge regarding the commonly performed cardiac interventions and surgical procedures and its complications, so that the patient may be monitored for the same.

RECOMMENDED READINGS

1. Saxena A. Congenital Heart Disease in India: A Status Report. Indian Pediatr. 2018 Dec 15;55(12):1075-82.
2. Manes A, Palazzini M, Leci E, Bacchi Reggiani ML, Branzi A, Galiè N. Current era survival of patients with pulmonary arterial hypertension associated with congenital heart disease: a comparison between clinical subgroups. Eur Heart J. 2014;35(11):716-24.
3. Murphy JG, Gersh BJ, McGoon MD, Mair DD, Porter CJ, Ilstrup DM, et al. Long-term outcome after surgical repair of isolated atrial septal defect. Follow-up at 27 to 32 years. N Engl J Med. 1990;323(24):1645-50.
4. Baumgartner H, De Backer J, Babu-Narayan SV, Budts W, Chessa M, Diller GP, et al. 2020 ESC Guidelines for the management of adult congenital heart disease. Eur Heart J. 2021;42(6):563-645.
5. Vongpatanasin W, Brickner ME, Hillis LD, Lange RA. The Eisenmenger syndrome in adults. Ann Intern Med. 1998;128(9):745-55.
6. Perloff JK, Rosove MH, Child JS, Wright GB. Adults with cyanotic congenital heart disease: hematologic management. Ann Intern Med. 1988;109(5):406-13.
7. Diller GP, Kempny A, Alonso-Gonzalez R, Swan L, Uebing A, Li W, et al. Survival prospects and circumstances of death in contemporary adult congenital

heart disease patients under follow-up at a large tertiary centre. Circulation. 2015;132(22):2118–25.
8. van Riel AC, Schuuring MJ, van Hessen ID, Zwinderman AH, Cozijnsen L, Reichert CL, et al. Contemporary prevalence of pulmonary arterial hypertension in adult congenital heart disease following the updated clinical classification. Int J Cardiol. 2014;174(2):299-305.
9. Regitz-Zagrosek V, Roos-Hesselink JW, Bauersachs J, Blomström-Lundqvist C, Cífková R, De Bonis M, et al. 2018 ESC Guidelines for the management of cardiovascular diseases during pregnancy. Eur Heart J. 2018;39(34):3165-241.
10. Presbitero P, Somerville J, Stone S, Aruta E, Spiegelhalter D, Rabajoli F. Pregnancy in cyanotic congenital heart disease. Outcome of mother and fetus. Circulation. 1994;89(6):2673-6.
11. Lui GK, Saidi A, Bhatt AB, Burchill LJ, Deen JF, Earing MG, et al. Diagnosis and management of noncardiac complications in adults with congenital heart disease: A Scientific statement from the American Heart Association. Circulation. 2017;136(20):e348-92.
12. Kristensen SD, Knuuti J, Saraste A, Anker S, Bøtker HE, Hert SD, et al. 2014 ESC/ESA Guidelines on non-cardiac surgery: cardiovascular assessment and management: The Joint Task Force on noncardiac surgery: Cardiovascular assessment and management of the European Society of Cardiology (ESC) and the European Society of Anaesthesiology (ESA). Eur Heart J. 2014;35(35):2383-431.
13. Habib G, Lancellotti P, Antunes MJ, Bongiorni MG, Casalta JP, Del Zotti F, et al. 2015 ESC Guidelines for the management of infective endocarditis: The Task Force for the Management of Infective Endocarditis of the European Society of Cardiology (ESC) Endorsed by: European Association for Cardio-Thoracic Surgery (EACTS), the European Association of Nuclear Medicine (EANM). Eur Heart J. 2015;36(44):3075-128.
14. Bhatt AB, Foster E, Kuehl K, Alpert J, Brabeck S, Crumb S, et al. Congenital Heart Disease in the Older Adult: A Scientific Statement From the American Heart Association. Circulation. 2015;131(21):1884-931.

CHAPTER 99

Pulmonary Artery Hypertension

Sandeep Bansal, Ashutosh Yadav, Anunay Gupta

ABSTRACT

Pulmonary artery hypertension (PAH) is Group 1 of World Health Organization (WHO) classification of pulmonary hypertension (PH). PH is a disease characterized by elevated pulmonary artery pressure (PAP) [mean PAP (mPAP) ≥20 mm Hg at rest with a pulmonary vascular resistance (PVR) ≥3 Wood units (WU)]. The WHO classifies patients with PH into five groups based upon etiology. In this review, we focus on evaluation and management of PAH patients. Nonetheless, we have discussed all other causes of PH also, which are more common and are managed differently.

"Measurement is the first step that leads to control and eventually to improvement"

—H James Harrington

INTRODUCTION

The pulmonary circulation is a low pressure, low resistant circuit as against the systemic circulation which is high pressure and high resistance. The relative pressures and vascular resistance in two circulations are shown in **Figure 1**. PH is a progressive disease characterized by an increase in PVR that occurs secondary to various underlying disorders. It results in right ventricular (RV) failure and death if left untreated. PH has been classified into five groups by the WHO. Group 1 is pulmonary arterial hypertension. Groups 2–5 are also called secondary luminary hypertension.

Group 1 PAH differs largely from PH Groups 2–5 in etiology, pathology, and response to treatment. Although we focus on PAH, several principles discussed, particularly those related to RV failure, apply to patients with all forms of advanced PH.

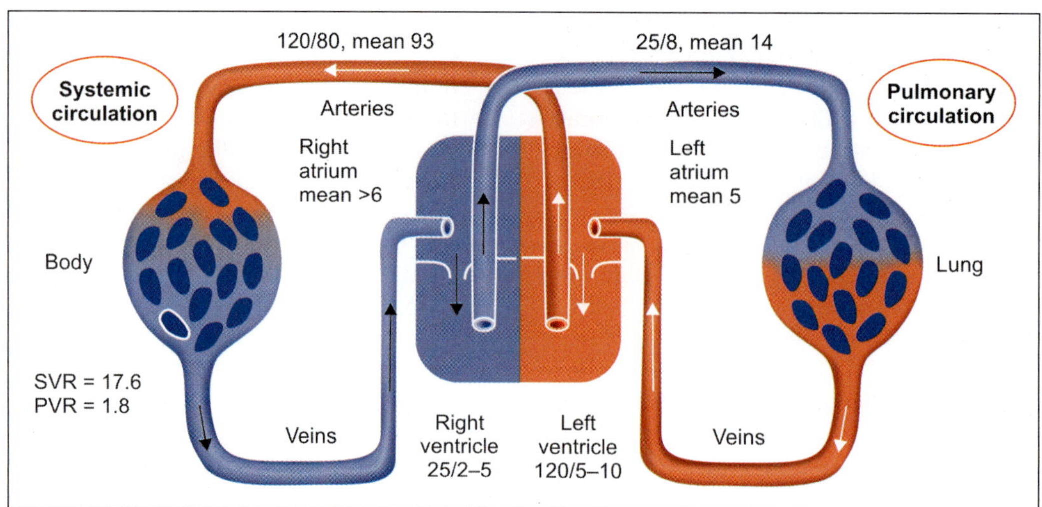

(PVR: pulmonary vascular resistance; SVR: systemic vascular resistance)

FIGURE 1: Pressure in various cardiac chambers and vascular systems with resistance in the two circulations.

DEFINITION

The normal range of mPAP is 14 ± 3.3 mm Hg resulting in the upper limit of normal as 20 mm Hg. Traditionally, the upper range of PH has been defined as mPAP ≥25 mm Hg. However, published multiple studies across different clinical types of PH documented poor outcomes in patients with mPAP between 20 and 25 mm Hg. In 2018, the sixth World Symposium on Pulmonary Hypertension (WSPH) held in Nice, France recommended changing the definition of PH to mPAP of >20 mm Hg as measured by right heart catheterization (RHC). However, this abnormal elevation of mPAP is not sufficient to define pulmonary vascular disease because it can be due to an increase in cardiac output (CO) or pulmonary arterial wedge pressure (PAWP). Therefore, this sixth WSPH task force included PVR of ≥3 WU in the definition of all forms of precapillary PH along with a mPAP of ≥20 mm Hg.

PATHOGENESIS OF PULMONARY ARTERY HYPERTENSION

The hallmark of PH is pulmonary vascular remodeling in medium to small vessels. Regardless of the underlying etiology of PH, pathological changes are similar in most of the patients including endothelial dysfunction, increased muscularization of small vessels, thickening of pulmonary arteriolar walls, neointimal formation, fibrinoid necrosis, in situ thrombosis with the formation of plexiform lesions. Remodeling involves all three layers of the vessel wall and is the consequence of cellular hyperplasia, hypertrophy, smooth muscle cell migration, inflammation, apoptosis, and accumulation of extracellular matrix. Progressive narrowing and loss of small vessels results in increased PVR, and RV failure and death.

There is a disruption of three signaling pathways: (1) The prostacyclin and thromboxane pathway, (2) The nitric oxide (NO) pathway, and (3) The endothelin-1 pathway. In PH there is impaired vasodilatation due to reduced prostacyclin and NO. The endothelin-1 action causes vasoconstriction and mitogenic effects.

WHO CLASSIFICATION OF PULMONARY HYPERTENSION (BOX 1)

GROUP 1

PAH is a relatively less common cause of PH and comprises diverse diseases resulting in pulmonary arterial remodeling resulting in intimal fibrosis, increased medial thickness, arteriolar occlusion, and plexiform lesions. Both endothelial dysfunction with inappropriate vasoconstriction and pulmonary vascular remodeling, and in situ thrombosis are the pathophysiological mechanisms in all types of PAH. As the disease develops and progresses, the cross-sectional area of the distal pulmonary vessels is reduced, causing a rise in PVR and PAP, which impacts the RV function. Without therapy, the progressive increase in afterload and strain on the RV is associated with significant morbidity and mortality.

This group includes idiopathic, familial, drug, and toxin-induced PAH and PAH associated with systemic sclerosis, portal hypertension, and human immunodeficiency virus (HIV). Idiopathic pulmonary arterial hypertension (IPAH) sometimes also known as primary pulmonary hypertension (PPH) is the most common type of Group 1 PH. Patients of IPAH need to be diagnosed with high index of suspicion since some studies have shown that they are often diagnosed late since some of these young women with sparse physical signs may be missed. Once IPAH is diagnosed we should rule out secondary causes like systemic sclerosis and other collagen vascular diseases and HIV-related PAH. IPAH is a progressive disease leading to right heart failure and death. It is primarily a disease of young women. Recently registry data has shown that its increasingly being identified in older individuals also. About 6–10% of patients have a heritable PAH. *BMPR2* gene is responsible for 80% of the heritable cases.

BOX 1	Simplified WHO classification of pulmonary hypertension.
Group 1 PAH	
• Idiopathic PAH • Heritable PAH • Drug-and toxin-induced PAH • PAH associated with other systemic diseasess—Connective tissue diseases, HIV, Portal hypertenision, Congenital heart disease • Persistent PH of the newborn syndrome	
Group 2	
PH due to left heart disease	
Group 3	
PH due to lung disease and/or hypoxia	
Group 4	
PH due to pulmonary artery obstructions including CTEPH	
Group 5	
• PH with unclear and/or multifactorial mechanisms • Hematological disorders • Systemic and metabolic disorders • Complex congenital heart disease	

(CTEPH: chronic thromboembolic pulmonary hypertension; HIV: human immunodeficiency virus; PAH: pulmonary artery hypertension; PH: pulmonary hypertension)

Compared to other causes of PH, Group I PAH is aggressive and associated with poor survival rates. The 5-year survival is 57% as shown by the REVEAL registry. The NIH registry shows 46% survival at 3 years and 38% at 4 years (**Fig. 2**).

Eisenmenger's syndrome (ES) is a type of Group 1 PAH which is still common in our country. ES results from flow reversal in some patients with left to right shunts (atrial septal defects, ventricular septal defect, patent ductus arteriosus, and admixture lesions) with PAH. The PAH is initially flow related and is reversible. Subsequently, when plexiform lesions develop in the pulmonary vasculature they become irreversible and right to left shunting occurs. These patients become inoperable and hemodynamically behave like IPAH. The prognosis in ES is better than in IPAH since the right side can decompress to the left side through the septal defect. The prognosis of collagen vascular and HIV-related PAH is worse than that of IPAH (**Fig. 3**).

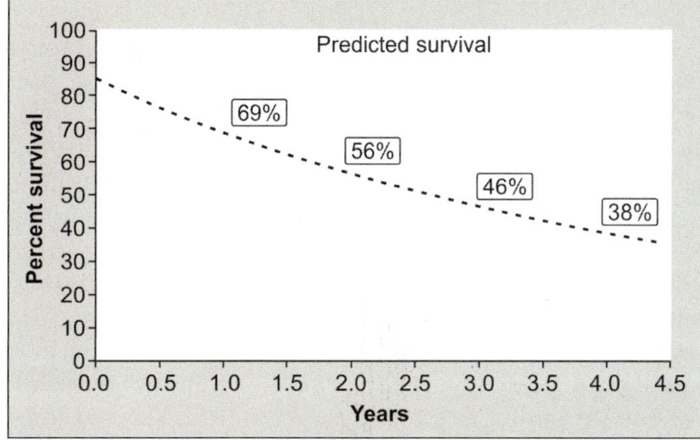

(NIH: National Institutes of Health; PAH: pulmonary artery hypertension)

FIGURE 2: Predicted survival of patients with PAH as seen in NIH registry.

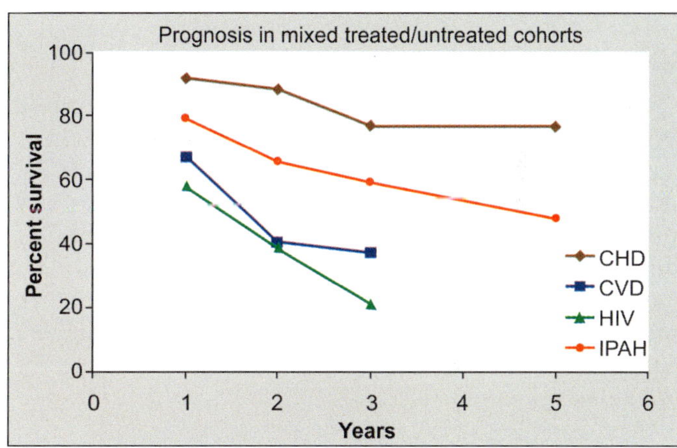

(CHD: congenital heart disease; CVD: collagen vascular disease; HIV: human immunodeficiency virus; IAPH: idiopathic primary artery hypertension; PAH: pulmonary artery hypertension)

FIGURE 3: Five-year survival in PAH due to various etiologies.

Source: McLaughin VV, Presberg KW, Doyle RL, Abman SH, McCrory DC, Fortin T, et al. Prognosis of pulmonary arterial hypertension: ACCP evidence-based clinical practice guidelines. Chest. 2004;126:78S-92S.

GROUP 2

Left heart disease is the most common cause of PH. Systolic or diastolic heart failure and valvular heart disease result in elevated left atrial (LA) pressure leading to passive transmission of pressure to the pulmonary circulation. Hemodynamic studies show mPAP >20 mm Hg, pulmonary capillary wedge pressure (PCWP) >15 mm Hg and PVR of <3 WU.

The presence of PH in patients with HF is associated with an overall poor prognosis. Chronic elevation of pulmonary arterial pressure can sometimes further lead to reactive pulmonary vasculopathy resulting in elevated transpulmonary gradient (mPAP-PAWP) >12 mm Hg and elevated PVR >3 WU. The pathologic changes in pulmonary vasculature are similar to Group 1 PH. The presence of a greater than expected rise in mPAP secondary to left heart failure led to the use of the term combined precapillary and postcapillary PH. However, unlike PAH in congenital heart diseases with left to right shunts the PH that develops in valvular heart disease is always reversible with correction of the lesion (like balloon mitral valvotomy in severe mitral stenosis with PAH).

GROUP 3

Lung disease is the second most common cause of PH. Although mPAP rise is modest in this group, it is associated with poor prognosis. PH should be suspected in patients with right heart failure and out of proportion hypoxemia related to the severity of the disease.

GROUP 4

Chronic thromboembolic pulmonary artery hypertension (CTEPAH) is an important cause of PH due to its curable nature with surgical intervention. It is characterized by precapillary PH with segmental perfusion defects detected by lung scanning or pulmonary angiography. A history of acute pulmonary embolism is present in 75% of patients with chronic thromboembolic pulmonary hypertension (CTEPH). The rest are secondary to asymptomatic pulmonary embolism. Contributing factors for CTEPH after acute pulmonary embolism are inadequate anticoagulation, large thrombus burden, residual thrombus, and recurrent embolism. Surgery with pulmonary endarterectomy is the mainstay of treatment followed by lifelong anticoagulation. Involvement of small pulmonary vessels results in suboptimal results after surgical intervention. Persistent PH after endarterectomy or patients not candidates for surgery should receive medical therapy.

GROUP 5

This group includes hematologic disorders, chronic myeloproliferative disorders, chronic myeloid leukemia, polycythemia vera, sickle cell disease, and beta thalassemia. Causative mechanisms include both precapillary (pulmonary vascular remodeling) and postcapillary (increased CO and fluid overload).

Other systemic disorders resulting in PH are sarcoidosis, pulmonary Langerhans histiocytosis, fibrosing mediastinitis, and end-stage renal disease with long-term maintenance hemodialysis.

PRE AND POSTCAPILLARY CLASSIFICATION

Pulmonary hypertension can be classified as precapillary PH and postcapillary PH (**Table 1**).

Precapillary PH is defined as mPAP >20 mm Hg, PCWP ≤15 mm Hg, and PVR >3 WU. Earlier definitions used to include diastolic pressure gradient, but the 2018 WSPH definitions have removed this. Precapillary PH includes groups 1, 3, 4, and 5.

Postcapillary PH is the elevation of mean PAP secondary to left heart causes, either left heart failure or valvular heart disease. It is defined as mPAP >20 mm Hg, PCWP >15 mm Hg and PVR <3 WU (**Fig. 4**).

In long-standing pulmonary venous hypertension, some patients can have reactive vasoconstriction with PAP beyond what can be expected by elevated LA pressure. These patients have combined precapillary and postcapillary PH and defined as mPAP >20 mm Hg, PCWP >15, and PVR ≥3 WU.

CLINICAL FEATURES

The clinical symptoms can be subtle and exertional dyspnea is invariably the presenting and the most common

TABLE 1 Updated hemodynamics definition based on the sixth WSPH.

Definition	Characteristics	Clinical group
Precapillary PH	• mPAP >20 mm Hg • PCWP = 15 mm Hg • PVR = 3 WU	Groups 1, 3, 4, and 5
Isolated postcapillary PH	• mPAP >20 mm Hg • PCWP >15 mm Hg • PVR <3 WU	Groups 2 and 5
Combined precapillary and postcapillary PH	• mPAP >20 mm Hg • PCWP >15 • PVR = 3 WU	Groups 2 and 5

(WSPH: World Symposium on Pulmonary Hypertension; mPAP: mean pulmonary artery pressure; PCWP: pulmonary capillary wedge pressure; WU: Wood units)

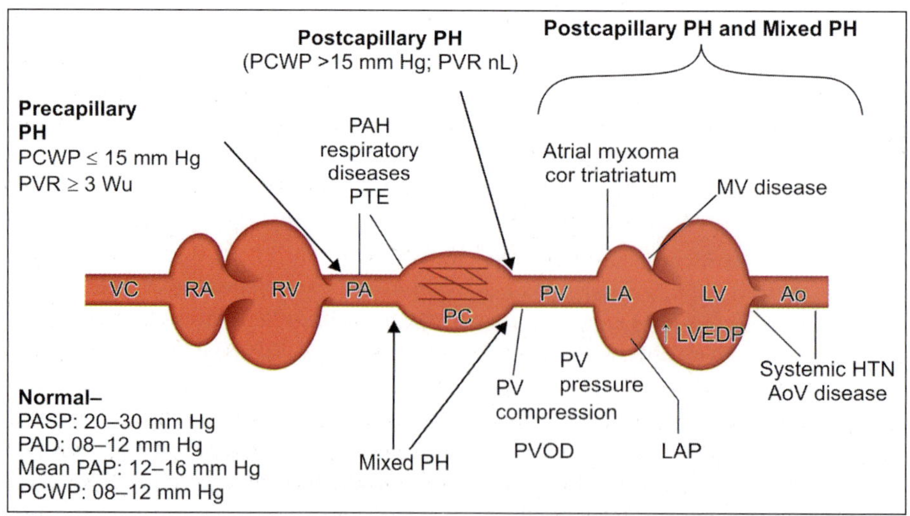

(PADP: pulmonary artery diastolic pressure; PASP: pulmonary artery systolic pressure; PCWP: pulmonary capillary wedge pressure; PV: pulmonary vein; PVOD: pulmonary veno-occlusive disease)

FIGURE 4: Site of obstruction in lesion in pre- and postcapillary hypertension.

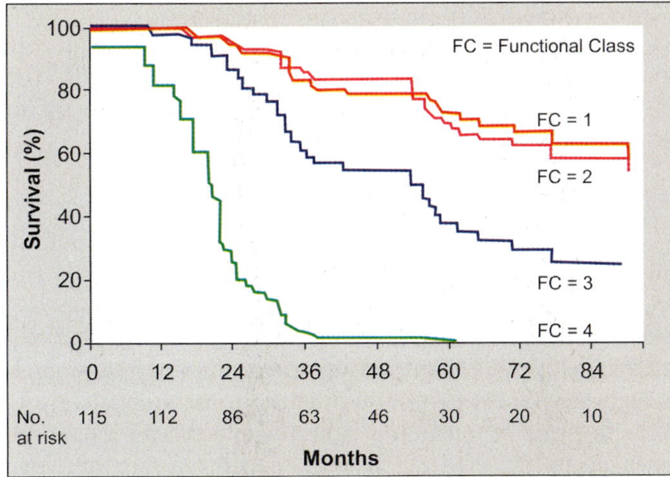

FIGURE 5: Impact of functional class on survival: Better survival in patients who are in functional classes I and II as compared to those in functional classes III and IV.

Source: McLaughin VV, Shillington A, Rich S. Survival in primary pulmonary hypertension: the impact of epoprostenol therapy. Circulation. 2002;106(12):1477-82.

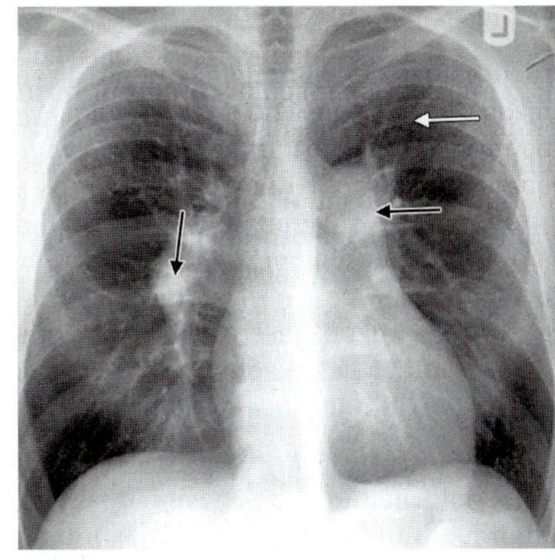

(IPAH: idiopathic pulmonary arterial hypertension)

FIGURE 6: Chest X-ray of patient with IPAH. Normal heart size with prominent main pulmonary artery (black arrow on left) and dilated right pulmonary artery (black arrow in right) and peripheral pruning (decreased vascular markings in the lateral one-third).

complaint. Fatigue, chest pain, and syncope can also occur. In late stages when right-sided heart failure (RHF) develops they can have abdominal distention, appetite loss, and pedal edema. The functional class of the patient is a simple and good prognostic marker of survival (**Fig. 5**).

On physical examination: The jugular venous pressure (JVP) shows a prominent "a" wave initially. Later when secondary tricuspid regurgitation (TR) and RHF develops, then can have raised JVP and prominent VY collapse. The heart size is initially normal. The subtle signs of PAH in idiopathic or primary PAH are often missed unless we pick up the loud P_2 component of S_2 and left parasternal heave. In very late stages they develop secondary TR and RHF.

In patients with pulmonary venous hypertension physical examination findings include signs of left heart failure or valvular involvement.

DIAGNOSIS

ELECTROCARDIOGRAPHY

Electrocardiography (ECG) has low sensitivity and specificity for PAH. A normal ECG does not exclude PH. Common features are right atrial enlargement, P pulmonale, right axis deviation, right bundle branch block (RBBB), RV enlargement with strain pattern, and prolongation of QTc.

CHEST X-RAY

Chest X-ray features of PAH are enlargement of main pulmonary artery (MPA) and hilar PA shadows, with peripheral pruning. Right atrial and ventricular enlargement can be seen. A specific etiologic diagnosis such as chronic obstructive pulmonary disease (COPD) (hyperinflation of lungs) and left-sided heart failure (pulmonary venous congestion), can be seen (**Fig. 6**).

BLOOD TESTS AND IMMUNOLOGY

All patients should undergo routine biochemistry and hematology. Those with clinical clues should be screened for connective tissue disease (CTD), hepatitis, and HIV as required. Elevations of brain natriuretic peptide (BNP) and N-terminal pro-BNP (NT-proBNP) are associated with RV overload and are predictors of worse outcome.

PULMONARY FUNCTION TESTS

Pulmonary function tests should be performed in all patients with pulmonary vascular disease. The earliest finding is a decrease in diffusing capacity of the lungs for carbon monoxide (DLCO). Routine spirometry measurements with forced expiratory volume, forced vital capacity, and total lung capacity measurement should be done. Most patients with PAH may show a mild restrictive component. A markedly lower DLCO (<60% of predicted), or marked exertional hypoxemia indicates pulmonary veno-occlusive disease (PVOD) or pulmonary capillary hemangiomatosis. DLCO <45% is associated with poor outcomes. Reduction in DLCO precedes PH in patients with scleroderma.

TRANSTHORACIC ECHOCARDIOGRAPHY

In all suspected patients, transthoracic echocardiography (TTE) is essential and the most important noninvasive test. Findings suggestive of PH are right atrial enlargement, RV enlargement, RV dysfunction, small left side chambers, flattening, and abnormal motion of interventricular septum, TR with elevated right ventricular systolic pressure (RVSP) (**Fig. 7**). A reduced tricuspid annular plane systolic excursion (TAPSE) is a sign of RV dysfunction (**Figs. 8 A** and **B**). Inferior vena cava (IVC) diameter and collapsibility on inspiration are abnormal in late stages when RHF develops.

Echocardiography can also detect left-sided cardiac lesions that can cause Group 2 PH. Left ventricular systolic and diastolic dysfunction, aortic or mitral valve involvement can be easily assessed. Enlarged LA is an important indicator of elevated left-sided filling pressures.

Right ventricular dysfunction is the most important echocardiographic prognostic indicator and the onset of RV dysfunction portends a subsequent poor prognosis.

Contrast echocardiography is needed when shunt lesions are suspected as a cause of PAH in those with ES.

VENTILATION/PERFUSION LUNG SCANNING

Chronic thromboembolic pulmonary hypertension should be considered in all patients with unexplained dyspnea and PH. CTEPH diagnosis is essential because a potentially curable surgical option is available. Ventilation/perfusion (V/Q) scan is the preferred and most sensitive 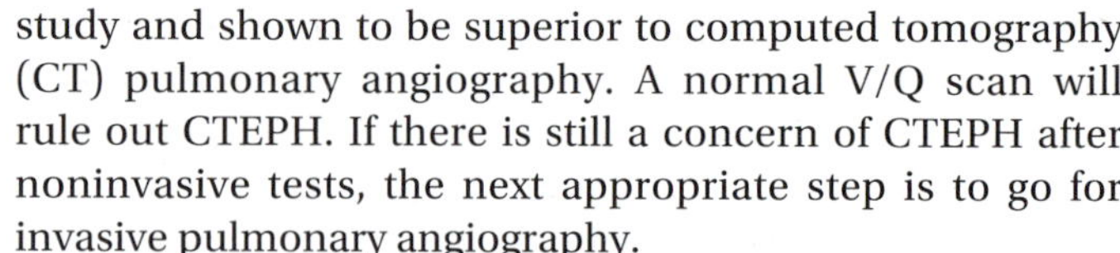 study and shown to be superior to computed tomography (CT) pulmonary angiography. A normal V/Q scan will rule out CTEPH. If there is still a concern of CTEPH after noninvasive tests, the next appropriate step is to go for invasive pulmonary angiography.

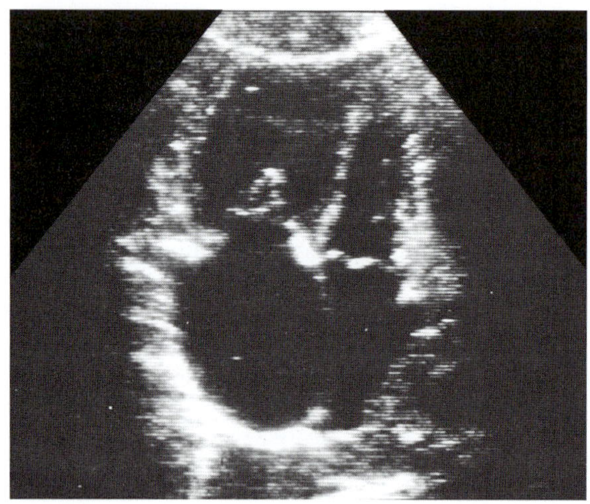

(IPAH: idiopathic pulmonary arterial hypertension)

FIGURE 7: Echocardiography: Apical four-chamber view showing dilated right ventricle and right atrium, interatrial septum bulging to the left atrium in a patient with severe IPAH.

CHEST COMPUTED TOMOGRAPHY

Chest CT is easily available and can provide important information about lung parenchyma, vasculature, and cardiac chambers. Findings suggestive of PH are RV dilatation, right atrial dilatation, enlarged MPA (diameter ≥29 mm), or MPA/ascending aorta diameter ratio ≥1 is suggestive of PH. Segmental artery to bronchus ratio of >1.1 in three or four lobes is highly specific for PH. High-resolution CT (HRCT) can also differentiate between parenchymal disease and IPAH and is diagnostic for interstitial lung disease (ILD), emphysema, and PVOD.

In suspected CTEPH, CT pulmonary angiography can be very helpful in identifying lesions amenable for pulmonary endarterectomy. Invasive pulmonary angiography is still the standard of care before surgical intervention.

CARDIAC CATHETERIZATION

Right heart catheterization may be done in some cases of PAH after noninvasive evaluation when there is need of additional information. RHC can confirm the diagnosis of PAH by direct measurement of pulmonary pressure, identification, and quantification of shunt lesions, calculation of PVR, and vasodilator reactivity test.

The data measured during the RHC is pressures in cardiac chambers and oxygen saturation. The CO PVR is calculated and vasoreactivity testing is done.

Vasoreactivity is performed with a short-acting vasodilator, most commonly 20–40 ppm of inhaled NO or intravenous epoprostenol. After 10–15 minutes, hemodynamics are assessed. Other agents that can be used are inhaled prostacyclin, inhaled milrinone, inhaled nitroglycerin, and intravenous adenosine.

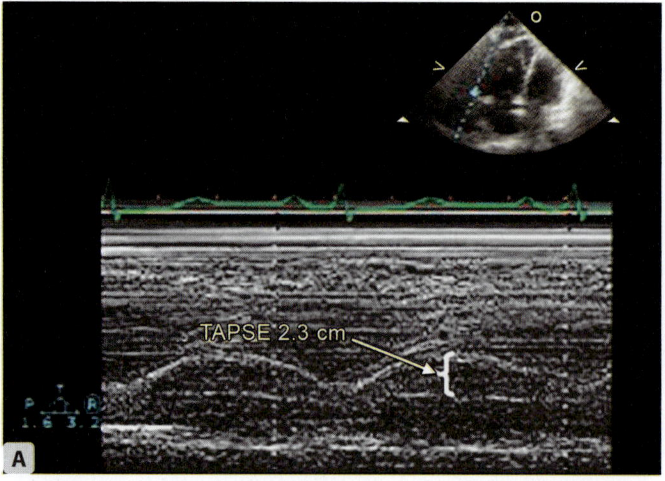

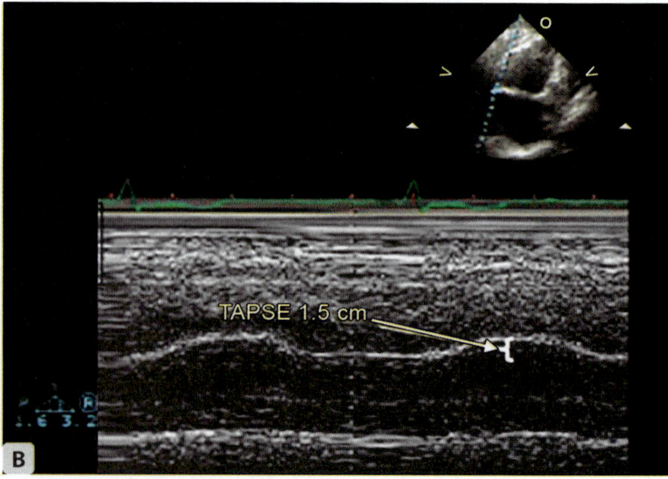

(IPAH: idiopathic pulmonary arterial hypertension; RV: right ventricular)

FIGURES 8 A & B: Tricuspid annular plane systolic excursion (TAPSE) is a marker of RV functions. **(A)** Normal TAPSE and **(B)** reduce TAPSE in a patient with IPAH and RV dysfunction.

A positive pulmonary vasodilator response is defined as a reduction in mPAP by ≥10 mm Hg to a value of ≤40 mm Hg, with unchanged or improved CO in response to administration of a rapidly active pulmonary vasodilator.

About 10% of patients with idiopathic and heritable PAH have a positive vasodilator response. These patients have a favorable response to treatment with calcium channel blockers (CCBs), amlodipine, and nifedipine and have a better long-term prognosis compared to patients without a positive response. However, since only a fraction of these patients shows vasoreactivity and response to these drugs it is done in frequently and these agents are often not used in PAH.

TREATMENT

Specific therapy is available for Group I PAH. The mainstay of management of Groups 2–5 is the treatment of underlying illness.

GROUP 1 PAH

General measures: Advise low-grade aerobic exercises. Heavy exertion and isometric exercises to be avoided in all patients. Oxygen supplementation is needed in a few patients in late stages to keep oxygen saturation above 92%. Restriction of sodium intake and management of fluid status in right heart failure are necessary. Routine immunizations are advised with influenza and pneumococcal vaccines. Current guidelines advise against pregnancy in patients with PAH. The use of epidural anesthesia is preferred to general anesthesia. Pregnancy is contraindicated in severe IPAH and Eisenmenger's since there is 30% maternal mortality and very poor fetal outcomes.

A risk stratification is done to define the management strategies (**Table 2**). Patients who are in low- and intermediate groups, should receive oral therapy (**Flowchart 1**). The combination therapy with an endothelin receptor antagonist (ERA) and a phosphodiesterase type 5 (PDE5) inhibitor is the treatment of choice. This recommendation is based on the outcomes of the AMBITION study where combination therapy with ambrisentan and tadalafil resulted in better outcomes than either agent alone. Patients who are at high risk should receive intravenous prostacyclin analog as first-line therapy and evaluation for lung transplantation.

There is inconclusive evidence regarding the benefit of anticoagulation, while earlier observational studies showing a benefit, no benefit was observed in the REVEAL registry. Still, oral anticoagulation can be considered in these patients. After initiation patients should be re-evaluated after 3–6 months. The goal of the treatment is the achievement of a low-risk status.

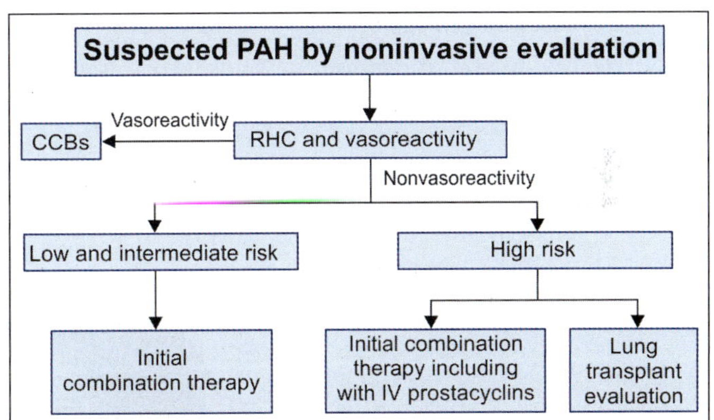

(CCBs: calcium channel blockers; RHC: right heart catheterization)

FLOWCHART 1: A simplified approach to treatment of Group 1 PAH.

TABLE 2 Risk assessment in pulmonary artery hypertension.

Determinants of prognosis	Low risk (<5%)	Intermediate risk (5–10%)	High risk (>10%)
Clinical signs of right heart failure	Absent	Absent	Present
Progression of symptoms	No	Slow	Rapid
Syncope	No	Occasional sncope	Repeated syncope
WHO functional class	I, II	III	IV
6MWD	>440 m	164–440 m	<165 m
• BNP • NT-ProBNP	• <50 ng/mL • <300 ng/mL	• 50–300 ng/mL • 300-1400 ng/mL	• >300 ng/mL • >1400 ng/mL
Imaging (echocardiography, CMR imaging)	• RA area <18 cm^2 • No pericardial effusion	• RA area 18–26 cm^2 • No or minimal pericardial effusion	• RA area >26 cm^2 • Pericardial effusion
Hemodynamics	• RAP <8 mm Hg • CI ≥2.25 L/min/m^2 • SvO_2 > 65%	• RAP 8–14 mm Hg • CI 2.0–2.4 L/min/m^2 • SvO_2 60% to 65%	• RAP >14 mm Hg • CI <2.0 L/min/m^2 • SvO_2 < 60%

(6MWD: 6-minute walking distance; NT-proBNP: N-terminal pro-brain natriuretic peptide; RA: right atrium; RAP: right atrial pressure; SvO_2: mixed venous oxygen saturation)

SPECIFIC MEDICAL THERAPY

Survival in PAH has been increased from a median survival of 2.8 years in 1980 to 7 years in the current era with the use of effective therapy. PAH secondary to congenital heart disease has a better prognosis as compared to idiopathic or hereditary PAH. PAH associated with CTD and HIV has the worst prognosis.

The three signaling pathways involved in the pathogenesis of IPAH are all utilized for management of these patients. We use PDE5 inhibitors, ERA, and prostanoids for the management of these patients (**Fig. 9**). Initially single class therapy was used in these patients. Now we often combined PDE5 inhibitors and endothelin antagonists as first line.

The prostanoids are available as parenteral infusions or as inhalers. These are used in patients with class IV symptoms. Also, they are more expensive and less easily available. The dosages of commonly used drugs are given in **Table 3**.

PHOSPHODIESTERASE TYPE 5 INHIBITORS

Nitric oxide in pulmonary vasculature acts by activating guanylyl cyclase, generating cyclic guanosine monophosphate (cGMP) in smooth muscles, and platelets with resulting pulmonary vasodilatation and inhibition of smooth muscle proliferation. cGMP is metabolized by PDE5. By inhibiting the degradation of cGMP, PDE5 inhibitors prolong the vasodilatory action of NO. Approved PDE5 inhibitors are sildenafil and tadalafil.

A soluble guanylyl cyclase (sGC) stimulator riociguat was approved for the treatment of PAH and CTEPH. It acts by stabilizing NO-sGC, sensitizing sGC to NO, and direct stimulation of sGC. All these results in an increase in cGMP synthesis.

The combination of PDE5 inhibitors and riociguat is contraindicated due to significant hypotension.

ENDOTHELIN RECEPTOR ANTAGONISTS

Endothelin-1 is a powerful vasoconstrictor and mitogenic effects are exerted by binding to endothelin-A (ET-A) receptors in the lungs. Endothelin antagonists exert their effects by binding to ET-A. These increases exercise capacity, quality of life, and prevent clinical worsening. Approved ERA for PAH are nonselective bosentan, macitentan, and selective ET-A antagonist ambrisentan.

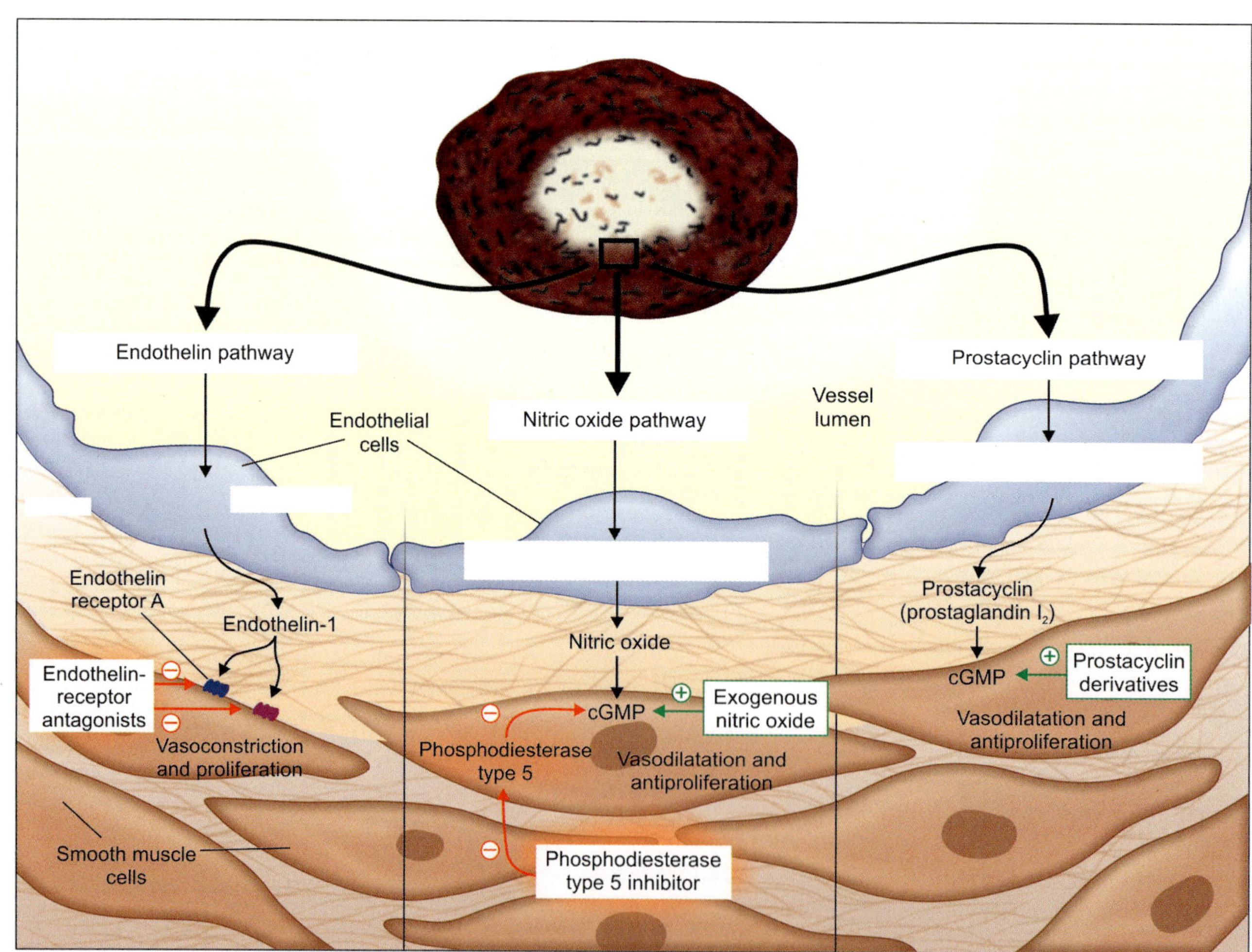

(cAMP: cyclic adenosine monophosphate; cGMP: cyclic guanosine monophosphate; PAH: pulmonary artery hypertension)

FIGURE 9: Drugs acting on the three pathways involved in the pathogenesis of PAH.

TABLE 3 Commonly used drugs for PAH along with dosages.

Class	Drugs	Dosages
CCB	• Amlodipine • Nifedipine ER • Diltiazem ER	• 20–30 mg/day • 120–240 mg/day • 240–960 mg/day
Endothelin receptor antagonists	• Ambrisentan • Bosentan • Macitentan	• 5–10 mg/day • <40 kg– Max 125 mg/day • >40 kg– Max 250 mg/day • 10 mg/day
Prostacycline analog	• Epoprostenol • Iloprost • Treprostanil	• IV – 1–2 ng/kg/min, titrate every 15 min to target dose of 20–40 ng/kg/min • INH: 2.5–5 μm inhaled 6–9 times/day; max 45 μm/day • SC/IV: 1.25 ng/kg/min titrate by 1.25 ng/kg/min every week for 4 weeks, than by 2.5 ng/kg/min per week up to 40 ng/kg/min • INH: 3–6 inhalations qid • Oral: ER tablet 0.25 mg every 12 h
Prostacycline receptor agonist	• Selexipag	• Max 3200 μm/day
Phosphodiestrase type 5 inhibitor	• Sildenafil • Tadalafil	• Max 60 mg/day • Max 40 mg/day
Soluble guanylate cyclase inhibitor	• Riociguat	• Max 2.5 mg tid

Note: Bosentan is given in two divided doses, Sildenafil is given in three divided doses per day. Tadalafil, Ambrisentan, and Macitentan are given once a day.

(CCB: calcium channel blockers; ER: extended release)

PROSTANOIDS

PAH is associated with reduced prostacyclin I_2. Prostanoids are potent vasodilators acting on prostacyclin receptors. Intravenous epoprostenol was the earliest prostanoid available and showed an improved quality of life, exercise capacity, 6-minute walking distance (6MWD), and mortality benefit.

Other available prostacyclin analogs include oral beraprost, intravenous and subcutaneous treprostinil, and iloprost, available in intravenous, oral, and nasal aerosol formulations.

ATRIAL SEPTOSTOMY

Graded balloon dilatation of atrial septum to create a right to left interatrial shunt has been tired but is not recommended now. It was done with the hope that it will reduce right-sided filling pressure and improve RV function and there will be increased left heart filling. However, a short-term symptomatic benefit occurs at the cost of systemic desaturation. Also, procedure is associated with high mortality. Hence, it is not done now.

CARDIAC TRANSPLANTATION

It is recommended after failure of medical therapy and patients who remain in WHO functional class III or IV. The overall survival rate after transplantation is 50% at 5 years. Single or double lung transplant can be done. Lung transplant is more difficult and has worse survival than heart transplant. For this reason, while heart transplant is being done in many centers in India, it is being done in just a few (2–3) centers in the country.

PROKERALA REGISTRY

PROKERALA is the only South Asian registry of PH, with enrolment of 2003 patients. Data was collected using standard questionnaire. The main inclusion criterion was echocardiographic RVSP >50 mm Hg. The mean age was age 56 ± 16.1 years, and 52% of patients were women. About 1 in 5 patients (18.5%) had evidence of right heart failure. New York Heart Association III (NYHA III) or greater class symptoms were present in more than one-third (36.5%) of the participants. The mean RVSP in the population was 68.2 ± 17.9 mm Hg. The most common cause of PH was secondary to LH disease (59%) cases. Group 1 was the etiologic cause in 21.2% cases. This group had female preponderance.

In patients with PH due to left heart disease the most common cause was valvular disease (27%), with coronary disease being a close second (23%).

Idiopathic pulmonary arterial hypertension was the etiologic factor in 6% cases, COPD in 11% cases, congenital heart disease in 15%, and chronic thromboembolic disease in 3.8% cases.

Hemodynamic and vasoreactivity testing was done in very few patients prior to be being initiated on PH specific therapy. Only 4.3% participants were on CCB therapy. The most common PH-specific therapies used were phosphodiesterase V in 17.1% cases and ERAs in 2.3% of cases. Combination therapy was used in negligible number of patients.

RECOMMENDED READINGS

1. Sahay S. Evaluation and classification of pulmonary arterial hypertension. J Thorac Dis. 2019;11(Suppl 14):S1789-99.
2. Kovacs G, Berghold A, Scheidl S, Olschewski H. Pulmonary arterial pressure during rest and exercise in healthy subjects: A systematic review. Eur Respir J. 2009;34(4):888-94.
3. Simonneau G, Montani D, Celermajer DS, Denton CP, Gatzoulis MA, Krowka M, et al. Haemodynamic definitions and updated clinical classification of pulmonary hypertension. Eur Respir J. 2019;53(1): 1801913.
4. Voelkel NF, Gomez-Arroyo J, Abbate A, Bogaard HJ, Nicolls MR. Pathobiology of pulmonary arterial hypertension and right ventricular failure. Eur Respir J. 2012;40(6):1555-65.
5. Machado RD, Southgate L, Eichstaedt CA, Aldred MA, Austin ED, Best DH, et al. Pulmonary arterial hypertension: A current perspective on established and emerging molecular genetic defects. Hum Mutat. 2015;36(12):1113-27.
6. Benza RL, Miller DP, Barst RJ, Badesch DB, Frost AE, McGoon MD. An evaluation of long-term survival from time of diagnosis in pulmonary arterial hypertension from the REVEAL registry. Chest. 2012;142(2):448-56.
7. Vachiéry JL, Tedford RJ, Rosenkranz S, Palazzini M, Lang I, Guazzi M, et al. Pulmonary hypertension due to left heart disease. Eur Respir J. 2019;53(1):1801897.
8. Lang IM, Pesavento R, Bonderman D, Yuan JX. Risk factors and basic mechanisms of chronic thromboembolic pulmonary hypertension: A current understanding. Eur Respir J. 2013;41(2):462-8.
9. Galiè N, Barberà JA, Frost AE, Ghofrani HA, Hoeper MM, McLaughlin VV, et al. Initial use of Ambrisentan plus Tadalafil in Pulmonary Arterial Hypertension. N Engl J Med. 2015;373(9):834-44.
10. Harikrishnan S, Sanjay G, Ashishkumar M, Menon J, Rajesh GN, Kumar RK, et al. Pulmonary hypertension registry of Kerala, India (PRO-KERALA) - Clinical characteristics and practice patterns. Int J Cardiol. 2018;265:212-7.
11. Galiè N, Humbert M, Vachiery JL, Gibbs S, Lang I, Torbicki A, et al. ESC/ERS Guidelines for the diagnosis and treatment of pulmonary hypertension: The Joint Task Force for the Diagnosis and Treatment of Pulmonary Hypertension of the European Society of Cardiology (ESC) and the European Respiratory Society (ERS): Endorsed by: Association for European Paediatric and Congenital Cardiology (AEPC), International Society for Heart and Lung Transplantation (ISHLT). Eur Respir J. 2015;46(4):903-75.
12. McLaughlin VV, Shah SJ, Souza R, Humbert M. Management of pulmonary arterial hypertension. J Am Coll Cardiol. 2015;65(18):1976-97.
13. Simonneau G, Montani D, Celermajer DS, Denton CP, Gatzoulis MA, Krowka M, et al. Haemodynamic definitions and updated clinical classification of pulmonary hypertension. Eur Respir J. 2019;53(1): 1801913.

CHAPTER 100

Infective Endocarditis: A Systemic Disease

Abhishek Goyal, Bishav Mohan, Jasvinder Singh

ABSTRACT

Infective endocarditis (IE) is uncommon but is associated with high morbidity and mortality. It disproportionately affects those with underlying structural heart disease and is increasingly associated with healthcare contact, particularly in patients who have intravascular prosthetic material. With an ageing population and increasing use of cardiac devices and heart valves, the epidemiology of IE has changed. In the setting of bacteremia with a pathogenic organism, an infected vegetation results on the surface of heart valves or holes when turbulence is there. It has varied clinical manifestations and once established it can affect almost any system of the body.

Hematological investigations, blood culture, and echocardiography are the mainstay for making the diagnosis. In case the blood cultures are negative IE, the diagnosis may be challenging. Novel microbiological and imaging techniques have been developed. These have been shown to reduce the rate of misdiagnosing IE, particularly in the setting of prosthetic valve endocarditis (PVE), paravalvular extension of infection, and cardiac implantable electronic devices. The diagnosis of IE may be difficult to establish and various clinical, microbiological, and echocardiography features have been included in modified Duke criteria. Once diagnosed, IE can be managed with multidisciplinary team with expertise in infectious disease, cardiology, and cardio surgery. Antibiotic prophylaxis for prevention of IE should be followed according to the latest guidelines.

"Sound judgement with discernment is the best of seers"

—Euripides

INTRODUCTION

Infective endocarditis is a complex multisystem disease caused by a microbial infection, usually bacterial, involving endothelial lining of heart mainly affecting heart valves but may also involve mural endocardium, chordal structures, deeper layer of myocardium, and/or pericardium. IE is associated with very high morbidity and mortality. Prompt diagnosis triggered by high index of clinical suspicion, aggressive and timely treatment helps to reduce complications and mortality. Management often requires multispecialty teamwork including at times cardiovascular surgery. Despite many advances in its diagnosis and treatment, IE continues to be a serious challenge.

EPIDEMIOLOGY AND RISK FACTORS

It is difficult to determine the exact incidence of IE, especially in developing countries. It is gradually increasing with more aging population and increased number of cardiac interventions. The estimated incidence is around 3–10 cases per 100,000 persons per year. No definite estimation of incidence of IE in India is available. The incidence of IE was 79.6 per 100,000 hospital admissions in a hospital-based study. More recently, the incidence of endocarditis has increased among the elderly. Median age of patient has gradually increased from fourth decade in early antibiotic era to sixth and seventh decade recently. Despite various diagnostic and therapeutic advances, prognosis remains dismal. The estimated in-hospital mortality is about 22% with 40% mortality at 5 years. Morbidity figures are also high. Almost 15–20% require surgical management in acute IE.

UNDERLYING DISEASE

Endocarditis can involve normal or more often diseased heart. In fact, the bacteremia settles at the site where turbulence causes endothelial roughness and break. It involves normal heart in those presenting with acute IE. Infection of underlying heart disease causes a presentation of subacute IE. The etiology of underlying disease in developed world has shifted from chronic rheumatic heart disease (RHD) (a common predisposition in developing countries till date) to degenerative valve disease, illicit intravenous (IV) drug use, and intracardiac devices.

Indian scenario: The incidence of RHD has declined in the last few decades in India. However, RHD is still the most frequent underlying disease and mitral valve (MV) is the most common site in India. Mitral valve prolapse (MVP) has been reported as a predisposing factor is 3–10% of native valve IE. **Table 1** highlights major Indian studies on IE. Most common predisposing condition was RHD accounting for 30–70% of cases. The varying incidence is partly attributed to regional variations, declining RHD incidence and referral bias as most of these studies are hospital based. In a recent study, intravenous drug abuse (IVDA) was responsible for 40.6% cases of IE. With changes in lifestyle and increasing addictions the IVDA-IE is expected to become more common in India.

Healthcare-related IE is defined as IE occurring in a healthcare setting with occurrence of symptoms after 48 hours of hospital admission. Prosthetic valves and cardiac devices are significant risk factors for IE. Rates of implantation of these devices have increased. IE associated with cardiovascular implantable electronic devices (CIEDs) occurs in 0.5–1.14 cases per 1,000 device recipients. Incidence of IE in transcatheter aortic valve implantation (TAVI) is 0.97%.

PRECIPITATING CAUSE

The most common entry site for bacteremia is cutaneous (40%) such as vascular access, surgical site, or site used for IV drug abuse. Second most common (29%) portal of entry was oral/dental. A history of invasive or dental procedure can be found in approximately 25% of patients within 60 days of clinical presentation with IE. A gastrointestinal source is found in 20% cases. A genitourinary or respiratory portal of entry is less common and is found in 5% cases.

MICROBIOLOGY

Only few bacterial species are responsible for vast majority of cases of IE. Staphylococci and streptococci are the most common organisms responsible for 80% of the cases. Recently *Staphylococcus aureus* has emerged as the most frequently isolated microbial agent worldwide pushing streptococci to second position. The emergence of healthcare-associated IE has been accompanied by an increase in the prevalence of *Staphylococcus aureus*. Enterococci are the third leading cause of IE. They are also linked to healthcare contact. Infections with gram negative

TABLE 1 Predisposing conditions in IE: Indian studies (values in percentage).

	Garg et al. (2003)	Senthil et al. (2010)	Gupta et al. (2013)	Subharaju et al. (2018)
Rheumatic heart disease	49	70	38	31
Congenital heart disease	29	10	23	16
Bicuspid aortic valve (BAV)	9	4	16	8
Mitral valve prolapse	3.1	6	3	24
Prosthetic valves	10	3	31	4
Implantable electronic devices	–	–	–	–
Degenerative valve disease	–	–	3	23

and fungal pathogens in IE are rare and primarily seen in immunocompromised individuals.

In approximately 10% of cases of IE, blood cultures are negative. Use of antibiotics prior to blood sampling is an important cause of culture negativity. True culture negative IE is caused by fastidious microorganism that are difficult to isolate with conventional technique. Highly specialized assays such as serologic testing and polymerase chain reaction (PCR) (using blood or valve biopsy) can detect causative organism in a significant number of cases. These tests should be utilized more frequently. Important etiological causes of true culture negative IE are *Coxiella burnetii*, *Bartonella* species, and *Brucella* species. Specific predisposing circumstances include people working in slaughterhouses (*Brucella* and *Coxiella*), homelessness or alcoholism (*Bartonella Quintana*), travel to Eurasia/Middle East (*Brucella*), contact with cats (*Bartonella henselae*) or healthcare exposure in patient with prosthetic valves (*Aspergillus*).

Beta-hemolytic streptococci are notorious to cause acute fulminant presentation of IE. *Streptococcus gallolyticus* is associated with gastrointestinal malignancies. Right-sided IE predominantly of tricuspid valve (TV) is seen in IVDA and is most commonly caused by *Staphylococcus aureus*. *Enterococcus faecalis* infection is associated with genitourinary tract abnormalities. HACEK (*Haemophilus parainfluenzae, Aggregatibacter aphrophilus, Aggregatibacter actinomycetemcomitans, Cardiobacterium hominis, Eikenella corrodens*, and *Kingella kingae*) group reside in oropharynx and respiratory tract and result in community acquired-IE. Among fungus, *Candida* is common in IV drug abusers and right-sided IE.

In Indian studies also, streptococci and staphylococci are the most common microbial isolates. Microbiology varies in different geographical area. In a recent study from Punjab, percentage of methicillin-resistant *Staphylococcus aureus* (42% vs. 17%) and pseudomonas-related IE (18% vs. 2%) was significantly higher among IVDA group compared to non-IVDA group. Pseudomonas seems to be common among IV drug abusers.

PATHOGENESIS

The primary prerequisite for the IE is underlying cardiac structural abnormality (valvular or nonvalvular) that results in endothelial injury by blood flow turbulence serving as a substrate for platelet and fibrin deposition. Subsequent bacteremia and fungemia (rarely) adheres and colonizes this damaged area resulting in IE. Valvular predisposition may be due to underlying valvular disease, mechanical injury by foreign such as CIED and direct injury of TV by injected particulate matter in IVDA. Certain bacteria such as *Staphylococcus* and beta-hemolytic streptococci can infect the normal valves too. Significant bacteremia is a prerequisite for the development of native valve IE. Transient and low-grade bacteremia is common in day-to-day life which usually does not result in IE.

Remote systemic manifestations are due to either systemic emboli or immune complex-mediated reactions. Embolism results in embolic stroke, limb gangrene, infarction of spleen, kidney, mesentery, and skin. Seeding and proliferation in local tissue creates visceral abscess which are often difficult to treat and need surgical drainage.

CLINICAL FEATURES

The clinical features of IE can be of three types: (1) Nonspecific evidence of systemic infection and/or inflammation, (2) Features of underlying cardiac condition and local complications in the heart, and (3) Systemic immunological and embolic complications in various systems in the body.

INFECTION/INFLAMMATION

Fever of >38°C is the most common presenting symptom in 80% of patients, but may be absent in 20% cases particularly in elderly, immune compromised patients, and previous treatment with antibiotics. Fever defervescence usually occurs with 5–7 days of antibiotic therapy. Persistence of fever may indicate progressive infection with perivalvular abscess, septic embolization, extracardiac site infection, inadequate antibiotics, or resistant organism. Other nonspecific constitutional symptoms of infection include chills, sweats, headache, malaise, and nausea. Myalgia and arthralgia may be noted in 20–40% cases.

CARDIAC MANIFESTATIONS

Dyspnea can occur in left-sided regurgitant lesions. Orthopnea and paroxysmal nocturnal dyspnea (PND) is predictor of poor prognosis. Congestive heart failure (CHF) complicates the course in 30–50% of patients with IE. Even with early surgical intervention, occurrence of heart failure (HF) doubles the in-hospital mortality to almost 25%.

Appearance of a new murmur or change in intensity/character of a previous murmur is the sign of valve damage due to the infection. A vegetation occurs usually in the line of closure of valve leaflet on atrial surface of mitral/TVs or ventricular surface of semilunar valves. Infection may lead to perforation of a valve leaflet or rupture of chordae tendineae, interventricular septum, or papillary muscles. Valve ring abscess with fistula formation in the myocardium or pericardial space may result. Angina pectoris or myocardial infarction can occur as an embolic complication of IE.

SYSTEMIC COMPLICATIONS

Neurological manifestations: The incidence of stroke is 4.8 cases per 1,000 patient-days in the first week of IE and drops rapidly after starting antibiotics. 20–30% patients have cerebral emboli. Mycotic aneurysm is localized enlargement of arteries caused by infection of arterial wall. These aneurysms can arise either by direct bacterial invasion of arterial wall with subsequent abscess formation or embolic occlusion of vasa vasorum or immune complex-mediated injury. The aneurysm may result in hemorrhage.

Pulmonary manifestations: Thromboembolic showers in which showers of tiny emboli occlude small vessel can lead to septic pulmonary infarct. This is usually seen in tricuspid valve infective endocarditis (TVIE). Pneumonia, pleural effusion, or empyema can occur. Sometime, rounded cannon ball lesions mimicking tumors can develop. Pleuritic chest pain can result from the septic pulmonary infarct.

Renal manifestations: Kidney may develop infarction due to emboli, abscess due to direct seeding by an embolus, or immune complex glomerulonephritis.

Splenic manifestations: Splenic infarct is frequently found in patients with IE. Splenic abscess presents with pain, fever, and leukocytosis. Splenomegaly is found in 10–20% of patients.

Skin manifestations: Skin findings include petechiae, Osler's nodes, and Janeway lesions. Petechiae occur most commonly on conjunctiva, oral mucosa, and extremities. Osler's node is immunologically induced. There is immune complex deposition and focal vasculitis. The Osler's nodes are painful, erythematous, and nodular lesions usually located in the pads of finger and toes. Janeway lesions are caused by septic emboli and have bacteria, neutrophils, necrosis, and subcutaneous hemorrhage. They are painless hemorrhagic macules with predilection for soles or palms and are sequel of peripheral septic embolization.

Ocular manifestations: The Roth spots are an immunological phenomenon and they appear on funduscopic examination as retinal hemorrhage with pale center. Microscopically they consist of fibrin platelet plugs or lymphocytes surrounded by edema and hemorrhage in nerve fiber layer of retina. Both Osler and Roth spots can also be observed in other conditions such as systemic lupus erythematosus (SLE), leukemia, and nonbacterial thrombotic endocarditis (NBTE).

The clinical signs and symptoms found in Indian patients are summarized in **Table 2**.

TABLE 2 Clinical manifestations of infective endocarditis (Indian studies).

Manifestation	Incidence
Fever	80–90%
Chills	70–75%
Dyspnea	60–70%
Weight loss	40%
Arthralgia	5–25%
Splenomegaly	5–40%
Clubbing	10–20
Arterial emboli	20–50
Cardiac murmurs	70–80%
New/worsened murmur	20–30%
Petechiae#	5%
Other peripheral manifestations*	10–15%

In Western studies, incidence is 10–40%. Low incidence in Indians is possibly due to dark complexion

* Osler notes, Janeway lesions, Roth spots, and subconjunctival/subungual hemorrhage

DIAGNOSIS

Diagnosis requires high index of suspicion. In patients with fever/septicemia, the presence of predisposing cardiac disease, new or changing murmurs, unexplained embolic phenomenon, and evolving HF or certain hemodynamic abnormalities should dictate for the evaluation of IE. Initial investigations are hematological. Blood cultures and echocardiography are integral part of evaluation. The diagnosis is made based on these three groups of investigations (sometimes newer diagnostic imaging modalities are also used) and then by applying the Duke criteria.

Hematological investigations: Complete blood count (CBC) is often abnormal in IE. Normocytic normochromic anemia often with low serum iron and total iron-binding capacity (TIBC) is detected. Leukopenia may occur in subacute IE and is usually associated with splenomegaly. Thrombocytopenia occurs in 10% of cases and is found to be a predictor of early adverse outcome. Erythrocyte sedimentation rate (ESR) is usually elevated. C reactive protein (CRP) is elevated in 60% of cases. Procalcitonin (PCT) is high but usually is not recommended as a routine biomarker.

Blood cultures: A minimum of three sets of blood cultures should be taken from separate venipuncture sites before starting antibiotic therapy. First and last blood culture should be taken at least 1 hour apart. Ideally, antibiotics should be started after blood culture reports in clinically stable patients. However, in routine clinical practice, antibiotics are started immediately after sampling, especially in sicker unstable patients.

Echocardiography allows assessment of vegetation (site, size, and number), periannular tissue destruction/abscess formation, leaflet perforation, aneurysm or fistula formation, or prosthetic valve dehiscence. The sensitivity of transesophageal echocardiogram (TEE) is much higher (85–95%) as compared to TTE (60–65%). TTE cannot detect smaller vegetations (<2 mm in diameter) and often is not helpful in mechanical PVE. TEE is also more useful in assessing complications (**Fig. 1**).

Newer diagnostic imaging modalities are needed when diagnosis is not made by routine methods. The 2015 European Society of Cardiology (ESC) guidelines have emphasized the role of additional diagnostic imaging modalities [cardiac computed tomography (CT), cardiac magnetic resonance imaging (MRI), and positron emission tomography-CT (PET-CT), or leukocyte labeled single photon emission CT], especially in PVE in patients with high level of clinical suspicion (**Box 1**). They are useful in certain scenarios such as abscess formation, paravalvular extension, extracardiac complications of IE, and when diagnosis is not confirmed by routine evaluation.

Modified Duke criteria are the current gold standard (**Box 1**). They stratify patients into three categories: Definite, possible, and rejected, on the basis of major or minor criteria.

By this diagnostic classification, a definite clinical diagnosis of IE is established in the presence of (1) two

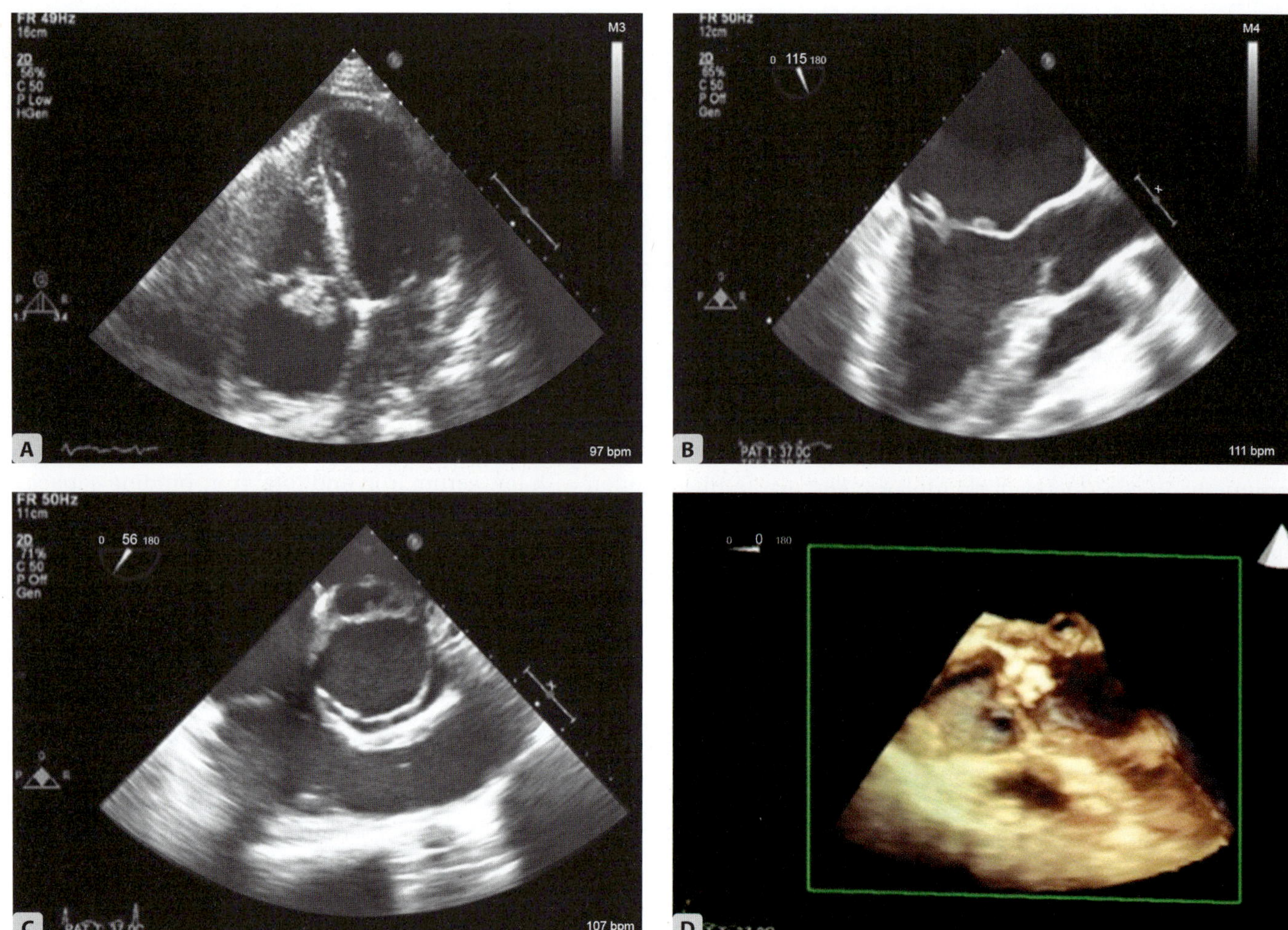

FIGURES 1 A to D: (A) Apical four chamber view showing large vegetation on anterior tricuspid leaflet; **(B)** Transesophageal echocardiogram (TEE) four chamber view showing vegetations on anterior mitral leaflet; **(C)** TEE short axis view showing bicuspid aortic valve with overlying abscess; **(D)** Three-dimensional (3D) TEE showing vegetation in a patient with bicuspid aortic valve endocarditis.

major criteria or (2) one major and three minor criteria, or (3) five minor criteria.

A possible clinical diagnosis of IE is appropriate in the presence of (1) one major and one minor criterion or (2) three minor criteria.

The diagnosis of IE is rejected if clinical evaluation (1) does not meet criteria for possible IE or (2) reveals complete resolution of suspected IE syndrome spontaneously or with antibiotic therapy of 4 days or less, or if (3) an alternative diagnosis explaining the initial presentation is confirmed.

PREVENTION

The substantial morbidity and mortality of IE has inspired efforts for prevention of IE. This leads to use of antibiotics in patients with wide range of cardiac conditions while they would undergo surgical procedures. Historically prevention efforts were focused on oral health because viridians streptococci are normal flora of oral cavity which is responsible for 20% cases of IE. However, such practice was not supported by scientific studies and advances in pathophysiological concepts. Low grade bacteremia is common during daily activities such as tooth brushing, flossing, or chewing. It is thought that IE may be the result of repeated and cumulative bacteremia rather than sporadic bacteremia related to dental or surgical procedures. Moreover, widespread irrational use of antibiotics is associated with risks of anaphylaxis and emergence of antibiotic resistance.

Hence, unlike the earlier practice of using antibiotic prophylaxis widely for various procedures its use is now restricted only to high-risk dental procedures in patients with very specific conditions. IE prophylaxis is not recommended outside these settings such as respiratory tract procedures, gastrointestinal or genitourinary procedures such as vaginal or caesarean delivery as well as all types of skin or musculoskeletal-related procedures. **Box 2** shows the indications of IE prophylaxis according to 2020 American College of Cardiology/American Heart Association (ACC/AHA) guidelines for the management of valvular heart disease.

MANAGEMENT

The duration and choice of antibiotic therapy should target to eradicate infection, as inadequate treatment can

BOX 1 Modified Duke criteria for the diagnosis of infective endocarditis.

Major criteria

Blood cultures positive for IE

- Typical microorganisms consistent with IE from two separate blood cultures:
    - Viridians streptococci, *Streptococcus gallolyticus (Streptococcus bovis)*, HACEK group, *Staphylococcus aureus*; or
    - Community-acquired enterococci, in the absence of a primary focus; or
- Microorganisms consistent with IE from persistently positive blood cultures:
    - More than or equal to two positive blood cultures of blood samples drawn >12 h apart; or
    - All of three or a majority of more than or equal to four separate cultures of blood (with and last samples drawn ≥1 h apart); or
- Single positive blood culture for *Coxiella burnetii* or phase I IgG antibody titer >1:800

Imaging positive for IE

- Echocardiogram positive for IE:
    - Vegetation
    - Abscess, pseudoaneurysm, and intracardiac
    - Valvular perforation or aneurysm
    - New partial dehiscence of prosthetic valve
    - Abnormal activity around the site of prosthetic valve implantation detected by ^{18}F-FDG PET/CT (only if the prosthesis was implanted for >3 months) or radiolabeled leukocytes SPECT/CT*
    - Definite paravalvular lesions by cardiac CT*

Minor criteria

- Predisposition such as predisposing heart condition, or injection drug use
- Fever as temperature >38°C
- Vascular phenomena (including those detected by imaging only): Major arterial emboli, septic pulmonary infarcts, infectious (mycotic) aneurysm, intracranial hemorrhage, conjunctival hemorrhages, and Janeway lesions
- Immunological phenomena: Glomerulonephritis, Osler's nodes, Roth's spots, and rheumatoid factor
- Microbiological evidence: Positive blood culture but does not meet a major criterion as noted above or serological evidence of active infection with organism consistent with IE

*Addition of these criteria was recommended by ESC guidelines (2015).

BOX 2 Recommendations of IE prophylaxis (2020 ACC guidelines).

- Antibiotic **prophylaxis is reasonable before dental procedures** that involve manipulation of gingival tissue, manipulation of the periapical region of teeth, or perforation of the oral mucosa in patients who have any of the following:
    - Prosthetic cardiac valves including transcatheter-implanted prostheses and homografts
    - Prosthetic material used for cardiac valve repair, such as annuloplasty rings, chords, or clips
    - Previous IE
    - Unrepaired cyanotic congenital heart disease or repaired congenital heart disease, with residual shunts or valvular regurgitation at the site of or adjacent to the site of a prosthetic patch or prosthetic device
    - Cardiac transplant with valve regurgitation attributable to a structurally abnormal valve
- Patients who are at high risk of IE, antibiotic prophylaxis is **not recommended for nondental procedures** (e.g., transesophageal echocardiography, esophagogastroduodenoscopy, colonoscopy, or cystoscopy) in the absence of active infection.

(ACC: American College of Cardiology; IE: infective endocarditis)

BOX 3A Treatment regimens for native valve endocarditis due to *Staphylococcus*.

- **Methicillin-susceptible strains**
    - AHA 2015
        - Nafcillin or oxacillin 12 g per 24 h, IV in four to six divided doses, for 6 weeks **Or**
        - Cefazolin 6 g per 24 h, IV in three divided doses, for 6 weeks
    - ESC 2015
        - Oxacillin or cloxacillin 12 g per 24 h, IV in four to six divided doses, for 4–6 weeks **Or**
        - Cefazolin 6 g per 24 h, IV in three divided doses, for 6 weeks **Or**
        - Cefotaxime 6 g per 24 h, in three divided doses
- **Methicillin-resistant strains**
    - AHA 2015
        - Vancomycin 30 mg/kg per 24 h, IV in two divided doses, for 6 weeks **Or**
        - Daptomycin 8 mg/kg per 24 h, IV once daily, for 6 weeks
    - ESC 2015
        - Vancomycin 30–60 mg/kg per 24 h, IV in two to three divided doses, for 4–6 weeks **Or**
        - Daptomycin 10 mg/kg per 24 h, IV once daily, for 4–6 weeks

result in relapse. Challenges are multifold, especially culture negative cases, antibiotic resistance, high bacterial density in vegetation with incomplete antibiotic penetration, especially in biofilms associated with prosthetic material and low microorganism metabolic activity which makes them less susceptible to antibiotics. As a result, extended course parenteral therapy is required. The therapy must be both bactericidal and prolonged. **Boxes 3** to **7** summarize ACC and ESC recommendations in various situations regarding the choice of antibiotics.

BOX 3B **Treatment regimens for prosthetic valve endocarditis due to *Staphylococcus*.**

Methicillin-susceptible strains

- AHA 2015
  - Nafcillin or oxacillin 12 g per 24 h, IV in six divided doses, for ≥6 weeks

  Plus
  - Rifampicin 900 mg per 24 h, IV or orally in three equally divided doses, ≥6 weeks

  Plus
  - Gentamycin 3 mg/kg per 24 h, IV or IM in two to three equally divided doses, for 2 weeks

Methicillin allergic patients or methicillin-resistant strain

- AHA 2015
  - Vancomycin 30 mg/kg per 24 h in two divided doses, for 6 weeks

  Plus
  - Rifampicin 900 mg/24 h, IV or orally in three divided doses, for ≥6 weeks

  Plus
  - Gentamycin 3 mg/kg/day, IV or IM in two to three doses, for 2 weeks
  - ESC 2015
  - Vancomycin 30–60 mg/kg/day, IV in two to three doses, for ≥6 weeks

  Plus
  - Rifampicin 900–1,200 mg, IV or orally in two to three divided doses

  Plus
  - Gentamycin 3 mg/kg/day, IV in one to two doses, for 2 weeks

(AHA 2015: American heart association 2015 guidelines; ESC 2015: European Society of Cardiology 2015 guidelines)

BOX 4 **Treatment regimens for endocarditis due to penicillin susceptible streptococci viridians and *Streptococcus gallolyticus (bovis)*.**

American Heart Association (AHA) 2015 (MIC ≤0.12 µg/mL)

- 4 weeks regimens
  - Aqueous penicillin G 12–18 million units per 24 h, IV either continuously or in four to six divided doses or (if penicillin is unavailable)
  - Ampicillin 2 g, IV every 4 h **Or**
  - Ceftriaxone 2 g per 24 h, IV or IM in one dose
  - For beta-lactam intolerant patients: Vancomycin 30 mg/kg per 24 h, IV in two divided doses
- 2 weeks regimens
  - Aqueous penicillin G 12–18 million units per 24 h, IV either continuously or in four to six divided doses **Or**
  - Ceftriaxone 2 g per 24 h IV or IM in one dose

  Plus
  - Gentamycin 3 mg/kg per 24 h, IV or IM in three divided doses

Continued...

Continued...

European Society of Cardiology (ESC) 2015 (MIC ≤0.125 µg/mL)

- 4 weeks regimens
  - Aqueous penicillin G 12–18 million units per 24 h, IV either continuously or in four to six divided doses **Or**
  - Amoxicillin 100–200 mg/kg per 24 h, IV in four to six divided doses **Or**
  - Ampicillin 12 g per 24 h, (or 100–200 mg/kg per 24 h) IV in six divided doses **Or**
  - Ceftriaxone 2 g per 24 h, IV or IM in one dose **Or**
  - Vancomycin 30 mg/kg per 24 h, IV in two divided doses
- 2 weeks regimens
  - Aqueous penicillin G 12–18 million units per 24 h, IV either continuously or in four to six divided doses **Or**
  - Amoxicillin 100–200 mg/kg per 24 h, IV in four to six divided doses **Or**
  - Ampicillin 12 g per 24 h, (or 100–200 mg/kg per 24 h) IV in six divided doses **Or**
  - Ceftriaxone 2 g per 24 h, IV or IM in one dose

  Plus
  - Gentamycin 3 mg/kg per 24 h, IV or IM in three divided doses

(MIC: minimum inhibitory concentration)

BOX 5 **Treatment regimens for strains of streptococci viridians and *Streptococcus gallolyticus (bovis)* relatively resistant to penicillin G.**

American Heart Association (AHA) 2015 (MIC >0.12 and <0.5 µg/mL)

Combination therapy:

Aqueous penicillin G 24 million units per 24 h IV either continuously or in four to six divided doses for 4 weeks **Or**

Ampicillin 2 g IV every 4 h for 4 weeks

Plus

Gentamycin 3 mg/kg per 24 h IV or IM in one dose for first 2 weeks

Monotherapy:

Vancomycin 30 mg/kg per 24 h IV in two divided doses for 4 weeks **Or**

Ceftriaxone 2 g per 24 h IV or IM in one dose for 4 weeks

European Society of Cardiology (ESC) 2015 (MIC >0.125 and <2 µg/mL)

Combination:

Aqueous penicillin G 24 million units per 24 h, IV either in four to six divided doses or continuous infusion, for 4 weeks **Or**

Amoxicillin 200 mg/kg per 24 h, IV in four to six divided doses, for 4 weeks **Or**

Ampicillin 12 g per 24 h (200 mg/kg per 24 h) in six divided doses, for 4 weeks **Or**

Ceftriaxone 2 g per 24 h, IV or IM in one dose, for 4 weeks

Plus

Gentamycin 3 mg/kg per 24 h, IV or IM in one dose, for first 2 weeks **Or**

Vancomycin 30 mg/kg per 24 h, IV in two divided doses, for 4 weeks

(MIC: minimum inhibitory concentration)

BOX 6	Treatment regimens for native or prosthetic valve endocarditis due to enterococcal strains.[A,B,C]
American Heart Association (AHA) 2015	
• Aqueous penicillin G 18 to 30 million units per 24 h, IV either continuously or in six divided doses, for 4–6 weeks **Or**	
• Ampicillin 2 g, IV every 4 h, for 4–6 weeks	
Plus	
• Gentamycin 3 mg/kg per 24 h, IV or IM in three divided doses, for 4–6 weeks	
• Ceftriaxone 2 g, IV every 12 h, for 6 weeks	
Plus	
• Ampicillin 2 g, IV every 4 h, for 6 weeks	
• Vancomycin 30 mg/kg per 24 h, IV in two divided doses, for 6 weeks	
Plus	
• Gentamycin 3 mg/kg per 24 h, IV or IM in three divided, doses for 4 weeks	
European Society of Cardiology (ESC) 2015	
• Amoxicillin 200 mg/kg per 24 h, IV in four to six divided doses, for 4–6 weeks **Or**	
• Ampicillin 12 g per 24 h, (200 mg/kg per 24 h) IV in four to six divided doses, for 6 weeks	
Plus	
• Gentamycin 3 mg/kg per 24 h, IV or IM in one dose, for first 4 weeks	
• Ceftriaxone 2 g, IV every 12 h, for 6 weeks	
Plus	
• Ampicillin 12 g per 24 h (200 mg/kg per 24 h), IV in four to six divided doses, for 6 weeks	
• Vancomycin 30 mg/kg per 24 h, IV in two divided doses, for 6 weeks	
Plus	
• Gentamycin 3 mg/kg per 24 h, IV or IM in one doses, for 4–6 weeks	

[A] High-level resistance to gentamicin (MIC 500 mg/L): If susceptible to streptomycin, replace gentamicin with streptomycin 15 mg/kg/day in two equally divided doses.

[B] Beta-lactam resistance: (1) If due to beta-lactamase production, replace ampicillin with ampicillin-sulbactam or amoxicillin with amoxicillin-clavulanate; (2) if due to PBP5 alteration, use vancomycin-based regimens.

[C] Multiresistance to aminoglycosides, beta-lactams, and vancomycin: Suggested alternatives are (i) daptomycin 10 mg/kg/day plus ampicillin 200 mg/kg/day IV in four to six doses; (ii) linezolid 2 × 600 mg/day IV or orally for ≥8 weeks (monitor hematological toxicity).

(MIC: minimum inhibitory concentration; PBP5: penicillin-binding protein 5)

DURATION OF THERAPY

Due to low penetrance of antibiotics into the vegetations, extended course of antibiotics is required. When bactericidal activity is rapid, shorter courses may be feasible. For example, a combination of penicillin or ceftriaxone with aminoglycoside is synergistic for viridians group streptococci. Uncomplicated right-sided endocarditis may require shorter course therapy as vegetations have lower bactericidal densities. Duration of therapy is calculated from first day of start of antibiotics. In native valve endocarditis (NVE), duration of treatment is usually 2–6 weeks, whereas for PVE duration of treatment is 6 weeks. The antibiotics are usually the same except for staphylococcal PVE, for which addition of rifampicin is recommended. In case of intracardiac device IE, or lead endocarditis, complete device removal is required.

In some patients we need to do cardiac surgery after a short course of antibiotics. The current recommendation of surgery is based on the results of observational studies and largely expert opinion. Surgery is indicated when patients develop HF or have features of uncontrolled infection despite optimal medical therapy. The indications for surgery in IE are given in **Table 3**.

BOX 7	Suggested regimens for therapy of native or prosthetic valve endocarditis due to HACEK microorganism.
AHA 2015	
• Ceftriaxone 2 g per 24 h, IV in one dose, for 4 weeks **Or**	
• Ampicillin 2 g, IV every 4 h, for 4 weeks **Or**	
• Ciprofloxacin 1,000 mg per 24 h, orally in two divided doses or 800 mg per 24 h, IV in two divided doses, for 4 weeks	
ESC 2015	
• Ceftriaxone 2 g per 24 h IV in one dose for 4 weeks **Or**	
• Combination therapy with: Ampicillin 12 g per 24 h, IV in six divided doses **Plus**	
• Gentamycin 3 mg/kg per 24 h, IV or IM in two or three divided doses, for 4–6 weeks **Or**	
• Ciprofloxacin 750 mg every 12 h orally or 400 mg every 8–12 h, IV for 4 weeks	

CONCLUSION

Infective endocarditis is a multisystem disease which is associated with significant morbidity and mortality. Despite improvement in diagnostic and microbiological techniques there are significant challenges. Routine hematological investigations especially ESR are helpful. Three to four blood cultures spaced over 1–2 hours drawn with aseptic techniques, transthoracic and where required transesophageal echocardiography help to establish the diagnosis.

Patients with IE need accurate clinical evaluation, high index of suspicion to establish early diagnosis. We need to identify the etiological agents and start early treatment with appropriate antimicrobial therapy. Surgery may be required in some patients with complications.

TABLE 3 Indications and timing of surgery in IE.

Indications for surgery	Timing
Heart failure	
Aortic or mitral NVE or PVE with severe acute regurgitation, obstruction or fistula causing refractory pulmonary edema or cardiogenic shock	Emergency
Aortic or mitral NVE or PVE with severe regurgitation or obstruction causing symptoms of HF or echocardiographic signs of poor hemodynamic tolerance	Urgent
Uncontrolled infection	
Locally uncontrolled infection (abscess, false aneurysm, fistula, and enlarging vegetation)	Urgent
Infection caused by fungi or multiresistant organisms	Urgent/ elective
Persisting positive blood cultures despite appropriate antibiotic therapy and adequate control of septic metastatic foci	Urgent
PVE caused by staphylococci or non-HACEK gram-negative bacteria	Urgent/ elective
Prevention of embolism	
Aortic or mitral NVE or PVE with persistent vegetations >10 mm after one or more embolic episode despite appropriate antibiotic therapy	Urgent
Aortic or mitral NVE with vegetations >10 mm, associated with severe valve stenosis or regurgitation, and low operative risk	Urgent
Aortic or mitral NVE or PVE with isolated very large vegetations (>30 mm)	Urgent
Aortic or mitral NVE or PVE with isolated large vegetations (>15 mm) and no other indication for surgery	Urgent

(NVE: native valve endocarditis; PVE: prosthetic valve endocarditis)

RECOMMENDED READINGS

1. Baddour LM, Wilson WR, Bayer AS, Fowler VG Jr, Tleyjeh IM, Rybak MJ, et al. Infective Endocarditis in Adults: Diagnosis, Antimicrobial Therapy, and Management of Complications: A Scientific Statement for Healthcare Professionals From the American Heart Association. Circulation. 2015;132:1435-86.
2. Habib G, Lancellotti P, Antunes MJ, Bongiorni MG, Casalta JP, Del Zotti F, et al. 2015 ESC Guidelines for the management of infective endocarditis: The Task Force for the Management of Infective Endocarditis of the European Society of Cardiology (ESC)Endorsed by: European Association for Cardio-Thoracic Surgery (EACTS), the European Association of Nuclear Medicine (EANM). Eur Heart J. 2015;36(44):3075-128.
3. Otto CM, Nishimura RA, Bonow RO, Carabello BA, Erwin JP 3rd, Gentile F, et al. 2020 ACC/AHA Guideline for the Management of Patients With Valvular Heart Disease: Executive Summary: A Report of the American College of Cardiology/American Heart Association Joint Committee on Clinical Practice Guidelines. Circulation. 2021;143(5):e35-71.
4. Gupta A, Gupta A, Kaul U, Varma A. Infective endocarditis in an Indian setup: Are we entering the 'modern' era? Indian J Crit Care Med. 2013;17(3):140-7.
5. Garg N, Kandpal B, Garg N, Tewari S, Kapoor A, Goel P, et al. Characteristics of infective endocarditis in a developing country: Clinical profile and outcome in 192 Indian patients, 1992-2001. Int J Cardiol. 2005;98:253-60.
6. Goyal A, Mohan B, Kumar P, Gupta D, Tandon R, Singla S, et al. Clinical characteristics and outcome of infective endocarditis among intravenous drug abusers in India. Indian Heart J. 2020;72(6):547-51.
7. Senthilkumar S, Menon T, Subramanian G. Epidemiology of infective endocarditis in Chennai, South India. Indian J Med Sci. 2010;64(4):187-91.
8. Subbaraju P, Rai S, Morakhia J, Midha G, Kamath A, Saravu K. Clinical-microbiological characterization and risk factors of mortality in infective endocarditis from a tertiary care academic hospital in Southern India. Indian Heart J. 2018;70(2):259-65.
9. Duval X, Delahaye F, Alla F, Tattevin P, Obadia JF, Le Moing V, et al. Temporal trends in infective endocarditis in the context of prophylaxis guideline modifications: three successive population-based surveys. J Am Coll Cardiol. 2012;59:1968-76.
10. Fournier PE, Thuny F, Richet H, Lepidi H, Casalta JP, Arzouni JP, et al. Comprehensive diagnostic strategy for blood culture-negative endocarditis: a prospective study of 819 new cases. Clin Infect Dis. 2010;51:131-40.
11. Murdoch DR, Corey GR, Hoen B, Miró JM, Fowler VG Jr, Bayer AS, et al. Clinical presentation, etiology, and outcome of infective endocarditis in the 21st century: the International Collaboration on Endocarditis-Prospective Cohort Study. Arch Intern Med. 2009;169:463-73.

CHAPTER
101

Pregnancy and Heart

Shibba Takkar Chhabra, Gurleen Kaur, Jyotsna Maddury

ABSTRACT

Pregnancy is a physiological state which is associated with hemodynamic alterations and stress especially in women with preexisting cardiac ailments. The present era witnesses elderly women, women with congenital heart disease, and those on infertility treatments getting pregnant with assisted reproductive techniques. Preconceptional counseling, an important component of cardio-obstetrics, should be considered by the physician. Hypertension in pregnancy, the most common cardiac ailment, could be pregnancy-induced or chronic hypertension per se. Prompt diagnosis and management are needed to prevent preeclampsia and eclampsia which cause significant morbidity and mortality.

Peripartum cardiomyopathy (PPCM) needs prompt recognition. It is encountered during last months of pregnancy and the early postpartum period. Valvular heart disease in pregnancy with decompensating lesions such as mitral stenosis and aortic stenosis and better tolerated regurgitant lesions need recognition and appropriate management. In congenital heart disease, usually atrial septal defect (ASD), smaller ventricular septal defect (VSD), and patent ductus arteriosus (PDA) are well tolerated in pregnancy. However, patients with severe pulmonary arterial hypertension (PAH) have significant mortality and morbidity and are a contraindication to pregnancy.

Besides intensive management of their underlying disease, a definitive plan regarding mode and timing of delivery is also imperative to prevent any decompensation especially in the second stage of labor. A multidisciplinary approach, close monitoring, and regular follow-ups are advocated in antepartum, peripartum, and postpartum period in pregnant cardiac patients so as to have favorable outcomes.

"There is no imprint too small to leave an imprint on this world"

—Anonymous

INTRODUCTION

Pregnancy is a physiological state associated with hemodynamic alterations and stress especially in women with preexisting cardiac ailments. The increasing number of women with congenital and valvular heart disease getting pregnant, the increasing maternal age with comorbidities (diabetes, hypertension, obesity etc.), infertility treatment, and assisted reproductive techniques make it imperative for a physician to be sensitive to cardiovascular issues during pregnancy. Maternal complications such as hypertensive disorders of pregnancy, gestational diabetes, materno-placental syndromes etc., can be a harbinger of future cardiovascular diseases. Cardiac causes of death are a significant proportion of maternal death world over and need to be recognized and prevented.

HEMODYNAMIC ALTERATIONS

Significant hemodynamic alterations occur during pregnancy, labor, and the postpartum period (**Table 1**). These initiate in the 5th to 8th week of gestation and reach a peak in late second trimester. The rise in plasma volume by 40–50% in the course of normal pregnancy surpasses the rise in red blood cell mass, hereby leading to decreased hemoglobin concentration also known as anemia of pregnancy. Likewise, cardiac output also increases 30–50% above baseline, peaking in late second trimester, and then plateaus till delivery. The factors responsible for the rise in cardiac output include increased preload because of a higher blood volume, reduced afterload because of a decline in systemic vascular resistance (SVR), and an elevation in the maternal heart rate by 10–15 beats/min. There is a rise in stroke volume in the first and second trimester which falls in the third trimester as inferior vena cava is compressed by the uterus.

Heart rate is the significant contributor to increased cardiac output in third trimester. Moreover, there is a decline blood pressure by around 10 mm Hg, which begins in first and peaks in the late second trimester. This is due to increase in uterine blood flow due to placental growth with subsequent fall in peripheral resistance.

At the time of labor and delivery, there are significant alterations in hemodynamics. Each uterine contraction pushes 500 mL of blood in circulatory system leading to an increase in cardiac output of 50% and an increase in blood pressure. In contrast to normal vaginal delivery where blood loss is around 500 mL, a cesarean section poses more hemodynamic stress to mother with blood loss of around 1,000 mL. A sudden increase in venous return follows the delivery owing to autotransfusion from uterus which continues for 24–72 hours. A release of compression over the

TABLE 1 Hemodynamic alterations during pregnancy.

Hemodynamic parameter	Increase	Hemodynamic parameter	Decrease
Blood volume	30–40%	RBC volume	18–30%
Cardiac output	40%	Hemoglobin	10–15%
Stroke volume	25%	Systemic vascular resistance	20%
Heart rate	15%	Blood pressure	5–10%
Pulmonary capillary wedge pressure	Slightly	Pulmonary vascular resistance	30%
Red cell mass	25%	Activity of protein C	–
Size of heart	30% (dilatation)	Protein S	–
Progesterone and estrogen	+	BP (during delivery)	–

inferior vena cava by the baby also contributes to increased venous return. These changes at the time of delivery in a susceptible patient can lead to pulmonary edema.

PRECONCEPTION COUNSELING

Preconception counseling by physician is desirable for women with heart disease. A baseline clinical examination, 12-lead electrocardiogram (ECG), and a transthoracic echocardiogram can be done for assessment of cardiac lesions. An exercise test is helpful in some of them. Family history of both the partners and genetic counseling may be required in some inherited single gene disorders.

Maternal and fetal risks need to be discussed with the mother. The need for regular follow-up during the pregnancy and combined obstetric and cardiovascular care should be explained. A modified WHO classification of maternal cardiovascular risk principles and application are shown in **Figures 1** and **2**.

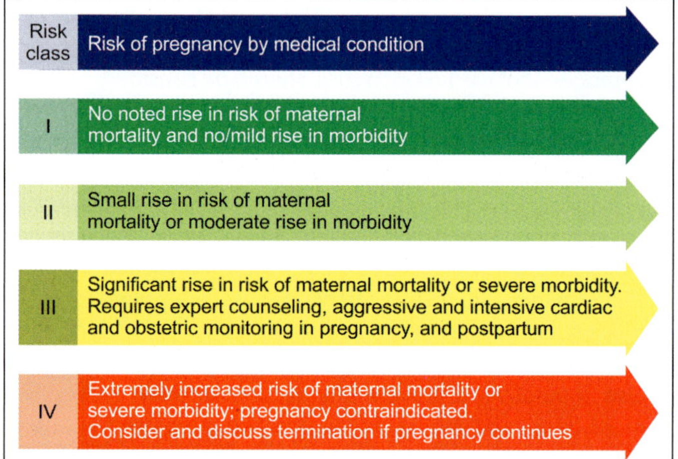

FIGURE 1: Risk class of maternal mortality and morbidity (Modified World Health Organization classification).

CARDIOVASCULAR EXAMINATION

The findings of cardiac examination in a pregnant female are consistent with an altered hemodynamics of a high output state. The patient usually has tachycardia with a bounding pulse volume. Peripheral edema is common as pregnancy advances. Jugular venous pressure (JVP) might be mildly elevated by the mid of second trimester with a brisk descent. This is usually consistent with the volume overload situation and decreased peripheral resistance. The apical impulse is prominent and the first and second heart sounds are loud. S3 is common and an ejection systolic murmur which is usually <3/6 intensity is common at the left parasternal area. Moreover, continuous murmurs like cervical venous hum or a mammary souffle are common, secondary to hyperdynamic circulation of pregnancy. The venous hum is usually best heard over the right supraclavicular fossa.

INVESTIGATIONS

Despite hyperdynamic state, women with normal pregnancy have a normal B-type natriuretic peptide (BNP level) which has a good negative predictive value for predicting any adverse cardiac outcome. *A chest radiograph* though usually not obtained with the concern of radiation exposure to fetus, whenever done might reveal a slightly prominent pulmonary artery with an elevated diaphragm leading to an increased cardiothoracic ratio. *A transthoracic echocardiogram* might reflect the features of a hyperkinetic state with raised left ventricular end-diastolic measurements, increased right ventricular size, and volumes of both the atria. Ejection fraction needs to be measured carefully especially when the preload gets reduced in supine position with a compressed inferior vena cava by the fetus. Valve area calculations are more relevant than measurement of valve gradient.

Serial echocardiography might be warranted in women with prosthetic mechanical valves who are prone to developing prosthetic valve thrombosis, women with aortic root dilatation, and in those with left ventricular dysfunction. Fetal echocardiogram might be done at 18–22 weeks gestation, in case the mother suffers from congenital heart disease so as to rule out any congenital cardiac anomaly.

MRI, whenever needed, can be done without gadolinium due to associated neonatal risks. MRI is indicated for baseline aortic imaging especially in women with high-risk aortopathies and to identify ectasia in Marfan syndrome. CT is best avoided because of significant radiation exposure to the fetus.

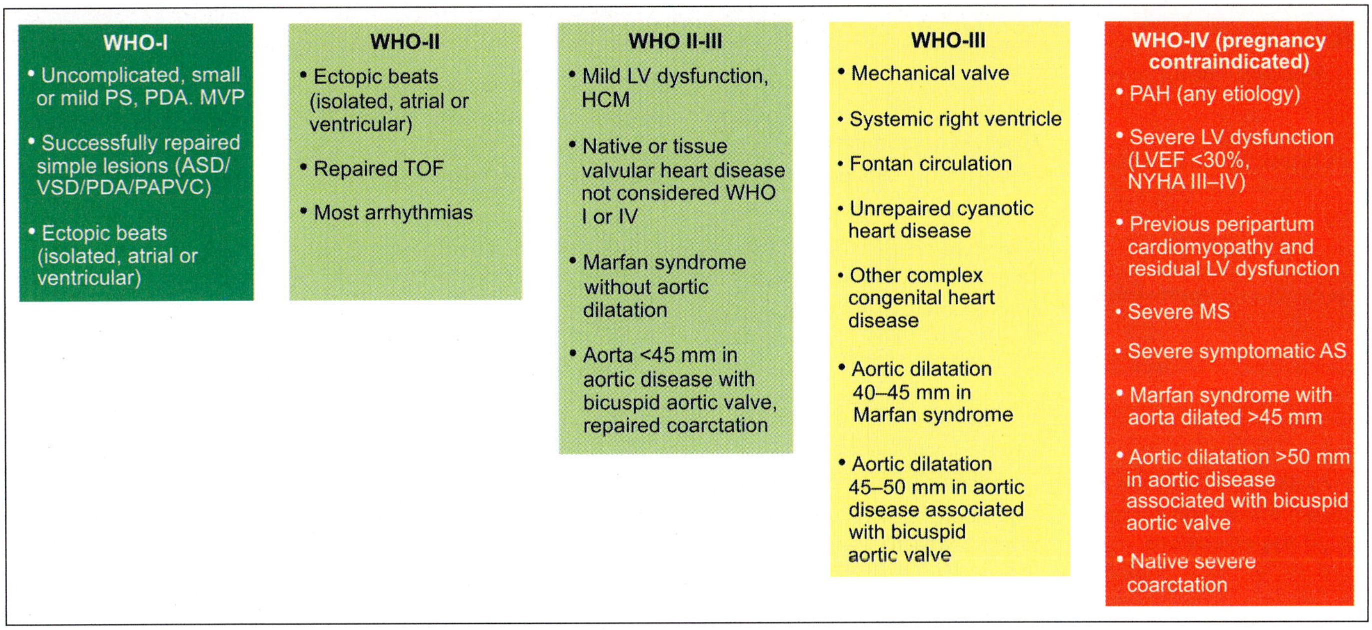

WHO-I	WHO-II	WHO II-III	WHO-III	WHO-IV (pregnancy contraindicated)
• Uncomplicated, small or mild PS, PDA. MVP • Successfully repaired simple lesions (ASD/VSD/PDA/PAPVC) • Ectopic beats (isolated, atrial or ventricular)	• Ectopic beats (isolated, atrial or ventricular) • Repaired TOF • Most arrhythmias	• Mild LV dysfunction, HCM • Native or tissue valvular heart disease not considered WHO I or IV • Marfan syndrome without aortic dilatation • Aorta <45 mm in aortic disease with bicuspid aortic valve, repaired coarctation	• Mechanical valve • Systemic right ventricle • Fontan circulation • Unrepaired cyanotic heart disease • Other complex congenital heart disease • Aortic dilatation 40–45 mm in Marfan syndrome • Aortic dilatation 45–50 mm in aortic disease associated with bicuspid aortic valve	• PAH (any etiology) • Severe LV dysfunction (LVEF <30%, NYHA III–IV) • Previous peripartum cardiomyopathy and residual LV dysfunction • Severe MS • Severe symptomatic AS • Marfan syndrome with aorta dilated >45 mm • Aortic dilatation >50 mm in aortic disease associated with bicuspid aortic valve • Native severe coarctation

(PAPVC: partial anomalous pulmonary venous connection)

FIGURE 2: Cardiac conditions in respective modified World Health Organization risk class.

Cardiac catheterization should be reserved for emergency situations. Whenever performed, the radiation exposure should be minimized by apt lead screening of the pregnant lady's abdomen and pelvis.

MANAGEMENT

Whenever indicated, the mother should not be deprived of the benefit of cardiovascular *medical drug therapy*. However, adverse side effects to the fetus and neonate are of utmost concern. Use of drugs with the long safety record, at the minimum possible dose, for the least number of days should be advocated.

Performance of *balloon mitral valvuloplasty* (BMV) should be done in centers with adequate experience and surgical backup because in pregnancy it might be fraught with the risks of worsening regurgitation, arrhythmias, cardiac tamponade, mortality, precipitation of labor, or fetal death. Usually BMV can be performed after 26 weeks of pregnancy.

Cardiothoracic surgery is best avoided at any phase of pregnancy especially with concerns of fetal malformation or fetal loss during the first trimester and concerns of precipitating a premature labor when in the third trimester. Hence, whenever feasible delivery should be performed prior to the cardiothoracic surgery. To improve the fetal outcomes, it is recommended to operate between 20 weeks and 28 weeks of gestation.

At the time of labor and delivery a team approach is warranted keeping in mind the hemodynamic changes in a cardiac patient with pregnancy. Vaginal delivery is the most feasible and preferred mode of delivery given lower complications and is usually best performed in left lateral recumbent position to avoid reduction in the venous return by a compressed inferior vena cava. In high-risk cases, the second stage must be supported and assisted by forceps or vacuum extraction to avoid a prolonged labor. A cesarean delivery is considered mostly for obstetric indications or in cases of dilated ascending aorta >45 mm, in Marfanoid patients with aortic diameter between 40 mm and 45 mm, in patients with severe aortic stenosis, preterm labor while receiving oral anticoagulation, or patients with severe heart failure or Eisenmenger's syndrome.

SPECIFIC CARDIAC CONDITIONS

HYPERTENSION

Hypertension is the most common medical problem in pregnancy and is known to attribute a significant amount of maternal mortality and morbidity. **Table 2** shows the varied types of hypertension seen in pregnancy. About 25% of patients with gestational and chronic hypertension develop preeclampsia. The factors predisposing to pre-eclampsia are obesity with body mass index (BMI) >30 kg/m^2, nulliparous, elderly >40 years, preexisting comorbidities such as kidney disease, diabetes mellitus, systemic lupus erythematosus (SLE), antiphospholipid antibody syndrome, history of preeclampsia in previous pregnancies, multifetal pregnancy and pregnancies after assisted reproductive techniques.

The antihypertensive medications used for treatment of chronic hypertension continue to be effective during pregnancy. Low-dose aspirin started at 16 weeks of gestation in those at high risk of preeclampsia reduces the likelihood. It is to be continued throughout pregnancy. Oral antihypertensives labetalol, nifedipine, and methyldopa are used in treatment of hypertension in pregnancy in that order. Renin-angiotensin-aldosterone system (RAAS)

TABLE 2 Classification of hypertension in pregnancy.

Hypertension type	Definition and/or description
Chronic hypertension	• HTN [BP ≥140/90 mm Hg (systolic) or ≥90 mm Hg (diastolic)] prior to pregnancy or detected prior to 20 weeks of gestation • Family history of hypertension or overweight or obesity may be present • Exclude secondary hypertension
Gestational hypertension	• Hypertension [BP ≥140 mm Hg (systolic) or ≥90 mm Hg (diastolic)] noted after the 20th week of pregnancy in absence of preeclampsia • Progression to preeclampsia in 25% • Usually normalizing by 12 weeks of post delivery
Preeclampsia (de novo or superimposed on chronic hypertension)	• Develops after 20 weeks of pregnancy with one or more of the following features: ◦ Proteinuria ◦ Renal insufficiency ◦ Liver involvement (transaminitis, pain epigastric and/or right hypochondrium) • Neurologic involvement (eclampsia, altered mental status, blindness, stroke, hyperreflexia (clonus), severe headaches, and persistent visual scotoma) • Hematologic complications (thrombocytopenia, disseminated intravascular coagulation, and hemolysis) • Uteroplacental dysfunction • Fetal growth retardation
White-coat hypertension	• ABPM confirms normal BP, seen in one of four outpatients

(ABPM: ambulatory BP monitoring; HTN: hypertension)

inhibitors are contraindicated in pregnancy due to their association with renal dysplasia, pulmonary hypoplasia, and growth restriction in the fetus.

If the systolic blood pressure is >160 mm Hg and diastolic pressure >110 mm Hg, this demands urgent treatment. A patient should be hospitalized when preeclampsia develops. Intravenous drugs such as labetalol and hydralazine can be used in this situation. Magnesium sulfate can be used to prevent any pre-eclamptic or eclamptic seizures and for fetal neuroprotection especially when prematurity is present. In patients with pulmonary edema nitroglycerin infusion is used.

Vaginal delivery is the preferred mode of delivery in the absence of any obstetrical or medical contraindications. Delivery is recommended at 37 weeks in uncomplicated patients. However, in patients with eclampsia, preeclampsia with visual or hemostatic disorders or hypertension, elevated liver enzymes, and low platelets (HELLP) syndrome, delivery should be considered at the earliest possible. Postpartum, the antihypertensive drugs should be continued with the knowledge that most of these drugs are secreted in milk in varying amounts. Methyldopa is best avoided due to the risk of postpartum depression. In gestational hypertension, usually the blood pressure normalizes rapidly after delivery.

CARDIOMYOPATHIES IN PREGNANCY

DILATED CARDIOMYOPATHY

The usual causes in a young woman with dilated cardiomyopathy could be idiopathic, secondary to drugs, toxins, or infection; occasionally, it could be a genetic where the transmission to fetus could be a concern. Women with left ventricular ejection fraction <30% or those who are in the New York Heart Association (NYHA) class 3 or 4 are usually recommended not to conceive. Preconception echocardiogram and exercise stress test for assessment of aerobic capacity is usually recommended in women with cardiomyopathy. In a patient of dilated cardiomyopathy and pregnancy the usual concerns are the worsening of left ventricular systolic function, pulmonary edema, or development of arrhythmias. Beta-blockers should usually be continued in women with cardiomyopathy, though angiotensin-converting enzyme (ACE) inhibitors and angiotensin-receptor blockers are contraindicated. When needed, hydralazine might be used for afterload reduction in patients who are symptomatic.

PERIPARTUM CARDIOMYOPATHY

Peripartum cardiomyopathy (PPCM) is the most common cardiomyopathy in pregnancy and usually develops in the month before or after partum. Although it can occur any time in the last peripartum months and the initial postpartum months. Black race, elderly pregnancy, and multiparous mothers are the predisposing factors. The women could present with heart failure, cardiogenic shock, arrhythmias or cerebrovascular accidents secondary to thrombi in left ventricle. Controversy exists as to whether this cardiomyopathy develops during pregnancy or it is unmasking of the preexisting cardiomyopathy.

It is believed that peripartum oxidative stress leads to cleavage of prolactin forming potent antiangiogenic, proapoptotic, and proinflammatory agents which lead to endothelial, cardiac vasculature, and myocyte dysfunction. This also forms the basis of the potential therapeutic strategy with bromocriptine which is a dopamine D2 receptor agonist. Prolactin, a thrombin scavenger when eliminated by bromocriptine might be associated by risk of thromboembolism hereby leading to an advice of concomitant anticoagulation with bromocriptine when used in PPCM, use of bromocriptine in PPCM is currently being evaluated in randomized trials. As in other patients of dilated cardiomyopathy, ACE inhibitors and angiotensin-receptor blockers are not advocated in pregnancy. Beta-blockers, digoxin, diuretics, inotropes, hydralazine, and nitrate can be used in women with PPCM. Aldosterone antagonists are best avoided with antiandrogenic effects reported in the fetus. Since left ventricular thrombi are well known in patients with severe left ventricular (LV) dysfunction and ejection fraction (EF) <35% anticoagulation with heparin might be considered in these patients.

The normalization of ventricular function was reported in 72% of patients with PPCM in a study. However, LVEF <30% or a LV end-diastolic dimension >6 cm at the time of presentation is usually associated with less chances of recovered LV functions. The usual improvement in the systolic functions is seen in the first 6–12 months of postpartum. There is always a possibility of recurrence of PPCM in a future pregnancy all the more in women who have incomplete recovery of the LV systolic functions. Recurrence of PPCM is usually associated with significant amount of maternal morbidity and mortality. Hence, in women who continue and persist to have LV dysfunction postpregnancy it is usually advocated not to conceive because of 20% maternal mortality rate in subsequent pregnancies.

HYPERTROPHIC CARDIOMYOPATHY

A preconceptional counseling of patient's personal and clinical history, family history, ECG, a transthoracic echocardiogram and exercise testing is advisable. The autosomal dominant inheritance pattern with variable penetrance of hypertrophic cardiomyopathy should be discussed with the prospective parents and adequate genetic counseling and family screening is recommended. It is reported that most of the patients with hypertrophic cardiomyopathy tolerate pregnancy well. In pregnancy, there occurs a decrease in after load leading to exacerbation of the gradient across the LV outflow tract. However, due to an increased maternal plasma volume this is largely offset.

Beta-blockers should be continued during the pregnancy. Avoid any hypotension for instance with use of epidural anesthesia or spinal block in a patient with hypertrophic cardiomyopathy which is obstruction. The blood losses in these patients should be replaced at the earliest possible. A cesarean section is to be done only when indicated for an obstetric cause. When a normal delivery is being conducted it is advocated to avoid any Valsalva maneuver and the second stage of labor should be facilitated in women with obstructive variety of hypertrophic cardiomyopathy.

VALVULAR HEART DISEASE

AORTIC STENOSIS

Bicuspid aortic valve and rheumatic heart disease are the usual causes of aortic stenosis in women of child-bearing age. While mild and moderate aortic stenosis is usually well tolerated, if the pregnant woman has a normal exercise capacity and is asymptomatic. Severe aortic stenosis (valve area of >1 cm^2 and mean gradient of >40 mm Hg) can present with an increased incidence of heart failure, arrhythmias, and premature labor. A woman with severe aortic stenosis and normal functional capacity and blood pressure response to exercise is usually able to tolerate pregnancy. In the other women with severe aortic stenosis usually aortic valve replacement is required prior to pregnancy. Associated aortic dilatation might be present in some patients with severe aortic stenosis. Abrupt hemodynamic changes with a reduction in after load immediately postpartum as the baby is delivered pose problems in a case of severe aortic stenosis. Blood loss at the time of delivery can precipitate maternal collapse.

MITRAL STENOSIS

In patients with mitral stenosis the pregnancy-related increased plasma volume and tachycardia cause a shortened diastolic filling time. This results in an increased left atrial pressure. Hence, they can present with acute pulmonary edema and atrial arrhythmias during pregnancy. It is advocated to have a valve intervention prior to pregnancy in patients with severe mitral stenosis. Once pregnant beta-blockers can reduce the heart rate and prolong the diastolic filling interval. This can reduce the symptoms in a patient of severe mitral stenosis and pregnancy. Diuretics and anticoagulants can be used in patients presenting with acute pulmonary edema and atrial fibrillation. Bed rest can also be advocated to reduce the exertion-related heart rate and increased cardiac demands. Balloon mitral valvotomy might be considered in case the patient has refractory symptoms and a pliable valve with favorable anatomy and no associated mitral regurgitation. In the patients in whom BMV is not feasible, surgical valvotomy might be performed when the symptoms are refractory.

MITRAL AND AORTIC REGURGITATION

Mitral and aortic regurgitation are well tolerated in pregnancy. The regurgitation volume decreases in pregnancy due to the decreased peripheral vascular resistance secondary to prostaglandin release. However, this usually stands true for the women with preserved LVEF.

PROSTHETIC VALVES

The choice of prosthetic valve in women planning pregnancy is pertinent to the final outcomes. While the tissue valves are less thrombogenic, they tend to degenerate after an average of 10–15 years, requiring reoperation. Whereas the mechanical valves which have greater longevity require anticoagulation. Anticoagulant strategy has its own risks with high chances of fetal loss, placental hemorrhage, and prosthetic valve thrombosis especially in the thrombogenic milieu of pregnancy. The maternal risk of valve thrombosis depends upon the chosen anticoagulation

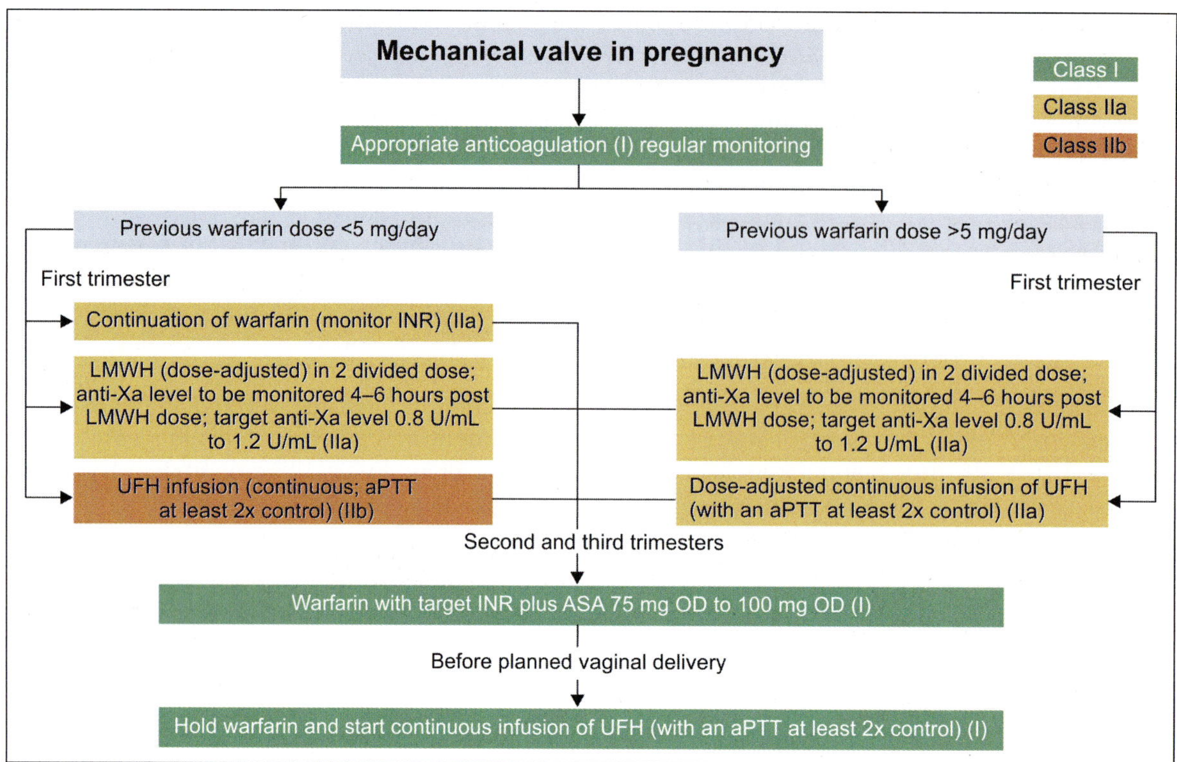

FLOWCHART 1: Anticoagulation regimen in prosthetic mechanical valve in pregnancy.

regimen, the maintenance of the anticoagulation control and the position of valve (mitral valve ≥ aortic valve).

Exposure to warfarin in the early gestation (6–9 weeks) can cause warfarin embryopathy with stippled epiphyses and nasal hypoplasia and central nervous system (CNS) abnormality. While the maternal risk is lowest with vitamin K antagonists, the fetal risk is lowest with heparin. The risk of embryopathy varies between 2% and 4% and can be reduced by initiation of heparin in the initial 6 weeks of gestation. The American College of Cardiology/American Heart Association (ACC/AHA) and the European Society of Endocrinology (ESE) guidelines for the advocated anticoagulation regimen for pregnant patients with mechanical valves are shown in **Flowchart 1**.

Unfractionated heparin is recommended since it can be started and stopped abruptly. Moreover, if epidural analgesia is planned the risk of spinal hematoma prevails with use of low molecular weight heparin.

CONGENITAL HEART DISEASE

Women with congenital heart disease even when post-operative might have residual lesion and sequelae which need adequate evaluations. The issue of inheritable disease and transmission of disease to the fetus is also there.

SHUNT LESION

Pregnancy in women with simple shunt lesions is well tolerated. Patients with secundum ASD are commonly seen. In the absence of coexisting pulmonary hypertension or atrial arrhythmias, pregnancy is usually well tolerated in these women even if uncorrected. The shunts in women with VSD and PDA are also well tolerated.

COARCTATION OF AORTA

Coarctation of aorta is usually repaired prior to pregnancy. Most of the women can have a successful pregnancy. In a woman with coarctation of aorta it is imperative to image the entire aorta due to associated aortopathy and the risk of residual or recurrent coarctation. The expected maternal complication is systemic hypertension which needs adequate treatment. However, aggressive antihypertensive therapy might lead to the placenta hypoperfusion and should be avoided. In presence of significant coarctation, impaired blood flow to uterus and fetus could result in small for date babies or even fetal loss.

PULMONARY STENOSIS

In presence of isolated valvular pulmonary stenosis (PS), pregnancy is usually well tolerated. Residual pulmonary regurgitation might be present in occasional woman who have undergone balloon pulmonary valvuloplasty. Even in these women pregnancy might be well tolerated if they have a good functional capacity and a preserved right ventricular systolic function.

EBSTEIN'S ANOMALY

The outcome of pregnancy in a woman with Ebstein's anomaly depends upon the right ventricular size, function, the degree of tricuspid regurgitation, and the presence or absence of any atrial defect. The presence of any atrial communication as seen in approximately 50% of patients and presence of any cyanosis at rest increase the risk of pregnancy multifold. Moreover, the presence of any atrial communication might predispose the patient to the risk of cerebrovascular accident secondary to a paradoxical embolus. A postoperative patient of Ebstein's anomaly with no residual lesions might tolerate pregnancy well.

CYANOTIC HEART DISEASE

Tetralogy of fallot: Cyanosis is an important determinant of risk to pregnancy especially in women with unrepaired tetralogy of Fallot (TOF). A fall in peripheral resistance in pregnancy can lead to an increased right to left shunting hereby, exacerbating maternal cyanosis. The issues of erythrocytosis can lead to an increased predisposition to thrombosis, paradoxical embolus, and cerebrovascular accidents can be seen in these women who develop deep venous thrombosis. Maternal hypoxemia is also associated with adverse fetal outcomes in women with cyanotic heart disease.

In the postoperative women of TOF with successful surgical repair, good exercise capacity with minimum residue, pregnancy is usually well tolerated. However, in postoperative women with significant right ventricular dilatation and dysfunction, volume overload of pregnancy might not be tolerated. These women can be at risk of atrial and ventricular arrhythmias during the course of gestation. The pregnant women with unrepaired TOF or palliative shunt surgeries can become symptomatic. The degree of risk during pregnancy is usually in proportion to the degree of cyanosis.

Fontan surgery: Fontan procedure is done for palliation in patients with tricuspid and mitral atresia, hypoplastic left or right heart syndrome or complex congenital heart disease when biventricular repair is not possible. Post-Fontan surgery, women usually have a single ventricle physiology without a subpulmonic ventricle. The issues in post-Fontan's surgery patients who are now pregnant could be atrial arrhythmias, heart failure, and thrombosis in Fontan circuit in presence of prothrombotic state of pregnancy or functional deterioration due to volume overload of pregnancy. Prematurity and low birth weight are common fetal and neonatal complications. At the time of delivery, women are cautioned not to push hard so as to avoid any fall in preload which is very important in driving the circulation across for the Fontan's circuit.

PULMONARY HYPERTENSION

The pregnant women with pulmonary hypertension might have idiopathic pulmonary hypertension or pulmonary hypertension secondary to cardiac shunt lesions or connective tissue disorders. Whatever be the cause, pulmonary arterial hypertension (PAH) is associated with high mortality rate when associated with pregnancy. Volume overload of pregnancy might compromise the functions of an already failing right ventricle hereby, precipitating heart failure. A decreased peripheral resistance in pregnancy might augment right to left shunt further worsening cyanosis. High caution is to be advocated during labor and delivery with highest maternal mortality noted during parturition and puerperium. Maternal mortality rate of up to 25% has been reported in women with PAH and pregnancy.

In women with PAH and pregnancy, termination of pregnancy has its own issues of a complex procedure needing anesthesia. When pregnancy is continued, cesarean section is the usually recommended option. When vaginal delivery is chosen epidural analgesia should be administered with utmost care to prevent any peripheral vasodilation. The second stage of labor should not be prolonged and if needed, be assisted.

MARFAN'S SYNDROME

Marfan syndrome an inherited autosomal dominant disease can pose cardiovascular complications in the mother and carries risks of getting transmitted to the offspring. Hence, an adequate preconceptional counseling is required in women with Marfan syndrome. In those with an aortic diameter of >4.5 cm, aortic replacement is advocated before pregnancy. An increased incidence of aortic complications in women with Marfan syndrome is associated with increased maternal mortality. Any associated aortic regurgitation and mitral valve prolapse should also be evaluated in these women. Beta-blockers should usually be continued during the pregnancy to prevent any worsening of aortic dilatation or dissection. Regular follow-up and monitoring of the aortic root size is recommended during pregnancy. The patient should be asked to report on onset of any chest pain, avoid pushing during labor and delivery. Assisted second stage of labor and conducting the delivery in a tertiary care center with adequate cardiac and hemodynamic monitoring is advocated in women with pregnancy and Marfan syndrome.

CORONARY ARTERY DISEASE

Coronary artery disease (CAD) is usually uncommon in women of child-bearing age. However, increasing maternal age, tobacco use, and presence of diabetes may lead to atherosclerotic CAD in these women. Coronary artery dissection, intracoronary thrombosis, and coronary artery spasm have also been reported in pregnancy. In presence of preexisting CAD, increased maternal mortality of up to 10%, myocardial infarction, heart failure, and acute coronary events are seen.

Acute myocardial infarction though rare in pregnancy has a mortality of 5–10%. Most common cause of myocardial infarction in pregnancy is coronary artery dissection. Left anterior descending (LAD) is the most involved artery. It occurs usually in the third trimester or early postpartum period. Primary percutaneous transluminal coronary angioplasty (PTCA) is preferred over thrombolysis as the preferred management strategy since thrombolysis may precipitate placental bleeding. The other standard drug therapies in myocardial infarction such as morphine, nitroglycerin, aspirin and clopidogrel, heparin, and beta-blockers can be used. ACE inhibitor and statins are not recommended due to the fetal risk.

ARRHYTHMIAS IN PREGNANCY

The physiological hemodynamic changes of pregnancy and increased catecholamines contribute to an arrhythmogenic potential in pregnancy. In those presenting with arrhythmias rule out any precipitating causes and associated comorbidities like thyroid disorders. Dyselectrolytemia should be ruled out and an echocardiogram performed to look for presence of underlying structural heart disease.

Supraventricular arrhythmias are the common arrhythmias seen during pregnancy. The management remains same as in nonpregnant women. However, the concerns of fetal toxicity of pharmacological drugs remain. Occurrence of *atrial fibrillation* would usually suggest an underlying structural heart disease like mitral stenosis. When accompanied with structural heart disease pregnant patient with atrial fibrillation need to receive an antiarrhythmic as well as an anticoagulant. Beta-blockers and digoxin have been used in pregnant patients safely. Electrical cardioversion needs to be considered only in case of hemodynamic instability.

Ventricular tachycardia is uncommon in a pregnant lady. Women with structurally normal hearts and idiopathic or outflow tract VT may present during pregnancy and usually respond to medical therapy. However, women with long QT syndrome can present with VT, syncope, or sudden cardiac death, especially in the postpartum period. During pregnancy as well as in postpartum period it should be ensured that all these women receive beta-blocker therapy.

CONCLUSION

Pregnancy is a vital stage of any woman's life with hemodynamic alterations. In presence of cardiac ailments these hemodynamic alterations can have a significant effect on the fetal and maternal health. It is imperative for a physician to adopt a multidisciplinary approach toward pregnant cardiac patients and to be prompt in diagnosing and managing cardiac ailments in pregnancy with aggression that it deserves.

RECOMMENDED READINGS

1. Clapp MA, Bernstein SN. Preconception counseling for women with cardiac disease. Curr Treat Options Cardiovasc Med. 2017;19(9):67.
2. Regitz-zagrosek V, Blomstrom Lundqvist C, Borghi C, Cifkova R, Ferreira R, Foidart JM, Gibbs JS, et al. ESC Guidelines on the management of cardiovascular diseases during pregnancy: The European Society of Cardiology (ESC). Eur Heart J. 2011;32:3147-97.
3. Baumgartner H, Hung J, Bermejo J, Chambers JB, Evangelista A, Griffin BP, et al. Echocardiographic assessment of valve stenosis: EAE/ASE recommendations for clinical practice. Eur J Echocardio. 2009;10(1):1-25.
4. John AS, Gurley F, Schaff HV, Warnes CA, Phillips SD, Arendt KW, et al. Cardiopulmonary bypass during pregnancy. Ann Thorac Surg. 2011;91(4):1191-6.
5. Magee LA, Pels A, Helewa M, Rey E, von Dadelszen P; Canadian Hypertensive Disorders of Pregnancy Working Group. Diagnosis, evaluation, and management of the hypertensive disorders of pregnancy: executive summary. J Obstet Gynaecol Can. 2014;36(5):416-41.
6. Fett JD, Christie LG, Carraway RD, Murphy JG. Five-Year Prospective Study of the Incidence and Prognosis of Peripartum Cardiomyopathy at a Single Institution. Mayo Clin Proc. 2005;80(12):1602-6.
7. Sliwa K, Blauwet L, Tibazarwa K, Libhaber E, Smedema JP, Becker A, et al. Evaluation of bromocriptine in the treatment of acute severe peripartum cardiomyopathy: a proof-of-concept pilot study. Circulation. 2010;121(13):1465-73. Erratum in: Circulation. 2010;121(21):e425.
8. Mahowald MK, Davis M. Case Series: Spontaneous Relapse After Recovery From Peripartum Cardiomyopathy. Clin Med Insights Case Rep. 2017; 10.1179547617749227.
9. Schinkel AF. Pregnancy in women with hypertrophic cardiomyopathy. Cardiol Rev. 2014;22(5):217-22.
10. Castrini AI, Lie ØH, Leren IS, Estensen ME, Stokke MK, Klæboe LG, et al. Number of pregnancies and subsequent phenotype in a cross-sectional cohort of women with arrhythmogenic cardiomyopathy. Eur Heart J Cardiovas Imag. 2019:20(2):192-8.
11. Ruiz S, Martinez-Marin M, Luque P, Nassar N, Oros D. Takotsubo cardiomyopathy after cesarean section: A case report and literature review. J Obstet Gynaecol Res. 2017;43(2):392-6.
12. van Hagen IM, Roos-Hesselink JW, Ruys TP, Merz WM, Goland S, Gabriel H, et al. Pregnancy in Women With a Mechanical Heart Valve: Data of the European Society of Cardiology Registry of Pregnancy and Cardiac Disease (ROPAC). Circulation. 2015;132(2):132-42.
13. Vitale N, De Feo M, De Santo LS, Pollice A, Tedesco N, Cotrufo M. Dose-dependent fetal complications of warfarin in pregnant women with mechanical heart valves. J Am Coll Cardiol. 1999;33(6):1637-41.
14. Nishimura RA, Otto CM, Bonow RO, Carabello BA, Erwin JP 3rd, Guyton RA, et al. 2014 AHA/ACC Guideline for the Management of Patients With Valvular Heart Disease: executive summary: a report of the American College of Cardiology/American Heart Association Task Force on Practice Guidelines. Circulation. 2014;129(23):2440-92.
15. Silversides CK, Dore A, Poirier N, Taylor D, Harris L, Greutmann M, et al. Canadian Cardiovascular Society 2009 Consensus Conference on the management of

adults with congenital heart disease: shunt lesions. Can J Cardiol. 2010;26(3):e70-9.
16. Greutmann M, Von Klemperer K, Brooks R, Peebles D, O'Brien P, Walker F. et al. Pregnancy outcome in women with congenital heart disease and residual haemodynamic lesions of the right ventricular outflow tract. Eur Heart J. 2010;31(14):1764-70.
17. Drenthen W, Pieper PG, Ploeg M, Voors AA, Roos-Hesselink JW, Mulder BJ, et al. Risk of complications during pregnancy after Senning or Mustard (atrial) repair of complete transposition of the great arteries. Eur Heart J. 2005;26(23):2588-95.
18. Elkayam U, Jalnapurkar S, Barakkat MN, Khatri N, Kealey AJ, Mehra A, et al. Pregnancy-associated acute myocardial infarction: a review of contemporary experience in 150 cases between 2006 and 2011. Circulation. 2014;129(16):1695-702.
19. Seth R, Moss AJ, McNitt S, Zareba W, Andrews ML, Qi M, et al. Long QT syndrome and pregnancy. J Am Coll Cardiol. 2007;49(10):1092-8.

CHAPTER 102

Ischemic Heart Disease: Risk Factors and Prevention

Rajeev Gupta

ABSTRACT

Ischemic heart disease (IHD) is the most common cause of death globally. It is the most important cause of premature deaths in India. In contrast to developed countries where IHD mortality and burden is decreasing, it is increasing in India and other Asian countries. Primary and primordial prevention have been responsible for half of the decline in its prevalence in developed countries. Primary prevention strategies focus on multiple risk factors control. Important are healthy lifestyles with smoking and tobacco-use cessation, ambient and indoor pollution control, regular aerobic physical activity, and promotion of healthy diet with control of saturated fats, trans fats and refined carbohydrates and greater intake of fruits, vegetables, lentils, nuts, and dairy products. Target-oriented control of blood pressure (BP) in hypertension (<130/85 mm Hg), low-density lipoprotein (LDL), cholesterol (<100 mg/dL, <70 mg/dL in high risk), non-high-density lipoprotein (non-HDL) cholesterol (<130 mg/dL, <100 mg/dL in high-risk), and glycemia in diabetes (HbA1c <7.0%) are important components of it. Risk stratification should guide physicians for targeted interventions. Promotion of lifelong adherence to therapies using technological innovations and shared decision-making is important.

Primordial prevention strategies are important to modify social determinants of health and avoid occurrence of risk factors. Improving health literacy in general population and medical literacy among medical professionals and other healthcare workers can provide sustained long-term reduction in risk factors and can ameliorate the IHD epidemic.

"He who cures a disease may be the skillfullest, but he that prevents it is the safest physician"

—Thomas Fuller

INTRODUCTION

Ischemic heart disease (IHD) is the most important cause of death and disease burden in India. Data from Million Death Study (India) and estimates in Global Burden of Diseases (GBD) study have reported that, in contrast to developed countries where IHD death rates are declining, the mortality and disability rate from IHD is increasing in India. Reasons for the decline of IHD in developed countries have been well studied and include prevention and control of risk factors, better acute and chronic IHD management, coronary interventions, and surgical procedures. These studies have determined that better risk factor control has been responsible for 40–50% of the decline in IHD. Lessons learnt from developed countries should be translated in India where the IHD epidemic is still evolving. In this chapter, I shall focus on risk factors of importance in India and highlight strategies for their prevention and control.

RISK FACTORS

Knowledge of IHD risk factors has evolved over the past century and, according to current understanding, the disease is due to a complex interaction of social, behavioral, biological, and genetic risk factors. Primacy of political and social factors and natural and structural environment in influencing behavioral, physical, and biological factors is fundamental to understanding causation. Although the

TABLE 1 Ischemic heart disease risk factors.

Social determinants of risk: Primordial factors	Lifestyle and biological proximate factors
• Low-quality urban and rural infrastructure • Social disorganization, stress • Illiteracy • Adverse early life events, maternal, and child health • Work environment, unemployment, and job stress • Transportation quality • Social support, lack of cohesion, and isolation • Food quality, agriculture • Unhealthy food promotion • Poverty, social exclusion, and minorities • Social patterning • Poor sanitation • Lack of facilities for physical activity, other health promotion behaviors • Lack of proper healthcare financing • Universal healthcare	• Ambient (outdoor, indoor) air pollution • Smoking and smokeless tobacco • Physical inactivity • Dietary factors (saturated fats, trans fats, and refined carbohydrates) • Excessive salt intake • Low fruit and vegetable intake • Psychosocial stress, anxiety, and depression • Alcohol abuse • High blood pressure and hypertension • High LDL and non-HDL cholesterol • Raised triglycerides • Lipoprotein(a) • Elevated glucose and diabetes • Family history • Genetics and genomics

concept of cardiovascular risk factors is decades old, there is still outdated thinking in scientific literature about causality. Risk factor is any attribute, characteristic, or exposure of an individual or group that increases the likelihood of developing a disease or injury. Bradford-Hill criteria to determine causality of a hypothesized risk factor are strength of association, consistency, specificity, temporality, biological gradient, plausibility, coherence, experiment, and analogy. These criteria can never be absolute, and causality is a matter of judgment based on totality of experimental and observational evidence. Studies have identified a range of IHD risk factors that can be addressed at the individual and population levels. Factors include individual level lifestyle, physical, biological and genetic factors (primary or proximate risk factors), and political, economic and social determinants of cardiovascular health (primordial or upstream risk factors) (**Table 1**).

MAJOR MODIFIABLE RISK FACTORS

The proximate or primary risk factors can be classified into modifiable and nonmodifiable. Modifiable risk factors include unhealthy lifestyles—tobacco use, ambient pollution, physical inactivity, unhealthy diet, alcohol, stress etc., and biological factors are hypertension, LDL cholesterol, non-HDL cholesterol, triglycerides, diabetes, obesity, and abdominal obesity etc. Most of these risk factors have been identified as important in Indian populations. Prospective Urban Rural Epidemiology (PURE) is the first

TABLE 2 Risk factors identified as important in the PURE study.

Cardiovascular diseases	Ischemic heart disease
• Hypertension (22%)	• High non-HDL cholesterol (17%)
• High non-HDL cholesterol (8%)	• Hypertension (13%)
• Household air pollution (7%)	• Tobacco use (12%)
• Tobacco use (6%)	• Abdominal obesity (11%)
• Poor diet (6%)	• Diabetes (8%)
• Low education (6%)	• Low education (7%)
• Abdominal obesity (6%)	• Low grip strength (7%)
• Diabetes (5%)	• Household pollution (5%)
• Low grip strength (3%)	• Poor diet (4%)
• Low physical activity (2%)	• Low physical activity (<1%)
• Depression (<1.0%)	• Depression (<1%)
• Excessive alcohol (<1.0%)	• Excessive alcohol (<1%)
• Cardiovascular diseases include IHD, stroke, and peripheral arterial disease • Numbers in parentheses are absolute population attributable fractions.	

(PURE: Prospective Urban Rural Epidemiology)

large-scale population-based prospective study in India and most developing countries. This study has identified that 12 common risk factors are responsible for 85–90% of incident IHD events and mortality (**Table 2**).

EMERGING RISK FACTORS

There are a number of IHD risk factors that do not fulfill the Bradford-Hill criteria for causality. These include political, economic, and social determinants of cardiovascular health and a few lifestyle, anthropometric, and biological factors (**Table 1**). All the social determinants of risk have not undergone rigorous evaluation similar to biological factors using randomized controlled trials. Data are purely observational. On the other hand a few biological factors that are emerging in importance are the metabolic syndrome, impaired glucose tolerance and raised fasting glucose, and insulin resistance; lipid fractions such as lipoprotein remnants, triglyceride remnants, small dense LDL; inflammatory markers including C-reactive proteins, cytokines, interleukins, vitamin E, and others; coagulation and thrombosis risk factors such as fibrinogen, plasminogen activator-1, homocysteine; and psychological factors, obstructive sleep apnea, and others. Evidence regarding prevention of IHD with control of these risk factors is weak and these factors shall not be discussed here.

NONMODIFIABLE RISK FACTORS

The risk factors that cannot be influenced by currently available interventions and therapies are called nonmodifiable factors and include age, sex, family history, and genetic factors. There is emerging evidence of reversal of aging processes at molecular level, but no outcome data exist. Genetic risk factors cannot be changed using current technologies, although certain molecular gene-modification methods and cell transplantation techniques have shown promise. Observational studies have reported that heightened genetic risk, identified using polygenic risk scores, can be reversed by leading a healthy lifestyle or use of statins for cholesterol lowering. These observations highlight interlinked importance of modifiable and nonmodifiable IHD risk factors and confirm multifactorial origin.

SOCIAL DETERMINANTS

Association of better and sustainable social development with lower IHD burden and mortality is well known. The GBD study reported that countries with higher socio-demographic index have lower IHD burden and mortality. It has been reported that countries that rapidly increased societal development in the early years of the last century had the largest mortality decline. Focus on social determinants and adoption of a health-in-all-policies approach have led to the lowest IHD rates in Scandinavian countries. In contrast, in many lower-middle and low-income countries, where there is poor focus on social determinants of health, IHD mortality and burden is increasing. World Health Organization (WHO) recommends this approach to achieve a significant reduction in communicable and noncommunicable disease burden and to achieve the sustainable development goals (SDGs). American Heart Association (AHA) has suggested more focus on the social determinants.

PRIMARY PREVENTION

The strategy for control of major cardiovascular risk factors for prevention of IHD events is known as primary prevention. This strategy focuses on control of important lifestyle factors (smoking and tobacco use, physical inactivity, unhealthy diet, and alcohol) and biological factors (hypertension, high LDL and non-HDL cholesterol, raised triglycerides, hyperglycemia, diabetes, and obesity). There is significant interaction amongst the interventions, for example, increased physical activity influences multiple biological risk factors including obesity, hypertension, lipid abnormalities, and diabetes. However, for sake of simplicity, we shall first focus on interventions for control of individual risk factors and then highlight important multifactorial interventions to reduce overall risk.

SMOKING AND TOBACCO CONTROL

An important population- and individual-level strategy for IHD prevention is smoking and tobacco control. Harmful effects of smoking and tobacco on cardiovascular system are well known and include direct vascular damage and augmentation of other risk factors. It has been estimated that a reduction of one-third in IHD risk could be achieved by doubling the inflation-adjusted cost of cigarettes, which in many low- and middle-income countries could be achieved by tripling the excise tax on tobacco. Other examples of community-based smoking control activities include adoption of smoking control ordinances, e.g., smoke-free restaurants, display bans, media advocacy to raise public awareness, paid counter-advertising, and sponsorship of stop-smoking events. A meta-analysis of 17 eligible studies reported that implementation of population-wide smoking cessation policies leads to 10% decline in the incidence of acute coronary syndromes.

At the individual level it must be emphasized that smoking and tobacco use is one of the most important risk factors for IHD, especially among the young in India. A number of factors are associated with smoking initiation and continued smoking including interpersonal influences by friends, coworkers, and family as well as individual factors (age, sex, race, beliefs and attitudes, and genetics). Poor social support is another determinant of tobacco use. Therefore, in adults who use tobacco, assistance and arrangement for individualized and group social support counseling are recommended. Medications are available for smoking cessation and approved ones are nicotine patch, nicotine gum, nicotine inhaler, nicotine nasal spray, varenicline, and bupropion.

AMBIENT AND INDOOR AIR POLLUTION

Outdoor and indoor air pollution have emerged as important IHD risk factors (**Table 2**). It has been estimated that 9 million deaths are directly attributable to environmental pollution, 4.2 million to ambient, and 2.9 million to household air pollution and >50% of these deaths are due to cardiovascular diseases. Well-characterized adverse cardiovascular effects of pollution are on all-cause mortality and cardiovascular mortality, emerging evidence of association is available for hypertension, diabetes, nonfatal coronary events, nonfatal strokes, and heart failure. Pollution leads to vascular damage, endothelial dysfunction, oxidation, and is thrombogenic. Although the relative risk for cardiovascular mortality of ambient particulate matter <2.5 microns ($PM_{2.5}$) is small 1.025, 95% confidence intervals (CI) 1.015–1.036 the absolute risk are high as over 90% of global population is exposed to pollution.

A number of interventions are available to reduce exposure. Important in global context are government and nongovernment organization-led publicity, shifting to clean fuels (public and household), emission trading programs, transportation reforms, reduction in traffic emissions, urban landscape reform, empowering civil society, and redirection of science and funding. Personal interventions include use of facemasks and air purifiers, reduction of in-house exposure of outdoor air pollution, home ventilation to eliminate kitchen pollution, reduction in traffic exposure time, and lifestyle changes.

PHYSICAL ACTIVITY

Regular physical activity is known to be associated with longer lifespan, better quality of life, and decreased incidence of IHD. Physical inactivity leads to a number of adverse consequences on cardiovascular health such as energy imbalance, oxidative stress, smooth muscle dysfunction, inflammation, and endothelial dysfunction. There is a dose-response relationship between sedentariness and premature mortality. Physical activity levels remain low worldwide and multiple factors are responsible. Community level hindrances are congested urban residences, poor access to open spaces, lack of enjoyable scenery and esthetics, poor street connectivity and street lighting, unsafe neighborhoods, safety of parks and trails, lack of sidewalks, cycle lanes and paths, unruly traffic and low walkability etc. Reviews have confirmed usefulness of mass media campaigns for physical activity promotion.

For a good health, WHO and other international guidelines recommend at least 150 minutes a week of moderate aerobic physical activity, 30 min/day for 5 days/week or 75 minutes a week of vigorous aerobic physical activity, 15 min/day for 5 days/week, or a combination thereof. In addition to the prescription of exercise it is important to assess neighborhood environment and access to facilities for physical activity. Healthcare providers should provide strong endorsement for promotion of physical activity. Apart from society level actions, it is important that physical activity education is disseminated at outpatient clinics and endorsed by community organizations. At personal level it is important to identify physical activity barriers and develop self-regulatory skills for lifelong adherence. Self-goal setting, self-monitoring (wearable devices or cellphone apps), feedback about progress, evaluation of activity levels, and fresh goal settings are important. Physicians, physician assistants, nurses, and physical activity counselors are important partners in this effort.

YOGA AND STRESS MANAGEMENT

Connections between psychological well-being and cardiovascular conditions may be mediated through biological, behavioral, and psychosocial pathways. Yoga-based exercises and relaxation techniques are promoted as useful approach for primary prevention. Meta-analyses of small randomized controlled trials reported that there is only a marginal evidence to suggest that such practices led to better regulation of sympathetic nervous system and hypothalamic-pituitary-adrenal system, decreased depressive and anxiety symptoms and lowered body mass index, systolic BP, total and LDL cholesterol, triglycerides, and heart rate. YOGACARE is one of the largest randomized trials that evaluated influence of breathing, meditation, and relaxation yogic exercises in 3,921 patients (yoga 1,953, controls 1,968) with known IHD. At end of median follow-up of 21.6 months there was a 10% reduction in major adverse coronary events in the overall group. However, evaluation in those adherent to yoga practices, a 25% significant risk reduction was observed.

European prevention guidelines emphasize psychosocial risk factor assessment in individuals at high cardiovascular risk. Implementation and integration of positive psychological well-being activities are important. Workplaces can be used for well-being-focused interventions to promote cardiovascular health.

DIETARY FACTORS

Food is an important aspect of IHD prevention. Three relevant domains of food composition are fats, carbohydrates, and micronutrients (e.g., salt). Emerging evidence suggests that instead of focus on individual nutrient, it is important to consider quality of the overall food patterns for IHD prevention.

Fats and saturated fats: Guidelines recommend curtailing saturated fats in the diet. Relationship of dietary fat to coronary risk has been evaluated using controlled feeding studies, surrogate plasma lipid-based end points, small- to medium-size randomized trials and large observational studies. Studies have shown that modest reduction in IHD by decrease in saturated fat is possible if replaced by combination of poly- and monounsaturated fats. However, little or no benefit results if saturated fat is replaced by carbohydrates. Because both N-6 and N-3 polyunsaturated fatty acids are essential and reduce IHD risk, the ratio of N-6 to N-3 is not useful. PURE study reported that greater saturated fat intake was associated with lower hazard of stroke with no influence on IHD mortality while total and unsaturated fats were associated with lower cardiovascular events. An AHA Advisory concluded that lower intake of saturated fat coupled with higher intake of polyunsaturated and monounsaturated fat is associated with lower rates of cardiovascular disease and recommended lowering intake of saturated fat and replacing it with unsaturated fats, especially polyunsaturated fats. In practice, reducing processed meats and increasing intakes of nuts, fish, soy products, and nonhydrogenated vegetable oils improves mix of fatty acids and have beneficial effect.

Trans fats: Trans fatty acids from partially hydrogenated vegetable oils have major adverse effects. A systematic review reported that policies aimed at reducing trans fats in the food supply are effective. Low socioeconomic status persons are more exposed to trans fats, especially in India and other lower income countries, as trans fat-laced foods are stable and cheaper. Although all policy approaches (voluntary self-regulation, mandatory labeling, voluntary reduction in restaurants, or their combination) lead to reduction of trans fats in foods, population-level trans fatty acid bans are the most effective approach.

Refined carbohydrates and sugar: Reviews have reported that high intake of refined carbohydrates is associated with greater cardiovascular risk. In a meta-analysis of 432,179 participants in eight cohort studies it was observed that both high- and low-carbohydrate diets were associated with increased IHD mortality, with minimal risk observed at 50–55% energy from carbohydrates. WHO has recommended that not >10% of calories should be from added sugar (refined sugars) in the diet. AHA recommends reductions in intake of added sugars, prudent upper limit of intake being <150 calories/day.

Sodium (salt) intake: There is incontrovertible evidence that high sodium in diet is associated with high BP and the relationship is linear. High sodium intake not only increases BP but also plays a role in endothelial dysfunction, cardiovascular structure and function, albuminuria and kidney disease progression, and cardiovascular morbidity and mortality. A Cochrane review concluded that a modest reduction in sodium intake causes significant and important fall in BP and supported limiting population-wide sodium intake to <1.5 g/day from the recommended 2 to 2.5 g/day. Many observational studies, on the other hand, have reported a U-shaped association of salt intake with all cause and cardiovascular mortality. In a meta-analysis of four studies, high sodium intake (>7 g/day) was associated with increased risk of cardiovascular events in hypertensive populations with no association in the normotensive. Low sodium intake (<3 g/day) was also associated with increased risk of cardiovascular events in those with or without hypertension. These data argue that moderate sodium intake 3–5 g/day should be recommended. A number of policy and community-based interventions exist for promoting sodium reduction in diet. Individual approaches are dietary counseling (for individuals, worksites, or communities), media campaigns, nutrition labeling, and voluntary and mandatory reformulation. Comprehensive strategy achieves larger reductions in salt consumption than individually focused interventions.

Healthy dietary patterns: The focus has now shifted to overall food quality rather than individual components. Multifactorial food-based dietary recommendations are most likely to succeed. Food choices must be strongly supported by clinical behavior change efforts, health systems reforms, novel technologies, and robust policy strategies targeting economic incentives, schools and workplaces, neighborhood environments, and the food system. Guidelines suggest complex interventions for changing food consumption habits. People eat food (and not nutrients) and changes in overall dietary patterns toward a healthy and sustainable diet are important. Diet recommended by EAT-Lancet Commission for sustainable health of planet and individuals is important. Dietary patterns that have been found to be beneficial in randomized trials are Dietary Approaches to Stop Hypertension (DASH), Franco-Mediterranean, Indo-Mediterranean, and Iberio-Mediterranean and have been incorporated in American and European guidelines (**Table 3**).

Alcohol: World Health Organization has reported that harmful use of alcohol is associated with violence, injuries, mental health problems, cancer, and cardiovascular diseases such as stroke and heart failure. Despite strong evidence of harm, most of the guidelines are ambiguous regarding safe limits for IHD prevention. A number of policy interventions have been suggested for curbing harmful use of alcohol which include leadership commitment, nationwide awareness raising activities, health services and community repose to alcohol ban, drink-driving countermeasures and penalties, regulating the availability of alcohol, marketing restrictions, pricing, reducing the negative consequences of drinking, addressing informal and illicit production, and continuous monitoring and surveillance. Similar to smoking bans, implementation of alcohol control recommendations is variable across countries and there is a need for a paradigm shift at national and subnational level.

HYPERTENSION

Hypertension is one of the most important risk factors for cardiovascular diseases (**Table 2**). Prevention and control of hypertension can be achieved through population-based as well as targeted strategies. In most countries of the world, hypertension treatment and control rates are suboptimal. Targeted strategy involves interventions to increase awareness, treatment, and control in individuals. Having a usual source of care, optimizing adherence, and minimizing therapeutic inertia are associated with better BP control. There is a need for a collaborative partnership among the patient, provider, and health system, which incorporates a multilevel approach for control of hypertension. Optimizing the prevention, recognition, and care of hypertension requires a paradigm shift to team-based care and the use of strategies known to control BP. Because other lifestyle habits can impact BP, access to healthy diet, physical activity options, and adequate sleep-duration are important.

Hypertension diagnostic criteria and classification have evolved over the past century. Current criteria recommended by leading societies are mentioned in **Table 4**. The US criteria are more stringent, based on multiple measurements using clinic, home, and ambulatory techniques. Other societies' guidelines rely on office BP measurements and hypertension is diagnosed when BP is ≥140 systolic and/or

TABLE 3 Recommendation for healthy food in various guidelines.

Mediterranean Diet (PREDIMED)	Lancet-EAT Commission Anthropocene Diet	American Heart Association	European Society of Cardiology
• Recommended: Olive oil, tree nuts or peanuts, fresh fruits, fatty fish, legumes, white meat, and wine • Discouraged: Soda drinks, commercial bakery goods, sweets, pastries, spread fats, and red and processed meats	• Diversity of plant-based foods • Low animal source • Balanced intake of unsaturated and saturated fats • Reduced amounts of refined grains, highly processed foods, and added sugars	• Greater intake of vegetables, fruits, legumes, nuts, whole grains, and fish • Low intake of refined grains, highly processed foods, and added sugars	• Recommendations for whole grain products, oily fish, and unsalted nuts • High intake of fruits and vegetables, >200 g each • Low intake of refined grains, highly processed foods, and added sugars

(PREDIMED: prevention with Mediterranean diet)

TABLE 4 Diagnosis and classification of hypertension based on BP levels in various guidelines.

Hypertension grade	ACC/AHA 2017	ESC/ESH 2018	NICE 2019	ISH 2020
Hypertension diagnosis				
Clinic (office BP, multiple)	130/80	140/90	140/90	140/90
Home (home BP, multiple)	130/80	135/85	135/85	135/85
Daytime (ambulatory BP)	130/80	135/85	135/85	135/85
Hypertension classification				
High normal	• Systolic 120–129 • Diastolic 75–79	• Systolic 130–139 • Diastolic 85–89	–	• Systolic 130–139 • Diastolic 85–89
Stage I	• Systolic 130–139 • Diastolic 80–89	• Systolic 140–159 • Diastolic 90–99	• Systolic 140–159 • Diastolic 90–99	• Systolic 140–159 • Diastolic 90–99
Stage II	• Systolic ≥140 • Diastolic ≥90	• Systolic ≥160 • Diastolic ≥100	• Systolic 160–179 • Diastolic 100–119	• Systolic ≥160 • Diastolic ≥100
Stage III	–	–	• Systolic ≥180 • Diastolic ≥120	–

(ACC/AHA: American College of Cardiology/American Heart Association; BP: blood pressure; ESC/ESH: European Society of Cardiology/European Society of Hypertension; NICE: National Institute of Clinical Excellence, UK; ISH: International Society of Hypertension)

TABLE 5 Evidence-based pharmacotherapy for BP control in various guidelines.

		ACC/AHA 2017	ESC/ESH 2018	NICE 2019	ISH 2020
Stage I	Monotherapy	A, C or D as monotherapy	A+C, A+D, or C+D as initial therapy as combination pill (SPC)	• A or C in young • C or D in older	A+C, A+D, or C+D as initial therapy as combination pill (SPC)
Stage II	Duotherapy	A+C, A+D, or C+D	High-dose combination pill	A+C, A+D, or C+D	A+C+D
Resistant hypertension	Polytherapy	Triple drug Spironolactone	Triple drug Spironolactone	Triple drug Spironolactone	Triple drug Spironolactone
Other classes	Context-specific polytherapy				
Comments	Add B at any stage if there is specific or compelling indication				

A: ACEI/ARB; B: Beta blockers; C: Calcium channel blockers; D: Diuretics

≥90 mm Hg diastolic. Slight differences in classification of various grades of hypertension are also present (**Table 4**). These levels are important for treatment strategies and prognostication. For example, in high-normal and Stage I hypertension initial management includes focus on healthy lifestyles—physical activity, weight management, alcohol abstinence, tobacco cessation, and salt restriction as described above. Drug therapy is indicated only after failure of sustained lifestyle modification efforts for 1–2 months.

Hypertension control targets have also evolved over the past century, initial focus being on very high systolic BP and targets varied from 160 to 180 mm Hg. The early US guidelines focused on the diastolic BP levels with target of <100 mm Hg. Multiple randomized controlled trials and large-scale meta-analysis have now shown that lowering systolic BP is more important than diastolic and current targets have been divided into two—the initial target being BP <140/90 mm Hg and final target <130/85 mm Hg in most guidelines. A panoply of drugs to supplement lifestyle interventions has been suggested (**Table 5**). In contrast to guidelines in early 21st century when beta-blockers and thiazide diuretics were the first-line treatment, current guidelines by almost all societies recommend a patient-specific approach with initiation of drug therapy with angiotensin-converting enzyme (ACE) inhibitors or angiotensin receptor blockers (ARBs), calcium channel blockers (CCBs) or a thiazide-like diuretic. Stepwise augmentation of therapy is suggested (**Table 5**). Control to targets is important to achieve cardiovascular benefit.

LDL CHOLESTEROL

There is plethora of evidence regarding epidemiological, genetic, and causal association of dyslipidemias with IHD incidence and mortality. High total cholesterol and its principal subtypes LDL cholesterol and non-HDL cholesterol are the most important. Additionally, recent epidemiological, Mendelian randomization, and clinical trials have confirmed importance of raised triglycerides and lipoprotein(a). The PURE study has identified raised non-HDL cholesterol as the most important CAD risk

TABLE 6 Targets for control of LDL and non-HDL cholesterol (mg/dL) in various risk categories. Risk estimated according to various guidelines.

	Low risk	Intermediate risk	High risk	Very high risk
LDL cholesterol targets	116	100	70	50
Non-HDL cholesterol targets	146	130	100	80

TABLE 7 Interventions for IHD prevention in diabetes.

Domains	Interventions	Targets
Lifestyle	Smoking/tobacco cessation; regular aerobic physical activity; muscle strengthening; healthy diet; alcohol avoidance; and pollution control	ACC/AHA and European guidelines
Diabetes control	Lifestyle and drugs, GLP-1 receptor agonists, SGLT-2 inhibitors, and metformin	HbA1c <7.0%
Hypertension management	• Lifestyle changes • Drugs: ACE inhibitors/ARBs, calcium channel blockers	BP <130/85 mm Hg in all diabetics; <120/80 mm Hg in high-risk individuals
LDL cholesterol management	Drugs: Statins	LDL cholesterol <100 mg/dL in all; <70 mg/dL in high risk
Triglycerides	Drugs: Fenofibrate, icosapent ethyl	Fasting triglyceride <150 mg/dL

(SGLT-2: sodium-glucose cotransporter-2; GLP-1: glucagon-like peptide-1)

factor in South Asians (**Table 2**). Regional and multisite epidemiological studies in India have reported increasing population level total cholesterol, LDL cholesterol, non-HDL cholesterol, and triglycerides in contrast to most developed countries where these are declining. LDL cholesterol is one of the most important targets for prevention. Targets for ideal LDL cholesterol for IHD primary prevention in low, intermediate, and high-risk individuals are shown in **Table 6**. These are based on European guidelines and Indian consensus statements. Non-HDL cholesterol has recently emerged as a strong target for intervention. This appears more promising as it summates all the atherogenic particles including LDL, very low-density lipoprotein (VLDL), intermediate-density lipoprotein (IDL), and lipoprotein remnants.

Dietary interventions and drugs (statins) are the mainstay of treatment. Focus on a healthy diet and greater physical activity is important and interventions are vide supra. Reviews and meta-analyses have highlighted the important role of these drugs for primary and secondary prevention. The targets of optimum LDL-cholesterol in low-risk individuals (general population with 1 or less risk factor) and other categories are given in **Table 6**. Healthy lifestyles have a limited role in achieving targets in high and very high-risk individuals and supplemental drug therapy, principally moderate to high dose statins (atorvastatin 20–80 mg/day or rosuvastatin 10–40 mg/day) are important in this regard. Nonstatin lipid-lowering drugs can be prescribed in statin-intolerant or statin nonresponders according to recent guidelines. Alternate drugs are ezetimibe, bempedoic acid, and PCSK9 inhibitors.

TRIGLYCERIDES

Serum triglycerides have been implicated as important risk factor for long. However, interventions to reduce it with lifestyle changes, niacin or fibric acid derivatives have not been successful in prevention. REDUCE-IT (Reduction of Cardiovascular Events with EPA-Intervention Trial) has demonstrated usefulness of high-dose fish oil supplement, icosapent ethyl, in reducing cardiovascular events in a mixed primary and secondary prevention cohort. More studies are needed in primary prevention before this strategy is widely recommended.

DIABETES

Primary prevention of macrovascular disease (IHD, stroke, and peripheral arterial disease) is a major goal in diabetes management. Guidance on BP and lipid control in diabetes to reduce cardiovascular risk in primary prevention is shown in **Table 7**. Control of hyperglycemia for preventing macrovascular disease has had a checkered history and short-term tight glucose control has been shown to have no benefit. Long-term benefits of initial tight control of glycemia (legacy benefits) have been reported. Metformin has been shown to be vasculoprotective in older studies but there are no recent outcome studies with this drug. Usefulness of new drug classes, sodium-glucose cotransporter-2 (SGLT-2) inhibitors and glucagon-like peptide-1 (GLP-1) receptor agonists, have been reported in secondary prevention and not in primary prevention. More studies are needed.

Studies have also reported that control of BP and LDL-cholesterol lowering are more important in diabetes than glycemic control and a target-based approach is important. Apart from these drugs, in diabetes patients interventions to control environmental and psychosocial factors including depression, stress, self-efficacy and social support, should be addressed to improve glycemic control and promote adherence.

RISK ASSESSMENT AND INTERVENTIONS

This approach is focused on the identification and management of individuals at high risk of developing IHD by using validated risk algorithms for a given population. Screening identifies those, based on a multifactorial risk assessment, at a high risk of developing IHD. Promoting healthy lifestyle and controlling associated risk factors reduce total risk in the high-risk individuals who would benefit the most. Strong evidence of benefit for this approach exists among moderate to high-risk individuals. Evidence from lower risk populations is still sparse.

RISK ASSESSMENT

National and international IHD prevention guidelines have recommended absolute risk assessment tools for decision-making regarding the intensity of lifestyle and pharmacologic interventions. Specialized risk-prediction models for different countries and diverse populations are necessary because risk-assessment tools developed for one population are often inaccurate when applied to another population, although recalibration is possible. Notable differences exist in risk-assessment recommendations between clinical guidelines issued by different regions and can affect decision-making in clinical practice.

A number of strategies could be used for risk prediction. These include traditional risk-prediction tools, vascular imaging-based tools, and gene-based polygenic risk scores (**Table 8**). Clinical risk-prediction tools are widely used in clinical practice. However, most of these tools have been developed in Caucasian populations and may not be applicable to global population. Three risk assessment tools—WHO, GLOBORISK-2, and INTERHEART risk scores—have region-specific risk-prediction charts. Coronary calcification-based risk assessment (coronary calcium score and calcium density) provides incremental positive predictive value. Ultrasound imaging-based risk assessment tools using plaque volume in carotid arteries, femoral arteries, and aorta also provide predictive value. A combination of clinical, imaging, and gene-based risk score using artificial intelligence algorithms could be useful.

MULTIPLE RISK FACTORS CONTROL

Using a risk scoring system, individuals can be divided into four groups: (1) very high risk-documented cardiovascular disease, diabetes with target organ damage, chronic kidney disease [glomerular filtration rate (GFR) <30] or very high score; (2) high risk markedly elevated single risk factor, diabetes, moderate chronic kidney disease (GFR 30–60) or intermediate risk score; (3) moderate risk; and (4) low risk. Therapeutic strategies vary according to the level of risk as well as presence or absence of risk enhancers. Risk enhancers include family history of premature IHD, primary hypercholesterolemia, elevated lipid biomarkers (lipoprotein(a), apolipoprotein B, VLDL, remnants), metabolic syndrome, chronic kidney disease, chronic inflammatory conditions [high-sensitivity C-reactive protein (hsCRP)], premature menopause, or high-risk ethnicity.

An important question is whether universal implementation of risk-assessment in clinical practice influences individual health behavior in primary prevention. As compliance to therapies is generally poor, both European and American guidelines emphasize clinical-patient risk discussion and shared decision-making for successful implementation. This process individualizes the therapeutic approach for a specific patient.

POLYPILLS

An important barrier for primary prevention of cardiovascular diseases is lack of lifelong adherence to drug therapies in moderate- and high-risk individuals. Fixed-

TABLE 8 Common cardiovascular risk assessment and prediction tools.

Validated for	Clinical	Imaging	Gene-based
North America	• Framingham • Reynolds • 2016 ACC/AHA	• Coronary calcium score • CT coronary angiogram • Ultrasound plaque imaging	• Gene risk score (50–150,000 SNPs) • Genome wide polygenic score
Europe	• SCORE • PROCAM • QRISK-2, QRISK-3/BHS-4	• Coronary calcium score • CT coronary angiogram • Ultrasound plaque imaging	• Gene risk score (10–150,000 SNPs) • Genome wide polygenic score
International	• WHO, GLOBORISK-2 • INTERHEART	• CT coronary angiogram • Ultrasound plaque imaging	• In development
India	• WHO • INTERHEART	• CT coronary angiogram • Ultrasound plaque imaging	• Genome wide polygenic score (India)

(SNP: single-nucleotide polymorphism)

dose combination therapy or polypills, using BP and LDL-cholesterol lowering drugs with aspirin, is an attractive strategy to promote lifelong compliance. Meta-analyses of polypill randomized controlled trials have reported significant decrease in BP and LDL cholesterol. In a systematic review of 67 trials that evaluated medication adherence, a significantly greater adherence to formulations of polypills was observed in 84%. Whether adherence to polypill leads to better cardiovascular outcomes has been studied in The International Polycap Study (TIPS-3). This is one of the first randomized trials that evaluated long-term effectiveness of a polypill on cardiovascular outcomes. In this study 5,713 participants were randomized to a polypill (ramipril, hydrochlorothiazide, atenolol, simvastatin, with or without aspirin) and followed up for 4.6 years. It was observed that those randomized to polypill alone had a significant 21% (95% CI 0–37%) lower hazard of cardiovascular outcomes while those randomized to polypill and aspirin had an even greater 31% (95% CI 3–50%) lower hazard. Implementation of this strategy requires more studies.

ADHERENCE

The final frontier for IHD prevention is sustaining lifelong adherence to a healthier lifestyle and drug therapies for all individuals. Adherence is defined as remaining attached to the medication regime and adequate adherence is use of therapies >80% of times. Studies have reported that in chronic diseases only 50% patients are adherent to therapies at 12 months and just 20% take medications in appropriate dose. Outcomes of interventions to promote adherence are limited. There is some evidence that technology-based interventions, pharmacists' level interventions, and health worker-based interventions are useful in promoting adherence and influence intermediate outcomes. Technology-based strategies to promote adherence to healthy lifestyles and drug therapy are available and given the universality of smartphone devices, the potential for this personalized approach is enormous.

PRIMORDIAL PREVENTION

The fundamental strategy to control IHD risk factors in populations is primordial prevention by addressing the political, economic, and social determinants of health (**Table 1**). This prevention strategy influences most of the proximate coronary risk factors that are focus for primary prevention. Influencing social determinants of health is not easy as our social world is complex and ever-changing.

UN-SUSTAINABLE DEVELOPMENT GOALS

The UN has promulgated 17 SDGs to address multiple social issues, WHO has added a health component to some of them (**Table 9**). We believe that every goal has potential to promote cardiovascular health. A major focus of SDGs is a health-in-all-policies approach which involves political and policy focus on disease prevention via interventions for healthcare financing, universal healthcare, urban infrastructure, agriculture, transportation, employment, sanitation, poverty, illiteracy, mother and child nutrition, smoking and tobacco, alcohol abuse, unhealthy food, physical activity, and healthy behaviors. System-wide efforts to improve the social determinants of health such as early childhood education and parenting skills, education and lifelong learning, working and employment conditions, poverty reduction, and ensuring a healthy standard of living, housing and environment are yet to take root in most countries. These population-wide interventions can favorably improve lifestyles and shift the distribution of risk factors with reduction in IHD incidence and mortality.

HEALTHCARE FINANCING

Life expectancy at birth is the highest for countries that have greater public health expenditure per capita and lowest in countries with high out-of-pocket expenditure. Healthcare financing should strive for high-quality primary, secondary, and tertiary care that is free at the point of delivery. Multiple models exist and political and bureaucratic inertia in implementation has to be overcome.

Nations with more robust and high-quality primary and secondary care systems have lower cardiovascular mortality despite a greater burden of risk factors. Universal healthcare with a focus on IHD primary prevention—health education, risk factor screening, appropriate lifestyle interventions, and treatments—can lead to changes in health behaviors in individuals and communities. Studies have reported that countries in the highest quintile of universal health coverage have lower smoking and tobacco consumption,

TABLE 9 UN sustainable development goals relevant for IHD prevention.

SDG number	SDG domain	WHO response
1	No poverty	Prioritizing the health needs of poor—smoking, unhealthy food, other factors
2	Zero hunger	Addressing the causes and consequences of all forms of malnutrition
3	Good health and well-being	Ensure healthy lives and promote well-being for all at all ages
4	Quality education	Supporting high-quality education for all to improve health and health literacy
5	Gender equality	Gender inequality in access for IHD prevention and management
8	Decent work and economic growth	Promoting health employment as a driver of inclusive economic growth
10	Reduced inequalities	Ensuring equitable access to health services through universal health coverage based on strong primary care; primary prevention

(SDG: sustainable development goal; UN: United Nations)

BP and hyperglycemia, and evidence of better risk factor control. Countries with the greatest IHD burden in absolute terms are China, India, and USA. China and USA have low while India has high out-of-pocket expenditure on health. The incidence of acute coronary events in China and USA is lower than India and the disease occurs 10 years later. System-wide interventional studies are needed to identify type of healthcare systems and healthcare financing models for cardiovascular disease prevention.

HEALTH LITERACY

Public health education, starting from schools, for adoption for healthy lifestyles and education regarding risk factors is crucial for prevention. Promotion of school-based health education has been shown to have lasting impact as healthy behaviors track into adulthood. Importance of healthy lifestyles should be emphasized and participation in outdoor activities and sports should be encouraged. In addition, intake of unhealthy foods, tobacco, alcohol, and other addictions should be continuously monitored, and remedial action should be taken.

MEDICAL EDUCATION

Change in medical school curriculum to incorporate preventive medicine in large countries, such as China and India, which have the largest IHD burden, is important. Suggested educational strategies to reorient undergraduate and postgraduate education are focused on healthy lifestyles and related domains. This could be performed using multidimensional curricula, pedagogies, technologies, and competency-based assessments. There is also a need for integrating formal learning with practical, heuristic, inquiry-driven, interprofessional, and population health management activities.

An important adjunct to change in physician education is training of nurses and allied professionals in general cardiovascular and preventive medicine and not just in specific areas such as nutrition, smoking/tobacco control, physical activity, or sports medicine. There is a need for nurses in assessment and management of hypertension, lipids, and diabetes. Education of community health workers for prevention is also important. In India and other lower income countries, where the IHD epidemic is evolving and physician shortage is widespread, task-sharing with health workers in public education, lifestyle improvement, and medication adherence can lead to better control of risk factors.

CONCLUSION

Ischemic heart disease is the most important cause of deaths globally as well as in India. In contrast to developed countries where mortality and burden is declining, it is increasing in India and other Asian countries. Primary prevention strategies should focus on multiple risk factors control with focus on healthy lifestyles (smoking/tobacco cessation, pollution control, regular physical activity, and promotion of healthy diet). Target-oriented control of BP in hypertension, LDL and non-HDL cholesterol, and glycemia in diabetes is important. Primordial prevention strategies are important to modify social determinants of health to avoid occurrence of risk factors. Improving health literacy in general population and medical literacy among medical professionals and other healthcare workers can lead to sustained long-term reduction in this disease.

RECOMMENDED READINGS

1. Arnett DK, Blumenthal RS, Albert MA, Buroker AB, Goldberger ZD, Hahn EJ, et al. 2019 ACC/AHA Guideline on the Primary Prevention of Cardiovascular Disease: A Report of the American College of Cardiology/American Heart Association Task Force on Clinical Practice Guidelines. Circulation. 2019;140(11):e596-e646.
2. Astrup A, Magkos F, Bier DM, Brenna JT, de Oliveira Otto MC, Hill JO, et al. Saturated Fats and Health: A Reassessment and Proposal for Food-Based Recommendations: JACC State-of-the-Art Review. J Am Coll Cardiol. 2020;76(7):844-57.
3. Collins DR, Tompson AC, Onakpoya IJ, Roberts N, Ward AM, Heneghan CJ. Global cardiovascular risk assessment in the primary prevention of cardiovascular disease in adults: Systematic review of systematic reviews. BMJ Open. 2017;7(3):e013650.
4. Roth GA, Mensah GA, Johnson CO, Addolorato G, Ammirati E, Baddour LM, et al. Global burden of cardiovascular diseases and risk factors, 1990–2019: Update from the GBD 2019 Study. J Am Coll Cardiol. 2020;76(25):2982-3021.
5. Gupta R, Gaur K. Epidemiology of ischemic heart disease and diabetes in South Asia: An Overview of the Twin Epidemic. Curr Diabetes Rev. 2020.
6. Gupta R, Wood DA. Primary prevention of ischaemic heart disease: populations, individuals, and health professionals. Lancet. 2019;394(10199):685-96.
7. Havranek EP, Mujahid MS, Barr DA, Blair IV, Cohen MS, Cruz-Flores S, et al. Social determinants of risk and outcomes for cardiovascular disease: A scientific statement from the American Heart Association. Circulation. 2015;132(9):873-98.
8. Musunuru K, Kathiresan S. Genetics of common, complex coronary artery disease. Cell. 2019;177(1):132-45.
9. Piepoli MF, Hoes AW, Agewall S, Albus C, Brotons C, Catapano AL, et al. 2016 European guidelines on cardiovascular disease prevention in clinical practice: The sixth joint task force of the European Society of Cardiology and other societies on cardiovascular disease prevention in clinical practice (constituted by representatives of 10 societies and by invited experts) developed with the special contribution of the European Association for Cardiovascular Prevention & Rehabilitation (EACPR). Eur Heart J. 2016;37(29):2315-81.
10. Puri R, Mehta V, Iyengar SS, Narasingan SN, Duell PB, Sattur GB, et al. Lipid Association of India Expert Consensus Statement on management of dyslipidemia in Indians 2020: Part III. J Assoc Physicians India. 2020;68(11[Special]):8-9.

11. Shah SN, Munjal YP, Kamath SA, Wander GS, Mehta N, Mukherjee S, et al. Indian guidelines on hypertension-IV (2019). J Hum Hypertens. 2020;34(11):745-58.
12. Unger T, Borghi C, Charchar F, Khan NA, Poulter NR, Prabhakaran D, et al. 2020 International Society of Hypertension global hypertension practice guidelines. J Hypertens. 2020;38(6):982-1004.
13. World Health Organization. HEARTS technical package for cardiovascular disease management in primary health care: Risk based CVD management. Geneva: World Health Organization. 2020.
14. Yusuf S, Joseph P, Rangarajan S, Islam S, Mente A, Hystad P, et al. Modifiable risk factors, cardiovascular disease, and mortality in 155 722 individuals from 21 high-income, middle-income, and low-income countries (PURE): a prospective cohort study. Lancet. 2020;395(10226):795-808.

CHAPTER 103

Hypertension: Epidemiology, Presentation, Causes, and Evaluation

Gurpreet S Wander, Sandhya Kamath

ABSTRACT

Hypertension is the most common noncommunicable disease. It effects 30% of adults >30 years. Since it remains silent the treatment and control rates are very low (10–20% in India). Due to this the hypertension-mediated organ damage (HMOD) occurs in the heart, kidneys, brain, eyes, and blood vessels. Most cases are due to environmental factors over a polygenic genetic predilection. There is no known cause, and it is called essential or primary hypertension. The autonomic nervous system (ANS) and renin–angiotensin–aldosterone system (RAAS) are involved in the pathogenesis of primary hypertension.

In 5–10% cases a known cause can be found (secondary hypertension) and treated. Secondary hypertension is uncommon and so most patients do not need detailed investigations.

Diagnosis and classification of blood pressure (BP) into stages is done based on multiple recordings since it is labile and often high readings are recorded when done in haste. The office BP recordings should be done in a quiet room after the patient has rested. Home BP recordings are useful for diagnosis and follow-up of patients.

Public education to improve compliance and better control of BP can make a major impact on reducing the incidence of atherosclerotic cardiovascular disease (ASCVD).

"One accurate measurement is worth a thousand expert opinions"

—Grace Hopper

INTRODUCTION AND PREVALENCE

Hypertension is the most common public health problem. Its prevalence is 28% in India, among adults more than 30 years. Prevalence is little less in rural than in urban areas. The global burden of disease (GBD) study has shown that while in 1990 it was responsible for 8% of all deaths, in 2017 it caused 16% of all deaths in India. Hypertension affects 1.13 billion people in the world, out of these 25 crores are from India. The BP continues to increase with age and in those ≥65 years, the prevalence is approximately 60%.

It is responsible for 50% of strokes and 25% of ischemic heart disease as it is a major risk factor for both. The problem is not only its prevalence but also that it often remains silent. It often remains undiagnosed for years and causes target organ damage (TOD). The awareness, treatment, and control rates of BP in India and USA are shown in **Table 1**. Public education is required to increase the awareness and control rates of hypertension.

Increased salt intake, obesity, smoking, sedentary lifestyle, and stress, all increase its prevalence. In India there has been a steady increase in its prevalence in last three decades. The special features of hypertension in Indians are shown in **Box 1**.

DEFINITION AND CLASSIFICATION

The latest Indian guidelines on hypertension (IGH-IV 2019) have defined hypertension as a pressure of ≥140/90 mm Hg. The European Society of Hypertension (ESH) and International Society of Hypertension (ISH) guidelines also use the same cut off level. The latest American College of Cardiology/American Heart Association (ACC/AHA) guidelines have defined a pressure of ≥130/80 mm Hg

TABLE 1	Awareness treatment and control rates of BP in India and USA.		
	USA	Urban India	Rural India
Awareness	81%	42%	25%
Treatment	74%	38%	25%
Control	53%	20%	11%

BOX 1 Special features of hypertension in India.

- Onset early in life
- Rising average BP of the general population
- Rural urban divide in prevalence
- Low awareness, treatment, and control rates
- Clustering of multiple CV risk factors
- Significant seasonal variation of BP
- Early HMOD—possibly due to poor control

(HMOD: hypertension-mediated organ damage)

TABLE 2	Classification of blood pressure for adults.		
Category	Systolic (mm Hg)		Diastolic (mm Hg)
Optimal	<120	and	<80
Normal	<130	and	<85
High-normal	130–139	or	85–89
Hypertension			
Stage 1	140–159	or	90–99
Stage 2	160–179	or	100–109
Stage 3	≥180	or	>110
Isolated systolic hypertension			
Grade 1	140–159	and	<90
Grade 2	>160	and	<90

as hypertension. However, this cut off level is not used in other parts of the world.

Within the normal range also, the BP is subclassified further. The stages of hypertension as mentioned in the Indian hypertension guidelines are shown in the **Table 2**. Systolic hypertension is more harmful than the diastolic. As we age the systolic hypertension becomes more important. The elderly often has isolated systolic hypertension.

MEASUREMENT

Blood pressure has been traditionally measured in the "**office**" **or** "**clinic**" for outpatients. The *mercury sphygmomanometer* was the first one to be developed by Riva Rocci in 1896. The mercury level is raised with the cuff applied on the upper arm. Initially palpation is done, till the pulse disappears and this indicates the systolic pressure. This is done to pick up the "auscultatory gap" (the Korotkoff sounds disappear for a gap of 15–20 mm Hg after they appear at the systolic pressure) which may be present in some. Then with a stethoscope on the brachial artery the cuff pressure is reduced and the five stages of Korotkoff sounds are heard. The pressure when the sounds appear is the systolic and the disappearance of sounds gives the diastolic pressure. These apparatuses are robust and reliable. However now, due to the environmental side effects of mercury the WHO has decided to do away with the mercury apparatus by 2025 from the world. Many countries have stopped its use for the last 10–15 years.

The other apparatus for manual BP recording is the "*aneroid sphygmomanometer*" which is usually in the form of a circular dial. It has a spring pressure gauge. There are no ecological issues since mercury is not being used here. However, they need 6 monthly calibration since the spring gets loose after some time.

The third one is the "*Oscillometric BP apparatus.*" This is being used most commonly now across the world. It is an automatic device which when applied raises the cuff pressure automatically and then by a company-specific algorithm gives the systolic and diastolic BP. This actually measures the mean BP and the systolic/diastolic pressures are derived. These devices are reliable, and so are used most commonly for office BP recording.

More recently an automatic office blood pressure (AOBP) apparatus has been used in the large SPRINT (Systolic blood PRessure INtervention Trial). This measures BP after a gap of 1–3 minutes. Mostly the recording is done unattended by the doctor in a quiet room. This is more reliable and corresponds to the daytime BP more closely. These devices are more expensive.

Since the office BP is recorded manually by the doctor, the patients have anxiety and higher pressures are recorded in some. This is known as "white coat hypertension." It needs to be recognized since we will be treating many patients unnecessarily.

The **Home BP Monitoring (HBPM)** is being relied upon and most guidelines advocate both for diagnosis and follow-up. It is a self-recording of the BP by the patient at home with the oscillometric devices. These are inexpensive and record the BP at home. The techniques of BP recording, posture of the patient, and other precautions to be taken for BP recording in the office and at home are shown in **Figure 1**.

The ambulatory blood pressure monitoring (ABPM) can be done with an equipment which is applied for 24 hours. It repeats readings every 30 minutes and, in the end, gives multiple readings during sleep, early morning, day, and night. This helps to pick up the "early morning surge" of BP which correlates with the increased stroke and coronary events in early morning. It also picks up the "nondippers," those who do not show the usual night-time decrease in BP of 10–20%. The nondippers are also at increased risk of TOD. The ABPM is indicated in resistant hypertension and especially when there is a disparity between home BP and office BP readings. BP readings in office and home settings may sometimes show a disparity.

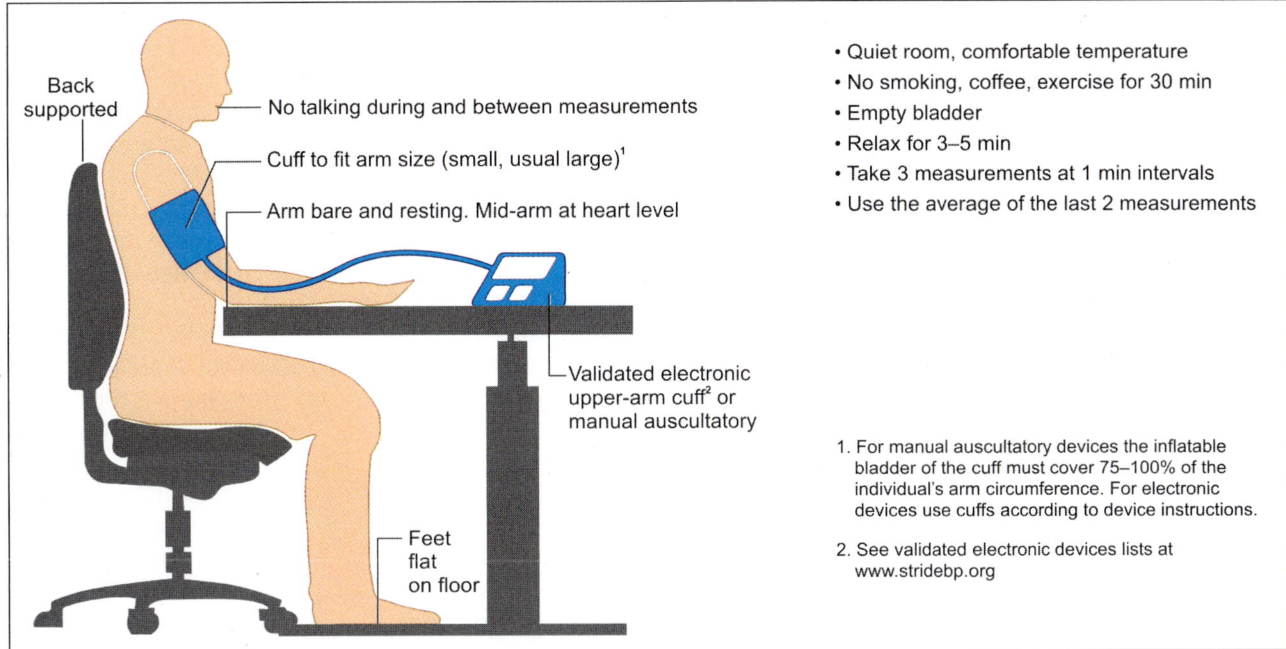

FIGURE 1: Correct technique for measurement of blood pressure with the oscillometric device.

True normotension (Normal home and office BP)	**Sustained hypertension** (High home and high office BP)
White coat hypertension (Normal home and high office BP)	**Masked hypertension** (High home and normal office BP)

FIGURE 2: Patterns of blood pressure (BP) based on office and home BP readings.

The masked hypertension and white coat hypertension are diagnosed on this basis. Their definitions are shown in **Figure 2**.

PATHOGENESIS

Most cases of hypertension are idiopathic or "primary hypertension." When a known cause is there hypertension is called secondary hypertension. Secondary hypertension constitutes approximately 7–10% of the total cases. The pathophysiology and mechanisms involved in primary hypertension are numerated in **Box 2** and discussed here.

BOX 2 Special features of hypertension in India.

- Hereditary and genetic factors
- Environmental and lifestyle factors
- Autonomic nervous system (ANS)
- Renin–angiotensin–aldosterone system (RAAS)
- Vascular mechanisms
- Intravascular volume
- Hemodynamic mechanisms

HEREDITARY AND GENETIC FACTORS

Hypertension is a polygenic disorder. There is a significant heritable component along with the environmental factors. Family studies has shown a 30–40% heritability. Genome-wide association studies (GWAS) have identified multiple genes that presently account for 1% of hypertension cases. More linked genes will be identified in future.

The epigenetic changes in deoxyribonucleic acid (DNA) provide the link between the environment and genetics. Epigenetics implies change in gene expression without any change in the DNA sequence. The environment causes changes in epigenome and not in the DNA sequence. Epigenetic dysregulation is the link between environment and genetics for multiple lifestyle diseases. There is also a genetic predilection for TOD [left ventricular hypertrophy (LVH) and nephropathy].

ENVIRONMENTAL AND LIFESTYLE FACTORS

Increased salt intake is an important risk factor for hypertension. It increases the age-related increase in BP. Low dietary calcium and potassium intake may also contribute. Obesity and overweight are independently related to hypertension. Reduced physical activity and psychological stress are other lifestyle factors. Environmental pollution, especially PM2.5 particulate level in the air, correlate with increased prevalence of hypertension and other noncommunicable diseases. Increased alcohol consumption is also important. These environmental and lifestyle factors contribute significantly toward development of hypertension.

AUTONOMIC NERVOUS SYSTEM

The adrenergic reflexes cause the short-term fluctuations in BP and the adrenergic tone and functions control BP on the long-term along with blood volume and RAAS system. The adrenergic hormones involved are norepinephrine, epinephrine, and dopamine. The adrenergic receptors are "α" and "β" receptors. The a receptors are activated more by norepinephrine and β receptors more by epinephrine. α_1 receptors are located in postsynaptic cells in smooth muscles and cause vasoconstriction. The α_2 receptors are located in presystolic membranes and by negative feedback cause inhibition of norepinephrine release. Drugs that inhibit α_1 receptors and agonists of α_2 receptors reduce BP. Prazosin and doxazosin are α_1 receptor blockers and reduce vascular tone. Clonidine is a central α_2 agonist and inhibits sympathetic outflow and so reduces pressure. β_1 receptors increase the rate and strength of cardiac contraction. β_2 receptor activation by epinephrine causes vasodilation.

The stretch sensitive baroreflexes are located in carotid sinus and aortic arch. These baroreflexes smoothen the fluctuations in BP, as occur during change in posture. Patients of autonomous neuropathy have very labile BPs and also postural hypotension.

There is increased sympathetic outflow in hypertension, specifically in obese and in obstructive sleep apnea (OSA) patients. Pheochromocytoma is the best example of hypertension due to excess catecholamines. Antisympathetic drugs (beta-blockers, α_1-blockers, and α_2-agonists) act as antihypertensive agents. Labetalol is an alpha and beta-blocker.

RENIN–ANGIOTENSIN–ALDOSTERONE SYSTEM

The RAAS and its participating hormones and their actions are shown in the **Flowchart 1**. The RAAS along with ANS is involved in the pathogenesis of hypertension and heart failure. The two systems are interlinked. Angiotensin-II is the most potent vasoconstrictor. The angiotensin-converting enzyme (ACE) inhibitors and the angiotensin receptor blockers (ARBs) are antihypertensive agents which are also used in heart failure. Since they act on the same system their actions are similar and are not used in combination. The ACE inhibitors also affect the bradykinin levels and so have a side effect of cough which is not seen with ARBs. Both these agents also have antiatherosclerotic effects and are used in individuals with high risk of ASCVD also.

Renin secretion depends on a feedback mechanism. Decreased renal perfusion causes an increase in renin secretion. Besides the systemic RAAS there is a local tissue angiotensin-II system also that augments atherosclerosis, cardiac hypertrophy, and renal failure.

Aldosterone is a mineralocorticoid. Even these receptors are present in various tissues and induce local structural and functional changes in the heart, kidneys, and blood vessels and cause myocardial fibrosis, nephrosclerosis, and vascular inflammation.

Aldosterone antagonists are used in resistant hypertension. These can be combined with ACE inhibitors or ARBs. However, the incidence of hyperkalemia is increased when they are used in combination and potassium needs to be monitored periodically.

VASCULAR MECHANISMS

Blood pressure depends on the structure and vascular tone of resistance arteries. Resistance to flow is inversely related to the fourth power of decrease in radius. Increased hypertrophy and reduced elasticity of vessels cause increase in pressure. Aging-related increased stiffness reduces the ability to accommodate flow. There is flow-related greater increase in pressure.

Ejection of blood in aorta generates a "pressure wave" (the percussion wave) which moves at a velocity. This generates "reflected waves" which travel toward aorta. The

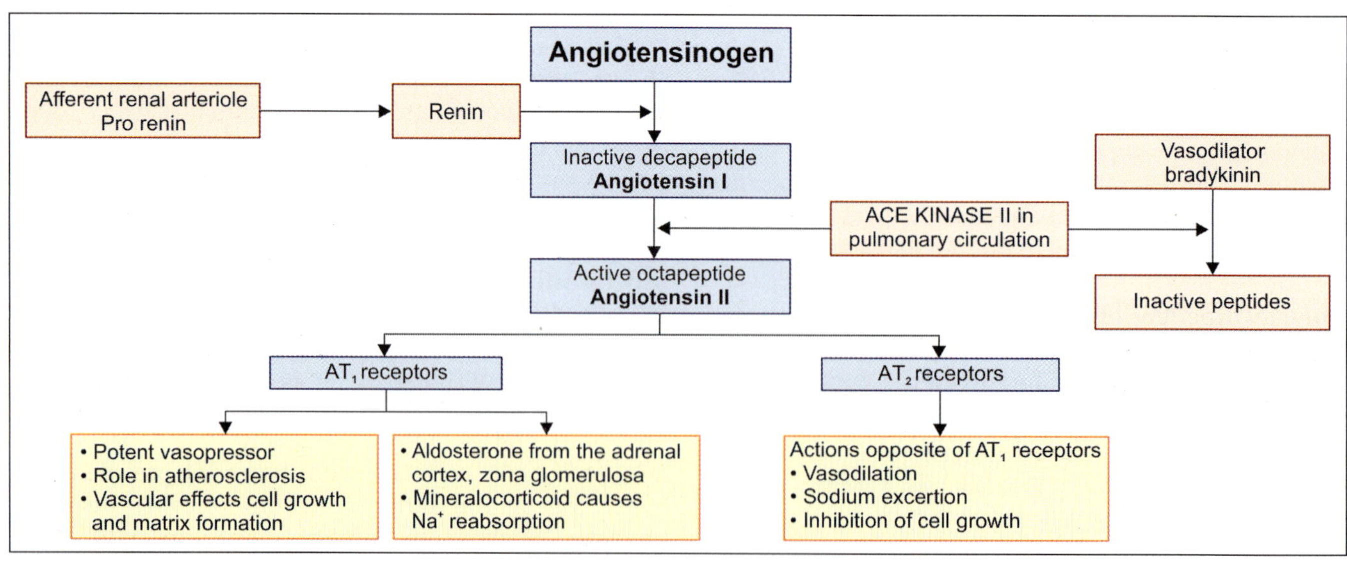

(ACE: angiotensin-converting enzyme; AT: angiotensin)

FLOWCHART 1: Mediators of renin–angiotensin–aldosterone system with their source and actions.

pulse pressure (difference between systolic and diastolic pressure) depends on the character of the vessel wall which determines the velocity of these waves. Increased stiffness causes increased pulse wave velocity and summation of both these waves causes a greater augmentation index and pulse pressure. The pulse wave velocity can be measured between the carotid and femoral arteries and is an index of arterial stiffness. Central aortic blood pressure (CABP) is often lower than the BP we measure from the brachial artery. It correlates better with the TOD. Some beta-blockers do not reduce the CABP as much as other antihypertensive agents. Hence, they are less effective in reducing TOD.

The vascular tone also depends on hormones released from the endothelium. Nitric oxide is a potent vasodilator release by endothelium. Endothelin is a potent vasoconstrictor peptide produced by the endothelin. Thus, vascular factors of structure, stiffness, tone, and locally released peptides all play a role in hypertension. Their cause-and-effect relationship is being evaluated as they are all interlinked.

HEMODYNAMIC MECHANISMS

The arterial BP depends on two factors, the peripheral resistance and blood volume. The cardiac output is a multiple of heart rate and stroke volume (blood ejected per beat). The peripheral resistance depends on the vascular bed structure, tone, and reactivity. The RAAS system and the ANS affect the vascular tone, heart rate, and stroke volume. The vascular mechanisms (stiffness and reactivity) depend on the aging process besides the RAAS and the ANS. Hypertension in younger patients (≤60 years) is associated with increased RAAS and sympathetic activity. The elderly (≥60 years) have a volume-dependent hypertension. This has implications on the choice of antihypertensive agents.

The above-mentioned mechanisms play a variable role in different patients. These are all interlinked and each one effects the other. They have a cumulative and cascading effect. Some of these factors play a role in cases of secondary hypertension also when there is a known cause.

BOX 3 Causes of secondary hypertension.

Renal causes

- Parenchymal: Glomerulonephritis, pyelonephritis, chronic renal failure, polycystic kidney disease, renal tumors, and obstructive uropathy
- Renovascular: Atherosclerosis, fibromuscular dysplasia, and aortoarteritis

Endocrine causes

- Adrenal:
  - Conn's syndrome (excess mineralocorticoid)
  - Medullary: Pheochromocytoma (excess catecholamines)
  - Cortex: Cushing's syndrome
- Thyroid: Hyperthyroidism and hypothyroidism
- Pituitary: Acromegaly
- Hyperparathyroidism

Neurological

- Psychogenic, porphyria, polyneuritis, lead poisoning, and raised intracranial pressure

Medications and external agents

- Oral contraceptive pills (OCP), steroids, nonsteroidal anti-inflammatory drugs (NSAIDs), cyclosporine, erythropoietin, appetite suppressants, tricyclic antidepressants (TCA), monoamine oxidase (MAO) inhibitors, and amphetamine cocaine
- Heavy metals (arsenic, lead), herbal products (yohimbine, St John's wort, and ephedra)

Single gene defects

- Glucocorticoids remedial hyperaldosteronism, Liddle syndrome, and pseudohypoaldosteronism (Gordon's syndrome)

Obstructive sleep apnea

SECONDARY HYPERTENSION

Although secondary hypertension is uncommon, it should always be kept in mind since the cause can be treatable. It is suspected when hypertension onset occurs at extremes of ages (≤30 years or ≥60 years), resistant hypertension, severe hypertension, or hypertension with symptoms indicative of a cause is present. The causes of secondary hypertension are given in **Box 3**.

Renal causes:

Renal parenchymal: There is a cause-and-effect relationship. Hypertension causes nephrosclerosis and thus causes renal damage and chronic renal failure (CRF). Hypertension is present in 80% cases of CRF. It is seen more in glomerular then in interstitial disease. The hypertension is more difficult to treat in patients with CRF.

Renovascular: Atherosclerosis causes renovascular hypertension in elderly (≥60 years) due to plaques at the origin of the renal arteries. Fibromuscular dysplasia occurs in young, more in women and affects distal part of the renal arteries in a beaded appearance. Aortoarteritis often causes hypertension and at times due to renal artery stenosis. Renal angioplasty with stenting was done earlier in renovascular hypertension. Recently two large trials the ASTRAL (Angioplasty and STenting for Renal Artery Lesions) study in 2009 and the CORAL (Cardiovascular Outcomes in Renal Atherosclerotic Lesions) study in 2014 have shown that medical therapy is as good as intervention in patients with renal artery stenosis. Hence, angioplasty is now done only in patients with bilateral renal artery stenosis who present with "flash pulmonary edema."

Endocrine causes: Two important endocrine causes of secondary hypertension are primary aldosteronism (PA) and pheochromocytoma. Others are Cushing syndrome and thyroid disorders.

Primary aldosteronism: It is a more common condition than it is being suspected. It is seen in the third to fifth decade. Patients have hypokalemic alkalosis with polyuria, polydipsia, and glucose intolerance in some. In a hypertensive patient with unprovoked hypokalemia or potassium level of ≤3.1 mmol/L even while on diuretics one should suspect PA.

The diagnosis is made on the basis of a plasma aldosterone to plasma renin activity (PRA) of ≥30:1 and plasma aldosterone levels of ≥20 mg/dL. When both these conditions are present, there is a 90% probability of primary aldosteronism. The two common causes of PA are aldosterone-producing adenoma and bilateral adrenal hyperplasia (idiopathic hyperaldosteronism). The adrenal adenomas are usually unilateral and are ≤3 cm in diameter. These can be picked up on adrenal computed tomography. Treatment is unilateral surgical adrenalectomy by laparoscopy. It cures hypertension in 60–70% patients. Patients with bilateral adrenal hyperplasia are treated medically with aldosterone antagonists.

Pheochromocytoma: Catecholamine-secreting tumors are located in adrenal medulla. Although an uncommon cause, it should not be missed since it is potentially curable with surgery. Hypertension is severe and resistance. There is wide fluctuation of BP with episodic rise and accelerated phases. Patients have palpitations, weight loss, and postural symptoms. 10% of pheochromocytomas are bilateral, 10% are malignant, 10% are extra adrenal, and 10% are familial (rule of 10% to remember). Sometimes it may be a part of syndromes like multiple endocrine neoplasia (MEN) type 2A or 2B. It is also associated with neurofibromatosis type 1 and Von Hippel–Lindau syndrome (renal angiomas, cerebral and spinal hemangioblastomas). The diagnosis is made based on 24-hour metanephrine levels in blood and urine. When elevated it raises a biochemical suspicion. The 24-hour urinary vanillylmandelic acid (VMA) levels are done less often now.

The pheochromocytomas can be localized on abdomen CT scan or a radionuclear MIBG (meta-iodobenzylguanidine) scan. The definite treatment is surgical removal of tumors. It needs surgical expertise and experience since complications can occur during surgery while handling the tumor. Patient are pretreated with alpha receptor antagonist phentolamine for 1–2 weeks and then beta-blockers are added for control of BP before surgery.

Other causes: *Obstructive sleep apnea* is an important cause of resistant hypertension. Weight loss helps to relieve both hypertension and sleep apnea. Use of continuous positive airway pressure (CPAP) also helps in better control of hypertension in these patients.

In some patient's hypertension may be due to *single gene defects*, although these are infrequent. Glucocorticoids remedial hyperaldosteronism is an autosomal dominant condition. Liddle syndrome is also an autosomal dominant condition with hypokalemia, low renin, and low aldosterone. Pseudohypoaldosteronism (Gordon's syndrome), another autosomal dominant condition, has hyperkalemia with normal glomerular filtration rate (GFR). These rare genetic disorders have definite gene linkages that are defined.

Drugs are an important cause of secondary hypertension and need to be kept in mind in patients with resistant hypertension. Sometimes withdrawal of these agents results in better control of BP with the same antihypertensive agents.

TABLE 3	Target organ damage due to hypertension.
Heart	Left ventricular hypertrophy, atrial fibrillation, coronary artery disease, acute coronary events, diastolic dysfunction, HFnEF, and HFrEF
Brain	Transient ischemic attacks, occlusive stroke, hemorrhagic stroke, vascular dementia, and hypertensive encephalopathy
Kidneys	Benign nephrosclerosis and chronic renal failure
Blood vessels	Aortic aneurysms, dissection
Eyes	Hypertensive retinopathy with exudates and hemorrhages, papilledema

TARGET ORGAN DAMAGE

Hypertension is usually silent and causes very little symptoms. It is treated since it causes long-term damage to various organs including the heart, kidneys, brain, eyes, and the peripheral vessels. Acute elevation of BP when beyond 200/120 mm Hg is known as accelerated hypertension. It can push patients into acute pulmonary edema, acute coronary syndrome, hemorrhagic stroke, and can cause aortic dissection. In the eyes it can cause papilledema when it is called "malignant hypertension."

The TOD generally occurs slowly over years and is seen in those with uncontrolled hypertension. In those with treated and controlled BP the target organs damage can be avoided. The terms TOD and HMOD are used interchangeably. **Table 3** shows the various target organs and the complications that occur.

Heart: Due to increased afterload LVH occurs over time. It is a marker of increased risk. LVH increases the risk of atrial fibrillation. The most common cause of atrial fibrillation in adults is hypertension. With increasing LVH, diastolic dysfunction sets in. It can be picked up on echocardiography by increased left ventricular (LV) mass, left atrial dilatation, and abnormal LV filling pattern on Doppler. Patients with increasing diastolic dysfunction start having dyspnea due to rise in left atrial pressure. Heart failure with normal ejection fraction (HFnEF) is diagnosed when patient have dyspnea, raised brain natriuretic peptide (BNP) levels, and normal ejection fraction on echo. Still later, they develop heart failure with reduced ejection fraction (HFrEF) when the LV dilates, and its contractility is reduced (evidenced by reduced EF).

Hypertension is a major risk factor for atherosclerosis. The ASCVD is increased in long-standing hypertension. Thus, the heart is affected in multiple ways if BP is not controlled.

Brain: Hypertension increases the risk of occlusive and hemorrhagic stroke. Stroke is the second most common cause of death after coronary artery disease. Up to 80% of strokes are ischemic and 20% are hemorrhagic. About 50% of strokes are due to hypertension. Good control of BP reduces the risk of stroke.

Sudden acute elevation of BP can result in failure of autoregulation of the cerebral blood flow and causes vasodilation and hyperperfusion. This can cause hypertensive encephalopathy, characterized with headache and vomiting. Later patient can get comatose, and it can even be fatal.

Long-standing hypertension has been linked with cognitive impairment and dementia in later life. This is due to beta amyloid deposition in hypertension. The other mechanism is multiple lacunar infarcts causing subcortical white matter ischemia.

Kidneys: Hypertension when long-standing causes a graded damage to the kidney resulting initially in albuminuria, reduced GFR, and subsequently end-stage renal failure. Microalbuminuria (urine albumin-creatinine ratio of 30–300 mg/g) and then macroalbuminuria (albumin-creatinine ratio ≥300 mg/g) are markers of kidney injury. They also correlate with cardiovascular complications.

The preglomerular arterioles are affected by vascular damage due to hypertension. Atherosclerosis also contributes to the development of ischemic changes in glomeruli. The autoregulation fails in afferent arteriole, exposing glomerulus to increased pressure. This causes hyperfiltration, hypertrophy, and focal glomerular sclerosis. The glomerulosclerosis progresses to involve the renal tubules which also become ischemic and sclerotic later.

During acute elevations in malignant hypertension, fibrinoid necrosis of afferent arterioles can cause renal damage.

Blood vessels: Hypertension is related to development of atherosclerosis in the aorta and aortic aneurysms. Subsequently aortic regurgitation can occur. Aortic dissection is seen more often in hypertensives. Vascular disease in the peripheral arteries presents with intermittent claudication. It is more common in diabetes and smokers.

Eyes: Fundus examination should be done in all hypertensive patients. The eye blood vessels are a reflection of arterioles in other parts of the body. Long-standing hypertension results in significant changes in the retinal arteries. These changes can be graded by the Keith and Wegner classification as shown in **Box 4**.

All these above-mentioned end-organ effects in hypertension are known as HMOD. These can be picked up early with the required investigations pertaining to the organ. When frank complications of hypertension occur in the form of stroke, myocardial infarction, renal failure, or retinal hemorrhages these are known as associated clinical conditions (ACC). The presence of these complications places the patient in a very high-risk category. Our effort should be to manage hypertension effectively, before the HMOD and ACCs occur.

BOX 4 Grading of retinal changes in hypertension as seen with fundus examination.

Keith and Wegner Grading

- **Grade 1:** Tortuosity (twisting) of retinal arteries with increased reflectiveness (silver wiring)
- **Grade 2:** Grade 1 + arteriovenous napping (thickened retinal arteries pass over retinal veins)
- **Grade 3:** Grade 2 + flamed shape hemorrhage and cotton wool exudates (due to small infarct)
- **Grade 4:** Grade 3 + papilledema (blurry margin of the optic disc due to swelling)

RECOMMENDED READINGS

1. Williams B, Mancia G, Spiering W, Agabiti Rosei E, Azizi M, Burnier M, et al. 2018 ESC/ESH Guidelines for the management of arterial hypertension. Eur Heart J. 2018;39(33):3021-104.
2. Whelton PK, Carey RM, Aronow WS, Casey DE Jr, Collins KJ, Dennison Himmelfarb C, et al. 2017 ACC/AHA/AAPA/ABC/ACPM/AGS/ APhA/ASH/ASPC/NMA/PCNA Guideline for the Prevention, Detection, Evaluation, and Management of High Blood Pressure in Adults. J Am Coll Cardiol. 2018;71(19): 2199-269.
3. Shah SN, Munjal YP, Kamath SA, Wander GS, Mehta N, Mukherjee S, et al. Indian guidelines on hypertension-IV (2019). J Hum Hypertens. 2020;34(11):745-58.
4. Wander GS, Ram CV. Blood Pressure-Methods to record & numbers that are significant: let's make a tailored suit to suit us. Indian J Med Res. 2018;147:435.
5. Kaul U, Wander GS, Sinha N, Mohan JC, Kumar S, Dani S, et al. Self-blood pressure measurement as compared to office blood pressure measurement in a large Indian population; the India Heart Study. J Hypertens. 2020;38(7):1262-70.
6. Mohan B, Kumar N, Aslam N, Rangbulla A, Kumbkarni S, Sood NK, et al. Prevalence of Sustained Hypertension and Obesity in Urban and Rural School Going Children in Ludhiana. Indian Heart J. 2004;56 :310-4.
7. Mohan B, Verma A, Singh K, Singh K, Sharma S, Bansal R, et al. Prevalence of sustained hypertension and obesity among urban and rural adolescents: a school-based, cross-sectional study in North India. BMJ Open. 2019;9(9):e027134.
8. Mohan B, Aslam N, Ralhan U, Sharma S, Gupta N, Singh VP, et al. Office blood pressure measurement practices among community health providers (medical and paramedical) in northern district of India. Indian Heart J. 2014;66(4):401-7.
9. Goyal A, Kahlon P, Jain D, Soni RK, Gulati R, Chhabra ST, et al. Trend in prevalence of coronary artery disease and risk factors over two decades in rural Punjab. Heart Asia. 2017;9(2):e010938.

CHAPTER

104 Management of Hypertension

Gurpreet S Wander, YP Munjal

ABSTRACT

The initial management involves confirmation of blood pressure with multiple readings taken in the office and at home. Evaluation is based on good history and some basic investigations in most. Overall assessment of patient includes presence of other risk factors, target organ effects and to rule out secondary causes. Patient compliance is very important. Counseling should be done, and patients made to participate in the treatment.

Lifestyle modifications can help reduce pressure and are supplementary to the drug treatment. Many pharmacological agents with different mechanisms of action are available. Long-acting agents in combination should be used dependently on the physician's experience. The most commonly used combination is an angiotensin-converting enzyme (ACE) inhibitor or angiotensin receptor blocker (ARB) with a calcium channel blocker (CCB). The target blood pressure to be achieved is 130–140/70–80 mm Hg. Good control results in greater reduction in hypertension-mediated organ damage (HMOD). The patients often have other risk factors and concomitant diseases. These can affect the choice of agent to be used. The approach is to control the blood pressure to the target levels with low pill burden (using fixed dose combinations) while maintaining good quality of life. The overall risk of the patient should be reduced along with the control of pressure. Good compliance and follow up are important since therapy is generally lifelong.

"We can't change what we are not aware of, and once we are aware, we can't help but change"

—Sheryl Sandberg

INTRODUCTION

Treatment of hypertension involves accurate measurement of blood pressure, assessment of the comorbidities, evaluation for complications, and looking for any secondary cause. It is important to know the pressure and the patient. Comprehensive management is to bring the pressure down to the target blood pressure, make the patient feel better, and to reduce the overall risk of the patient. Patients need to understand that lifestyle modification is an important component of the management and drug therapy will usually be lifelong.

CLINICAL EVALUATION

Accurate and reliable measurement of blood pressure is most important. The technique is simple but should not be done in a crowded outpatient with haste. All due precautions for blood pressure recording should be adhered to. At times we need multiple readings in office and have to make an overall assessment of the pressure. Detailed clinical evaluation and some basic baseline investigations should be done in all. Further investigations are done only when there are clinical pointers.

The overall risk assessment of the patient should be done. This includes looking for the other risk factors, HMOD and the associated clinical conditions (ACCs) which are the complications due to hypertension. The factors that are associated with the increased risk of these patients are summarized in **Table 1**. The risk stratification into low risk, medium, high, and very high risk is done based on the above-mentioned factors and is shown in **Table 2**.

Risk assessment scales are available in other countries, like the atherosclerotic cardiovascular disease (ASCVD) risk score in USA. The SCORE risk for Europeans. The Framingham risk score is one of the oldest. The major factors that are included in the scoring systems are age, sex, diabetes, lipids, and the level of systolic blood pressure. These scores highlight the value of these five factors in increasing the risk of an individual.

Symptoms and signs: Hypertension often causes minimal symptoms and unless checked it can remain undiagnosed for years. Symptoms, when present, may be headache and vertigo. History of smoking, alcohol use, and other drug intake is important. Symptoms of episodic palpitations and surges in pressure can point toward pheochromocytoma. Ask for history of renal disease, gout, and diabetes as these are common associations. History of response to prior drug treatment can be helpful.

EXAMINATION

Blood pressure should be recorded in both arms. A difference of 10 mm Hg may be normal. The arm with the higher pressure is taken as the true pressure. All pulses should be felt since atherosclerotic disease, aortoarteritis,

TABLE 1 Factors that determine the risk of an individual who is hypertensive.

Risk factors (RF) for coronary artery disease	Hypertension-mediated organ damage (HMOD)	Associated clinical conditions (ACCs)
• Age >55 years • Male sex • Smoking and tobacco use • Diabetes mellitus • Family history of premature CAD • Increased waist: Hip ratio • Obesity and obstructive sleep apnea (OSA) • High LDL or total cholesterol • Low HDL and high triglycerides • Estimated GFR	• Left ventricular hypertrophy detected by ECG and/or echocardiogram • Microalbuminuria/proteinuria and/or elevation of serum creatinine (1.2–2.0 mg/dL) • Urinary ACR (albumin creatinine ratio) increased • Ultrasound or radiological evidence of atherosclerotic plaques in the carotids • Hypertensive retinopathy • Ankle brachial index (<0.9)	• Cerebrovascular disease: ∘ Ischemic stroke ∘ Cerebral hemorrhage • Heart disease: ∘ CAD ∘ Atrial fibrillation ∘ Congestive heart failure • Renal disease: ∘ Renal failure (serum creatinine >2.0 mg/dL) • Vascular disease: ∘ Peripheral arterial disease ∘ Aortic dissection • Advanced hypertensive retinopathy: ∘ Papilledema

TABLE 2 Risk stratification of patients with hypertension.

Stages	Risk factors and disease	Stage 1 140–159/90–99	Stage 2 160–179/100–109	Stage 3 >180/>110
I	No other risk factors	Low risk	Medium risk	High risk
II	1–2 risk factors	Medium risk	Medium risk	Very high risk
III	3 or more risk factors or HMOD	High risk	High risk	Very high risk
IV	ACCs	Very high risk	Very high risk	Very high risk

(ACC: associated clinical conditions; HMOD: hypertension-mediated organ damage)

and coarctation of aorta can have disparity in pulses. Kidneys may be palpable in polycystic kidney disease. Renal bruit may be audible in the back at the renal angle in renal artery stenosis. Arcus senilis in the cornea may indicates dyslipidemia. Ankle brachial index of ≤0.9 indicates peripheral vascular disease. The fundus should be examined for hypertensive retinopathy.

INVESTIGATIONS

There are some investigations which should be done in every patients with hypertension; additional investigations are done when there is a clinical indication. These are shown in **Box 1**.

BOX 1 Laboratory investigations.

- **Routine**
  - Urine examination for protein and glucose and microscopic examination for red blood cells (RBCs) and other sediments
  - Hemoglobin, fasting blood glucose, serum creatinine, potassium, and total cholesterol
  - 12-lead electrocardiogram
- **Additional investigations in special circumstances**
  - Fasting lipid profile and uric acid
  - Urine albumin creatinine ratio
  - Echocardiogram
  - Ultrasound of abdomen
- **Other specific tests to rule out secondary causes**

TREATMENT

The goal of treatment is to control the blood pressure to target blood pressure whenever, it is above the threshold level of 140/90 mm Hg. The effort is to control blood pressure to normal range without causing any side effects. Patients with stage II and III hypertension need to be started on treatment at the first visit with multiple readings or within a week. In patients with stage I hypertension we can try nonpharmacological treatment for 4–6 weeks. In case pressure remains high then drugs are started.

NONPHARMACOLOGICAL TREATMENT

The nonpharmacological treatment is the initial therapy and has to be continued along with the pharmacological therapy for lifelong period. Lifestyle modification helps to control blood pressure and reduce complications. Patients need to be emphasized the value of these changes. The various lifestyle interventions for control of blood pressure are summarized in **Table 3**.

TABLE 3 Lifestyle interventions for blood pressure reduction.

Intervention	Recommendation	Expected SBP reduction (range)
Weight reduction	Maintain ideal BMI (20–25 kg/m^2)	5–20 mm Hg per 10 kg weight loss
DASH eating plan	Eat diet rich in fruits, vegetables, low-fat dairy products. Eat less saturated and total fat	8–14 mm Hg
Dietary sodium restriction	Reduce dietary sodium intake to <100 mmol/day <2.4 g sodium or <6 g salt (sodium chloride)	2–8 mm Hg
Physical activity	Regular aerobic physical activity, e.g., brisk walking for at least 30 minutes on most days	4–8 mm Hg
Alcohol moderation	Total abstinence preferred and recommended. If must then MEN ≤20 units per week, Women ≤14 units per week	4–8 mm Hg
Tobacco	Total abstinence	4–8 mm Hg

(DASH: dietary approaches to stop hypertension)

TABLE 4 Sodium content of foods per 100 g-common Indian diets.

<25 mg Low		25–50 mg Moderate	≥50 mg High
• Bitter gourd (*Karela*) • Bottle gourd (*Laukee*) • Brinjal (*Baingan*) • Cabbage • Lady finger (*Bhindi*) • French beans • Peas • Onion • Tomato ripe	• Cow pea (*Lobiya*) • Vermicelli (*Saviyan*) • Wheat • Milk • Grapes • Papaya • Orange • Sapota (*Chikoo*)	• Raisins • Carrots • Black gram (*Urad*) dal • Green gram (*Moth*) dal • Red gram (*Arhar*) dal • Bengal gram (*Chana*) • Banana • Apple	• Cauliflower • Fenugreek (*Methi*) • Lettuce (*Salad patta*) • Beetroot • Water melon • Prawns • Chicken • Amaranth (*Rajgira*) • Bacon • Egg

Weight reduction is a very important component of lifestyle change. Excess salt intake results in hypertension. Total daily intake should be ≤6 g (3–4 g of sodium). An ICMR (Indian Council of Medical Research) study shows that we consume 10–12 g/day of salt in India. The salt content of commonly used food items in India is shown in **Table 4**. Food items with high-salt content that need to be avoided in hypertension, so as to reduce the overall risk are given in **Table 5**. Vegetarians have lower blood pressure. Also, saturated fat needs to be reduced to ≤10% of the total calories. The recent PURE (Prospective Urban Rural Epidemiology) study shows that high carbohydrate intake forming ≥60% of the total calories, is harmful. In India we take a high carbohydrate diet. It needs to be reduced and replaced with proteins.

Smoking cessation is very important. Tobacco chewing is common in some regions and is equally harmful. Yoga and meditation help to relieve stress and by a biofeedback mechanism help to reduce the blood pressure.

TABLE 5 Food items to be avoided in hypertensives.

A	B
• Table salt • Monosodium glutamate (ajinomoto) • Baking powder • Fried foods • Alcohol • Bakery products • Biscuits, cakes, breads, and pastries	• Salt preserved foods • Pickles • Canned foods • Papads • Ketchup and sauces • Potato chips • Cheese, peanut butter, and salted butter

PHARMACOLOGICAL THERAPY

The goals of drug treatment are to reduce blood pressure to target levels of approximately 130/80 mm Hg on a long-term basis without causing any side effects to the patient. The associated risk factors are to be controlled to reduce the risk of ASCVD. Good control of blood pressure helps to reduce the chances of HMOD and ACCs.

Basic principle is to use multiple drugs in low doses, with synergistic actions rather than using a single agent in high dose. This helps to reduce the toxicity and better control of blood pressure. The choice of antihypertensive drugs for a patient depends on the following factors: Age, concomitant risk factors, presence of HMOD, socioeconomic considerations, availability of the drug, and experience of the patient and physician. In 70% of patients blood pressure is controlled with combination of drugs. To improve compliance, fixed dose formulations are encouraged in the form of single-pill combination. Drugs with long duration of action are preferred since they can be given once a day. The antihypertensive therapy is usually lifelong. Sometimes therapy needs to be stepped down. Due to seasonal variation therapy needs to be up regulated in winters and downregulated in summers. Drug compliance is important, and patients should be explained the advantages of regular use of medicines.

There are five class of agents which are considered first-line agents for management. The ACE inhibitors, ARBs, CCBs, diuretics, and beta-blockers (BBs). The BBs and diuretics are the older drugs and are known as the "conventional agents." The ACE inhibitors, ARBs, and CCBs are the "newer agents." The conventional agents had metabolic side effects like new onset diabetes and dyslipidemias. The newer agents are metabolically neutral and are so preferred. Salient features of each class of agents are discussed here.

ACE inhibitors: They are first-line agents for hypertensive with diabetes, metabolic syndrome, and in postmyocardial infarction (MI), and heart failure patients. They retard the onset and progression of renal disease. In the HOPE (Heart Outcomes Prevention Evaluation) trial use of ramipril reduced mortality and cardiovascular events even in those with high normal pressure. ACE inhibitors are agents with good "quality of life" of the patient. The most common side effect is cough. Uncommon ones are skin rash, and rarely angioedema. Angioedema usually occurs early when ACE inhibitors are started especially in smokers. We need to monitor renal functions and potassium levels when patients are on ACE inhibitors or ARBs. ACE inhibitors and ARBs are contraindicated in pregnancy. ACE inhibitor and ARB should never be combined.

ARBs: They act on the angiotensin (AT) receptors and block the actions of AT-II which is a potent vasoconstrictor. In the LIFE (Losartan Intervention For Endpoint) trial losartan was found to be better than atenolol in reducing stroke and MI. The ARBs like ACE inhibitors are preferred in younger individuals (≤60 years), have no metabolic side effects, and very few side effects. Telmisartan and olmesartan are once a day drugs and used very commonly. ARBs reduce albuminuria better than other agents.

CCBs: The two type of CCBs are dihydropyridine (amlodipine and cilnidipine) and nondihydropyridines (verapamil and diltiazem). Amlodipine is the most commonly used. CCBs are particularly preferred in hypertension with asthma, peripheral vascular disease, angina, and in the elderly. Pedal edema is seen in 5–10% patients with its use. They are often used in combination with ACE inhibitors and ARBs.

Diuretics: They have been used as first-line agents for a long time. Chlorthalidone is preferred over hydrochlorothiazide since it has longer action. Indapamide is a vasodilator diuretic which has less metabolic side effects. Diuretics can cause new onset diabetes, hypokalemia, and dyslipidemia. Due to this, they are used in low doses now. The ALLHAT (Antihypertensive and Lipid-Lowering Treatment to Prevent Heart Attack Trial), one of the largest hypertension treatment trials, showed that chlorthalidone is as effective as lisinopril and amlodipine. Due to this trial, there has been a revival in their use. They are often used in combination with ACE inhibitors or ARBs.

The mineralocorticoid receptor antagonists (spironolactone and eplerenone) are often used as add-on therapy in resistant hypertension as the fourth agent after a combination of ACE inhibitor/ARB with CCB and diuretic has not controlled blood pressure. The PATHWAY-2 (Prevention And Treatment of Hypertension With Algorithm-based therapY-2) study (2015) showed that spironolactone is to be preferred over α_1 blocker (doxazosin) and β-blockers (bisoprolol) as the fourth agent. They are especially useful in hypertensives with heart failure.

Beta-blockers: Beta-blockers have been used for long in treatment of hypertension. Atenolol was the agent used most commonly. Since they do not reduce the central blood pressure as effectively as other agents, have metabolic side effects (dyslipidemia and impaired glucose tolerance), and were shown to be less effective in clinical trials, they are no longer used as first-line agents. In fact, in most guidelines β-blockers have been relegated to fifth add-on agents. However, newer β-blockers like the most cardioselective nebivolol and α-β-blockers carvedilol and labetalol are good agents. β-blockers are used as first-line agents in hypertension with heart failure and coronary artery disease. In young patients with increased sympathetic activity and palpitations they are the preferred agents. Labetalol is the agent of choice in pregnancy with hypertension.

Other agents: *Alpha-1 blockers* (prazosin, terazosin, and doxazosin) can be used in hypertension with benign prostate hyperplasia and chronic renal failure. However, they increase the risk of new onset heart failure and so are used in less frequency now.

Centrally acting drugs (alpha methyldopa, clonidine, and moxonidine) are still used in resistant hypertension especially in renal failure. They have side effects of postural hypertension, anticholinergic effects, and rebound hypertension on withdrawal.

Direct vasodilators, hydralazine and minoxidil, are used less often as they can cause reflex tachycardia, headache, and retention of salt and water. They are used as add-on agents in resistant hypertension in renal failure.

The ABCD algorithm for use of antihypertensive agents as given in the Indian guidelines on hypertension-IV (IGH-IV) is shown in **Figure 1**. We use a stepped care approach and drug combinations are made as shown in **Figure 1**. Younger age hypertension is high renin and ACE inhibitors or ARBs are preferred. The hypertension in old age is volume dependent and so CCBs and diuretics are preferred. Generally, we follow this simple algorithm for choosing the drug. However, the concomitant diseases, risk factors, and

HMODs can affect the choice of agents. These are shown in **Tables 6** and **7**.

Some drug combinations are preferred while others are not used. The combinations that act synergically and do not cause side effects are good combinations. The desirable and undesirable combinations are shown in **Table 8**.

Interventional therapies: The *renal sympathetic denervation therapy* evolved around a decade back. Ablation of nerves in the wall of renal arteries is done. It is based on the premise that this will reduce the afferent and efferent sympathetic activity from the kidneys and will reduce the blood pressure. Initial results showed promise. However, a sham-controlled randomized trial, the SIMPLICITY-III, showed that it had no benefit in blood pressure control. The procedure is no longer advocated as a routine and is under evaluation now.

A *baroreceptor activation implanted device* that reduces blood pressure by stimulation of baroreceptors has been developed and is being evaluated. It is not yet approved for clinical application.

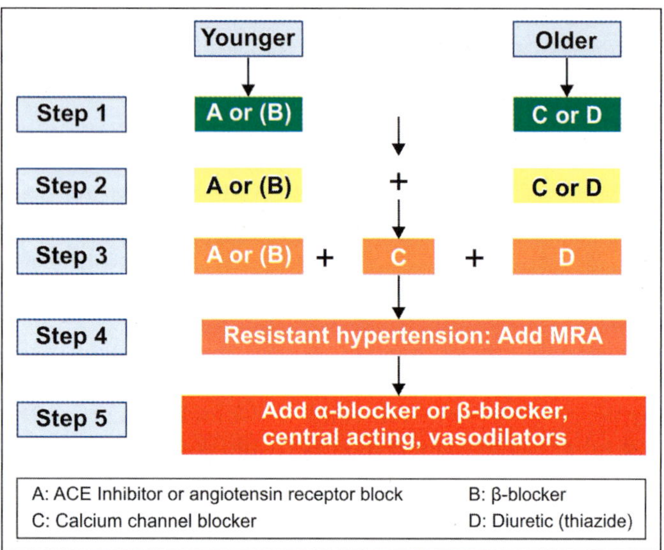

(MRA: mineralocorticoid receptor antagonist)

FIGURE 1: ABCD algorithm for use of antihypertensive agents.

Associated therapies: So as to reduce the overall risk of the patient other risk factors need to be controlled. A recent large trial, the HOPE-III trial, showed that 10 mg of rosuvastatin results in significant benefit in hypertensive patients with mild hypercholesterolemia.

Aspirin has not been shown to be of any benefit in hypertensive patients to reduce the overall CVD risk. Three large primary prevention trials, the ASCEND (A Study of Cardiovascular Events iN Diabetes), ARRIVE (Aspirin to Reduce Risk of Initial Vascular Events), and the ASPREE (Aspirin in Reducing Events in the Elderly) trials, all showed no benefit of using aspirin for primary prevention of CAD.

HYPERTENSION IN SPECIAL SITUATIONS

Hypertension in pregnancy: It affects 5–10% of pregnancies. It increases the risk of stroke, placental abruption, and multiorgan failure in the mother and prematurity, intrauterine growth retardation and intrauterine death in the fetus. It is defined as a blood pressure of ≥140/90 mm Hg in pregnancy also. It is classified mild from 140–159/90–109 mm Hg. Severe hypertension in pregnancy is ≥160/100 mm Hg.

"Chronic hypertension" is present before pregnancy and usually present before 20 weeks gestation. *"Gestational hypertension"* develops after 20 weeks. It usually resolves by 6 weeks after delivery. *Preeclampsia* is defined as hypertension with significant proteinuria of ≥0.3 g/24 hours

TABLE 6 Guidelines for selecting the most appropriate first-line antihypertensive drugs.

Class of drugs	Definite indication/s	Possible indication/s	Definite contraindication/s	Relative contraindication/s
Diuretics	• Heart failure • Elderly • Systolic HT	• Diabetes	• Gout	• Dyslipidemia
CCBs	• Metabolic syndrome • Angina • Elderly • Systolic HT • Diabetes	• PVD • CVA	• Heart block	• Congestive heart failure
ACE inhibitors	• Metabolic syndrome • Heart failure • Post MI • Proteinuria • Diabetes	• CVA	• Pregnancy and lactation • Bilateral RAS • Hyperkalemia	• CKD (creatinine levels >3 mg/dL)
ARBs	• Metabolic syndrome • Diabetes • Proteinuria • ACE inhibitors—cough	• Heart failure • CVA	• Pregnancy and lactation • Bilateral RAS • Hyperkalemia	• CKD (creatinine levels >3 mg/dL)

(PVD: peripheral vascular disease; RAS: renal artery stenosis)

TABLE 7 Guidelines for other drugs used as add-on agents.

Class of drugs	Definite indication/s	Possible indication/s	Definite contraindication/s	Relative contraindication/s
Beta-blockers	• Angina • Post-MI • Tachyarrhythmias • Heart failure	• Pregnancy • Diabetes	• Heart block	• Dyslipidemia • Physically active • PVD • COPD
α-blockers (doxazosin and prazosin)	• Prostatic hypertrophy • CKD	• IGT • Dyslipidemia	• Orthostatic hypotension • CHF	
α-methyldopa	• HT in pregnancy	• Resistant HT	• CLD	
Clonidine	• Resistant HT	• CKD	• Pregnancy and lactation	
Vasodilators (hydralazine)	• Resistant HT • HT in pregnancy			• CAD

TABLE 8 Desirable and undesirable combinations.

Desirable combinations	Undesirable combinations
• ACE inhibitors + CCBs	• BBs and ACE inhibitors
• ARBs + CCBs	• BBs and ARBs
• ACE inhibitors + diuretics	• BBs and verapamil/diltiazem
• ARBs + diuretics	• ACE inhibitors and ARBs
• Amlodipine + BBs	• Two drugs from the same class

or protein creatinine ratio of ≥30 mg/mmol and/or evidence of maternal organ dysfunction. There is evidence of uteroplacental dysfunction. HELLP (hemolysis, elevated liver enzymes, and low platelet count) can occur in some patients and we should look for it. *Eclampsia* is diagnosed when seizures occur in a patient with preeclampsia.

Hypertension in pregnancy is diagnosed by recording phase IV of Korotkoff sounds. Manual equipment are preferred over the automatic devices in pregnancy. Ambulatory blood pressure recording can be useful.

Women with moderate to high risk for preeclampsia (diabetes mellitus, chronic hypertension, multiple pregnancy, maternal age ≥40 years, previous history of preeclampsia, and chronic kidney disease) should we given prophylactic aspirin, 100–150 mg/day from 12th to till birth of the baby to prevent it.

In mild hypertension treatment is initiated in those with blood pressure ≥140/90 mm Hg. The target is 135/85 mm Hg. The agent of choice is labetalol. Alpha-methyldopa is the agent of second choice. CCBs, nifedipine, and amlodipine can be used as third choice.

The ACE inhibitors and ARBs are contraindicated in pregnancy. Diuretics are avoided since pregnancy is a volume-depleted state. Severe elevation of ≥160/110 mm Hg needs to be reduced rapidly. Parenteral labetalol or hydralazine may need to be used. Intravenous (IV) magnesium sulfate is the agent of choice for prevention and treatment of eclampsia.

Hypertension with diabetes: About 30–35% of hypertensive patients have diabetes. Their coexistence results in a manifold increased risk of CVD. The HOPE trial with ramipril and ONTARGET (Ongoing Telmisartan Alone and in Combination with Ramipril Global Endpoint Trial) trial with telmisartan showed that RAAS blockers reduce the micro and macrovascular complications of diabetes especially in hypertensive patients although these trials were primary prevention trails and had many nonhypertensive patients also.

The ACE inhibitors and ARBs are the drugs of choice in hypertension with diabetes, especially in the presence of microalbuminuria. Patients with long-standing diabetes can have autonomic neuropathy which can cause postural hypotension. Blood pressure should be checked in lying and standing position. A fall of ≥20 mm Hg systolic and ≥10 mm Hg diastolic 1 minute after standing signifies postural hypertension. The patients can have falls and so need to be counseled.

Hypertension and cerebrovascular accidents: In acute cerebrovascular disease (hemorrhagic or occlusive) sudden reflex increase in blood pressure can occur for the first 24 hours. Also, the cerebral autoregulation is affected in acute stroke. For this reason, blood pressure is not reduced in acute state. In occlusive stroke, it is appropriate to withhold treatment for the first 24 hours unless pressure is >220/120 mm Hg. Beyond this level we should reduce pressure by 10–15% only. In patients receiving IV thrombolysis blood pressure should be lowered and maintained below 180/105 mm Hg for at least 24 hours after thrombolysis.

In hemorrhagic stroke also acute elevations occur and it should be treated when systolic pressure is ≥220 mm Hg. Here it should be maintained below 180/105 mm Hg.

In poststroke patients on a long-term basis, blood pressure is maintained between 120–130/70–80 mm Hg. Blood pressure control reduces the risk of stroke recurrence by 50%.

Resistant hypertension: Around 10–15% hypertension patients have resistant hypertension. It is defined as failure

TABLE 9 Preferred parenteral drugs for selected hypertensive emergencies.

Hypertensive emergency	Preferred drugs
Hypertensive encephalopathy	Sodium nitroprusside, nicardipine, and labetalol
Malignant hypertension	Labetalol, sodium nitroprusside, and enalaprilat
Stroke	Nicardipine, labetalol, and nitroprusside
Myocardial infarction/ unstable angina	Nitroglycerin, nicardipine, labetalol, and esmolol
Acute left ventricular failure	Nitroglycerin, enalaprilat, and loop diuretics
Aortic dissection	Nitroprusside, esmolol, and labetalol
Adrenergic crisis	Phentolamine and nitroprusside
Postoperative hypertension	Nitroglycerin, nitroprusside, and labetalol
Preeclampsia/eclampsia of pregnancy	Hydralazine, labetalol, and nicardipine

to reach the target blood pressure with three drugs in adequate dose with one of them being a diuretic. We should rule out white coat hypertension and pseudohypertension (falsely high readings due to noncompressible vessels) before making a diagnosis of resistant hypertension. The drug compliance should be checked. Sometimes high-salt intake, alcohol use, and nonsteroidal anti-inflammatory drugs (NSAIDs) are responsible for lack of response. Prevalence of secondary hypertension is high in those with true resistant hypertension and they should be evaluated for secondary causes.

Hypertensive urgencies and emergencies: *Hypertensive urgency* denotes a severe elevation of blood pressure of ≥220/120 mm Hg without any acute target organ damage. These patients have long-standing hypertension and acute precipitous reduction of blood pressure is not required. They are best managed with rapid-acting oral medications.

Hypertensive emergency is a situation when patient has acute target organ damage due to severe hypertension. This requires rapid reduction of blood pressure with IV medications in an intensive care unit (ICU) setting. Often patients need an intra-arterial line for continuous pressure monitoring. The different parenteral agents that are used in hypertensive emergencies are given in **Table 9**.

Malignant hypertension term is used when acute elevation of blood pressure is associated with diffuse necrotizing vasculitis, arterial thrombi, and fibrin deposition in arteriolar wall. Clinically, this is recognized with papilledema on fundus examination. However, the fibrinoid necrosis occurs in other arteries in the brain and kidney also.

CONCLUSION

The management of hypertension should generally be kept simple. Patient's participation is very important to improve drug compliance. Since it is often asymptomatic proper counseling is important. Drug combinations in single pills are useful. Target blood pressure levels should be achieved since the SPRINT has shown that good control of blood pressure helps to reduce the complications in a better manner. Overall risk assessment of patient is done and besides control of blood pressure other risk factors should also be controlled as part of comprehensive care of the patient.

RECOMMENDED READINGS

1. Wright JT Jr, Williamson JD, Whelton PK, Snyder JK, Sink KM, Rocco MV, et al. A Randomized Trial of Intensive versus Standard Blood-Pressure Control. N Engl J Med. 2015;373(22):2103-16.
2. Yusuf S, Lonn E, Pais P, Bosch J, López-Jaramillo P, Zhu J, et al.; HOPE-3 Investigators. Blood-Pressure and Cholesterol Lowering in Persons without Cardiovascular Disease. N Engl J Med. 2016;374(21):2032-43.
3. Wander GS, Ram CV. Global impact of 2017 American Heart Association/American College of Cardiology hypertension guidelines: a perspective from India. Circulation. 2018;137:549-50.
4. Wander GS, Gupta R, S Ram CV. Western guidelines bring in cardiovascular risk prediction along with blood pressure levels for initiation of antihypertensive drugs: Is the pitch ready for Indians. J Hum Hypertens. 2019;33(8):566-7.
5. Wander GS, Ram CV. Optimal blood pressure goals recommended by the latest hypertension guidelines: India may benefit the most. Eur Heart J. 2018;39: 3012-6.
6. Goyal A, Narang K, Ahluwalia G, Sohal PM, Singh B, Chhabra ST, et al. Seasonal variation in 24 h blood pressure profile in healthy adults- A prospective observational study. J Hum Hypertens. 2019;33(8):626-33.
7. Unger T, Borghi C, Charchar F, Khan NA, Poulter NR, Prabhakaran D, et al. 2020 International Society of Hypertension Global Hypertension Practice Guidelines. Hypertension. 2020;75(6):1334-57.
8. Goyal A, Aslam N, Kaur S, Soni RK, Midha V, Chaudhary A, et al. Factors affecting seasonal changes in blood pressure in North India: A population based four-seasons study. Indian Heart J. 2018;70(3):360-7.

CHAPTER 105 Dyslipidemias and Drugs Used for Management

Debabrata Roy, Navanil Biswas, Saurabh Dhumale

ABSTRACT

Dyslipidemia is one of the most important modifiable risk factors for atherosclerotic cardiovascular diseases (ASCVD). The Framingham Heart Study established the role of blood cholesterol as a significant risk factor for atherosclerosis and coronary heart disease (CHD). Since then, countless observational studies, randomized clinical trials and other research work have been performed in this field. Abnormality in any fraction of lipids is called as dyslipidemia. However, the most important one is raised total cholesterol (TC) which reflects in raised low-density lipoprotein (LDL) levels. Statins are the mainstay of treatment for high cholesterol and LDL. All patients with ASCVD should be put on high-intensity statins irrespective of the lipid levels. For primary prevention the benefits are in selected patients [those with LDL >190 mg/dL or even lower levels (160 mg/dL)] when multiple risk factors are present or even LDL of 130 in those with diabetes. Triglycerides (TGs) and very-low-density lipoprotein (VLDL) correlate less with ASCVD and the benefits of reducing these have not been shown in clinical trials. Recently molecular biology is exposing newer targets thereby leading to the development of novel drugs.

"There is always going to be need for new medications, better medications"

—Anthony Fauci

INTRODUCTION

Dyslipidemia implies abnormality in any of the lipid fractions. It is one of the most important modifiable risk factors for ASCVD. The prevalence of dyslipidemia is very high in Indians—79% of subjects have at least one lipid abnormality, 72.3% have decreased high-density lipoprotein (HDL), 29.5% hypertriglyceridemia, and 11.8% of subjects have elevated LDL. This is sometimes labeled as "Indian pattern of dyslipidemia."

The first lipid-lowering medication, developed in 1955 was cholestyramine, a bile acid sequestrant and the first statin developed was lovastatin. Application of molecular biology is exposing hitherto unknown aspects of dyslipidemia thereby leading to the development of newer drugs.

LIPIDS: A BRIEF OVERVIEW

Lipids are a complex group of organic compounds that provide essential fuel for our body and serve a host of other important functions including: storage, mobilization and utilization of energy, growth and differentiation of cells, formation of the structure of cell membranes, transmission of various biochemical signals, synthesis of various hormones, and synthesis of bile acids.

However, when these same lipids build up in excess inside the body, they give rise to a whole gamut of deleterious cardiovascular effects.

Cholesterol and TG, the two lipids, cannot move freely in blood. So, they are tagged to apoproteins and the combination is in the form of lipoproteins. The lipoproteins are nothing, but hydrophobic lipid particles packed inside a hydrophilic core made of apoproteins. They are divided into seven classes based on their ultracentrifugation density and electrophoretic mobility (**Fig. 1**).

In a traditional lipid profile measurement, we get the TC, TGs, LDL, HDL, and the VLDL levels along with some ratios.

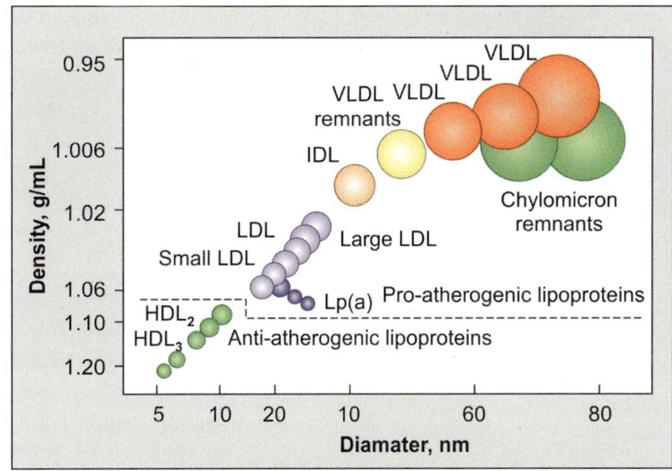

(IDL: intermediate-density lipoprotein; Lp(a): lipoprotein(a))

FIGURE 1: Classes of lipoproteins based on ultracentrifugation density.

Source: Adapted from Feingold KR, Anawalt B, Boyce A, Chrousos G, de Herder WW, Dungan K, et al. Introduction to lipids and lipoproteins. Endotext. South Dartmouth (MA): MDText.com, Inc.; 2000. Also available from https://www.ncbi.nlm.nih.gov/books/NBK305896/

The TC and LDL levels are directly related to occurrence of ASCVD. HDL levels are inversely related and higher values are protective. The relationship of TG and VLDL with ASCVD is less consistent. TGs are considered as a marker of ASCVD rather than a cause-and-effect relationship.

These values were earlier generally measured in the fasting state. This is because LDL cholesterol (LDL-C) was derived from the Friedewald formula instead of being directly measured. This Friedewald formula is only accurate at low levels of TGs (especially at levels <150 mg/dL), which usually occurs in the fasting state. However, since now LDL levels are measured directly, the lipid profile is now done in a nonfasting state also. Any deviation from the normal range of these values is designated as dyslipidemia (**Table 1**). Classically LDL has been termed as "bad cholesterol" and HDL as "good cholesterol."

Mostly lipid abnormalities are polygenic and multiple genes are responsible for the risk of lipid abnormalities. This is shown in single nucleotide polymorphism (SNP) studies done on population basis. However, some of them (lipid abnormalities) are single gene related. The most common one is heterozygous hypercholesterolemia which has a prevalence of 1:500 in the general population. These individuals have TC in the range of 280–320 mg/dL and LDL levels in the range of 180–220 mg/dL. On family survey, other members of the family often have high lipids and it should always be done in them. The incidence of homozygous hypercholesterolemia is much less common. They have cholesterol levels in range of 450–600 mg/dL and have tendon xanthomas. These individuals have premature coronary artery disease (CAD) and do not respond to statins.

The above mentioned (familial hypercholesterolemia) and other genetic mutations responsible for causing other dyslipidemias are classified according to the Fredrickson classification (**Table 2**).

A brief description of LDL-C, HDL, lipoprotein(a) [Lp(a)], TGs, and VLDL is given below.

LOW-DENSITY LIPOPROTEIN CHOLESTEROL

Low-density lipoprotein is derived from the sequential metabolism of VLDL and then intermediate density lipoprotein (IDL). LDL constitutes 90% of atherogenic

TABLE 1 Laboratory values of commonly measured lipids.

	Optimal	Intermediate	High
Total cholesterol	<200 mg/dL	200–239 mg/dL	>239 mg/dL
LDL cholesterol	<130 mg/dL	130–159 mg/dL	>159 mg/dL
HDL cholesterol	>60 mg/dL	40–60 mg/dL	<40 mg/dL
Triglycerides	<150 mg/dL	150–199 mg/dL	>199 mg/dL
Non-HDL cholesterol	<130 mg/dL	130–159 mg/dL	>159 mg/dL
TG to HDL ratio	<3	3–3.8	>3.8

TABLE 2 Fredrickson classification of primary dyslipidemia.

Type	Synonym	Defect	Serum abnormality	Clinical features	Treatment	Serum appearance
Type 1	Familial hyperchylomicronemia	Low LDL Altered ApoC2	Chylomicron ↑	Pancreatitis, lipemia retinalis, skin eruptions, xanthoma, and hepatosplenomegaly	Diet	Creamy top layer
Type IIa	Familial hypercholesterolemia	↓LDL receptor	LDL↑	Xanthelasma, arcus senilis, and tendon xanthomas	Cholestyramine or colestipol, Statins, niacin	Clear
Type IIb	Familial combined hypercholesterolemia	↓LDL receptor and ↑ApoB	LDL and VLDL↑		Statins, niacin, fibrate	Clear
Type III	Familial dysbetalipoproteinemia	ApoE2 synthesis defect	IDL↑	Tuboeruptive xanthomas, palmar xanthoma	Fibrate, statins	Turbid
Type IV	Familial hyperlipemia	↑VLDL production, ↓elimination	VLDL↑		Statins, niacin, fibrate	
Type V	Endogenous hypertriglyceridemia	↑VLDL production, ↓LPL	VLDL and chylomicron↑		Niacin, fibrate	Creamy top layer and turbid bottom

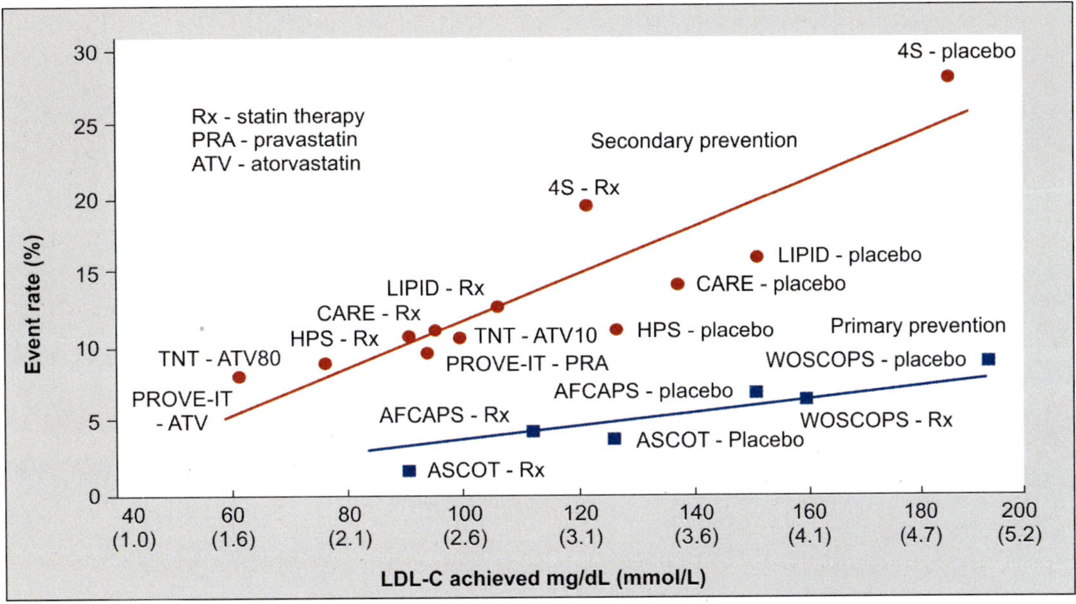

FIGURE 2: **Primary and secondary prevention trials showing lower MACE with lower LDL-C levels.**

Source: Rosenson RS. Statins: Can the new generation make an impression? Expert Opin Emerg Drugs. 2004;9(2):269-79. LaRosa JC, Grundy SM, Waters DD, Shear C, Barter P, Fruchart JC, et al. Intensive lipid lowering with atorvastatin in patients with stable coronary disease. N Engl J Med. 2005;352:1425-35.

lipoprotein particle and is related most significantly to major adverse cardiovascular events (MACE). A number of primary and secondary prevention trials established the "lower is better" concept as regards LDL (**Fig. 2**). Hence, these form the primary target of lipid-lowering therapy.

A few more important points to note about LDL-C levels are:

- The effect of LDL-C on the cardiovascular system is additive to other risk factors and proportional to the duration of exposure to its high level (**Fig. 3**).
- Low-density lipoprotein cholesterol, even at levels currently considered normal, is independently associated with the presence and extent of early systemic atherosclerosis in the absence of major cardiovascular risk factors. These findings support more effective LDL-C lowering for primordial prevention, even in individuals conventionally considered at optimal risk.
- At lower levels (<1.4 mmol/L or 50 mg/dL), the LDL particles may even reverse cholesterol deposition in atherosclerotic plaque and may result in their regression.

LDL cholesterol pathways: Under physiological conditions, LDL particles circulate in plasma and supply cholesterol esters for cell membrane synthesis. After performing its task, the particles are taken up by the liver with the help of LDL-receptors (LDLRs), where the cholesterol esters are again repackaged for another run through the VLDL pathway or excreted as bile acids.

However, in energy excess states, or in metabolically dysfunctional individuals, these LDL particles, on account of their increased number, are less readily removed from circulation by the hepatic LDLR and circulate in plasma for longer periods. This leads to greater removal of cholesterol from them by peripheral tissues making them more small and dense. As a result of their small size, increased number,

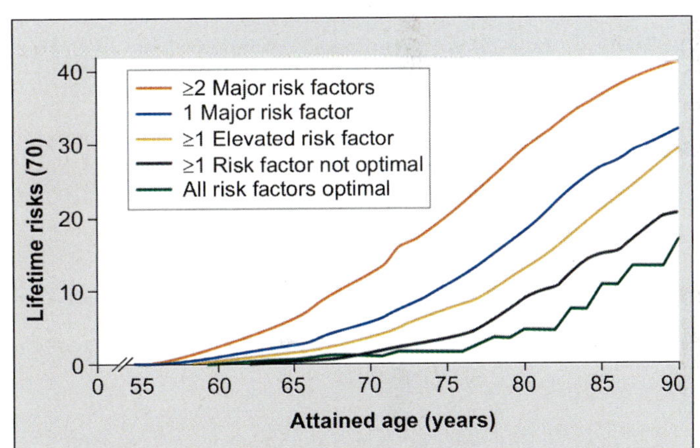

FIGURE 3: Cardiovascular mortality due to high cholesterol levels combined with other risk factors, and younger age of development.

Source: Berry JD, Dyer A, Cai X, Garside DB, Ning H, Thomas A, et al. Lifetime Risks of Cardiovascular Disease. N Engl J Med. 2012;366:321-9.

longer duration of exposure as well as a combination of the three, these LDL particles readily penetrate the vascular endothelium. This process is facilitated by endothelial dysfunction which makes the endothelium more porous. Once they are in the intimal space, these LDL particles are prone to oxidation and thus initiate atherosclerotic process (**Fig. 4**).

Residual risk of atherosclerosis: It was seen in PROVE-IT TIMI trial, that despite reducing the LDL levels to around 60 mg/dL, a quarter of post-ACS patients within two-and-a-half years suffered from death or MACE. Since the recognition of this fact, a lot of research has gone into finding out the components of this "residual risk." This showed that other components of lipid network, especially Lp(a), should be targeted as well. Even among LDL particles, an important

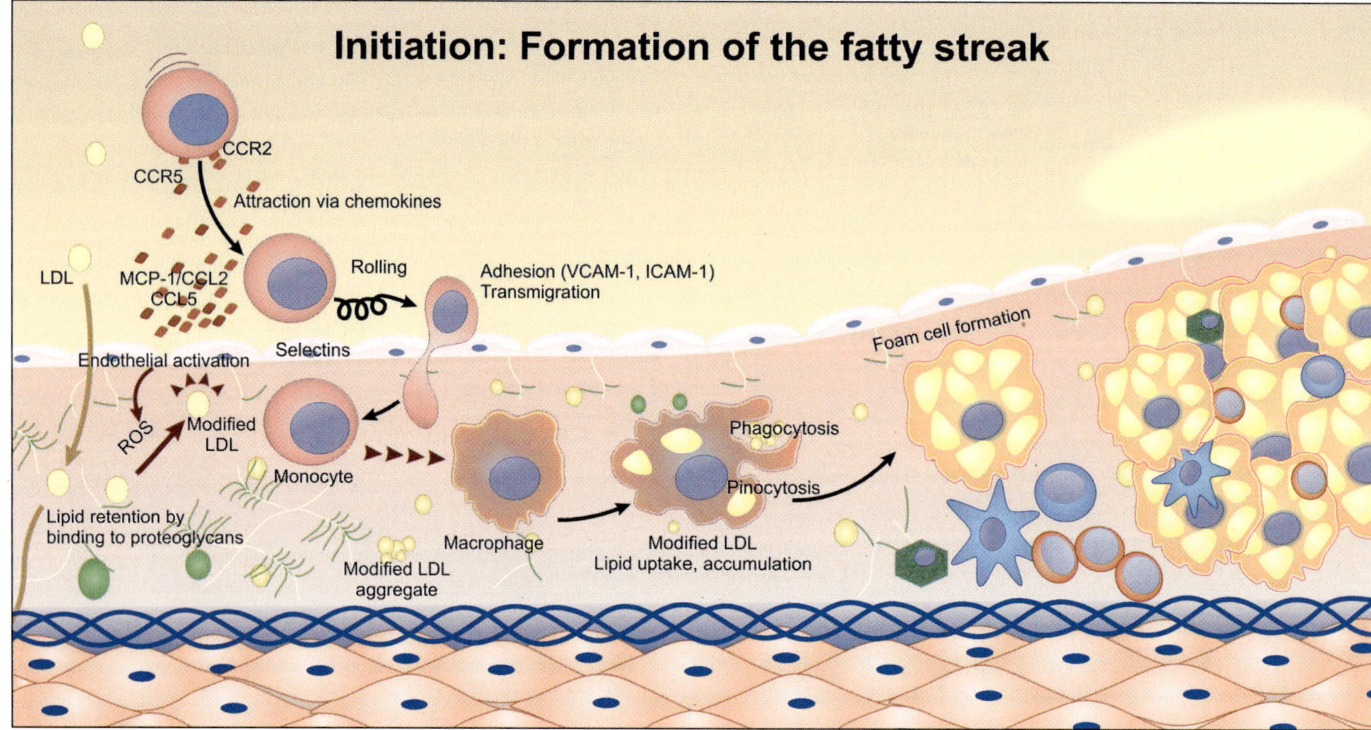

(CCR: creatinine clearance; ROS: reactive oxygen species)

FIGURE 4: Low-density lipoprotein cholesterol and initiation of atherosclerosis.

TABLE 3 Advantages and disadvantages of non-HDL-C and ApoB measurement.

	Advantages	Disadvantages
Non-HDL-C	• Low cost of screening • Rapid turnaround of results • High-level consensus for its clinical value	• Accurate definition and characterization are not possible
ApoB	• Measurement of ApoB, TC, and TG allows classification of all the dyslipidemias • Those with persistently high levels of ApoB may be candidates for intensive statin therapy	• Increased cost • Lack of universal availability

(ApoB: apolipoprotein-B; non-HDL-C: non-high-density lipoprotein cholesterol)

subgroup "small dense LDL (sdLDL)" also forms a part of this residual risk.

NON-HDL CHOLESTEROL AND APOLIPOPROTEIN-B

High-density lipoprotein cholesterol (HDL-C), which is responsible for reverse cholesterol transport, has been described as the "good cholesterol" and all others can be described as "bad" or "atherogenic" cholesterol. This led to the concept of measuring "non-HDL-cholesterol (non-HDL-C) levels" as a more accurate marker of residual risk. Non-HDL-C goal is 30 mg/dL above LDL-C goal, that is, if the LDL-C goal is <70 mg/dL, the non-HDL-C goal should be <100 mg/dL.

Another important marker that can be used as a measure of atherogenic lipoproteins is apolipoprotein-B (ApoB). ApoB-48 is a component of chylomicrons, whereas ApoB-100 is present in LDL. Though both non-HDL-C and ApoB are markers of atherosclerotic risk, their measurements are associated with some disadvantages (**Table 3**). The non-HDL-C is considered as important target, as LDL-C for lipid-lowering therapy by the Lipid Association of India.

SMALL DENSE LOW-DENSITY LIPOPROTEIN

Small dense LDL is a distinct subgroup of LDL particles, that is much more atherogenic than normal LDL particles (**Fig. 5**). Its concentration significantly increases in patients with metabolic disorder and is closely related to the TG level in the body. Its harmful effect is affected by:

- Very low affinity of LDLRs for sdLDL particles
- Increased circulation time compared to normal LDL particles (2–3 times)
- Increased propensity to penetrate the endothelial barrier

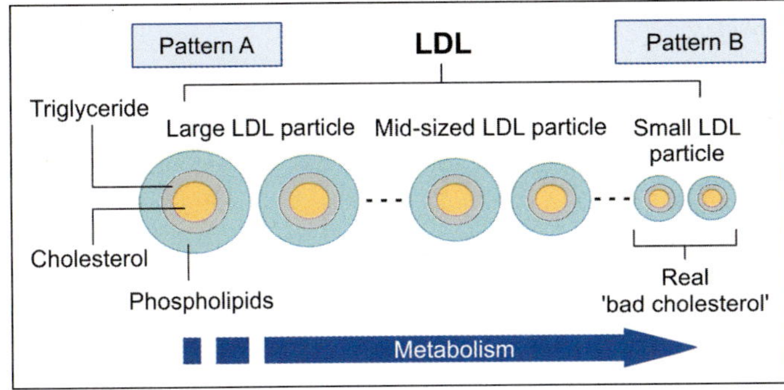

FIGURE 5: Small dense LDL (sdLDL) particles (pattern B) and normal LDL particles (pattern A).

- More vulnerability to oxidation and glycation, increasing chances of retention in the vascular intima, and progression to atherosclerosis
- It is not yet clear whether statins are efficient for specific lowering of sdLDL.

The size of LDL particles is inversely proportional to their numbers. Thus, besides sdLDL concentration, LDL particle number can also serve as a valuable marker of residual risk.

HIGH-DENSITY LIPOPROTEIN CHOLESTEROL

Besides participating in reverse cholesterol transport, HDL has a number of pleiotropic effects, all of which make it a "highly desirable cholesterol" (**Fig. 6**).

LIPOPROTEIN(A)

Another very important subclass of LDLC is Lp(a), discovered in 1963. It is an LDL particle containing ApoB and Apo 'a' and has emerged in the last decade as a genetic, independent, and likely causal risk factor for cardiovascular disease (CVD) and calcific aortic vascular disease (CAVD). It has homogeneity with the plasminogen molecule and has been seen to be the most prevalent monogenic disorder globally. It does not depend much on lifestyle factors and is independent of other risk factors. Prevalence of Lp(a) >50 mg/dL is estimated to be >1.4 billion people worldwide, i.e., 20–30% of the world's population.

Lipoprotein(a) has atherogenic, proinflammatory, prothrombotic, and prooxidant properties (**Fig. 7**). For a given level of LDL-C the proportion of Lp(a) varies and this determines the response to statins as Lp(a) itself is resistant to statins (**Fig. 8**). It can present with varying clinical phenotypes:

- Stroke in pediatric age group
- ST-elevation myocardial infarction (STEMI) in young males
- Calcific aortic vascular disease in elderly population

Measurement of Lp(a) has following challenges:

- Wide concentration range
- Apo(a) isoform size variation
- ApoB and plasminogen like components
- Lack of assay standardization
- No uniform cutoff point for CVD risk

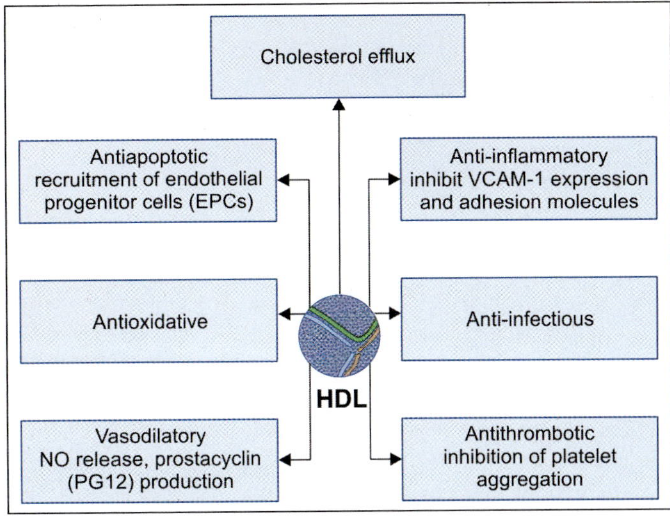

(HDL: high-density lipoprotein; VCAM: vascular cell adhesion molecule)

FIGURE 6: Pleiotropic effects of HDL.

TRIGLYCERIDES

Failure of increasing HDL levels to achieve appreciable cardiovascular risk reduction in AIM-HIGH (Atherothrombosis Intervention in Metabolic Syndrome with Low HDL/High TG: Impact on Global Health Outcomes) trial paved the way for investigation for other potential targets. The Copenhagen General Population Study (CGPS) brought to light the importance of TGs and triglyceride-rich lipoproteins (TRLs) as important markers of atherosclerotic cardiovascular risk.

High TG is often accompanied by low HDL levels and increased proportion of sdLDL, a pattern known as atherogenic dyslipidemia.

VERY-LOW-DENSITY LIPOPROTEIN

Very-low-density lipoprotein is the parent lipoprotein giving rise to both IDL and LDL. It also contains the largest proportion of TGs among lipoproteins. The CGPS revealed the importance of this little studied fraction of lipoprotein.

Both, the TG and the cholesterol content of VLDL particles, are associated with increased cardiovascular risk. This gave rise to the concept of "remnant cholesterol." Remnant cholesterol = TC – LDL-C – HDL-C.

The mechanisms behind the atherogenic nature of VLDL particles are:

- VLDL or remnant lipoproteins can penetrate the arterial wall, just like LDL.
- The lipoprotein lipase located at the surface of endothelial cells or in the intima, hydrolyzes the TG, and releasing the toxic-free fatty acids causing inflammation.
- The TG-rich remnants may get trapped within the intima due to their larger size.
- They can be directly taken up by the macrophages, converting them to foam cells, which in turn gives rise to atherosclerotic plaque.

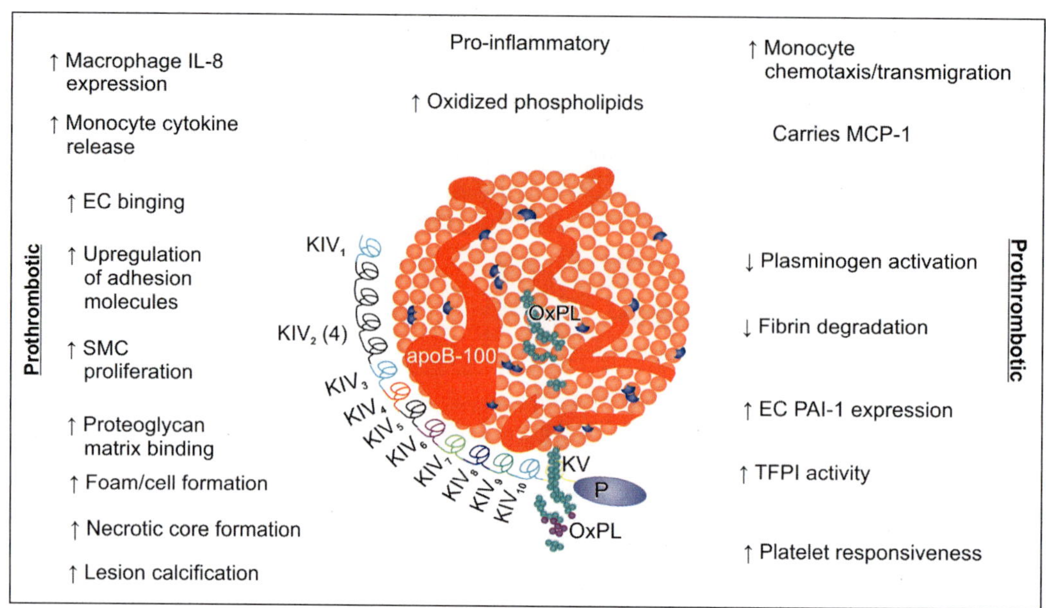

(EC: endothelial cell; Lp(a): lipoprotein(a); MCP: monocyte chemotactic protein; PAI-1: plasminogen activator inhibitor-1; SMC: smooth muscle cell; TFPI: tissue factor pathway inhibitor)

FIGURE 7: Lp(a) and its pro-inflammatory, prothrombotic and proatherogenic nature.

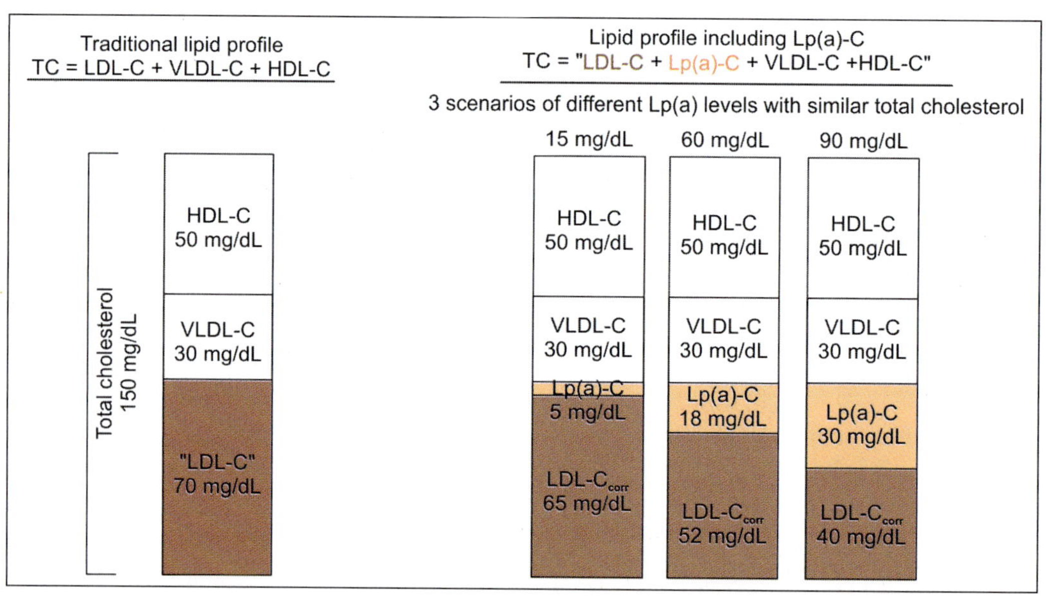

(LDL-C: low-density lipoprotein-cholesterol; Lp(a): lipoprotein(a); HDL-C: high-density lipoprotein-cholesterol; TC: total cholesterol; VLDL-C: very-low-density lipoprotein cholesterol)

FIGURE 8: Diagram showing how for similar values of total and LDL-C, the relative proportion of true LDL-C and Lp(a) cholesterol varies, hence resulting in varying responses to statins.

MANAGEMENT

DIETARY MODIFICATIONS

Nutrition and smoking cessation form the cornerstone of lifestyle modification in ASCVD risk reduction. Effects of diet on lipid levels and ASCVD risk are:

- Some food items are best consumed more; while others including alcohol are best avoided (**Table 4**).
- Dietary Approach to Stop Hypertension (DASH) diet and the Mediterranean diet are both effective in reducing ASCVD risk as well as atherogenic dyslipidemia and CHD.

TABLE 4: Various food products and their recommended consumption.

Consume more	Consume less
• Fruits • Vegetables and beans • Whole grains • Nuts • Fish and shellfish • Dairy products • Vegetable oils	• Food containing partially hydrogenated (transfats) oils • Refined grains and carbohydrates • Processed meats • Alcohol

- Dietary carbohydrates have no net effect on plasma LDL-C levels, though excess consumption has an unfavorable effect on plasma TG and HDL-C levels.
- In individuals with normal TG levels, moderate (1 unit/day) alcohol consumption is acceptable, while complete cessation of smoking has a clear benefit in reducing cardiovascular (CV) risk.

PHARMACOTHERAPY

The mainstay of pharmacotherapy is use of statins, since these are the agents which have shown reduction of ASCVD events and mortality reduction. All individuals with evidence of ASCVD [CAD, stroke, and peripheral artery disease (PAD)] should be given "high-intensity statins" for lifelong period. For primary prevention (those with no ASCVD), we need to look at the lipid level and associated risk factors to decide regarding need for statins. For primary preventions, LDL levels of ≥190 mg/dL should be treated with statins. In the presence of other risk factors even lower levels of LDL (130–160 mg/dL) need treatment especially in presence of diabetes.

Risk estimation: Risk stratification followed by a goal-directed medical therapy is the cornerstone of the lipid management. Risk factor screening including the lipid profile should be considered in men >40 years old, and in women >50 years of age or postmenopausal.

However, none of the risk estimators are derived from or accurately predict risk in South Asians. The traditional tools that are used include the Framingham Risk Score, American Heart Association/American College of Cardiology ASCVD Risk Estimator Plus, the ESC (European Society of Cardiology) SCORE (Systematic COronary Risk Evaluation) charts. A few key points to keep in mind—younger patients without traditional risk factors are at lower risk, the risk increases to moderate to high with increasing LDL-C levels, age and addition of another risk factor like diabetes, hypertension and/or smoking, patients with documented ASCVD constitute the very high-risk group, age is a driving factor in the estimation of absolute risk in most risk scores, and thus, South Asians tend to have underestimated risk, although they have multiple risk factors at younger ages, and the target LDL-C levels correspond with the risk as shown in the **Figure 9**.

STATINS

Statins inhibit the enzyme hMG-CoA (3-hydroxy-3-methyl-glutaryl-coenzyme A) reductase and thus prevent the formation of mevalonate, a rate-limiting step in sterol synthesis. The reduction in LDL levels is dose-dependent. Statins also reduce TG values by 10–20% from the baseline and elevate HDL by 1–10% in various meta-analyses. This overall benefit of statins is attributable to the overall lipid-lowering efficacy as well as their "pleotropic effects."

The usual lipid-lowering regimen should be individualized and nuanced based on individual risk score followed by starting the suited intensity viz. low-, moderate-, or high-intensity statin therapy (**Tables 5** and **6**). An addition of ezetimibe and/or PCSK9 inhibitor is advised if the target LDL or the percent reduction is not achieved with maximum tolerated statin dose (**Fig. 10**).

Adverse effects of statins: Statins are generally tolerated very well. Statin-associated muscle symptoms (SAMS) are the most clinically relevant side effect of statins. Myalgia with or without elevated creatine kinase (CK) levels has an

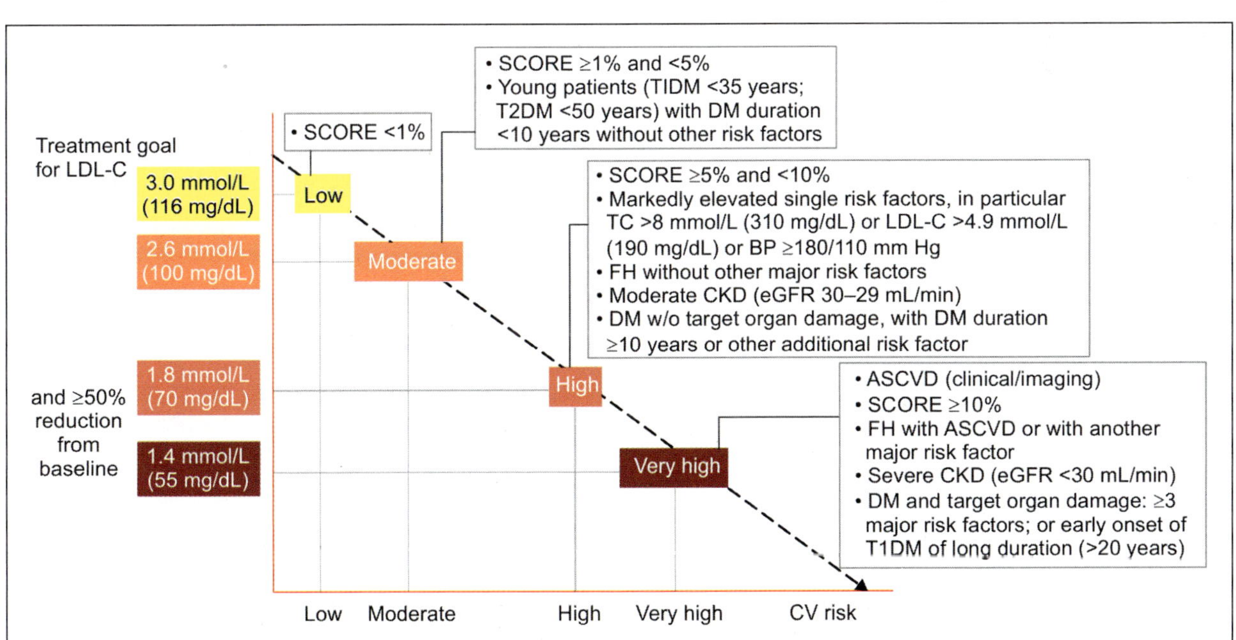

(ESC/EAS: European Society of Cardiology/ European Atherosclerosis Society; SCORE: systematic coronary risk estimation)

FIGURE 9: Treatment goals for LDL-C across categories of total cardiovascular disease risk.

Source: Adapted from 2019 ESC/EAS guidelines for the management of dyslipidemias: Lipid modification to reduce cardiovascular risk.

TABLE 5 Classification of intensity of statin regimen.

	High intensity	Moderate intensity	Low intensity
LDL-C Lowering*	≥50%	30%–49%	<30%
Statins	• Rosuvastatin 20 mg (40 mg) • Atorvastatin 40 mg (80 mg)	• Rosuvastatin 10 mg • Atorvastatin 20 mg • Simvastatin 40 mg • Pravastatin 40 mg (80 mg) • Lovastatin 40 mg (80 mg) • Fluvastatin 80 mg • Pitavastatin 1–4 mg	• Atorvastatin 10 mg • Simvastatin 20 mg • Pravastatin 10–20 mg

* LDL-C lowering that should occur with the dosage listed below each intensity.

TABLE 6 Expected clinical benefits of low-density lipoprotein cholesterol (LDL-C)-lowering therapies.

Treatment	Average LDL-C reduction
Moderate-intensity statin	≈30%
High-intensity statin	≈50%
High-intensity statin plus ezetimibe	≈65%
PCSK9 inhibitor	≈60%
PCSK9 inhibitor plus high-intensity statin	≈75%
PCSK9 inhibitor plus high-intensity statin plus ezetimibe	≈ 85%

Source: Adapted from 2019 ESC/EAS guidelines for the management of dyslipidemias: Lipid modification to reduce cardiovascular risk.

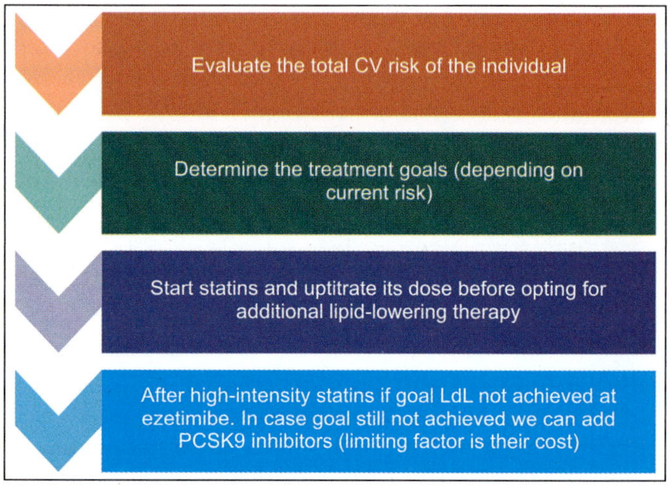

FIGURE 10: The approach to lipid-lowering regimen.

incidence of 10–15%. Rhabdomyolysis is the most severe form of statin-induced muscle damage, characterized by severe muscular pain, muscle necrosis, and myoglobinuria potentially leading rarely to renal failure. Its diagnosis is made when severe muscle symptoms are associated with a CK elevation by ≥10 times, and often ≥40 times, the upper limit of normal (ULN). The frequency of rhabdomyolysis has been estimated to be 1–3 cases/100,000 patient-years. SAMS can be dealt as follows:

- Acknowledge patients symptoms, if significant, stop the statin
- After resolution of symptoms, if the myopathy is not severe, rechallenge; a lower dose, less frequent dosing (1–3/week), or change in the choice of statin can be considered.
- Consider adding a nonstatin adjuvant such as ezetimibe or PCSK9 inhibitor in order to offset statin dose.

Mild elevation of alanine aminotransferase (ALT) occurs in 0.5–2.0% of patients on statin treatment, more commonly with potent statins or high doses. The common definition of clinically relevant ALT elevation is an increase of three times the ULN on two consecutive occasions. Statin-induced liver failure is exceedingly rare. Hence, monitoring of liver enzymes is no longer advised. The statins use *CYP3A4* and 2C9 enzyme systems in liver for its metabolism, hence other drugs using the same pathway may potentiate the toxicity of statins (**Table 7**). Statins can be used to treat dyslipidemia in patients with nonalcoholic fatty liver disease (NAFLD) without any increased risk of hepatotoxicity. However, treatment of NAFLD with statins is debatable and cannot be recommended at present.

TABLE 7 Drugs potentially interacting with statins metabolized by cytochrome P450 3A4 leading to increased risk of myopathy and rhabdomyolysis.

Anti-infective agents	Calcium antagonists	Others
• Itraconazole • Ketoconazole • Erythromycin • Clarithromycin • HIV protease inhibitors	• Verapamil • Diltiazem • Amlodipine	• Cyclosporine • Danazol • Amiodarone • Ranolazine • Grapefruit juice • Gemfibrozil

Patients on statin treatment have been shown to harbor an increased risk of dysglycemia and development of new-onset type 2 diabetes mellitus (T2DM). However, the benefit of CVD risk reduction clearly outweighs the minor increase in diabetes incidence. There is conflicting evidence from various meta-analyses about statin and its role in paradoxical increase in TG levels. There is no clear evidence of statins adversely affecting kidney function. Statins should be initiated at a lower dose in patients with eGFR <30 mL/min, and gradually escalated to recommended dose with monitoring for adverse events.

EZETIMIBE

- Ezetimibe inhibits intestinal uptake of dietary and biliary cholesterol at the brush border of the intestine.
- A meta-analysis of randomized controlled trials (RCTs) showed 18.5% reduction in LDL-C with ezetimibe as compared with placebo. In addition, there was 3% increase in HDL-C, 8% reduction in TGs, and a 13% reduction in TC.
- Ezetimibe has arguably the safest side effect profile and is generally well tolerated.

As a result of this significant efficacy and good tolerability, ezetimibe has become a pivotal part of all major lipid-lowering guidelines, either as an adjunct to the statins or as a monotherapy in statin intolerant individuals.

PCSK9 INHIBITORS

- Elevated concentration or function of PCSK9 protein in plasma reduces LDLR expression by promoting LDLR lysosomal catabolism and a subsequent increase in plasma LDL concentrations.
- Alirocumab in ODYSSEY trial (**Fig. 11**) and evolocumab in FOURIER trial—either alone or in combination with statins, and/or other lipid-lowering therapies—have been shown to significantly reduce LDL-C levels on average by 60%, depending on dose.
- In phase II trials, evolocumab lowered TG levels by 26%, and raised HDL-C and apolipoprotein A-I (ApoA-I) by 9% and 4%, respectively; similar findings have been reported for alirocumab. This class of drugs also reduces plasma Lp(a) levels and confer greater reduction in CV risk.
- No major side effects are recorded. Minor side effects like itching at the injection site and flu-like symptoms are infrequent. Being monoclonal antibodies, there are virtually no drug interactions.

However, its incredibly high cost and lack of oral formulation preclude its widespread usage.

OTHER AGENTS

Bile acid sequestrants: Cholestyramine and colestipol are both bile acid-binding exchange resins (synthetic drug colesevelam). These bind with the bile acids, preventing its reabsorption into the blood. The liver, depleted of bile, synthesizes more bile acids from hepatic cholesterol, therefore increasing the hepatic demand for cholesterol which results in a decrease of circulating LDL. They cause a reduction in LDL-C of 18–25%. However, they are not used these days due to their gastrointestinal (GI) side effects like flatulence, constipation, and dyspepsia are common.

Fibric acid derivatives: Fenofibrate and gemfibrozil are the earlier members of this class which acts as an agonist of peroxisome proliferator-activated receptor alpha (PPAR-α). They have shown good efficacy in lowering fasting and postprandial TGs. They achieve 50% reduction in the TG levels and a 10–20% reduction of the LDL-C level. The recent PROMINENT study showed efficacy of pemafibrate, a selective PPAR-α modulator in reducing TRLs. Fibrates can increase plasma concentrations of statins and so can increase risk of toxicity. Currently, fibrates are recommended for use

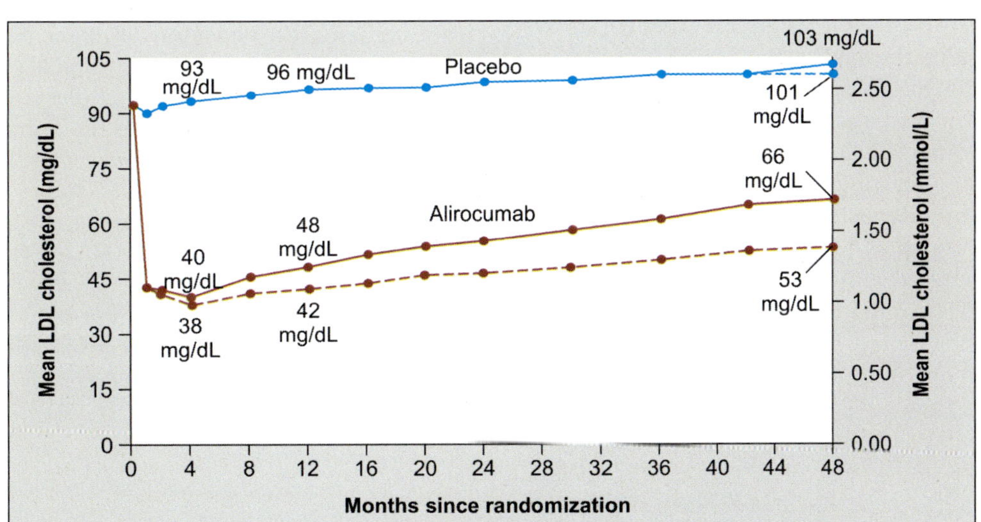

FIGURE 11: Low-density lipoprotein cholesterol lowering achieved with alirocumab in the ODYSSEY trial.

in the treatment of severe hypertriglyceridemia (TG >400 mg/dL) and as an add-on to statin in combined dyslipidemia (when not corrected with statins alone).

The omega-3 and icosapent ethyl: There are contradicting evidence from various trials on beneficial effect of consumption of omega-3 polyunsaturated fatty acids {PUFAs [eicosapentaenoic acid (EPA) and docosahexaenoic acid (DHA)]}. Icosapent ethyl, the more widely used Food and Drug Administration (FDA)-approved EPA, had shown significant reduction in plasma TG levels as well as significant reduction in primary cardiovascular endpoints in the REDUCE-IT trial. However, it failed to show any significant reduction in primary MACE events despite significant TG levels in STRENGTH and OMEMI trials.

Nicotinic acid inhibits diacyl-glycerol acyltransferase-2 resulting in decreased VLDL particles, which also reflects in reduced IDL and LDL particles. It primarily raises HDL-C by increasing ApoA-I production in the liver.

Lomitapide is an MTP inhibitor designed for oral treatment of homozygous familial hypercholesterolemia (HoFH) and is shown to decrease frequency of apheresis in HoFH patients.

Mipomersen is an antisense oligonucleotide capable of binding to the mRNA of ApoB-100, in turn reducing plasma LDL-C and Lp(a) levels.

Cholesteryl ester transfer protein (CETP) inhibitors like torcetrapib, dalcetrapib, and anacetrapib have been evaluated and have shown to increase HDL-C levels by as much as 100%. However, this increase in HDL-C has not translated into a comparable reduction in CV risk.

FUTURE PERSPECTIVES

Newer approaches to reduce LDL-C include drugs like inclisiran, a small interfering ribonucleic acid (siRNA) molecule that inhibits the synthesis of PCSK9. It is being tested in HPS4/TIMI65/ORION4 trials and has shown promise in the form of sustained LDL-C control without any significant adverse effects. Bempedoic acid is a novel oral small molecule that inhibits cholesterol synthesis by inhibiting the enzyme adenosine triphosphate (ATP) citrate lyase. Novel targets such as TRLs with their proven role in CV risk are being targeted with novel drugs like evinacumab which is an ANGPTL3 antibody and volanesorsen which is an antisense oligonucleotide targeting apolipoprotein C-III (ApoC-III) messenger ribonucleic acid (mRNA) which is critical in TRL clearance.

RECOMMENDED READINGS

1. Iyengar SS, Puri R, Narasingan SN. Lipid Association of India Expert Consensus Statement on Management of Dyslipidemia in Indians 2016: Part 1 - Executive summary. J Clin Prev Cardiol. 2016;5(2):51-61.
2. Iyengar SS, Puri R, Narasingan SN, Nair DR, Mehta V, Mohan JC, et al. Lipid Association of India (LAI) expert consensus statement on management of dyslipidaemia in Indians 2017: part 2. Clin Lipidol 2017;12(1):56-109.
3. Rosenson RS, Brewer Jr HB, Chapman MJ, Fazio S, Hussain MM, Kontush A, et al. HDL measures, particle heterogeneity, proposed nomenclature, and relation to atherosclerotic cardiovascular events. Clin Chem. 2011;57(3):392-410.
4. Balling M, Langsted A, Afzal S, Varbo A, Smith GD, Nordestgaard BG. A third of nonfasting plasma cholesterol is in remnant lipoproteins: Lipoprotein subclass profiling in 9293 individuals. Atherosclerosis. 2019;286:97-104.
5. Mach F, Baigent C, Catapano AL, Koskinas KC, Casula M, Badimon L, et al. 2019 ESC/EAS Guidelines for the management of dyslipidaemias: lipid modification to reduce cardiovascular risk. Eur Heart J. 2020;41(1): 111-88.
6. Zipes DP, Libby P, Bonow RO, Mann DL, Tomaselli GF. Braunwald's heart disease: A textbook of cardiovascular medicine 2-volume set 11th edition. Elsevier. 2018.
7. Bhatt DL. REDUCE-IT. Eur Heart J. 2019;40(15):1174-5.
8. Nicholls SJ, Lincoff AM, Garcia M, Bash D, Ballantyne CM, Barter PJ, et al. Effect of high-dose omega-3 fatty acids vs corn oil on major adverse cardiovascular events in patients at high cardiovascular risk: The STRENGTH randomized clinical trial. JAMA. 2020;324(22):2268-80.
9. Schwartz GG, Steg PG, Szarek M, Bhatt DL, Bittner VA, Diaz R, et al. Alirocumab and cardiovascular outcomes after acute coronary syndrome. N Engl J Med. 2018;379(22):2097-107.
10. Giugliano RP, Pedersen TR, Park JG, De Ferrari GM, Gaciong ZA, Ceska R, et al. Clinical efficacy and safety of achieving very low LDL-cholesterol concentrations with the *PCSK9* inhibitor evolocumab: a prespecified secondary analysis of the FOURIER trial. Lancet. 2017;390(10106):1962-71.
11. Grundy SM, Stone NJ, Bailey AL, Beam C, Birtcher KK, Blumenthal RS, et al. 2018 AHA/ACC/AACVPR/AAPA/ABC/ACPM/ADA/AGS/APhA/ASPC/NLA/PCNA guideline on the management of blood cholesterol: A report of the American College of Cardiology/American Heart Association Task Force on Clinical Practice Guidelines. J Am Coll Cardiol. 2019;73(24):e285-350.

CHAPTER
106

Chronic Stable Angina

Artur Lopes, Rajesh G Nair, Boban Thomas

ABSTRACT

Chronic stable angina (CSA) is predominantly caused by atherosclerotic coronary artery disease (CAD), leading to obstructive or nonobstructive stenotic epicardial lesions. A significant burden of the plaque is detected in the proximal segments of the coronary arteries. Assessment of these lesions can be done, nowadays, by anatomical or functional approaches. Usually, a combination of both is required. However, in the foreseeable future, coronary computed tomography angiography (CCTA) will transform our understanding and the therapeutic approach to CSA.

"It is not the delicate neurotic person who is prone to angina, but the robust, the vigorous in mind and body, the keen and ambitious man, the indicator of whose engines is always at full speed ahead"

—William Osler

INTRODUCTION

Coronary artery disease is characterized by atherosclerotic plaque deposition in the epicardial arteries, and can be defined as obstructive or nonobstructive, based on the severity of the stenosis of the lesions.

The dynamic nature of the CAD process results in various clinical presentations, which can be conveniently categorized as either acute coronary syndrome (ACS) or chronic coronary syndrome (CCS).

In ACS, the rupture or erosion of the atherosclerotic plaque can lead to thrombus formation and vessel occlusion with ensuing myocardial ischemia and infarction. Most patients with CAD have chronic ischemic heart disease (CIHD), often causing CSA which is a CCS. The distinction between these two forms of clinical presentation, acute and chronic, is fundamental because prognosis and management of these patients are different. Both the syndromes, ACS and CCS, are more often associated with obstructive CAD, but in a few cases, these can be due to normal or nonobstructive CAD as shown in **Flowchart 1**.

Current understanding of CIHD is moving away from an ischemia-centered approach to an understanding of the total atherosclerotic burden in the coronary arteries. Presence and extent of CAD better predict the risk of future events than ischemia itself. Ischemia is probably a surrogate for the burden of CAD but not the main driver in prognosis. Some variation in terminologies used to describe patients of CSA exits and these terminologies are shown in **Table 1** with the year when they were used in the American and European guidelines.

The goal of this chapter is to provide a bird´s eye view on the relevant concepts and recent advances in our understanding and management of CSA due to CAD. We include a brief perspective on the recent ISCHEMIA (International Study of Comparative Health Effectiveness With Medical and Invasive Approaches) trial and its major contribution to this field.

Every attempt is made to avoid redundancy in information that can be easily accessed through freely available publications and web-based platforms. For more detailed information on the diagnostic approaches including exercise stress test (EST), stress echocardiography, CCTA, stress cardiac magnetic resonance and nuclear

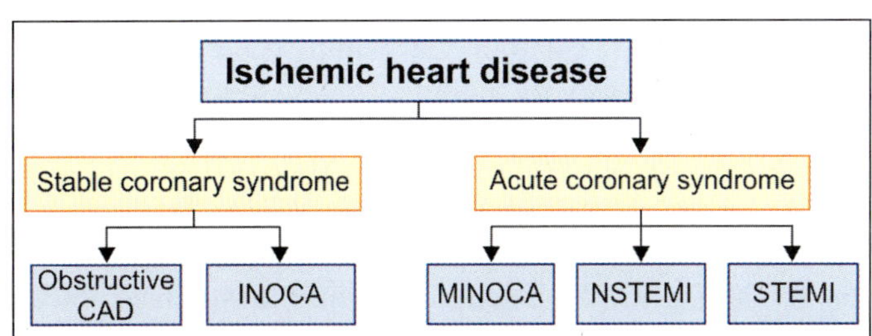

(INOCA: ischemia and no obstructive coronary artery disease; MINOCA: myocardial infarction with nonobstructive coronary arteries)

FLOWCHART 1: Modes of presentations of ischemic heart disease (IHD) and terminologies used when there are obstructive or nonobstructive findings on coronary angiography.

TABLE 1 Terminologies used from time to time for patients with chronic stable angina.

American guidelines	European guidelines
• Chronic Stable Angina (2002) • Stable Ischemic Heart Disease (2012)	• Stable coronary artery disease (2013) • Chronic coronary syndrome (2019). Includes six situations of patients with stable IHD

medicine studies, as well as optimal doses of medications, the reader should refer to the relevant chapters in this book, the ESC and the American College of Cardiology/American Heart Association (ACC/AHA) guidelines and premier books in cardiovascular medicine.

KEY MESSAGES

- Ischemic heart disease is mainly due to CAD.
- It has two clinical presentations with different prognosis and management:
  - Acute coronary syndromes
  - Chronic ischemic heart disease also designated as CCS often causing CSA or anginal equivalents.

PATHOPHYSIOLOGY

Myocardial ischemia is caused by an imbalance between myocardial O_2 requirements and myocardial O_2 supply.

Enhanced O_2 requirements are caused by (1) tachycardia, (2) increased contractility, and (3) increased left ventricular (LV) wall stress, as in the case of LV hypertrophy due to hypertension, aortic stenosis, or hypertrophic cardiomyopathy.

Diminished O_2 supply comes from (1) diminished arterial O_2 content, such as in severe anemia or hypoxia, and (2) diminished coronary blood flow, usually due to CAD.

The natural history of CAD atherosclerotic plaques includes long periods of "stability," punctuated by episodes of "instability" caused by micro-ruptures with enhanced thrombotic and inflammatory activity, followed by a healing phase that ends up in plaque growth. Many of these events are clinically unnoticed, but occasionally they may evolve to significant thrombus formation with vessel obstruction, causing prolonged ischemia and an ACS. Healing of plaques eventually involves calcification and the finding of coronary artery calcium (CAC) in many individuals with no previous history of a clinical ACS, suggests that they have had clinically silent plaque ruptures that have healed without any catastrophic outcomes. These calcified plaques are detected on CCTA and are reported as a CAC score.

The mechanism behind CAD causing myocardial ischemia is not only the degree of luminal stenosis. Recent CCTA studies using invasive fractional flow reserve (iFFR) demonstrated that plaque characteristics, namely low-attenuation plaques (LAPs) are associated with ischemia, independently of the degree of luminal stenosis.

Additionally, high-risk plaque characteristics such as LAP, spotty calcification, positive remodeling, and thin fibrous cap are better predictors of future ACS than the simple degree of luminal stenosis.

These high-risk plaque characteristics cannot be detected on invasive coronary angiography (ICA) as they are extraluminal features highlighting the fact that prognosis is determined by more than just the degree of luminal stenosis or even ischemia detected by functional testing.

Coronary artery disease also affects endothelial and vasomotor response, impairing coronary artery autoregulatory mechanisms, even in the absence of significant (>70%) luminal stenosis.

Myocardial perfusion can also be compromised by microvascular dysfunction as in the case of patients with angina, evidence of ischemia on noninvasive testing, but no signs of functionally significant epicardial CAD. Specific testing in these patients shows diminished coronary flow reserve and/or increased microcirculatory resistance. This is particularly important in women.

Finally, myocardial perfusion can also be transiently impaired, causing angina and ischemic electrocardiogram (ECG) changes, due to coronary vasospasm, as in the case in Prinzmetal angina.

KEY MESSAGES

- Ischemia results from a mismatch between myocardial oxygen supply and demand.
- Major determinants of oxygen demand are heart rate, contractility, and LV wall stress.
- In epicardial CAD, plaque characteristics (LAPs) contribute to impaired blood flow, in addition to and independent of luminal stenosis.
- Microvascular dysfunction and coronary vasospasm can cause ischemia in the absence of functionally significant epicardial CAD.

CLINICAL FEATURES

Chronic ischemic heart disease can manifest in different forms. Typical angina is the most specific symptom, but many patients present with atypical angina, nonanginal chest pain or anginal equivalents, such as dyspnea and fatigue, particularly women (**Flowchart 2**).

Symptom type and severity are useful for (1) predicting the likelihood of CAD, the so called pretest probability (PTP) and, hence, decide the need of further investigation, and (2) adjust treatment. The age, sex, and symptoms when used in combination suggest the PTP since the same symptom has different connotations regarding probability of obstructive CAD as shown in **Flowchart 3**. When we combine the PTP with risk factors and exercise ECG and

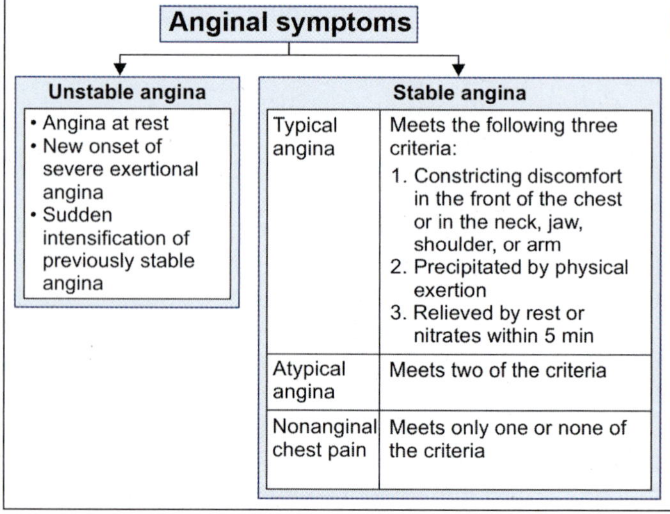

FLOWCHART 2: Clinical definitions of anginal syndromes.

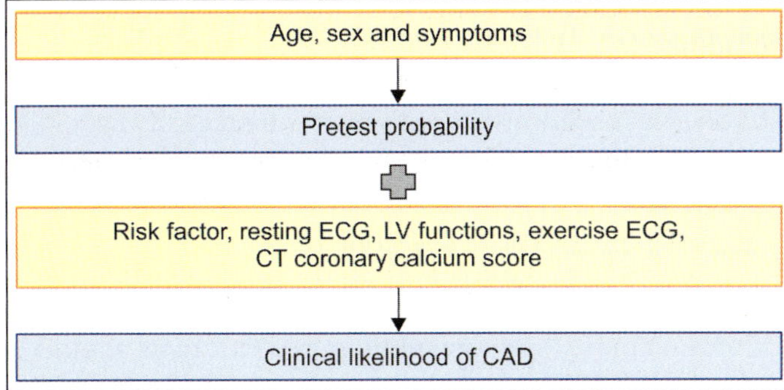

FLOWCHART 3: Pretest probability (PTP) is used for interpretation of exercise ECG and when PTP is combined with noninvasive tests one looks more recently at the clinical likelihood of CAD.

sometimes CCTA we can look at the "clinical likelihood" of CAD. Such a clinical approach is recommended and used these days.

There are different systems for grading symptom severity and impact on quality of life, the most common being the Canadian Cardiovascular Classification.

MANAGEMENT

The central objectives in the management of CSA include:

- Confirming the presence and extent of CAD
- Establishing symptom severity
- Identifying high-risk features by risk stratification
- Using the right therapeutic strategy to relieve symptoms and improve outcomes

The aim of all medical intervention is improving wellbeing and prognosis. For years, the paradigm of CAD management has been centered on detecting ischemia, identifying the potential cause of the detected ischemia through identification of the so-called culprit stenotic lesions and correcting it with revascularization.

The first step in patient management consists of evaluating the probability of patient's symptoms being due to ischemia (the PTP) and deciding on the need for further investigation. The PTP can be calculated from various tables that are specifically available. In patients with very low and low PTP it is usually considered safe to defer further testing, as the prognosis is good. For higher PTP patients, further testing is advised, usually to document and quantify ischemia (EST, stress echocardiography, nuclear medicine studies, stress cardiac magnetic resonance) or, alternatively, to directly detect obstructive CAD (CCTA). **Figures 1** to **3** are representative of images from a current-generation CT scanner.

Coronary computed tomography angiography is slowly becoming the preferred method to identify and characterize CAD. CAC score has proven very useful at identifying low and very low PTP patients, ruling out the need for further testing when the CAC score is zero. Clinical decisions cannot be made just on a simple absolute number alone.

After diagnosis of CSA caused by epicardial atherosclerotic CAD and risk stratification, therapeutic

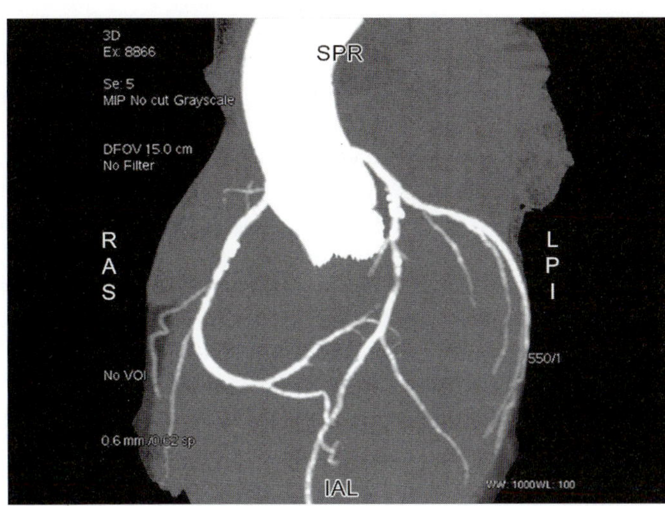

FIGURE 1: Angiography-type reformatted image on CCTA with obstructive calcified lesions in the LAD and a nonobstructive calcified lesion in the RCA.

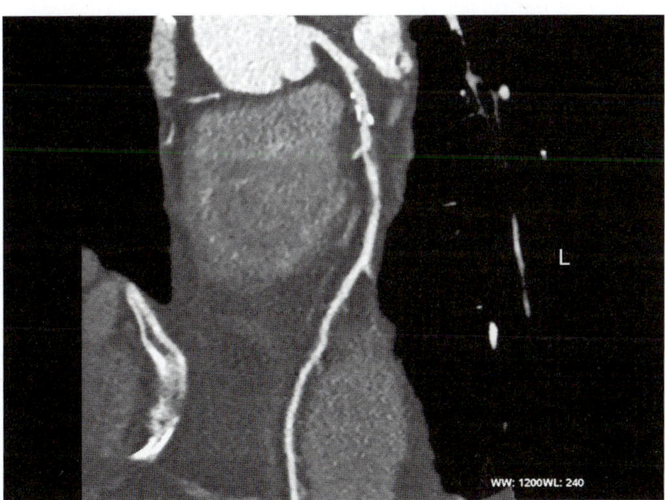

(CCTA: coronary computed tomography angiography)

FIGURE 2: Enhanced view of the LAD detailing the obstructive lesions in the LAD. It is easier to evaluate noncalcified lesions on CCTA. In the proximal LAD one of the three calcifications noted is a spotty calcification, an adverse prognostic feature.

options include lifestyle changes, therapeutic control of modifiable risk factors, optimal medical therapy (OMT), and revascularization techniques such as percutaneous coronary intervention (PCI) and coronary artery bypass grafting (CABG).

RISK STRATIFICATION

All patients with CAD and CSA should undergo risk stratification based on objective data and clinical judgment for the choice of therapies.

High-risk patients include those with:

- Resting LV dysfunction (hence the need for an echocardiography as a routine study in the evaluation of these patients)

- Significant ST segment changes early on and with low workload on an EST and/or ventricular arrhythmias (hence the need for an ECG and EST if potentially indicated).
- Extreme perfusion abnormalities (>10% of myocardium), or stress-induced LV dilation or dysfunction on nuclear medicine or cardiac MR studies (if available and indicated)
- Left main (LM) disease, multivessel CAD in proximal segments, or high-risk plaque features and extensive nonobstructive CAD found on CCTA (hence the seminal future role of CCTA)
- Wall motion abnormalities on stress echocardiography that involve multiple segments and/or segments in multiple coronary artery territories (if available but often hampered by logistic and time constraints). *The sensitivity and specifically of various noninvasive tests for CSA patients are given in **Table 2**.*

Low-risk patients include those with none of these abnormalities or with changes on EST occurring at high levels of exercise. *The findings suggestive of high risk, on various noninvasive tests, are shown in **Table 3**.*

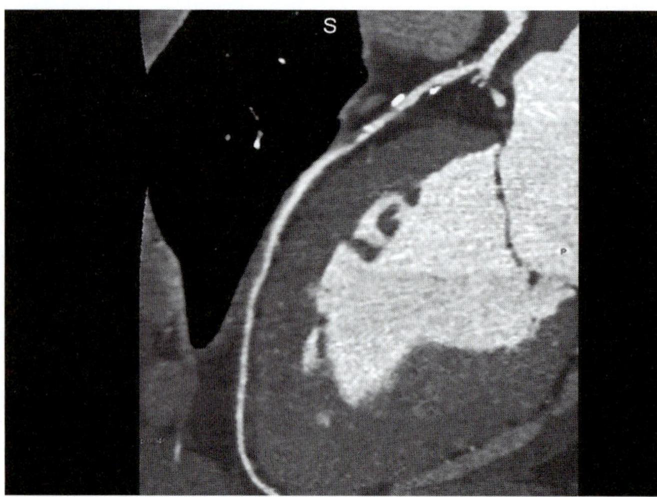

(FFR: fractional flow reserve)

FIGURE 3: The calcified lesions in the proximal LAD were nonobstructive on invasive coronary angiography while the subsequent lesion was hemodynamically significant by FFR and was stented. The stented lesion also had a high-risk feature called positive remodeling making it a relatively unstable lesion while the more proximal lesion being calcified is probably more stable.

After risk stratification, the following approaches should be adopted:

- *Lifestyle changes* including (1) smoking cessation, (2) dietary modifications with higher intakes of vegetables, fruits and whole grains and restricted consumption of saturated fats, processed foods, refined carbohydrates and sugar, and (3) regular physical exercise.
- *Risk factor control* including management of dyslipidemia, hypertension, diabetes, and obstructive sleep apnea. Established therapeutic targets should be the goal. *Risk factor modification should include all as shown in **Box 1**.*

Environmental hazards in the form of air and noise pollution are increasingly recognized risk factors in cardiovascular disease and are of particular concern in India. Not only do they directly promote CAD, but they also pose significant barriers to regular physical exercise which is a cornerstone in the management of the disease. Physical inactivity and dietary practices in India, including the high intake of saturated fats, trans fats, processed foods, high carbohydrate, and sugar content in regional cuisines contribute to the increasing incidence of type 2 diabetes mellitus in India.

- *Optimal medical therapy* including the use of medications that improve prognosis and symptoms. Those that improve prognosis include statins and antiplatelet agents. *The symptom-reducing angina therapy and secondary prevention strategy are shown in **Figure 4**. The choice of antianginal medications for symptom relief may depend on heart rate and LV functions as shown in **Table 4**.*
  - Medications that improve symptoms include beta-blockers, calcium channel blockers, nitrates, and long-acting nitrates. The second-line agents are nicorandil, trimetazidine, ivabradine, and ranolazine.
  - Treatment should be optimized in stages, starting with beta-blockers and followed by calcium channel blockers. If angina persists nitrates can be added, followed by *the second-line agents.*
  - The exact sequence of the initiation and escalation of therapy should be guided by clinical judgment and efficacy in relief of symptoms paying attention to side effects which can hinder compliance.
  - The management of hypertension also relieves symptoms of angina.

TABLE 2 The sensitivity, specificity, positive predictive value (PPV), and negative predictive value (NPV) of various noninvasive tests for diagnosis of chronic stable angina (CSA).

Test	Sensitivity	Specificity	PPV	NPV
Exercise electrocardiography	62%	68%	57%	72%
Stress echocardiography	88%	89%	93%	80%
Single photon emission computed tomography	83–84%	77–85%	79–85%	79–85%
Positron emission tomography	90–91%	82–91%	94%	75–84%
Stress magnetic resonance imaging	81%	87%	93%	70%
Coronary computed tomography angiography	98.2%	81.6%	90.5%	99%

TABLE 3 Findings that indicate a high-risk patient with each test.

Test	Findings indicating high-risk subjects
Exercise ECG	Cardiovascular mortality >3% per year according to duke treadmill score
SPECT or PET perfusion imaging	Area of ischemia ≥10% of the left ventricle myocardium
Stress echocardiography	≥3 of 16 segments with stress-induced hypokinesia or akinesia
CMR	≥2 of 16 segments with stress perfusion defects or ≥3 dobutamine-induced dysfunctional segments
Coronary CTA or ICA	Three-vessel disease with proximal stenoses, LM disease, or proximal anterior descending disease
Invasive functional testing	FFR ≥0.8, iwFR ≥0.89

(FFR: fractional flow reserve; ICA: invasive coronary angiography; iwFR: instantaneous wave-free ratio)

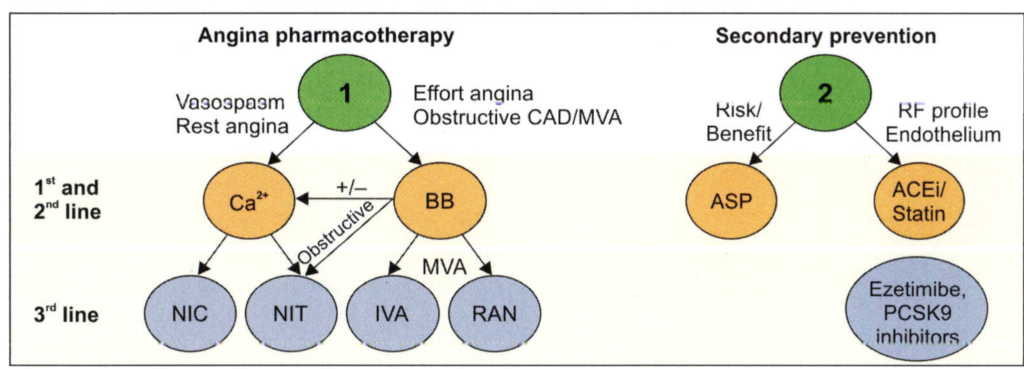

* For secondary prevention initially use high intensity statins. For those targets LDL <55 not achieved and Ezetimibe. In case still high add PCSK9 inhibitor

(ACEi: angiotensin-converting enzyme inhibitor; BB: beta blocker; ASP: aspirin; NIC: nicorandil; NIT: longacting nitrates; IVA: ivabradine; RAN: ranolazine; MVA: microvascular angina)

FIGURE 4: Pharmacotherapy in patients with chronic stable angina. Secondary prevention agents reduce mortality. Angina pharmacotherapy is for symptom relief only.

BOX 1 Factors that need to be controlled for risk reduction in patients of chronic stable angina (CSA).

- Physical activity
- Weight management
- Smoking cessation counseling
- Management of psychological factors
- Lipid management
- Blood pressure management
- Diabetes management

- *Revascularization*: As demonstrated by the results of the ISCHEMIA trial, after an initial approach with OMT and adequate attempts at optimization, revascularization should be considered, either with PCI or CABG, mainly to relieve poorly controlled symptoms and to decrease antianginal medications, especially in the case of side effects. An increased quality of life with revascularization was observed in ISCHEMIA for those with severe angina or frequent episodes.

The ideal modes of revascularization are (1) PCI, using current generation stents and guided by FFR, and (2) CABG, always using a left internal mammary artery graft and preferentially using only arterial grafts such as the right internal mammary artery and the radial artery. Both methods, PCI and CABG, should attempt to achieve complete revascularization.

- Percutaneous coronary intervention when indicated is extremely efficacious in providing symptom relief and will allow for reduction in medications to treat symptomatic angina.
- For patients with single vessel disease or two vessel disease with ongoing frequent angina, despite OMT, PCI is a reasonable option.
- Even those with three vessel disease and a SYNTAX score <22, PCI is an option.
- Current generation stents are virtually devoid of the problem of in-stent restenosis and technology keeps improving.
- PCI is also an option for whom CABG is contra-indicated if the targets are amenable to stenting.

The risks of stroke and other complications seen with CABG are much less with PCI.

TABLE 4 The choice of angina pharmacotherapy agents for symptom relief depends on heart rate, blood pressure, and left ventricular (LV) functions of the patients.

	Standard therapy	High heart rate (e.g., >80 beats/min)	Low heart rate (e.g., <50 beats/min)	LV dysfunction or heart failure	Low blood pressure
1st Step	BB or CCB	BB or non-DHP-CCB	DHP-CCB	BB	Low-dose BB or low-dose non-DHP-CCB
2nd Step	BB + DHP-CCB	BB + CCB	Switch to LAN	BB + LAN or BB + ivabradine	Switch to ivabradine, ranolazine, or trimetazidine
3rd Step	Add second-line drug	BB + ivabradine	DHP-CCB + LAN	Add another second-line drug	Combine two second-line drugs
4th Step			Add nicorandil, ranolazine, or trimetazidine		

(BB: beta-blockers; CCB: calcium channel blockers; DHP: dihydropyridine; LAN: long-acting nitrates)

However an analysis of data comparing PCI to CABG reveals the following:

- There is data suggestive of improved survival over the long term with CABG compared to PCI.
- The Achilles heel of CABG is the early procedural mortality and morbidity, while for PCI it is the need for repeat revascularization.
- Coronary artery bypass grafting is superior to PCI for cases of complex and extensive CAD, as quantified by a high SYNTAX score.
- Coronary artery bypass grafting provides flow distal to all, obstructive or nonobstructive, proximal lesions. For this reason, it can be considered a form of myocardial protection. PCI treats the most stenotic lesion, while not affording protection against other nonstenotic lesions elsewhere. Conceptually, OMT is also a form of myocardial protection, regardless of the method of revascularization, because it impacts the course of CAD and for that reason it is always indicated.
- Coronary artery bypass grafting is still preferable to PCI for LM lesions, for those with LV dysfunction and diabetes.

IMPORTANT CLINICAL TRIALS IN CSA

COURAGE: Among patients with stable CAD, *treatment with PCI was not associated with a difference in death or myocardial infarction (MI) compared with treatment with medical therapy through 15 years of follow-up*. Relief of angina occurred slightly more frequently with PCI early in the trial, but not differently from OMT at 5 years, with both arms showing marked reductions in angina throughout the trial.

BARI-2D: Among patients with diabetes and stable CAD, *revascularization by PCI or CABG failed to demonstrate superiority to OMT* over a mean of 5.3 years.

ORBITA: Among patients with stable angina, *PCI does not result in greater improvements in exercise times or anginal frequency compared with a sham procedure*, despite the presence of anatomically and functionally significant stenoses even though PCI resolved ischemia more effectively. Patients with more severe ischemia were more likely to show improvement in angina, a finding confirmed in ISCHEMIA.

PROMISE: This was the first randomized controlled trial to compare clinical outcomes in patients receiving functional stress testing or anatomic CCTA to investigate new-onset stable chest pain in those with no prior diagnosis of CAD. The study showed no difference between patients receiving a CCTA and those receiving functional heart tests in terms of the study's primary endpoint.

SCOT-HEART: The goal of the trial was to evaluate CCTA compared with standard care among low- to intermediate-risk patients with chest pain suggestive of obstructive coronary disease. At a median follow-up of nearly 5 years, CCTA was associated with a reduction in coronary heart disease (CHD) death or MI compared to standard care due to a reduction in nonfatal MI. *Long-term benefit from CCTA may have been due to lifestyle modification and statin therapy. LAP burden was the strongest predictor for MI compared with cardiovascular risk score, CAC score, and coronary artery area stenosis.*

SCOT-HEART and PROMISE showed that CCTA is an alternative to standard care (including conventional stress testing) in the evaluation of patients with chest pain.

The ISCHEMIA trial: The recent publication of the ISCHEMIA trial has practical relevance to the Indian scenario. Approximately 20% of the 5,179 randomized patients were from India. The trial compared two strategies of management in patients with stable CAD and moderate-to-severe ischemia on stress testing: (1) an early or initial invasive strategy including OMT and appropriate revascularization, and (2) OMT alone (**Fig. 5**). There were no differences in the primary outcomes or secondary outcomes including cardiovascular death, MI, cardiac arrest, or stroke, between the two management strategies. The trial data indirectly leads credence to the hypothesis that atherosclerotic burden in the form of both obstructive and nonobstructive CAD, and not ischemia may be the main driver of clinical events and outcomes. It is important to emphasize that patients with LM disease as detected by CCTA or LV dysfunction with LV ejection fraction (LVEF) <35% were excluded from the study. One

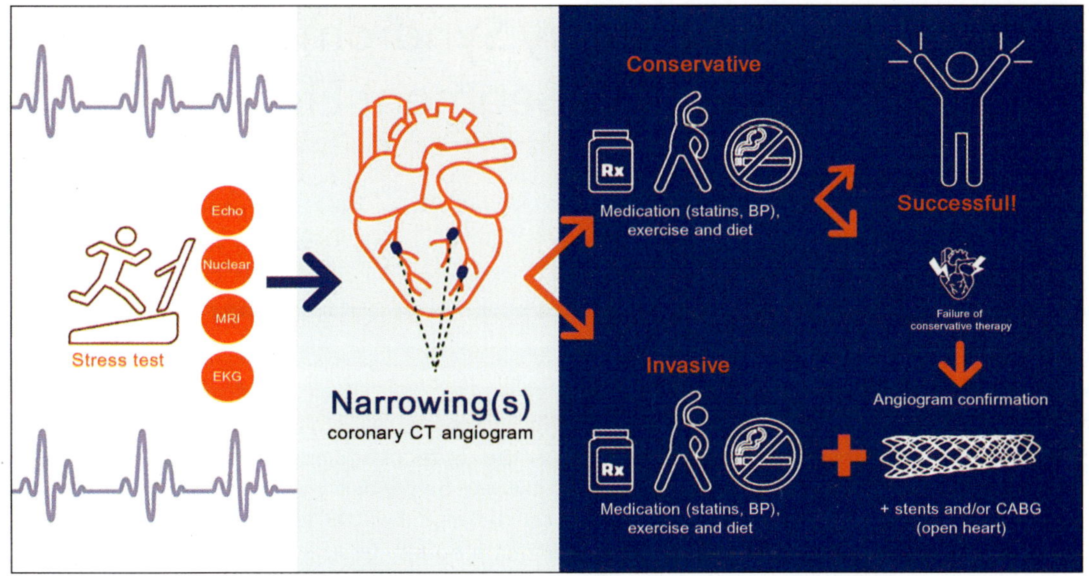

FIGURE 5: The design of the ISCHEMIA study with the two therapeutic arms.

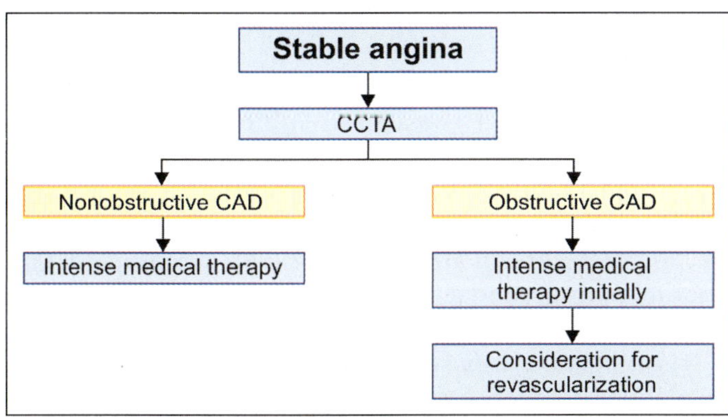

FLOWCHART 4: Simplified diagnostic algorithm that will probably become the standard in the future. Ischemia imaging or exercise stress testing can be applied after initial detection of CAD by CCTA to adopt the optimal therapeutic approach.

of the major strengths of the study was that randomization occurred prior to angiography and CCTA enriched the trial with patients with real ischemia as it weaned out the false positives (those who were diagnosed as having ischemia but no epicardial atherosclerotic significant stenotic disease detected on CCTA). Those with significant LM disease detected by CCTA were excluded in the trial because according to current recommendations OMT alone probably is inappropriate. Important lessons can be gleaned for us from this trial. The EST is the predominant mode of detecting ischemia in India and CCTA is increasingly available. The management algorithm in the trial is transferrable to the practical clinical setting in India remarkably well. Also, OMT has improved considerably leading to low event rates, even in Indian patients.

In summary, management decisions in CSA should be based on clinical judgment, robust evidence from clinical trials, and clinical guidelines respecting patient preferences and encouraging discussion within a Heart Team if indicated. Most patients can be managed with OMT initially and revascularization can be considered for ongoing symptoms, intolerance of medication, or in specific circumstances such as disease of the LM or those with significant LV dysfunction (**Flowchart 4**).

ACKNOWLEDGMENTS

The authors wish to thank Drs Silvia Aguiar and Imad Hassan for helpful comments on the chapter.

RECOMMENDED READINGS

1. Thomas B, Hassan I. The wisdom in ISCHEMIA. Indian Heart J. 2020;72(6):623-4.
2. Ferraro R, Latina JM, Alfaddagh A, Michos ED, Blaha MJ, Jones SR, et al. Evaluation and Management of Patients With Stable Angina: Beyond the Ischemia Paradigm: JACC State-of-the-Art Review. J Am Coll Cardiol. 2020;76(19):2252-66.
3. Doenst T, Haverich A, Serruys P, Bonow RO, Kappetein P, Falk V, et al. PCI and CABG for Treating Stable Coronary Artery Disease: JACC Review Topic of the Week. J Am Coll Cardiol. 2019;73(8):964-76.
4. Knuuti J, Wijns W, Saraste A, Capodanno D, Barbato E, Funck-Brentano C, et al. ESC Scientific Document Group. 2019 ESC Guidelines for the diagnosis and management of chronic coronary syndromes. Eur Heart J. 2020;41(3):407-77.
5. Singh T, Bing R, Dweck MR, van Beek EJR, Mills NL, Williams MC, et al. Exercise Electrocardiography and Computed Tomography Coronary Angiography for Patients With Suspected Stable Angina Pectoris: A Post Hoc Analysis of the Randomized SCOT-HEART Trial. JAMA Cardiol. 2020;5(8):920-8.

CHAPTER 107 Acute Coronary Syndrome: Unstable Angina and Non-ST-Segment Elevation Myocardial Infarction (NSTEMI)

Mohanan Padinhare

ABSTRACT

The management of acute coronary syndrome (ACS) has been at the center of an impressive amount of research leading to a significant improvement in outcomes over the last 50 years. ACS can be divided into subgroups of ST-segment elevation myocardial infarction (STEMI), non-ST-segment elevation myocardial infarction (NSTEMI), and unstable angina. ACS carries significant morbidity and mortality and the prompt diagnosis and appropriate treatment are essential. NSTEMI and unstable angina are very similar, with NSTEMI having positive cardiac biomarkers. The presentation, diagnosis, and management of unstable angina and NSTEMI are discussed below.

"In the confrontation between the stream and the rock, the stream always wins, not through strength but by perseverance"

—H Jackson Brown

INTRODUCTION

Acute coronary syndrome occurs when atherosclerotic coronary plaque becomes unstable, leading to a series of events that eventually result in partial or total thrombotic occlusion of a coronary artery. ACSs are categorized into unstable angina, NSTEMI, and STEMI. The terms "transmural," "nontransmural," "Q wave MI," and "non-Q wave MI" are no longer recommended.

Unstable angina: Three kinds of presentations of unstable angina exist:

1. Exertional angina of new onset (even if relieved with rest and requiring a consistent amount of exertion to produce symptoms, angina is considered unstable when it first occurs)
2. Exertional angina that was previously stable and now occurs with less physical exertion
3. Anginal symptoms at rest without physical exertion

In unstable angina, the cardiac enzymes remain normal.

Non-ST-segment elevation myocardial infarction: Anginal symptoms at rest that result in myocardial necrosis as identified by elevated cardiac biomarkers with no ST-segment elevation on the 12-lead electrocardiogram (ECG).

ST-segment elevation myocardial infarction: Anginal symptoms at rest that result in myocardial necrosis, as identified by elevated cardiac biomarkers with ST-segment elevation on the 12-lead ECG.

PATHOPHYSIOLOGY

Atherosclerotic plaques in the coronary arteries are responsible for coronary artery disease (CAD). Some atherosclerotic plaques have a more stable fibrous cap. Others are thin and considered vulnerable. Vulnerable plaque is responsible for ACSs. Rupture or erosion of a vulnerable plaque causes coronary artery thrombosis. A substance known as "tissue factor" is located within the necrotic core of the plaque. When exposed to the bloodstream, tissue factor activates the clotting cascade, and thrombosis occurs (**Fig. 1**).

Tissue factor is exposed when the fibrous cap that covers the plaque becomes disrupted or ulcerated. This disruption of the fibrous cap is called "plaque rupture" or "plaque erosion." Surprisingly, plaque rupture and thrombosis frequently occur at the site of modest coronary stenosis (<50% luminal narrowing); therefore, even if stress test results are normal, the risk for an ACS is still present. Of course, stress testing is a useful method to detect stenosis of 70% or greater.

Unstable angina has a lower incidence of coronary thrombosis compared with NSTEMI or STEMI and is more often the result of fixed atherosclerotic stenosis. Plaque rupture or erosion resulting in coronary occlusion is the predominant mechanism in NSTEMI and STEMI.

SYMPTOMS

The symptoms of occlusive CAD can manifest as chronic stable angina pectoris or angina as a part of an ACS. Both of which are similar, with the latter frequently occurring at rest. Substernal chest pressure with radiation to the medial portion of the left arm or left jaw is the classic description.

Angina can be described as a "tightness," "discomfort, not pain," "squeezing," "indigestion," "heaviness," or an "elephant sitting on my chest." Levine sign is when a patient places his or her fist in the center of the chest to describe the sensations of squeezing and tightness with angina.

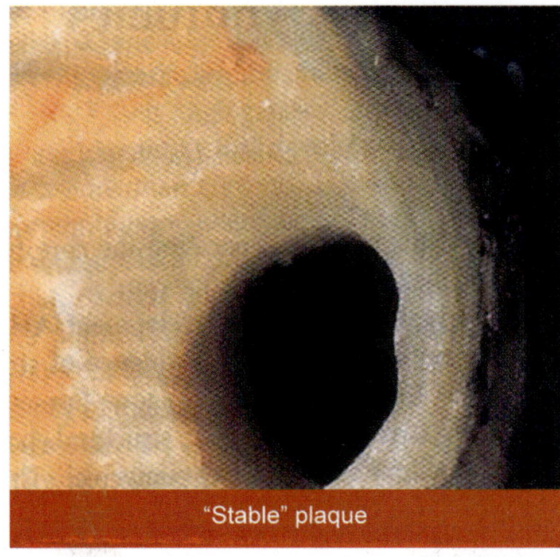

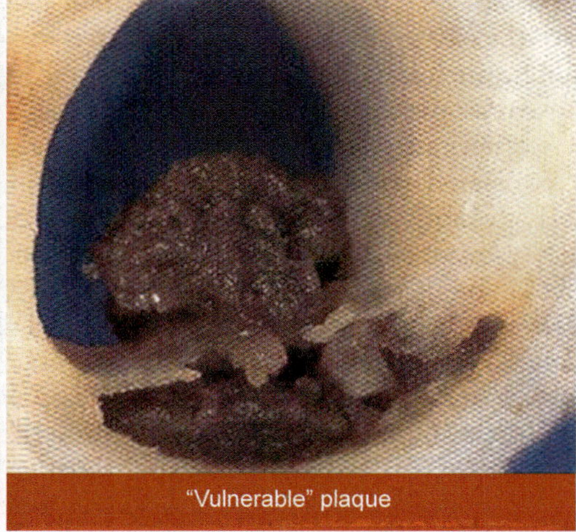

FIGURE 1: Stable plaque with thick fibers cap (patient presents as chronic stable angina) on the left and a ruptured vulnerable plaque with formation of intracoronary thrombosis (patient presents with ACS).

The pain from angina is gradual in onset and must last for at least 5 minutes. Also, the pain is diffuse and difficult to localize to one part of the chest; the description of a large versus small area of pain can help distinguish from musculoskeletal issues.

Less common presentations include only shoulder pain, pain down both arms, left wrist pain, right-sided chest or jaw pain, radiation to the right arm, mid-thoracic back pain, and only dyspnea without chest pain. Rarely, the pain of angina is described as sharp.

Some associated symptoms that occur simultaneously with the classic anginal symptoms above include dyspnea, diaphoresis (cold sweats), fatigue/weakness, nausea, and dizziness. Women, elderly patients, and patients with diabetes tend to have more atypical presentations of angina.

Many noncardiac disease states can cause chest pain, as well. Important features that would suggest noncardiac causes of chest pain include worsening with inspiration (pleuritic pain), the duration of the pain (<5 min), a small pinpoint area of pain (angina is more diffuse), and no relief with nitroglycerine. Esophageal spasm—a relatively uncommon cause of chest pain—can be relieved with nitroglycerine, causing it to mimic symptoms of angina. Sharp, shooting chest pains lasting a few seconds to a minute are common and usually musculoskeletal.

When an atherosclerotic plaque ulcerates and thrombosis occurs, an ACS develops and the above-mentioned anginal symptoms can occur at rest. In this setting, the pain is frequently more severe and has a longer duration.

PHYSICAL EXAMINATION

Physical examination findings are relatively nonspecific. They are usually only present during the anginal episode, making this a less helpful means of diagnosis. When examined during an anginal attack, the heart rate and blood pressure may be elevated due to increased sympathetic tone.

A fourth heart sound (S4) may be present during myocardial ischemia due to the lack of adenosine triphosphate (ATP) production impairing left ventricular relaxation. Myocardial relaxation is an active process requiring ATP, which is reduced during ischemia, and a S4 occurs when a noncompliant, stiffened left ventricle receives blood after atrial contraction because it is unable to relax adequately.

During inferior ischemia, posteromedial papillary muscle dysfunction can cause mitral regurgitation, resulting in a holosystolic murmur at the cardiac apex radiating to the axilla. This rarely occurs during anterior or lateral ischemia because the anterolateral papillary muscle has dual supply from the left anterior descending and circumflex coronary artery.

When the left ventricular end-diastolic pressure (LVEDP) increases during myocardial ischemia, that pressure can be transmitted backward to the pulmonary veins and into the pulmonary vasculature, causing transient pulmonary edema that results in dyspnea and rales on lung examination.

Cardiac auscultation in patients with acute chest pain is more helpful to rule out other conditions that can cause chest pain and have cardiac murmurs. Aortic stenosis and hypertrophic cardiomyopathy, both will have systolic murmurs. A quiet and silent precordium helps to exclude these conditions.

DIAGNOSIS

The diagnosis of unstable angina and NSTEMI is predominantly based on the ECG and cardiac enzymes. Physical examination, as previously described, is nonspecific.

- *Electrocardiogram*: ECG tracing can have multiple abnormalities, but, by definition, there is no ST-segment elevation. The most common finding is ST-segment depression. This ST-segment depression is horizontal or down-sloping in shape. The T waves may be inverted, usually symmetrically (**Fig. 2**).

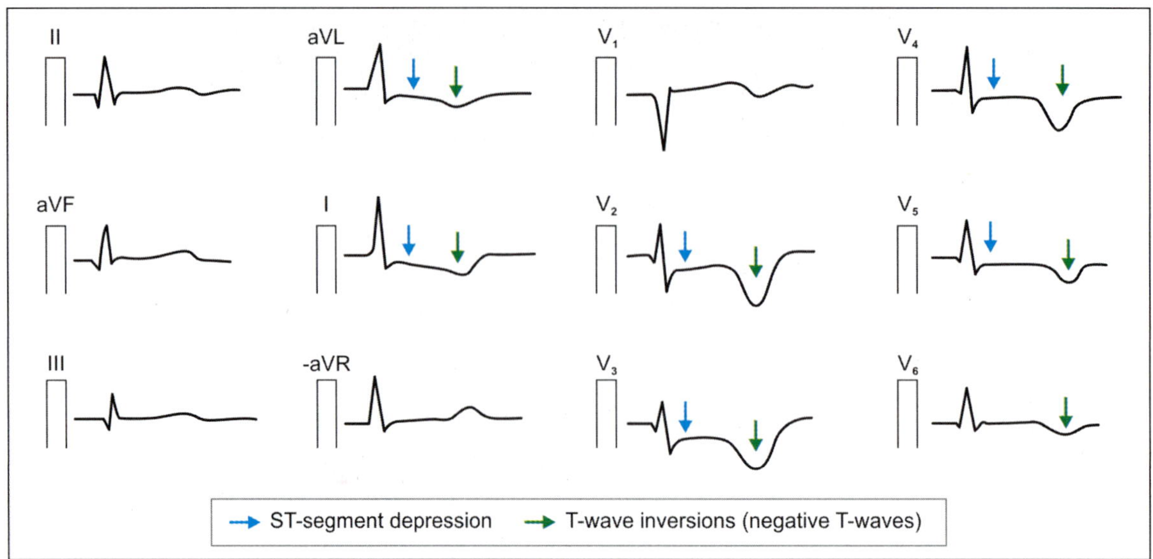

FIGURE 2: ST-T wave changes in patients with ACS. The ST-segment depression is usually horizontal or downsloping in shape. The T waves may be inverted and it is typically symmetrical.

Surprisingly, unstable angina and NSTEMI both can occur, even with a completely normal ECG; this makes diagnosis quite a challenge. Observation in the hospital for cardiac enzymes in context of serial ECGs (usually 6–8 hours apart) is required to completely exclude unstable angina and NSTEMI, as the ECG changes can be dynamic (come and go) and may be normal initially. Also, cardiac enzymes (troponin) require 3–4 hours after the injury before significant elevation in the blood.

- *Cardiac enzymes*: During NSTEMI, there will be elevation of the cardiac enzymes, indicative of myocardial necrosis. During unstable angina, however, there is no—or only very minimal—elevation. This is the main distinguishing feature between the two diagnoses. The vast majority of cardiac troponin assays that are run on automated platforms in the central laboratory are sensitive (i.e., allow for detection of cardiac troponin in ~20–50% of healthy individuals) or high-sensitivity (detection in ~50–95% of healthy individuals) assays. Due to the higher sensitivity and diagnostic accuracy for the detection of MI at presentation, the time interval to the second cardiac troponin assessment can be shortened with the use of high-sensitive cardiac troponin (hs-cTn) assays. This seems to substantially reduce the delay to diagnosis, translating into shorter stays in the emergency department, and lower costs. Natriuretic peptides may provide incremental prognostic information and may help in risk stratification.

Many cardiac pathologies other than MI also result in cardiomyocyte injury and, therefore, cardiac troponin elevations. Tachyarrhythmias, heart failure (HF), hypertensive emergencies, critical illness, myocarditis, Takotsubo syndrome, and valvular heart disease are the common ones.

Among the multitude of *additional biomarkers* evaluated for the diagnosis of NSTE-ACS, only creatine kinase-myocardial band (CK-MB), myosin-binding protein C, and copeptin may have clinical relevance in specific clinical settings when used in combination with cardiac troponin T/I. Compared with cardiac troponin, CK-MB shows a more rapid decline after MI and may provide added value for the timing of myocardial injury and the detection of early reinfarction.

Serum creatinine and estimated glomerular filtration rate (eGFR) should also be determined in all patients with ACS because they affect prognosis.

- *Coronary CT angio (CCTA)* may be an option in patients who present to the emergency with chest pain and have a low-to-modest clinical likelihood of CAD since a normal scan excludes CAD. In addition, upfront imaging with CCTA reduces the need for invasive coronary angiography in some high-risk patients also.

The diagnostic algorithm for distinguishing patients presenting with acute chest pain into noncardiac pain, unstable angina, NSTEMI, and STEMI as given by the latest ESC guidelines of 2020 is shown in **Figure 3**. One must make an integrated opinion based on history of chest pain, serial changes in ECG, and biomarkers. It is important clinically so that patients with CAD are not sent back from the emergency with a missed diagnosis of ACS. This can prove to be risky. On the other hand, those with noncardiac chest pain need to be diagnosed within 6–12 hours so that they can be sent back with surety that it is not due to CAD.

TREATMENT

After evaluation, these patients need to be admitted in the coronary care unit (CCU) for at least 48–72 hours. The progress of symptoms can be variable. Some patients can have recurrent pain, arrhythmias, and left ventricular failure. High risk markers in ACS patients are old age, recurrent chest pain, known multivessel disease, prolonged pain, ectopics, elevated troponins, and diffuse ST change in ECG. Recurrent arrhythmias (ventricular ectopics and ventricular tachycardia), reduced ejection fraction

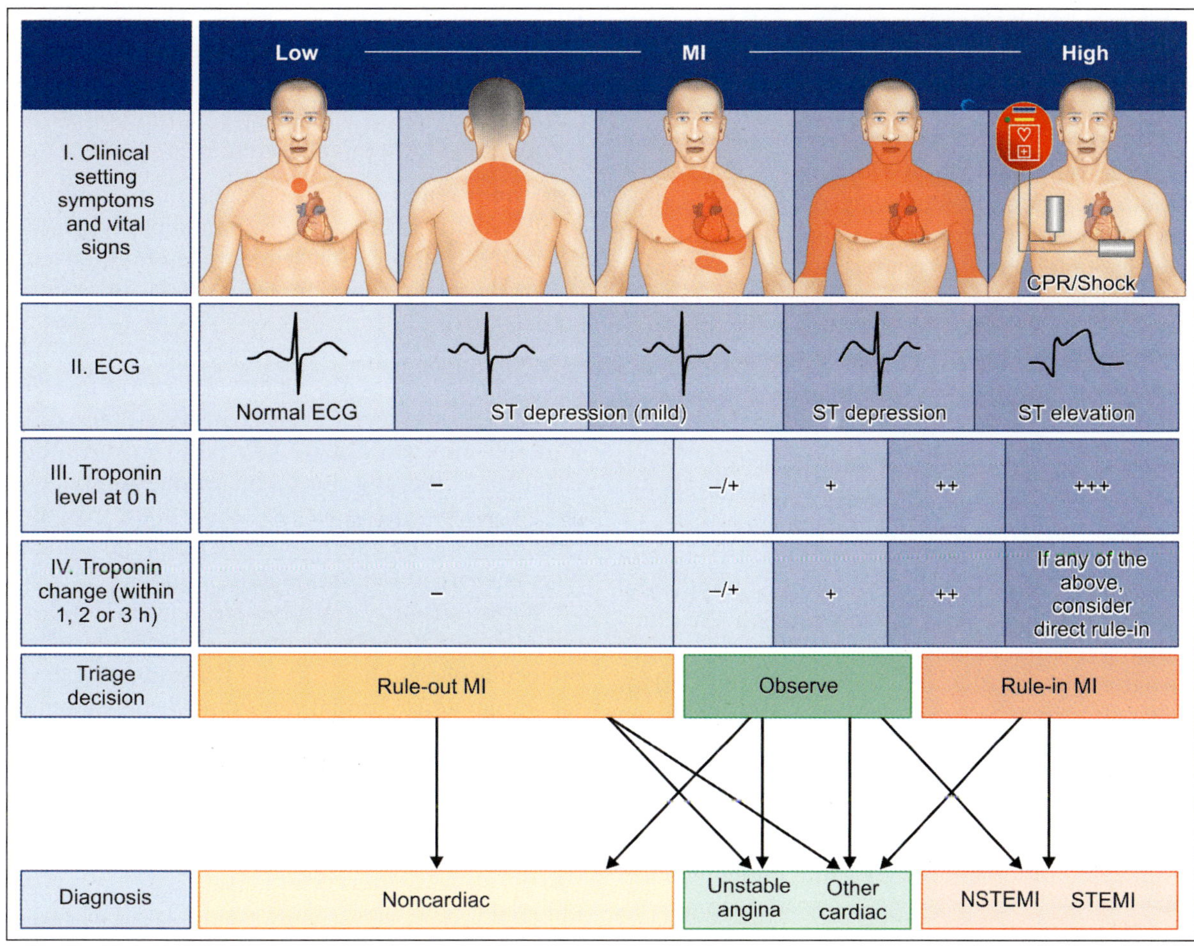

FIGURE 3: Diagnostic algorithm and triage in acute coronary syndrome.

Source: Adopted from ESC guidelines 2020 on ACS.

(EF) of <40%, and history of intervention [percutaneous transluminal coronary angioplasty/coronary artery bypass grafting (PTCA/CABG)] in the preceding 6 months are also markers of high risk. These factors determine whether, patients of ACS are to be managed with initial invasive or conservative strategy.

Early invasive strategy refers to proceeding to coronary angiography with possible percutaneous coronary intervention (PCI) within 4–24 hours of hospital admission. Invasive coronary angiography helps in evaluation of these patients and need of intervention. Intracoronary imaging methods, IVUS and OCT, also help and allow real-time tomographic assessment of vessel size, lumen area, plaque composition and volume, as well as stent coverage and expansion. Patients with unstable plaque respond well to early PCI. Approximately 5–10% of ACS patients require CABG and these represent a challenging subgroup given their high-risk characteristics compared with patients undergoing elective CABG. In the absence of randomized data, optimal timing for nonemergency CABG in ACS patients should be determined individually.

Radial access is recommended as the preferred approach in ACS patients undergoing invasive assessment with or without PCI. Multivessel disease is frequent in ACS. The timing and completeness of revascularization should be decided according to functional relevance of all stenoses, age, general patient condition, comorbidities, and left ventricular function.

Initial conservative management involves management of patients with medicines, both injectable and oral. Most of these patients have no elevation in troponins and do not have any complications like recurrent pain, arrhythmias, or HF. Once they are stabilized, after a few days additional risk stratification must be done by evaluation of left ventricular systolic function either by echocardiography or myocardial perfusion imaging. If the EF is <40%, the patient is at high risk and invasive coronary angiography should be performed. If the EF is >40%, a stress test with imaging should be performed later. Only those with high-risk stress imaging need to be sent for intervention.

Initial therapy focuses on stabilizing the patient's condition, relieving ischemic pain, and providing anti-thrombotic therapy (antiplatelet drugs and anticoagulants).

Antiplatelet therapy: There are three main categories of antiplatelet drugs.

Aspirin: This acts by blocking the enzyme cyclooxygenase resulting in decreased thromboxane A2 production and platelet inhibition. The dose is 75–150 mg once daily.

Thienopyridines: It is also known as P2Y12 receptor blockers, these agents include clopidogrel, prasugrel, and ticagrelor. Clopidogrel has delayed onset of action, no means of reversing the effects, and a significant percentage of people simply do not respond to this therapy. Prasugrel and ticagrelor have fast onsets of action and few if any nonresponders, but carry a higher risk for bleeding. Prasugrel is not recommended if there is a prior history of transient ischemic attack (TIA) or stroke, as it may cause harm (class III).

In patients with ACS the newer agents, ticagrelor and prasugrel, are preferred. All patients of ACS should be put on dual antiplatelet therapy (DAPT) with aspirin and one of the three P2 Y12 receptor antagonist. A loading dose of thienopyridines is given when they are started (clopidogrel 300 mg, ticagrelor 180 mg, and prasugrel 60 mg). Then they are continued in regular maintenance dose (clopidogrel 75 mg OD, ticagrelor 90 mg BID, and prasugrel 10 mg OD) for at least 1 year after an ACS. Ticagrelor and prasugrel are the preferred agents in ACS patients when they undergo PCI with stenting. Patients on conservative strategy are generally treated with clopidogrel along with aspirin as a component of the DAPT. Every patient must be assessed for bleeding risk since they are put on antiplatelets and anticoagulants at the same time.

Glycoprotein IIb/IIIa inhibitors: This category includes abciximab, eptifibatide, and tirofiban. These agents very strongly inhibit platelet function by blocking the binding of fibrinogen to the activated glycoprotein IIb/IIIa receptor complex. They are rarely used now.

Anticoagulants: Full anticoagulation should be started in all patients with unstable angina and NSTEMI, unless a contraindication exists. The choice of anticoagulant used differs between early invasive and initial conservative strategy groups.

When initial conservative management is undertaken, anticoagulation with either unfractionated heparin, low-molecular-weight heparin (e.g., enoxaparin), or fondaparinux should be started. The duration of anticoagulation therapy should be for minimum 48 hours, but guidelines based on clinical trials state that they can be continued for the entire length of hospitalization, especially if invasive treatment is not contemplated.

When an early invasive strategy is employed, anticoagulation should be with unfractionated heparin, low-molecular-weight heparin, or bivalirudin. Bivalirudin is not recommended for initial conservative management (**Fig. 4**).

Other agents in medical management: The other agents used are statins, beta blockers, angiotensin-converting enzyme (ACE) inhibitors/angiotensin receptor blockers (ARBs), aldosterone antagonists, calcium channel blockers, and nitrates. Treatment with fibrinolytic agent is not recommended for unstable angina and NSTEMI management.

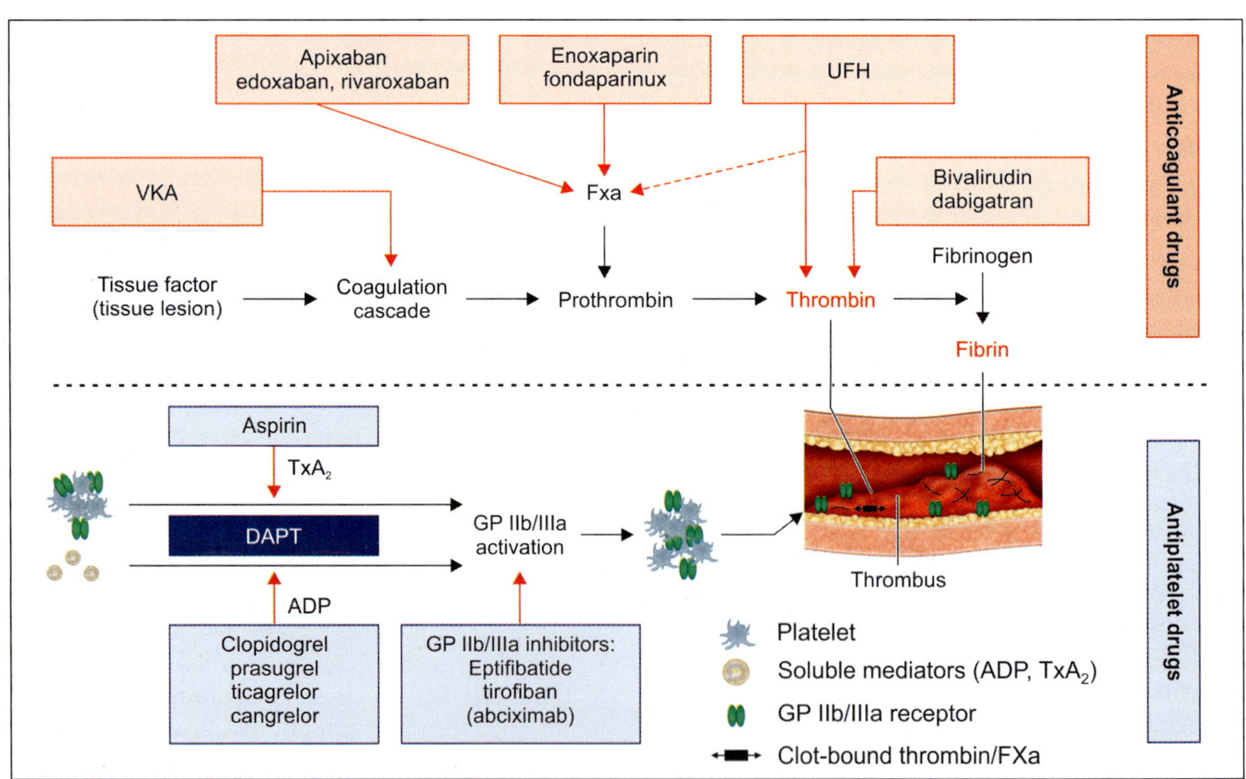

(ADP: adenosine diphosphate; DAPT: dual antiplatelet therapy; FXa: factor Xa; GP: glycoprotein; TxA_2: thromboxane A_2; UFH: unfractionated heparin; VKA: vitamin K antagonist)

FIGURE 4: The type of antiplatelet and anticoagulant drugs used in ACS. The sites of action of various agents are also shown.

β-hydroxy β-methylglutaryl-CoA (HMG-CoA) reductase inhibitors (statins): Every patient with unstable angina and NSTEMI should receive high-dose statin therapy. The Multicenter InSync Randomized Clinical Evaluation (MIRACLE) and Pravastatin or Atorvastatin Evaluation and Infection Therapy–Thrombolysis in Myocardial Infarction 22 (PROVE-IT TIMI 22) trial used atorvastatin (80 mg/day) with good results. Statin therapy should be lifetime after a person has an ACS, unless a contraindication exists.

Beta-blockers: Although little data exists regarding the efficacy of beta-blockers during unstable angina and NSTEMI, there are an abundance of data for their use during STEMI. American College of Cardiology/American Heart Association (ACC/AHA) guidelines recommend early intravenous beta blockers when no contraindication exists and there is angina, hypertension, or tachycardia not related to HF. Long-term (lifetime) therapy has been shown to reduce MI incidence and improve mortality.

ACE inhibitors/ARBs: There are also less data to support using ACE inhibitors during unstable angina and NSTEMI than during STEMI, where definite benefit is seen. The ACC/AHA guidelines recommend that ACE inhibitors be given upon hospital discharge in patients with hypertension, diabetes, LV systolic dysfunction (EF < 40%), and/or HF symptoms. There may be a benefit to all patients, but the data are limited; thus, a recommendation to use ACE inhibitors in all patients following unstable angina and NSTEMI is yet to be made. When a patient does not tolerate an ACE inhibitor due to cough, an ARB is a good alternative.

Aldosterone antagonists: The aldosterone antagonist eplerenone was evaluated in the Eplerenone Post-Acute Myocardial Infarction Heart Failure Efficacy and Survival (EPHESUS) trial, leading to the recommendation for use of the agents with an ACE inhibitor prior to hospital discharge after unstable angina and NSTEMI if there is left ventricular systolic dysfunction (EF < 40%) and either diabetes or symptomatic HF and no contraindication (serum creatinine > 2.5 mL/min and or potassium > 5.0 mEq/L). A class effect is likely present; therefore, spironolactone is frequently used instead of eplerenone due to cost concerns, though there are no direct data to support this practice.

Calcium channel blockers: The nondihydropyridine calcium channel blockers diltiazem and verapamil can be used when there is a contraindication to beta blockers, such as in asthma, and no HF or significant left ventricular systolic dysfunction is present. Sublingual nifedipine is contraindicated due to a reflexive increase in the sympathetic nervous system, which can be harmful.

Nitrates: Nitrates are helpful to treat angina symptoms, hypertension, and HF during unstable angina and NSTEMI; however, no clinical data exists to show a mortality benefit and thus their use is individualized. The use of nitrates should not preclude using drugs that do show a mortality benefit.

Treatment of arrhythmias: Ventricular tachycardia and ventricular fibrillation can occur in patients with ACS. Although less common, atrial fibrillation and atrial flutter can also be seen. To prevent arrhythmias during an ACS we should use beta blockers and maintain electrolytes (potassium and magnesium) within normal limits.

Treatment of anemia: There are no official guidelines regarding the threshold for transfusion in patients who are anemic during an ACS. In general, the hematocrit should be maintained at >21% and preferably above 30%. Given that the treatment of NSTE-ACS and unstable angina includes antithrombotic therapy (which may exacerbate bleeding), it is important to identify the cause of anemia and occult bleeds.

RECOMMENDED READINGS

1. Jneid H, Anderson JL, Wright RS, Adams CD, Bridges CR, Casey DE Jr, et al. 2012 ACCF/AHA focused update of the guideline for the management of patients with unstable angina/Non-ST-elevation myocardial infarction (updating the 2007 guideline and replacing the 2011 focused update): a report of the American College of Cardiology Foundation/American Heart Association Task Force on practice guidelines. Circulation. 2012;126(7):875-910.
2. Braunwald E, Morrow DA. Unstable angina: is it time for a requiem? Circulation. 2013;127(24):2452-7.
3. Kumar A, Cannon CP. Acute Coronary Syndromes: Diagnosis and Management, Part 1. Mayo Clin Proc. 2009;84(10):917-38.
4. Collet JP, Thiele H, Barbato E, Barthélémy O, Bauersachs J, Bhatt DL, et al.; ESC Scientific Document Group. 2020 ESC Guidelines for the management of acute coronary syndromes in patients presenting without persistent ST-segment elevation. Eur Heart J. 2021;42(14):1289-1367.
5. Xavier D, Pais P, Devereaux PJ, Xie C, Prabhakaran D, Reddy KS, et al.; CREATE registry investigators. Treatment and outcomes of acute coronary syndromes in India (CREATE): a prospective analysis of registry data. Lancet. 2008;371(9622):1435-42.
6. Antman EM, Cohen M, Bernink PJ, McCabe CH, Horacek T, Papuchis G, et al. The TIMI risk score for unstable angina/non-ST elevation MI: A method for prognostication and therapeutic decision making. JAMA. 2000;284(7):835-42.

CHAPTER

108 Acute ST-elevation Myocardial Infarction

Srinivasan Narayanan, Ajit S Mullasari, Thomas Alexander

ABSTRACT

One of the most serious forms of acute coronary syndrome (ACS) is ST-elevation myocardial infarction (STEMI). It is a life-threatening and time-sensitive emergency which must be promptly diagnosed and treated early with either thrombolysis or revascularization of the culprit artery with primary percutaneous coronary intervention (PPCI), if available. Most STEMI occurs due to rupture of an atheromatous plaque with formation of a thrombus over it. The patients present with acute severe chest pain which is distinct and is accompanied with perspiration, tachypnea, and sympathetic overactivity.

Electrocardiogram (ECG) and echocardiography are important first investigations for the diagnosis. The current Fourth 2018 Universal Definition of Myocardial Infarction (MI) emphasize the role of biomarker cardiac troponin (cTn) along with documentation of myocardial ischemia for the diagnosis of MI. Rise in troponin without ischemia indicates myocardial injury only. Early diagnosis and rapid institution of reperfusion therapy have reduced the mortality significantly. Dual antiplatelet and antithrombotic agents should be given along with reperfusion therapy. Relief of pain and continuous rhythm monitoring are important.

"A heart can be broken, but it will keep beating, just the same"

—Fannie Flagg

INTRODUCTION

ST-elevation myocardial infarction is an acute event that occurs due to occlusion of one or more coronary arteries supplying the heart resulting in myocardial injury and necrosis. Occlusive luminal thrombosis is the mechanism underlying most STEMI. Total of 75% of autopsy studies after fatal STEMI relate thrombotic occlusion to atherosclerotic plaque rupture. Most of the remainder involves plaque erosion. STEMI comprises of 30–40% of ACS cases. STEMI incidence ranges from 66 to 77/100,000/year according to various registries. In India, one-fourth of cases of STEMI occur in the age group under 45 years. STEMI is the leading cause of death in both, the developed and developing world. Early diagnosis with prompt reperfusion of the infarct-related artery by either thrombolysis or PPCI is very importance in saving lives in STEMI. Due to this and other factors there has been a study decline in STEMI mortality in the last two decades. About 30% of patients with STEMI still do not get acute reperfusion therapy.

RISK FACTORS

Data from the INTERHEART study showed that nine modifiable risk factors accounted for 90% of the population attributable risk (PAR) in men and 94% in women for MI as shown in **Box 1**.

Nonmodifiable risk factors include age, male sex, postmenopausal period in females, and people with family history of first-degree blood relative having coronary artery disease (CAD) less than, 55 years in male relative and 65 years for female relative. The current lifestyles of young people characterized by smoking, drinking alcohol with fast food snack diet coupled with lack of physical exercise, and high work stress contributes to the increasing incidence of young MI.

BOX 1	Modifiable risk factors for ST-elevation myocardial infarction (STEMI).
• Lipids (apolipoprotein levels)	
• Smoking	
• Systemic hypertension	
• Diabetes mellitus	
• Abdominal obesity	
• Psychosocial factors such as depression and stress	
• Dietary factors	
• Lack of physical exercise	
• Alcohol consumption	

CLASSIFICATION

The type of MI as classified in the 2013 Third Universal Definition of MI is showed in **Box 2**.

The current 2018 updated Fourth Universal Definition of MI expert document updates the definition of MI to accommodate the increased use of high-sensitivity cardiac troponin (hs-cTn). The detection of an elevated cTn value above the 99th percentile upper reference limit (URL) is

BOX 2 Classification of myocardial infarction.
Type 1: Spontaneous MI
Spontaneous MI related to atherosclerotic plaque rupture, ulceration, fissuring, erosion, or dissection with resulting intraluminal thrombus in one or more of the coronary arteries leading to the decreased myocardial blood flow or distal platelet emboli with ensuing myocyte necrosis. The patient may have underlying severe CAD but on occasion nonobstructive or no CAD
Type 2: MI secondary to an ischemic imbalance
In instances of *myocardial injury with necrosis* where a condition other than CAD contributes to an imbalance between myocardial oxygen supply and/or demand, e.g., coronary endothelial dysfunction, coronary artery spasm, coronary embolism, tachy-/brady-arrhythmias, anemia, respiratory failure, hypotension, and hypertension with or without LVH
Type 3: MI resulting in death when biomarker values are unavailable
Cardiac death with symptoms suggestive of myocardial ischemia and presumed new ischemic ECG changes or new LBBB, but death occurring before blood samples could be obtained, before cardiac biomarker could rise, or in rare cases when cardiac biomarkers were not collected
Type 4a: MI related to PCI
MI associated with PCI is arbitrarily defined by elevation of cTn values >5 x 99th percentile ULN in patients with normal baseline values (≤99th percentile ULN) or a rise of cTn values >20% if the baseline values are elevated and are stable or falling. In addition, 1 of the following are required: (1) symptoms suggestive of myocardial ischemia; (2) new ischemic ECG changes or new LBBB; (3) angiographic loss of patency, of a major coronary artery or a side branch of persistent slow-or-no-flow or embolization; or (4) imaging demonstration of new loss of viable myocardium or new regional wall motion abnormality
Type 4b: MI related to stent thrombosis
MI associated with stent thrombosis is detected by coronary angiography or autopsy in the setting of myocardial ischemia and with a rise and/or fall of cardiac biomarkers values with ≥1 value above the 99th percentile ULN
Type 5: MI related to CABG
MI associated with CABG is arbitrarily defined by elevation of cardiac biomarker values >10 x 99th percentile ULN in patients with normal baseline cTn values (≤99th percentile ULN). In addition, 1 of the following are required: (1) new pathological Q waves or new LBBB; (2) angiographic documented new graft or new native coronary artery occlusion; or (3) imaging evidence of new loss of viable myocardium or new regional wall motion abnormality

(ULN: upper limit of normal)

defined as myocardial injury. The injury is considered acute if there is a rise and/or fall of cTn values.

The clinical definition of MI as per the Fourth Universal Definition denotes the presence of acute myocardial injury detected by abnormal cardiac biomarkers in the setting of evidence of acute myocardial ischemia. For diagnosis of STEMI there should be evidence of myocardial injury [increased troponin and/or other biomarkers creatine phosphokinase-MB (CPK-MB)] with myocardial ischemia. Most STEMI cases are type I (80%) and are due to rupture of an atheromatous plaque. Type II cases are due to supply and demand mismatch. This needs to be recognized since there long-term mortality is higher than in the usage type I MI. Also, thrombolysis may not be helpful in these cases. Their presentation is often atypical and based on associated diseases (**Box 3**).

Thus, STEMI is a clinical condition that includes the following:

- Characteristic clinical features of myocardial ischemia;
- Persistent J-point ST-segment elevation in ≥2 contiguous leads (≥2 mm in men or ≥1.5 mm in women in leads V_2 and V_3 or ≥1 mm in other precordial or limb leads) in the absence of left bundle branch block (LBBB) or left ventricular (LV) hypertrophy; and
- Elevated biomarkers of myocardial cell death (cTn is the preferred biomarker).

BOX 3 Type I and type II myocardial infarction (MI).
Type I MI
Myocardial injury related to acute myocardial ischemia due to atherosclerotic plaque disruption with thrombosis
Type II MI
Myocardial injury related to acute myocardial ischemia because of oxygen supply/demand imbalance
Reduced supply (myocardial perfusion)
• Coronary artery spasm
• Microvascular dysfunction
• Coronary embolism
• Coronary artery dissection
• Sustained bradyarrhythmia
• Hypotension or shock
• Respiratory failure
• Severe anemia
Increased demand (myocardial oxygen)
• Sustained tachyarrhythmia
• Severe hypertension with or without left ventricular hypertrophy

Source: Adapted from the Fourth Universal Definition of Myocardial Infarction (JACC 2018).

It is increasingly being recognized that there is a group of MI patients with no angiographic obstructive CAD (≥50% diameter stenosis in a major epicardial vessel), and the term "MI with nonobstructive coronary arteries (MINOCA)" has been coined for this entity.

Patients may have elevated cTn values and marked decreases in ejection fraction due to sepsis caused by endotoxin, with myocardial function recovering completely with normal ejection fraction once the sepsis is treated.

Hence, arriving at a diagnosis of MI requires integration of clinical findings, patterns on the ECG, laboratory data, observations from imaging procedures, and on occasion pathological findings, all viewed in the context of the time horizon over which the suspected event unfolds.

CLINICAL PRESENTATION

Patients present with severe diffuse, retrosternal excruciating tightness, or heaviness. Pain and discomfort is very severe and accompanied with tachypnea, sweating, and symptomatic overactivity. Sometimes there may be burping and burning sensation in retrosternal and epigastric area (misdiagnosed as gas and acidity). Pain radiates to both arms and is severe. It persists for more than half to 1 hour. Around 20% cases, especially in diabetes and elderly the MI can be painless also.

DIAGNOSIS

ELECTROCARDIOGRAM

Electrocardiogram is an important tool in the evaluation of a patient with suspected MI. ST-segment elevation suggests coronary occlusion. The initial ECG is neither sensitive nor specific for MI. When presentation is suggestive of MI and ECG is normal, serial tracings must be obtained every 10 minutes to detect development of ST-segment elevation to ensure early use of reperfusion therapies.

Electrocardiogram changes in STEMI evolve through three overlapping phases that include: (1) Early hyperacute or acute phase; (2) Evolved acute phase; and (3) Chronic stabilized phase. The first changes are tall T waves and concave upwards ST-segment elevation in leads representing an area of infarction. Within few hours (2–3) the ST segment becomes convex (coved) upwards and T waves become inverted. ST-T changes revert to normal by 6 weeks to 3 months. Q waves are formed in 6–12 hours and persist for entire life.

Early reperfusion therapy tends to accelerate the reversion of ECG changes accompanying MI and persistence of ST-segment elevation by >50–70% 1–2 hours after fibrinolysis, indicates failed thrombolysis and it should prompt consideration for coronary angiography and possibly "rescue angioplasty". The ECG can help in localization of the infarct-related artery in STEMI. Changes in V_1 to V_4 indicate anteroseptal infarct (**Fig. 1**). The presence of right bundle branch block with q (qRBBB) with anterior wall STEMI points to a proximal left anterior descending (LAD) occlusion (**Fig. 2**).

In inferior wall STEMI, there is ST-segment elevation in inferior limb leads (leads II, III, and aVF) (**Fig. 3**). It is desirable to obtain right-sided precordial leads (V_3R and V_4R) to seek ST-segment elevation associated with right ventricular (RV) infarction. Criteria for RV MI include ST-segment elevation of >0.05 mV in V_4R.

ECHOCARDIOGRAPHY

Echocardiography may be useful when patient has severe ischemic symptoms, but the regular 12-lead ECG does not manifest ST elevation but changes such as hyperacute T waves. In such instances, echocardiography may reveal wall motion abnormalities due to ischemia—the sensitivity and specificity is greater than 90%. Echocardiography is particularly useful in the diagnosis of posterior wall infarction when the ECG shows only precordial ST depression. Wall motion abnormality of the posterior or posterolateral wall is confirmatory of STEMI and usually involves the circumflex artery. However, lesser degrees of infarction may not

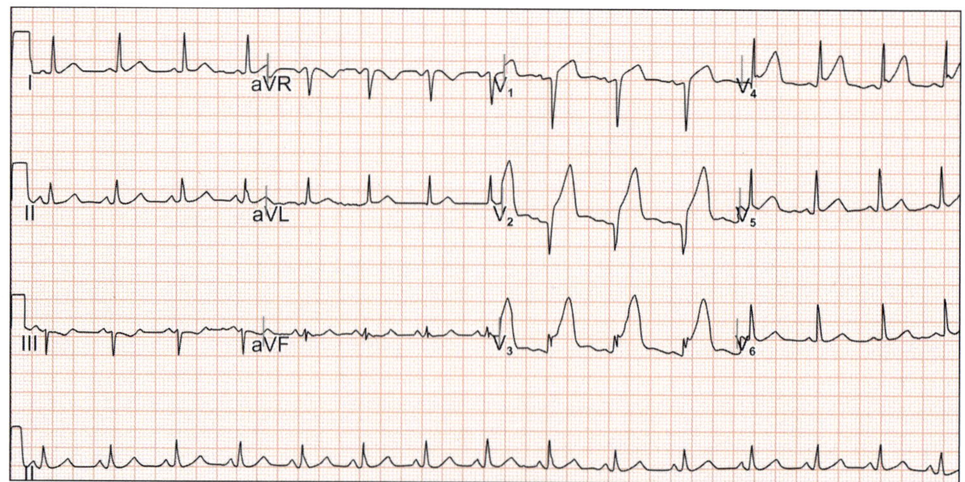

FIGURE 1: Acute anteroseptal myocardial infarction (MI) with ST elevation in V_1 to V_4. ST is concave upward, T wave is tall, and Q waves have started forming. Indicates acute infarction of <6–8 hours duration.

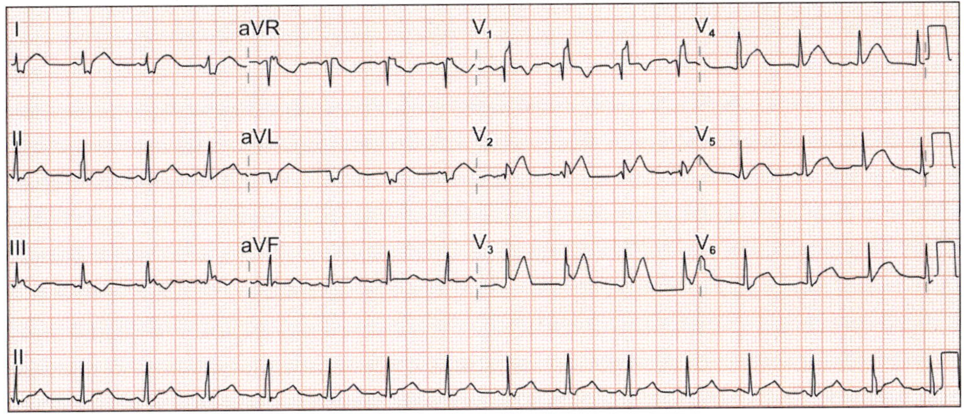

FIGURE 2: Right bundle branch block with q (qRBBB) with anterior wall ST elevation with ST elevation in V_1 to V_4 again shows acute infarction of few hours only.

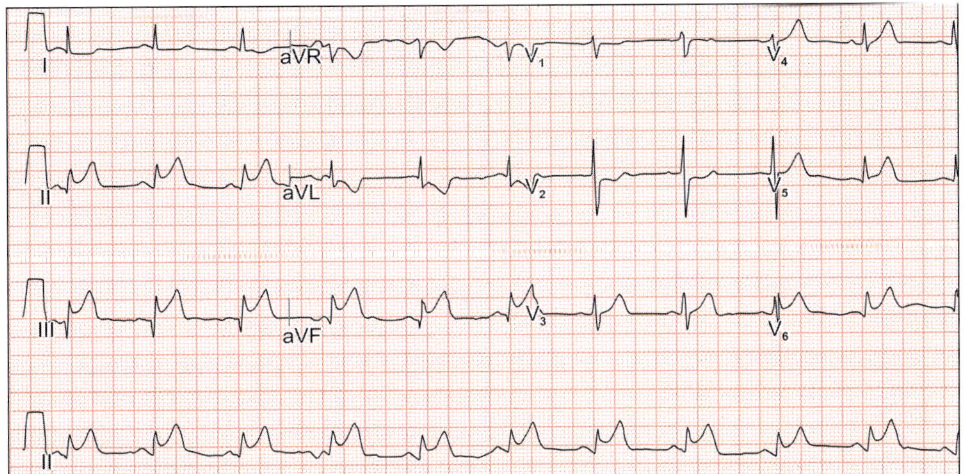

FIGURE 3: ECG showing ST elevation in II, II, and aVF (inferior wall STEMI). Concave upward ST elevation in II, III, and aVF indicates hyperacute inferior MI.

produce any wall motion changes whereas older MIs can cause similar abnormalities. Echocardiogram is useful to diagnose the mechanical complications of MI including mitral regurgitation (MR) due to papillary muscle rupture and ventricular septal rupture.

DIFFERENTIAL DIAGNOSIS

Sometimes, acute chest pain can be due to other causes. Aortic dissection, acute pericarditis, pulmonary thromboembolism and pneumothorax, esophageal spasm, acute cholecystitis, and pancreatitis can all have overlapping presentation with severe diffuse pain in the chest and epigastrium. These differentials need to be kept in mind while managing patients presenting with severe chest discomfort in the emergency.

Other conditions that can cause ST-segment elevations include myocarditis, pericarditis, stress cardiomyopathy (takotsubo cardiomyopathy), benign early repolarization, acute vasospasm, spontaneous coronary artery dissection, various channelopathies, and electrolyte abnormalities. All these have to be considered in the differential diagnosis.

COMPLICATIONS

There are multiple complications of STEMI. These can be broadly divided into rhythm related and mechanical complications. In arrhythmias, there can be tachyarrhythmias including atrial fibrillation, ventricular ectopics, ventricular tachycardia, and ventricular fibrillation which are fatal. Bradyarrhythmias can be in the form of sinus bradycardia or atrioventricular (AV) blocks up to complete heart block (CHB). CHB is more common in inferior wall infarct. However, when it occurs in anterior wall infarction it carries the very high mortality of 40–50%. Advent of continuous monitoring has helped in early diagnosis of arrhythmias and has reduced mortality.

Left heart failure is common and clinically it is judged by the **Killip class**. Killip class I indicates MI with no heart failure, class II is MI with mild heart failure (basal crepitations), class III is MI with pulmonary edema, and class IV is MI with cardiogenic shock. This bedside classification can help in prognostication of the patients. The mortality in class I, II, III, and IV is 5%, 15%, 25%, and 45%, respectively. The mechanical complications such as

MR and ventricular septal defect (VSD) can cause heart failure and often need surgical correction. The various complications are as follows:

- Arrhythmias
- Heart failure/left ventricular failure (LVF)
- Cardiogenic shock
- Sudden death
- Reinfarction, extension, and expansion of infarction
- Infarction of papillary muscle of mitral valve—MR
- Rupture of interventricular septum leading to VSD
- Thrombus in LV causing peripheral embolism
- Cardiac rupture
- Deep vein thrombosis in legs causing pulmonary embolism
- Pericarditis during massive infarction
- Aneurysm of ventricle with thrombosis and thrombo-embolic phenomenon
- Dressler's syndrome (post-MI syndrome)

MANAGEMENT

Patients with STEMI need to be managed immediately in the emergency. They should be put on a monitor to diagnose arrhythmias which are common in acute phase. Relief of pain and other measures are important. Immediate ECG and decision regarding reperfusion needs to be taken and then implemented as fast as possible. Some of the important components of management are described here, although they should all start simultaneously.

SUPPLEMENTAL OXYGEN

Scant data exist to support or refute the value of the routine use of oxygen in the acute phase of STEMI. A 3-fold higher risk of mortality associated with oxygen therapy (compared with room air) in acute MI was reported by a pooled Cochrane report of three clinical trials. It has been reported that oxygen can induce coronary vasoconstriction resulting in increased vascular resistance. Therefore, oxygen should not be routinely administered for prolonged periods when arterial oxygen saturation is normal. Supplemental oxygen should be administered in patients with arterial oxygen saturation <90%. Caution is advocated in chronic obstructive pulmonary disease (COPD) and carbon dioxide retention.

RELIEF OF PAIN AND ANXIETY

Nitroglycerine: Sublingual nitroglycerin should be administered to patients with ongoing chest discomfort as follows: 0.4 mg every 5 minutes for a total of three doses. Intravenous (IV) nitroglycerine should be initiated in those with continuing chest pain, hypertension, or for management of pulmonary congestion. Nitrates should be avoided when systolic blood pressure (SBP) is <90 mm Hg, in suspected RV infarction, severe bradycardia (<50 beats/min), or tachycardia (>100 beats/min). There is no role for the routine use of oral nitrates in the convalescent phase of STEMI.

Analgesia: Morphine sulfate is the drug of choice for pain relief in patients with STEMI, especially those whose course is complicated by acute pulmonary edema. It can reduce anxiety and favorably affect ventricular loading conditions. The dose is 2–4 mg administered IV with increments of 2–4 mg IV repeated at 5–15 minutes intervals. Nonsteroidal anti-inflammatory drugs and selective cyclooxygenase-2 enzyme (COX-2) inhibitors are not used for pain relief since they may be associated with an increased risk of death, reinfarction, cardiac rupture, hypertension, and death.

BETA-BLOCKERS

Oral beta-blocker therapy should be initiated in the first 24 hours in the absence of contraindications such as reactive airways disease, PR interval >0.24 second or high-degree AV block, cardiogenic shock, acute pulmonary edema, or low output state. IV beta-blockers may be used only when there is significant hypertension (SBP >150 mm Hg). Dose of beta-blockers should be up-titrated to maximum tolerated dose or target dose and should be continued long term in those with LV systolic dysfunction.

STATINS

High-intensity (dose) statins have both immediate pleiotropic benefit and long-term cardiovascular risk reduction. It should be given as early as possible. Atorvastatin 80 mg or rosuvastatin 40 mg per day can be used.

ANTIPLATELET AGENTS

Aspirin: The initial dose of aspirin at the start of STEMI treatment should be 150–325 mg chewable (nonenteric) aspirin with maintenance dose of 150–162 mg. Chewing the nonenteric-coated aspirin provides more rapid absorption through buccal than gastric mucosa. When aspirin is contraindicated or not tolerated due to allergy or dyspepsia, then clopidogrel monotherapy is an alternative.

P2Y12 antagonists (thienopyridines): Clopidogrel, prasugrel, or ticagrelor in combination with aspirin should be recommended for up to 12 months. Clopidogrel should be added to aspirin for STEMI patients treated with fibrinolytic therapy or when no reperfusion therapy is administered. A loading dose of a thienopyridine is recommended for STEMI patients. For thrombolysis patients loading of 300 mg clopidogrel is given, patients ≥75 years of age are not given any loading dose. For patients undergoing percutaneous coronary intervention (PCI), 600 mg loading dose of clopidogrel is given. When coronary artery bypass graft (CABG) is planned, it is recommended that clopidogrel should be discontinued for 5 days before surgery.

Ticagrelor and prasugrel are more effective than clopidogrel. For PCI in ACS, ticagrelor and prasugrel are preferred. For patients undergoing thrombolysis, the P2Y12 inhibitor used is clopidogrel. Ticagrelor and prasugrel are not used along with thrombolysis. Ticagrelor, a reversible and direct-acting oral antagonist, provides faster, greater, and more consistent P2Y12 inhibition than does clopidogrel. The loading dose is 180 mg and this is followed by a dose of 90 mg twice daily. Prasugrel is used in a loading dose of 60 mg and then 10 mg daily dose. It is avoided in patients <60 kg and those ≥70 years of age.

Dual antiplatelet therapy (DAPT) with aspirin and P2Y12 inhibitors should be continued for 12 months in STEMI patients receiving a drug-eluting stent (DES). In patients with first-generation DES, DAPT can be continued for beyond 12 months if bleeding risk is low and multiple stents have been used.

ANTITHROMBOTICS

The benefits of administering anticoagulant therapy in STEMI patients include reducing the incidence of deep vein thrombosis, pulmonary embolism, ventricular thrombus formation, and cerebral embolism. In addition, it assists in the establishment and maintenance of patency of the infarct-related artery. Anticoagulants that have been demonstrated to be efficacious in STEMI patients undergoing fibrinolysis include unfractionated heparin (UFH) and low-molecular-weight heparin (LMWH). Enoxaparin is the most commonly used LMWH. The other LMWH dalteparin is preferred in patients with renal failure. Patients who receive fibrinolytic therapy should receive anticoagulants for a minimum of 48 hours and preferably for the duration of index hospitalization. In those undergoing PCI, UFH is used before the procedure to achieve the activated clotting time of ≥ 250 seconds. Enoxaparin or UFH can be used perithrombolysis and PCI.

Unfractionated heparin is beneficial in STEMI—for every 1,000 patients treated with UFH compared with aspirin alone—there are five fewer deaths and three fewer recurrent infarctions at the expense of three more major bleeds. Other benefits of UFH include possibly maintaining the patency of the infarct-related artery and possibly reducing the burden of LV thrombus. Therefore, it is considered prudent to administer heparin after thrombolysis for ≥48 hours with a goal of maintaining activated partial thromboplastin time (aPTT) at 1.5–2 the control time. LMWHs are comparable to heparin in ensuring early (60–90 min) reperfusion of the infarct artery, but they are better in reducing the rates of reocclusion of the infarct artery, reinfarction, and recurrent ischemic events.

Besides UFH and LMWH, two other antithrombotic agents can be used in STEMI patients. Fondaparinux an indirect factor Xa inhibitor can be used after thrombolysis in those with high bleeding risk. Fondaparinux is not used in patients for PCI, since it is a weaker antithrombotic and there is risk of thrombosis of the cardiac guide catheter. Direct thrombin inhibitors, such as bivalirudin has been used in patients undergoing PCI. However, it is expensive and so is being used infrequently in some centers only during primary PCI.

THROMBOLYTICS

Thrombolytic therapy is the main reperfusion strategy in STEMI. The other one is PPCI. The reperfusion therapy is useful only when administrated and within 12 hours of onset of MI. The CREATE registry showed that approximately 60% patients of STEMI receive thrombolytic therapy in India. About 10% patients get primary PCI. Some patients who reach the hospital after 12 hours cannot be reperfused and so have a higher mortality.

Public education about benefits of reaching the nearest hospital at the earliest can help a lot. Time is a very important factor. Those thrombolyzed within 3 hours of symptom onset derive maximum benefit. Hospitals have to develop protocols to shorten the "door-to-needle" time in thrombolysis and "door-to-balloon" time in PCI strategy. There is no debate that PCI is better than thrombolysis as a reperfusion strategy, but the latter is more practical. All patients who get thrombolysis therapy should get coronary angiography and PCI in 3–24 hours. This strategy is called pharmacoinvasive strategy and is a practical approach since all patients cannot reach a PCI capable center in 6–12 hours. With fibrinolytic therapy 30–40% of patients may not achieve infarct artery reperfusion. In these patients, *rescue PCI* for failed thrombolysis has to be done. There are some contraindications to thrombolytic therapy, these are given below.

Absolute contraindications for fibrinolytic use in STEMI include the following:

- Prior intracranial hemorrhage (ICH)
- Known structural cerebral vascular lesion
- Known malignant intracranial neoplasm
- Ischemic stroke within 3 months
- Suspected aortic dissection
- Active bleeding or bleeding diathesis (excluding menses)
- Significant closed head trauma or facial trauma within 3 months
- Intracranial or intraspinal surgery within 2 months
- Severe uncontrolled hypertension (unresponsive to emergency therapy)
- For streptokinase, prior treatment 5 days to within the previous 6 months

Relative contraindications for fibrinolytic use in STEMI include the following:

- History of chronic, severe, and poorly controlled hypertension
- Significant hypertension on presentation (SBP >180 mm Hg or diastolic blood pressure >110 mm Hg)
- Traumatic or prolonged (>10 min) cardiopulmonary resuscitation (CPR) or major surgery <3 weeks previously
- History of prior ischemic stroke not within the last 3 months
- Dementia
- Recent (within 2–4 weeks) internal bleeding
- Pregnancy
- Active peptic ulcer

The fibrinolytics differ in various properties as shown in **Table 1**. Streptokinase, which is the cheapest, is still the most commonly used thrombolytic agent in India. The fibrin-specific agents, i.e., tenecteplase and reteplase are being increasingly used now. Tenecteplase is given as a weight-adjusted single-bolus injection. So there is convenience of administrations. Reteplase is given in two boluses 30 minutes apart. Alteplase is expensive and is used in infusion. For this reason, its use has been replaced by tenecteplase. Dual antiplatelet (aspirin + clopidogrel) and antithrombotic agent (UFH or LMWH) should be both

TABLE 1 The characteristics of commonly used thrombolytic agents.

	SK (Streptokinase)	tPA (Alteplase)	tPA (Reteplase)	TNK (Tenecteplase)
Dose	1.5 million units (MU) in 30–60 min	100 mg in 90 min	10 u + 10 u 30 min apart	30–50 mg over 5 s
Circulating half-life (minute)	20	6	18	20
Antigenic	Yes	No	No	No
Allergic reactions	Yes	No	No	No
Systemic fibrinogen depletion	Severe	Mild moderate	Moderate	Minimal
Intracerebral hemorrhage	0.4%	0.7%	0.8%	0.7%
Patency (TIMI-2/3) rate, 90 min	51%	73–85%	83%	77–88%
Lives saved per 100 treated	3	4	4	4

(TIMI: thrombolysis in myocardial infarction)

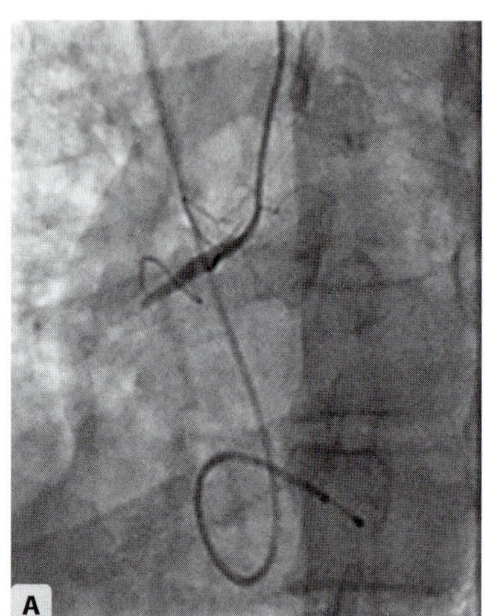

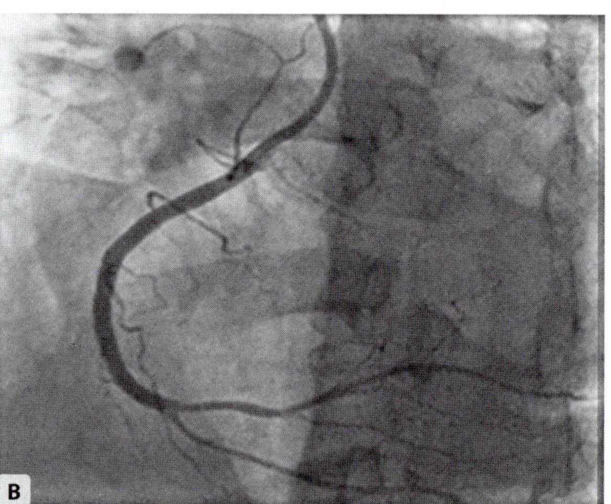

FIGURES 4 A & B: Primary percutaneous coronary intervention (PCI) to right coronary artery (RCA). **(A)** Occluded RCA; **(B)** Poststenting.

administrated as early as possible along with thrombolytic therapy.

PRIMARY ANGIOPLASTY

Primary angioplasty or PPCI is the preferred reperfusion strategy for patients with STEMI if it can be performed in a timely manner and by experienced operators due to immediate restoration of thrombolysis in MI (TIMI) 3 flows (**Fig. 4**).

The definitive goal in STEMI management is early, complete, and sustained reperfusion, which in turn results in better short-term and long-term outcomes.

CAPTIM and PRAGUE trials have shown that there is no strong preference between PCI and thrombolysis in STEMI patients who present within 3 hours after symptom onset, as the mortality is similar and low in both groups. An analysis of 21 trials showed that as PCI-related time delay increased the advantage of absolute mortality reduction is decreased. STEMI guidelines indicate that thrombolysis is generally preferred over PPCI when the door-to-balloon time minus door-to-needle time exceeds 1 hour. According to the American College of Cardiology/American Heart Association (ACC/AHA) 2013 guidelines, in non-PCI capable hospitals, it is indicated to thrombolysis when >120 minutes time delay is expected from point of first medical contact (FMC) to PPCI. The guidelines strongly recommend that all PCI hospital systems achieve a median door-to-balloon time for PPCI of 90 minutes.

CURRENT STATUS OF CARE IN INDIA

Primary PCI is the gold standard for treatment for STEMI the world over, but is available to <10% STEMI patients in India. Data from the National Informatics Centre (NIC) database shows that PPCI comprises of just 17% of all interventional cardiac procedures in India in 800 interventional centers across India. Only about half of these centers provide round the clock services and more than half of them had no surgical capability. There are several challenges unique to the Indian context. These include long-time delay in reaching the hospital due to initial patient lack of awareness and traffic congestion/lack of transfer facilities. The third delay is possible within the tertiary care hospital due to various factors viz. finances, obtaining consent, round the clock manpower, and availability of PCI laboratory in busy hours. Inadequate private and public insurance results in patients having to self-finance and hence resulting in underutilization of therapy.

2017 ESC GUIDELINES

Recently the European Society of Cardiology (ESC) updated the 2012 guidelines in STEMI. The salient features of which are as follows:

- Selection of reperfusion strategy for all STEMI patients is based on anticipated time from "STEMI diagnosis" to PCI-mediated reperfusion. If ≤120 minutes, refer to primary PCI, if >120 minutes, immediate fibrinolysis (administered within 10 minutes from STEMI diagnosis) and transfer to a PCI center.
- Cardiac arrest survivors with ST elevation on postresuscitation ECG must undergo a PPCI strategy. In cases without ST-segment elevation on postresuscitation ECG but with a high suspicion of ongoing myocardial ischemia, urgent angiography should be done within 2 hours after a quick evaluation to exclude noncoronary causes.
- Oxygen is only recommended when arterial saturation is <90% or partial pressure of oxygen (PaO_2) <60 mm Hg based on findings of the DETOX2 trial.
- Primary PCI state-of-the-art technique includes reperfusion within 90 minutes from STEMI diagnosis, routine radial access (data from MATRIX study), and routine DES implant should be preferred over bare-metal stent (BMS). Preload with aspirin and prasugrel/ticagrelor and anticoagulation with UFH.
- Complete revascularization with stenting of noninfarct-related artery is class IIA indication in patients with cardiogenic shock based on PRAMI and COMPARE trials. Treatment of severe noninfarct artery stenosis (evaluated either by angiography or fractional flow reserve) should be considered for staged angioplasty before hospital discharge.
- State-of-the-art fibrinolysis strategy includes fibrin-specific lytic agent, aspirin and clopidogrel, and anticoagulation with enoxaparin. Dose adjustment of tenecteplase and loading clopidogrel should be made in patients ≥75-year-old. Maximum time from STEMI diagnosis to administration of fibrinolytic ≤10 minutes in patients unable to meet PPCI target times.

  Even in cases of successful reperfusion, routine angiography must be done between 2 and 24 hours after bolus of lytic.
- Patients should be monitored for at least 24 hours after reperfusion. Early ambulation and early discharge are the best options in uncomplicated patients.
- 1 year of DAPT (aspirin plus prasugrel/ticagrelor) is the standard maintenance regimen. In patients at high bleeding risk, reduction to 6 months should be considered (aspirin monotherapy thereafter). Conversely, in patients who tolerate 1 year of DAPT and are at high ischemic risk, extension of DAPT may be considered.
- Early high-dose statin therapy is indicated with a low-density lipoprotein (LDL) goal of <70 mg/dL. If this target is not met, additional lipid lowering therapy should be considered.
- In patients with MI with nonobstructive coronary arteries (MINOCA), it is important to perform additional diagnostic tests to identify the etiology and tailor appropriate therapy, which may be different from typical STEMI.
- It is important to measure established quality indicators to audit practice and improve outcomes in real life. This will help filling the gap between best evidence-based recommendations and daily practice.

RECOMMENDED READINGS

1. Thygesen K, Alpert JS, Jaffe AS, Chaitman BR, Bax JJ, Morrow DA, et al. Fourth Universal Definition of Myocardial Infarction (2018). J Am Coll Cardiol. 2018;72(18):2231-64.
2. Ibanez B, James S, Agewall S, Antunes MJ, Bucciarelli-Ducci C, Bueno H, et al. 2017 ESC Guidelines for the management of acute myocardial infarction in patients presenting with ST-segment elevation: The Task Force for the management of acute myocardial infarction in patients presenting with ST-segment elevation of the European Society of Cardiology (ESC). Eur Heart J. 2018;39.119-77.
3. O'Gara PT, Kushner FG, Ascheim DD, Casey DE Jr, Chung MK, de Lemos JA, et al. 2013 ACCF/AHA guideline for the management of ST-elevation myocardial infarction: Executive summary a report of the American College of Cardiology Foundation/American Heart Association Task Force on Practice Guidelines. Circulation. 2013;127:529-55.
4. Thygesen K, Alpert JS, Jaffe AS, Simoons ML, Chaitman BR, White HD. Third universal definition of myocardial infarction. Glob Heart. 2012;7:275-95.
5. Dalal JJ, Alexander T, Banerjee PS, Dayasagar V, Lyengar SS, Kerkar PG, et al. 2013 consensus statement for early reperfusion and pharmaco-invasive approach in patients presenting with chest pain diagnosed as STEMI (ST elevation myocardial infarction) in an Indian setting. J Assoc Physicians India. 2014;62:473-83.
6. Pakshirajan B, Subban V, Mullasari AS. Pharmacoinvasive Management. Interv Cardiol Clin. 2012;1:409-19.
7. Alexander T, Mehta S, Mullasari A, Nallamothu BK. Systems of care for ST-elevation myocardial infarction in India. Heart. 2012;98:15-7.
8. Alexander T, Mullasari AS, Joseph G, Kannan K, Veerasekar G, Victor SM, et al. A System of care for Patients with ST-Segment elevation myocardial infarction in India: The Tamil Nadu-ST-Segment Elevation Myocardial Infarction Program. JAMA Cardiol. 2017;2:498-505.
9. Dharma S, Kedev S, Jukema JW. Thrombus management in the catheterization laboratory in the setting of primary percutaneous coronary intervention: what is the current evidence? Heart. 2013;99:279-84.
10. Shah N, Cox D. Controversies in the management of ST Elevation Myocardial Infarction: Thrombin Inhibition. Interv Cardiol Clin. 2016;5:497-511.

CHAPTER
109 Diseases of the Myocardium

Ajay Bahl

ABSTRACT

Heart muscle diseases or cardiomyopathies are disorders that primarily involve the myocardium. Myocardial dysfunction secondary to coronary artery or valvular heart disease is not included in the standard definitions of cardiomyopathies. Hypertrophic cardiomyopathy (HCM) is the most common heart muscle disease followed by dilated cardiomyopathy (DCM). Most cardiomyopathies are genetic disorders with a Mendelian pattern of transmission. Most of the pathogenic variants found in Indians have also been reported from other populations. However, several genetic variations are unique to Indians. Genetic counseling and family screening form an important part of management. Many of these disorders are associated with risk of sudden death. Risk stratification and prevention of sudden death using implantable cardioverter defibrillator (ICD) should be considered in most cardiomyopathies. Advances in management have resulted in improved outcomes for many of these disorders.

"Our own genomes carry the story of evolution written in DNA, the language of molecular genetics and the narrative is unmistakable"

—Kenneth R Miller

INTRODUCTION

Heart muscle diseases or cardiomyopathies were defined by World Health Organization in 1995 as diseases of myocardium of unknown etiology associated with cardiac dysfunction. Now, we have better understanding of the etiopathogenesis of these disorders and the etiology of most cardiomyopathies is now known. Cardiomyopathies include primary disorders of myocardium. Disorders in which the ventricular dysfunction is secondary to other conditions like coronary artery or valvular heart disease are labelled secondary cardiomyopathies and not included in traditional definitions of cardiomyopathies. Most cardiomyopathies have a genetic origin. Thus, a detailed family history and screening are important components in management of these patients.

> Most cardiomyopathies are genetic disorders and follow a Mendelian pattern of inheritance.

CLASSIFICATION

The initial 1995, World Health Organization/International Society and Federation of Cardiology Task Force classification was morphological and included HCM, DCM, restrictive cardiomyopathy (RCM), arrhythmogenic right ventricular cardiomyopathy (ARVC), and put all the remaining into a basket called unclassified cardiomyopathies. Since these early attempts at classification, etiology of many cardiomyopathies has been identified. The two commonly used classifications are the European Society of Cardiology working group etiological classification (2008) which is clinically oriented and the American Heart Association classification (2006) which is primarily based on the etiology. American Heart Association classification additionally includes cardiac channelopathies like Brugada syndrome in the ambit of cardiomyopathies.

The European Society of Cardiology working group classification is based on the clinical phenotype and thus may be more intuitive for the physician. In this classification, cardiomyopathies are divided into HCM, DCM, RCM, ARVC, and unclassified cardiomyopathies that form a miscellaneous group. These are then subdivided into familial and nonfamilial (**Table 1**). In contrast, the American Heart Association divides primary cardiomyopathies into genetic, mixed, and acquired disorders. Each of these three groups is then subclassified into specific cardiomyopathies depending on the morphology and hemodynamics. A mere glance at these classifications highlights the importance of genetics. Many cardiomyopathies are Mendelian disorders most commonly transmitted in an autosomal dominant pattern. Purely genetic cardiomyopathies include HCM, ARVC, ion channel disorders, mitochondrial myopathies, left ventricular noncompaction, and glycogen storage disorders. Disorders with no genetic basis are classified as acquired cardiomyopathies. These include peripartum cardiomyopathy, myocarditis, takotsubo cardiomyopathy, and tachycardia induced cardiomyopathy. Mixed disorders may either have a genetic basis or may be due to acquired

TABLE 1 Etiological classification of cardiomyopathies (adapted from the position statement of the European Society of Cardiology working group on myocardial and pericardial diseases 2008).

HCM		DCM		RCM		ARVC	Unclassified
Familial	**Nonfamilial**	**Familial**	**Nonfamilial**	**Familial**	**Nonfamilial**	**Familial**	**Familial**
• With sarcomeric gene mutations ◦ B myosin heavy chain ◦ Myosin binding protein C ◦ Cardiac troponin I ◦ Cardiac troponin T ◦ α tropomyosin • Mitochondrial myopathies • Friedreich's ataxia • Unknown mutations • Noonan, leopard, and Costello syndromes	• Athlete's heart • Infants of diabetic mothers • Obesity • Acromegaly • Pheochromocytoma • Amyloidosis • Drugs-anabolic steroids, tacrolimus	• Sarcomeric gene mutations—as in HCM • Cytoskeletal gene mutations ◦ Dystrophin ◦ Desmin • Nuclear membrane mutations ◦ Lamin A/C • Mitochondrial myopathies • Fabry disease • Unknown mutations	• Alcohol • Hyperthyroidism • Myocarditis • Pheochromocytoma • Peripartum cardiomyopathy • Cocaine • Drugs • Nutritional including beriberi	• Sarcomeric gene mutations—as in HCM ◦ B myosin heavy chain ◦ Troponin I • Desminopathy • Familial amyloidosis • Fabry disease • Hemochromatosis • Unknown mutations	• Amyloidosis • Endomyocardial fibrosis • Hypereosinophilia • Radiation • Metastatic cancer • Carcinoid	• Intercalated disc protein mutations ◦ Desmoplakin ◦ Plakophilin 2 ◦ Plakoglobin ◦ Desmoglein 2 ◦ Desmocollin 2 • Cardiac ryanodine receptor mutations	• Left ventricular noncompaction • Nonfamilial • Takotsubo cardiomyopathy

causes. Mixed disorders include DCM and RCM. Thus, an understanding of genetics, genetic counseling, and family screening form an important aspect of cardiomyopathy management.

HYPERTROPHIC CARDIOMYOPATHY

Hypertrophic cardiomyopathy is the most common inherited cardiac disorder caused by mutations in sarcomeric proteins encoding genes and is the most common cause of sudden death in young individuals. The prevalence is thought to be 1 in 500 in the general population. Diagnosis is based on left ventricular hypertrophy that cannot be explained by an underlying lesion or any hemodynamic stress like hypertension. Hypertrophy is usually asymmetrical and can involve any segment (**Fig. 1**). Basal anteroseptal and anterior segments are most commonly involved.

Hypertrophic cardiomyopathy has an age-related penetrance. The disease typically manifests initially during adolescence at the time of the growth spurt. HCM can rarely manifest in infancy and childhood. The disease penetrance increases with age and it may manifest as late as the seventh decade. Individuals carrying mutations in myosin binding protein C gene *(MyBPC3)* often have late onset disease.

Mutations are detected in around 50–60% of cases. Genotype-phenotype correlation is poor. Mutation in the same gene may give rise to several different HCM phenotypes. Some manifestations may be more common with mutations in specific genes, e.g., mild hypertrophy with mutations in troponin T gene (*TNNT2*) and

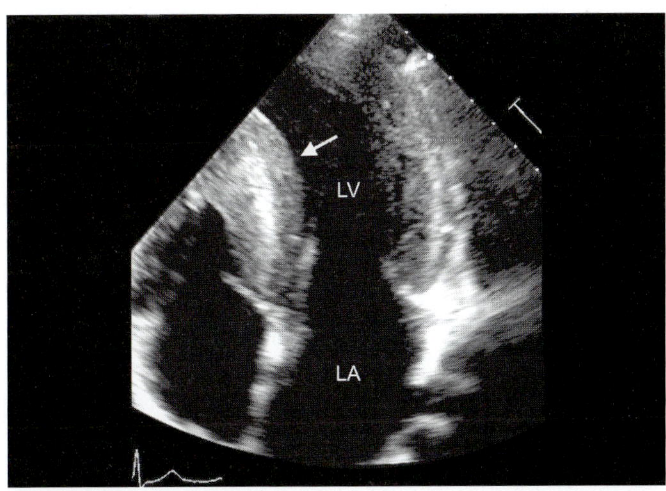

(LA: left atrium; LV: left ventricle)

FIGURE 1: Asymmetrical septal hypertrophy (arrow) in a patient with hypertrophic cardiomyopathy.

overrepresentation of restrictive phenotype with mutations in troponin I (*TNNI3*) gene.

> Mutations in genes encoding myosin heavy chain (*MYH7*) and myosin binding protein C (*MyBPC3*) are the most common in patients with HCM.

The fascinating hallmark of HCM is a dynamic left ventricular outflow tract obstruction (LVOTO) which is usually due to the systolic anterior motion of mitral valve. Around a third of patients have LVOTO at rest while another third have a provocable gradient. Some patients have a midcavity gradient due to papillary muscle or myocardial hypertrophy. Some of these individuals with midcavity obstruction develop an apical aneurysm (**Fig. 2 A**). Patients with apical aneurysms are at increased risk of thrombus formation in the aneurysm and thus systemic embolism and stroke (**Fig. 2 B**). They are also at increased risk of ventricular tachyarrhythmias and sudden death. Around 3% HCM patients develop end-stage disease characterized by left ventricular ejection fraction (LVEF) <50%.

CLINICAL FEATURES

The clinical presentation is variable. Many patients are asymptomatic being detected only on routine medical examination or family screening while others may have severe symptoms. Usually, patients with LVOTO are more symptomatic. Common symptoms include breathlessness, chest pain, palpitations, fatigue, and giddiness. Syncope is an important symptom and is multifactorial. Important causes are abnormal neutrally mediated vascular reflexes, LVOTO, or sustained ventricular tachyarrhythmias. Unexplained recent syncope is a risk factor for sudden death. However, remote syncope episodes >5 years back are not associated with increased sudden death risk.

On examination, the distinctive features are the findings of dynamic LVOTO. Carotid pulse is brisk and bifid and the jugular venous pulse has prominent "a" waves. Apex is normal in location but may have double or triple impulse. A dynamic ejection systolic murmur at the left sternal border is the hallmark. LVOTO gradient and hence intensity of the murmur increases with reductions of preload and afterload and also with increased myocardial contractility (**Table 2**). Dynamic auscultatory findings distinguish the LVOTO murmur from those with fixed aortic gradients as in valvular aortic stenosis. Mitral regurgitation may occur either because of systolic anterior motion of mitral valve or intrinsic mitral valve abnormalities. Pansystolic murmur may be present at the apex in these patients. In patients without LVOTO, the findings are less remarkable. Brisk carotid upstroke, sustained apex, and a left ventricular fourth heart sound may be present.

INVESTIGATIONS

Electrocardiogram (ECG) abnormalities usually precede the development of left ventricular hypertrophy and the ECG is abnormal in over 95% patients. ECG abnormalities include left ventricular hypertrophy, q waves, atrial enlargement and ST segment, and T wave abnormalities. Deep T wave inversions defined as ≥10 mm in precordial leads and ≥5 mm in limb leads is found in patients with apical hypertrophy (**Fig. 3**). Conduction defects like heart block and short PR interval with preexcitation are more common in storage disorders or mitochondrial myopathy.

Echocardiography is the most important investigation and usually confirms the diagnosis. Echocardiography provides important information like pattern and severity of hypertrophy, systolic and diastolic ventricular function, systolic anterior motion of mitral valve, and LVOTO and midcavity obstruction. LVOTO may not be present at rest. In that case, maneuvers like exercise and Valsalva maneuver

TABLE 2 Maneuvers that increase intensity of the dynamic LVOTO murmur in patients with HCM.

Reduction in preload	Reduction in afterload	Increased contractility
• Standing up from squatting position • Valsalva maneuver • Nitrates	• Amyl nitrate	• Postventricular extrasystolic beat • Beat after a long cycle in atrial fibrillation • Exercise

(HCM: hypertrophic cardiomyopathy; LVOTO: left ventricular outflow tract obstruction)

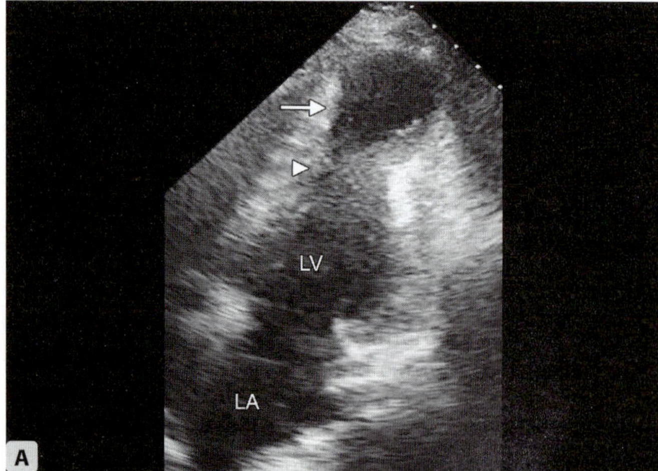

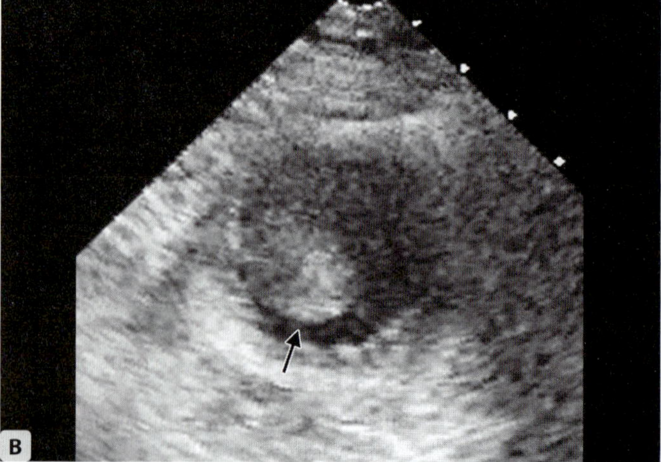

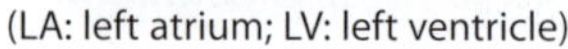

(LA: left atrium; LV: left ventricle)

FIGURES 2 A & B: (A) Left ventricular (LV) apical aneurysm (arrow) in a patient with midcavity obstruction (arrowhead); **(B)** Thrombus (black arrow) in an apical aneurysm in a patient with hypertrophic cardiomyopathy and midcavity obstruction.

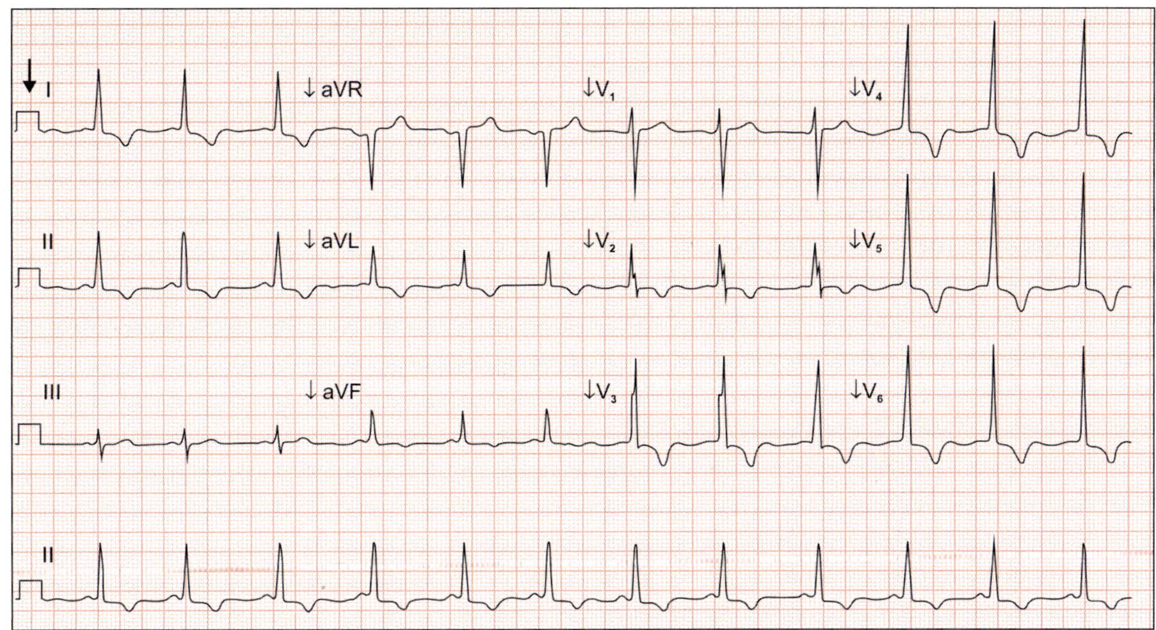

FIGURE 3: ECG of a patient with apical hypertrophic cardiomyopathy showing left ventricular hypertrophy with deep T wave inversions. Note that due to high voltages the ECG calibration has been set to 5 mm/mV (arrow).

should be used to provoke the gradient. Mitral regurgitation is usually present in patients with LVOTO even in absence of associated mitral valve abnormalities. These jets are usually directed laterally and subside with relief of LVOTO using myectomy or alcohol septal ablation. It is important to identify mitral regurgitation due to intrinsic mitral valve disease since this will require additional mitral valve repair or replacement. Left atrial enlargement, especially dimension above 50 mm, puts a patient at higher risk of atrial fibrillation. Other causes of ventricular hypertrophy like valvular aortic stenosis and coarctation of aorta can also be excluded by echocardiography.

Holter monitoring is useful for assessing risk for sudden cardiac death (SCD) and at least 24 hour monitoring should be carried out. Nonsustained ventricular tachycardia is a risk factor for SCD. Abnormal blood pressure response on exercise testing is a marker for SCD risk only in young individuals ≤40 years of age. Abnormal blood pressure response is defined by fall in systolic blood pressure or failure to rise ≥20 mm Hg. Genotyping using next-generation sequencing should be offered to identify disease causing mutations in the family.

Cardiac magnetic resonance (CMR) imaging is currently the gold standard imaging modality. It is especially useful in diagnosing apical hypertrophy and aneurysms which may be missed on echocardiography. Late gadolinium enhancement indicates scarring and it is useful in prognostication. Extensive late gadolinium enhancement ≥15% is a risk factor for SCD.

Stress imaging or coronary angiography may be needed to exclude coronary artery disease in patients with chest pain. Patients with apical HCM have a spade-shaped left ventricle on ventriculography.

DIFFERENTIAL DIAGNOSIS

Hypertensive heart disease also produces left ventricular hypertrophy and may be difficult to differentiate from HCM. The pattern of hypertrophy in hypertensive heart disease is usually concentric. Elderly patients especially women with long-standing hypertension may occasionally have sigmoid septum, systolic anterior motion of mitral valve, and LVOTO. Other conditions that increase afterload like valvular aortic stenosis and coarctation of aorta also produce left ventricular hypertrophy. These potentially treatable conditions should not be missed.

An important differential diagnosis in young active individuals is athlete's heart. However, athlete's heart has only mild LVH, left ventricular cavity size is mildly increased or on the upper side of normal. Abnormalities seen in athlete's heart reverse with physical deconditioning.

Other causes of LVH include Noonan syndrome, Friedreich's ataxia, amyloidosis, chronic renal failure, Fabry disease, mitochondrial myopathies, glycogen storage disorders, acromegaly, and drugs like androgenic steroids and tacrolimus.

MANAGEMENT

Management of HCM has few important aspects—management of symptoms, LVOTO, prevention of thromboembolism, and sudden death prevention. Most patients with HCM remain asymptomatic or have only mild symptoms. Genetic counseling and family screening of first-degree relatives clinically is also important. Genotyping can be offered to relatives if a disease-causing mutation is identified in the proband. Recommendations on exercise should be individualized. Moderate exercise like brisk walking, cycling, jogging, and light sports can be carried out by most patients. Strenuous physical activities and competitive sports should be avoided.

Asymptomatic individuals do not need any drug therapy. Common symptoms of breathlessness and chest pain can initially be treated with beta-blockers or verapamil. Beta-blockers are preferred in presence of LVOTO. If beta-blockers are not effective, then verapamil can be tried. Patients with HCM are at risk of atrial fibrillation. All patients with even a single-documented atrial fibrillation are candidates for lifelong oral anticoagulation irrespective of the CHA_2DS_2-VASc score.

Sudden cardiac death prevention: Sudden cardiac death is a dreaded complication and ICD is the only intervention that prevents sudden death. Antiarrhythmic drugs have not been shown to be effective in preventing SCD. Decision regarding ICD implantation is probably the most important aspect of the management especially since SCD is unpredictable and may be the first manifestation of the disease. All patients with sustained ventricular tachycardias and SCD survivors have a high risk of subsequent events and should be advised ICD implantation for secondary prevention. Event rate in these individuals is approximately 10% per year.

Implantable cardioverter defibrillator should also be considered for primary prevention in individuals at high risk of SCD (**Box 1**). Most HCM patients with one or more risk factor do not experience SCD since some individual risk factors have a low positive predictive value. Electrophysiological studies do not predict SCD risk.

European Society of Cardiology online risk calculator (http://doc2do.com/hcm/webHCM.html) can be used for SCD risk stratification. The calculator divides adult patients into low-, intermediate-, and high-risk groups with 5-year SCD risks of <4%, ≥4–6%, and ≥6%, respectively. Another approach is to follow the 2020 American College of Cardiology guidelines. Individuals with family history of premature SCD, unexplained recent syncope, or maximal LV wall thickness ≥30 mm should be recommended ICD implantation. ICD may be considered in patients with nonsustained VT or abnormal exercise blood pressure response if other risk factors are also present. Late gadolinium enhancement on magnetic resonance imaging (MRI) or left ventricular apical aneurysm also increases the risk of SCD and can be used for decision making in individuals at intermediate risk. Decisions regarding ICD implantation should always be individualized and taken after discussion with the patient.

Management of left ventricular outflow tract obstruction: The treatment options are listed in **Box 2**. Beta-blockers are the initial drug of choice for symptomatic patients. Beta-blockers reduce the LVOTO during exercise but are not effective under basal condition. Due to its negative inotropic effects disopyramide relieves both resting as well as exercise gradients in two-thirds of patients. It is used in patients who remain symptomatic despite beta-blocker therapy. Disopyramide enhances atrioventricular node conduction due to its anticholinergic effects. This can result in fast ventricular rates if the patient develops atrial fibrillation. Thus, disopyramide must always be combined with either beta-blockers or verapamil. Due to its anticholinergic effects, prostatic hypertrophy and glaucoma are relative contraindications. It also prolongs the QT interval which should be monitored. Disopyramide should not be combined with drugs like amiodarone that prolong the QT interval. Mavacamten, a cardiac myosin ATPase inhibitor, showed benefit in HCM patients with LVOTO in the EXPLORER-HCM trial. This is a promising drug, though not commercially available at present.

Drugs that reduce preload or afterload result in an increase of the gradient in HCM. Angiotensin-converting enzyme inhibitors (ACEIs), angiotensin receptor blockers (ARBs), nifedipine, and diuretics should be avoided in patients of HCM.

If patients continue to be symptomatic despite drug therapy, either alcohol septal ablation or myectomy may be considered. Even though myectomy is considered the gold standard, alcohol septal ablation is the more commonly performed procedure since it is less invasive. Myectomy has excellent long-term data, does not result

BOX 1 Risk factors for SCD in patients with HCM.

- Aborted cardiac arrest
- Sustained ventricular tachycardia
- Unexplained recent syncope (within past 5 years)
- Family history of premature SCD
- Maximal LV wall thickness ≥30 mm
- Nonsustained ventricular tachycardia on Holter monitoring (three or more beats at rate of ≥120 beats/min)
- Abnormal blood pressure response to exercise in individuals <40 years of age
- Late gadolinium enhancement on MRI

Potential risk factors:

- Left ventricular apical aneurysm
- LVOTO
- Double or compound mutations

BOX 2 Treatment options for left ventricular outflow tract obstruction (LVOTO) in patients with hypertrophic cardiomyopathy.

- Beta-blockers—drugs of first choice
- Disopyramide—always used along with beta-blockers
- Mavacamten
- Alcohol septal ablation
- Septal myectomy
- Dual chamber pacemaker—only in selected elderly individuals where other treatment options cannot be used

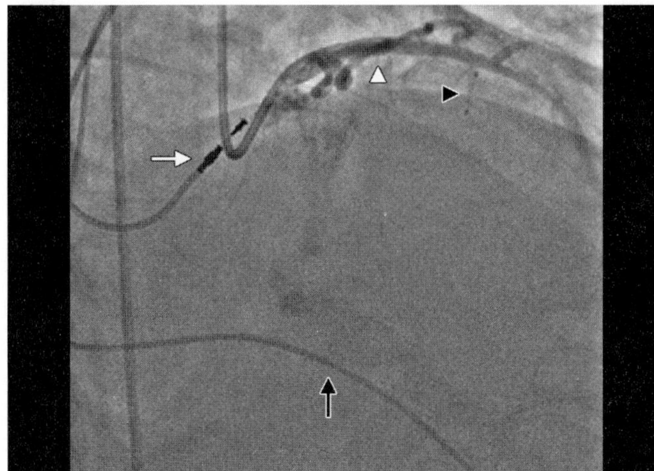

FIGURE 4: Alcohol septal ablation being carried out in a patient with hypertrophic obstructive cardiomyopathy. Balloon is placed in the septal branch (black arrowhead) of the left anterior descending artery (white arrowhead). A dual chamber permanent pacemaker with ventricular lead (black arrow) and atrial lead (white arrow) are also seen.

in a myocardial scar, if needed associated mitral valve repair can also be carried out and risk of heart block is low. Alcohol septal ablation involves selective injection of absolute alcohol into a septal branch of left anterior descending artery (**Fig. 4**). Alcohol causes infarction resulting in septal thinning thus relieving the obstruction. Right bundle branch block is common after alcohol septal ablation whereas left bundle branch block (LBBB) frequently occurs after septal myectomy. Heart block is the most common complication of alcohol septal ablation with 5–10% patients requiring permanent pacemaker implantation. Dual chamber pacing with short atrioventricular (AV) delay has become a less popular treatment option for LVOTO since this has not been found to be beneficial in randomized trials. Dual chamber pacing may still be considered in elderly patients with LVOTO in the absence of other treatment options.

DILATED CARDIOMYOPATHY

Dilated cardiomyopathy is characterized by dilatation and impaired contraction of left or both ventricles in the absence of secondary causes like coronary or valvular heart disease. DCM has a prevalence of around 1 in 2,500–5,000 in general population. DCM occurs at all ages but is most common in the third and fourth decades.

ETIOLOGY

Common causes of DCM are genetic (20–35%), alcoholic cardiomyopathy, chemotherapeutic drugs, and a sequela of myocarditis. Mutations in gene encoding titin (*TTN*) are common and has been found in 25% of familial and 18% of sporadic idiopathic DCM patients. Etiological causes of DCM are listed in **Box 3**. Despite complete evaluation a definite cause is not detected in a majority of the patients.

BOX 3	Causes of dilated cardiomyopathy.

- Familial
- Alcohol
- Drugs— anthracyclines
- Cocaine
- Myocarditis:
  - Viral—coxsackie B, adenovirus, parvovirus B19, HIV, and hepatitis C
  - Bacterial—diphtheria, meningococcus
  - Rickettsial—typhus
  - Parasitic—Chagas disease
- Endocrine disorders:
  - Hypothyroidism/hyperthyroidism
  - Pheochromocytoma
  - Cushing's disease
- Tachycardia induced cardiomyopathy
- Collagen vascular disorders
- Sarcoidosis
- Nutritional deficiencies:
  - Thiamine—beriberi
  - Selenium
- Metabolic disturbances:
  - Hypocalcemia
  - Hypophosphatemia
- Neuromuscular disorders:
  - Duchenne/Becker muscular dystrophies
  - Emery–Dreifuss muscular dystrophy
- Radiation
- Heavy metals—cobalt, lead, mercury, and arsenic
- Idiopathic

CLINICAL PRESENTATION

The presentation is variable with most patients presenting with insidious onset and gradually progressive symptoms although presentation with acute heart failure is not infrequent. Some patients are asymptomatic, being incidentally detected on routine examination. Symptoms of left heart failure like breathlessness on exertion, paroxysmal nocturnal dyspnea, and orthopnea often predominate. Right heart failure symptoms like pedal edema generally occur later in the disease course. Patients may also complain of fatigue, giddiness, and palpitations. Though the risk is lower than in ischemic cardiomyopathy, patients with LVEF <30–35% are at risk of SCD usually due to ventricular tachyarrhythmias. Alcoholic cardiomyopathy occurs in individuals with heavy alcohol intake for at least 5 years.

Clinical findings include laterally displaced and diffuse apex, soft first heart sound, third heart sounds, and features of pulmonary hypertension. Reverse splitting of the second heart sound is prominent in patients with LBBB or severe left ventricular dysfunction. Mitral and tricuspid regurgitation murmurs are usually soft. Features of heart failure are present in most patients.

INVESTIGATIONS

Electrocardiogram usually shows nonspecific abnormalities including atrial enlargement, intraventricular conduction defects, bundle branch blocks, and ST-T waves changes. LBBB is common (**Fig. 5**). Echocardiography shows impaired systolic function and dilatation of the left ventricle. Pulmonary hypertension, severe left ventricular enlargement, right ventricular dysfunction, and severe mitral and tricuspid regurgitation are poor prognostic markers.

Cardiac MRI is being increasingly used because it allows tissue characterization which is useful in assessing myocarditis and fibrosis. In addition, MRI allows accurate assessment of right ventricular function. Radionuclide imaging can also be used to document left and right ventricular ejection fraction. Endomyocardial biopsy has a limited role. It is indicated in patients with fulminant heart failure, amyloidosis, or suspected myocarditis. Genotyping using next-generation sequencing may be especially useful in those with family history of DCM or sudden death. Patients with mutations in lamin A/C can be identified. It is important because they are at high risk of SCD and ICD implantation should be considered.

DIFFERENTIAL DIAGNOSIS

It is important not to miss secondary causes of left ventricular dysfunction. Coronary artery disease is by far the most common cause of left ventricular dysfunction. Coronary artery disease should be excluded by stress test or coronary angiography. Coarctation of aorta and silent aortic stenosis can also cause left ventricular dysfunction. Evaluation for underlying conditions enumerated in **Box 3** should be carried out. It is especially important not to miss potentially treatable causes like alcoholism, hyperthyroidism, pheochromocytoma, sarcoidosis, tachycardia induced cardiomyopathy, and beriberi.

TREATMENT

Advances in therapy have produced remarkable improvements in survival of DCM patients. Drugs that improve survival include ACEIs, ARBs, beta-blockers, aldosterone receptor antagonists, angiotensin receptor–neprilysin inhibitors (ARNIs), and sodium-glucose cotransporter-2 inhibitors (dapagliflozin or empagliflozin). It should be ensured that all DCM patients receive ACEIs, beta-blockers, and aldosterone receptor antagonists unless they are not tolerated or contraindicated. ARBs are as efficacious and can be used instead of ACEIs but both should not be combined. Isosorbide dinitrate/hydralazine combination may be used in those unable to use ACEI/ARB either due to renal dysfunction or pregnancy.

Sacubitril-valsartan an ARNI is more efficacious and should be used instead of ACEIs/ARBs in patients with persistent left ventricular dysfunction. Sacubitril-valsartan should only be started at least 36 hours after the last dose of ACEIs. Sodium-glucose cotransporter-2 inhibitors also reduce mortality even in nondiabetic patients and may be added to standard therapy. Spironolactone is the preferred aldosterone receptor antagonist because of its low cost. Eplerenone may be substituted in patients who develop gynecomastia with spironolactone. All beta-blockers do not have the same efficacy. Carvedilol, metoprolol succinate, and bisoprolol have been shown to reduce mortality in clinical trials. Only one of these three

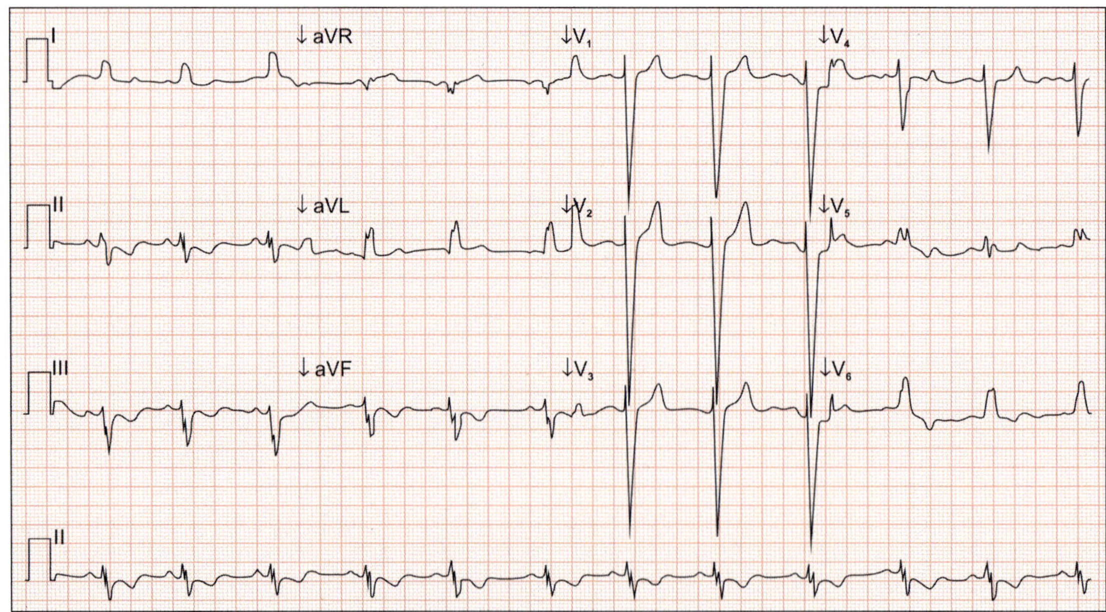

FIGURE 5: ECG of a patient with DCM and left bundle branch block (LBBB). It is important to recognize LBBB since these patients benefit from cardiac resynchronization therapy.

TABLE 3	Target doses of drugs in dilated cardiomyopathy.
Drug	**Target dose**
Ramipril	10 mg OD
Enalapril	20 mg BID
Carvedilol	25 mg BID
Bisoprolol	10 mg OD
Metoprolol succinate	200 mg OD
Losartan	150 mg OD
Valsartan	160 mg BID
Candesartan	32 mg OD
Sacubitril-valsartan	200 mg BID

(BID: twice a day; OD: once daily)

should be used. Starting these drugs is not enough. It is important to uptitrate the dose gradually every 2–3 weeks to reach target doses (**Table 3**). If target doses cannot be reached due to side effects, then maximally tolerated doses should be used. Patients on ACEI, ARBs, or aldosterone antagonists should be monitored for renal dysfunction and hyperkalemia.

With above drugs, left ventricular function will return to normal or near normal in around a third of patients. These patients may relapse even years later. Lifelong beta-blocker and ACEI/ARB therapy should probably be continued even in recovered patients.

In addition, drugs are important for symptom relief. Most important among these are loop diuretics. Digoxin may be used in patients who remain symptomatic despite optimal drug therapy. Only low-dose digoxin should be used. Ivabradine may also be used in symptomatic patients in sinus rhythm with resting heart rates >70 beats/min. Oral anticoagulant should be used in patients with history of thromboembolism, atrial fibrillation, or cardiac thrombus.

Sudden death is an important cause of mortality in DCM patients. Patients at the highest risk of sudden death of around 11% per year are those with history of sustained ventricular tachycardia or cardiac arrest. ICD should be advised. Even though the risk of SCD is lower in patients with DCM as compared to ischemic cardiomyopathy, guidelines recommend ICD implantation for SCD primary prevention in DCM patients with LVEF < 35%. The risk of SCD should be discussed with patients. Patients like with lamin A/C mutations and cardiac sarcoidosis are at high risk of sudden death and ICD should be advised. Patients with wide QRS >120–130 ms, LBBB, and LVEF <35%, who remain symptomatic despite medical therapy should be advised cardiac resynchronization therapy (CRT) using a biventricular pacemaker. Patients with QRS width of ≥150 derive maximal benefit. Ideally, CRT should be combined with a defibrillator (CRT-D). Patients with end-stage heart failure should be considered for heart transplant or left ventricular assist device implantation.

MYOCARDITIS

Inflammation of myocardium with cellular infiltration with or without associated myocyte necrosis characterizes myocarditis. Myocarditis may be due to infections or noninfective inflammatory disorders. Among infective causes, viruses are the most common. A number of viruses can cause myocarditis. These are enteroviruses including coxsackie B virus, adenovirus, human immunodeficiency virus (HIV), hepatitis C, parvovirus B19, influenza, and herpes virus 6. Other infections that may cause myocarditis include diphtheria, rickettsial infections, Lyme disease, Chagas disease, and helminthic infestations. Noninfective causes of myocarditis include sarcoidosis, collagen vascular disorders, Takayasu disease, Kawasaki disease, celiac disease, inflammatory bowel disease, and hypersensitivity drug reactions.

The diagnosis of myocarditis requires a high index of suspicion. Myocarditis may present with acute heart failure, chronic heart failure with a DCM like picture, chest pain, arrhythmias, or rarely sudden death. This may be preceded by a prodrome of gastrointestinal or respiratory febrile illness. Features that suggest underlying myocarditis include fulminant or acute presentation, ventricular tachyarrhythmias, heart blocks, raised cardiac biomarkers, eosinophilia, raised erythrocyte sedimentation rate (ESR), and history of a preceding prodrome.

Electrocardiogram may show sinus tachycardia, arrhythmias, and nonspecific changes. Occasionally ECG changes can mimic myocardial infarction. Heart blocks may be seen in diphtheria, sarcoidosis, and Lyme disease. Cardiac biomarkers like troponins may be raised in patients with recent onset of symptoms.

Echocardiographic picture resembles DCM with reduced left and/or right ventricular contractility. The advantage of cardiac MRI over echocardiography is that it allows tissue characterization and is being increasingly used now for diagnosis.

Magnetic resonance imaging provides a global picture and is more sensitive as compared to endomyocardial biopsy which often may not sample areas of active inflammation.

Endomyocardial biopsy is especially important in patients with fulminant myocarditis. The classical picture is lymphocytic infiltration. Histological examination is important in picking up granulomas, giant cells, or eosinophilia due to therapeutic implications. Use of immunohistochemistry along with the classical Dallas criteria on histology is important to increase sensitivity of endomyocardial biopsy. Positron emission tomography (PET) scan is useful in patients with suspicion of sarcoidosis.

Patients with myocarditis are at risk of sudden death. They should avoid heavy physical activities for at least 3–6 months. Standard heart failure therapy similar to that of DCM patients should be instituted. Patients with hemodynamic instability may need inotropes. Immunosuppressive and antiviral therapy do not have a proven role in lymphocytic myocarditis. Lymphocytic myocarditis constitutes around 90% cases of myocarditis.

Myocarditis associated with connective tissue disorders granulomatous myocarditis, giant cell myocarditis, and eosinophilic myocarditis however are treated with immunosuppressive drugs. Left ventricular assist device and heart transplant are options in patients in refractory heart failure or shock.

RESTRICTIVE CARDIOMYOPATHY

Unlike HCM and DCM which are diagnosed on morphological criteria, diagnosis of RCM is based on hemodynamic features of severe diastolic dysfunction. RCM is characterized by restrictive features with normal or near normal ventricular wall thickness. Initially, the systolic function is normal or near normal. Later in the course, systolic dysfunction may become prominent in conditions like amyloidosis. Due to poor ventricular compliance, even small increases in ventricular volume cause marked rise in ventricular diastolic pressures. Both ventricles are usually involved. However, in endomyocardial fibrosis (EMF) only one ventricle may be predominantly affected.

ETIOLOGY

Idiopathic RCM, amyloidosis, EMF, and hypereosinophilia are the common causes of RCM in Indians. Other causes of RCM are listed in **Box 4**. Idiopathic RCM is etiologically similar to HCM with around half the cases being caused by sarcomeric gene mutations. These are transmitted in an autosomal dominant pattern. RCM is most commonly due primary amyloidosis also called AL variety. Cardiac amyloid deposition is also seen in multiple myeloma. Secondary amyloidosis rarely involves the heart. Familial amyloidosis may rarely be caused by deposition of mutant type transthyretin.

Endomyocardial fibrosis is a tropical disease of unknown etiology and has been most commonly reported from Kerala. The dense endocardial fibrosis most commonly affects the apices and inflow region of the ventricles and also involves the underlying myocardium (**Fig. 6**). A preceding inflammatory phase has been reported in some patients. Most patients present in the fibrotic phase. Mitral and tricuspid regurgitation may occur due to involvement of the subvalvular apparatus. Cardiac involvement in hypereosinophilia resembles EMF.

CLINICAL FEATURES

Patients with RCM usually present with progressive heart failure. Symptoms include breathlessness, pedal edema, anasarca, palpitations, and giddiness. On physical examination jugular venous pressure is often raised with a positive Kussmaul sign. Features of right heart failure like pedal edema, tender hepatomegaly, and ascites may be present. The apex is ill sustained and normally located. Third and fourth heart sounds may be present. The fourth heart sound is absent in atrial fibrillation, or if amyloid infiltration is causing impaired atrial contraction. Murmurs of mitral and tricuspid regurgitation are usually soft.

BOX 4	Causes of restrictive cardiomyopathy.
• Idiopathic restrictive cardiomyopathy	
• Familial restrictive cardiomyopathy (usually autosomal dominant)	
• Amyloidosis	
• Endomyocardial fibrosis	
• Hypereosinophilic syndrome	
• Desminopathy	
• Radiotherapy	
• Metastatic cancer	
• Hemochromatosis	
• Sarcoidosis	
• Carcinoid heart disease	
• Noonan syndrome	
• Storage disorders like Fabry disease and glycogen storage disorders	
• Drugs—anthracyclines, chloroquine, and methysergide	
• Scleroderma	

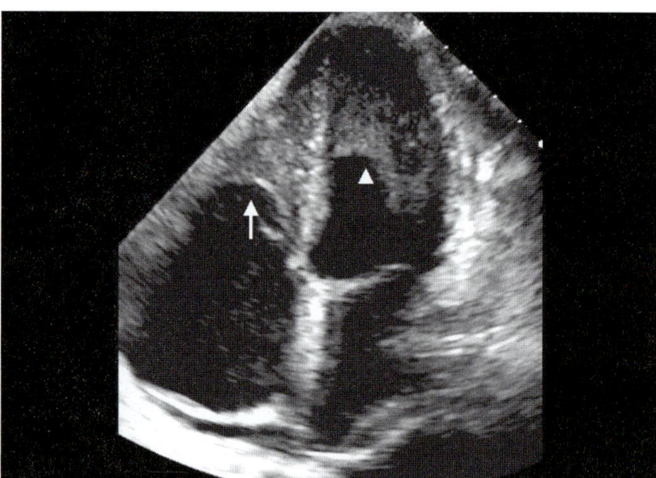

FIGURE 6: Transthoracic echocardiogram in the apical four-chamber view in a patient with endomyocardial fibrosis shows obliteration of the left (arrowhead) and right ventricular (arrow) apex.

INVESTIGATIONS

Electrocardiogram abnormalities are commonly seen. QRS voltage is usually normal but increased voltages may be present in some patients with idiopathic RCM. In amyloidosis, low limb lead voltage defined as QRS voltage ≤5 mm in all limb leads may be present (**Fig. 7**). This low QRS voltage despite increased left ventricular wall thickness is typical of amyloidosis. In addition, atrial enlargement may be seen in patients with sinus rhythm. Due to raised atrial pressures and atrial enlargement patients with RCM are at risk of atrial fibrillation. Patients with amyloidosis or desminopathy may show conduction defects. Cardiomegaly is seen on chest X-ray and is due

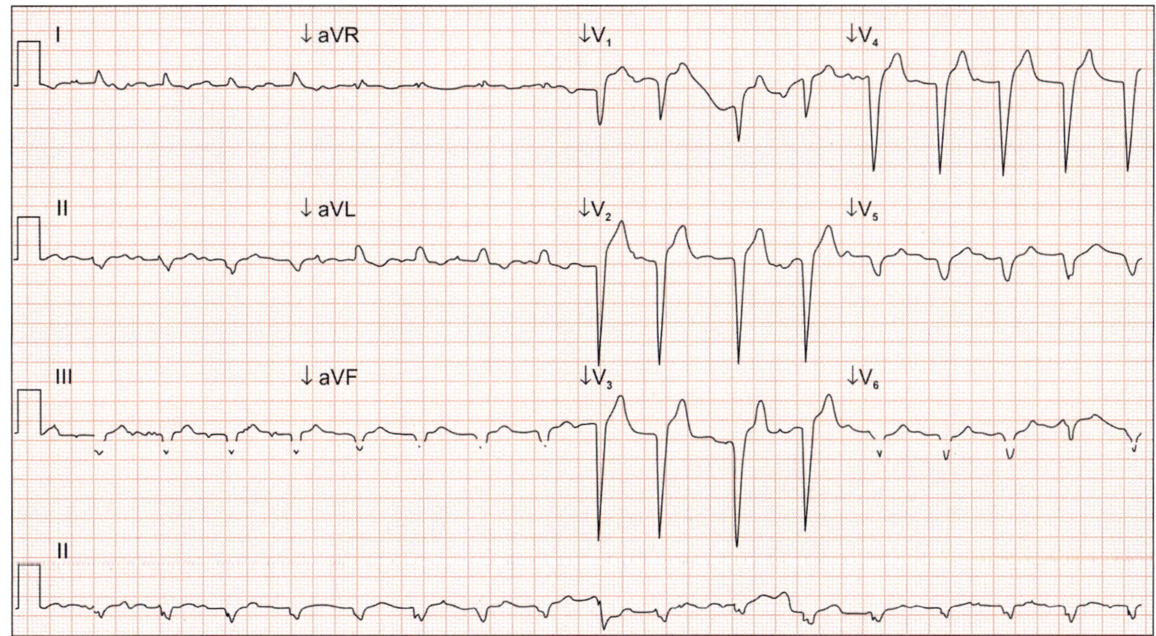

FIGURE 7: ECG of a patient with amyloidosis with increased left ventricular wall thickness on echocardiography. Limb leads show low QRS voltage.

to atrial enlargement. Features of pulmonary venous and arterial hypertension are common.

Echocardiography usually confirms the presence of RCM. Additional investigations are needed to confirm the etiology. Biatrial enlargement with normal-sized ventricles is a typical feature of restrictive physiology. Doppler shows restrictive filling pattern. Mitral and tricuspid regurgitation may be seen in all forms of RCM. These are particularly common in EMF due to involvement of subvalvular apparatus. Apical obliteration may be seen in EMF. Thickened ventricular walls and interatrial septum and impaired ventricular contractility may be seen in amyloidosis (**Fig. 8**). Evaluation for underlying cause includes serum-free light assay for amyloidosis and genotyping for idiopathic RCM.

Magnetic resonance imaging allows tissue characterization and is also useful in establishing the etiology, especially in amyloidosis and EMF.

Cardiac catheterization is useful in assessing the hemodynamics. Raised ventricular end-diastolic pressure with dip and plateau pattern is seen. Endomyocardial biopsy may be required to establish the diagnosis. It is particularly useful in infiltrative disorders like amyloidosis.

Constrictive pericarditis is the most important differential diagnosis. Constrictive pericarditis should not be missed since it is a surgically treatable condition. It is important to realize that 15–20% patients with constrictive pericarditis have normal pericardial thickness. Thus, a normal pericardial thickness does not rule out constrictive pericarditis.

TREATMENT

Loop diuretics are used for relief of dyspnea and fluid overload. Patients with RCM are at high risk of atrial

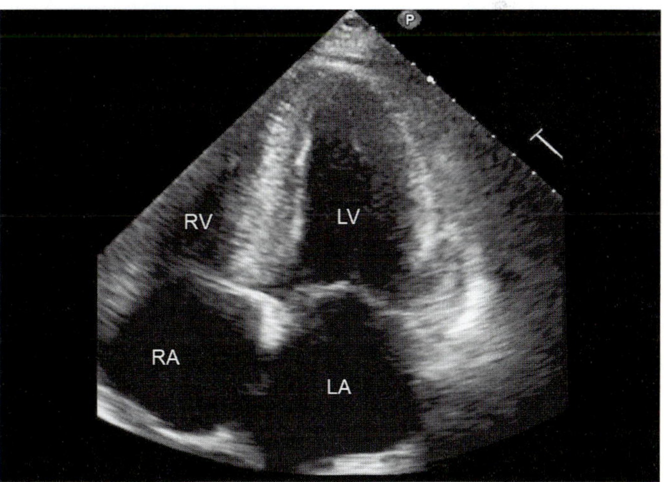

FIGURE 8: Transthoracic echocardiogram four-chamber view in a patient with cardiac amyloidosis showing biatrial enlargement with increased left ventricular wall thickness.

fibrillation and systemic embolism. Patients with even a single episode of atrial fibrillation should receive long-term oral anticoagulation (in absence of contraindications) even if the CHA_2DS_2-VASc score is 0. Specific treatment includes chemotherapy including bortezomib for amyloidosis and iron chelation therapy for hemochromatosis.

Pacemaker implantation is indicated in patients with high grade heart blocks that may occur in amyloidosis and sarcoidosis. ICD implantation should be considered in patients with history of cardiac arrest or sustained ventricular tachycardias.

Digoxin, verapamil, and diltiazem bind to amyloid fibrils and may have an exaggerated effect. These should be avoided or used only in low doses in patients with amyloidosis.

ARRHYTHMOGENIC RIGHT VENTRICULAR CARDIOMYOPATHY

Arrhythmogenic right ventricular cardiomyopathy is an inherited cardiomyopathy caused by mutations in genes encoding cardiac desmosomes. These are proteins responsible for cell-to-cell adhesion and include desmoplakin, plakophilin 2, desmoglein 2, and desmocollin 2. The right ventricle is almost always involved. However, biventricular involvement is also common. Histologically, the disease is characterized by loss of cardiomyocytes and their replacement with fibrous and fatty tissue. These changes result in right ventricular wall thinning and sometimes aneurysm formation.

Arrhythmogenic right ventricular cardiomyopathy most commonly presents in the second to fourth decade. The most common presentation is palpitations, due to ventricular arrhythmias. Right heart failure is a late manifestation. ARVC is an important cause of sudden death in young individuals and sudden death may be the first presentation in an asymptomatic individual. Establishing the diagnosis may be difficult in early cases with subtle manifestations. A combination of family history, ECG manifestations, documentation of arrhythmias, imaging, and genotyping can help. Endomyocardial biopsy may be diagnostic. However, biopsy is usually not carried out because of risk of perforation of the thin-walled right ventricle. The ECG may show repolarization changes like T inversions in leads V_1–V_3 and epsilon waves (**Fig. 9**). T inversions are significant in individuals >14 years of age in the absence of right bundle branch block. Sustained or ill-sustained ventricular tachycardia is of LBBB pattern may be seen on Holter monitoring. Imaging using echocardiography, MRI or ventriculography may show right ventricular dysfunction and regional akinesia or aneurysms.

All patients with ARVC should avoid intense sporting activities. Beta-blockers are recommended for all patients, even though evidence for benefit is sparse. Most important aspect of management involves prevention of sudden death using ICD. ICD should be recommended in patients with history of unexplained syncope, sustained or non-sustained ventricular tachycardia, ventricular fibrillation or ventricular dysfunction. Catheter ablation may be tried in individuals with recurrent sustained monomorphic ventricular tachycardia. These unfortunately tend to recur from another focus since ARVC is a progressive disease. Patients with ventricular dysfunction are managed with standard heart failure therapy. Heart transplant is an option in patients with end-stage heart disease.

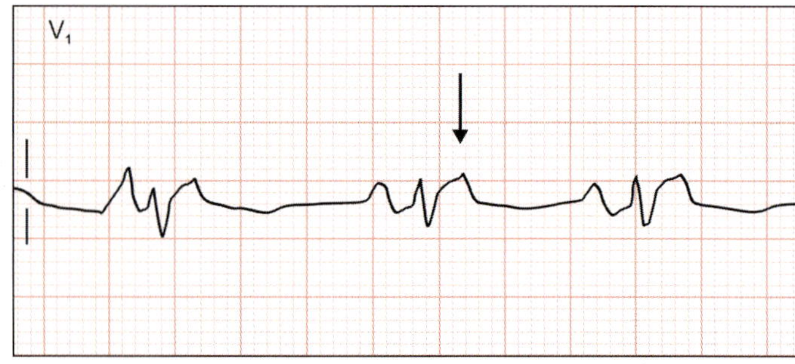

(ARVC: arrhythmogenic right ventricular cardiomyopathy)

FIGURE 9: ECG showing epsilon waves (arrow) in lead V_1 in a patient with ARVC.

INDIAN CONTEXT

Even though epidemiological data on Indian patients with cardiomyopathies is lacking, certain specific features stand out. As emphasized earlier cardiomyopathies are genetic disorders. All ethnic groups have some differences in their genetic makeup. A few such variations that are unique to Indians contribute to development of cardiomyopathies. These variations occur de novo in an individual and over the generations may spread to thousands or millions of individuals. The most common variation that is unique to South Asia is a 25-base pair deletion in intron 32 of the cardiac myosin binding protein C gene (*MyBPC3*). It first occurred in a person in India around 23,000–33,000 years back and has spread to involve 4% of the Indian population over this period of time. This variation increases the heart failure risk with an odds ratio of around 7. Another common variation unique to Indians *MyBPC3* p.Asp389Val is found in around 10% individuals with the 32 base pair deletion. This variation is also associated with abnormal cardiac contractility. In addition, EMF is a tropical cardiomyopathy and has been reported all over the country but is most common in Kerala.

> Common genetic variants that predispose to cardiomyopathies and are unique to South Asians are a 32 base pair deletion in intron 32 of *MyBPC3* and a missense mutation *MyBPC3* p.Asp389Val.

RECOMMENDED READINGS

1. Richardson P, McKenna W, Bristow M, Maisch B, Mautner B, O'Connell J, et al. Report of the 1995 World Health Organization/International Society and Federation of Cardiology Task Force on the definition and classification of cardiomyopathies. Circulation. 1996;93(5):841-2.
2. Elliott P, Andersson B, Arbustini E, Bilinska Z, Cecchi F, Charron P, et al. Classification of the cardiomyopathies: a position statement from the European Society of Cardiology working group on myocardial and pericardial diseases. Eur Heart J. 2008;29(2):270-6.
3. Maron BJ, Towbin JA, Thiene G, Antzelevitch C, Corrado D, Arnett D, et al. Contemporary definitions and classification of the cardiomyopathies: An American Heart Association Scientific Statement from the Council on Clinical Cardiology, Heart Failure and Transplantation Committee; Quality of Care and Outcomes Research and Functional Genomics

and Translational Biology Interdisciplinary Working Groups; and Council on Epidemiology and Prevention. Circulation. 2006;113(14):1807-16.

4. Maron BJ, Gardin JM, Flack JM, Gidding SS, Kurosaki TT, Bild DE. Prevalence of hypertrophic cardiomyopathy in a general population of young adults. Echocardiographic analysis of 4111 subjects in the CARDIA Study. Coronary Artery Risk Development in (Young) Adults. Circulation. 1995;92(4):785-9.
5. Mogensen J, Murphy RT, Kubo T, Bahl A, Moon JC, Klausen IC, et al. Frequency and clinical expression of cardiac troponin I mutations in 748 consecutive families with hypertrophic cardiomyopathy. J Am Coll Cardiol 2004;44(12):2315-25.
6. Kubo T, Gimeno JR, Bahl A, Steffensen U, Steffensen M, Osman E, et al. Prevalence, clinical significance, and genetic basis of hypertrophic cardiomyopathy with restrictive phenotype. J Am Coll Cardiol. 2007;49(25):2419-26.
7. Gersh BJ, Maron BJ, Bonow RO, Dearani JA, Fifer MA, Link MS, et al. 2011 ACCF/AHA guideline for the diagnosis and treatment of hypertrophic cardiomyopathy: executive summary: a report of the American College of Cardiology Foundation/American Heart Association Task Force on practice guidelines. Circulation. 2011;124(24): 2761-96.
8. Elliott PM, Anastasakis A, Borger MA, Borggrefe M, Cecchi F, Charron P, et al. 2014 ESC Guidelines on diagnosis and management of hypertrophic cardiomyopathy: The task force for the diagnosis and management of hypertrophic cardiomyopathy of the European Society of Cardiology (ESC). Eur Heart J. 2014;35(39):2733-79.
9. Ommen SR, Mital S, Burke MA, Day SM, Deswal A, Elliott P, et al. 2020 AHA/ACC Guideline for the diagnosis and treatment of patients with hypertrophic cardiomyopathy: Executive Summary: A Report of the American College of Cardiology/American Heart Association Joint Committee on clinical practice guidelines. J Am Coll Cardiol. 2020;76(25):3022-55.
10. Olivotto I, Oreziak A, Barriales-Villa R, Abraham TP, Masri A, Garcia-Pavia P, et al.Mavacamten for treatment of symptomatic obstructive hypertrophic cardiomyopathy (EXPLORER-HCM): a randomised, double-blind, placebo-controlled, phase 3 trial. Lancet. 2020;396(10253):759-69.
11. Herman DS, Lam L, Taylor MR, Wang L, Teekakirikul P, Christodoulou D, et al. Truncations of titin causing dilated cardiomyopathy. N Engl J Med. 2012;366(7):619-28.
12. Taylor MR, Fain PR, Sinagra G, Robinson ML, Robertson AD, Carniel E, et al. Natural history of dilated cardiomyopathy due to lamin A/C gene mutations. J Am Coll Cardiol. 2003;41(5):771-80.
13. McMurray JJV, Solomon SD, Inzucchi SE, Køber L, Kosiborod MN, Martinez FA, et al. Dapagliflozin in patients with heart failure and reduced ejection fraction. N Engl J Med. 2019;381(21):1995-2008.
14. Gupta A, Goyal P, Bahl A. Frequency of recovery and relapse in patients with nonischemic dilated cardiomyopathy on guideline-directed medical therapy. Am J Cardiol. 2014;114(6):883-9.
15. Caforio ALP, Pankuweit S, Arbustini E, Basso C, Gimeno-Blanes J, Felix SB, et al. Current state of knowledge on aetiology, diagnosis, management, and therapy of myocarditis: A position statement of the European Society of Cardiology Working Group on myocardial and pericardial diseases. Eur Heart J. 2013;34(33):2636-48.
16. Bahl A, Saikia UN, Khullar M. Idiopathic restrictive cardiomyopathy - perspectives from genetics studies. Is it time to redefine these disorders? Cardiogenetics. 2012;2(1):15-8.
17. Kubo T, Gimeno JR, Bahl A, Steffensen U, Steffensen M, Osman E, et al. Prevalence, clinical significance, and genetic basis of hypertrophic cardiomyopathy with restrictive phenotype. J Am Coll Cardiol. 2007;49(25):2419-26.
18. Rai TS, Ahmad S, Ahluwalia TS, Ahuja M, Bahl A, Saikia UN, et al. Genetic and clinical profile of Indian patients of idiopathic restrictive cardiomyopathy with and without hypertrophy. Mol Cell Biochem. 2009;331(1-2):187-92.
19. Dhandapany PS, Sadayappan S, Xue Y, Powell GT, Rani DS, Nallari P, et al. A common MYBPC3 (cardiac myosin binding protein C) variant associated with cardiomyopathies in South Asia. Nat Genet. 2009;41(2):187-91.
20. Viswanathan SK, Puckelwartz MJ, Mehta A, Ramachandra CJA, Jagadeesan A, Fritsche-Danielson R, et al. Association of cardiomyopathy with MYBPC3 D389V and MYBPC3Δ25bpIntronic deletion in South Asian descendants. JAMA Cardiol. 2018;3(6):481-8.

CHAPTER

110 Pericardial Diseases

Sandeep Seth, SS Kothari

ABSTRACT

Pericardial diseases can occur due to multiple causes. Acute pericarditis is most often viral and usually it resolves without any residual effects. Some cases can have recurrence. Treatment is usually anti-inflammatory drugs. Pericardial effusion can develop in some cases with pericarditis. When effusion exerts pressure effects on the heart and impairs venous filling, we diagnose cardiac tamponade. This is an emergency and needs pericardial tapping. Constrictive pericarditis is a chronic condition due to thickening of the pericardium. The most common cause is tuberculosis (TB) in our country. It needs to be differentiated from restrictive cardiomyopathy (RCM). The treatment is surgical pericardiectomy.

"My powers are ordinary, only my application brings me success"

—Isaac newton

INTRODUCTION

The pericardium is the outer most layer of the heart. It has visceral and parietal layer with minimal (5–10 mL) fluid between them. Pericardium helps to preserve the heart from friction with surrounding tissues during contraction.

Diseases of the pericardium include acute pericarditis, pericardial effusion and tamponade, and chronic pericarditis including constrictive pericarditis. Rarely the pericardium may be absent congenitally. Absent pericardium is a rare condition. Left-sided absence is more common. It is generally asymptomatic and harmless condition although the heart shows increased mobility and it is displaced. There is minimal increased risk of aortic dissection in this condition. Acute pericarditis can sometime result in pericardial effusion. Cardiac tamponade can occur in large pericardial effusions or sometimes when it occurs rapidly even in smaller collections. Chronic constrictive pericarditis is characterized by a shell around the heart due to thickening of the pericardium. It can gradually develop as a consequence of pericardial effusion with thickening, or it may be the first presentation in some cases.

ACUTE PERICARDITIS

It is an inflammation of the pericardium and is the most common type of pericardial disease. Generally, patients present acutely. The various causes of acute pericarditis are listed in **Box 1**. Majority of the cases are idiopathic and presumed to be viral. Other causes include TB, neoplasia, and systemic diseases.

The clinical features include a sharp localized retrosternal chest pain on inspiration which may vary with posture. There is accompanying fever, malaise, and shortness of breath. Sometimes pain is severe and can mimic acute coronary syndrome (ACS). Pain more often radiates to the back.

BOX 1 Causes of pericarditis.

- **Infections**
  - Viral (coxsackie, mumps)
  - Bacterial (pneumococcal, tubercular)
  - Fungal
  - Parasitic
- **Autoimmune diseases**
  - Systemic lupus
  - Rheumatoid arthritis
- **Immune reactions**
  - Postsurgery
  - Rheumatic fever
- **Metabolic**
  - Uremic
  - Myxedema
- **Miscellaneous**
  - Myocardial infarction
  - Myocarditis
- **Trauma**
  - Blunt trauma chest
- **Neoplastic**
  - Lung carcinoma
  - Breast carcinoma
  - Leukemia
  - Lymphoma

On examination, a pericardial friction rub is often audible. It may be monophasic, biphasic, or more typically and less frequently triphasic in character. Rub is distinguished from murmur by its superficial character (appears to be close to diaphragm of the stethoscope). It can be transient and can vary in intensity over few hours. Generally, when more fluid accumulates the rub disappears. Most acute pericarditis of viral etiology disappears over 2–3 weeks and do not result in significant fluid accumulation. In some cases, acute pericarditis can reoccur, sometimes even multiple times.

On investigations the electrocardiogram shows diffuse ST-segment elevation which is not limited to any vessel territory. There is associated PQ segment depression which is suggestive of pericarditis. There is concave upward ST elevation which does not evolve (as it does in ACS) and stays the same. Later there can be T wave inversion.

Since it is an inflammatory condition marker such as total leukocyte count, erythrocyte sedimentation rate (ESR) and C-reactive protein (CRP) are elevated. A collagen profile may be required in patients with other systemic features like joint pains. In India, TB can also present with acute pericarditis although it more often presents with pericardial effusion. Bacterial infections also present more often with pericardial effusion rather than with features of acute pericarditis. In case the pericarditis extends to the myocardium, then the troponins and other myocardial enzymes may go up although this is uncommon.

Chest X-ray will reveal a normal size heart in acute pericarditis. When significant effusion occurs, there may be a water bottle heart without any significant pulmonary venous or pulmonary artery hypertension. Echocardiogram shows pericardial collection which is initially mild, but can go on to develop effusion. The inferior vena cava (IVC) must always be seen and commented upon. Pericardiocentesis is usually not done in patients with pericarditis.

Treatment: Patients with acute pericarditis may need to be admitted. Nonsteroidal anti-inflammatory drugs are the first drugs started. Ibuprofen up to 800 mg thrice a day is given, sometimes for weeks, till the effusion disappears and inflammatory markers in the blood settle. Colchicine can be used as initial treatment or to prevent recurrences (0.5 mg twice a day). Steroids are used in the setting of a systemic autoimmune disease. Most patients of acute pericarditis are of viral etiology and thus stabilized over 2–3 week's time.

TYPES

The three common types of acute pericarditis are viral, bacterial, and tubercular. They have different presentations and thus different management principles. They are described individually here.

Viral pericarditis: This is a common cause of pericarditis. It may be due to a direct viral invasion or an immune response. Viral pericarditis usually resolves but if it persists, specific etiologies can be looked for and treated. For cytomegalovirus (CMV) (hyperimmune globulin), Coxsackie B virus (interferon alpha or beta) or adenovirus and parvovirus B19 (immunoglobulin)-specific immune therapies can be done. Pericardial manifestations of human immunodeficiency virus (HIV) can be due to local HIV infection and bacterial or tubercular infection. In 85%, it resolves without leaving any effects. In a small fraction, there can be repeated episodes.

Bacterial pericarditis: Bacterial involvement of the pericardium is rare, but has a high mortality of 30–40%. Complications include tamponade and constriction. It can be due to hematogenous or contiguous spread. It is an acute fulminant illness. Pericardiocentesis, high-end antibiotics, intrapericardial instillation of streptokinase, or urokinase are necessary. Often surgical pericardial drainage is needed for treatment and to prevent constriction.

Tubercular pericarditis: Tubercular pericarditis is seen in the setting of TB at other sites or it can be de novo. Patients present with acute pericarditis, cardiac tamponade, effuso-constrictive pericarditis, or constrictive pericarditis. The diagnosis is a combination of clinical history plus trying to find acid-fast bacilli (AFB) in the pericardial fluid (pericardiocentesis) or tissue (pericardial biopsy) and caseous granulomas in the pericardial biopsy. Polymerase chain reaction (PCR) can pick up TB deoxyribonucleic acid (DNA) from the pericardial fluid. In the pericardial fluid, adenosine deaminase (ADA) levels are elevated. The pericardial fluid protein levels are high and the white blood cell (WBC) count is predominantly lymphocytic. Since the presentation is usually subacute, the fluid should be screened for malignant cells. If clinical and bacteriological evidence suggests TB, the patient is started on antitubercular therapy. This is usually the two stages standard therapy with a minimum of three drugs. In the first 2–3 months, steroids are usually given. A meta-analysis of various studies has shown that giving steroids in the initial phase of therapy is associated with fewer deaths, faster resolution of pericardial fluid, and less chances of constriction. The duration of therapy varies from 6 to 12 months though most centers in India prefer to give longer regimens.

PERICARDIAL EFFUSION AND CARDIAC TAMPONADE

Pericardial effusions occur with neoplasms, TB, uremia, and sometimes with myxedema. Other causes include postsurgical, post-trauma, and postinfection. Some cases of acute pericarditis can also go on to develop effusion and later present as pericardial effusion. Acute bleeding in the pericardial space presents with cardiac tamponade even when small-to-moderate amount of blood accumulates rapidly in the pericardial. The causes for bleeding in pericardial space are shown in **Box 2**.

Large collections in the pericardium cause cardiac chamber compression and fall in blood pressure (BP) and cardiac output. This can happen with less amount of fluid in a rapid collection as discussed above in conditions causing bleeding in the pericardial space. In chronic collections, it occurs with large amount of fluid when it collects slowly as in tubercular involvement. Cardiac tamponade implies impaired cardiac filling due to effusion which compresses upon the heart and impedes venous filling. It is a cardiac emergency and needs early management.

BOX 2	Causes of bleeding in the pericardial space.
• Blunt and penetrating trauma	
• Post-MI rupture of LV free wall	
• Complication of cardiac procedures (BMV)	
• Retrograde bleeding in aortic dissection	
• Perioperative bleeding	

Clinical presentation in chronic pericardial effusion is with chest discomfort, exertional dyspnea, fever, and fatigue. Sometimes it is picked on echocardiogram or ultrasound during workup in a case of pyrexia of unknown origin (PUO). As more fluid accumulates the breathlessness and fatigue increase. In cardiac tamponade, patients become class III or IV dyspneic and have hypotension causing extreme weakness. In acute pericardial effusion (periprocedural and perioperative), presentation is more dramatic with hypotension, features of collapse, and difficult breathing. It needs immediate relief. The presence of Beck's triad of hypotension, muffled heart sounds, and elevated jugular venous pressure (JVP) suggests severe tamponade.

On examination, patients at stage of pericardial effusion may have normal findings with some tachycardia and dull precordial percussion note. The heart sounds may be soft. As tamponade develops, they have increasing tachycardia. The jugular venous pulse is raised. Kussmaul's sign (rise in JVP with inspiration) is more often seen is constrictive pericarditis although may be there in cardiac tamponade.

Pulsus paradoxus is a typical feature of cardiac tamponade. It is picked up while measuring BP initially. There is a fall in systolic BP of ≥10 mm Hg in inspiration as compared to expiration. It is best appreciated if we bring down the pressure gradually and stop at the systolic pressure. Later, when the paradox is more, it may even be palpable. It can be seen on bedside monitor if patient has an arterial line in place. Respiratory rate is increased. Cardiac examination shows increased precordial dullness, soft heart sounds, and no murmurs.

INVESTIGATIONS

Electrocardiogram shows low voltages, P wave, ST changes, and electrical alternans. *Chest X-ray* shows large cardiac shadow ("water bottle" heart) with clear lung fields. There is cardiomegaly with no evidence of pulmonary venous or arterial hypertension. The superior vena cava (SVC) is slightly prominent. Associated pleural effusions are common. Lung fields might give a clue if due to TB. The differentials for an X-ray with marked cardiomegaly are Ebstein's anomaly, severe tricuspid regurgitation, and dilated cardiomyopathy (**Fig. 1**).

Echocardiogram helps to diagnose pericardial effusion easily. It shows an echo free space around heart. Amount of fluid can be estimated from anterior and posterior echo-free space. In tubercular etiology, there may be septations in the space. In bacterial infection, there are dense echoes in the space due to pus. Sometimes effusion can be localized to one segment. When tamponade occurs, there is diastolic collapse of the right atrium and right ventricular (RV) free wall. Impaired filling can be documented on Doppler. The subcostal view is the best view to pick up a large pericardial collection. If the IVC is dilated with hypotension and there is a pulsus paradoxus, this combination suggests a diagnosis of cardiac tamponade (**Fig. 2**).

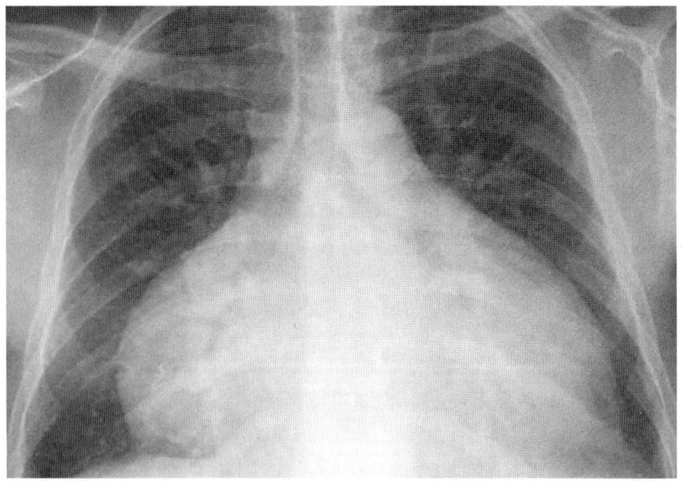

FIGURE 1: X-ray of chest showing "water bottle heart" due to a large pericardial effusion. Such marked cardiomegaly with clear lung field and no pulmonary venous hypertension is a feature of slowly accumulating chronic pericardial effusion.

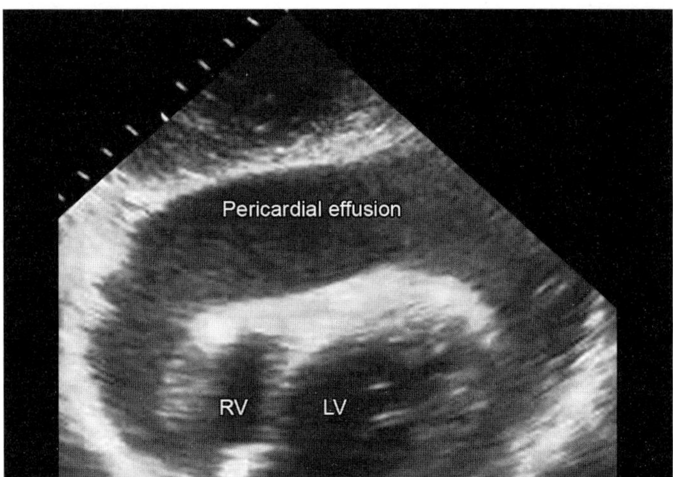

FIGURE 2: Subcostal veiw showing a large pericardiul fluid causing tamponade.

A *computed tomography (CT) scan* of thorax helps to look at lung fields and pericardial thickness when it occurs in long-standing effusions. Such patients have an effuso-constrictive pathology.

TREATMENT

On diagnosing a pericardial effusion, we must risk at its etiology. Effusions in myxedema resolve with treatment soon. Tubercular patients respond to antitubercular treatment (ATT) and steroids. Prednisolone 40–60 mg daily can be given for 8–12 weeks in tubercular pericardial effusion. Uremic effusion responds to more frequent dialysis. Malignant effusions need treatment of basic cause. Irradiation and steroids can also help in resolution of fluid.

Cardiac tamponade is an emergency. When patients are hypotensive then fluid needs to be tapped and sent for evaluation. Most pericardial effusions are hemorrhagic and exudative when tapped.

An indwelling pig tail catheter is put in the pericardial space under echocardiographic guidance. The catheter is removed after about a week when the fluid analysis report is available, and the patient has been started on definite treatment according to the cause. If the pericardial fluid cannot be drained by percutaneous methods, a limited surgical pericardial window can also be created to drain the fluid.

Analysis of pericardial fluid: The analysis is aimed at establishing a diagnosis for bacterial, tubercular, malignant, or viral effusion. The fluid protein levels help to separate exudative and transudate fluids. Gram stain and cultures should be done for bacterial infections. For malignant effusions, a malignant cell cytology should be done on the fluid. It can also be tested for tumor markers such as carcinoembryonic antigen (CEA), alpha fetoprotein (AFP), and cancer antigen 125 (CA125) according to the presentation. For TB, acid-fast bacillus staining and culture, BACTEC cultures, ADA, and PCR can be done. A high CEA and low ADA helps diagnose a malignant effusion. Viral cultures can be done.

CONSTRICTIVE PERICARDITIS

INTRODUCTION

Constrictive pericarditis occurs due to chronic inflammation of the pericardium making the pericardium stiff, impairing the diastolic filling of the heart, and sometimes the systolic ventricular function. The pericardium is thickened in most of the patients.

CAUSES

The causes include TB, bacterial pericarditis, previous cardiac surgery, or radiation to the chest. The most common cause is idiopathic in Western literature while in developing countries it is TB. The presentation of constrictive pericarditis can vary from transient, effuso-constrictive to chronic constrictive pericarditis.

Transient constrictive pericarditis: In about 20% of patients, the constriction resolves with therapy and therefore, it is advisable to treat most patients who have just developed constriction, for a period of 2–3 months before considering surgical options.

Effuso-constrictive pericarditis: This is usually diagnosed when a patient has pericardial effusion, undergoes a pericardiocentesis, and then has features of constriction with elevated right atrial (RA) pressures. Pericardiocentesis provides some relief. In these patients if they need early surgery, it can be difficult because they need removal of the visceral pericardium which is difficult.

Chronic constrictive pericarditis: Typical constrictive pericarditis is chronic and there is no fluid in pericardial space. It develops if the symptoms persist for more than 3 months and there is restricted diastolic filling due to a thickened pericardium.

CLINICAL PRESENTATION

On examination, patients have systemic congestion with raised JVP, pedal edema, hepatomegaly, ascites, and often bilateral pleural effusions. This happens due to generalized pericardial constriction and a high preload is required to maintain cardiac output. The pulse is usually normal although 20–30% patients can have pulsus paradoxus which is a feature of cardiac tamponade. The JVP is typical and grossly raised. It shows prominent "a" and "v" waves with a M or W pattern. Kussmaul's sign is often present and is characterized by a rise in mean JVP with inspiration. The increased venous return with inspiration cannot be accommodated due to a fixed shell around the heart and so there is a rise.

On cardiac examination, heart sounds are soft and distant. There are no murmurs. A pericardial knock may be heard. It is little earlier than the third heart sound in diastole and is at the end of the rapid filling phase. There are no precordial murmurs. In fact, clinical examinations are typical with high JVP, gross systemic venous congestion with quiet precordium, no cardiomegaly, and no cardiac murmurs.

PATHOPHYSIOLOGY

The thickened pericardium forms a fixed shell around the heart and restricts its ability to accommodate blood. The preload rises and so they have raised RA and left atrial (LA) pressures. Features of systemic venous congestion predominate. They have dyspnea but orthopnea and paroxysmal nocturnal dyspnea (PND) do not occur in cardiac catheterization procedure (CCP). The RA, LA, and diastolic pressures in RV and LV are within 5 mm Hg. The septum gets pushed to the left side due to the fixed space. The heart is not able to receive more blood and so the cardiac output does not increase with exercise.

The ventricular filling is impeded by pericardial pressure in both CCP and cardiac tamponade. In CCP, the initial part of ventricular filling is rapid due to high filling pressure and comes to an abrupt halt (so the pericardial knock). While in cardiac tamponade the ventricular filling is impeded throughout the diastole. For this reason, while the Y descent in JVP is prominent in CCP it is indistinct in cardiac tamponade.

Initially, the ventricles fill rapidly and then filling comes to a halt. This is seen on ventricular pressure recording in catheterization laboratory as a "square root" sign in ventricular diastolic tracing.

INVESTIGATIONS

Electrocardiogram shows low voltages. Atrial fibrillation is present in 20–25% patients.

Chest X-ray can sometimes show pericardial calcification. Pleural effusions are commonly seen and are often bilateral. Pericardial calcification is better seen on fluoroscopy. Once present, it helps to distinguish CCP from RCM. The heart size is usually normal.

Echocardiography shows pericardial thickening, features of restrictive ventricular filling, and dilated IVC suggestive of elevated RA pressures. The ventricular systolic functions are normal and the atria are usually normal in size. Mild dilatation of LA may be present. Major findings are pericardial thickening and calcification [better seen in transesophageal echocardiography (TEE)], abrupt displacement of interventricular septum (IVS) in early diastole (septal bounce), and signs of systemic venous congestion. There is exaggerated respiratory variation in mitral and tricuspid inflow on Doppler evaluation.

Imaging with computed tomography and magnetic resonance imaging: A CT scan is useful if only the pericardial thickness needs to be measured but an magnetic resonance imaging (MRI) is more useful if the diagnosis has to be established for the cause of systemic congestion as it gives information about myocardial function as well as clues regarding possible inflammation or fibrosis in the myocardium. MRI is less useful to image the pericardium (**Fig. 3**).

Pericardial biopsy can be done as part of the diagnostic workup. It can be done by the surgeon if there is pericardial fluid, by a limited incision while creating a pericardial window.

DIFFERENTIAL DIAGNOSIS

The main differential diagnosis is from RCM. Sometimes cor pulmonale and tricuspid stenosis can also have similar presentation. Both CCP and RCM present with features of gross systemic venous congestion. Sometimes it is difficult to distinguish even after all the investigations and cases have happened when surgery is done with diagnosis of CCP and on opening one finds the normal pericardium and a diagnosis of RCM. The main differentiating features between these two conditions are summarized in **Table 1**.

TREATMENT

Patients with CCP need treatment based on etiology. Most cases are idiopathic and no definite cause can be ascertained. If it is not due to irradiation, malignancy, or renal failure than patients are put on ATT empirically. There three conditions can be ruled out on history and investigations. After 4–6 weeks of ATT, they are taken for pericardiectomy surgically by mid-sternotomy incision. Surgical treatment of constrictive pericarditis is total pericardiectomy. Usually, surgery is rewarding although it is a bit messy since the pericardium is attached to the myocardium. Surgery has a mortality of 10%. The report of histopathology sample after pericardiectomy is invariably nonspecific fibrosis. However, still the ATT is continued for its full course.

Before surgery since these patients present with gross systemic congestion and edema, one is tempted to use diuretics. These should be used in minimal doses only as they can cause hypotension and low cardiac output. There is no role of digitals.

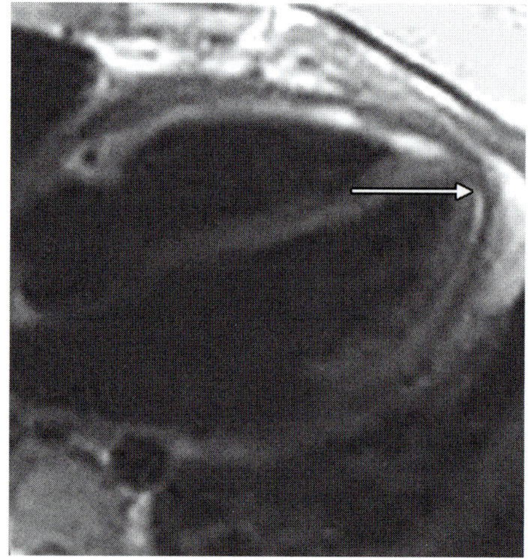

FIGURE 3: Magnetic resonance imaging (MRI) of the heart. The white arrow shows the thickened pericardium.

TABLE 1 Differences in clinical features and investigations between chronic constrictive pericarditis (CCP) and restrictive cardiomyopathy (RCM).

	CCP	RCM
Clinical		
• History of tuberculosis and pericardial effusion	++	–
• Chest pain of pericarditis	±	–
Examination		
• Apex beat	Ill defined	Localized
• Precordium	Silent	Pulsations present
• Pericardial knock	+	– (S4 present)
• Cardiac murmur	–	+
• JVP	• Prominent Y descent • Inspiratory increase	• Absent Y descent • Inspiratory fall

Continued...

Continued...

	CCP	RCM
Investigations		
• Chest X-ray—shaggy heart borders	±	–
• Echocardiography		
◦ Left atrial enlargement	–	++
◦ Pericardial effusion	+	±
◦ Mitral regurgitation or tricuspid regurgitation	–	+ (mild)
◦ Ventricular wall thickening	–	+
• CT scan		
◦ Pericardial thickening	+	–
◦ Pericardial calcification	±	–
• Cardiac catheterization		
◦ Difference in RA, LA, RVEDP, and LVEDP	≤5 mm Hg	≥5 mm Hg
◦ Pulmonary artery systolic pressure	≤50 mm Hg	≥50 mm Hg
◦ Square root sign in the trace	Present	Absent

(LA: left atrial; LVEDP: left ventricular end-diastolic pressure; RA: right atrial; RVEDP: right ventricular end-diastolic pressure)

RECOMMENDED READINGS

1. Maisch B, Seferović PM, Ristić AD, Erbel R, Rienmüller R, Adler Y, et al. Guidelines on the diagnosis and management of pericardial diseases executive summary; The Task force on the diagnosis and management of pericardial diseases of the European society of cardiology. Eur Heart J. 2004;25,587-610.
2. Vistarini N, Chen C, Mazine A, Bouchard D, Hebert Y, Carrier M, et al. Pericardiectomy for Constrictive Pericarditis: 20 Years of Experience at the Montreal Heart Institute. Ann Thorac Surg. 2015;100(1):107-13.
3. Lotan D, Wasserstrum Y, Fardman A, Kogan M, Adler Y. Usefulness of Novel Immunotherapeutic Strategies for Idiopathic Recurrent Pericarditis. Am J Cardiol. 2016;117(5):861-6.
4. LeWinter MM. Clinical practice. Acute pericarditis. N Engl J Med. 2014;371(25):2410-6.
5. Garcia MJ. Constrictive pericarditis versus restrictive cardiomyopathy? J Am Coll Cardiol. 2016;67(17):2061-76.
6. Adler Y, Charron P, Imazio M, Badano L, Barón-Esquivias G, Bogaert J, et al. ESC Scientific Document Group. 2015 ESC Guidelines for the diagnosis and management of pericardial diseases: The Task Force for the Diagnosis and Management of Pericardial Diseases of the European Society of Cardiology (ESC) Endorsed by: The European Association for Cardio-Thoracic Surgery (EACTS). Eur Heart J. 2015;36(42):2921-64.

CHAPTER 111

Diseases of the Aorta

Gurbhej Singh, George Joseph

ABSTRACT

The aorta is the largest artery in the human body and is the major conduit carrying blood from the left ventricle to the rest of the body. Its elastic properties play a vital role in the maintenance of optimal blood pressure by reducing systolic and raising diastolic pressures. Diseases of the aorta range from aneurysm formation, acute aortic syndromes (aortic dissection, intramural hematoma, penetrating ulcer), thrombosis, vasculitis, traumatic injury, congenital anomalies to involvement in systemic disorders. With improved imaging modalities, the diagnosis of aortic diseases has been simplified in the recent past. The evolution of aortic disease management strategies in the form of advanced surgical techniques and endovascular therapies has been remarkable. In this chapter, we briefly discuss the diseases of the aorta and the current status of management options available.

"Without knowledge action is useless and knowledge without action is futile"

—A Bakr

INTRODUCTION

Aortic diseases have long been recognized as potentially having serious outcomes and find mention in the ancient Indian literature work *Sushruta Samhita* where the aortic aneurysm was said to have a poor outcome on rupture. The aorta is the largest artery in the human body and performs the vital functions of delivering blood to the entire systemic circulation and maintaining optimal systemic blood pressure. *Congenital aortic diseases* include coarctation of the aorta and anomalies of aortic origin. Acquired diseases of the aorta may be broadly classified as acute and chronic. *Acute aortic diseases* include aortic dissection, aortic rupture, penetrating ulcer, intramural hematoma, and trauma-induced aortic injury. *Chronic aortic diseases* include aneurysms, atherosclerosis, vasculitis, thromboembolism, infections, and tumors. Management of aortic diseases requires a thorough knowledge of its anatomy, the natural history of its diseases, the various treatment options available, and the complications associated with them.

EMBRYOLOGY AND ANATOMY

The aorta develops starting from the 3rd week of gestation from vascular islands that coalesce to form a ventrally located aortic sac that continues from the truncus arteriosus emerging from the heart and is connected to a pair of dorsal aortae through six pairs of aortic arches that develop progressively and supply blood to the developing fetus. The formation of aorta and its branches is the result of the retention or disappearance of parts of these six pairs of aortic arches. Abnormalities in this process result in congenital anomalies of the aorta and its branches.

The aorta is the conduit that receives oxygenated blood pumped out by the left ventricle and delivers the same via the systemic circulation for perfusion of the organs of the human body. Histologically, it is formed by an innermost layer, the tunica intima (that is lined internally by the endothelium), a middle layer, the tunica media (comprising smooth muscle cells limited by the internal and external elastic laminae), and the outermost layer, the tunica adventitia (made predominantly of connective tissue). The aortic wall receives its own blood supply from the vasa vasorum which arise from the aorta.

Anatomically, the aorta begins from the aortic valve annulus as the sinuses of Valsalva and continues sequentially as the ascending aorta, arch of aorta, descending thoracic aorta and abdominal aorta, before bifurcating into the common iliac arteries. The aortic root comprises of sinuses of Valsalva from which arise the coronary arteries. The ascending aorta lies in the anterior mediastinum beginning from the sinotubular junction till the origin of the innominate (or brachiocephalic) artery. The aortic arch gives rise to the arm and neck vessels.

The descending aorta is the continuation of the aorta beyond the left subclavian artery origin, where it is located posteriorly along the left side of the spine and passes through the diaphragmatic aortic hiatus to continue as abdominal aorta. The abdominal aorta may be divided into suprarenal and infrarenal parts in relation to the origin of renal arteries. Normally, the aorta does not exceed 40 mm in diameter at any point in its entire length and it downsizes as the branches arise along its course. A detailed knowledge of the anatomy of the aorta and its branches is essential to plan the management of aortic diseases.

PHYSIOLOGY OF AORTA

In addition to being a conduit, the aorta performs important functions that maintain systemic circulation and organ perfusion. The aorta regulates blood pressure in the human body by acting as a compliant expansile chamber with elastic recoil. The aorta expands during ventricular ejection storing some of the ejected blood which, during diastole, is forced out into the peripheral circulation by the elastic recoil of the aorta (Windkessel effect), thus damping large pressure fluctuations and converting pulsatile aortic blood flow to a more constant peripheral perfusion. This "Windkessel" property, seen especially in the ascending aorta, may reduce with aging owing to stiffening and calcification, leading to increased systolic blood pressure and end-organ damage.

Most of the mechanical properties of the aorta are determined by the media, and to some extent, the adventitia. Elastic fibers are an important component of the extracellular matrix in the aortic wall and are macromolecules made of an elastin core surrounded by a covering of fibrillin-rich microfibrils. Fibrillin is a glycoprotein and has three isoforms, of which fibrillin-1 persists throughout the life of an individual. Elastic fibers contribute significantly to the "Windkessel" property of the aorta. Collagen fibers, on the other hand, are highly organized structures that have opposite mechanical properties to elastic fibers. Any defect in the structural components of the aortic wall could be pathological and leads to overt disease. Although not absolute, dissection is a defect of collagen fiber function and aneurysm formation a defect in elastin.

AORTIC ANEURYSMS

An aneurysm is a pathological dilatation of a blood vessel and is defined as dilatation of >50% of the normal arterial diameter. A true aneurysm is dilatation of the entire wall thickness. A false or pseudoaneurysm has a breach in the aortic wall which is contained by the surrounding structures. Aortic aneurysms are one of the most frequent aortic diseases encountered in clinical practice. Abdominal aortic aneurysms (AAAs) are more common than thoracic aortic aneurysms (TAAs). Among abdominal aneurysms, infrarenal aneurysms are encountered more often. It is interesting to note that patients with aortic aneurysms have an increased risk

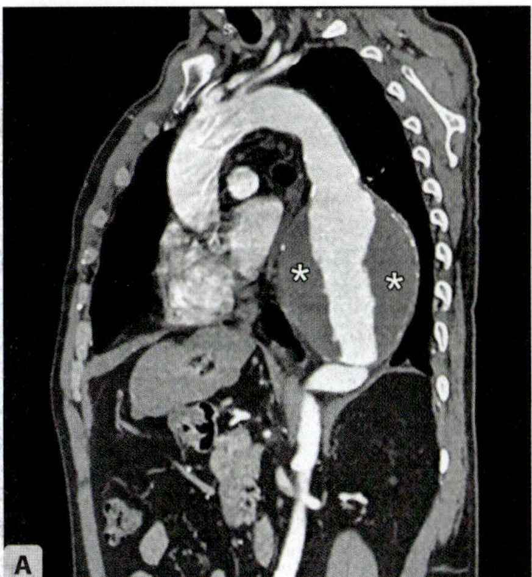

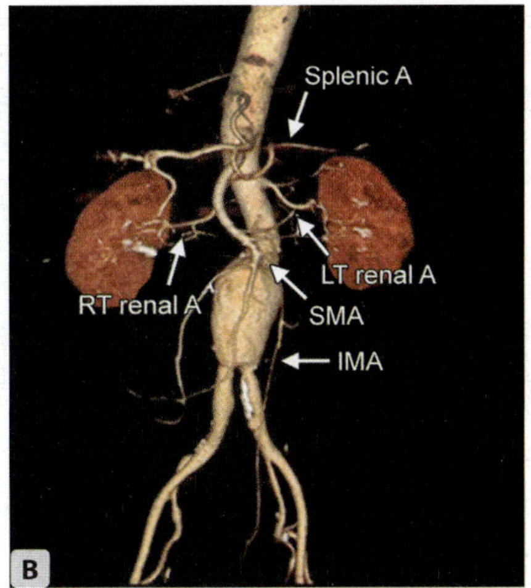

(A: artery; IMA: inferior mesenteric artery; LT: left; RT: right; SMA: superior mesenteric artery)

FIGURES 1 A & B: (A) CT aortic angiogram showing descending thoracic aorta aneurysm with thrombus (asterisk); **(B)** Three-dimensional reconstruction of infrarenal aortic aneurysm.

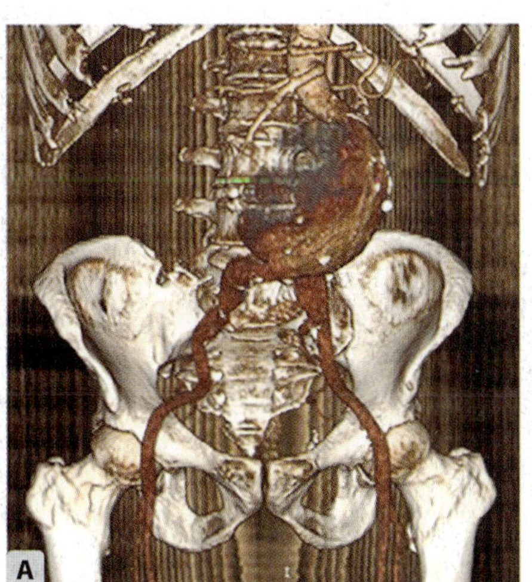

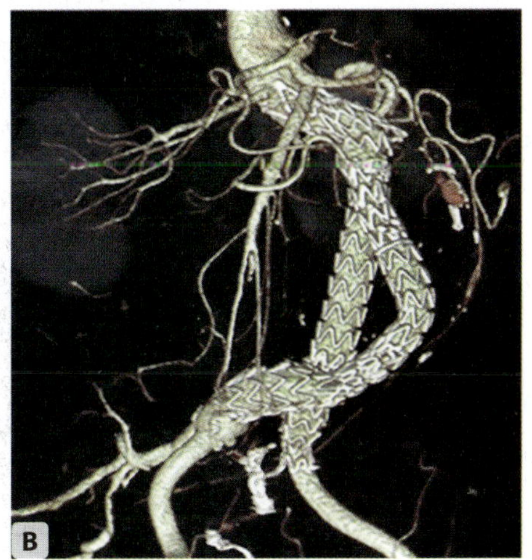

FIGURES 2 A & B: Three-dimensional reconstruction from CT angiography—abdominal aortic aneurysm. **(A)** Preprocedure; **(B)** Postendovascular graft placement.

of cardiovascular events owing to shared risk factors (**Figs. 1** and **2**).

THORACIC AORTIC ANEURYSM

Thoracic aortic aneurysms are more common in males. Ascending aortic aneurysms are more frequently seen than arch and descending aortic aneurysms. Most TAAs are detected during imaging and evaluation for other diseases or screening for congenital diseases like Marfan's syndrome.

The main causes for TAA include age-related degeneration, congenital syndromes, and infectious and noninfectious inflammatory disorders. The ascending aorta contains more elastin than the abdominal aorta hence is more distensible. This is thought to be responsible for increased susceptibility to age-related degeneration seen in ascending aorta. Degeneration of the extracellular matrix by matrix metalloproteinases and cathepsins leads to fragmentation of the elastic tissue in the media and adventitia. Apoptosis of smooth muscle cells and associated inflammation, production of reactive oxygen species, and endoplasmic reticulum stress lead to degeneration of the aortic media. This loss of structural integrity leads to progressive weakening of the aortic wall, and due to the pressure of blood resulting from left ventricular contraction, progressive expansion.

In congenital syndromes like *Marfan's syndrome*, the defect in the gene encoding the glycoprotein fibrillin is responsible. Also, increased levels of transforming growth factor-beta (TGF-β) are thought to play a major role in the pathogenesis of Marfan's syndrome. All patients with Marfan's syndrome should undergo screening for aortic size annually. *Ehlers-Danlos syndrome (EDS)* occurs due to a defect in type III collagen. Type IV EDS comprises vascular involvement in the form of aortic root dilatation or rupture, carotid artery rupture, or mitral valve prolapse. *Loeys-Dietz syndrome (LDS)* is an autosomal-dominant disorder due to alteration in TGF-β signaling leading to a severe elastogenesis defect and a marked excess of aortic wall collagen. The aneurysm expansion is at a rapid rate as compared to other pathologies and hence requires intervention at smaller diameters. Bacterial infections have been seen to cause mycotic aneurysms. Syphilis was a common cause of aneurysms before the extensive use of antibiotics. Noninfectious *inflammatory causes* of aneurysms include large-vessel vasculitides like giant cell arteritis, Takayasu's arteritis, connective tissue diseases like systemic lupus erythematosus (SLE), rheumatoid arthritis, and Wegener's granulomatosis.

Clinical presentation: Usually, TAAs are asymptomatic and diagnosed during imaging for other structures. Patients may have complaints due to compression of surrounding structures by the aneurysm like hoarseness of voice, dysphagia, chest pain, or neurological deficit. Patients may develop heart failure symptoms from aortic regurgitation when the aortic root dilates. Patients with an aortic aneurysm may develop aortic dissection or rupture and present with associated complications.

Investigations: The ascending aorta can be visualized during a transthoracic echocardiogram performed in the parasternal long-axis or suprasternal views. A transesophageal echocardiogram can also be useful except for the visualization of descending thoracic aorta. For planning interventions and to have a better visualization of the aorta in three dimensions, computed tomography (CT) angiography or magnetic resonance (MR) angiography is more useful as it allows measurement of dimensions in multiple planes with accuracy.

Management: Management of TAA is based on the aneurysm size and the growth rate. All ascending aorta aneurysms should be monitored regularly for size and complications. *Ascending aortic aneurysm of size > 5.5 cm is an indication for intervention.* However, this may be lower for specific cases: More than 4.5 cm for a patient undergoing an aortic valve replacement, >5 cm for Marfan's syndrome/familial TAA syndromes/bicuspid aortic valve aneurysm, 4.2–4.4 cm for LDS, >3.5 cm or 2.5 cm/m^2 for Turner's syndrome.

The growth rates of aneurysms have marked individual variability and usually they grow at 0.1–0.2 cm/year. Ascending aorta aneurysm growth is 0.07 cm/year as compared to descending aorta aneurysm rate of 0.19 cm/year. Besides, larger aneurysms grow at a faster pace than smaller ones. Risk factors associated with increased growth and rupture are advanced age, smoking, female sex, family history, and dissection. Aortic size index (ASI) takes into consideration the body surface area. ASI <2.75 cm/m^2 has complication rate of 4%, 2.75–4.25 cm/m^2 of 8%, and >4.25 cm/m^2 has event rates as high as 20–25%.

Surgical treatment for thoracic aneurysms involves resection of aneurysm and replacement with a prosthetic graft. For ascending aortic aneurysms, this may involve aortic valve replacement also (Bentall procedure). For arch aneurysms, arch or hemiarch replacement may be necessary. With the advance of endovascular techniques, surgical repair (arch debranching) can now be combined with thoracic endovascular aortic repair (TEVAR) as a hybrid procedure. Frozen elephant trunk procedure involves ascending and arch replacement with vascular graft attached to endovascular graft positioned in the descending thoracic aorta. These complex procedures are performed at highly specialized centers. For descending thoracic aorta and thoracoabdominal aneurysms, endovascular repair may be preferable.

Medical management of TAA includes blood pressure control with angiotensin receptor blockers, angiotensin-converting enzyme inhibitors, beta-blockers, and/or a calcium channel blocker. Risk factor modification includes smoking cessation. Lifestyle modification is necessary like avoidance of strenuous physical activity and weightlifting. Pregnancy may be considered high risk for patients with aneurysms. Family screening for TAA is recommended in affected individuals of familial congenital syndromes.

ABDOMINAL AORTIC ANEURYSM

The abdominal aorta begins at the level of the diaphragm and extends till the lumbar 4 vertebra where it bifurcates into the common iliac arteries. It is a retroperitoneal structure and gives branches that include celiac trunk, superior mesenteric, inferior mesenteric, suprarenal and renal arteries, gonadal arteries, lumbar arteries, and iliac arteries. Depending on the location, AAAs may be classified as suprarenal, pararenal, or infrarenal aneurysms. The risk factors for abdominal aneurysms include advanced age, family history, smoking, hypertension, chronic obstructive airway disease, coronary artery disease, and peripheral artery disease. In addition, many infectious and inflammatory disease may be causative.

Clinical presentation: It may be with abdominal or back pain or a pulsating mass in the abdomen. Frequently, AAAs are diagnosed during ultrasound evaluation for other diseases. New onset of severe pain which is persistent in a patient known to have an aneurysm is indicative of impending rupture. Patients with rupture present with pain, hypotension, and a pulsatile abdominal mass. Rarely, the aneurysm may rupture into adjacent structures such as the gastrointestinal tract causing blood in stools, urinary bladder causing hematuria, or even inferior vena cava leading to the formation of an aortocaval fistula.

Investigations: Imaging forms the main modality for the diagnosis of aneurysms in patients with suggestive clinical features. Abdominal ultrasound may define the length and diameter of the aneurysm. However, it is operator-dependent and needs proper preparation due to acoustic shadowing from intestinal gas. CT angiography or MR angiography defines the extent of involvement along with branch vessel involvement. These also define the nature of the wall of the aneurysm, presence of thrombus, or dissection. CT images need to be carefully looked at for signs of rupture like extravasation of contrast, retroperitoneal collection, or pseudoaneurysm formation.

The annual risk of AAA rupture is <1% per year in aneurysm size <5.5 cm, 9.4% for 5.5–5.9 cm, 10.2% for 6.0–6.9 cm, and 32.5% for aneurysms of >7 cm.

Management: *Intervention for an abdominal aneurysm is recommended for aneurysm size >5.5 cm* and surveillance is recommended for <4 cm. Patients with aneurysm size 4.0–5.4 cm should have therapeutic interventions performed if there are risk factors for rupture present. Endovascular repair of infrarenal AAAs has been shown to have outcomes comparable to that of open surgery in large randomized trials. The European Society for Vascular Surgery recommends open repair for patients with reasonable prospects of long-term survival. In contrast, those with shorter life expectancy are likely to benefit from EVAR rather than open repair, particularly if their surgical risk is higher than average.

AORTIC DISSECTION

It is a dangerous condition characterized by intimal disruption and separation of the aortic wall into a true lumen and a false lumen. Diagnosis of acute aortic dissection continues to be a clinical challenge despite advances in imaging methods.

CLASSIFICATION

Aortic dissection may be classified depending on the site of origin of the dissection in the aorta. There are two major classification criteria followed. *According to DeBakey classification*, aortic dissection is divided into types I, II, and III. Type I starts from ascending aorta and may extend up to iliac arteries. Type II has only ascending aortic involvement, whereas type III starts in the descending aorta and could extend beyond. Type III aortic dissection is subclassified into IIIa that is confined above the diaphragm or IIIb that extends below the diaphragm. *According to the Stanford classification*, type A aortic dissection originates in the ascending aorta and type B aortic dissection originates in the descending aorta. Both may extend distally, even up to the iliac arteries. Dissections involving the aortic arch but not the ascending aorta are classified as type B dissections with arch involvement (**Fig. 3**).

TYPE A AORTIC DISSECTION

Type A aortic dissection is a life-threatening condition involving the ascending aorta. The exact incidence is unknown as many patients with type A aortic dissection are unable to reach the hospital. The incidence reported varies from 3.5–6/100,000, with a male predominance.

Causes and associations: In the younger age group, genetic conditions like Marfan's syndrome (FBN1), Turner's syndrome (*XO* karyotype), LDS (*TGFBR1 and TGFBR2*), EDS (*COL3A1*), and other mutations affecting structural proteins are commonly seen. Patients with bicuspid aortic valve also have a higher risk of aortic dissection as compared to the general population. Patients with hypertension, chronic kidney disease, smoking, prior history of stroke are also at higher risk. Recently, the use of fluoroquinolones has been seen to predispose to aortic dissection.

Clinical presentation: Type A dissection usually presents with tearing or stabbing chest pain, hypertension, back pain, hypotension, or syncope. A neurological presentation may be seen with syncope, stroke, seizure, limb weakness, or encephalopathy. Some patients may have myocardial infarction due to coronary artery involvement. Malperfusion of vital organs may occur as the dissection flap compromises their blood supply. The presence of malperfusion needs early identification and repair at the time of surgical intervention. On examination, pulse deficit may be present, a narrow or wide pulse pressure may be secondary to pericardial effusion or aortic regurgitation, respectively.

Investigations: An *electrocardiogram* (ECG) may show ST-T changes due to coronary involvement or changes

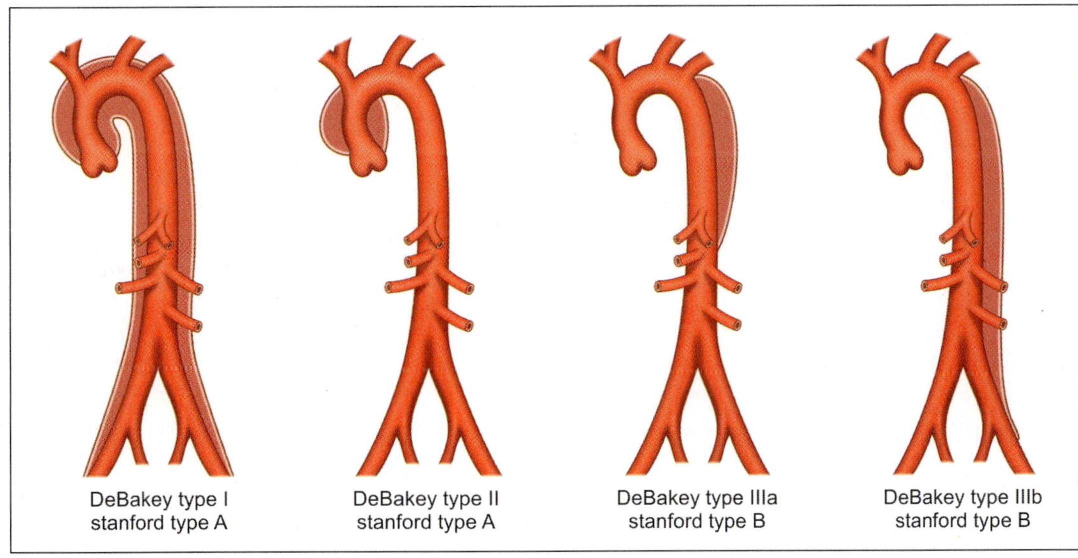

FIGURE 3: Classification of aortic dissection.

secondary to left ventricular hypertrophy in patients with systemic hypertension. ST-elevation indicates coronary artery involvement and is seen in 5–15% of patients.

Chest X-ray may show a dilated aortic border or calcification.

Two-dimensional echocardiography may help visualize the ascending aorta, arch, and descending aorta if clinical suspicion of dissection is present. Transesophageal echocardiography may better define the false lumen, aortic regurgitation, and extent of dissection in the thoracic aorta.

Computed tomography angiography defines the origin and extent of dissection, true and false lumen, and branch involvement, which may help risk stratification and planning of management strategy.

Magnetic resonance angiography may also define the extent of dissection, however, it takes a long time for image acquisition, making it unsuitable in sick patients. Also, this imaging modality may not be widely available.

Management: Treatment of type A aortic dissection is usually needed promptly as it has high mortality of 1–2% every hour in the initial time period after diagnosis. *Treatment of type A dissection is usually surgical.* Some patients may be considered inoperable due to comorbidities, stroke, advanced age, or poor neurological status. Medical management involves stabilization of the patient. For hypertension control, beta-blockers and calcium channel blockers are often used. Surgical repair aims to excise and replace the aorta at the entry point of dissection and to maintain patency of the true lumen and branch vessels. Besides, in case there is an aneurysm, to repair it. Replacement of the ascending aorta with prosthetic graft is sometimes combined with aortic valve replacement (Bentall procedure) if there is significant aortic regurgitation. In case the arch or descending aorta has significant dissection or aneurysm, simultaneous repair of the same is undertaken. This may involve a hybrid endovascular approach, especially in the descending aorta.

On follow-up, imaging should be done at 1 month, 6 months, 12 months, and annually if clinically stable. Medical management to control blood pressure aggressively should be undertaken.

TYPE B AORTIC DISSECTION

Type B aortic dissection (**Figs. 4 A** and **B**) does not involve the ascending aorta. There is intimal layer disruption leading to a tear in the media (entry tear) creating a false lumen that extends antegrade or retrograde and causes malperfusion of branch vessels. In the absence of distal communication with the true lumen (exit tear), the false lumen may expand and even rupture. Also, it exerts pressure on the true lumen causing it to narrow or even get obliterated. Type B aortic dissection is seen to have lower mortality as compared to type A aortic dissection. The risk of mortality is higher in patients with complications like branch vessel occlusion, hypotension, and visceral hypoperfusion like the renal, spinal cord, or mesenteric ischemia. Advanced age and comorbidities are also risk factors for poor survival.

Clinical presentation: It varies depending on the site of dissection, but most commonly patients present with chest or back pain which may be severe. Pulse deficit, if present, is associated with poor outcome. Neurological symptoms may include syncope, paraparesis, or paraplegia. Symptoms of visceral hypoperfusion like reduced urine output abdominal pain and ischemic pain in limbs may be seen.

Investigations: *Electrocardiogram and chest X-ray* may be abnormal but are not sensitive for diagnosis. Abdominal ultrasonography (USG) or echocardiography may show a dissection flap in the abdominal or lower descending aorta.

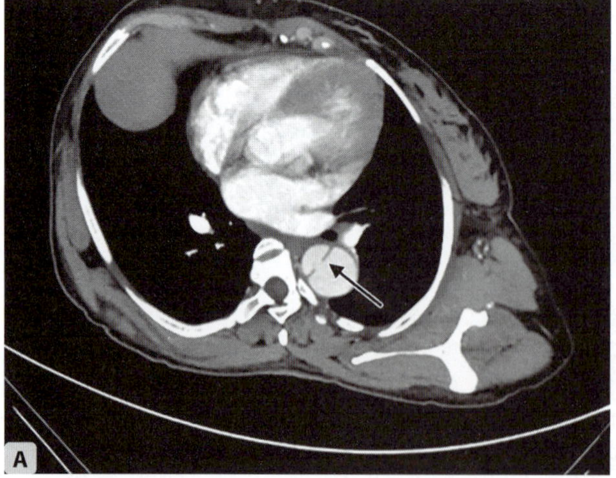

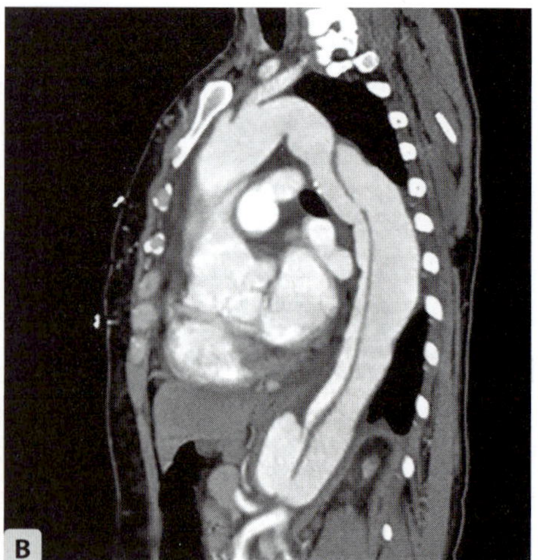

FIGURES 4 A & B: CT images of type B dissection showing the dissection flap dividing the aortic lumen to true and false lumen with small communication.

Computed tomography angiography and MR angiography are sensitive and specific and define the aortic dissection extent and branch vessel involvement accurately.

Management: Treatment of type B aortic dissection depends on the clinical presentation and presence of complications. Indications for surgery are persistent pain, visceral hypoperfusion, impending rupture as visualized by imaging, rapid expansion of the false lumen, or presence of genetic aortic diseases like Marfan's syndrome.

Medical stabilization involves drugs to control heart rate and blood pressure. A short-acting beta-blocker like esmolol may be used initially, followed by an alpha- and beta-antagonist like labetalol. Vasodilators should be introduced after heart rate control as they could otherwise increase heart rate. Other useful antihypertensive medications include angiotensin receptor blockers, angiotensin-converting enzyme inhibitors, and sodium nitroprusside.

Definitive intervention is indicated in patients with high-risk features. TEVAR has evolved greatly in the last decade giving the benefit of a less invasive modality with mortality benefit compared to surgical repair. This procedure involves the placement of an endovascular graft in the true lumen across the entry tear of the dissection, thus expanding the true lumen, compressing the false lumen and preventing entry of blood into the false lumen. Thorough imaging-based knowledge of the anatomy of dissection, especially branch vessel involvement and location of true and false lumina is necessary before attempting this type of intervention. The INSTEAD trial showed that in patients with uncomplicated type B aortic dissection, TEVAR was associated with lower all-cause mortality at 5 years compared to medical treatment alone. Mortality at 5 years for medically treated type B is nearly 40%, hence these patients need to be on close follow-up for false-lumen growth or development of complications and undergo interventional treatment if necessary.

OTHER ACUTE AORTIC SYNDROMES

Aortic dissection is the most common form of acute aortic syndrome. Besides it, the other acute aortic syndromes are intramural hematoma, penetrating aortic ulcer, and aortic pseudoaneurysm. These are discussed here.

INTRAMURAL HEMATOMA

Intramural hematoma arises secondary to rupture of vasa vasorum without intimal tear and communication with the lumen of the aorta. It is classified similar to aortic dissection as type A or type B depending on the location. It progresses to dissection in 15–45% of the patients. Clinically, patients present commonly with chest pain. Diagnosis is confirmed with CT or MR angiography. Management of intramural hematomas is usually conservative but may require surgery especially if type A and there are radiological features indicating risk for dissection or rupture.

PENETRATING AORTIC ULCER

Penetrating aortic ulcer is the term used when there is intimal layer disruption and erosion of atherosclerotic plaque leading into the media. It is more likely than type A dissection to cause aortic rupture. It is commonly seen in the descending aorta. Risk factors include systemic hypertension, age, male sex, and comorbidities for atherosclerosis. For ascending aortic penetrating atherosclerotic ulcers, surgery is considered at the earliest (**Figs. 5 A** and **B**).

AORTIC PSEUDOANEURYSM

Aortic pseudoaneurysm is dilatation of the aorta secondary to disruption of the wall and may be surrounded by the periaortic connective tissue. Any increase in the pressure in the pseudoaneurysm may lead to rupture which is most of the time life-threatening. Other complications may

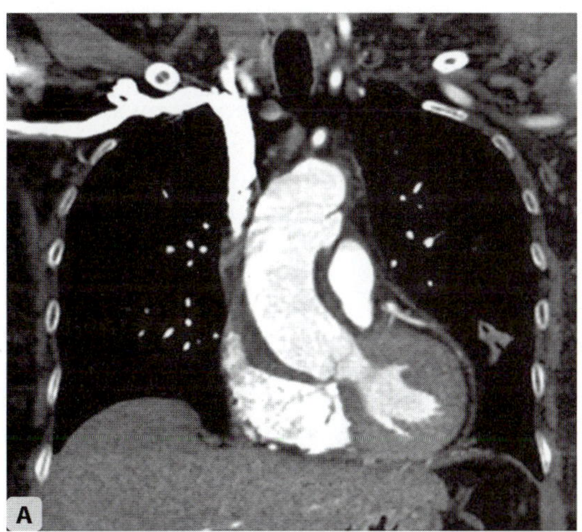

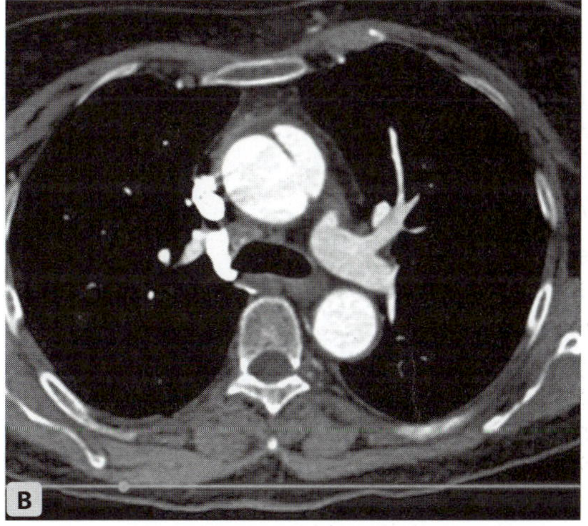

FIGURES 5 A & B: A CT aortogram showing a penetrating aortic ulcer in ascending aorta.

arise due to expansion and compression on surrounding structures, fistula formation, infection, or erosion into adjacent viscera. An aortic pseudoaneurysm needs urgent intervention with endovascular or surgical repair.

INFLAMMATORY DISEASES OF AORTA

Aorta may be involved in systemic inflammatory disorders which may include connective tissue disorders. It is worth describing few inflammatory diseases involving aorta which are commonly encountered in clinical practice.

TAKAYASU'S ARTERITIS

It is an inflammatory disease of large- and medium-sized arteries more commonly affecting females during young age (second to forth decade). Also called the pulseless disease.

Pathogenesis: The pathogenesis is not clearly understood, however, it is characterized by inflammatory cells leading to disruption of media and elastic lamina. What triggers this inflammatory response in still not known, but there is geographical variation noted for this disease.

Invovlement: Proximal thoracic aorta (reversed coarctation) involvement is predominantly seen in Japanese population, whereas abdominal aorta involvement with renal artery lesions (middle aortic syndrome) is seen in Southeast Asians. The involvement may be in the form of stenosis, occlusion, or aneurysm formation.

Based on the site of involvement, Takayasu's arteritis may be classified into type I—branches of aortic arch; type IIa—ascending aorta, arch, and their branches; type IIb—ascending aorta, arch, and branches with descending thoracic aorta; type III—thoracic descending aorta, abdominal aorta, and/or renal arteries; type IV—abdominal aorta and/or renal arteries; and type V—combined features of types IIb and IV.

Diagnosis: According to the *American College of Rheumatology, any three of the following six criteria* when present lead to a diagnosis of Takayasu's arteritis: (1) the onset of disease <40 years of age; (2) blood pressure difference >10 mm Hg in upper extremities; (3) presence of claudication; (4) reduced brachial artery pressure; (5) bruit in subclavian artery or aorta; and (6) documentation of narrowing or complete occlusion which is not due to atherosclerosis or fibromuscular dysplasia.

Clinical presentation: There are two clinical phases described for the disease, first phase consists of constitutional symptoms like fever, myalgias, arthralgias, and malaise. Vascular symptoms are seen in the chronic phase of the disease. Clinical suspicion arises when all peripheral pulses are examined and a difference in pulse or blood pressure is found. Hypertension may be seen secondary to renal artery stenosis or reduced elasticity of the aorta. Heart failure may be due to hypertension or aortic regurgitation. Radiological imaging helps to diagnose, localize the disease, and plan intervention.

Management: The medical management consists of drugs to suppress inflammation. Corticosteroids are the first-line drugs and almost 60% patients show clinical evidence of inflammation suppression after initiation. Steroid-sparing drugs like methotrexate and azathioprine are also used to control disease activity. Newer biological agents are being investigated in the management with partial success so far. Patients with stenotic or flow-limiting lesions may need intervention in the form of percutaneous or surgical techniques.

GIANT CELL ARTERITIS

It is one of the most common large-vessel vasculitides affecting the elderly females more often than males. Aortic involvement is reported from 10 to 25% cases. The American College of Rheumatology gives the criteria for diagnosis of giant cell arteritis if three of the following are fulfilled: Age of disease onset ≥50 years, new-onset headache, temporal artery with decreased pulsation or tenderness to palpation, elevated erythrocyte sedimentation rate (ESR) >50 mm/h, biopsy evidence of vasculitis, predominance of mononuclear cell infiltration and granulomatous inflammation, usually with multinucleated giant cells. The presentation may mimic that of Takayasu's arteritis. Management consists of corticosteroids to which majority of patients respond. Methotrexate has been studied as a steroid-sparing drug, however, with limited success. Newer drug interleukin-6 (IL-6) inhibitor tocilizumab has been evaluated in giant cell arteritis and suggested a role in management. Use of low-dose aspirin has shown to reduce the risk of stroke, visual loss, or transient ischemic attack.

Aorta may be involved in ankylosing spondylitis, Behçet's disease, rheumatoid arthritis, immunoglobulin G4 (IgG4)-related disease, and other rheumatic diseases like SLE. Aorta being the largest vessel of human body may be involved in many systemic diseases and need to be managed early as diseases involving aorta may be life-threatening.

COARCTATION OF AORTA

Coarctation of aorta is congenital narrowing of the aorta and may be diagnosed at any age. It is seen in 5–7% of all congenital heart diseases. Coarctation may refer to a localized discrete narrowing mostly juxtaductal in location or diffuse long-segment narrowing.

ASSOCIATIONS

It may be diagnosed alone or in association with other cardiac defects such as bicuspid aortic valve, hypoplastic left heart disease, ventricular septal defect, patent ductus arteriosus, or left ventricular outflow obstruction. It is sometimes associated with genetic syndromes like Turner's syndrome and Down's syndrome. There is a male preponderance seen in coarctation. Multiple congenital left-sided obstructive lesions, referred to as Shone's complex, may involve coarctation of the aorta. More than half of these patients have a bicuspid aortic valve and structural abnormality in the media layer.

EMBRYOLOGY

Abnormality in the development of the left 4th and 6th arch leads to the thoracic aortic coarctation. Two theories are proposed for the coarctation of the aorta: (1) the ductal theory and (2) the hemodynamic theory. The ductal theory proposes the migration of the ductal smooth muscle cells to the periductal aorta leading to the narrowing of the aorta. The hemodynamic theory says that coarctation develops secondary to alteration in blood flow through the developing fetal arch. During fetal life, coarctation does not cause a disturbance in blood flow as only 10% of ventricular output traverses the aortic isthmus; however, after birth, this flow suddenly increases thus leading to hemodynamic changes.

CLINICAL DIAGNOSIS

If the coarctation is severe, it manifests clinically as left ventricular dysfunction and heart failure in the newborn after the closure of the ductus. Collateral circulation develops to supply the descending aorta by childhood or adolescence. The epigastric arterial system forms the anterior part of collateral circulation and intercostal arteries form the posterior part. In 3–5% of the patients, there are associated aneurysms of the circle of Willis. During childhood, coarctation is usually diagnosed by a murmur or upper extremity hypertension. The arterial pulses below the level of coarctation are usually diminished in amplitude and may have delayed timing. The blood pressure difference in the upper and lower extremities may define the severity of coarctation.

INVESTIGATIONS

An ECG may be normal in an infant. During later childhood, ECG shows evidence of left ventricular hypertrophy and strain. Chest X-ray in an infant may show increased pulmonary markings with cardiomegaly. Rib notching from collaterals is evident during later years. The aortic arch may be prominent and descending aorta may be dilated just distal to the coarctation. Echocardiographic examination in an infant must includes views to see the aortic arch and descending aorta. Color flow Doppler defines the site of coarctation and the gradient across it is measured. Coarctation may be imaged with MR angiography or CT angiography.

MANAGEMENT

It depends on the severity of coarctation and age of presentation. During infancy with severe coarctation, medical therapy to keep the ductus open may be vital to improve distal perfusion. This should be followed by the definitive repair once the child is stable. During childhood, surgical repair of the coarctation may be done. Percutaneous balloon angioplasty for native coarctation is not preferred for the risk of recurrence of stenosis or formation of an aneurysm at the dilatation site. Long-term effectiveness of balloon angioplasty for the postoperative recurrence of coarctation is established from many studies. Coarctation stenting is a good definitive treatment option in older children and adults. However, in growing children, the sizing of the stent might be a challenge as the growth of native aorta may outgrow the stent diameter necessitating additional procedures later.

CONCLUSION

The aorta is the largest blood vessel of the human body and plays crucial functions in systemic blood supply, regulation of heart rate, and blood pressure. Diseases of the aorta are often life-threatening. Knowledge of normal and pathological aortic structure and function is crucial for management. Imaging has helped to better understand the anatomy and pathology of various aortic diseases.

RECOMMENDED READINGS

1. Bhishagratna KK. An English Translation of the Sushruta Samhita. Calcutta: Self Published; 1916.
2. Nienaber CA, Rousseau H, Eggebrecht H, Kische S, Fattori R, Rehders TC, et al. Randomized comparison of strategies for type B aortic dissection: the INvestigation of STEnt Grafts in Aortic Dissection (INSTEAD) trial. Circulation. 2009;120(25):2519-28.
3. Nienaber CA, Kische S, Rousseau H, Eggebrecht H, Rehders TC, Kundt G, et al. Endovascular repair of type B aortic dissection: long-term results of the randomized investigation of stent grafts in aortic dissection trial. Circ Cardiovasc Interv. 2013;6(4):407-16.
4. Hagan PG, Nienaber CA, Isselbacher EM, Bruckman D, Karavite DJ, Russman PL, et al. The International Registry of Acute Aortic Dissection (IRAD): new insights into an old disease. JAMA. 2000;283:897-903.
5. Isselbacher EM. Diseases of the aorta. In: Braunwald E, Zipes DP, Libby P, Bonow RO (Eds). Braunwald's Heart Disease: A Textbook of Cardiovascular Medicine, 7th edition. Philadelphia: WB Saunders; 2004.
6. Dieter RS, Dieter RA Jr, Dieter RA III. Diseases of the Aorta. Switzerland: Springer Nature Switzerland AG; 2019.
7. Mukhtyar C, Guillevin L, Cid MC, Dasgupta B, de Groot K, Gross W, et al. EULAR recommendations for the management of large vessel vasculitis. Ann Rheum Dis. 2009;68(3):318-23.

CHAPTER

112 Peripheral Vascular Disease

NN Khanna, Sushant Mishra, Swati Singh

ABSTRACT

Atherosclerosis can affect any part of the vascular tree. When it affects the coronary vessels, it causes ischemic heart disease. Involvement of the cerebral vessels results in stroke. In the splanchnic vessels, it can cause mesenteric vessel occlusion and gut ischemia. In the renal vessels, it causes renal artery stenosis (RAS) and consequently hypertension and renal insufficiency. These are discussed in the respective Gastrointestinal (GI) and Nephrology sections. Involvement of the pudendal artery can cause vascular impotence.

The arterial occlusion of peripheral limb vessels generally causes acute or chronic lower limb ischemia. The upper limbs have good collaterals and so vascular occlusions are less common in the upper limbs. Generally, the acute and chronic occlusions of the lower limb vessels have different presentation and management plan. Diabetics and smokers are especially prone to vascular disease of the lower limb. Acute occlusion causes impending gangrene and it needs emergent evaluation and management since time is a big factor. In chronic occlusions, patients present with intermittent claudication (IC) and nonhealing leg ulcers. These have been discussed in detail in this chapter.

The venous disorders can be in the form of deep vein thrombosis (DVT) of the legs and varicose veins. These need to be recognized and managed effectively. Peripheral lymphatic occlusion can cause lymphedema. It is not so common.

"He who has health has hope, he who has hope has everything"

—Arabian Proverb

INTRODUCTION

It was not very long ago, when a patient presenting with leg ulcer, not improving with a few weeks of medical/conservative management would be treated with amputation. Advances in endovascular therapies during the past decade have broadened the options for treating noncoronary vascular diseases percutaneously. The physician who cares for the patient with peripheral vascular disease (PVD) should have a broad understanding of atherosclerotic disease involving all vascular beds including arterial, venous, and lymphatic. This chapter attempts to summarize the most common and few rarer PVDs that we come across these days and offer appropriate guideline-directed medical therapy and intervention when needed.

The term "peripheral artery disease (PAD)" generally refers to a disorder in which blood supply to the extremities is obstructed. The term PVD is broader, less specific because it encompasses a group of diseases affecting blood vessels (including other atherosclerotic conditions such as renal artery disease and carotid artery disease) as well as vasculitis, vasospasm, venous thrombosis, venous insufficiency, and lymphatic disorders (**Table 1**).

Although the most common cause is atherosclerosis, it may also result from thrombosis, embolism, vasculitis, or entrapment. PVD strongly correlates with risk for major adverse cardiovascular (CV) events because it associates frequently with coronary atherosclerosis. Additionally, symptoms of PVD adversely affect quality of life for many patients. PVD is commonly underdiagnosed and undertreated.

When compared with open surgical revascularization for PAD, peripheral vascular intervention (PVI) offers slightly lower periprocedural risk, but it is limited by lower initial success with occlusive disease. Although significant progress has been made, further challenges remain such as restenosis after PVI. Endovascular therapy is performed

TABLE 1 Types and causes of vascular disease.

Arterial	Venous	Lymphatic
• Atherosclerosis • Vasculitis • Takayasu's arteritis • Thromboangiitis obliterans • Coarctation of aorta • Raynaud's disease	• Deep vein thrombosis • May–Thurner syndrome • Pulmonary embolism • venous reflux, varicose veins • AV malformation • Central vein occlusions • Occluded dialysis access	• Lymphedema

(AV: arteriovenous)

by a wide variety of operators, including interventional cardiologists, CV radiologists, neuroradiologists, and vascular surgeons trained in endovascular techniques. Improvements in the hardware including catheter, sheath, wire, balloon and stent design, and the introduction of embolic protection devices and other novel technologies have led to the safe and durable treatment of peripheral vascular disorders. Endovascular techniques available for the management of PVD ranges from plain old balloon angioplasty (POBA), drug-coated balloons (DCBs) to bare-metal stents (BMS), and drug-eluting stents (DES), as well as numerous atherectomy devices. Stent implantation increases the patency rate compared to POBA. Thus, it is often used, DES these days especially in long and/or calcified lesions.

The vascular disorders common in India are: diabetic foot and Berger's disease presenting as critical limb ischemia (CLI), Takayasu's arteritis (TA), inflammatory and atherosclerotic aneurysmal disease of aorta, and central vein obstruction secondary to long duration of indwelling catheters and venous reflux disease because of sedentary lifestyle. The PVD shares the same traditional risk factors for atherosclerotic disease; namely, smoking, diabetes mellitus, high blood pressure (BP), dyslipidemia, and older age.

HISTORICAL PERSPECTIVE

Gangrene was the first manifestation that was attributed to peripheral arterial disease. Quesnay, in 1771, was the first to ascribe distal gangrene to proximal arterial obstruction. In 1831, Bouley first described the syndrome of IC albeit horse. Brodie described similar disease in man in 1846.

The US interventional radiologist Charles Theodore Dotter in 1863, "accidentally" percutaneously recanalized an occluded right iliac artery retrogradely while performing an abdominal aortogram in a patient with RAS. On 16 January 1964, Dotter with his pupil, Melvin Judkins, 1st did "intentional" percutaneous transluminal angioplasty of an 82-year-old woman with a nonhealing ulcer and gangrenous toes.

Charles Dotter is known as the "Father of Interventional Radiology" and was nominated for the "Nobel Prize in medicine in 1978". Mathias in 1979 did the first carotid angioplasty and did first stent deployment in 1989. Grüntzig in 1978 performed the first angioplasty in patients with RAS. World's first aortic endovascular aneurysm repair (EVAR) was performed by Nicholas Volodos in Kharkov, Soviet Union, in 1987.

EPIDEMIOLOGY

The prevalence of PAD rises with age and affects a significant proportion of the elderly population (>20% in >80-year-old individuals).

India has more than 10 million people with PAD. A 40% patients of coronary artery disease (CAD) have associated PVD, 14% have carotid artery stenosis, and 17% have associated RAS in India. The incidence of death from atherosclerotic vascular diseases and stroke is estimated to rise from 19% in 2003 to 36% by 2030. In Indian PAD patients, the prevalence of CAD is 52%. Some important features about the significance and risk due to PAD are mentioned in **Box 1**. The Chennai Urban Rural Epidemiology Study (CURES III) reported 8.3% prevalence of PAD in South Indian patients of type 2 diabetes mellitus.

BOX 1	Evidence-based facts related to peripheral arterial disease.
• The risk of PAD increases substantially with age	
• >50% of PAD is asymptomatic	
• Twofold increase in incidence of heart failure	
• One-third of PAD has diabetes mellitus	
• Diabetic patients have two to four times the risk of developing PAD, CAD, and ischemic stroke	
• Smokers have 2.5 times the risk of developing PAD	
• Atherosclerosis accounts for more than 90% of cases of PAD	
• The prevalence of amputation in PAD patients is 3%	
• The femoral and popliteal arteries are affected in 80–90% of PAD patients	

Contrary to earlier belief, the incidence of venous thromboembolism (VTE) in India is comparable to that in Western countries. The prevalence of varicose veins and venous reflux disease in India is alarmingly high and is estimated to be about 47 million. According to another estimate, its prevalence is 15% in Indian population.

PERIPHERAL ARTERY DISEASE OF LOWER LIMBS

The lower limb arterial disease can present with chronic arterial occlusion and insufficiency. It causes significant morbidity due to nonhealing diabetic foot wounds. The disease is often diffuse and not amenable to interventions. Acute occlusion of a lower limb vessel can cause acutely threatened limb and risk of gangrene. It needs rapid evaluations and management. The two are discussed below.

LOWER EXTREMITY ARTERY DISEASE

Most patients of lower extremity artery disease (LEAD) are asymptomatic and are detected by ankle-brachial index (ABI) of <0.9. Even asymptomatic patients are at high risk of CV events and will benefit from most CV preventive strategies of strict control of risk factors. Additionally, a subset of these asymptomatic LEAD may be having severe disease, labeled as "masked LEAD" will be at higher risk of limb emergencies. In symptomatic patients, the most typical presentation is IC. The Edinburgh Claudication Questionnaire is a standardized method to screen and diagnose typical IC.

Chronic limb-threatening ischemia (CLTI) is defined by the presence of ischemic rest pain, with or without tissue loss (ulcers and gangrene) or infection. CLTI is a clinical diagnosis and is often associated with an ankle pressure of

<50 mm Hg or toe pressure of <30 mm Hg. It is also a marker for severe atherosclerosis with a threefold increased risk of myocardial infarction (MI), stroke, and vascular death as compared to patients with IC.

Diagnostic evaluation:

Ankle-brachial index: ABI is indicated as the first-line noninvasive test for screening and diagnosis of LEAD. In the case of incompressible ankle arteries or ABI of >1.40 alternative methods such as the toe-brachial index, Doppler wave form analysis or pulse volume recordings are indicated (ESC guidelines 2017).

The ABI is measured in supine position with cuff placed just above the ankle, avoiding wounded zones. After 5–10 minutes rest, the systolic blood pressure (SBP) is measured by a Doppler probe (5–10 MHz) on the posterior and anterior tibial (or dorsalis pedis) arteries of each foot and on the brachial artery of each arm. Automated BP cuffs are mostly not valid for ankle pressure and may display overestimated results in case of low ankle pressure. The ABI of each leg is calculated by dividing the highest ankle SBP by highest arm SBP. The method of cuff replacement for measurement of ABI is shown in **Figure 1**. The interpretation of ABI for diagnosis of LEAD is done separately for each leg. For calculating the CV risk, we take the lower of the toe ABI. The interpretation of ABI, as suggested by European Guidelines of 2017, is shown in **Figure 2**.

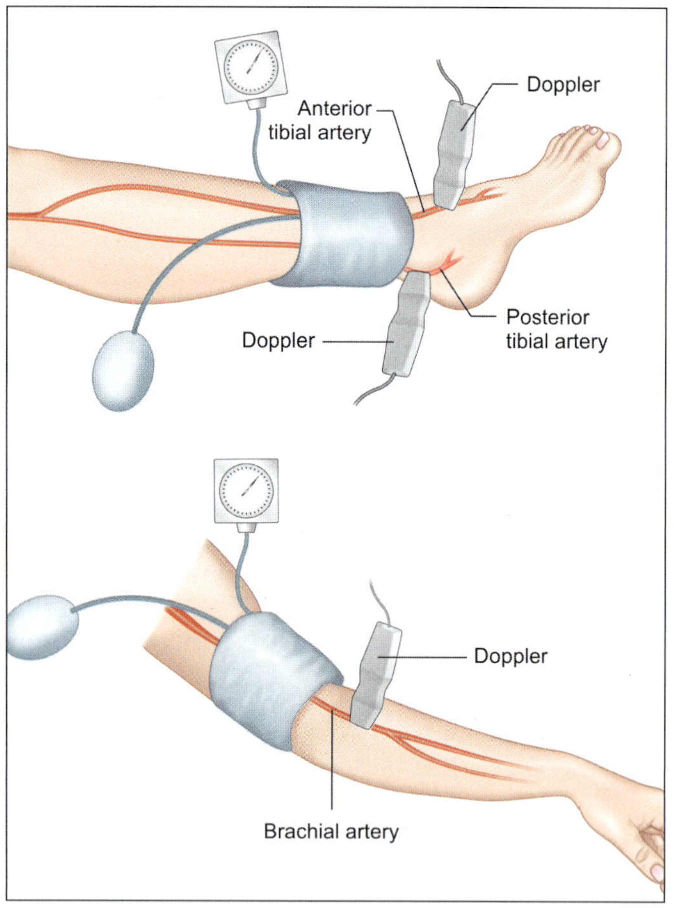

FIGURE 1: Method of cuff placement in upper and lower limb for measurement of ankle-brachial index (ABI).

When a postexercise ankle SBP decreases by >30 mm Hg or a postexercise ABI decreases by >20%, it is diagnostic for LEAD.

Ultrasound and intravascular ultrasound: It must be combined with ABI measurement. It presents 85–90% sensitivity and >95% specificity to detect stenosis >50%. The role of imaging in evaluation of PVD is emerging. It can be done with intravascular ultrasound (IVUS) or by optical coherence tomography (OCT). The flow can be evaluated by fractional flow reserve (FFR).

Angiography has been the traditional gold standard for evaluation of PVD. However, it has many limitations compared with the above-mentioned newer imaging modalities. Angiography depicts two dimensional representations of vascular structures with findings highly dependent on the projection. The relative merits of IVUS as compared to angiography are shown in **Table 2**.

The IVUS helps in guiding arterial interventions. IVUS can subclassify plaques into four major categories: (1) fibrous, (2) fibro-fatty, (3) necrotic-lipid, and (4) calcific. There is sufficient evidence to suggest that calcification as well as degree of stenosis can be more accurately assessed by IVUS than angiography alone. With the help of IVUS, proper lesion preparation can be done, e.g., atherectomy, predilatation etc. to improve outcome of calcific lesion. Proper expansion and need for postdilatation can be subsequently assessed well after the procedure. However, there is paucity of consensus guidelines justifying use of IVUS in peripheral intervention.

Optical coherence tomography: OCT provides high-quality cross-sectional images of arterial structure and pathology. Unlike IVUS, it is not limited by calcification. It has additional potential to characterize the nature of atherosclerotic plaque. Information on plaque composition may lead to more advanced and specific treatment options.

Fractional flow reserve: Analogous to coronary FFR, peripheral fractional flow reserve (pFFR) measures baseline and hyperemic pressure gradients. It is useful in the diagnosis of borderline stenosis and to decide the need of intervention.

Computed tomography angiography: The main advantages of computed tomography angiography (CTA) are

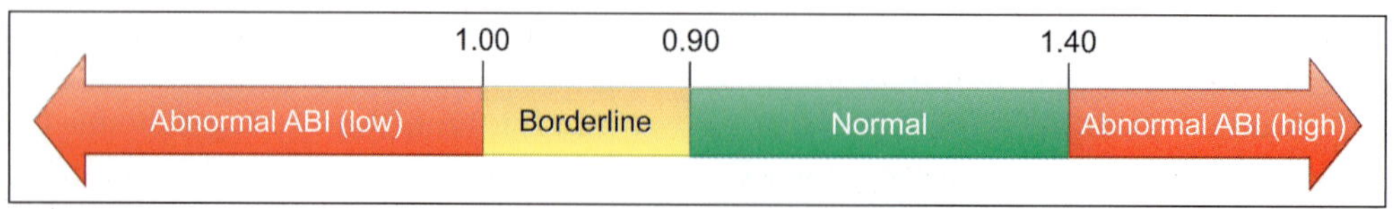

FIGURE 2: Interpretation of ankle-brachial index (ABI) as normal border line and abnormal as per the European Society of Cardiology (ESC) guidelines of 2017.

TABLE 2 **Comparison of intravascular ultrasound (IVUS) and angiography for evaluation of plaque characteristics.**

Characteristics	IVUS	Angiography
Stenosis	+++	++
Plaque morphology	+++	–
Adherent thrombus	+++	+
Dissection	+++	++
Flow	–	+++
Extrinsic compression	+++	++
Stent apposition	+++	++

+: Fair; ++: Good; +++: Excellent; –: Not applicable

visualization of calcifications, clips, stents, bypasses, and concomitant aneurysm.

Management: Exercise therapy improves symptoms and quality of life and increases maximal walking distance (WD). Some antihypertensive drugs (e.g., verapamil), statins, antiplatelet agents, and prostanoids have some favorable effects on WD and leg functioning. The drugs mostly studied are cilostazol and pentoxifylline.

Aortoiliac lesions:

- Occlusion up to the renal arteries and iliac arteries—aortobifemoral bypass surgery is indicated. Endovascular therapy may be an option, but has very high perioperative risk and long-term occlusion.
- In occlusion extending to the infrarenal aorta—covered endovascular reconstruction of an aortic bifurcation is done.
- In short stenosis/occlusions (<5 cm) of iliac arteries—endovascular therapy gives good long-term patency.
- In iliofemoral lesions—hybrid procedure, i.e., endarterectomy or bypass at the femoral level combined with endovascular therapy of iliac arteries is preferred.

Femoral-popliteal lesions:

- For stenosis/occlusions of <25 cm, endovascular therapy is the first choice if repair is needed.
- For occlusions/stenosis of >25 cm, endovascular recanalization is still possible but surgical bypass is preferable especially using the great saphenous vein (GSV).
- For IC, endovascular therapy is advocated only for severe, disabling system, and those who do not respond to exercise therapy for minimum three months.

Chronic limb-threatening ischemia: All patients with CLTI must have best medical therapy with correction of risk factor. Proper wound management and glycemic control is very important. The BASIL (Bypass versus Angioplasty in Severe Ischaemia of the Leg) trial was a randomized control trial comparing endovascular therapy with surgical bypass. It showed no significant difference in amputation free survival at 2 years between the two therapies. This is the reason that endovascular treatment is gaining popularity.

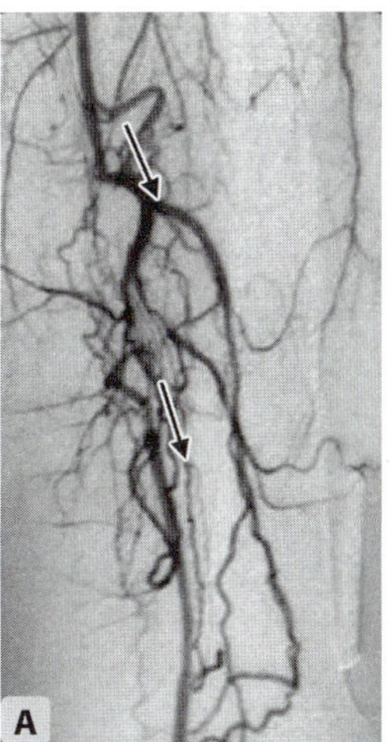

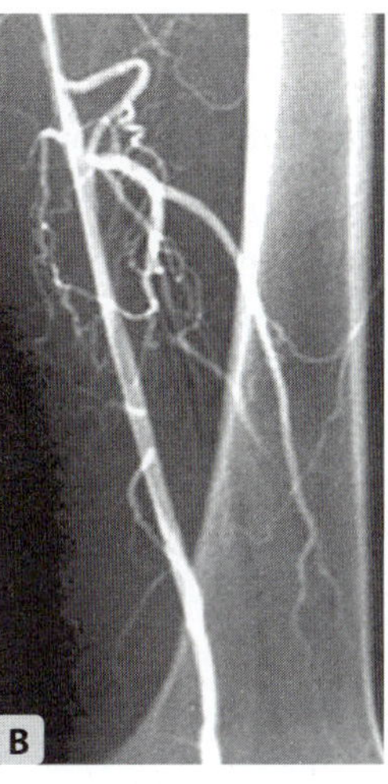

FIGURES 3 A & B: Angiogram of long segment mid femoral occlusion before and after intervention.

The aortoiliac disease often has downstream disease. Hybrid procedures (e.g., aortoiliac stenting and distal bypass) are therefore promising. The femoropopliteal disease is seldom isolated. A concomitant aortoiliac or below-the-knee disease is found commonly. In more than one-third of cases, inflow treatment is needed. If endovascular therapy is chosen first, landing zones for potential bypass grafts should be preserved (**Fig. 3**). When bypass surgery is decided, the bypass should be as short as possible, using the saphenous vein. The infrapopliteal disease is also often associated with superficial femoral artery (SFA) lesions (inflow disease). Full-leg digital subtraction angiography (DSA) down to the plantar arches is mandatory to explore all revascularization options. In stenotic lesions and short occlusions, endovascular therapy can be the first choice. In long occlusions of crural arteries, bypass with an autologous vein gives superior long-term patency and leg survival.

Acute limb ischemia: *Acute limb ischemia (ALI) is caused by* an abrupt cessation of perfusion usually caused by atherosclerotic artery disease progression, cardiac embolization, aortic dissection or embolization, entrapment syndrome, trauma, phlegmasia cerulea dolens, ergotism etc. Prompt diagnosis and management is needed to prevent limb loss.

Findings on physical examination can include absence of pulses distal to the occlusion, cold skin, pallor, delayed capillary venous refilling, diminished or absent sensory perception, and muscle weakness or paralysis often recalled as the six Ps: pain, paresthesia, pallor, pulselessness, poikilothermia, and paralysis. Once the clinical diagnosis is made, appropriate anticoagulant and analgesic should be started. The treatment depends on clinical presentation and neurologic involvement. Any neurologic deficit warrants immediate revascularization.

The diagnosis of ALI based on symptoms and signs and its common causes are shown in **Table 3**.

The clinical categories of ALI and its diagnosis based on physical findings and Doppler as per the Rutherford classification are shown in **Table 4**.

Management: The options available are percutaneous catheter-directed thrombolytic therapy, mechanical thrombus extraction or thromboaspiration and surgical thrombectomy, bypass and/or arterial repair. Owing to lesser morbidity, endovascular approach is preferred these days. The concept of the combination of intra-arterial thrombolysis and catheter-based clot removal has decreased the 6-month amputation rates off 10%. It is important to realize that systemic thrombolysis has no role in the treatment of patients with ALI. **Flowchart 1** shows the algorithm for management of ALI.

TABLE 3 Diagnosis of acute limb ischemia based on symptoms and physical signs.

Potential causes	Symptoms	Signs
1. Thrombosis of artery or bypass graft 2. Embolism from heart or proximal vessel 3. Dissection 4. Trauma	1. Pain 2. Paresthesia 3. Weakness or paralysis 4. Decreased strength 5. Limb blood pressure <50 mm Hg	1. Absent pulses 2. Pallor 3. Cool skin 4. Decreased sensation

OTHER PERIPHERAL VESSEL OCCLUSIONS

CAROTID ARTERY STENOSIS

Carotid artery stenosis refers to a >50% stenosis of the extracranial internal carotid artery (ICA), with stenosis severity estimated using the NASCET (North American Symptomatic Carotid Endarterectomy Trial) method. Carotid stenosis is defined as "symptomatic" if associated with symptoms in the preceding 6 months and "asymptomatic" if no prior symptoms can be identified or when symptoms occurred >6 months ago.

Evaluation: Doppler ultrasound (DUS) as first-line imaging and CTA and/or magnetic resonance angiography (MRA) for evaluating the extent and severity of extracranial carotid stenosis.

TABLE 4 Clinical categories of acute limb ischemia (Rutherford classification).

	Description	Findings		Doppler signals	
Category	**Prognosis**	**Sensory loss**	**Muscle weakness**	**Arterial**	**Venous**
Viable	Not immediately threatened	None	None	Audible	Audible
Threatened a. Marginally	Salvageable if treated promptly	Minimal (toes) or none More than toes, rest Pain	None	(Often) Inaudible	Audible
b. Immediately	Salvageable with immediate revascularization	Minimal (toes) or none More than toes, rest Pain	Mild and moderate	(Usually) inaudible	Audible
Irreversible	Major tissue loss or permanent nerve damage inevitable	Profound anesthetic	Profound paralysis (rigor)	Inaudible	Inaudible

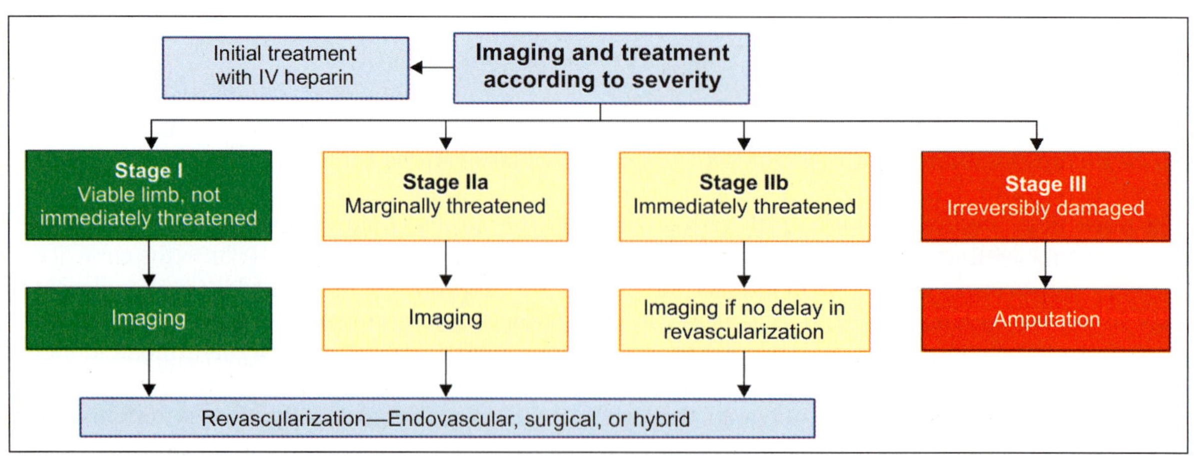

(IV: intravenous)

FLOWCHART 1: Algorithm for diagnosis and treatment of acute limb ischemia.

Management: Of all strokes, around 15% follow thromboembolism from a 50 to 99% ICA stenosis. Most symptomatic patients will gain maximum benefit when carotid interventions are performed within 14 days of symptom onset. With improvement in medical management, the treatment of asymptomatic carotid disease is controversial.

Antiplatelet therapy: Lifelong low-dose aspirin should be started treatment to reduce the risk of stroke. So far, the only strong recommendation for dual antiplatelet therapy (DAPT) is for patient undergoing carotid artery stenting (CAS). DAPT may be considered within 24 hours of a minor ischemic stroke or transient ischemic attack (TIA) and may be continued for 1 month in patients treated conservatively.

Intervention: It is recommended to perform revascularization of symptomatic 50–99% carotid stenosis as soon as possible, preferably within 14 days of symptom onset. Symptomatic patients with >70% occlusion benefit from carotid endarterectomy (CEA). Those with favorable anatomy and high risk for CEA can be subjected to CAS (**Fig. 4**).

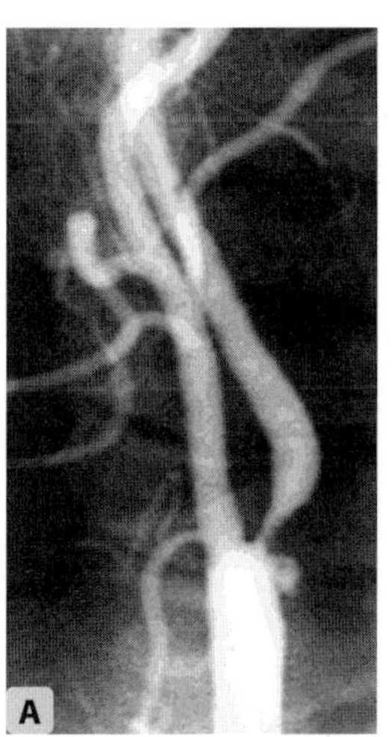

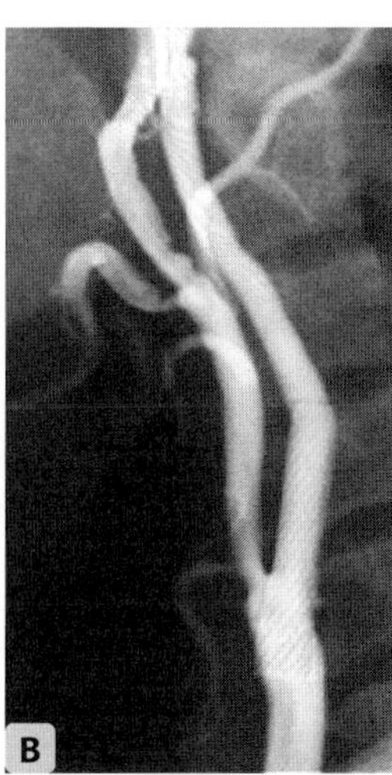

FIGURES 4 A & B: Carotid artery stenting for bifurcation lesion in left internal carotid artery before **(A)** and after **(B)** stenting.

TAKAYASU'S ARTERITIS

Takayasu's arteritis is systemic large vessel chronic inflammatory granulomatous vasculitis affecting the aorta and its main branches and pulmonary arteries. The disease is more common in Asians and Africans. Patients with TA, more commonly young females present with constitutional symptoms early in course of disease which later progress to segmental stenosis, occlusion or dilatation and aneurysm. Endovascular techniques are now the treatment of choice for stenotic lesions although they are used for aneurysmal lesions too (**Fig. 5**).

Indications of endovascular intervention in TA are as follows:

- End-organ ischemia or peripheral limb ischemia
- Cerebral ischemia
- Coronary ischemia
- Mesenteric ischemia
- Aortic aneurysm or severe aortic regurgitation (AR)
- Hypertension from stenotic coarctation of aorta or renovascular disease

MESENTERIC ARTERY OCCLUSION

Acute mesenteric ischemia is a medical emergency and it most commonly involves superior mesenteric artery (SMA). It is more commonly due to embolic phenomenon leading to proximal mesenteric artery occlusion rather than *in situ* thrombosis. High-resolution CTA is the most preferred modality of diagnosis. Most patients will need revascularization. There is a controversy whether bowel exploration or revascularization should be done first, but most data suggest that revascularization should be attempted first unless there is septic shock and severe peritonitis. In embolic occlusion, endovascular revascularization performs as good as open surgical revascularization while in cases of thrombotic occlusion, endovascular therapy is preferred over surgery. Intra-arterial catheter-directed thrombolysis (CDT) of SMA has also shown promising results and is not associated with severe bleeding complications in most patients without intestinal gangrene.

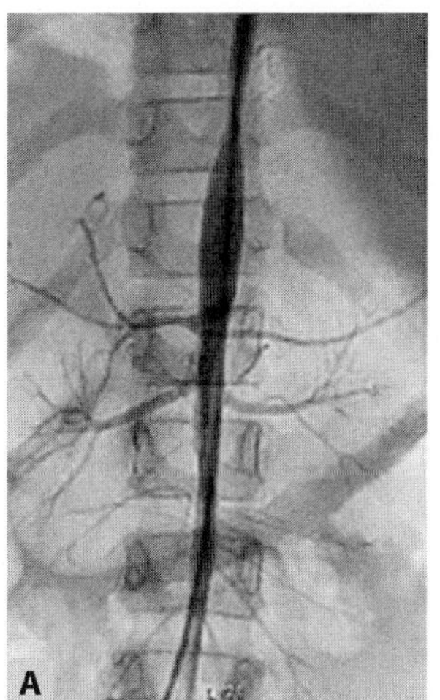

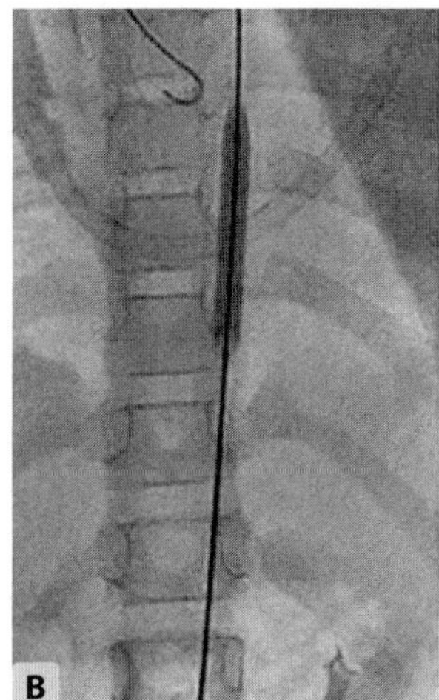

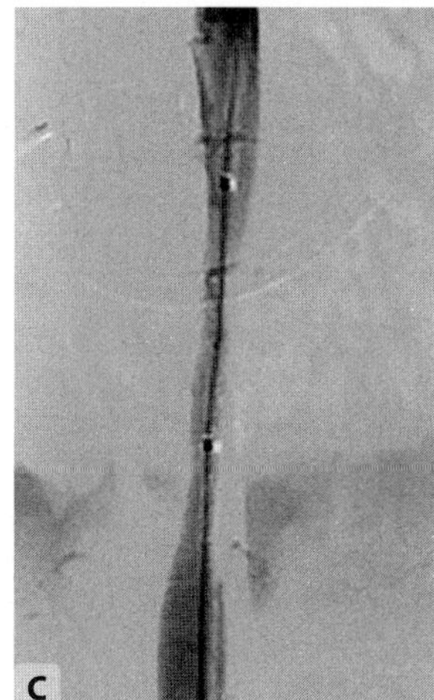

FIGURES 5 A to C: Percutaneous transluminal angioplasty in a case of Takayasu's arteritis. **(A)** Thoracoabdominal aorta before the procedure; **(B)** Ballooning with noncompliant balloon; **(C)** Digital subtraction angiography postprocedure.

Chronic mesenteric ischemia is a part of generalized atherosclerotic disease involving other vascular beds also and its prevalence increases with age. Generally, two or more mesenteric arteries are involved. Duplex ultrasonography (USG) is first-line investigation tool. However, CTA is usually needed for proper anatomical mapping. MRA or DSA can also be done. Intervention is not indicated in asymptomatic patients and at the same time revascularization should not be delayed in symptomatic patients. Surgical revascularization with reimplantation of mesenteric arteries is associated with high mortality and morbidity (10–15%), but has higher patency and lower reintervention rates. On the other hand, endovascular revascularization has shown lower morbidity and mortality and high success rates. There are no randomized controlled trials (RCTs) with head-to-head comparison of both modalities.

VENOUS DISEASES AND INTERVENTIONS

Venous disease consists of a host of diseases including deep venous thrombosis and pulmonary thromboembolism, chronic venous insufficiency, and central venous occlusions. VTE, varicose veins had traditionally been managed by conservative measures until recently when there is a notable progress in endovascular interventions and these treatments become more available, feasible, and safer.

VENOUS THROMBOEMBOLISM

Venous thromboembolism comprising of DVT and pulmonary embolism (PE). It is the third most common CV disease. Traditional management had been conservative by anticoagulation and thrombolysis. Nowadays, inferior vena cava (IVC) filters can be implanted in a subgroup of patients in whom anticoagulation is contraindicated or failed. Also, preoperative prophylactic IVC filter placement in patients at high risk of PE has also been talked widely but is still controversial (**Fig. 6**).

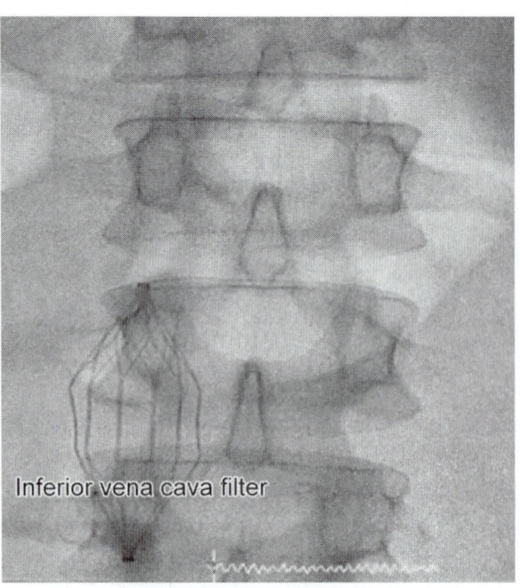

FIGURE 6: An inferior vena cava (IVC) filter.

Apart from that, it has been seen that in long term, 40% patients with DVT develop post-thrombotic syndrome (PTS) despite anticoagulation which adversely affect quality of life. It implies persistent leg swelling due to chronic blockage of leg veins. This causes long-term discomfort. Usually, elastic compression stockings are used for prevention of PTS, but studies have shown it to be equal to sham, however, it can help in some symptomatic relief. It has been seen in studies that decreasing the amount of residual thrombus decrease the chances of PTS (Open Vein Theory). Catheter-based techniques have direct access to thrombus and decrease thrombus burden to a greater extent. These include CDT, pharmacomechanical catheter-directed thrombolysis (PCDT), and percutaneous mechanical thrombectomy (PMT). Once a PTS has already established, the approach would be different. In iliofemoral chronic venous occlusions due to DVT or any other cause as May–Thurner syndrome needs wiring and stenting of affected segment up to or extending into IVC. Angioplasty of isolated chronic femoropopliteal lesions is more controversial due to unpredictable long-term patency rates.

VARICOSE VEINS

Varicose veins due to incompetence of superficial, deep, and perforator vein of lower limbs have long been mistaken as only a cosmetic problem.

Pain, swelling, paresthesia, and venous stasis ulcers have high-treatment cost and adversely affect work efficiency and quality of life. Asymptomatic patients may be treated for cosmetic reasons by sclerotherapy and surface laser therapy; however, this does not decrease future development of venous reflux disease. For symptomatic patients, initial treatment is nonoperative only and includes skin care, leg elevation, avoiding prolonged standing, exercise, and compression therapy. Patients who do not respond to conservative therapy and develop venous ulcers and significant symptoms are candidates for ablative procedure as sclerotherapy and endovascular heat ablative procedures [endovascular laser ablation (EVLA), endovascular radiofrequency ablation (EVRA), and endovascular steam ablation (EVSA)]. Phlebectomy and surgical vein stripping can also be done.

Endovenous laser ablation: Endovenous laser ablation (EVLA) works on principle of selective photothermolysis and used to ablate incompetent varicose veins by inducing permanent venous wall damage. In it a laser catheter with laser fibers is placed at desired location in vein and then pulled back slowly while delivering thermal energy evenly to blood and vessel wall causing localized blood clotting and irreversible venous tissue damage. This is cheap and office-based procedure with minimal complications and good results. EVLA is contraindicated in acute DVT and pregnant females. **Figure 7** shows varicose veins before and after EVLA. Personal experience of 6,018 cases of EVLA is shown in **Table 5**.

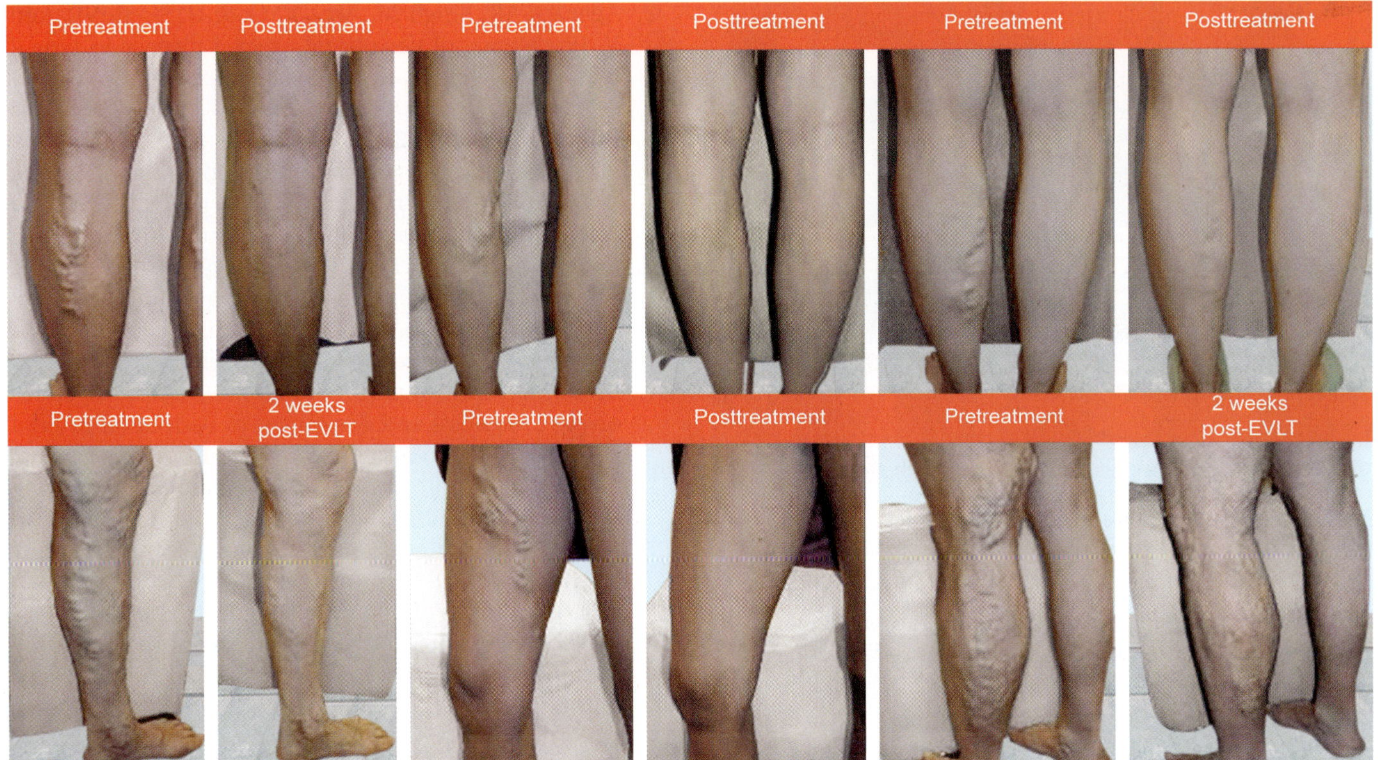

(EVLA: endovenous laser ablation; EVLT: endovenous laser treatment)

FIGURE 7: Clinical images showing effect of EVLA.

TABLE 5 Personal experience of 6,018 cases of endovenous laser ablation therapy (EVLA).

Number	6,018
Great saphenous vein (GSV)	3,948
Short saphenous vein (SSV)	1,520
Both (GSV + SSV)	1,428
Perforators	783
Wavelength of LASER	810 μm
Average laser time	3–5 min
Average procedural time	62 min
Procedural success	6,018 (100%)
Immediate mobilization	6,018 (100%)
Complications	
• Deep vein thrombosis (DVT)	17
• Pain	1,268
• Swelling	78

CENTRAL VENOUS OCCLUSIONS

There is a growing body of literature and experience in venous interventions. These interventions are safer and have lesser morbidity compared to surgery and are preferred over it. Central venous occlusions are seen frequently in patients with indwelling central venous catheters as for chemotherapy and maintenance hemodialysis and dialysis patients with autogenous fistula or prosthetic graft arteriovenous access. It can also be seen in patients with transvenous pacemaker leads. Routine bedside examination can give an idea of access integrity. In cases of access obstruction, continuous medium pitch bruit is replaced by short high-pitched bruit. Patient may present with superior vena cava (SVC) syndrome. Dialysis is also not possible due to access obstruction.

Imaging is needed to assess exactly the site and extent of obstruction. DSA is gold standard for diagnosis. Proper preprocedural imaging by duplex USG, MR venography, CT venography, or conventional angiography is needed for finer anatomic details as site, length, thrombus load, presence of collaterals to plan access, and hardware. Access can be taken from SCV, brachial, and femoral vein. A venovenous loop is created to provide adequate support for passage of balloons and stents. Balloon angioplasty is rarely sufficient due to risk of recoil and stenting is often needed. Focal lesions can be tackled with balloon expandable stents with high radial force and precision in placement while larger lesions need self-expanding stents taking the advantage of their flexibility. Thrombosis usually accompanies stenosis and CDT or thrombus aspiration may be needed alongside angioplasty. Stents are needed to be oversized by ~10–20% compared to normal reference vein and extended above and below the lesion to avoid stent migration. DAPT is given for 1 month followed by aspirin 150 mg. Success rate is ~80% and clinical relief of symptoms is immediate within hew hours to days. Patients can resume dialysis immediately (**Fig. 8**).

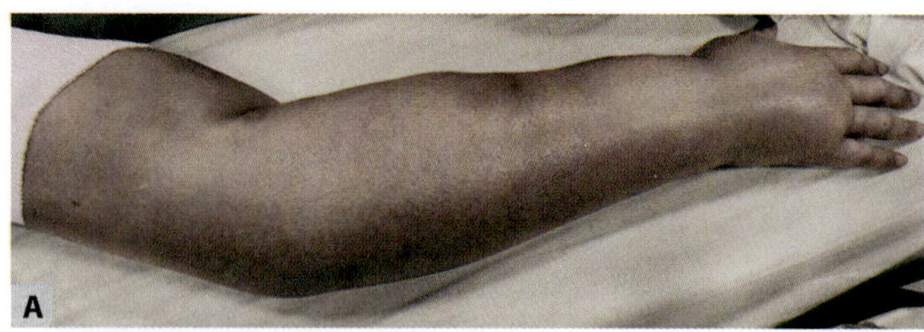

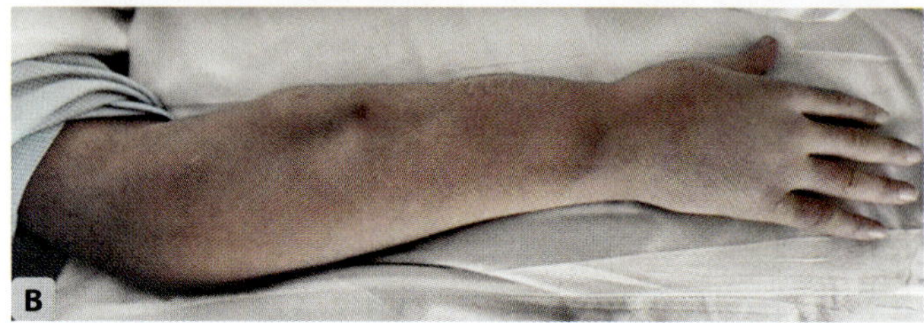

FIGURES 8 A & B: Clinical images showing effect of percutaneous intervention in a patient with superior vena cava (SVC) syndrome.

Lymphatic system interventions: Traumatic lymphorrhagia, especially postoperative, is a rare but potentially life-threatening situation. Leak occurs usually from aortoiliac lymphatics and less commonly from hepatic lymphatics. Percutaneous thoracic duct embolization is a good alternative to surgical ligation in these cases.

RECOMMENDED READINGS

1. Shu J, Santulli G. Update on peripheral artery disease: Epidemiology and evidence-based facts. Atherosclerosis. 2018;275:379-81.
2. Agarwal AK, Singh M, Arya V, Garg U, Singh VP, Jain V. Prevalence of peripheral arterial disease in type 2 diabetes mellitus and its correlation with coronary artery disease and its risk factors. J Assoc Physicians India. 2012;60:28-32.
3. Pradeepa R, Chella S, Surendar J, Indulekha K, Anjana RM, Mohan V. Prevalence of peripheral vascular disease and its association with carotid intima-media thickness and arterial stiffness in type 2 diabetes: the Chennai urban rural epidemiology study (CURES 111). Diab Vasc Dis Res. 2014;11(3):190-200.
4. Aboyans V, Ricco JB, Bartelink MEL, Björck M, Brodmann M, Cohnert T, et al. 2017 ESC Guidelines on the Diagnosis and Treatment of Peripheral Arterial Diseases, in collaboration with the European Society for Vascular Surgery (ESVS): Document covering atherosclerotic disease of extracranial carotid and vertebral, mesenteric, renal, upper and lower extremity arteries Endorsed by: the European Stroke Organization (ESO)The Task Force for the Diagnosis and Treatment of Peripheral Arterial Diseases of the European Society of Cardiology (ESC) and of the European Society for Vascular Surgery (ESVS). Eur Heart J. 2018;39(9): 763-816.
5. Gloviczki P, Comerota AJ, Dalsing MC, Eklof BG, Gillespie DL, Gloviczki ML, et al. The care of patients with varicose veins and associated chronic venous diseases: clinical practice guidelines of the Society for Vascular Surgery and the American Venous Forum. J Vasc Surg. 2011;53(5 Suppl):2S-48S.

MULTIPLE CHOICE QUESTIONS

To access the multiple choice questions of this Section online, kindly scan the QR code.

CHAPTER 113

Disorders of the Hypothalamus and Pituitary Gland

Liza Das, Kirti Gupta, Pinaki Dutta

ABSTRACT

The pituitary-hypothalamus unit functions as the central regulator of multiple endocrine glands and determines several physiological functions. Disorders of the hypothalamus-pituitary unit can be secondary to congenital or developmental causes, genetic syndromes, or acquired causes. Functionally, any of these can lead to under- or overfunctioning of a single cell type or multiple cell subtypes of the pituitary. Underfunctioning of the pituitary is termed hypopituitarism, which may be a result of transcription factor defects, trauma including birth trauma, tumors and nontumoral causes (infective, inflammatory, traumatic, and degenerative).

Pituitary overfunctioning is usually due to tumoral causes (monoclonal or polyclonal proliferation of cells) or pituitary hyperplasia (in case of certain syndromic causes of acrogigantism). Rarely, the hormonal production is from an ectopic source causing acromegaly or Cushing's syndrome due to ectopic secretion of growth hormone-releasing hormone (GHRH) or corticotropin-releasing hormone (CRH), respectively. Over 90–95% pituitary adenomas are sporadic while the rest 5–10% have an underlying genetic background. Identification of a genetic cause warrants surveillance for other organ involvement, which may appear over time or perform cascade screening to identify relatives at a presymptomatic or early symptomatic stage.

"Be like Pituitary gland, be master of all (glands), size does not matter but most importantly, do follow your supreme master (Hypothalamus)"

—Anonymous

INTRODUCTION

The pituitary gland is a midline structure located within the sella turcica recess of the sphenoid bone at the base of the brain. It is regarded as the master endocrine gland, which controls a multitude of physiological processes, such as growth, puberty, metabolism, energy regulation, fluid balance, and fertility. It integrates signals from the central nervous system which are relayed to it from the hypothalamus and secretes various hormones from different cell populations. These hormones then act on target organs and regulate physiological processes. In some instances, the hormone is also trophic for the target gland.

The unifying feature of all hormone axes (hypothalamus-pituitary-target organ) is a negative feedback system in all cases, except estrogen which works in a feed-forward cycle for luteinizing hormone (LH) in the preovulatory phase of the menstrual cycle. This principle of feedback not only governs physiology but has clinical relevance in terms of diagnostic tests in various pituitary tumor associated endocrinopathies. Therefore, stimulation tests with appropriate pharmacological agents are used to diagnose hormone deficiencies while suppression tests are used to identify autonomous hormone excess states.

ANATOMY AND ONTOGENY

The pituitary is composed of adenohypophysis which develops from the oral ectoderm (or Rathke's pouch) and grows cranially to meet the neurohypophysis which develops from the neural ectoderm and grows caudally. The intermediate lobe develops from the Rathke's pouch and the infundibulum (stalk), which connects the hypothalamus to the pituitary as well as the posterior pituitary develops from the diencephalon. The anterior lobe comprises about two-thirds of the pituitary and the rest is constituted by the posterior lobe.

A sequence of tightly regulated cellular and molecular events subsequently begins to guide the formation of differentiated cell types within the anterior pituitary. They secrete specific hormones; prolactin (PRL) from lactotrophs, growth hormone (GH) from somatotrophs, LH and follicle-stimulating hormone from gonadotrophs, adrenocorticotropic hormone (ACTH) from corticotrophs, and thyroid-stimulating hormone (TSH) from thyro-trophs. Other cells in the anterior pituitary include the folliculostellate cells, which are regarded as the stem cells, enabling pituitary plasticity in case of physiological conditions like enlargement of the pituitary during pregnancy and lactation. The intermediate lobe contains melanotrophs, which secrete pro-opiomelanocortin (POMC). The stalk consists of a neurovascular bundle (axons from the hypothalamus and hypophyseal portal system) and transmits releasing hormones to act on the pituitary. This stalk traverses the dura mater to join the pituitary, which is an extradural structure. The neurons (magnocellular) from the hypothalamus include the supraoptic and paraventricular nuclei that secrete vasopressin and oxytocin, respectively. These neurons project to the posterior lobe, which acts as a reservoir for these hormones. The posterior pituitary also contains pituicytes, specialized glial cells, which account for a variety of posterior pituitary tumors. The median eminence, at the base of the hypothalamus, contains a capillary bed into which the parvocellular neurons secrete hypophysiotropic (releasing hormones), which pass through the portal system to reach and stimulate the anterior and intermediate lobes. Thus, the pituitary gland synchronizes multiple physiological processes including growth, reproduction, and homeostasis through central hypothalamic and peripheral hormonal signals.

PHYSIOLOGY

The major physiological functions of the anterior, intermediate, and posterior lobes and distribution of the different cell populations are summarized in **Tables 1** & **2** and **Figure 1**.

TABLE 1 Hormones of the pituitary gland with their role in normal physiology.

Hormone	Target organ/cell	Effects on target organ	Downstream endocrine effects
Anterior lobe			
GH	Liver, skeleton, and soft tissues	• IGF-1 generation (from the liver) • Nutrient metabolism	• Linear growth directly and via IGF-1 • Protein synthesis • Lipolysis • Anti-insulin, causing glucose intolerance • Water, sodium, and phosphate retention
ACTH	Adrenal cortex	• Cortisol production • Adrenocortical development	• Resistance to physiologic stress • Fuel metabolism • Maintenance of vascular tone • Immunity
LH/FSH	Testis/ovaries	• Secretion of testosterone and estrogen/ progesterone • LH—ovulation, maintenance of corpus luteum in females, and testosterone production in males • FSH—follicular development in females and spermatogenesis in males	• Onset and progression of sexual development in puberty • Adult sex steroid production • Fertility
TSH	Thyroid gland	• Induction of T4 secretion • Trophic for thyroid follicles	• Homeostasis including BMR • Cellular metabolism • Growth
PRL	Breast	• Galactopoiesis • Lactation	
Intermediate lobe (rudimentary in humans)			
POMC	• CLIP • γ-LPH • β- endorphin • α-MSH • β-MSH	Only some amount of β-endorphin is secreted	
Posterior lobe			
ADH/AVP	Renal collecting ducts	• V1a (vascular smooth muscle) • V1b (anterior pituitary) • V2 (renal collecting ducts)	• Principal action is on water homeostasis and maintenance of osmolality • Pressor action • ACTH secretion
Oxytocin	Suckling breast	Lactation	Myoepithelial cell contraction in the breast for milk "let-down", bonding, and love

(ACTH: adrenocorticotropic hormone; ADH: antidiuretic hormone; AVP: arginine vasopressin; BMR: basal metabolic rate; CLIP: corticotropin-like intermediate lobe peptide; FSH: follicle-stimulating hormone; GH: growth hormone; LH: luteinizing hormone; LPH: lipotropin hormone; MSH: melanocyte-stimulating hormone; POMC: pro-opiomelanocortin; PRL: prolactin; TSH: thyroid-stimulating hormone)

TABLE 2	Distribution of cells in the pituitary.	
Cell type	**Proportion of cells in the pituitary**	**Location and distribution**
Somatotrophs	~40–50%	Lateral aspect
Lactotrophs	~20–25%	Posterolateral aspect
Corticotrophs	~10–20%	Posteromedial aspect
Thyrotrophs	~5%	Anteromedial aspect
Gonadotrophs	~10%	Distributed all throughout the pituitary

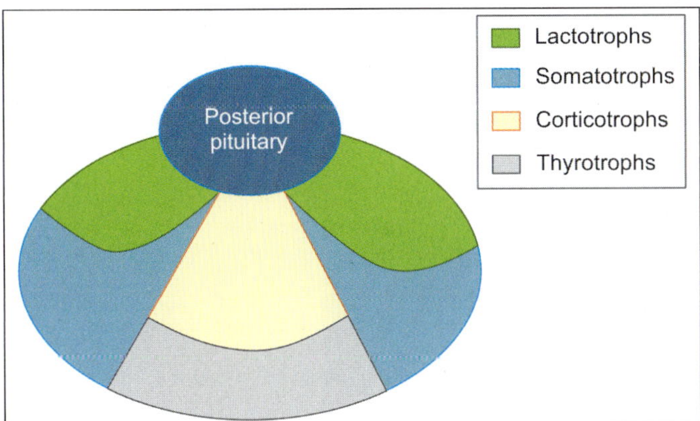

FIGURE 1: Schematic representation of distribution of cells in the pituitary.

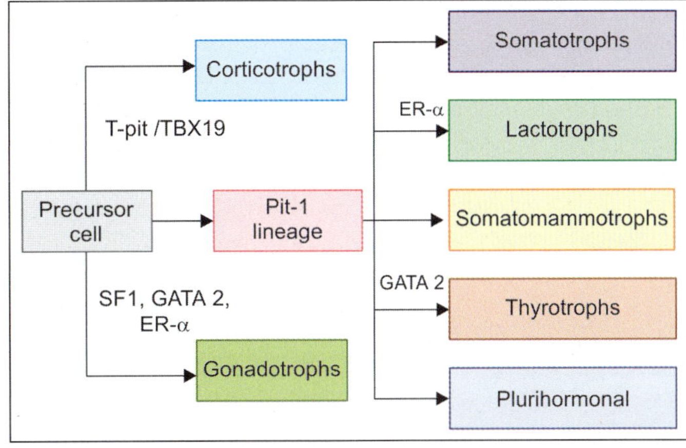

FIGURE 2: Lineage of pituitary cell development and role of transcription factors.

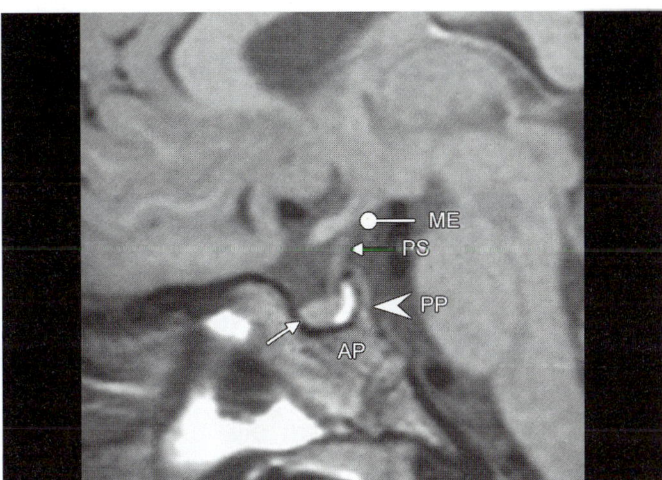

(AP: anterior pituitary; ME: median eminence; MRI: magnetic resonance imaging; PP: posterior pituitary; PS: pituitary stalk)

FIGURE 3: Normal landmarks of the sellar-suprasellar region on sagittal section MRI.

PATHOLOGY

Disorders of the hypothalamus and pituitary gland include congenital/developmental and acquired causes. Congenital/developmental disorders of the hypothalamus-pituitary unit are predominantly caused by defects in the various transcription factors involved in the development of the pituitary and its constituent cells (**Fig. 2**). Acquired causes including infective, inflammatory, infiltrative, degenerative, traumatic, or neoplasms can cause hypopituitarism. On the other hand, endocrinopathies associated with pituitary tumors result in clinical syndromes associated with the excess of one or multiple hormones.

CONGENITAL DISORDERS

Defects in the orchestrated development of the pituitary gland, primarily of the transcription factors, result in hypopituitarism. Depending upon the involved factor, it may result in isolated or multiple pituitary hormone deficiency (MPHD). Risk factors for hypopituitarism include breech presentation and birth asphyxia. Clinical presentation may include hypoglycemia, pathological jaundice, and micropenis. The radiological tetrad of empty sella, hypoplastic anterior pituitary, redundant or absent stalk, and ectopic or absent posterior pituitary bright spot is the characteristic feature. GH deficiency is the most common and other hormone deficiencies in the absence of GH deficiency (except TBX19/T-Pit) are undescribed. Moreover, there is a correlation between radiological abnormalities and severity of GH deficiency.

Normal anatomic landmarks of the pituitary are shown in **Figure 3**. Magnetic resonance imaging (MRI) of a neonate depicting physiological T1 hyperintensity of the entire gland is shown in **Figure 4**. Individual cases of MPHD with clinical and radiological aspects of diagnosis are shown in **Figures 5** and **6**.

Apart from transcription factor defects, other congenital anomalies of the hypothalamus-pituitary unit include hypothalamic malformations such as hamartoma which can manifest as precocious puberty with or without gelastic seizures (**Fig. 7**). It may be seen in association with GLI3 mutations as part of the Pallister–Hall syndrome which also includes polydactyly and cleft lip/palate. Congenital defects also include other hamartomas and persistent craniopharyngeal canal (**Fig. 8**).

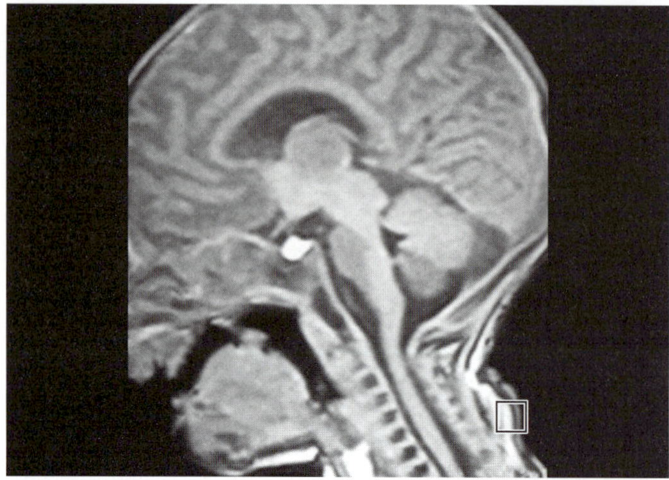

FIGURE 4: This sagittal magnetic resonance image of a neonate highlights that unlike adult pituitary where T1 hyperintensity is restricted to the posterior pituitary, the entire gland (including anterior pituitary) shows T1 hyperintensity.

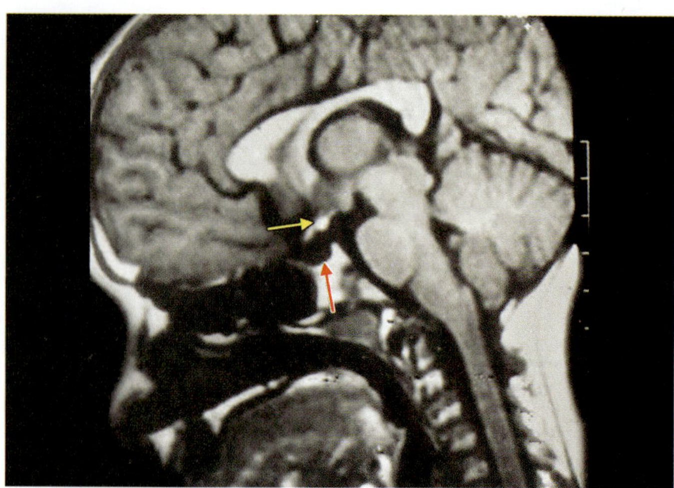

FIGURE 5: Magnetic resonance imaging (MRI) tetrad in transcription factor defects depicting small sella, hypoplastic anterior pituitary (red arrow), absent stalk, and ectopic posterior pituitary bright spot (yellow arrow).

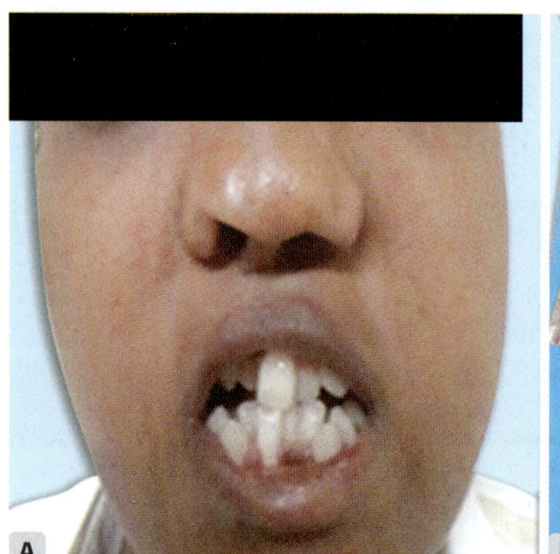

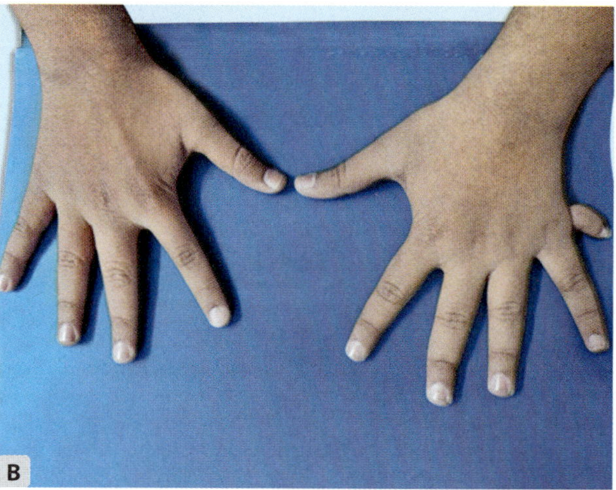

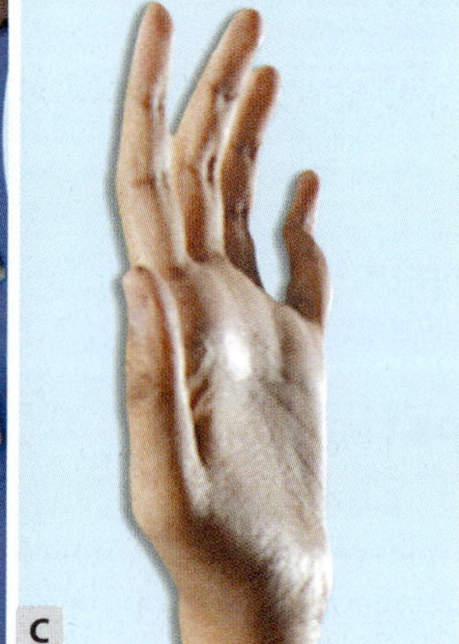

FIGURES 6 A to C: Clinical defects noted in children with multiple pituitary hormone deficiency (MPHD). Depicted here are the **(A)** single central incisor, **(B)** hexadactyly, and **(C)** clinodactyly in different patients with MPHD.

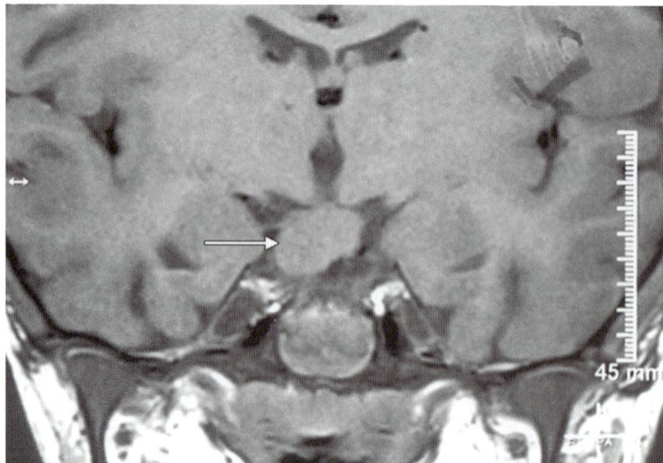

FIGURE 7: Magnetic resonance imaging (MRI) showing a hypothalamic mass consistent with hypothalamic hamartoma. He was treated with gonadotropin-releasing hormone (GnRH) agonist (leuprolide) monthly injections and letrozole (aromatase inhibitor).

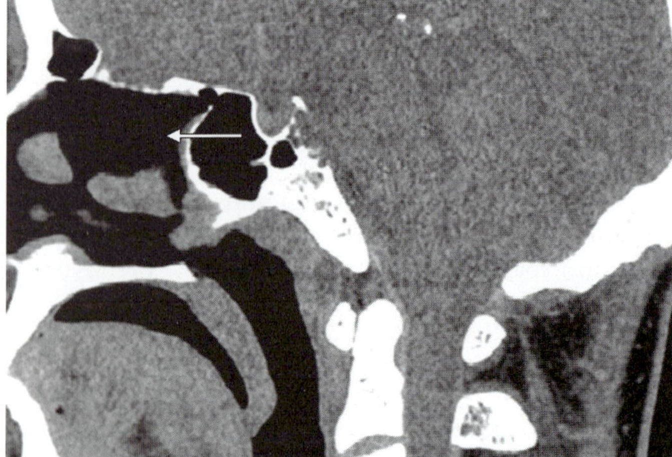

FIGURE 8: Sagittal computed tomography (CT) scan: Erosive lesion is appreciated on the dorsum sella in the retroclival location (arrow) reaching up till the posterior pituitary typical of ecchordosis physaliphora (a congenital benign hamartomatous lesion derived from notochord remnants).

ACQUIRED DISORDERS

Among acquired causes of hypopituitarism, infective, inflammatory (primary or secondary to mass lesion or systemic inflammation), traumatic, and degenerative causes may lead to hypopituitarism in varying degrees. The degree and type of hormone deficiencies are variable and there may be discordance between clinical and radiological findings.

INFECTIVE

The risk factors for infections are meningitis, paranasal sinusitis (direct spread), immunocompromised host (hematogenous spread), and surgery. Tuberculosis may involve the pituitary gland either directly by tuberculomas or indirectly by hypophysitis (**Figs. 9** and **10**). Nearly 80% patients of tubercular meningitis are reported to have hypopituitarism at presentation with hyperprolactinemia and secondary hypoadrenalism being the most common patterns of presentation. Persistence of these abnormalities in nearly half of those following completion of antituberculous therapy suggests evaluation of hypothalamic–pituitary–adrenal (HPA) axis in all patients. Among other infections, syphilis (gumma), parasitic involvement by neurocysticercosis, *Pneumocystis carinii* and toxoplasma, viruses [herpes simplex virus (HSV), Varicella-zoster virus (VZV), and cytomegalovirus (CMV)] and fungi (*Candida* and *Aspergillus*) are also described.

INFLAMMATORY

Primary hypophysitis: Primary inflammatory involvement of the pituitary is termed hypophysitis, which is of four types, as summarized in **Table 3**. **Figure 11** depict individual case of primary hypophysitis.

Secondary hypophysitis: Hypophysitis may be secondary to a number of conditions, including tumors, drugs, and hematopoietic malignancies, including lymphoma. Emerging causes include drug-induced inflammation secondary to drugs viz. immune checkpoint inhibitors (ICP) (anti-PD-1/anti-PD-L1). They cause an idiosyn-

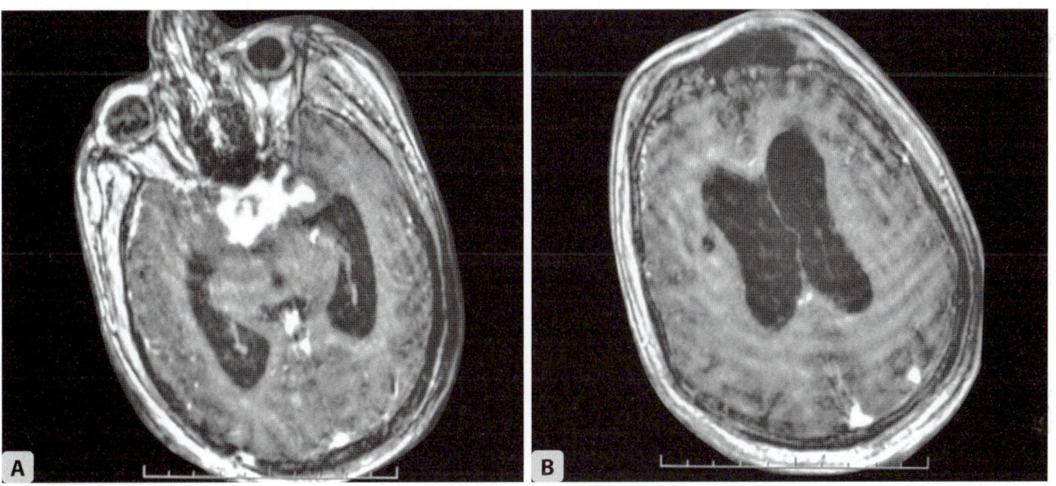

FIGURES 9 A & B: **Basal exudates, hydrocephalus, and hypophysitis in tuberculous meningitis (TBM).**

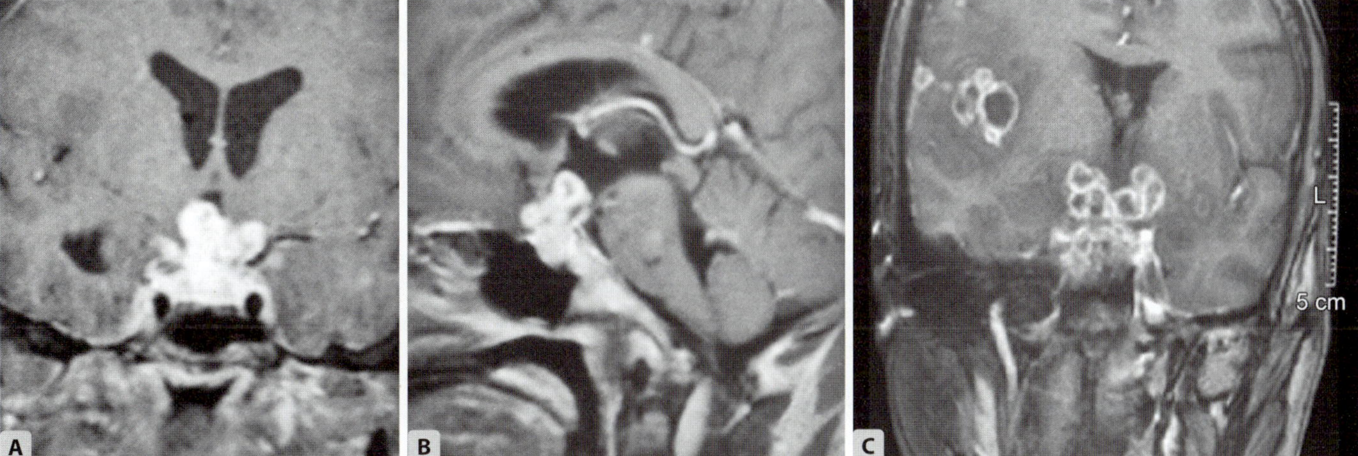

FIGURES 10 A to C: **(A and B)** Gadolinium-enhanced magnetic resonance imaging (MRI) in the coronal and sagittal planes show suprasellar tuberculomas causing compression and encasement of the infundibulum and chiasma leading to vision loss; **(C)** MRI in the coronal plane in another patient shows conglomerate tuberculomas in the sellar-suprasellar region.

TABLE 3 Patterns and spectrum of primary hypophysitis with diagnostic and management aspects.

Type of hypophysitis	Characteristic finding(s)	Imaging findings	Age and gender	Extrapituitary involvement	Management
LYH/ autoimmune hypophysitis	• ACTH, LH/FSH deficiency • Associated with pregnancy • Diffuse involvement of pituitary by lymphocytes and other inflammatory cells, later causing pituitary fibrosis and atrophy	• Diffuse pituitary enlargement (isointense on T1) • Stalk thickening • Contrast enhancement	• F:M 3:1 3rd to 4th decade • 75–85% of cases	• Hashimoto's • APS II • GD	• High-dose glucocorticoids • Surgery in nonresponders
IgG4/ plasmacytic	• Variable • Mononuclear infiltrate of plasma cells and lymphocytes and at least 10 IgG4 positive plasma cells/ high-power field (HPF) along with storiform fibrosis	Simultaneous involvement of sinuses and/or skull base can point towards IgG4 subtype	• M:F 2:1 • 6th to 7th decade • 30% of cases	• Retroperitoneal fibrosis • Exophthalmos	• High-dose glucocorticoids • AntiCD20 therapy (rituximab), mycophenolate or surgery in nonresponders
Granulomatous	Infiltration of gland by granulomas composed of multinucleated giant cells and histiocytes	• Diffuse pituitary enlargement (isointense on T1) • Stalk thickening	• F:M 3:1 • 5th decade • 20% of cases	-	• Glucocorticoids less effective • Surgery is preferred
Xanthomatous	Variable infiltrate of lipid laden foamy macrophages, histiocytes without granulomas	Hypointense on T1	• F:M 3:1 • 4th decade • 3–5% of cases		• Glucocorticoids less effective • Replacement of hormone deficiencies • Data is scarce
Necrotizing	Diffuse nonhemorrhagic necrosis with inflammatory infiltrate	Enlarged gland without contrast enhancement	<1% of cases		Replacement of hormone deficiencies
ICP induced (anti CTLA4 and anti PD-1/ PD-L1)	• ACTH, LH/FSH uncommon deficiency • PRL excess • Idiosyncratic reaction • Complement fixation • Hypersensitivity reactions (type II, IV)	Diffuse enlargement of the pituitary, contrast enhancement		• Thyroiditis or hypo/ hyperthyroidism • Hypoadrenalism (primary) • Fulminant diabetes • Nonendocrine associations like hepatitis	• Hormone replacement in mild cases • High-dose glucocorticoids in moderate-to-severe cases • In most cases, the drug can be continued

(ACTH: adrenocorticotropic hormone; APS: autoimmune polyglandular syndrome; FSH: follicle-stimulating hormone; GD: Graves' disease; ICP: immune checkpoint inhibitor; LH: luteinizing hormone; LYH: lymphocytic hypophysitis; PD-1/PD-L1: programmed death 1/programmed death ligand 1)

cratic pattern of hypophysitis, predominantly with hypocortisolism, hypogonadism, and hypothyroidism. Hyperprolactinemia and diffuse enlargement as well as contrast enhancement of the pituitary are classical of lymphocytic hypophysitis (LYH). Diabetes insipidus (DI) is also more common with LYH than with ICP-induced hypophysitis. Some cases of hypophysitis secondary to primary conditions like tumors or systemic inflammation are shown in **Figures 12** and **13**.

Isolated hypothalamic involvement, though rare, is also reported, leading to deficiencies of trophic hormones and consequently hypopituitarism (**Fig. 14**).

Among other causes of hypophysitis due to secondary or systemic causes, sarcoidosis, Langerhans cell histiocytosis, Wegener's granulomatosis, and lymphomatous involvement are rare but reported.

NEOPLASTIC

Pituitary adenomas are the third most common intracranial tumors, accounting for nearly 15–25% of all cases. A change in nomenclature to pituitary neuroendocrine tumors (PitNETs) has been recently suggested. Nonfunctioning pituitary adenomas (NFPAs) are the most common subtype and include gonadotropinomas, silent pituitary adenomas, or null cell adenomas. After the proposition of the transcription factor-based classification, it has been suggested that PitNETs form a continuum, varying from null cell adenomas to silent and whispering

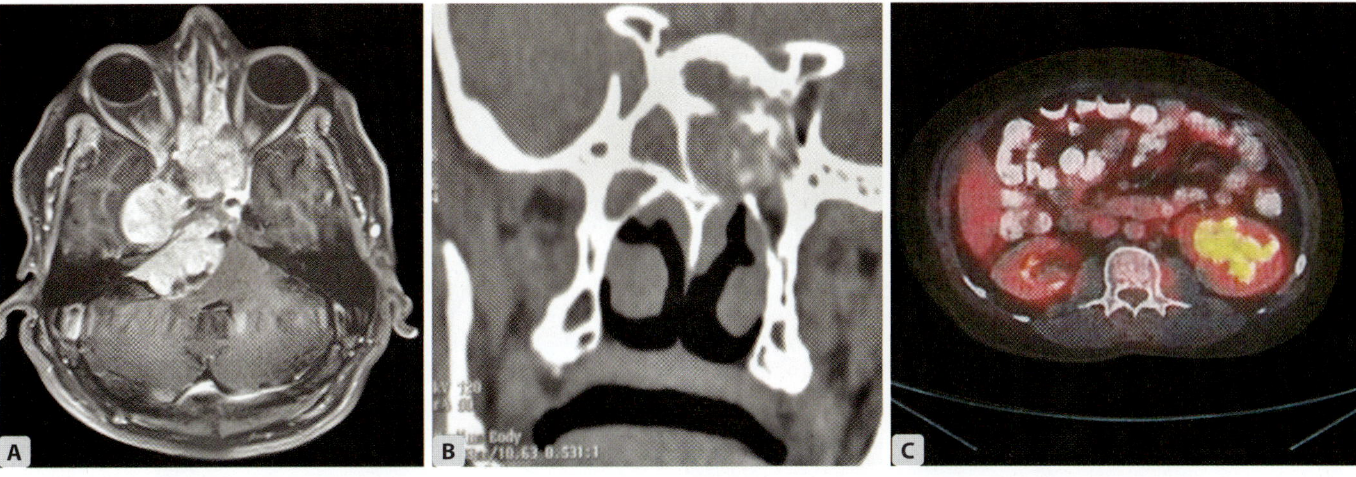

FIGURES 11 A to C: A 50-year-old man who presented with hemiparesis and involvement of multiple lower cranial nerves (VII, VIII, IX, and XI) was found to have an infiltrating mass in the sellar region on magnetic resonance imaging (MRI) with concomitant sinus involvement. Biopsy revealed immunoglobulin G4 (IgG4)-related disease and fluorodeoxyglucose positron emission tomography (FDG PET) showed focal lesion in the right kidney.

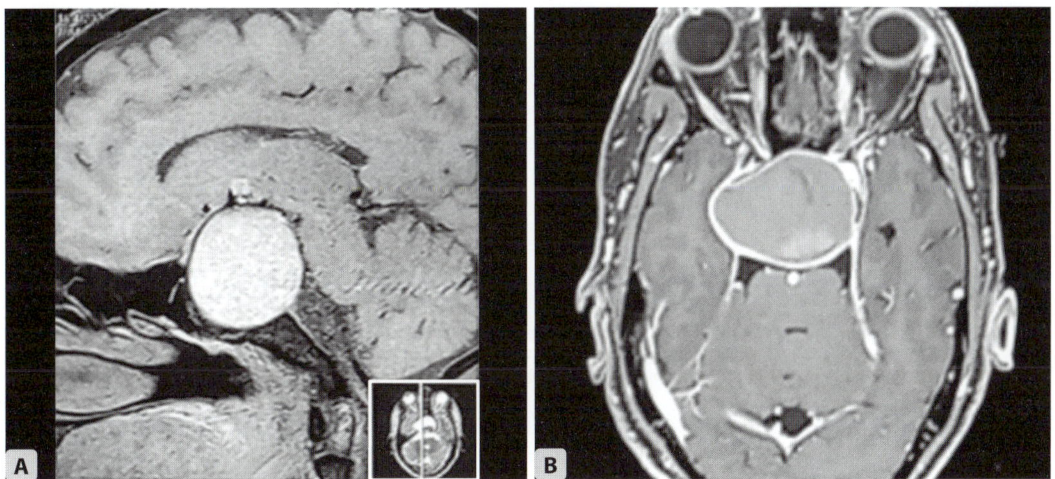

FIGURES 12 A & B: A 45-year-old male presented with headache, blurring of vision, and was found to have panhypopituitarism on evaluation. Magnetic resonance imaging (MRI) sagittal image depicts a large, cystic mass compressing the optic chiasma and extending up to the floor of the third ventricle with peripheral rim enhancement noted in the axial section. Following replacement with hydrocortisone, thyroid hormone, and testosterone, he was subjected to excision of the mass by transsphenoidal route and histopathology revealed xanthgranulomatous hypophysitis.

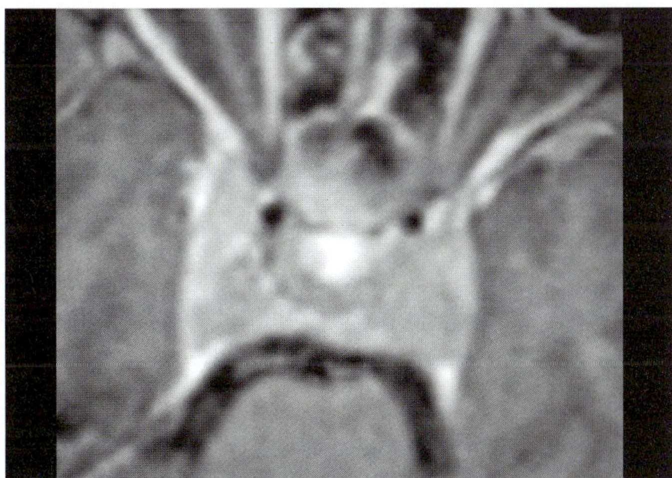

FIGURE 13: Diffuse sheet-like sellar-parasellar soft tissue extending on either side and partly encasing the internal carotid artery (ICA) without luminal compromise on this postcontrast T1 magnetic resonance (MR) image suggests a pliable tumor typically seen in lymphoma.

tumors to functional tumors (**Fig. 15**). Among the functional tumors, prolactinomas are the most common followed by somatotropinomas, corticotropinomas, and thyrotropinomas.

Various endocrinopathies are associated with these PitNETs due to hormonal hypersecretion associated with proliferation of specific subtypes of cells (**Table 4**). Mixed or multiple hormone production may also be present, for example, PRL hypersecretion in acromegaly (due to acidophil stem cell adenoma, mammosomatotroph adenoma, or mixed GH and PRL secreting adenoma). In case of other tumors, immunohistochemistry helps in diagnosis of multiple hormone positivity in a given tumor.

All tumors with macroadenomas should be subjected to assessment of visual acuity, visual fields at baseline, and at follow-up to determine remission for planning adjuvant therapy and/or surveillance for recurrence.

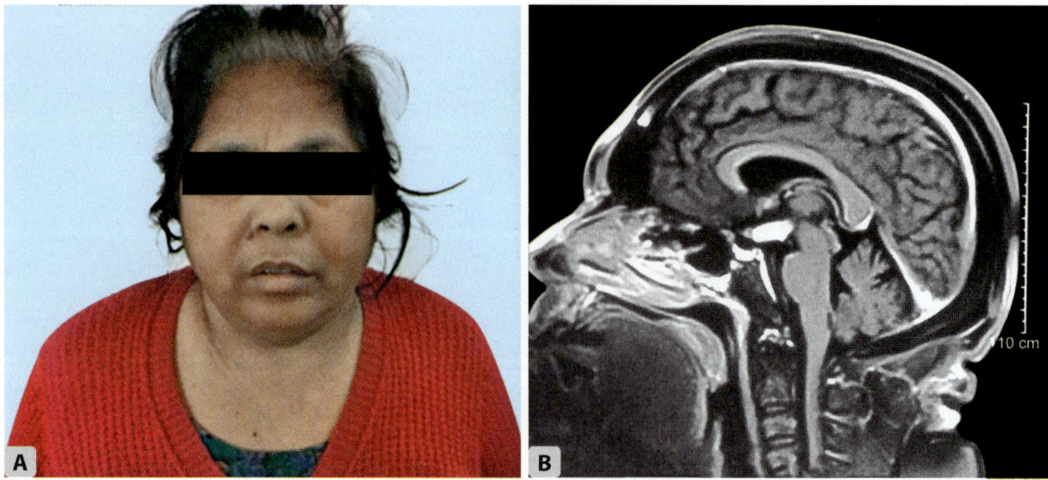

FIGURES 14 A & B: A 50-year-old female presented with cognitive dysfunction and diencephalic syndrome. She had past history of bronchial asthma for which she was on inhaled steroids intermittently. She was found to have multiple pituitary hormone deficiency (MPHD) and central diabetes insipidus. Magnetic resonance imaging (MRI) T1-weighted sagittal section showing an intensely enhancing lesion in the hypothalamus with sparing of the pituitary. She was managed with high-dose glucocorticoids, which were tapered, besides hormone replacement for MPHD and oral desmopressin.

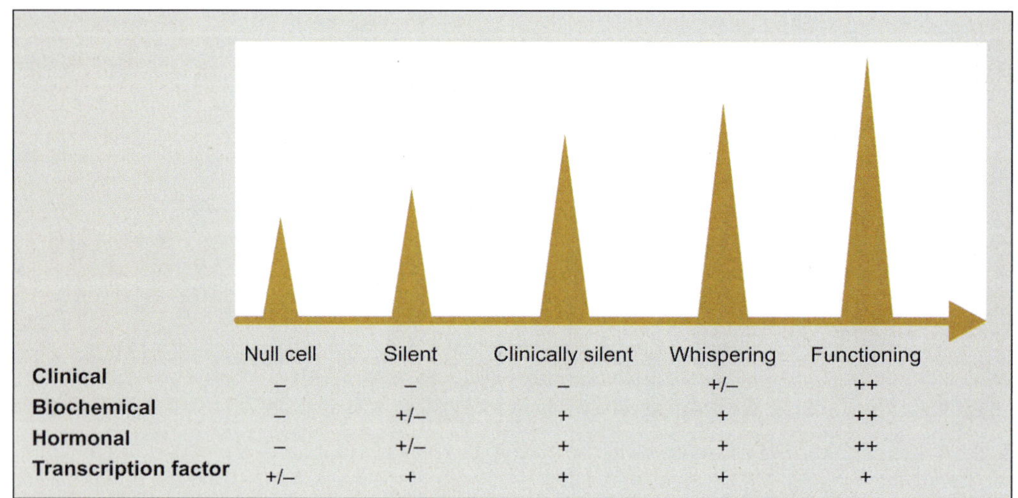

FIGURE 15: Proposed spectrum of pituitary neuroendocrine tumors (pituitary adenomas) based on clinical and biochemical features, hormonal immunohistochemistry, and transcription factors.

Source: Adapted from Drummond J, Roncaroli F, Grossman AB, Korbonits M. Clinical and pathological aspects of silent pituitary adenomas. The Journal of Clinical Endocrinology and Metabolism. 2019;104(7):2473-89.

TABLE 4 Investigations for hormone hypersecretion syndromes in pituitary adenomas.

PitNET-associated endocrinopathy	Screening/Confirmatory test and further testing
Prolactinoma	• Prolactin (in dilution), pooled sample preferable • CEMRI sella • Rule out secondary causes in case of equivocal prolactin elevation (<200 ng/mL)
Acromegaly	• IGF-1 (above the age matched range) • GH not suppressible to 1 ng/mL on 75 g OGTT • CEMRI sella
Cushing's disease	• Screening tests (two of four including UFC, ONDST, LNPC/LNSC, LDDST) • ACTH dependency • CEMRI sella • IPSS (+/-) • CECT chest and abdomen, Ga68 DOTANOC (to rule out ectopic source of ACTH excess)

Continued...

PitNET-associated endocrinopathy	Screening/Confirmatory test and further testing
Thyrotropinoma	• High total or free T3, high total or free T4 with nonsuppressed or elevated TSH • CEMRI sella
Nonfunctioning pituitary adenoma	• Basal hormones; rarely stimulation tests to determine deficiencies of various hormone axes • CEMRI sella

(CEMRI: contrast-enhanced magnetic resonance imaging; GH: growth hormone; IGF-1: insulin-like growth factor-1; IPSS: inferior petrosal sinus sampling; LNPC: late night plasma cortisol; LNSC: late night salivary cortisol; LDDST: low-dose dexamethasone suppression test; OGTT: oral glucose tolerance test; ONDST: overnight dexamethasone suppression test; PitNET: pituitary neuroendocrine tumor)

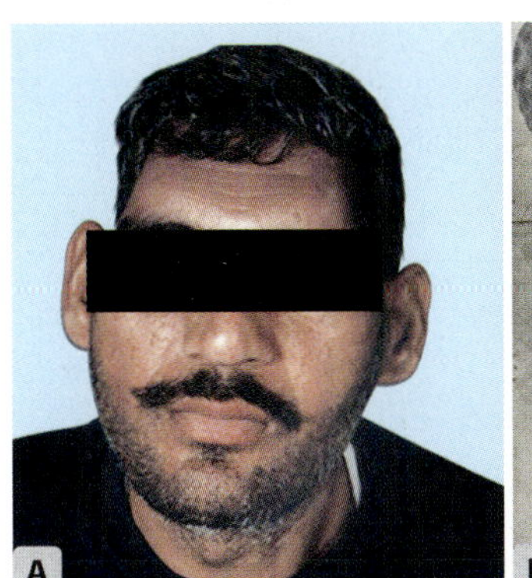

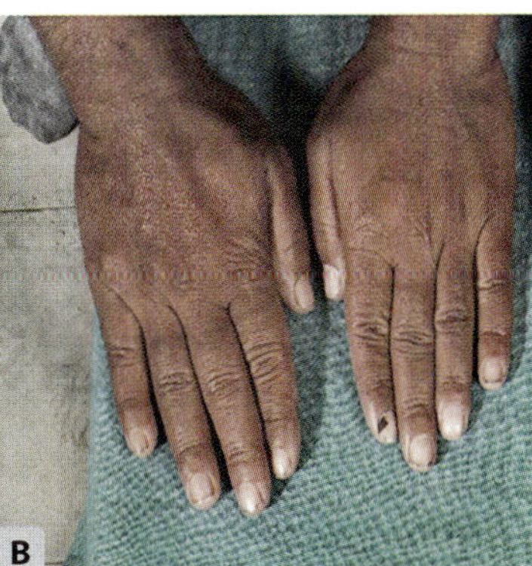

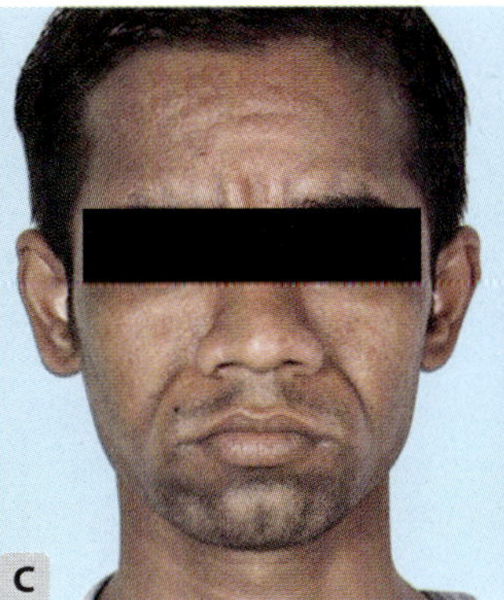

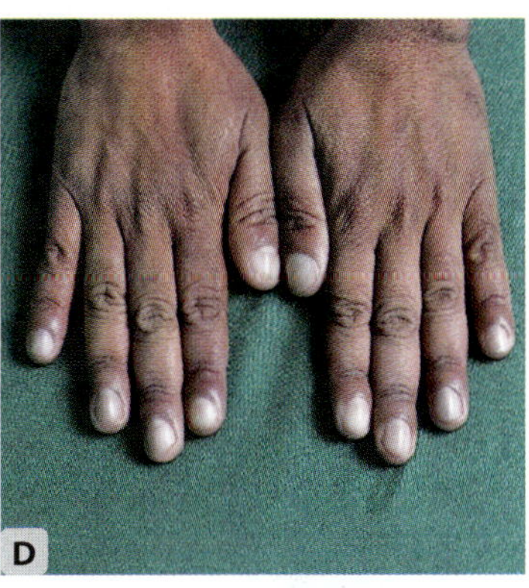

FIGURES 16 A to D: The upper panel showing a patient with acromegaly showing coarse features, prominent forehead, and supraorbital ridges and hands showing acral enlargement but no clubbing. The bottom panel shows another patient with similar coarse features, and cutis verticis gyrata over the forehead along with clubbing of all digits, consistent with pachydermoperiostosis, a cause of pseudoacromegaly.

ENDOCRINOPATHIES ASSOCIATED WITH HORMONE-SECRETING ADENOMAS

Prolactinomas: Prolactinomas are the most common subtype of functioning PitNETs. It is more common in females. The most common *presentation* is with amenorrhea and galactorrhea in females and compressive features (headache, visual acuity, and/or field disturbances) in males. This sexual dimorphism is due to the fact that females more commonly harbor microadenomas and males harbor macroadenomas, probably owing to the lack of specific features in case of males. However, there is also some evidence to suggest that males have more proliferative tumors.

The diagnosis of prolactinomas is confirmed by unequivocally raised PRL (>200 ng/mL) in case of macroadenomas corroborated by MRI findings. Values of PRL under 100 ng/mL may be due to other secondary causes such as drugs, chronic kidney disease, hypophysitis, stalk-related hyperprolactinemia, pregnancy and lactation, and stress. Rarely, some drugs like risperidone may be associated with high levels of serum PRL (up to 500 ng/mL). Occasionally, macroprolactin (polymeric PRL) may lead to falsely elevated PRL, but usually without clinical symptomatology (amenorrhea and galactorrhea) which can be circumvented by polyethylene glycol (PEG) precipitation. In other instances, "hook effect" can occur in the presence of a macroadenoma due to saturation of both the capture and signal antibodies used in chemiluminescent assays, especially in patients having PRL levels between 20 and 200 ng/mL, which can be circumvented by serial dilution.

Acromegaly: Acromegaly is a clinical syndrome characterized by excessive secretion of GH, which leads to insulin-like growth factor-1 (IGF-1) generation. The most common cause is a somatotropinoma, but rarely, ectopic sources of GHRH and GH including gangliocytoma, choristoma, lymphoma, or neuroendocrine tumor (NET). It is an insidious onset disease with interval from onset to time of diagnosis being 10–12 years. Clinical features are due to excess of both GH and IGF-1 as well as compressive features (**Figs. 16** and **17**). Concurrent hyperprolactinemia is seen in nearly 20–30% patients.

Common comorbidities include dysglycemia, hypertension, cardiomyopathy, obstructive sleep apnea (OSA), central sleep apnea (CSA), arthropathy, fractures, colonic polyps, and increased risk of neoplasia. Acromegaly in young patients is characterized by acrogigantism in nearly one-third of all adolescent acromegaly patients. The common causes of acrogigantism include multiple endocrine neoplasia type 1 (MEN1), McCune–Albright syndrome (MAS), Aryl hydrocarbon receptor-interacting protein (AIP), X-linked acrogigantism (X-LAG), and Carney complex.

Diagnosis of acromegaly rests on the demonstration of IGF-1 and nonsuppressible GH on oral glucose tolerance test (OGTT) (to <1 ng/mL) and MRI corroboration

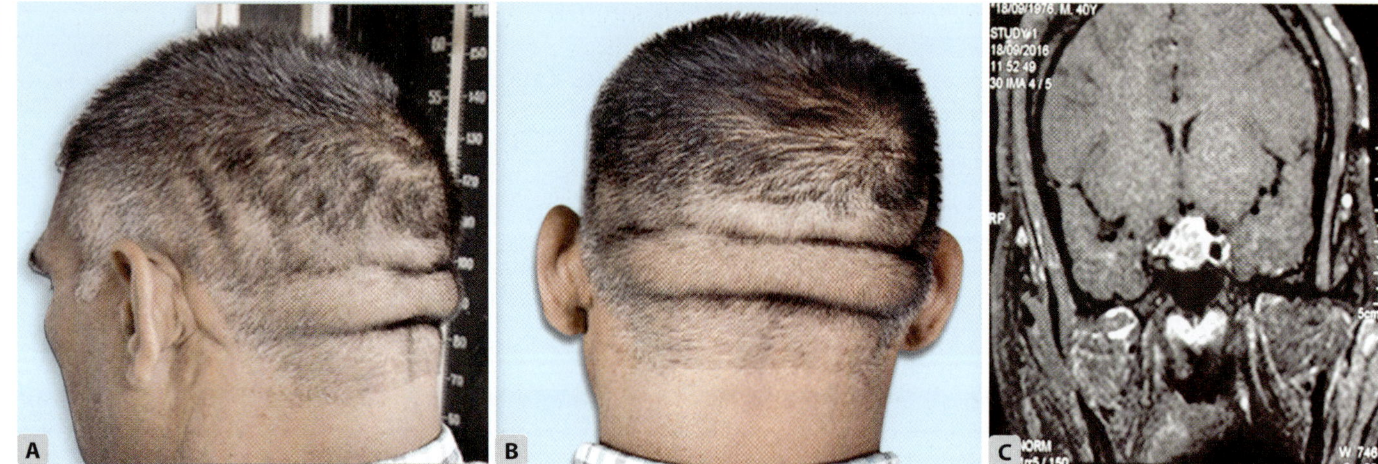

FIGURES 17 A to C: **(A and B)** A 48-year-old male presented with headache and visual field deficits. In addition to the classical features of acromegaly, he was found to have cutis verticis gyrata all over the scalp; **(C)** magnetic resonance imaging (MRI) showed a macrosomatotropinoma.

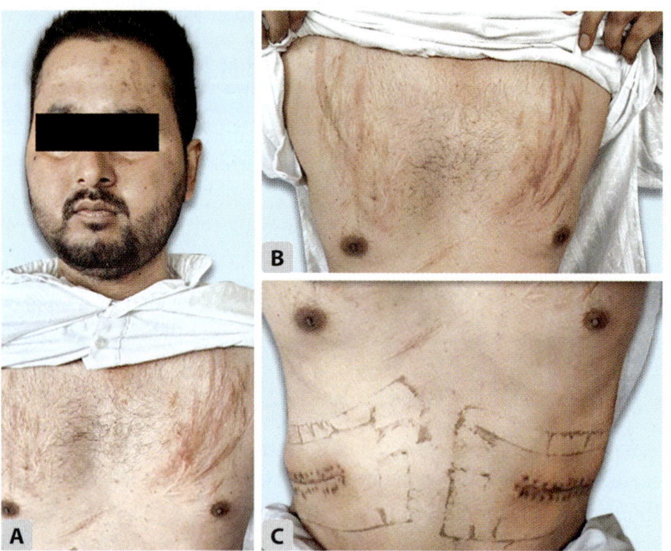

FIGURES 18 A to C: A 26-year-old male who presented with weight gain and hypertension, had moon facies, acne, hyperpigmentation, and wide and violaceous striae on the chest wall. However, investigations revealed adrenocorticotropic hormone (ACTH)-dependent Cushing's syndrome and these were deemed as typical stretch marks of Cushing's syndrome due to protein catabolism located in atypical site.

Courtesy: Dr Momin, SKIMS.

of adenoma. The treatment of choice is surgery [transsphenoidal surgery (TSS)]. However, remission is up to 50–70% in case of macroadenomas and 80–90% in microadenomas. Adjuvant therapy includes radiotherapy and medical management [including octreotide long-acting release (LAR), cabergoline, pegvisomant, or pasireotide).

Cushing's disease: Cushing's disease (CD) is the most common cause of endogenous hypercortisolism. It is frequently caused by a microadenoma in nearly 80% of cases and is more common in women (F:M 2–3:1).

Clinical features at presentation include weight gain, fat redistribution (central obesity, dorsocervical fat pad, and supraclavicular fat pad), hyperpigmentation, and features of protein catabolism (broad, violaceous striae, proximal myopathy, cuticular atrophy/Liddle's sign, pulp atrophy, bruising, and thinning of hair) which are the specific features of the disease (**Fig. 18**).

Other clinical features include androgen excess (acne, hirsutism, and oligomenorrhea), secondary diabetes mellitus, hypertension, cardiomyopathy, osteoporosis, and neuropsychiatric manifestations. Newer and less frequently described features include spinal epidural lipomatosis and central serous retinopathy. Around one-third to one-half of patients are estimated to harbor the somatic ubiquitin-specific peptidase 8 (USP8) mutations leading to its constitutive action and overexpression of epidermal growth factor receptor (EGFR) on corticotropes.

Diagnosis of CD: The tenets of diagnosis of CD depend on demonstration of loss of circadian rhythm of cortisol, nonsuppressibility of cortisol with dexamethasone and ACTH dependence with evidence [radiological using MRI or biochemical using inferior petrosal sinus sampling (IPSS)] of localization to the pituitary. Late night (2,300 h) serum cortisol (>207 nmol/L in awake or 50 nmol/L in sleeping state) or late night salivary cortisol, nonsuppressible cortisol to ≤50 nmol/L with 1 mg dexamethasone overnight or with 0.5 mg dexamethasone q6hrly for 48 hours and 24 hours urinary-free cortisol exceeding the upper limit of normal on two occasions are all screening tests to demonstrate endogenous hypercortisolism. Any two of these screening tests positive with ACTH >20 pg/mL indicates ACTH-dependent Cushing's syndrome and MRI (with dynamic cuts) is used for localization of the mass. In event of nonvisualization of the adenoma, visualized adenoma <6 mm or nonsuppressibility of cortisol to 50% of baseline value with 2 mg dexamethasone q6hrly, IPSS should be performed to localize the lesion to the pituitary and possibly lateralize it. The first line of treatment of CD is surgery. However, disease recurrence and persistence can occur in about one-half of all cases. In these patients, adjuvant radiotherapy and/or medical management (using adrenal-directed drugs such as ketoconazole and low-dose mitotane or pituitary-directed drugs such as pasireotide, octreotide, and cabergoline or EGFR inhibitors like gefitinib in USP8-mutated adenomas) can help in remission of the hypercortisolic state. In case of failed surgery, severe comorbidities including parasuicide or catastrophic Cushing's, bilateral adrenalectomy is used as it is the only therapeutic modality which can offer complete resolution of the hypercortisolism. However, these patients need to be offered hydrocortisone, fludrocortisone replacement lifelong, and be under regular surveillance for the development of Nelson's syndrome.

Thyrotropinomas: Thyrotropinomas account for under 1–2% of all PitNETs. The TSH secretion is autonomous and refractory to the negative feedback of thyroid hormones (inappropriate TSH secretion) and this stimulates the thyroid gland and the consequent hyper-secretion of T4 and T3. Thus, the biochemical picture resembles a central hyperthyroidism characterized by elevated T3, T4, and nonsuppressed or high TSH. The other condition with this biochemical picture is the entity of peripheral resistance to thyroid hormone. Thyrotropinomas can *present with* signs/symptoms of thyroid hormone excess (weight loss, palpitations, sweating, and tremors), TSH excess (diffuse goiter), or compressive features due to macroadenomas. Patients with these tumors sometimes have history of inadvertent treatment for Graves' disease with thyroid ablation or surgery or rarely, treatment with thyroid hormone supplement for an isolated high TSH, both of which can potentially worsen the primary condition.

Diagnosis of thyrotropinomas is made on the basis of the classical biochemical thyroid profile, technetium scan suggestive of diffuse uptake in the thyroid gland, and MRI demonstration of an adenoma. The first line of management is surgical removal of the adenoma following optimization with beta blockers and/or octreotide.

Nonfunctioning pituitary adenomas/nonfunctioning pituitary neuroendocrine tumors: NFPAs are the most common tumor subtype of PitNETs and are not associated with hormonal hypersecretion. They consist of different histological subtypes: Gonadotropinomas, silent pituitary adenomas or null cell adenomas. Presenting features include compressive features due to mass effect or in some cases due to concurrent hyperprolactinemia (stalk effect) and varying degrees of hypopituitarism. Patients with NFPAs should undergo hormonal, clinical, and laboratory evaluation for hyper- and hypopituitarism.

The primary treatment for NFPAs with neuro-ophthalmologic compromise is surgical resection. Visual deficits may improve following surgery but hormone deficits are likely to persist or new deficiencies may develop. High rates of recurrence is observed in up to one-half of all cases over a period of 5–10 years, especially in cases of invasive macroadenomas and those with high proliferation indices but clinically significant tumor growth is noted in up to one-fifth. Adjuvant radiotherapy is generally offered for residual tumors or those that progress during follow-up. Medical management including cabergoline may offer some respite in selected cases.

In terms of anatomical and morphological characteristics, an adenoma with maximum dimension under 10 mm is a microadenoma, that equal to 10 mm is a mesoadenoma and any one dimension exceeding 10 mm is a macroadenoma. An invasive adenoma is one which has either dural, sphenoid, or mucosal invasion. A proliferative adenoma is one which has any two of the following out of three parameters positive: Ki-67 ≥ 3%, p53 positivity, or mitotic count exceeding 2/10 high-power field (HPF). Invasive tumors may not be proliferative and vice versa. Aggressive tumors are defined based on the clinical course of the tumor in a given patient as large, invasive lesions with high proliferation with clinically relevant tumor regrowth or recurrence despite standard therapies, and are usually associated with resistance to standard therapies including surgery, requiring multimodality therapy (**Fig. 19**).

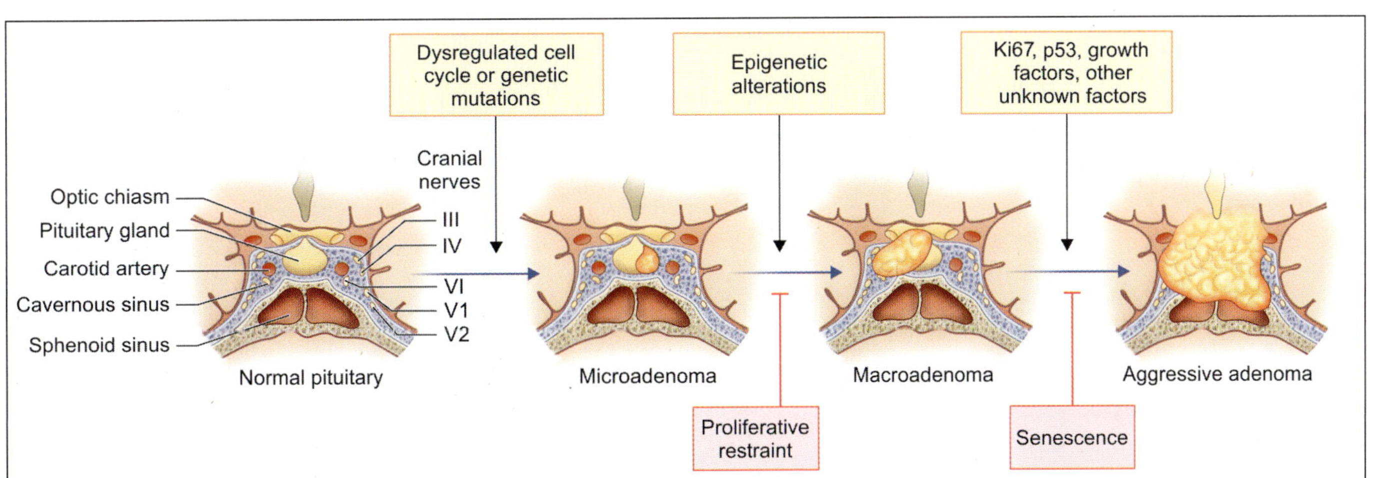

FIGURE 19: Schematic diagram of the normal anatomical landmarks of the pituitary and events involved in transition to micro, macro, or aggressive adenomas.

Source: Adapted from Melmed S. Pituitary–Tumor Endocrinopathies. N Engl J Med. 2020;382(10):937-50.

Clinicopathological classification: There is a recent clinicopathological classification of PitNETs based on these parameters of invasiveness and proliferation (**Table 5**). Depending on these, tumors can be subdivided into various grades as follows into a five-tiered classification including tumor diameter, tumor type, and grade based on invasion and proliferation. This clinicopathological classification has been validated for predicting recurrence and prognosis following surgery.

Treatment of pituitary adenoma: Except for a prolactinoma, surgery is the treatment of pituitary adenoma. Surgery remains the treatment of choice for pituitary adenomas, both functional and nonfunctional. Surgical intervention leads to maximum tumor resection, decompression of the optic apparatus, and rapid hormonal normalization. For a nonfunctional adenoma, gross total surgical resection provides the optimal chances of long-term tumor control with correction of endocrinopathy. Endoscopic transnasal transsphenoidal route is preferred to transcranial approaches. With better armamentarium inside the operation theatres, chances of gross total resection are high; however, it decreases to nearly 67–70% with tumor's lateral extension into the cavernous sinuses. Transcranial approaches are limited to tumors with significant supra and parasellar extension, and recurrent tumors with prior radiotherapy.

The ideal strategy is to attempt maximum safe resection followed by adjuvant radiosurgery to the residual tumor, if any. For a residual nonfunctional adenoma, Gamma Knife radiosurgery (GKRS) may be offered as proactive treatment or any evidence of radiological growth of the tumor. Proactive GKRS is advocated for any residual functional adenoma to ensure long-term tumor control and hormonal normalization. Alternative radiation techniques such as intensity-modulated radiotherapy (IMRT) should be preferred to GKRS for tumors with no safe margin from the optic apparatus or large residual volume.

In conclusion, management of a pituitary adenoma needs a multimodality coordinated approach to ensure long-term tumor control with hormonal correction.

TABLE 5 Trouillas classification to define tumor grade of pituitary neuroendocrine tumors (PitNETs).

Criteria for determining tumor grade	
Invasion	Histological and/or radiological evidence of sphenoid or cavernous sinus invasion
Proliferation	Two of the following three markers: • Mitoses >2/10 high-power field (HPF) • p53 positive • Ki-67 ≥3%
Tumor grade	
Ia	Noninvasive, nonproliferative
Ib	Noninvasive, proliferative
IIa	Invasive, nonproliferative
IIb	Invasive, proliferative
III	Metastatic tumor (spinal or noncontiguous cranial or distant metastases)

Pituitary carcinomas: They are rare entities (<0.5% of all sellar neoplasms) characterized by the presence of distant metastasis, usually noncontiguous. Commonly, metastases involve the craniospinal region via dissemination through the subarachnoid space, lymph, or blood vessels. Prolactinomas and CD have the highest propensity to become malignant. Clinical clues to suspect malignancy include an acute transformation from a silent or easy-to-manage tumor to a functional or resistant-to-standard-therapy phenotype.

Apart from the rare pituitary carcinomas, metastases from various solid-organ malignancies can also be seen in the pituitary. Commonly the posterior pituitary is involved owing to its rich vascular supply. The characteristic features of metastases include destruction of the sellar floor and DI and hypopituitarism, which are common (**Fig. 20**). Breast cancer and lymphomas are the most common primary sources and rarely, thyroid and lung.

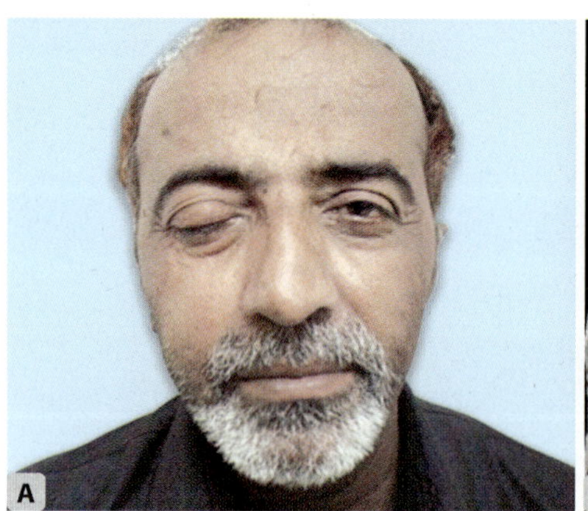

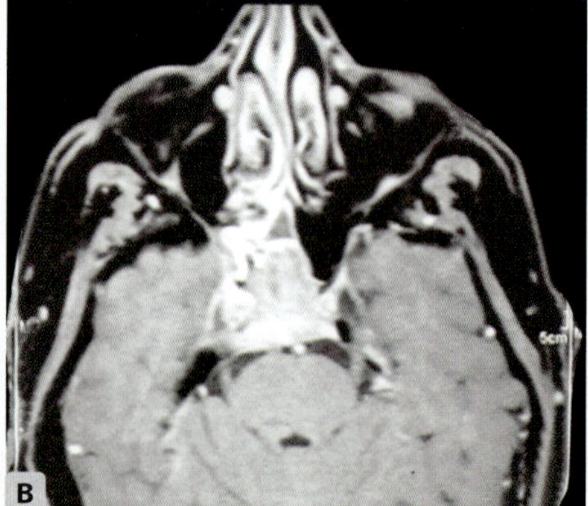

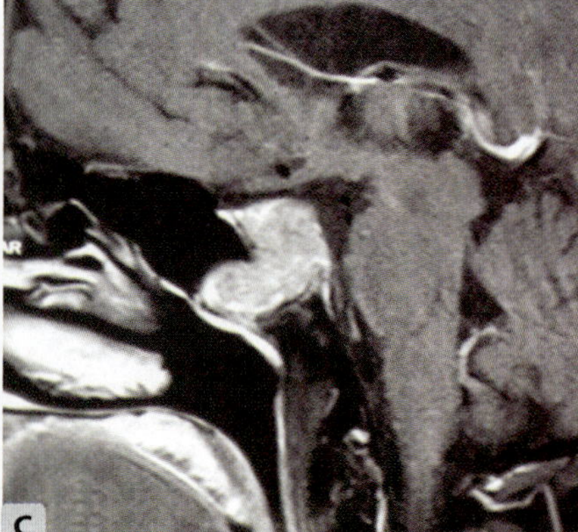

FIGURES 20 A to C: A 47-year-old male presented with acute onset ptosis. He had deficiency of multiple pituitary hormones and diabetes insipidus. Magnetic resonance imaging (MRI) showed a large sellar-suprasellar mass with contrast enhancement, destruction of the sellar floor suggestive of malignancy. He underwent biopsy of the lesion which revealed metastatic transitional cell carcinoma. Fluorodeoxyglucose positron emission tomography (FDG PET) did not reveal any primary focus. He was administered chemotherapy and radiotherapy, but succumbed to the disease.

Other unusual sellar masses include chordoma, meningioma, chondrosarcoma, paraganglioma, and nasopharyngeal carcinoma.

DEGENERATIVE

Sheehan's syndrome: It is a cause of postpartum pituitary infarction and necrosis characterized by secondary amenorrhea and lactational failure, usually preceded by an event of postpartum hemorrhage (PPH) and shock. Pituitary, being highly susceptible to vascular insults, can be involved in event of PPH, vasospasm, thrombosis, and hypophyseal vessel compression. Varying degree of anterior pituitary dysfunction is common with somatotrophs and lactotrophs being most frequently affected, but DI has been reported. MRI usually reveals a partially empty sella at diagnosis due to long diagnostic delay, but in early stages, may show central ischemic necrosis (**Fig. 21**).

Snakebite: It is an important yet less recognized cause of hypopituitarism in our country. It can cause both early and delayed hypopituitarism of which anterior pituitary hormone deficiencies are the most common, especially corticotropes and somatolactotropes. Pituitary involvement is common in cases with vasculotoxic envenomation which leads to acute kidney injury warranting hemodialysis. Posterior pituitary involvement is exceedingly rare, however reported both with and without absent posterior pituitary bright spot. There are rare reports of ectopic posterior pituitary bright spot without DI, possibly due to the involvement of the anterior pituitary by disseminated intravascular coagulation leading to anterior pituitary hypoplasia and reorganization of the posterior pituitary at an ectopic site.

Trauma: It is yet another cause of late-onset pituitary degeneration and hypopituitarism. The risk factors for post-traumatic hypopituitarism include low Glasgow Coma Scale (GCS) (<10), skull fracture, severity of the injury, diffuse brain edema, and raised intracranial tension. Gonadotropins and GH are the most commonly affected axes (**Fig. 22**). DI is less common than anterior hypopituitarism, but is more commonly transient. If persistent and severe, it portends poor prognosis in these patients.

PITUITARY APOPLEXY

Pituitary apoplexy is a clinical syndrome resulting from abrupt hemorrhage or infarction in a pre-existing adenoma. Rarely, it can occur in the normal pituitary or in physiological hyperplastic conditions such as pregnancy and lactation.

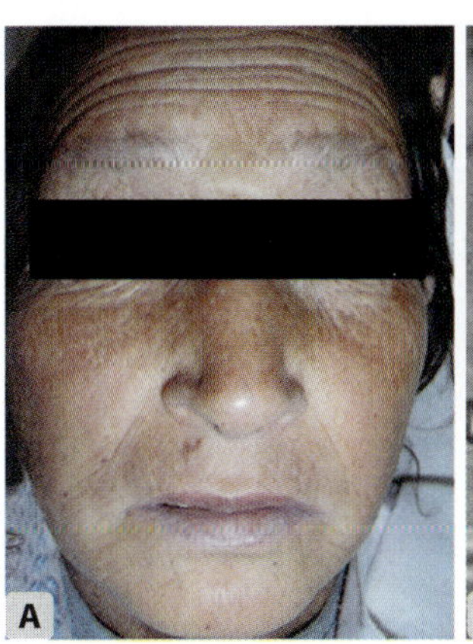

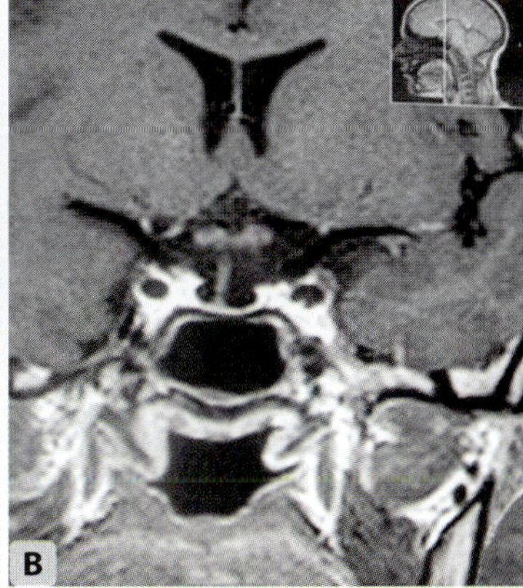

FIGURES 21 A & B: (A) A 35-year-old female presented with secondary amenorrhea with facial features suggestive of multiple pituitary hormone deficiencies [puffy face consistent with hypothyroidism, facial hypopigmentation, especially on the lower half suggestive of hypocortisolism due to adrenocorticotropic hormone (ACTH) deficiency and facial wrinkling due to growth hormone (GH) deficiency]. **(B)** Magnetic resonance imaging (MRI) shows an empty sella with stalk prolapse.

Courtesy: Dr Bashir Laway, SKIMS.

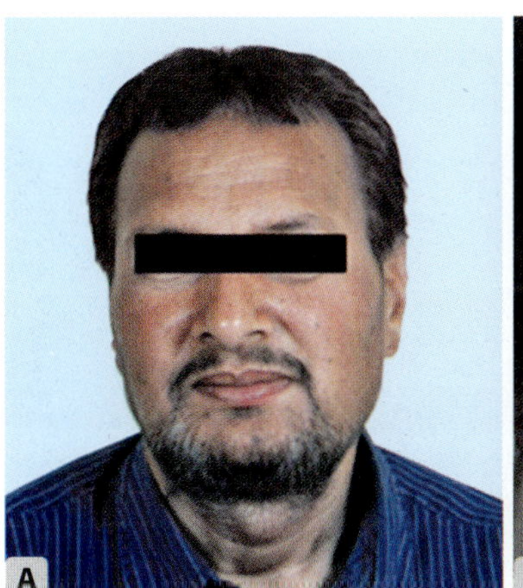

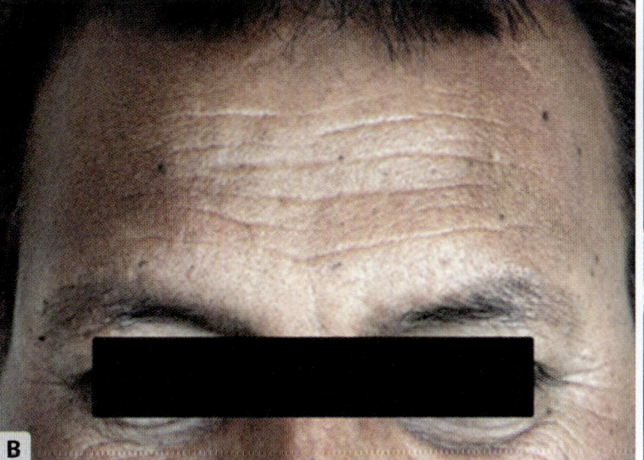

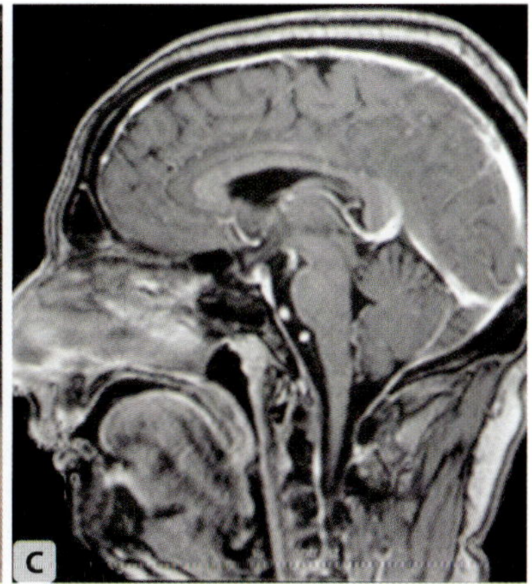

FIGURES 22 A to C: A 43-year-old male presented to the emergency with hyponatremic encephalopathy. On evaluation, he was found to have euvolemic hyponatremia due to secondary hypoadrenalism and hypothyroidism. Clinical photographs of the patient show premature wrinkling on forehead and at the lateral corners of his eyes, suggestive of hypogonadism and growth hormone (GH) deficiency. He was investigated further and indeed, found to have deficiency of GH and secondary hypogonadism. On probing, he revealed history of traumatic brain injury 6 years back in a road traffic accident, without any skull fracture or loss of consciousness. However, he was not evaluated for pituitary hormones at that time or subsequently. Magnetic resonance imaging (MRI) showed empty sella, thereby confirming the diagnosis of post-traumatic hypopituitarism.

Sudden, severe headache with or without cranial nerve (CN) palsies (commonly CN III, IV, and VI) are the most common presentations of an apoplectic event (**Table 6**). Rarely, the event may be radiological alone, without clinical symptoms or signs severe enough to be noted by the patient, termed "radiological apoplexy". Common risk factors for apoplexy include major surgery including coronary artery bypass grafting, hypertension, macroadenoma, trauma, dynamic tests [gonadotropin-releasing hormone (GnRH) and CRH], dopamine agonists, anticoagulant use, coagulopathies, and pregnancy. Although apoplexy has more commonly been described in NFPAs, this may be due to a longer latency and consequently greater prevalence of macroadenomas (**Fig. 23**). Hypocortisolism is the most common pattern of hormone deficiency, but other hormones are also affected. DI is rare.

TABLE 6 Pituitary apoplexy score.

Variable	Points
Level of consciousness	
GCS 15	0
GCS 8–14	2
GCS <8	4
Visual acuity	
Normal or no change from baseline	0
Reduced, unilateral	1
Reduced, bilateral	2
Visual field	
Normal	0
Unilateral	1
Bilateral	2
Ocular paresis	
Absent	0
Present, unilateral	1
Present, bilateral	2

(GCS: Glasgow Coma Scale)

Management of apoplexy involves the mandatory use of steroids immediately. Hydrocortisone 50–100 mg intravenous (IV) q6hrly is a reasonable protocol. Patients in shock may benefit from early administration of normal saline and 5% dextrose to prevent and treat hypoglycemia. Dexamethasone 4–6 mg IV q6–8 hourly is preferred in some settings as it can reduce vasogenic edema and help improve neurological deficits, including consciousness. Worsening visual acuity or fields or nonimprovement of consciousness with medical management are indications for surgery.

DEVELOPMENTAL

Developmental malformational lesions of the pituitary include craniopharyngiomas and Rathke's cleft cysts.

Craniopharyngiomas are tumors arising from the Rathke's pouch (remnant of the craniopharyngeal duct epithelium), an invagination at the roof of the developing mouth. Anatomically, they can be purely sellar, purely suprasellar, or mixed sellar-suprasellar. The two main subtypes include adamantinomatous and papillary varieties. The adamantinomatous variety is more common, may occur in any age group (but predominantly in children aged 5–15 years) and is driven by somatic mutations in catenin beta 1 (CTNNB1) that activates the Wnt pathway. In contrast, papillary craniopharyngiomas (PCPs) are usually limited to adults (50–60 years old) and are characterized by $BRAF^{V600E}$ mutations that activate the mitogen-activated protein kinase (MAPK) pathway (**Figs. 24**). The clinical features in children include headache, visual impairment, and hormone deficiencies whereas adults present with varying degrees of hypopituitarism and psychiatric abnormalities. Central DI may be present in

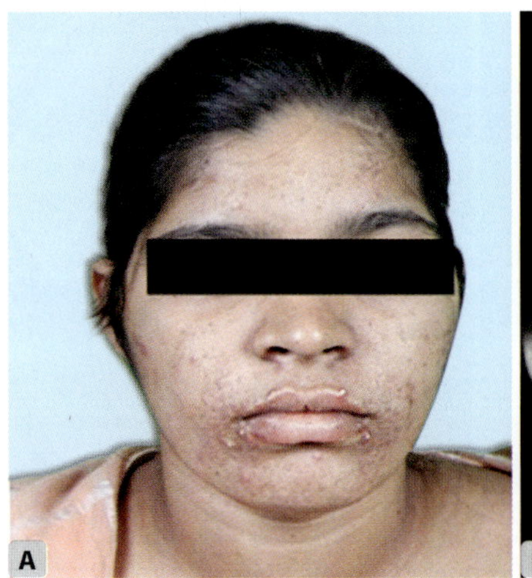

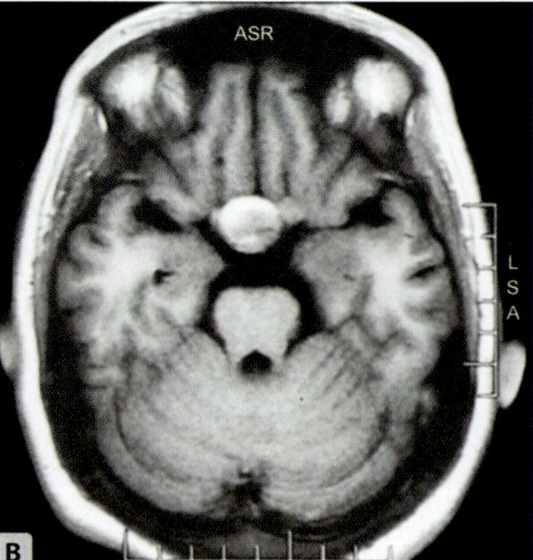

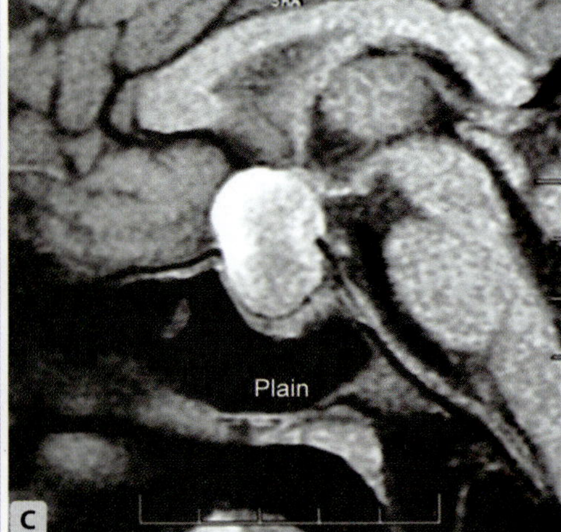

FIGURES 23 A to C: A 25-year-old girl presented with acute worsening of pre-existing headache without any cranial nerve palsies or deterioration in consciousness. She was found to have acral enlargement, coarse facial features, acne and seborrhea and on investigation, was found to have acromegaly with a macrosomatotropinoma. Magnetic resonance imaging (MRI) axial and sagittal images depicting the T1 hyperintensity on noncontrast images, consistent with a diagnosis of pituitary apoplexy at presentation of acromegaly in this young patient.

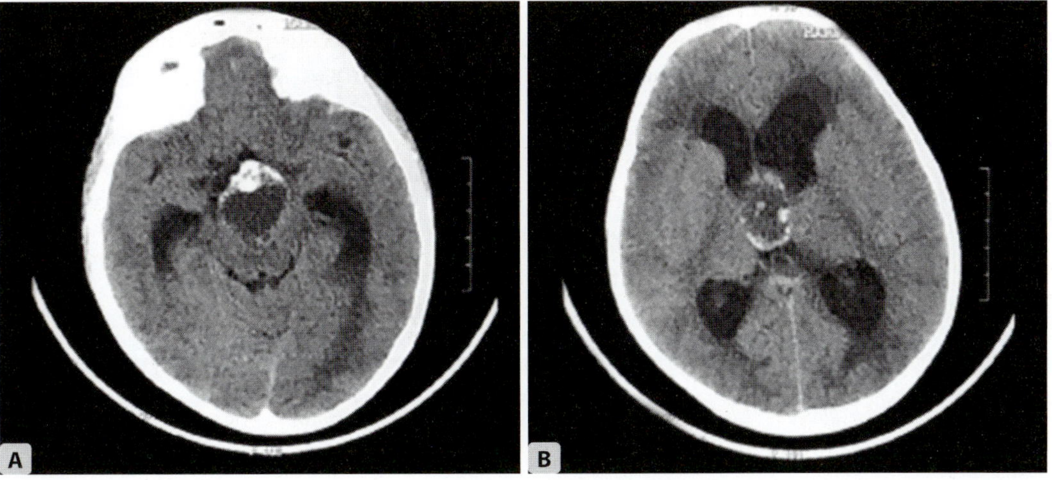

FIGURES 24 A & B: An 8-year-old girl who presented with progressive diminution of vision in her left eye with intermittent headache was found to have a sellar-suprasellar mass with computed tomography (CT) showing a heterogenous mass, central hypodensity representing necrotic/cystic area, and peripheral flocculent calcification. The adjacent CT image depicts hydrocephalus and dilation of lateral ventricles due to the mass.

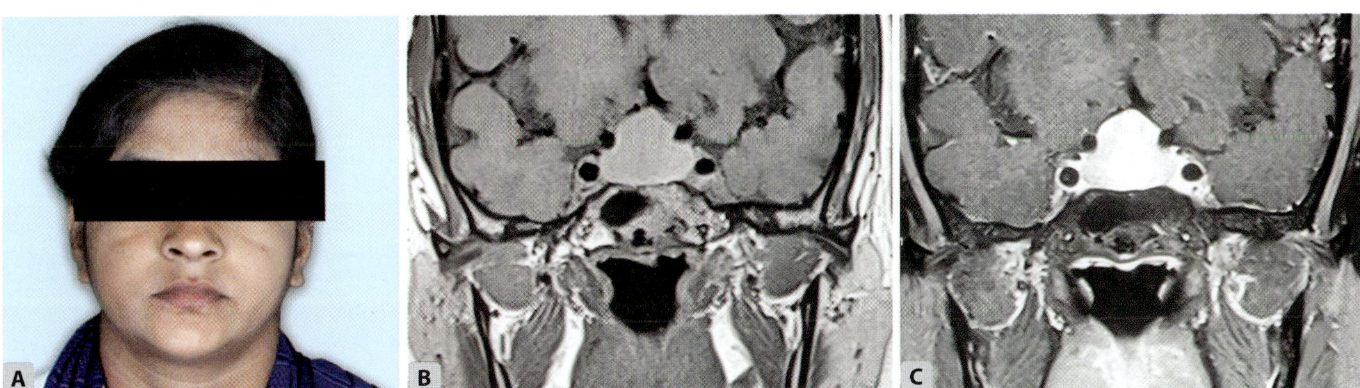

FIGURES 25 A to C: A 19-year-old girl who presented with oligomenorrhea and galactorrhea with breast engorgement. She underwent fine-needle aspiration cytology (FNAC) of breasts outside which was normal. Later, she consulted and was found to have myxedematous features and dry, lusterless skin. Investigations revealed the presence of primary hypothyroidism due to Hashimoto's disease and hyperprolactinemia. Magnetic resonance imaging (MRI) coronal section shows a T1 iso- to hyperintense diffuse enlargement of the pituitary showing intense contrast enhancement of the enlargement.

up to one-fourth of patients prior to surgery, but it is much more common after surgery. Radiological clues include a heterogeneous solid-cystic mass (cystic due to the presence of cholesterol-rich oily fluid) and calcifications. Treatment entails the use of surgery for subtotal to gross total resection with adjuvant radiotherapy. Medical therapy for craniophayngiomas involves the use of inhibitors of the MAPK and MEK pathways and use of intracystic interferon-α (IFN-α), bleomycin or systemic interleukin-6 (IL-6) inhibitors, all with variable efficacy.

Rathke's cleft cysts are benign, sellar suprasellar lesions arising from epithelial remnants of the Rathke's pouch. They contain gelatinous material encapsulated by a thin cyst wall containing pseudostratified cuboidal or columnar epithelium. Commonly, they present with compressive features but rarely, they may be associated with hormone excess. The aim of treatment is to drain the cyst contents and remove the capsule.

HYPERPLASIA

Hyperplasia of the pituitary can occur in multiple physiological conditions such as pregnancy and lactation. There are pathological conditions that can cause hyperplasia, including thyrolactotrope hyperplasia seen in primary hypothyroidism (**Fig. 25**). Other pathological situations include Nelson's syndrome following total bilateral adrenalectomy done for CD.

GENETIC ANALYSIS IN PITUITARY NEUROENDOCRINE TUMORS

The vast majority (95%) of pituitary adenomas are sporadic characterized by somatic or mosaic mutations. The rest 5% cases occur in familial settings. The likelihood of finding a germline mutation in sporadic tumors is low; hence select patients should undergo genetic screening. Common clinical correlates that should arouse a

TABLE 7 Familial causes of pituitary neuroendocrine tumors.

Etiology	Mutation	Presentation/Spectrum of involvement	Clinical clues
MEN1	MEN1 (menin tumor suppressor gene-11q13) CDKN1B, CDKN2C	• Pituitary adenomas (30–40%), prolactinomas most common • PHPT • PNETs • Carcinoids, adrenocortical tumors/nonfunctional adrenomegaly, rarely pheochromocytomas	• Most common and earliest presentation is with PHPT • Other lesions that may be associated include collagenomas, lipomas, angiofibromas, and meningiomas
MEN4	CDKN1B (12p13)	• Pituitary adenomas • PHPT • GEP-NETs • Angiomyolipomas of the kidney, testicular and cervical tumors	No specific clinical findings
Carney complex	PRKAR1A (17q23-24) PDE	• Acromegaly • Prolactinomas • Thyroid adenomas, rarely carcinomas • PPNAD • Sertoli cell tumors • Breast and uterine myxomas	Lentigines, atrial or cutaneous myxomas, blue nevi
SDH	SDH B, SDH D, SDH C, SDH A	• Pituitary adenomas • Pheochromocytoma/paraganglioma • "3P" syndrome	None
FIPA	AIP (11q13)	• Isolated pituitary adenomas • Acromegaly most common	None
XLAG	Gain of function of GPR101	• Acrogigantism • (pituitary hyperplasia)	None
MAS	GNAS (gain of function of α-subunit of GPCR)	• Acrogigantism • Thyroid hyperplasia (nonautoimmune hyperthyroidism) • Rarely, PHPT	• Fibrous dysplasia • Café-au-lait macules

(AIP: Aryl hydrocarbon receptor-interacting protein; FIPA: familial isolated pituitary adenoma; GEP-NETs: gastroenteropancreatic neuroendocrine tumors; GPCR: G protein coupled receptors; MAS: McCune–Albright syndrome; MEN1: multiple endocrine neoplasia type 1; PDE: phosphodiesterase; PHPT: primary hyperparathyroidism; PNETs: pancreatic neuroendocrine tumors; PPNAD: primary pigmented nodular adrenocortical disease; SDH: subdural hematoma; XLAG: X-linked lissencephaly with abnormal genitalia)

suspicion for investigation for underlying genetic causes include:

- Young age
- Syndromic disease
- Positive family history
- Neurocutaneous markers (café-au-lait macules, lipomas, collagenomas, angiofibromas, lentigines, and cutaneous myxomas)

Sporadic causes include GNAS mutations (most common), PKC, PI3K, and USP8 mutations (seen in up to 50% of all patients with CD) (**Table 7**).

Familial causes include syndromic etiologies such as MEN1, MEN4, PKC/PRKAR1A, Carney complex, subdural hematoma (SDH) and familial isolated pituitary adenoma (FIPA) syndromes (most commonly due to AIP mutations) and X-linked acrogigantism (XLAG) mutation (**Table 7**). Nonfamilial postzygotic syndromic cause of pituitary involvement is seen in MAS characterized by fulfillment of any two of the following three criteria: Endocrinopathy (precocious puberty, acrogigantism, nonautoimmune hyperthyroidism, or rarely primary hyperparathyroidism), polyostotic fibrous dysplasia, and café-au-lait macules (not crossing the midline).

ACKNOWLEDGMENTS

We are thankful to Dr Manjul Tripathi, Associate Professor, Department of Neurosurgery, and Dr Chirag Kamal Ahuja, Assistant Professor of Radiology, PGIMER, Chandigarh for helping us prepare this chapter.

RECOMMENDED READINGS

1. Melmed S, Polonsky KS, Larsen PR, Kronenberg HM. Williams Textbook of Endocrinology E-Book. Elsevier Health Sciences.
2. Jameson JL, De Groot LJ. Endocrinology-E-Book: Adult and Pediatric. Elsevier Health Sciences.
3. Katznelson L, Laws Jr ER, Melmed S, Molitch ME, Murad MH, Utz A, et al. Acromegaly: an endocrine society clinical practice guideline. The Journal of Clinical Endocrinology & Metabolism. 2014;99(11):3933-51.
4. Nieman LK, Biller BM, Findling JW, Newell-Price J, Savage MO, Stewart PM, et al. The diagnosis of

Cushing's syndrome: an endocrine society clinical practice guideline. The Journal of Clinical Endocrinology & Metabolism. 2008;93(5):1526-40.

5. Melmed S, Casanueva FF, Hoffman AR, Kleinberg DL, Montori VM, Schlechte JA. Diagnosis and treatment of hyperprolactinemia: An Endocrine Society clinical practice guideline. J Clin Endocrinol Metab. 2011;96(2): 273-88.
6. Barry S, Korbonits M. Update on the genetics of pituitary tumors. Endocrinol Metab Clin North Am. 2020;49(3):433-52.
7. Kaltsas GA, Kolomodi D, Randeva H, Grossman A. Nonneuroendocrine neoplasms of the pituitary region. J Clin Endocrinol Metab. 2019;104:3108-23.
8. Dworakowska D, Grossman AB. The pathophysiology of pituitary adenomas. Best Pract Res Clin Endocrinol Metab. 2009;23:525-41.
9. Melmed S. Pituitary-Tumor Endocrinopathies. N Engl J Med. 2020;382(10):937-950.
10. Joshi MN, Whitelaw BC, Carroll PV. Mechanisms in endocrinology: hypophysitis: Diagnosis and treatment. Eur J Endocrinol. 2018;179:R151-63.

CHAPTER

114

Thyroid Disorders

Suresh Vaikkakara, Avinash Patil

ABSTRACT

Diseases of the thyroid gland are some of the most common endocrine disorders. They may be, by and large classified into three main categories: (1) Hypothyroidism, characterized by reduced thyroid hormone action caused, either by low levels or by resistance to thyroid hormones; (2) Hyperthyroidism with increased thyroid hormone action related either to increased hormone production, or due to excessive release of preformed hormone; (3) Euthyroid patients presenting with diffuse or nodular thyroid enlargement, i.e., goiter. These latter patients may have either benign thyroid enlargement or may harbor a malignancy (papillary, follicular, medullary, anaplastic thyroid carcinoma, or lymphoma as histology).

Primary hypothyroidism may be caused by autoimmunity (Hashimoto's thyroiditis), and prior surgical or radioactive iodine ablation or drugs. Thyroxine replacement, titrated to maintain thyrotropin in the normal range, is the treatment of choice.

Hyperthyroidism due to autoimmune disease (Graves' disease) or due to autonomous thyroid nodules in toxic multinodular goiter (MNG) or toxic adenoma may be managed by medical therapy followed by either surgery or radioactive iodine ablation (in nonremitting cases). Patients with release of preformed hormone (subacute thyroiditis, chronic thyroiditis with transient toxicosis etc.) have self-limited thyrotoxicosis; hence a wait-and-watch appearance is warranted with only symptomatic management in the interim period.

In euthyroid nodular thyroid disease, ultrasound and needle cytology are the key to either diagnose or to assess the risk of malignancy. Benign lesions rarely merit surgery, while malignant lesions require surgery and a structured follow-up with additional radioiodine ablation or chemotherapy/targeted therapy as per well-established guidelines.

"Our entire personality, our energy level, and how we cope is hormonal"

—Sandra T Loh

INTRODUCTION

The thyroid gland is a vital endocrine gland situated in the anterior aspect of the neck that secretes the two thyroid hormones, (1) thyroxine (T4) and (2) triiodothyronine (T3). These hormones released into the blood stream circulate in association with a number of binding proteins including thyroxine-binding globulin (TBG), transthyretin, and albumin to virtually all tissues of the body. After specific uptake into the cells, T4, the inactive form is converted to T3 (by deiodinases), which then binds to the tissue-specific thyroxine receptors (TRα and TRβ), translocates to the nucleus and exerts its effects through the modulation of gene expression via the regulation of their transcription and translation to proteins.

The thyroid hormones enhance a number of physiological processes including but not limited to heat production, energy expenditure, bone turnover, erythropoiesis, gastrointestinal motility, cardiac contractility, heart rate, and free water clearance. In childhood, thyroid hormones promote growth, maturation, and pubertal development. In preschool years, they play a role in arborization and myelination of neurons and the development of the brain including that of intelligence and cognitive functions.

Like many other endocrine glands, the thyroid gland is controlled by the central nervous system by a hypothalamo–pituitary–thyroid (HPT) hormone axis that is influenced both by higher centers in the brain and by the negative feedback of thyroxine on the hypothalamus and the pituitary. The hypothalamus secretes thyrotropin-releasing hormone (TRH) into the hypothalamo–hypophyseal portal circulation, which then stimulates thyrotroph cells in the anterior pituitary to secrete thyrotropin [also known as thyroid-stimulating hormone (TSH)]. The latter in turn stimulates the thyroid gland to produce and release T4 and T3. Circulating T4 is primarily responsible for exerting a negative feedback on the secretion of TRH and TSH by acting on the hypothalamus and pituitary, respectively.

Diseases of the thyroid gland are, by far, some of the most common disorders in the field of Endocrinology. These can be divided into three large categories:

1. *Hypothyroidism*: It is characterized by reduced thyroid hormone action on the body either due to low levels of thyroid hormones or rarely due to resistance of the body tissues to thyroid hormone action.
2. *Thyrotoxicosis/Hyperthyroidism*: It is characterized by an enhanced thyroid hormone action on the body, which may be due to increased thyroid hormone production by the thyroid gland or increased release of preformed stored hormone.
3. *Goiter*: It is an enlargement of the thyroid gland, which includes diffuse enlargement or nodules that may be benign or malignant. Patients with goiter may be metabolically hyperthyroid, hypothyroid, or euthyroid.

In an epidemiological study, from Kochi, Kerala, the prevalence of overt hypothyroidism was 3.9%, that of overt hyperthyroidism was 1.3%, and of goiter was 12% in adults. The age-adjusted incidence of thyroid cancer in the Mumbai cancer registry was 1 per 100,000 in males and 1.8 per 100,000 in females per year.

The metabolic state of thyroid function can best be defined by direct measurement of thyroid hormones in serum by various types of immunoassays including enzyme-linked immunosorbent assays (ELISA), radioimmunoassay (RIA), and chemiluminescence immunoassay (CLIA). Thyroid hormones are elevated in thyrotoxicosis and are low in hypothyroidism. As only the unbound or free thyroid hormones are biologically active, assays have been developed to estimate free T3 and free T4. They are useful, when the levels of binding proteins are altered. Marwaha et al. studied 1,916 adult Indians without any evidence for thyroid disorder and determined that in them, FT3 and FT4 values ranged from 2.4 to 8.8 pmol/L and 10.1 to 24.8 pmol/L, respectively. TSH range in this population was 2.2 ± 0.9 mIU/L.

When the thyrotoxicosis is primarily due to disease of the thyroid gland (i.e., autonomous overproduction or excessive release of preformed stored hormone); negative feedback on hypothalamus and pituitary ensures that the TSH will be low. However, in the rare instance when excessive TSH production from the pituitary is the cause of the thyroid hyperfunction, TSH levels will be either high or will be inappropriately normal relative to the elevated level of thyroid hormones.

TABLE 1 Alterations in Free T4 and thyrotropin in various thyroid states.

Metabolic state	Free thyroxine (T4)	Thyrotropin (TSH)
Primary hypothyroidism	Low	High
Primary hyperthyroidism	High	Low
Subclinical hypothyroidism	Low but still in normal range	High
Subclinical hyperthyroidism	High but still in normal range	Low
Central (secondary) hypothyroidism	Low	Low or inappropriately normal (relative to the low T4) or mildly elevated (but with low bioactivity)
Thyrotropinoma	High	High or inappropriately normal (i.e., nonsuppressed)

In hypothyroidism due to primary thyroid disease, TSH will be high due to reduced thyroid hormone negative feedback. However, in diseases of the pituitary or hypothalamus causing low stimulation of thyroid gland, the low T3 and T4 may be accompanied by no or only minimal elevations of TSH (secondary hypothyroidism). In subclinical hypo- or hyperthyroidism, the thyroid hormones levels per se are normal, while the TSH is high (subclinical hypothyroidism) or low (subclinical hyperthyroidism), respectively.

The usual pattern of thyroid function test alterations in various thyroid disorders is summarized in **Table 1**.

PRIMARY HYPOTHYROIDISM

This is one of the most prevalent endocrine disorders.

ETIOLOGY

Common causes include:

- *Autoimmune destruction of the thyroid gland*: Often associated with a diffuse firm rubbery goiter (Hashimoto's thyroiditis) or with thyroid atrophy (primary myxedema or atrophic thyroiditis), this is by far the most common cause of hypothyroidism in iodine-sufficient areas. In a few cases, the autoimmune destruction follows a use of newer anticancer-targeted therapies such as sunitinib, ipilimumab, pembrolizumab, and nivolumab. In the majority, the autoimmune process is related to genetic susceptibility combined with a favorable environmental influence.
- *Severe iodine deficiency*: With universal iodine supplementation (in salt) program, this is now much less

prevalent than in the past. Less severe deficiency may cause goiter without hypothyroidism.

- *Post thyroidectomy* for treatment of diffuse autoimmune hyperthyroidism (Graves' disease), multinodular goiter, or for thyroid cancer
- *Postradioactive iodine ablation* for hyperthyroidism
- *Drug-induced hypothyroidism*: Excessive exposure to iodine through seaweed consumption, iodinated radiocontrast media, amiodarone etc., can induce hypothyroidism in susceptible persons through persistent inhibition of organification of iodine and coupling of iodotyrosine residues; steps involved in thyroid hormone biosynthesis (persistent Wolff-Chaikoff effect) leads to a condition called iodide myxedema. Lithium, para-aminosalicylicacid, phenylbutazone, aminoglutethimide, and ethionamide are other drugs which interfere with thyroid hormone biosynthesis.
- *Congenital hypothyroidism*: This may be due to inadequate thyroid tissue at birth as seen in agenesis, hemiagenesis, and ectopic thyroid tissue (e.g., lingual thyroid see **Fig. 1**). Congenital disorders associated with defects in thyroid hormone synthesis are usually associated with the presence of goiter, caused by elevation of TSH (dyshormonogenic goiter). These include defects in the sodium-iodine symporter (NIS) that concentrates iodine in the thyroid, thyroid peroxidase (TPO)—the enzyme for organification and coupling processes, pendrin (Pendred syndrome—sensory neural deafness with dyshormonogenic goiter), thyroglobulin, and iodotyrosine dehalogenase. Inactivating mutations in *TSH receptor* gene cause hypothyroidism without goiter.

A more detailed list of causes of primary hypothyroidism is given in **Table 2**.

CLINICAL FEATURES

The consequences of hypothyroidism are different for adults and children. System-wise clinical features of hypothyroidism are given in **Table 3**.

Congenital hypothyroidism if not detected and treated at birth is associated with poor feeding, lethargy, hoarse cry, puffy face, protruded tongue, constipation, and prolonged neonatal jaundice. Further delay in diagnosis is associated with delayed closure of fontanelles, flat nasal bridge, delayed appearance of teeth, poor growth, global delay in milestones, distension of abdomen, and everted umbilicus ultimately resulting in short stature and severe mental retardation—a condition known as cretinism.

Hypothyroidism developing in childhood but after the preschool years (juvenile hypothyroidism) is associated with short stature and delayed puberty.

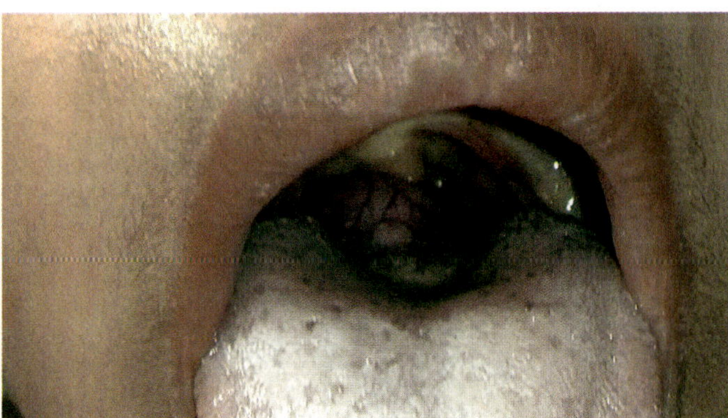

FIGURE 1: Ectopic thyroid tissue at the base of the tongue—lingual thyroid.

DIAGNOSIS

The diagnosis of primary hypothyroidism is made when the T4 levels are low and the TSH is elevated. Central

TABLE 2 Causes of primary hypothyroidism.

Broad mechanism	Specific etiology
Autoimmune	• Hashimoto's thyroiditis • Hypothyroid phase of chronic thyroiditis with transient toxicosis
Postinfectious (viral)	Hypothyroid phase of subacute thyroiditis
Postsurgery	• Total, near-total thyroidectomy • Some cases of subtotal thyroidectomy
Postirradiation	• Postradioactive iodine ablation • Post external beam irradiation for neck malignancies
Nutrient deficiency	Severe iodine deficiency
Dietary and environmental goitrogens	• Iodide excess due to seaweed consumption • Thiocyanates in vegetables of *Cruciferae/Brassica* family (cabbage, turnip, and mustard) • Linamarin in cassava meal
Drugs	• Multiple actions: Iodine, amiodarone, lithium, iodine-containing radio-contrast media • Synthesis: Para-aminosalicylic acid, phenylbutazone, aminoglutethimide, ethionamide • Autoimmunity: Ipilimumab, pembrolizumab, nivolumab, sunitinib, interferon α, interleukin-2
Congenital	• Agenesis • Hemiagenesis • Ectopic thyroid (including lingual thyroid) • Hypoplasia (inactivation mutation of TSH receptor) • Sodium/iodide symporter defect • Thyroid peroxidase defect • Pendred syndrome • Thyroglobulin defect • Iodotyrosine dehalogenase defect
Infiltrative disorders	Amyloidosis, hemochromatosis, Riedel's thyroiditis

TABLE 3 Clinical features and findings on investigation in patients with hypothyroidism.

System	Symptom	Sign	Investigation abnormality
Skin	• Dry skin • Puffiness of face • Increased scalp hair loss	• Dry, cold, pale or yellow skin • Brittle lusterless hair • Generalized nonpitting edema (myxedema)	• Accumulation of glycosaminoglycans (GAG) in the dermis in skin biopsy
Nervous system	• Lethargy • Fatigue • Increased sleepiness • Poor memory • Headache • Hearing loss • Numbness and tingling of hands and feet • Night blindness	• Cerebellar ataxia • Slowness of activity and speech • Delayed relaxation of deep tendon reflexes (hung up reflexes) • Apparent enlargement of muscles particularly calf muscles (pseudohypertrophy) • Both sensorineural and conductive deafness	• Electrophysiology may show compression of median nerve at the carpal tunnel (carpal tunnel syndrome) • Elevated creatine kinase (CK)
Gastrointestinal system	• Constipation • Reduced appetite • Minor weight gain	Gaseous distension of abdomen	• Imaging findings of fatty liver, ascites and megacolon • Elevated carcinoembryonic antigen (CEA) • Elevated aspartate aminotransferase
Hematological system	• Poor wound healing • Increased bruisability	Pallor	• Typically normocytic normochromic anemia • Concomitant iron, B12 and folate deficiency anemias also common
Cardiovascular	Unmasking or worsening of angina pectoris after initiation of treatment	• Bradycardia • Diastolic hypertension • Narrow-pulse pressure • Cardiac enlargement • Muffled heart sounds and signs of tamponade (in case of pericardial effusion)	• Sinus bradycardia in ECG • Cardiomegaly on chest X-ray PA view • Pericardial effusion with or without tamponade on echocardiography • Elevated homocysteine ,C-reactive protein (CRP) • Elevated cardiac enzymes: Creatine kinase, lactate dehydrogenase, aspartate transaminase
Respiratory	• Hoarseness of voice • Snoring	Enlarged tongue: Macroglossia	• Obstructive sleep apnea on polysomnography • Hypercapnia in severe cases
Renal			Hyponatremia
Reproductive and endocrine	• Reduced libido • Erectile dysfunction • Infertility • Menorrhagia • Spontaneous abortion	Galactorrhea (rare)	• Oligospermia • Anovulation • Reduced sex hormone binding globulin (SHBG) • Hyperprolactinemia • Reduced GH and IGF-1 • Increased total cholesterol, LDL cholesterol and triglycerides

(IGF-1: insulin-like growth factor-1; PA: posteroanterior)

hypothyroidism due to pituitary/hypothalamic disease is diagnosed when the TSH is low, normal, or only minimally elevated in the context of a low T4. In patients with receptor level resistance to thyroid hormones (loss of function mutation in TRβ), T3 and T4 are both elevated, while TSH is moderately elevated or inappropriately normal.

Autoimmune thyroid disease should be looked for in patients with acquired hypothyroidism who do not give a history of surgery, radioiodine ablation or use of relevant drugs. It can be confirmed by detecting elevated levels of antithyroid peroxidase and/or antithyroglobulin antibodies.

TREATMENT

The treatment of hypothyroidism is to replace the thyroid hormone deficiency with levothyroxine. This may require a dose of 1.6 μg/kg body weight of thyroxine—usually taken in an empty stomach. Young adults may receive the estimated full dose from the very beginning. Older individuals with underlying heart disease require slowly escalating doses, starting with 25 μg/day and gradually increasing with small increments (12.5–25 μg) at monthly intervals to maximally tolerated doses. Starting at full dose or escalating rapidly may lead to palpitation or precipitation of angina. Patients with severe, long-standing hypothyroidism, and those with central hypothyroidism having documented adrenal insufficiency must receive glucocorticoid replacement before starting thyroxine to avoid precipitation of crisis due to adrenal insufficiency.

Dose of thyroxine is titrated by monitoring the TSH—to keep it in the normal range for the given laboratory. As thyroxine has a half-life of 1 week, TSH levels should be tested at around 6 weeks after every dose change. Once the dose has been stabilized, TSH done annually may suffice to monitor patients in the long term. Target TSH is <2.5 mIU/L in pregnant women with hypothyroidism receiving thyroxine.

HYPERTHYROIDISM

This could be further classified into two broad categories: Hyperthyroidism due to increased hormone production and that due to excessively rapid release of preformed hormone (release toxicosis).

ETIOLOGY

Causes of thyrotoxicosis due to increased production are chiefly three:

1. **Graves' disease:** This is an autoimmune disease characterized by the presence of an antibody in circulation that binds to and stimulates the TSH receptor. Like many other autoimmune disorders, it is nearly four times commoner in women than men and affects individuals in their youth or middle age. It is a multisystem disease with involvement of eyes (Graves' ophthalmopathy) and skin (Graves' dermopathy) as well. The goiterous enlargement seen in around 50% of the patients is diffuse and soft.
2. **Toxic MNG:** This is a long-standing thyroid enlargement that over time becomes nodular and functionally autonomous of pituitary control. It occurs in middle-to-older age groups.
3. **Toxic adenoma:** This single nodule in an otherwise normal gland represents a true benign monoclonal neoplasm, often due to an activating mutation in the TSH receptor and therefore produces thyroid hormones autonomously. It presents in the fourth to fifth decades of life.

Toxicosis due to release of preformed hormone: Inflammation in the thyroid gland following a viral illness (subacute thyroiditis) or as a consequence of an autoimmune process (chronic thyroiditis with transient toxicosis) often occurring postpartum (postpartum thyroiditis) or inflammation caused by drugs [sunitinib, sorafenib, granulocyte-macrophage colony-stimulating factor (GM-CSF), interferon α etc.] can result in release of preformed T4 with transient toxicosis. The toxicosis resolves rapidly as the thyroid hormone stores get depleted and may be followed by a phase of hypothyroidism, which ultimately gives way to final euthyroid state in most cases. Permanent hypothyroidism can occur in some patients on long-term follow-up.

A more detailed potential list of causes of thyrotoxicosis is given below in **Table 4**.

TABLE 4 Causes of thyrotoxicosis.

Broad category	Mechanism	Disease
Overproduction of thyroxin	Overstimulation by hCG	• Trophoblastic disease • Hyperemesis gravidarum • Familial gestational thyrotoxicosis
	Overstimulation by TSH	Thyrotropinoma
	Overstimulation by stimulating anti-TSH receptor antibody	Graves' disease
	Autonomous thyroid hyperfunction	• Toxic multinodular goiter • Toxic adenoma
	Extrathyroidal production of excess thyroid hormone	• Functional thyroid cancer metastasis • Struma ovarii
Excessively rapid release of stored preformed hormone	Autoimmune thyroiditis	Chronic thyroiditis with transient toxicosis including postpartum thyroiditis
	Postviral thyroiditis	Subacute thyroiditis
	Drug induced thyroiditis	• Amiodarone-induced thyrotoxicosis (type 2) • Interferon α
Excessive oral consumption of thyroid hormones	Thyroxine tablets	• Iatrogenic hyperthyroidism • Thyrotoxicosis factitia (deliberate or accidental)
	Consumption of animal thyroid-containing products in foodstuffs	E.g., Hamburger toxicosis

(hCG: human chorionic gonadotrophin)

TABLE 5 Clinical features and findings on investigation in hyperthyroidism.

System	Symptoms	Signs/Investigation abnormalities
Skeletal	Increased susceptibility to fractures	Hypercalcemia, osteoporosis, increased bone turnover markers
Skin	Heat intolerance, sweating, alopecia	Plethora, perspiration, fine skin texture, palmar erythema, onycholysis
Nervous system	Anxiety, insomnia, tremulousness, periodic paralysis	• Fine action tremor of hands, eyelids, tongue • Exaggerated deep tendon reflexes
Gastrointestinal system	• Increased appetite • Weight loss • Frequent passage of formed stools (hyperdefecation)	Increased liver enzymes and hyperbilirubinemia in severe cases
Cardiovascular	• Palpitation • Dyspnea • Onset or worsening of angina pectoris • Mild swelling of feet	• Tachycardia • Atrial fibrillation • Systolic hypertension and diastolic hypotension and thus a wide-pulse pressure • Flow murmurs • High-output congestive cardiac failure
Eyes	Prominent stare	• Lid retraction with exposure of sclera • Lid lags behind globe on looking down exposing upper sclera • Globe lags behind lid on looking up
Reproductive and endocrine	• Frequent menstruation • Amenorrhea • Infertility • Gynecomastia • Erectile dysfunction	Hyperglycemia, reduced cholesterol

CLINICAL FEATURES

These are summarized below in **Table 5**.

A diffuse soft goiter with a palpable thrill and an audible bruit is typical of Graves' disease. Graves' ophthalmopathy is characterized by forward protrusion of eyes (exophthalmos), redness of eyelids, and conjunctiva and diplopia due to extraocular muscle weakness. Severe cases may have sight-threatening disease due to corneal exposure or due to compression of the optic nerve (dysthyroid optic neuropathy). On occasion, such eye disease may also be seen in euthyroid or in hypothyroid individuals with Hashimoto's thyroiditis.

Dermopathy may consist of itching and nonpitting edema over the shins and feet (pretibial myxedema)—see **Figure 2**. A clubbing-like phenomenon on the digits in Graves' is called thyroid acropachy.

These additional features in the eyes and skin are lacking in toxic MNG or in toxic adenoma. The architecture of the goiter (multinodular or solitary nodule) serves to differentiate them from Graves' disease.

Subacute thyroiditis, occurs in the aftermath of a viral upper respiratory infection and is associated with a tender thyroid gland, low-grade fever, malaise, and an elevated erythrocyte sedimentation rate (ESR). Chronic thyroiditis with transient toxicosis occurs usually in the postpartum setting (postpartum thyroiditis) and is by and large painless.

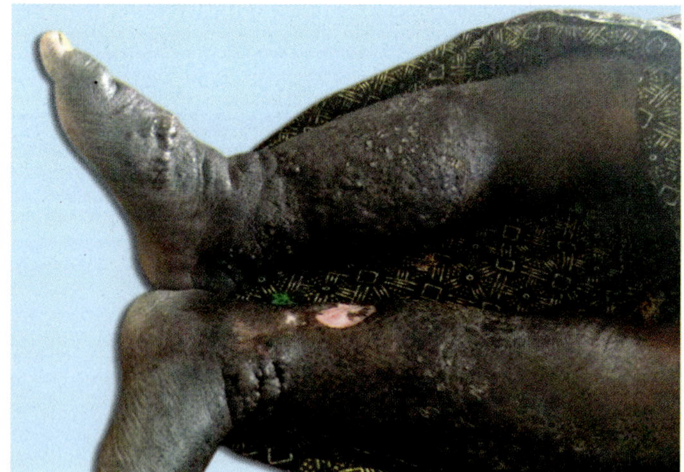

FIGURE 2: Thickened, hyperpigmented plaques on the skin of both shins and feet—pretibial myxedema.

INVESTIGATIONS

In overt primary hyperthyroidism, the thyroid hormones T3 and T4 are elevated, while the TSH is suppressed (due to the negative feedback of the elevated T3 and T4 on HPT axis). An ultrasound of the thyroid may reveal diffuse thyroid architecture in Graves, multiple thyroid nodules of various sizes in toxic MNG, and a solitary nodule in toxic adenoma.

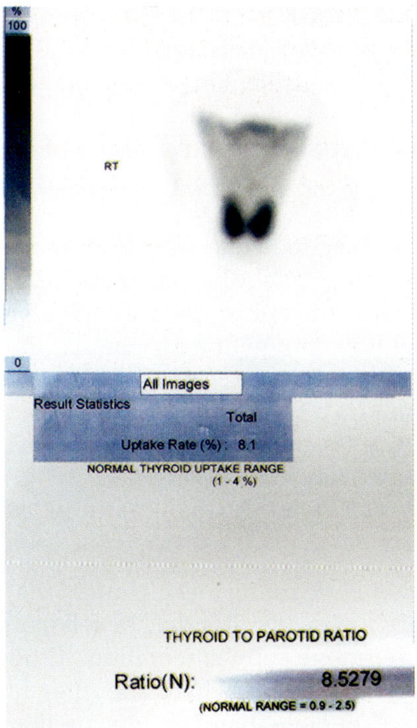

(Tc^{99m}: technetium-99m)

FIGURE 3: Tc^{99m} thyroid scintigraphy showing diffuse increased uptake in a patient with thyrotoxicosis suggestive of Graves' disease.

Uptake studies of radioactive isotopes of iodine (I^{123} or I^{131}) or technetium-99m (Tc^{99m}) into the thyroid (via the Na/I symporter on the thyroid cell surface) are useful nuclear medicine imaging modalities to directly quantify the function of the thyroid. While uptake is high in Graves', toxic MNG, and toxic adenoma, it is low or virtually undetectable in subacute thyroiditis, chronic thyroiditis with transient toxicosis, and other forms of release toxicosis.

The pattern of uptake as seen on thyroid scintigraphy is diffuse in Graves' (see **Fig. 3**), patchy in MNG, and confined to the solitary nodule in toxic adenoma (rest of the gland having reduced uptake).

TREATMENT

Medical management of Graves' disease revolves around the use of thionamides—carbimazole, methimazole, and propylthiouracil (PTU). These drugs inhibit organification and coupling steps in thyroid hormone synthesis and may also have immunomodulatory properties. These are started at higher doses (10–40 mg methimazole per day or 50–150 mg PTU thrice a day) till the patient becomes euthyroid—usually at 6 weeks to 3 months. The doses are then down titrated to the lowest dose required to maintain euthyroidism, with frequent monitoring of serum T4, aiming to keep it in the normal range. Treatment may be continued thus for 12–18 months after which attempts are made to withdraw the medication. Only one third of Graves' disease patients enter into lasting remission, not needing further management, other than annual estimation of T4.

When palpitation, tremor, or hypokalemic periodic paralysis are troublesome issues for the patient, the nonspecific beta-blocker propranolol may relieve these symptoms in the initial stages, while the patient is still hyperthyroid.

Common side effects of thionamides include skin rash and joint pains. Rarely patients may develop agranulocytosis, necessitating drug withdrawal. Because PTU is associated with fulminant hepatic failure on rare occasions, use of this drug is reserved for pregnant women in early pregnancy (due to its lower fetal mutagenic potential than carbimazole/methimazole) and for those with severe thyrotoxicosis with impending metabolic decompensation (due to the property of PTU to impair conversion from T4 to T3 at high doses, it acts more rapidly than methimazole).

In the patients where the disease does not remit or when recurrence occurs, consideration may be given for a lasting relief by *ablation of thyroid tissue either by surgery (near total thyroidectomy) or by the administration of radioactive iodine* (10–15 mCi of I^{131}), enough to render the patient hypothyroid. Radioactive iodine is concentrated in thyroid tissue by the action of Na/I symporter. It destroys the thyroid gland by radiation damage (necrosis and fibrosis) over the next 3–6 months. Subsequently patients are given thyroxine replacement as mentioned above in the section on hypothyroidism.

Near-total thyroidectomy is associated with the long-term risk of permanent hypoparathyroidism and of recurrent laryngeal nerve injury. These complications are rare (<2%) in expert hands. Likewise, radioactive iodine ablation is associated with the risk of developing or worsening of eye disease (around 15%). Conception must be postponed by at least 6 months after an ablative dose of radioactive iodine.

Toxic MNG and toxic adenoma do not have a natural history of remission. Hence after controlling the thyrotoxicosis with drugs, these patients are subjected to either surgery (near-total thyroidectomy for MNG and adenoma removal for toxic adenoma) or radioactive iodine ablation.

The choice of ablative therapy; surgery versus radioactive iodine ablation depends on several factors. Large goiters (>80 g) in MNG and Graves' and adenoma >5 cm diameter and goiters suspected to be harboring a malignancy are usually operated upon. Likewise, surgery is the choice for patients with active, moderate-to-severe eye disease and when the couple desires a pregnancy within the next 6 months.

EUTHYROID GOITER

Euthyroid goiterous enlargement of the thyroid gland may be diffuse (simple goiter), multinodular, or a solitary thyroid nodule.

A prior simple goiter is believed to evolve over time into a MNG. These enlargements may be caused by iodine deficiency or local environmental factors including local dietary goitrogens and then tends to occur in certain geographical areas (endemic goiter), e.g., in mountainous locales such as the Himalayas or Andes regions where soil is deficient in iodine. Other goiters occur in a familial manner or sporadically and may be due to subtle defects in thyroid

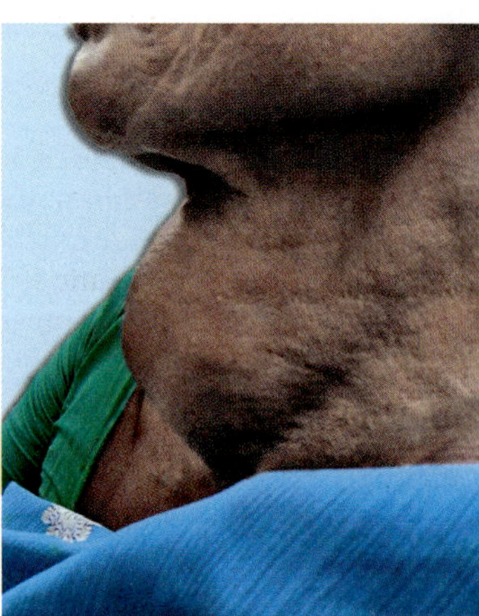

FIGURE 4: Large thyroid swelling on the anterior aspect of neck—a goiter.

hormone biosynthesis, dietary goitrogens, genetic factors, drugs, or unknown factors.

Goiters present as swellings in the neck (**Fig. 4**) that may be unsightly or when massive cause compression of trachea or esophagus or the superior vena cava as they extend down retrosternally. Nontoxic MNGs may evolve into toxic MNG over time as the nodules gain autonomy. Any nodule in the neck may raise the suspicion of malignancy and cause the patient to seek medical attention.

Once blood investigations confirm that T4 and TSH are normal, an ultrasound of the neck supplements the clinical examination to determine the true architecture of the thyroid gland (diffuse vs. MNG vs. solitary nodule) and the extent of the goiter. In nodular goiter, it helps to select out nodules for cytological evaluation.

The high-risk features on ultrasonography in a nodule are irregular margins, microcalcifications, greater anterio-posterior than transverse diameter, rim calcifications with small extrusion of soft-tissue component, and evidence of extrathyroidal extension. Solid hypoechoic nodules or solid hypoechoic component of partially cystic nodules with above features (highly suspicious) or without these features (intermediate suspicion) are subjected to fine-needle aspiration cytology (FNAC) when they are >1 cm in diameter. Iso- or hyperechoic solid nodules without any suspicious features are considered to be at low risk and are subjected to FNAC if nodules > 1.5 cm in diameter. Partially cystic nodules and spongiform nodules without any high-risk features are considered to have very low suspicion and should be cytologically assessed only above a threshold of 2 cm. Pure cystic lesions do not need to undergo FNAC. This sonological risk stratification is as per the American Thyroid Association guidelines of 2015 on thyroid nodules.

Once the nodules are selected for FNAC based on ultrasound, the risk of malignancy is again assessed based on FNAC using the Bethesda classification system (latest revision 2017).

- Category I consists of those FNACs which are nondiagnostic or unsatisfactory.
- Category II is clearly benign (malignancy risk 0–3%)
- Category III is known as atypia of undetermined significance (AUS) or follicular lesion of undetermined significance (FLUS) and may carry a 10–30% risk of malignancy.
- Category IV, i.e., follicular neoplasm or suspicious for follicular neoplasm may be malignant in 25–40%. FNAC alone is not sufficient to resolve follicular neoplasms into follicular adenoma or carcinoma, the distinction depends on blood vessel or capsule invasion and is defined only on a biopsy specimen.
- Category V is "Suspicious of malignancy." It is associated with a 50–75% risk of malignancy.
- Category VI is clearly malignant (97–99% risk of malignancy).

Management of euthyroid goiters: Goiters that are diffuse or harbor only benign nodules may be left alone or treated with thyroid hormone supplementation. Although around 60% may reduce in size on thyroxine, they tend to recur on stopping treatment—thereby reducing the enthusiasm to treat in this manner. Unsightly nodules or those with compressive symptoms may be treated with surgery—either removal of nodule or lobectomy or near-total thyroidectomy depending on extent of the disease. Management of toxic nodules has already been discussed in the earlier text.

Malignancy of the thyroid could be follicular, cell derived, C-cell derived (medullary carcinoma) or a lymphoma. The former are further divided into well-differentiated (papillary, follicular or Hurthle cell types) or poorly differentiated (including the anaplastic type).

Management of malignant nodules is surgery (either lobectomy or near-total thyroidectomy) with appropriate lymph node management based on histology and stage of the disease. Postsurgery, selected patients receive radioactive I^{131} ablation. They are then followed up with tumor markers (thyroglobulin for follicular cell-derived carcinomas and calcitonin/carcinoembryonic antigen (CEA) for medullary thyroid cancers) for presence of residual disease. Details of surgery and follow-up are beyond the scope of this chapter.

Lesions in Bethesda categories I, III, and IV require close follow-up, repeated FNACs, and additional diagnostic procedures including molecular diagnostics. Category V patients are usually subjected to surgery (near-total thyroidectomy or lobectomy) followed by histopathology.

RECOMMENDED READINGS

1. Usha Menon V, Sundaram KR, Unnikrishnan AG, Jayakumar RV, Nair V, Kumar H. High prevalence of undetected thyroid disorders in an iodine sufficient adult south Indian population. J Indian Med Assoc. 2009;107(2):72-7.
2. Unnikrishnan AG, Usha Menon V. Thyroid disorders in India: An epidemiological perspective. Indian J Endocrinol Metab. 2011;15 (Suppl 2):S78-81.

3. Marwaha RK, Tandon N, Ganie MA, Mehan N, Sastry A, Garg MK. Reference range of thyroid function (FT3, FT4 and TSH) among Indian adults. Clin Biochem. 2013;46(4-5):341-5.
4. Alexander EK, Pearce EN, Brent GA, Brown RS, Chen H, Dosiou C, et al. 2017 Guidelines of the American Thyroid Association for the Diagnosis and Management of thyroid disease during pregnancy and the postpartum. Thyroid. 2017;27(3):315-89.
5. Ross DS, Burch HB, Cooper DS, Greenlee MC, Laurberg P, Maia AL, et al. 2016 American Thyroid Association Guidelines for Diagnosis and Management of Hyperthyroidism and Other Causes of Thyrotoxicosis. Thyroid. 2016;26(10):1343-421.
6. Haugen BR, Alexander EK, Bible KC, Doherty GM, Mandel SJ, Nikiforov YE, et al. 2015 American Thyroid Association Management Guidelines for adult patients with thyroid nodules and differentiated thyroid cancer: The American Thyroid Association Guidelines Task Force on Thyroid Nodules and Differentiated Thyroid Cancer. Thyroid. 2016;26:1-133.
7. Cibas ES, Ali SZ. The 2017 Bethesda System for Reporting Thyroid Cytopathology. Thyroid. 2017;27(11): 1341-46.

CHAPTER 115

Disorders of Adrenal Gland

Rama Walia, Rajat Gupta

ABSTRACT

This chapter discusses the disorders of adrenal glands. To begin with, adrenal steroidogenesis and its feedback mechanisms are discussed. Later on, this chapter includes very important endocrine disorders such as Cushing syndrome, adrenal insufficiency, adrenal incidentalomas, primary hyperaldosteronism, and pheochromocytoma (PCC). The precise and latest information about etiopathogenesis, diagnostic approach, and treatment is given about each of these topics.

"Symptoms are the body's mother tongue; signs are a foreign language"

—John Brown

THE ADRENAL GLAND

ANATOMY

The adrenal glands (two in number) are pyramidal-shaped structures lying on the posteromedial surface of each kidney. Adrenal gland has outer adrenal cortex and inner adrenal medulla.

FUNCTIONS

Adrenal cortex: From outward to inward, adrenal cortex has three distinct zones:

1. *Zona glomerulosa*: Produces glucocorticoids (cortisol) under the stimulation of adrenocorticotropic hormone (ACTH)
2. *Zona fasciculata*: Produces mineralocorticoids (aldosterone) under the stimulation of angiotensin II
3. *Zona reticularis*: Produces androgen precursors [dehydroepiandrosterone (DHEA), dehydroepiandrosterone sulfate (DHEAS), androstenedione] and small amount of testosterone

Details of adrenal steroid synthesis and enzymes involved are mentioned in **Figure 1**.

Adrenal medulla: It produces catecholamines (epinephrine, norepinephrine, and dopamine).

GLUCOCORTICOID SECRETION

The hypothalamic–pituitary–adrenal axis: Corticotropin-releasing hormone (CRH), a 41-amino acid peptide secreted from the paraventricular nucleus of hypothalamus, stimulates ACTH secretion from the anterior pituitary. ACTH, a 39-amino acid peptide, in turn stimulates adrenal glucocorticoid biosynthesis and secretion. Secretion of CRH and ACTH is inhibited by cortisol in a negative feedback manner. Various physical stressors, acute psychological stress, and depression lead to increased cortisol secretion by stimulating CRH secretion. Arginine vasopressin (AVP) and various proinflammatory cytokines (interleukin 1, interleukin 6, TNF-α) increase cortisol secretion by stimulating ACTH secretion.

Circadian rhythm: ACTH, and hence cortisol, are secreted in a pulsatile manner with a circadian rhythm, levels being highest on awakening (5 AM to 9 AM) and then declining throughout the day to reach a nadir at midnight.

Cholesterol
↓
Pregnenolone -3βHSD → Progesterone -21α Hy →11-DOC -11β Hy → Corticosterone – AS → Aldosterone
↓17α Hy ↓17α Hy
17 OH Pregnenolone -3βHSD → 17 OH Progesterone-21α Hy → 11-Deoxycortisol -11β Hy → Cortisol
↓17, 20 Lyase ↓ 17, 20 Lyase
DHEA -3βHSD → Androstenedione -17βHSD → Testosterone -5α reductase → Dihydrotestosterone
↓Sulfotransferase ↓Aromatase ↓Aromatase
DHEAS Estrone -17βHSD → Estradiol

(AS: aldosterone synthase; DHEA: dehydroepiandrosterone; DHEAS: dehydroepiandrosterone sulfate; DOC: deoxycorticosterone; Hy: Hydroxylase; 3βHSD: 3β-hydroxysteroid dehydrogenase/Δ5→Δ4 isomerase)

FIGURE 1: Adrenal steroidogenesis.

MINERALOCORTICOID SECRETION

The renin–angiotensin–aldosterone axis: Renin secreted from juxtaglomerular cells in the kidney converts angiotensinogen (from liver) to angiotensin I. Angiotensin I is converted in the lungs by angiotensin-converting enzyme (ACE) into angiotensin II. Renin release is stimulated by low tubular sodium content and low renal perfusion pressure. Angiotensin II stimulates aldosterone synthesis and secretion. In addition to angiotensin II, potassium also directly stimulates aldosterone secretion. ACTH has very little impact on aldosterone secretion, only in acute setting.

ADRENAL ANDROGEN SECRETION

Adrenocorticotropic hormone stimulates adrenal androgen secretion. Adrenal androgens constitute >50% of circulating androgens in premenopausal females. This fraction is much smaller in males. Adrenal glands secrete DHEA, DHEAS, androstenedione, and a very small amount of testosterone.

CORTICOSTEROID HORMONE ACTION

More than 90 % of circulating cortisol is bound to corticosteroid-binding globulin (CBG). Changes in CBG results in parallel change in total cortisol concentration but free hormone concentration remains same. Glucocorticoid and mineralocorticoid exert their effects via binding to nuclear receptor, termed glucocorticoid receptor (GR) and mineralocorticoid receptor (MR), respectively. GR and MR share considerable homology. Steroid binds to the receptor in cytosol and then the steroid–receptor complex translocates to the nucleus. The nucleus receptor binds to the specific DNA sequences in the promoter region of target gene (glucocorticoid response element) to stimulate or inhibit gene transcription.

Effects of glucocorticoids:

- Increase blood glucose concentration: By increasing gluconeogenesis and insulin resistance
- Increase visceral obesity: By promoting adipogenesis
- Muscle and skin atrophy: By inhibiting muscle protein synthesis and inhibiting epidermal cell division and collagen synthesis
- Osteopenia and osteoporosis: By inhibiting osteoblast function
- Osteonecrosis/avascular necrosis: Primarily affects femoral head by inducing osteocyte apoptosis
- Inhibit intestinal calcium absorption and increases renal calcium excretion
- Inhibit linear skeletal growth by its catabolic effects on bone, muscle, and connective tissues and through inhibition of the effects of insulin-like growth factor-1 (IGF-1)
- Suppress the secretion of TSH and growth hormone and reduces pulsatility of gonadotropin-releasing hormone (GnRH) and hence luteinizing hormone/follicle-stimulating hormone (LH/FSH) release.
- In kidneys, glucocorticoids cause sodium retention and potassium loss (via action on MR) and free water clearance (via antagonism of vasopressin).
- Increase neutrophil counts, and decrease lymphocyte and eosinophil counts. Inhibit lymphocytes cytokine production [by inhibiting nuclear factor kappa B (NF-κ B) action] and immunoglobulin synthesis
- Cause euphoria, psychosis, depression, and apathy
- Raise intraocular pressure by increase in aqueous humor production and inhibiting its drainage
- Long-term use can cause peptic ulcer disease and pancreatitis.

GLUCOCORTICOID EXCESS

CUSHING SYNDROME

Cushing syndrome (CS) is a group of signs and symptoms caused by chronic exposure to excess glucocorticoids (endogenous/exogenous). The first ever case was published by Harvey Cushing in 1932 (a case of basophil adenoma of the pituitary). The term *Cushing disease* is reserved for pituitary-dependent Cushing syndrome. While endogenous Cushing syndrome is a rare disease (incidence—two to three cases per 1 million population per year), exogenous Cushing syndrome is common. The clinical features of Cushing syndrome are summarized in **Table 1**.

Causes of Cushing syndrome (Box 1):

Endogenous cushing syndrome:

ACTH-dependent causes:

- *Cushing disease (pituitary dependent)*: Cushing disease accounts for about 70% of all cases of endogenous Cushing syndrome. ACTH-secreting pituitary adenoma (microadenoma 90% and macroadenoma 10%) is the cause of Cushing disease in most of the cases; with very few are caused by basophil hyperplasia alone.
- *Ectopic ACTH syndrome*: Ectopic ACTH-secreting tumors account for about 15% of all cases of endogenous Cushing syndrome. Small-cell lung carcinoma, pancreatic neuroendocrine tumors with high proliferative rate, and bronchial neuroendocrine tumors with low proliferative rate (carcinoids) are the most common tumors associated with ectopic ACTH syndrome. While ACTH-secreting indolent tumors present such as classical Cushing syndrome, malignant tumors present with hyperpigmentation, myopathy, weight loss, hypokalemic alkalosis, and peripheral edema.
- *Macronodular adrenal hyperplasia*: Few patients with long-standing Cushing disease, bilateral adrenal hyperplasia is associated with one or more autonomous adrenal adenoma formation. So adrenals secrete more cortisol for a given ACTH level, which ultimately can lead to autosuppression.

ACTH-independent causes:

- *Adrenal adenoma and carcinoma*: Adrenal adenomas account for about 10–15% and adrenal carcinomas account for about 5% of all cases of endogenous Cushing syndrome. However in children, adrenal carcinomas and adenoma cause about 50 and 15% all cases of endogenous Cushing syndrome, respectively. Adrenal carcinoma sometimes cosecrete adrenal androgens, so females may present with hirsutism and clitoromegaly.
- *Primary pigmented nodular adrenal hyperplasia (PPNAD) and Carney syndrome*: ACTH-independent bilateral pigmented nodular hyperplasia of adrenal glands accounts for <2% of endogenous Cushing

BOX 1 Causes of Cushing syndrome.

- **Exogenous:**
    - Iatrogenic/surreptitious steroid intake (oral/injection/percutaneous/inhaled)
- **Endogenous:**
    - ACTH-dependent causes:
        - Cushing disease (Pituitary-dependent)
        - Ectopic ACTH syndrome
        - Macronodular adrenal hyperplasia
    - ACTH-independent causes:
        - Adrenal adenoma and carcinoma
        - Primary pigmented nodular adrenal hyperplasia and Carney syndrome
        - McCune–Albright syndrome

(ACTH: adrenocorticotropic hormone)

TABLE 1 Symptoms and signs for the diagnosis of Cushing syndrome.

Symptoms	Signs	Overlapping conditions
Features that best discriminate Cushing syndrome; most do not have a high senstivity		
	• Easy bruising • Facial plethora • Proximal myopathy • Striae (especially if reddish purple and >1cm wide) • In children, weight gain with decreasing growth velocity	
Features in the general population that are common and/or less discriminatory		
• Depression • Fatigue • Weight gain • Back pain • Change in appetite • Decreased concentration • Decreased libido • Impaired memory • Insomnia • Irritability • Menstrual abnormalities • In children, slow growth	• Dorsocervical fat pad (buffalo hump) • Facial fullness • Obesity • Supraclavicular fullness • Thin skin • Peripheral edema • Acne • Hirsutism or female balding • Poor skin healing • In children, abnormal genital virilization, short stature, pseudoprecocious puberty or delayed puberty	• Hypertension • Incidental adrenal mass • Vertebral osteoporosis • Polycystic ovary syndrome • Type 2 diabetes mellitus • Hypokalemia • Kidney stones • Unusual infections

syndrome. Nodules are 2–4 mm in diameter and colored black/brown in cut section. Patients are mostly <30 years of age. Some cases of PPNAD are associated with atrial myxoma and spotty skin pigmentation (Carney syndrome), a familial autosomal dominant disease.

- *McCune–Albright syndrome*: McCune–Albright syndrome (MAS) results from somatic-activating mutation of *GNAS1* gene, encoding α subunit of GTP-binding protein (Gsα). This leads to constitutive ligand-free activation of G protein. Typical features are polyostotic fibrous dysplasia, café-au-lait macules, and GnRH-independent sexual precocity. Other endocrine disorders include acromegaly [via growth-hormone-releasing hormone (GHRH) receptors] and Cushing syndrome (via ACTH receptors).

Exogenous Cushing syndrome: This is by far the most common cause of Cushing syndrome. It is due to iatrogenic or surreptitious use of synthetic steroids (**Table 2**) (oral/injection/percutaneous/inhaled). Detailed drug history is required to exclude exogenous Cushing syndrome. Some clinical features such as cataract, raised intraocular pressure, benign intracranial hypertension, osteonecrosis, osteoporosis, and pancreatitis are more common than endogenous Cushing syndrome while hypertension, hirsutism, hyperpigmentation, and oligomenorrhea are less common.

Investigations:

There should be high clinical index of suspicion for Cushing syndrome before proceeding for biochemical testing. Exogenous steroid exposure should be excluded beforehand. Certain clinical conditions mimic Cushing syndrome biochemically and to some extent clinically also (**Box 2**). During biochemical evaluation first goal is to establish the diagnosis of Cushing syndrome and then to evaluate for the cause (**Table 3**). Various caveats of tests should be considered while interpreting the results (**Table 3** and **Box 3**).

Tests to establish the cause of Cushing syndrome

- *ACTH-dependent versus independent*: Morning plasma ACTH levels (Drawn at 9 AM, in ice cold tubes) of <10 pg/mL suggest ACTH-independent Cushing syndrome and CT (computed tomography) of adrenals should be next step to complete the workup. Occasionally ACTH levels can be low in mild Cushing disease, so measurement of at least two values is recommended. ACTH levels >10 pg/mL suggest ACTH-dependent cause.
- *Pituitary versus ectopic ACTH secretion*: Plasma ACTH values in ectopic Cushing syndrome are high (usually >90 pg/mL), nevertheless, overlap values are seen in Cushing disease in 30% of cases. Tests needed to locate ACTH source are:
  - High-dose dexamethasone suppression test (2 mg dexamethasone q6h): Up to >50% suppression in serum cortisol value at 48 hours from the basal value suggests pituitary source.
  - CRH stimulation test (intravenous CRH—1 µg/kg body weight): Serum cortisol and ACTH are measured at baseline and then every 15 minutes for 1–2 hours after CRH injection. ACTH rise of 100% or a cortisol rise of 50% over baseline value suggests pituitary source.
  - Inferior petrosal sinus sampling: Blood from each half of the pituitary drains into ipsilateral inferior petrosal sinus. Simultaneously blood is drawn for plasma ACTH estimation from petrosal sinus and peripheral vein at baseline and post 2, 5, and 15 minutes of CRH administration (100 µg ovine/human CRH intravenous). ACTH petrosal sinus/peripheral ratio >3 has a sensitivity of 95% and specificity of nearly 100% for the diagnosis of Cushing disease.

Radiology and nuclear imaging: Imaging should always be based on biochemical results, as pituitary and adrenals incidentalomas are not uncommon. MRI pituitary is the investigation of choice, if biochemical tests suggest Cushing

BOX 2 Examples of hypercortisolism not associated with Cushing syndrome (Pseudo-Cushing syndrome).

- Alcoholism, especially withdrawal
- Depression
- Obesity
- Pregnancy
- Sleep apnea
- Obligate exercise
- Uncontrolled diabetes
- Stress

TABLE 2 Relative potencies of synthetic steroids.

Steroid	Anti-inflammatory action	Hypothalamic–pituitary–adrenal suppression	Salt retention
Cortisol	1	1	1
Prednisolone	4	4	0.75
Methylprednisolone	6	4	0.5
Fludrocortisone	12	12	125
Dexamethasone	25	17	0

TABLE 3 Tests to establish a diagnosis of Cushing syndrome.

Biochemical test	Cutoff point	Sensitivity	Specificity	Caveats
Bedtime or late night salivary cortisol	2 ng/mL	100%	96%	Older age, smoking, hypertension, diabetes
Serum cortisol (1 mg overnight dexamethasone suppression test, given at 11 PM to 12 midnight) (ONDST)	1.8 µg/dL (at 7 AM to 8 AM, next morning)	98–100%	88%	Abnormal dexamethasone metabolism/CBG abnormalities
24 hours urinary free cortisol	Upper limit of normal	–	–	Incomplete/overcollection, excess fluid intake
Serum cortisol (0.5 mg low-dose dexamethasone suppression test, q6h × 8 doses) (LDDST)	1.8 µg/dL (6 hours after last dose)	98–100%	97–100%	Abnormal dexamethasone metabolism/CBG abnormalities
Bedtime or late night serum cortisol	7.5 µg/dL (if awake)	–	–	CBG abnormalities

(CBG: corticosteroid-binding globulin)

BOX 3 Various drugs affecting steroid metabolism.

- **Drugs causing induction of CYP 3A4 (accelerate dexamethasone metabolism leading to false positive results)**: Phenobarbitone, phenytoin, carbamazepine, rifampicin, pioglitazone
- **Drugs causing inhibition of CYP 3A4 (decrease dexamethasone metabolism leading to false negative results)**: Ritonavir, itraconazole, fluoxetine, diltiazem
- **Drugs increasing cortisol binding globulin levels leading to false positive results in serum cortisol assays**: Estrogen, mitotane

disease. About 90% of ACTH-secreting pituitary tumors are microadenoma, which appear as hypointense lesion on gadolinium (Ga)-enhanced T1-weighted images. Adrenals are better seen on CT. If biochemistry suggests ectopic ACTH secretion, CT scan of thorax, abdomen and pelvis is done. Nuclear imaging studies such as ^{68}Ga-DOTATATE and ^{18}F-FDG (Fluorodeoxyglucose) PET (positron emission tomography)/CT have greatly enhanced the chances of locating ectopic ACTH-secreting neuroendocrine tumors, not otherwise seen on radiological imaging. Recently, ^{68}Ga-DOTA-CRH PET CT correctly localized pituitary lesion in 14/15 patients of Cushing's disease.

Treatment of Cushing syndrome:

Cushing disease: Transsphenoidal hypophysectomy is the treatment of choice for Cushing disease. Remission rates are 70–90% for microadenomas and 50% for macroadenomas at best centers. As the corticotrophs surrounding the ACTH secreting adenoma are suppressed, successful removal of adenoma is indicated by 9-AM serum cortisol levels of <2 µg/dL on postoperative days 2–5. As suppressed HPA (hypothalamic-pituitary-adrenal) axis may take months to a year to recover after successful surgery, such patients are given glucocorticoid replacement therapy till that time. Predictors of remission include low cortisol levels measured postoperatively, histological identification of an ACTH-secreting adenoma and visualization of microadenoma on preoperative imaging. Long-term recurrence rate for patients in remission after pituitary surgery is up to 30%. Treatment options for recurrent cases are repeat pituitary surgery, gamma knife radiosurgery, medical therapy (metyrapone, ketoconazole), and bilateral adrenalectomy.

Ectopic ACTH syndrome: Treatment is directed to the cause of ectopic ACTH syndrome. Removal of localized tumor can be curative. Sometimes bilateral adrenalectomy is performed, if ectopic source of ACTH is not localized.

Adrenal causes: Unilateral adrenal adenoma is removed by adrenalectomy, with cure rate close to 100%. As pituitary corticotrophs and opposite adrenal gland are suppressed, postoperative 9-AM serum cortisol levels of <2 µg/dL indicate successful surgery. Patients are then replaced with glucocorticoids till the recovery of HPA axis. Prognosis of adrenal carcinomas is bad and treatment usually involves removal of primary tumor followed by chemotherapy.

GLUCOCORTICOID DEFICIENCY

Glucocorticoid deficiency as a result of direct adrenal disease is called primary hypoadrenalism (Addison's disease), while that occurring due to ACTH deficiency is called as secondary/central hypoadrenalism. Thomas Addison described first ever, a case of primary hypoadrenalism in 1855. Various causes of adrenal insufficiency are detailed in **Box 4**.

PRIMARY HYPOADRENALISM

Addison disease is a rare disease with an estimated incidence of 0.8 cases per 100,000 population per year.

Autoimmune adrenalitis accounts for >70% of the cases in the west; while in India, tuberculosis remains the most common cause. Up to 50% cases of autoimmune adrenal disease have associated other autoimmune disease; APS I and APS II syndrome. APS I is a rare autosomal recessive disease, characterized by chronic mucocutaneous candidiasis and ectodermal dystrophy [APECED (autoimmune polyendocrinopathy-candidiasis-ectodermal dystrophy)], Addison disease, and hypoparathyroidism. The much more common APS II has polygenic inheritance and may

BOX 4	Causes of glucocorticoid deficiency.

Primary causes:

- Autoimmune: Isolated, autoimmune polyendocrine syndrome type I (APS I), autoimmune polyendocrine syndrome type II (Schmidt syndrome)
- Infections: Tuberculosis, histoplasmosis, cryptococcosis, coccidioidomycosis, cytomegalovirus, HIV
- Metastatic tumor: Breast, lung, stomach
- Infiltrations: Amyloidosis, hemochromatosis, sarcoidosis, lymphoma
- Intra-adrenal hemorrhage: Waterhouse–Friderichsen syndrome (meningococcal septicemia), *Pseudomonas aeruginosa*
- Congenital adrenal hyperplasia: *CYP21A2, CYP11B1, CYP17A1, HSD3B2, POR* gene defect
- Congenital lipoid adrenal hyperplasia: *StAR, CYP11A1* gene defect
- Adrenal hypoplasia congenital: *DAX-1, SF-1* mutation
- X-linked adrenoleukodystrophy
- ACTH resistance syndrome: *MC2R* gene, *MRAP* gene, *AAS* gene mutation (Triple A syndrome, Allgrove's syndrome)
- Bilateral adrenalectomy
- Drug induced: Mitotane, abiraterone, suramin, ketoconazole, RU486

Secondary causes:

- Exogenous glucocorticoid therapy
- Autoimmune hypophysitis
- Pituitary tumors and other mass lesion involving hypothalamic pituitary lesion: Craniopharyngioma, meningioma, metastasis (breast, lung)
- Pituitary irradiation
- Pituitary apoplexy
- Postpartum pituitary infarction (Sheehan syndrome)
- Pituitary infiltration (tuberculosis, sarcoidosis, eosinophilic granuloma)
- Isolated ACTH deficiency: Idiopathic, lymphocytic hypophysitis, *PCSK 1* gene mutation, *POMC* gene mutation
- Multiple pituitary hormone deficiency: *HESX1 gene, LHX4* gene, *SOX3* gene, *PROP1* gene mutation

comprise Addison disease, hypothyroidism, primary gonadal failure, type 1 diabetes mellitus, and vitiligo. X-linked adrenoleukodystrophy results from mutation in *ABCD1* gene encoding for ABC peroxisomal membrane protein leading to failure in import of very long-chain fatty acids (VLCFAs) into the peroxisome and hence accumulation of VLCFAs.

SECONDARY HYPOADRENALISM

Adrenocorticotropic hormone suppression by exogenous glucocorticoids is the most common cause of hypoadrenalism overall. Dose, duration, route, timing, and type of exogenous steroid determines the overall suppression of HPA axis. In any person who has taken more than the equivalent of 30 mg of hydrocortisone per day orally for >3 weeks, adrenal insufficiency should be anticipated. Recovery of HPA axis should be ensured before stopping steroids in such cases (short Synacthen test).

Other causes of secondary hypoadrenalism are described in **Box 4**.

CLINICAL FEATURES

Symptoms vary considerably depending upon rapidity/severity of disease. Common symptoms are weakness, tiredness, fatigue, anorexia, weight loss, and low-grade fever. Few symptoms seen only in primary adrenal insufficiency are skin hyperpigmentation (sun-exposed areas, recent scars, nipples, buccal mucosa) and salt craving (nausea, vomiting, abdominal pain, and postural dizziness). Loss of function of adrenal androgens can manifest in females as loss of axillary and pubic hairs, dry and itchy skin, and loss of libido. In acute adrenal insufficiency/Addisonian crisis, patient can present with shock, acute abdominal pain, nausea, vomiting, stupor, and coma.

BIOCHEMICAL CONFIRMATION

Diagnosis of adrenal insufficiency is established by plasma cortisol value of <18–20 µg/dL, 30–60 minutes after intravenous or intramuscular administration of 250 µg cosyntropin/Synacthen (Synacthen stimulation test). This test, however may fail to detect recent-onset (<4–6 weeks) secondary adrenal insufficiency. Random serum cortisol value is rarely helpful in making diagnosis. Once diagnosis of adrenal insufficiency is established, differentiation is done between primary and secondary causes. Primary adrenal insufficiency is associated with high ACTH, high plasma renin activity (PRA), and low aldosterone levels. Patients with secondary adrenal insufficiency have low-normal ACTH, normal PRA, and aldosterone levels. In primary hypoadrenalism, further testing include CT adrenals, autoantibodies to 21-hydroxylase, chest X-ray, serum 17-hydroxy progesterone, plasma VLCFAs depending on the clinical presentation. In secondary hypoadrenalism, MRI of pituitary and hypothalamic area is indicated, if there is no conclusive history of exogenous steroids intake.

OTHER INVESTIGATIONS

Common laboratory findings in primary hypoadrenalism are hyponatremia (90%) and hyperkalemia (65%), and raised blood urea due to aldosterone deficiency. Hyponatremia can be seen in secondary hypoadrenalism also, due to loss of feedback inhibition by cortisol on AVP release. Other findings related to glucocorticoid deficiency are anemia, lymphocytosis, eosinophilia, and slightly elevated serum TSH and calcium levels.

TREATMENT

Acute adrenal insufficiency: In adults, intravenous bolus of 100 mg hydrocortisone is given immediately followed by 100 mg every 6–8 hourly. One liter of normal saline with 5% dextrose is given by intravenous route over 1 hour. After the first 24 hours, hydrocortisone dose can be reduced to 50 mg every 6 hours for 1–2 days and subsequently to oral hydrocortisone. It is important to treat the cause of acute adrenal insufficiency simultaneously.

Long-term replacement therapy:

Glucocorticoid replacement: It involves oral administration of 15–25 mg of hydrocortisone per day in two to three divided doses (10–15 mg on awakening—5 mg at 12 noon and 5 mg at 4 PM). All the patients should be told to increase the replacement dose by two to three folds during minor illness. Major trauma/stress/surgery might necessitate intravenous/intramuscular 100 mg hydrocortisone. Adequacy of replacement is judged clinically, as there are no reliable laboratory markers.

Mineralocorticoid replacement: It is needed only in primary adrenal insufficiency. Oral fludrocortisone 100–150 µg per day given as a single dose in the morning is the usual replacement. Adequacy of the therapy is judged by measuring supine and erect blood pressure and serum sodium, potassium, and PRA.

Adrenal androgen replacement: Females with primary or secondary adrenal insufficiency can get improvement in sexual function and wellbeing with 25–50 mg/day of DHEA replacement.

ADRENAL INCIDENTALOMAS

Incidentally discovered adrenal masses can be seen in up to 4% of patients imaged for nonadrenal disease. These are more common in females and increases with age. Evaluation is needed in every case to decide whether lesion is functional and whether lesion is malignant. The radiological imaging helps in diagnosis to a certain extent (**Table 4**). The biochemical testing should include 8-AM serum cortisol following 1 mg overnight dexamethasone suppression test, plasma fractionated metanephrines, DHEAS, and for those with hypertension PRA and aldosterone also. Role of adrenal biopsy is restricted to suspected lymphoma, sarcoma, infiltrative infection such as tuberculosis/fungal or metastasis. It does not differentiate between adrenal adenoma and adrenocortical carcinoma. Management depends on the cause of adrenal incidentaloma.

PRIMARY ALDOSTERONISM

This disease entity was first described in 1955 by Jerome W Conn in a 34-year-old woman with hypertension, severe hypokalemia, metabolic alkalosis, and right adrenal adenoma. Primary aldosteronism accounts for about 5–10% of all hypertensive patients. Clinical suspicion of primary aldosteronism is done in any patient with hypertension which is severe, requiring more than three drugs to control or associated hypokalemia or adrenal mass or family history of early-onset hypertension or cerebrovascular accident at <40 years of age. Hypokalemia, if severe can cause muscle weakness/cramps and polyuria. Periodic paralysis can be seen, particularly in patients from Asian descent. Serum sodium tends to be high normal or slightly above normal. Edema is not a common finding because of mineralocorticoid escape. However, there may not be any typical clinical feature to suggest primary aldosteronism. About 70% of patients with primary aldosteronism are normokalemic!! Target organ damage is much more common than other causes of hypertension.

LABORATORY EVALUATION

Screening: It involves paired hormone measurement of plasma aldosterone concentration (PAC) and PRA, done in the morning seated ambulant patient. Patient should be made normokalemic and spironolactone or eplerenone should be stopped for 4–6 weeks before doing tests. Other antihypertensive drugs can be continued but results should be interpreted accordingly (**Table 5**). Various other similar causes of hypertension must also be considered (**Box 5**). Primary aldosteronism should be suspected if the PRA is suppressed (<1 ng/mL/h) and PAC is increased (>10 ng/dL). This should be followed by confirmatory aldosterone suppression test. However, confirmatory tests are not required if hypertensive patient is having spontaneous hypokalemia and markedly elevated PAC (>20 ng/dL) and PRA is suppressed (<1 ng/mL/h).

Confirmation: It involves intravenous 2 L of isotonic saline infusion over 4 hours. The test is done in the seated position after an overnight fast. Blood is withdrawn at the completion of the infusion. In normal subjects, PAC level

TABLE 4 Radiological features of adrenal mass.

Tumor type	Characteristics	CT	MRI
Adrenal adenoma	<4 cm, homogeneous with smooth margins	Noncontrast HU value <10, >50% contrast washout at 10 minutes	Isointense on T2-weighted images
Adrenal carcinoma	>4 cm, inhomogeneous with irregular margins	Noncontrast HU value >10, <50% contrast washout at 10 minutes	Hyperintense on T2-weighted images
Pheochromocytoma	Size variable, inhomogeneous with smooth margins	Noncontrast HU value >10, <50% contrast washout at 10 minutes	Hyperintense on T2-weighted images
Metastasis	Size variable, inhomogeneous with irregular margins	Noncontrast HU value >10, <50% contrast washout at 10 minutes	Hyperintense on T2-weighted images

(HU: hounsfield units)

TABLE 5 Effect of various drugs on RAAS.

Drug	Effect on renin	Effect on aldosterone	Effect on ARR
β-blockers/central α2 agonist	↓↓	↓	↑
ACE inhibitors	↑	↓	↓
AT1R blockers	↑	↓	↓
Diuretics	↑	↑	↔/↓
Calcium antagonists/ α1 blockers	↔	↔	↔

(ACE: angiotensin-converting enzyme; ARR: aldosterone/renin ratio; AT1R: angiotensin 1 receptor)

BOX 5 Various causes of primary aldosteronism and its differential diagnosis.

- **Low renin, high aldosterone:**
    - Primary aldosteronism
    - Aldosterone-producing adenoma (Conn's) (APA) – 30%
    - Bilateral idiopathic (micronodular) hyperplasia (IHA) – 60%
    - Familial hyperaldosteronism (FH)
    - Aldosterone-producing adrenocortical carcinoma
- **Low renin, low aldosterone:**
    - Congenital adrenal hyperplasia (11β hydroxylase/17α hydroxylase deficiency)
    - Syndrome of apparent mineralocorticoid excess (AME)
    - Glucocorticoid resistance
    - Deoxycorticosterone producing tumor
    - Cushing syndrome
- **High renin, high aldosteronism:**
    - Renovascular disease

is suppressed to <5 ng/dL while in most patients with primary aldosteronism, PAC level remains >10 ng/dL. Oral sodium loading and fludrocortisone suppression tests are alternatives. Hypertension and hypokalemia must be corrected before doing these tests.

Computed tomography adrenals: After biochemical confirmation, CT adrenals should be done. If a typical unilateral adrenal adenoma (>1 cm) is seen in a patient <35 years of age with severe primary hyperaldosteronism, no further testing is required and unilateral laproscopic adrenalectomy can be performed. But if CT adrenal is normal or shows bilateral micronodularity (<1 cm) or age is >35 years, adrenal vein sampling is required for lateralization before desired surgery.

TREATMENT

Treatment for idiopathic hyperaldosteronism (IHA) is pharmacological and for confirmed aldosterone-producing adenoma (APA) treatment options are both surgical (unilateral laproscopic adrenalectomy) and pharmacological. Goal of treatment is not only to normalize the blood pressure but also to ensure complete MR blockade (high normal serum potassium). A sodium-restricted diet (sodium <100 mEq/2.4 g or 6 g salt) is a must. Pharmacological drug of choice is spironolactone, a MR antagonist. Dose of spironolactone is 12.5–25 mg bid and can be increased to 400 mg/day if necessary to achieve a high normal serum potassium concentration without oral potassium chloride supplementation. The more selective MR antagonist, eplerenone can also be used. Dosage is 25 mg bid and can be increased to 200 mg/day.

PHEOCHROMOCYTOMA AND PARAGANGLIOMAS

Pheochromocytomas and paragangliomas (PGLs) are catecholamines-producing neuroendocrine tumors, arising from chromaffin cells of adrenal medulla and sympathetic ganglia, respectively. Approximately 25 % of PCC/PGLs are malignant, 25% are extra-adrenal, and up to 40% are hereditary. The association between adrenal medullary tumors and symptoms was first recognized by Frankel in 1886. Annual incidence of catecholamine-producing tumors is 2–8 cases per 1 million people. Most cases present in third to fifth decade of their life with equal gender distribution.

CLINICAL PRESENTATION

Palpitations, headache, diaphoresis, syncope or presyncope, pallor, anxiety, weight loss, and constipation are common symptoms. At times, patients can be asymptomatic and normotensive detected as an adrenal incidentaloma. Symptoms and hypertension can be chronic or episodic (paroxysm/spells/catecholamine crisis). Spells can be spontaneous or precipitated by postural change, medications (β-blockers, anesthetic agents), exercise, or changes in intra-abdominal pressure and usually lasts for 15–20 minutes. During paroxysm, patient can have accelerated hypertension, heart failure, pulmonary edema, cardiac arrhythmias, or intracranial hemorrhage. Various genetic disorders associated with PCCs/PGLs are mentioned in **Table 6**.

BIOCHEMICAL TESTING

Patients with resistant hypertension, hyperadrenergic spells, incidentally detected adrenal mass with image characteristics suggestive of PCC, family history of PCC or associated genetic syndromes should be evaluated for PCCs/PGLs. Either the measurement of plasma-fractionated metanephrines (sensitivity: 96–100%, specificity: 85–89%) or 24 hours urinary metanephrines (sensitivity: 92–97%, specificity: 86–95%) can be used as case detection strategy. Test, if normal, should be repeated during a hyperadrenergic spell in a patients with high clinical suspicion. Any interfering medication should be discontinued for at least 2 weeks prior to the evaluation (**Table 7**).

LOCALIZATION

Computed tomography or MRI of the abdomen and pelvis should be the first localization test (sensitivity 89%

TABLE 6 Pheochromocytoma and paragangliomas – Associated genetic syndromes.

Syndrome	Gene	Tumor location	Malignancy rate	Other features
Von Hippel–Lindau disease	*VHL*	Adrenal (bilateral)	5%	Renal cell carcinoma, retinal angiomas, pancreatic cyst
Multiple endocrine neoplasia type 2A	*RET*	Adrenal (bilateral)	<5%	Medullary thyroid carcinoma, primary hyperparathyroidism
Multiple endocrine neoplasia type 2B	*RET*	Adrenal (bilateral)	<5%	Medullary thyroid carcinoma, Marfanoid habitus, mucosal neuroma
Neurofibromatosis type 1	*NF1*	Adrenal (bilateral)	12%	Neurofibromas, café-au-lait spots, iris hamartomas
Familial paraganglioma syndrome	• SDHA • SDHB • SDHC • SDHD • SDHAF2	• Any location • Primarily extraadrenal • Head and neck • Head and neck • Head and neck	• Low • 23% • Low • <5% • Low	Renal cancers, gastrointestinal stromal tumors, pituitary adenomas

TABLE 7 Medications associated with false-positive results.

Medication	False high metabolite
α-blockers, tricyclic antidepressants	Norepinephrine, normetanephrine
Sympathomimetics (ephedrine, albuterol, amphetamines)	Norepinephrine, normetanephrine epinephrine, metanephrine
Caffeine, cocaine	Norepinephrine, epinephrine
Levodopa	Norepinephrine
MAO inhibitors	Metanephrine, normetanephrine

(MAO: monoamine oxidase)

and 98%, respectively). Typical image characteristics of PCC are mentioned in **Table 4**. If CT/MRI fail to detect the tumor in biochemically proven PCCs/PGLs, additionally Ga^{68} -DOTATATE PET/CT or ^{123}I-MIBG scintigraphy can be performed. Also if adrenal PCC is >10 cm or paraganglioma is discovered on CT/MRI, Ga^{68} -DOTATATE PET/CT or ^{123}I-MIBG scintigraphy should be done to look for metastatic disease.

TREATMENT

The treatment of choice for PCCs is complete surgical resection. Preoperative adequate α-adrenergic blockade should be achieved to avoid hypertensive crisis during surgery. It usually requires 7 days. Because these patients are volume constricted, liberal salt (>5 g sodium/12.5 g salt) and fluid replacement is ensured to avoid orthostasis. Prazosin is most commonly used agent, in a daily dose of 2–15 mg in three to four dividing doses. Preoperatively β-blockers are indicated to control the tachycardia, but should be initiated only after achieving adequate α-blockade. Propranolol 40–240 mg/day in two to three divided doses or metoprolol 50–400 mg/day in two divided doses can be used. Target blood pressure should be low normal for the age and target heart rate 60–80 beats/minute. Calcium channel blockers (nicardipine/verapamil/amlodipine) can be added preoperatively if blood pressure control is inadequate with maximally tolerable α-blockers. About 1–2 weeks after surgery urine/plasma metanephrines are tested to confirm the complete resection. Afterward, annual biochemical screening is done lifelong to look for any recurrence.

RECOMMENDED READINGS

1. Nieman LK, Biller BM, Findling JW, Newell-Price J, Savage MO, Stewart PM, et al. The diagnosis of Cushing's syndrome: an Endocrine Society Clinical Practice Guideline. J Clin Endocrinol Metab. 2008;93(5):1526-40.
2. Shukla J, Walia R, Kumar R, Singh H, Vatsa R, Chhabra A, et al. Ga-68 DOTA-CRH: A novel radiopharmaceutical for diagnosis of ACTH dependent Cushing's syndrome. J Nucl Med. 2020;61(supplement 1):51.
3. Bornstein SR, Allolio B, Arlt W, Barthel A, Don-Wauchope A, Hammer GD, et al. Diagnosis and Treatment of primary adrenal insufficiency: An Endocrine Society Clinical Practice Guideline. J Clin Endocrinol Metab. 2016;101(2):364-89.
4. Sherlock M , Scarsbrook A, Abbas A, Fraser S, Limumpornpetch P, Dineen R, et al. Adrenal Incidentaloma. Endocr Rev. 2020;41(6):775-820.
5. Vaidya A, Mulatero P, Baudrand R, Adler GK. The expanding spectrum of primary aldosteronism: Implications for diagnosis, pathogenesis, and treatment Endocr Rev. 2018;39(6):1057-88.
6. Lenders JWM, Duh QY, Eisenhofer G, Gimenez-Roqueplo AP, Grebe SKG, Murad MH, et al. Pheochromocytoma and paraganglioma: An Endocrine Society Clinical Practice Guideline. J Clin Endocrinol Metab. 2014;99(6):1915-42.

CHAPTER 116 Gonadal and Pubertal Disorders

Aashima Dabas, Rekha Ramot, Rajesh Khadgawat

ABSTRACT

Puberty is a developmental stage in the life cycle, characterized by physical and psychosocial maturation of an individual. The physical changes of puberty are a result of gonadal sex hormone production (gonadarche), triggered by the pulsatile release of gonadotropin-releasing hormone (GnRH), which in turn activates the hypothalamic-pituitary-gonadal (HPG) axis. Pubertal onset is initiated as thelarche in girls and gonadarche in boys. A deviation in growth and puberty (delayed or precocious) warrants a detailed assessment. Gonadotropin-dependent and -independent causes of precocious puberty and incomplete forms should be recognized early and treated. Systemic illness and constitutional delay in growth and puberty (CDGP) are the most common causes of delayed puberty. Adequate nutrition and prevention of micronutrient deficiencies are important during puberty.

Hypogonadism in adults is a clinical syndrome resulting from malfunctioning of the HPG axis. Primary hypogonadism/hypergonadotropic hypogonadism is caused by dysfunction of gonads (testes in men and ovaries in women), resulting in infertility which is usually nontreatable. The secondary hypogonadism/hypogonadotropic hypogonadism results from dysfunction of the hypothalamus and/or pituitary gland and is characterized by isolated GnRH deficiency. Hypogonadism in males manifests as a failure of testes to secrete adequate levels of serum testosterone, decreased sperm counts, or both. Female hypogonadism results from ovarian failure, leading to insufficient production of sex steroids. The most common clinical feature in prepubertal girls with hypogonadism is delayed pubertal onset and primary amenorrhea. Secondary amenorrhea is the most common finding in women with hypogonadism. Because of the complicated nature of hypogonadism due to nonspecific clinical features, appropriate medical management requires interprofessional collaboration.

"Other than dying, I think puberty is probably about as rough as it gets"

—Rick Springfield

INTRODUCTION

Gonadal functions are essential for the propagation of life in any organism. They not only produce sperm and ova but also produce a variety of hormones and cytokines, essential for both reproduction and general health. The functions of the gonads are under the control of the pituitary [gonadotrophs secret luteinizing hormone/follicle-stimulating hormone (LH/FSH)], which in turn controlled by the hypothalamus by secretion of GnRH. Any disease affecting the hypothalamus, pituitary, or gonad may lead to altered functions of the gonad. Decreased secretion of gonadal sex steroid hormones produces a state of hypogonadism. It may occur before the start of puberty (delayed puberty) or during the adult age group (hypogonadism). Since, altered gonadal function at different age groups (children and adults) has causes, clinical features, and treatment that are not common, so they are discussed separately.

DISORDERS IN CHILDREN

Puberty is a stage of physical, psychosocial, and gonadal maturation that usually spans adolescence. Puberty is defined as "a transitional period between childhood and adulthood, during which a growth spurt occurs, secondary sexual characteristics appear, fertility is achieved, and profound psychological changes take place". These pubertal changes are under close regulation by the hypothalamic-pituitary axis, which in turn are modulated by intrinsic factors, gender, race, and genetics, and extrinsic factors such as diet, exercise, and chemicals. Recent understanding of the pathophysiology of puberty has indicated the role of leptin from adipose tissue and neurotransmitters such as kisspeptin, gamma-aminobutyric acid (GABA), and glutamate on the pubertal onset. The neurons in the arcuate nucleus of the hypothalamus, which coexpress kisspeptin, neurokinin B, and dynorphin, may act as the pulse generator for pubertal onset.

PUBERTAL TIMING AND ONSET

Pubertal onset and maturation follow a sequence and pattern specific for both genders, as shown in **Box 1**. The usual timing of initiation of these pubertal changes is approximately 9–11 years in girls and 10–12 years in boys. However, this age range is variable as per genetic and racial differences and shows a secular trend worldwide.

BOX 1	Abnormalities of puberty.

- **Deviations of puberty:**
  - Premature thelarche
  - Premature adrenarche
  - Premature menarche
- **Diseases of puberty:**
  - *Precocious puberty*: Appearance of secondary sexual characteristics before 8 years in girls and 9 years in boys
  - *Delayed puberty*: Absence of any secondary sexual characteristics till 13 years in girls and by 14 years in boys, and/or menarche by 16 years of age

A small proportion of children may show deviant pubertal onset or progression, which is discordant to the timing as per normative data of the population. It is defined as precocious puberty when it occurs earlier and delayed when it does not start or progress by a certain age. Abnormalities of puberty are given in **Box 1**.

Deviations of puberty: These are self-limited, more or less exaggerated physiological deviations of the normal pubertal process which do not lead to any permanent disadvantage to the child. Most of the time, they do not progress and do not require treatment; however, they are an important cause of concern for the family.

Premature thelarche: This is a self-limiting benign condition usually seen as isolated unilateral or bilateral breast enlargement around 1–2 years of age in girls. The anthropometry is usually within the normal range without any significant increase in bone age. The basal LH levels are normal with a prepubertal response on GnRH stimulation. Treatment is reassurance as the condition regresses on follow-up.

Premature adrenarche: This is defined as a transient increase in adrenal androgens, which may be accompanied by the premature appearance of pubic and axillary hair. The growth velocity is usually normal with normal bone age. The onset of puberty is usually normal with near-normal final adult height in affected children.

Premature menarche: Rarely, girls may present with an isolated complaint of vaginal bleeding. There is an absence of other associated secondary sexual characters with no pubertal height spurt. The causes that should be investigated are infection, trauma, foreign body, and sexual abuse. An abdominal ultrasound should also be performed. The cycles usually stop after 2–3 cycles and do not need active treatment.

The two disorders of puberty are precocious puberty and delayed puberty. These are discussed below.

PRECOCIOUS PUBERTY

Premature or early development of puberty has major consequences on the health of a developing child. The major concern in precocity is 2-fold. One is early exposure to sex steroid leading to acceleration of growth, but the premature fusion of epiphysis will lead to short stature in final height. The second is a dichotomy between mental and physical maturation, their cognitive maturation is according to age, but sexual development is advanced, so they are at very high risk for sexual abuse. Causes of precocity can be divided into two major groups, central and peripheral, based on gonadotropins levels.

CAUSES

Central precocious puberty (CPP): This is, in the actual sense, the start of a normal pubertal process, occurring at an early age. All sequences of normal puberty are followed and, if untreated, can lead to the achievement of fertility. It is also known as complete precocious puberty; CPP or gonadotropin-dependent precocious puberty (GDPP). All cases of early pregnancy reported in <10 years aged girls are cases of CPP, who were abused. CPP is much more common in girls than boys. Causes of CPP are given in **Table 1**.

Peripheral precocious puberty (PPP): It is also known as gonadotropin-independent precocious puberty (GIPP) or pseudoprecocity. Here, all sequences of the normal pubertal process are not followed, so the achievement of fertility is not seen in most of the cases. PPP is much less common than CPP, but more difficult to diagnose and treat. Causes of PPP are given in **Table 1**.

CLINICAL PRESENTATION

Usually, parents notice early development of secondary sexual characters in the form of development of breast or pubic hair (girls) and increase in penile length, pubic hair, and change in behavior in boys. Both boys and girls show rapid gain in height, so they appear taller than their peers at the time of presentation. An increase in sex steroid, especially estradiol, causes premature fusion of epiphyses, leading to short stature.

DIAGNOSTIC WORKUP

Workup of all cases with precocity should include a detailed history with the systemic examination. Investigations should include basal gonadotropins measurement with a caveat that below normal LH concentrations do not exclude central precocity. A GnRH stimulation test may be required for those cases where serum LH levels are not elevated. The measurement of random estradiol or testosterone is required for diagnosis. Pelvic ultrasound in girls with increased uterine length and ovarian volume is supportive of the diagnosis, but not always seen as they are operator-dependent parameters with large variation in the measurement. Another important investigation is an assessment of bone age. An increase in bone age over chronological age (gap of >1 year) is very much supportive of a diagnosis of precocity. In all cases of CPP, magnetic resonance imaging (MRI) brain is required to rule out an intracranial lesion, especially in children younger than 6 years of age.

TABLE 1 Causes and difference between central precocious puberty (CPP) and peripheral precocious puberty (PPP).

Feature	Central precocious puberty	Peripheral precocious puberty
Definition	Increase in gonadotropins (LH/FSH) (gonadotropin dependent) leading to increased sex steroids	Increased sex steroid production from peripheral causes which is independent of gonadotropin secretion
Cause	• Idiopathic (most common in girls) • Organic (most common in boys) ◦ Tumors: Hypothalamic hamartoma, glioma, and astrocytoma ◦ Congenital: Cerebral dysgenesis and hydrocephalous ◦ CNS insult: Infection, head trauma, and radiation	• Adrenal tumors ◦ CAH: Virilizing type ◦ Adrenal carcinoma and adenoma • Gonadal tumors: ◦ Ovarian tumors ◦ Leydig cell tumor ◦ Familial testotoxicosis: Activating mutation of LH receptor • hCG secreting tumors: Central (CNS) or peripheral (teratoma) • Idiopathic • Untreated primary hypothyroidism
Pattern	Follows sequence of normal puberty	May have an isolated event like pubarche or thelarche alone
Laboratory investigations	• Basal LH elevated (>0.3 IU/L) • Response on GnRH stimulation: Both LH and FSH increase (LH > FSH with levels >5–8 IU/L)	• Basal LH: Suppressed or normal • GnRH stimulation: Does not increase serum LH

(CAH: congenital adrenal hyperplasia; GnRH: gonadotropin-releasing hormone; hCG: human chorionic gonadotropin)

TREATMENT

Treatment is targeted at the identification and management of the underlying cause. In central causes of precocious puberty (like idiopathic), the primary cause should be treated if possible, like removal of the tumor. However, all tumors or lesions may not be amenable to curative therapy. The use of GnRH analogs is recommended in central precocity as a continuous administration of GnRH suppresses the release of LH. The cessation of puberty also halts the growth velocity and progression of secondary sexual characters. However, improvement in final height outcomes is seen only if GnRH analogs are started before the age of 6 years.

Treatment with GnRH analog (leuprolide or triptorelin) is highly successful in decreasing features as well as elevated sex steroids. These analogs are available as depot preparations, given as once in a month or 3 months injections; however, the cost is the major limitation (one 3 monthly injection costs approximately Rs. 7,000–10,000). After the age of 6–7 years, the effect of treatment with GnRH analogs may not be able to improve the predicted final adult height. However, treatment is still required to address the issue of elevated sex steroid. It is also recommended that girls who present with thelarche after 7 years of age may be kept under observation for 3–6 months before deciding to treat as most untreated girls with CPP in this age would achieve normal adult height. Treatment with GnRH can be discontinued once the age of normal onset of puberty is reached; however, most of the families continue treatment till 10–11 years.

Treatment of PPP is usually aimed at the treatment of underlying causes. Oral agents to suppress puberty such as anastrazole/letrozole (aromatase inhibitor), ketoconazole, or tamoxifen/fulvestrant (selective estrogen receptor inhibitor) have been used in congenital adrenal hyperplasia (CAH) and McCune–Albright syndrome. In boys with testotoxicosis, oral agents such as ketoconazole, spironolactone, medroxyprogesterone, and bicalutamide have been used. However, treatment of PPP is not as successful as of CPP, and end results are not very rewarding.

DELAYED PUBERTY

Delayed puberty is the failure to attain secondary sexual characters by the age of 13 years in the girls and 14 years in boys. The delay in the start of puberty may be because of physiological or pathological reasons. As the process is controlled by the pituitary, it may be due to a primary defect in the pituitary/hypothalamus (hypogonadotropic hypogonadism) or maybe due to diseases of gonads (hypergonadotropic hypogonadism). Physiological causes are much more common than pathological causes.

PHYSIOLOGICAL CAUSES

As reproduction is a secondary process, the presence of severe disease of any system or severe psychological/mental stress would cause a delay in the start of the pubertal process, or even if puberty has started, it can be arrested also. Similarly, whenever there is a scarcity of energy and a lack of critical fat mass in the body, the onset of puberty is delayed, as seen in anorexia nervosa, athletes with very high physical activity like gymnasts. Once they gain critical fat mass, the process starts spontaneously.

Constitutional delay in growth and puberty: This is the most common cause of delay in puberty seen in clinical practice. It is more common in boys than girls.

These patients usually present around the age of 13–14 years with the complaint of short stature and failure to develop secondary sexual characters. The bone age is delayed by >2 years compared to chronological age. A child with CDGP will usually grow at a lower centile for his age with a normal height velocity. The growth remains poor during adolescence with delayed puberty, which is the cause of referral. Most of these children usually have a positive family history of delayed puberty. CDGP, however, is a diagnosis of exclusion after underlying systemic causes of delayed puberty have been excluded. The closest differential diagnosis for CDGP is isolated hypogonadotropic hypogonadism (IHH). Once diagnosed, reassurance of the family without any treatment is required in most cases. In some cases, with psychological concerns and low self-esteem in the child/family, puberty is initiated with low doses of gonadal steroids (injection testosterone 50–100 mg monthly for three doses) for 2–3 months and stopped. This results in the maturation of the axis with the spontaneous start of puberty.

Pubertal delay may be consonant when it is delayed in the sequence of normal puberty. In few cases, isolated delay in secondary sexual characters may be seen. Rarely, these may be the only clue of an underlying sinister disorder like complete androgen insensitivity syndrome, where the gender of rearing is usually female with absent pubarche or menarche.

PATHOLOGICAL CAUSES

Hypogonadotropic hypogonadism: Here, defect lies either in the hypothalamus or pituitary, resulting in failure of secretion of gonadotropins (LH/FSH), leading to delay. As testes are normal, fertility is possible with LH/FSH therapy in the future. The causes are hypogonadotropic hypogonadism given in **Box 2**.

Hypergonadotropic hypogonadism: This results from diseases of gonads leading to low levels of sex steroids. Therefore, loss of negative inhibition by sex steroids at the pituitary and hypothalamus would result in elevated levels of serum LH and FSH. As the primary defect/disease of testes also affects germ cells, fertility is not possible in most cases. The causes of hypergonadotropic hypogonadism differ between boys and girls and are given in **Table 2**.

Klinefelter syndrome: It is the most common genetic cause of delayed puberty in boys. The affected males have XXY or multiple copies of X chromosome and are usually tall with eunuchoid body proportions. They have gynecomastia with small firm testes. Affected boys have learning disabilities, behavioral issues, and anxiety or depression. They are at higher risk of metabolic syndrome, diabetes, osteoporosis, thromboembolic events, cardiovascular diseases, and male breast cancer.

Turner syndrome (TS): This is the most common cause of hypergonadotropic hypogonadism in girls with an incidence of 1:2,500 births. The genetic defect results from partial or complete loss of X chromosome (mosaic or complete XO, respectively). The affected patients may present with characteristic physical features such as a webbed neck, short stature, cubitus varus, nevi, short 4th metacarpal, broad chest, low hairline, and lymphedema in the newborn period (physical stigmata). The loss of a distal segment of the short arm of X chromosome (Xp-) is associated with haploinsufficiency of the short stature homeobox (SHOX), which is associated with short stature, skeletal defects, and hearing difficulty. Intrinsic abnormalities which should be screened in TS include hearing loss, bicuspid aortic valve, horseshoe kidneys, autoimmune thyroiditis, and learning disability. Around 10–20% of these children may enter spontaneous puberty and rarely may be fertile also. Treatment is aimed at early correction of height deficit with recombinant growth hormone use and timely pubertal induction.

BOX 2 Causes of hypogonadotropic hypogonadism in both boys and girls.

- **Congenital causes:**
  - Kallmann syndrome: Associated with anosmia or hyposmia
  - Isolated hypogonadotropic hypogonadism: Normal olfaction
  - Hypopituitarism: Associated with deficiency of other pituitary hormones
  - With associated syndromes: Prader–Willi syndrome (PWS) and Laurence-Moon-Bardet-Biedl (LMBB) syndrome
- **Acquired causes:**
  - Central nervous system (CNS) tumors: Especially in vicinity of hypothalamus/pituitary
  - Pituitary surgery or cranial/pituitary irradiation
  - Infections and postinfections process: Tubercular meningitis and encephalitis
  - Trauma: Traumatic brain injury

TABLE 2 Causes of hypergonadotropic hypogonadism in children.

Girls	Boys
• Chromosomal/Genetic: ◦ Turner syndrome ◦ Mixed gonadal dysgenesis • Disorders of steroid synthesis: ◦ Luteinizing hormone (LH) resistance ◦ Congenital adrenal hyperplasia • Primary ovarian failure (POF): ◦ Autoimmune ◦ Pelvic/spinal irradiation ◦ Chemotherapy ◦ Pseudohypoparathyroidism	• Chromosomal/Genetic: ◦ Klinefelter syndrome ◦ Mixed gonadal dysgenesis • Disorders of steroid synthesis: ◦ LH resistance ◦ Congenital adrenal hyperplasia ◦ Partial or complete androgen resistance • Primary testicular failure: ◦ Leydig cell failure ◦ Anorchia—post trauma or surgery ◦ Cryptorchidism ◦ Irradiation ◦ Infections—mumps ◦ Chemotherapy

DIAGNOSIS

A thorough history for underlying systemic causes, any neurological complaints and family history of pubertal delay should be taken. The examination should include interpretation and corroboration of anthropometry with pubertal staging. One of the essential parts of the examination is to look for features of any systemic disease where delayed puberty may be the only presenting complaint. A bone age assessment and screening blood tests such as hemogram, liver, kidney functions, and thyroid function tests are an essential part of workup and should be done in all cases to rule out systemic disease. Measurement of basal LH/FSH along with gonadal steroid is required in all cases. In cases where a diagnosis cannot be reliably confirmed by basal LH/FSH levels (especially differentiating CDGP from hypogonadotropic hypogonadism), a stimulation test with GnRH analog is very useful. A karyotype analysis for TS should be performed in all girls with delayed puberty, and short stature irrespective of any physical stigmata of TS as mosaics may have Y-cell line, which increases the risk of malignancy in the future and should be removed. In all cases of hypogonadotropic hypogonadism, MRI imaging of the hypothalamus and pituitary region is a must to rule out any mass or operable lesion.

TREATMENT

Treatment of delayed puberty is to initiate puberty with gonadal steroid supplementation. As the normal pubertal process takes 2–4 years for completion of puberty, puberty induction is started at very low doses, gradually increased to mimic physiological puberty.

Treatment in boys is started with supplementation of testosterone. Injectable testosterone enanthate is the commonly used agent, started in the dose of 50 mg, intramuscular (IM), every month for 6–12 months, and then, gradually increased over 6 months interval to reach an adult replacement dose of 250 mg once in 3 weeks, by the end of 2–3 years.

In girls, the oral and transdermal route has been used for estrogen supplementation. Commonly used preparations are estrogen valerate 0.5 mg alternate day for 6 months with dose escalation to reach an adult dose of 2 mg. Another option is ethinylestradiol started at 2 µg/day, increased to reach an adult dose of 20 µg/day. Conjugated equine estrogen preparation should never be used for puberty induction. Once the endometrium is well developed and estrogenized, it sheds on regular supplementation (called "breakthrough bleeding"). At this time, progesterone (medroxyprogesterone acetate, 10 mg/day for the last 10 days of estrogen supplementation) is added to regular estrogen supplementation in a cyclical fashion to have regular bleeding (called "withdrawal bleeding"). Although, the transdermal route has certain advantages over the oral route of estrogen administration but not commonly used because of the cost and nonavailability.

CONCLUSION

Pubertal onset is heralded by thelarche in girls and gonadarche in boys. The timing and tempo of pubertal onset vary in different populations. Pubertal signs should be interpreted with growth patterns. A deviation in growth and puberty (delayed or precocious) mandates further assessment and workup. Gonadotropin-dependent and -independent causes of precocious puberty and incomplete forms should be recognized early and treated. Systemic illness and CDGP are the most common causes of delayed puberty. Adequate nutrition and the prevention of micronutrient deficiencies are important during puberty.

HYPOGONADISM IN ADULTS

Hypogonadism is a state of decreased functional activity of sex steroids produced from the gonads. Both ovaries and testes produce various sex steroids, predominantly testosterone in males and estrogen in females. Production of sex steroids by gonads is under the control of gonadotropins secretion (LH/FSH) from the anterior pituitary, which is under the control of secretion of GnRH from the hypothalamus. The absence of sex steroids affects not only sexual health but also deleterious for physical and mental health. Loss of gonadal function is associated with an increased risk of sarcopenia, adiposity, osteoporosis, fragility fractures, and coronary artery disease. Causes of hypogonadism, as well as treatment, are entirely different in males and females, hence described separately.

HYPOGONADISM IN MALES

The clinical diagnosis of androgen deficiency acquired in adults is very challenging, particularly in older men. Hypogonadism is common, but most of the time, it is not recognized or even diagnosed very late because clinical manifestations of hypogonadism are nonspecific and depend upon the age of onset, severity, and duration of androgen deficiency. The social stigmas associated with clinical features are lack of privacy and confidence in treating physicians. Associated comorbidities are other important contributors for late diagnosis. It can occur at all stages of life, starting from infancy to old age. As age increases, the risk of development of hypogonadism also increases; with the highest prevalence seen in later life (sixth to ninth decade). Hypogonadism in males is a clinical syndrome comprised of symptoms and signs and biochemical evidence of testosterone deficiency. The primary functions of testes are testosterone production (by the Leydig cells) and spermatogenesis (by the spermatogenic and Sertoli cells in the seminiferous tubules). It may occur because of pathology/defect in testes (primary hypogonadism) or because of pathology/defect in the pituitary gland leading to failure of LH/FSH production (secondary hypogonadism).

TABLE 3 Causes of hypogonadism in males.

Primary hypogonadism	Secondary hypogonadism
Congenital:	
• Klinefelter syndrome • Down syndrome • Androgen synthesis disorders • Follicle-stimulating hormone (FSH) receptor gene mutation • Cryptorchidism (undescended testes) • Varicocele • Myotonic dystrophy	• Isolated gonadotropin deficiency: ∘ Kallmann syndrome ∘ Normosmic isolated gonadotropin deficiency ∘ Leptin or leptin receptor mutation ∘ Prader–Willi syndrome ∘ Gonadotropin subunit mutation • Deficiency of combined pituitary hormones: ∘ Hypopituitarism
Acquired:	
• Cirrhosis • Chronic renal failure • Human immunodeficiency virus (HIV) • Drugs—glucocorticoids, alkylating/neoplastic agents, and ketoconazole • Autoimmune damage • Infections—mumps • Radiation-induced orchitis • Trauma • Testicular torsion	• Diseases causing gonadotropin suppression: ∘ Hyperprolactinemia ∘ Drugs—gonadal steroids, glucocorticoids, opiates, and gonadotropin-releasing hormone (GnRH) analogs ∘ Critical illness/severe systemic illness ∘ Diabetes mellitus • Gonadotropic cell damage: ∘ Benign or malignant tumors and cysts ∘ Infiltrative diseases ∘ Infections ∘ Pituitary apoplexy ∘ Trauma ∘ Surgery/radiation of sellar region

TYPES OF HYPOGONADISM

Primary hypogonadism: Here, low testosterone levels result from primary disease of testes with normal pituitary functions. In an attempt to stimulate testosterone production, the pituitary secretes more gonadotropins (LH/FSH), resulting in elevated levels; hence, it is also known as "hypergonadotropic hypogonadism". Since, the primary defect is in testes, not only testosterone production but sperm production is also affected by the same testicular disease. Hence, fertility is not possible in most cases. Causes of primary hypogonadism can be divided into two categories, congenital and acquired. Important causes are listed in **Table 3**.

Klinefelter syndrome is the most common chromosomal disorder associated with primary hypogonadism. It results from an extra X chromosome (karyotype 47XXY).

Secondary hypogonadism: It results from a primary defect of gonadotropin production from the pituitary (gonadotropin deficiency) with normal testes; hence also known as "hypogonadotropic hypogonadism". As there is no primary testicular-defect, fertility is possible with spermatogenesis induction by exogenous administration of LH/FSH. It can result from diseases of the pituitary (loss of LH/FSH secretion) or diseases of the hypothalamus (loss of GnRH secretion). It can occur as an isolated condition (only loss of LH/FSH secretion; a condition known as "IHH") or may be associated with loss of other pituitary hormone secretion (hypopituitarism). Secondary hypogonadism results from any disease process affecting functions of either pituitary or hypothalamus, which could be congenital or acquired (**Table 3**).

Congenital causes: Congenital hypogonadotropic hypogonadism can result from either decreased gonadotropin secretion (pituitary cause) or impaired function of the GnRH pulse generator (hypothalamic cause). Mutations in genes regulating the development and migration of GnRH neurons or genes involved in the GnRH secretion have been reported. Since fertility can be induced with treatment, the familial transmission of hypogonadotropic hypogonadism has been reported (as an autosomal dominant trait in 50% cases, X-linked in 20%, or could be autosomal recessive inheritance in 30%).

During fetal development, GnRH neurons originate from the olfactory placode and then they migrate along the fetal olfactory neurons to reach their final location in the hypothalamus. Defects in transcription factors/genes controlling the development of olfactory placode or migration of GnRH neurons can result in loss of activity of these neurons. Failure of the early development of olfactory placode results in both anosmia/hyposmia and hypogonadism. This syndrome of hypogonadism and anosmia is known as "Kallmann syndrome" (mutations in *KAL1, FGF8, FGFR1, NELF, PROK2, PROK2R*, and *CHD7* genes). However, defects occurring in the later part of development result in hypogonadism without affecting smell [normo-osmic hypogonadotropic hypogonadism; normosmic IHH (nIHH), mutations in *GnRHR, GNRH1, KISS1R, TAC3, TACR3*, and *NROB1* genes]. In both of these cases, Kallmann syndrome as well as nIHH, the rest of the pituitary hormones are secreted normally.

Acquired causes: The common acquired causes are trauma, tumor, and infection, affecting the hypothalamus or pituitary gland (**Table 3**). Head injury of any severity is known to cause hypogonadism, where it is most neglected. It has been reported that approximately 50% of survivors of severe traumatic brain injury develop hypogonadism on long-term follow-up.

CLINICAL FEATURES

The development of clinical features is so gradual that it gets neglected most of the time. Sexual dysfunctions (reduced sexual thoughts, desire/libido, erections, erectile dysfunction, difficulty in attaining orgasm, reduced night-time or morning spontaneous erections, reduced ejaculate, and infertility) are the most common features; however, not easily recognized. Hypogonadism persisting over a long period will lead to regression of secondary sex characteristics such as decreased facial hair manifesting as reduced frequency of shaving, decreased pubic and axillary hair, reduced energy/stamina, weakness, decreased physical performance, depressed mood, increased irritability, and difficulty in concentrating. A decrease in testosterone level would result in an imbalance in testosterone to estradiol level and result in gynecomastia which may be the only finding of hypogonadism. Hence, all cases of gynecomastia should be investigated for hypogonadism. As testosterone is an anabolic hormone, the long-term deficiency would lead to anemia, reduced muscle mass, abdominal adiposity, and a decrease in bone mineral density with an increased risk of osteoporosis later in life.

DIAGNOSIS

Measurement of serum testosterone level is the usual first-line test for diagnosis of hypogonadism. Most laboratories measure total testosterone, while some laboratories also measure free or bioavailable testosterone levels. Measurement of total testosterone is always preferable over free or bioavailable as it is easy, direct, and robust measurement. Most of the diagnostic methodology and guidelines are based on serum total rather than free or bioavailable testosterone. Interpretation of free or bioavailable has always remained controversial and would only be helpful when the interpretation of total is affected by some condition or disease state. Total serum testosterone can be determined by enzyme immunoassays or mass spectroscopy, later being more sensitive and reliable but expensive and not widely available.

Method and timing of testosterone measurement: The preferred and best time for sample collection for serum testosterone is morning, between 8–10 AM and in a fasting state. As testosterone secretion follow a circadian rhythm, reaching a peak at 8 AM with a nadir around 10 PM. This circadian secretion is more important while collecting a sample in young patients. As age increases, the circadian rhythm becomes less marked. It is always better to take the sample on 2–3 occasions in place of one for a better understanding of secretion pattern. The testes usually produce 3–10 mg of testosterone daily, which results in serum levels between 300 and 1,000 ng/dL. The cutoff for diagnosis of hypogonadism has always remained controversial, varying between 200 and 350 ng/dL. The various guidelines suggest a cutoff of 300 ng/dL as the threshold level for diagnosis of hypogonadism. This is based on studies showing that below this level, there is evidence of bone loss and increased fat accumulation. However, normal ranges differ between laboratories, assay kits, and populations.

Measurement of gonadotropins: It is the second step once the diagnosis of hypogonadism is confirmed. Measuring serum levels of LH/FSH in the morning is helpful in differentiating the cause of hypogonadism. Low testosterone level accompanied by elevated gonadotropin levels suggests primary hypogonadism. In secondary hypogonadism, low testosterone level is accompanied by low, normal, or inappropriately elevated levels. Low testosterone level accompanied by low or inappropriately normal gonadotropin levels suggests secondary hypogonadism (**Flowchart 1**). In secondary hypogonadism, other pituitary hormone deficiencies should be ruled out. In addition, MRI of the pituitary can be performed to rule out a mass lesion in the sellar or hypothalamic area. Semen analysis is required for those planning for fertility.

TREATMENT

Starting treatment with testosterone replacement is a debatable issue. The Endocrine Society Clinical guidelines recommend reserving treatment for those patients with clinical symptoms rather than those with just low testosterone levels. Once decided to start treatment, testosterone replacement therapy is the primary treatment option. The aim of testosterone supplementation is to relieve symptoms of androgen deficiency and prevention of long-term complications of androgen deficiency. It can be started by various methods such as IM injections, transdermal

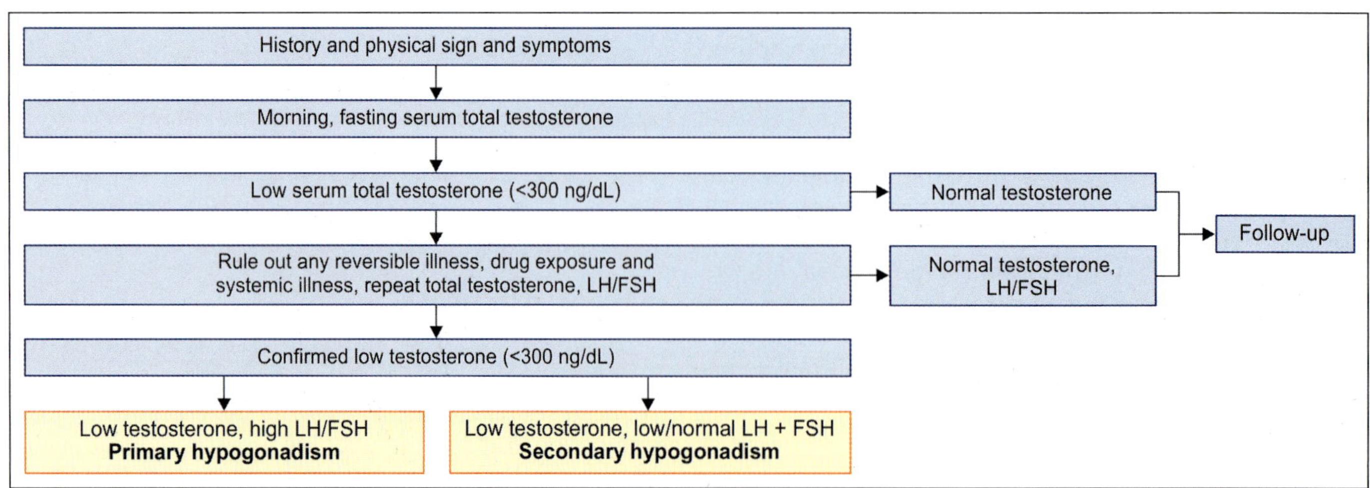

FLOWCHART 1: Diagnostic workup of a suspected case with hypogonadism (males).

TABLE 4 Causes of hypogonadism in females.

Primary hypogonadism	Secondary hypogonadism
Congenital primary ovarian insufficiency: • Chromosomal abnormalities: Turner syndrome, fragile X syndrome, and galactosemia • Ovarian dysgenesis or agenesis • Congenital adrenal hyperplasia **Acquired primary ovarian insufficiency:** • Medications: Chlorambucil, cyclophosphamide, and alkylating agents • Radiotherapy to ovarian region • Autoimmune disorders: Autoimmune polyglandular syndrome type 1 • Viral infections: Mumps oophoritis, tuberculosis (TB), malaria, and varicella • Bacterial infections: *Shigella* • Iatrogenic diseases: Post oophorectomy (surgical removal of ovaries)	**Congenital secondary hypogonadism:** • Genetic mutations: Kallmann syndrome • Isolated hypogonadotropic hypogonadism (IHH) **Acquired secondary hypogonadism:** • Intracranial space occupying lesions • Infiltrative diseases: Sarcoidosis and hemochromatosis • Infection: Meningitis and TB • Pituitary apoplexy • Trauma **Acquired causes of gonadotropin suppression:** • Chronic diseases • Strenuous exercise • Critical or severe illness of any system • Chronic exposure to opiates, glucocorticoids, and anabolic steroids

patch, topical gel, transbuccal tablets, implantable pellet, and oral capsules. However, of all these options, IM injections are most widely used and are most cost-effective. These injections are a combination of 2–4 esters (enanthate and cypionate) of testosterone with different duration of action (immediate and long-acting esters). These injections are to be given once in 2–3 weeks. The standard dose for an adult male is 250 mg IM once in 3 weeks.

A longer-acting ester (testosterone undecanoate) to be used once in 3 months is also available, but not much in clinical use. In comparison, oral capsules are to be given thrice a day and gel is to be applied daily (1-month treatment cost is 10–20 times of injections). Testosterone supplementation is contraindicated in men with metastatic prostate cancer or breast cancer because of concern of stimulation of growth of these androgen or estrogen-dependent neoplasms. Before starting testosterone supplementation, routine screening with hematocrit, liver function test, and serum prostate-specific antigen (PSA) should be carried out, and after starting supplementation, it should be repeated annually.

In case of secondary hypogonadism, where fertility is required, testosterone supplementation is stopped, and spermatogenesis induction therapy is started with human chorionic gonadotropin (hCG) therapy (subcutaneous injections, thrice a week, starting dose is 75 IU) for 3–6 months followed by addition of 3-hydroxymethyl-3-methylglutaryl (HMG) or synthetic FSH (subcutaneous injections, thrice a week, starting dose is 75–150 IU) to ongoing hCG therapy for another 6–12 months. The success rate of this therapy (outcome—live birth) is 30–40%. Fertility is not possible in primary hypogonadism.

HYPOGONADISM IN FEMALES

Female hypogonadism is defined as a deficient or abnormal function of the hypothalamic-pituitary-ovarian axis causing estrogen deficiency and menstrual cycle disturbances. It may be caused due to gonadal (primary hypogonadism or hypergonadotropic hypogonadism or primary ovarian insufficiency) or failure of adequate production of gonadotropins (LH/FSH) by the hypothalamus or pituitary gland (secondary hypogonadism or hypogonadotropic hypogonadism).

TYPES AND CAUSES

Primary hypogonadism (hypergonadotropic hypogonadism): It is characterized by abnormal function of gonads leading to ovarian insufficiency. Since the primary defect lies in the ovary, fertility is not possible. The etiological factors could be congenital or acquired. Congenital hypergonadotropic hypogonadism could be a result of ovarian dysgenesis (TS) or a rare enzyme deficiency (CAH caused by enzyme 17-α hydroxylase deficiency). The acquired causes are gonadal toxins, including radiation, chemotherapy, or certain infections.

Premature ovarian failure (POF): Cessation of ovarian function before the age of 40 years results in premature menopause. Ovarian insufficiency leads to the disruption of negative-feedback restraint on the hypothalamus/pituitary gland leading to increased LH/FSH. Serum FSH is a better marker of ovarian failure as its levels are less variable than those of LH. POF should be suspected in any woman who is younger than 40 years and presents with menstrual irregularity, and has elevated serum FSH and low estradiol levels. The diagnosis of POF requires further evaluation to find out the cause of premature cessation of the function. Details of causes are given in **Table 4**. TS is the most common chromosomal abnormality resulting from primary or POF. It results from a deletion or the nonfunctioning of one X chromosome in females.

Secondary hypogonadism/hypogonadotropic hypogonadism: Secondary hypogonadism results from an abnormality in secretion of GnRH from the hypothalamus

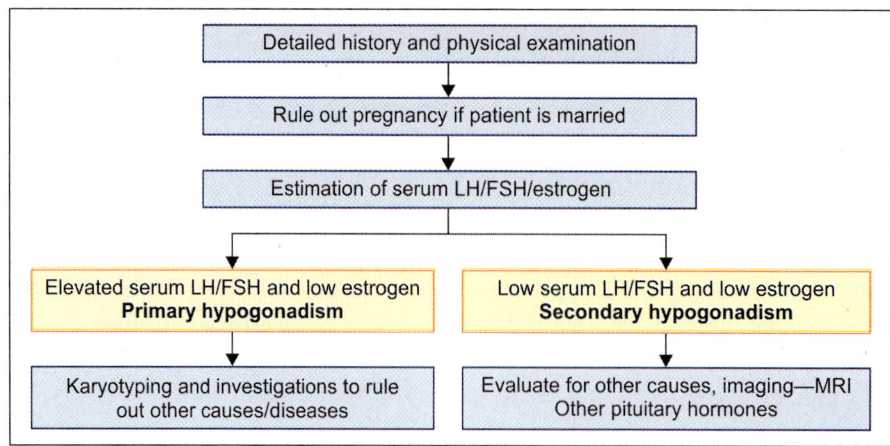

FLOWCHART 2: Diagnostic workup for a suspected case of hypogonadism (females).

or gonadotropins secretion from the pituitary. Low serum estrogen levels along with normal or low or inappropriately elevated LH and FSH levels are seen with anatomic, genetic, or functional abnormalities disturbing the hypothalamic GnRH secretion or pituitary responsiveness to GnRH. Although relatively uncommon, tumors and infiltrative diseases may be an underlying cause of hypogonadotropic hypogonadism manifesting with primary or secondary amenorrhea. It can occur as an isolated abnormality of LH/FSH secretion (Kallmann syndrome and idiopathic hypogonadotropic hypogonadism) or as a part of hypopituitarism with deficiencies of other pituitary hormones (postpartum pituitary necrosis or Sheehan's syndrome and lymphocytic hypophysitis).

Functional hypothalamic amenorrhea (HA): It is caused by a mismatch between energy expenditure and energy intake. Leptin secretion plays a key role in transducing the signals from the periphery to the hypothalamus. The hypothalamic-pituitary-adrenal axis may also play a role. In patients with leptin deficiency, clinical manifestations include hyperphagia, obesity, and secondary hypogonadism. The diagnosis is generally based on a careful history, detailed physical examination, and the presence of low gonadotropins and normal prolactin levels. Eating disorders such as anorexia nervosa and chronic disease must be specifically excluded while diagnosing HA.

Isolated hypogonadotropic hypogonadism: It generally presents with primary amenorrhea, although some patients may have initiation of breast development, and only a few may have few menstrual cycles. When IHH is associated with anosmia/hyposmia, it is called Kallmann syndrome. A defective GnRH neuron migration leads to Kallmann syndrome, which is characterized by secondary hypogonadism due to GnRH deficiency and anosmia. Genetic causes of IHH have been identified in approximately 60% of patients. Mutations in KISS1 and KISS1 receptors (KISS1R alias GPR54), which have a critical role in hypothalamic GnRH signaling and release have been identified in IHH.

CLINICAL FEATURES

In contrast to males, identification of hypogonadism in females is very easy as it would lead to abnormalities of menstrual cycles. Any subject having spontaneous, regular, predictable menstrual cycles in the last 6 months practically rules out the diagnosis of hypogonadism. Absent or irregular, unpredictable menstrual cycles are the main presenting features. Depending on the underlying cause, the clinical presentation may include headaches or vision loss (in case of tumor), milky breast discharge (hyperprolactinemia), symptoms of other hormonal deficiencies (such as hypothyroidism and hypocortisolism), and congenital anomalies (in congenital GnRH deficiency). Some patients may undergo some degree of pubertal development which does not progress normally. In secondary amenorrhea, menstrual cessation occurs after its normal initiation. In long-standing cases of hypogonadism, regression of secondary sexual characters such as a decrease in pubic/axillary hair and breast size also occurs.

DIAGNOSIS

Diagnosis of female hypogonadism is based on the age of onset, comorbidities, and severity of the dysfunction (**Flowchart 2**). Differentiation of hypogonadism from other causes of menstrual irregularity or amenorrhea is easy. Progesterone challenge test (PCT) reliably differentiates hypogonadism from causes. In any female presenting with amenorrhea, pregnancy should be ruled out first by pregnancy test because it may be possible that even without visible menstrual bleed, pregnancy can occur. Once pregnancy is ruled out, PCT can be carried out to differentiate. In PCT, progesterone preparation (medroxyprogesterone acetate, 10 mg daily, once a day for 10 days and stop and observe for any bleeding for the next 10 days) is given for a short period and withdrawn. Sudden withdrawal of high progesterone would result in the shedding of endometrium and menstrual bleed (withdrawal bleed). If the withdrawal of progesterone does not result in bleed in the next 10 days suggests that there is not sufficient estrogen levels, thereby confirming the diagnosis of hypogonadism. It reliably differentiates from the most common cause of nonhypogonadism menstrual abnormality caused by polycystic ovarian disease (PCOD). However, PCT cannot differentiate between hypo- or hypergonadotropic hypogonadism. To differentiate between these two, serum LH/FSH measurement is required. A low serum estrogen with elevated LH/FSH would confirm hypergonadotropic hypogonadism, while low or normal LH/FSH would suggest hypogonadotropic hypogonadism. Once the diagnosis of hypogonadism is confirmed, additional investigations are required to find out the cause of hypogonadism such as systemic biochemical workup, MRI of hypothalamic/pituitary area, evaluation of other pituitary hormones, and karyotype.

TREATMENT

Treatment of hypogonadism is required in all patients as it has been shown that absence of treatment is associated with psychosexual dysfunction, increased risk of coronary artery disease, and osteoporosis, and many other dysfunctions.

The treatment of hypogonadism depends upon the requirement of fertility as it is possible in cases of hypogonadotropic hypogonadism. Ovulation induction with synthetic LH/FSH is possible and can be carried out with a success rate of 20–30% with live birth is possible. Patients not requiring fertility and all cases of hypergonadotropic hypogonadism should be started on sequential estrogen-progesterone therapy to have a regular withdrawal bleed. One of the common methods is to start combined oral contraceptive pills (OCPs) for 21 days and then stop to have a progesterone withdrawal bleed and then again started. Duration of OCP therapy is a highly debatable issue. Usually, menopause occurs between the ages of 45–55 years, therapy may be continued till that time in discussion with the patient. As prolonged estrogen-progesterone administration is associated with adverse effects such as increased risk of thromboembolism, increased incidence of carcinoma breast, and endometrium, it should be explained to the patients and regular annual monitoring for these side effects are required. Those subjects who have undergone hysterectomy along with oophorectomy would require only continuous estrogen therapy (estradiol valerate 2 mg daily with no progesterone). For patients who have hypergonadotropic hypogonadism, fertility can be achieved by ovum donation and in vitro fertilization.

RECOMMENDED READINGS

1. National Research Council (US) and Institute of Medicine (US) Forum on Adolescence, Kipke MD. Adolescent Development and the Biology of Puberty. Washington (DC): National Academies Press (US); 1999.
2. Delemarre-van de Waal HA. Regulation of puberty. Best Pract Res Clin Endocrinol Metab. 2002;16:1-12.
3. Farello G, Altieri C, Cutini M, Pozzobon G, Verrotti A. Review of the Literature on Current Changes in the Timing of Pubertal Development and the Incomplete Forms of Early Puberty. Front Pediatr. 2019;7:147.
4. Sultan C, Gaspari L, Maimoun L, Kalfa N, Paris F. Disorders of puberty. Best Pract Res Clin Obstet Gynaecol. 2018;48:62-89.
5. Surana V, Dabas A, Khadgawat R, Marwaha RK, Sreenivas V, Ganie MA, et al. Pubertal Onset in Apparently Healthy Indian Boys and Impact of Obesity. Indian J Endocrinol Metab. 2017;21:434-8.
6. Khadgawat R, Marwaha RK, Mehan N, Surana V, Dabas A, Sreenivas V, et al. Age of Onset of Puberty in Apparently Healthy School Girls from Northern India. Indian Pediatr. 2016;53:383-7.
7. Vizmanos B, Martí-Henneberg C, Clivillé R, Moreno A, Fernández-Ballart J. Age of pubertal onset affects the intensity and duration of pubertal growth peak but not final height. Am J Hum Biol. 2001;13:409-16.
8. Khera M, Broderick GA, Carson CC 3rd, Dobs AS, Faraday MM, Goldstein I, et al. Adult-Onset Hypogonadism. Mayo Clin Proc. 2016;91:908-26.
9. Marcelli M, Mediwala SN. Male hypogonadism: a review. J Investig Med. 2020;68:335-56.
10. Bhasin S, Brito JP, Cunningham GR, Hayes FJ, Hodis HN, Matsumoto AM, et al. Testosterone Therapy in Men With Hypogonadism: An Endocrine Society Clinical Practice Guideline. J Clin Endocrinol Metab. 2018;103:1715-44.
11. Buvat J, Maggi M, Guay A, Torres LO. Testosterone deficiency in men: systematic review and standard operating procedures for diagnosis and treatment. J Sex Med. 2013;10:245-84.
12. Mulhall JP, Trost LW, Brannigan RE, Kurtz EG, Redmon JB, Chiles KA, et al. Evaluation and Management of Testosterone Deficiency: AUA Guideline. J Urol. 2018;200:423-32.
13. Irena I. Etiology of Central (Hypogonadotropic) Female Hypogonadism: Genetic, Organic and Functional Causes. Glob J Reprod Med. 2017;2:96-102.
14. Rothman MS, Wierman ME. Female hypogonadism: evaluation of the hypothalamic-pituitary-ovarian axis. Pituitary. 2008;11:163-9.

CHAPTER

117 Obesity

Ashu Rastogi

ABSTRACT

Obesity is a multifactorial complex disease with increasing incidence across the globe. The pathogenesis of obesity includes a state of calorie excess and reduced energy expenditure unless due to endogenous causes such as endocrine or monogenic disorders. Definition of obesity encompasses the measurement of body mass index (BMI), waist circumference (WC) and regional adiposity (visceral) evaluation. Obesity is the harbinger of various metabolic disorders including diabetes, dyslipidemia, hypertension, nonalcoholic fatty liver disease (NAFLD), osteoarthritis, malignancy, and even higher mortality compared to lean individuals. Management of obesity should involve behavioral intervention, dietary change with restriction of calorie intake, increased physical activity, and restricting sedentary time. Pharmacotherapy for weight loss is required in scenario of lack of benefits with lifestyle interventions. Bariatric surgery including sleeve gastrectomy (SG) and Roux-en-Y gastric bypass (RYGB) is a reliable option for weight loss and remission of obesity-associated comorbid disorders.

"Obesity affects every aspect of people's lives, from health to relationships"

—Jane V Mitchell

INTRODUCTION

Human species have evolved from hunter-gatherer that hunted food, and human body stored it as fat for times of food scarcity. Unfortunately, the present modern era of food abundance and calorie excess propounded by technological advancements limiting calorie consumption because of decreased physical activity has led to an epidemic of obesity. Obesity is a chronic disease that occurs because of imbalance in the calorie intake and expenditure unless endogenous in nature. Obesity is not a new disorder as it has been described much earlier by Hippocrates and Galen underscoring the significance of diet in individuals with excess weight. Presently, more than 1.9 billion adults are overweight and 650 million are supposedly obese on the planet making it most prevalent disorder affecting the mankind.

According to the World Health Organization (WHO) World Health Statistics Report 2012, globally one in six adults are obese and approximately 2.8 million deaths are reported because of being overweight or obese. Obesity is associated with an increased risk of mortality as compared to normal-weight individuals with a twice the risk of death from all causes. Life expectancy of obese individuals could be shortened by 2–5 years and even more if complicated with obesity-associated metabolic diseases. Thus, obesity is considered as the most significant public health problems contributing to burden on heath infrastructure. Metabolic syndrome (MetS) encompasses the physical characteristics and laboratory parameters into a single definition to define individuals who are likely to have adverse consequences, mainly atherosclerotic cardiovascular disease (ASCVD) and cardiovascular events (CVEs) because of obesity.

DEFINITIONS

Obesity is practically a state of excess fat that is determined by BMI, calculated as weight (in kilogram) divided by height square (in cm) and/or WC. Ideally, both should be measured for epidemiology or risk characterization of the population. However, BMI is an imperfect measure of excess fat as it is not a factor for metabolically active fat [visceral adiposity (VA)] or muscle mass, and many people with higher BMI may be metabolically healthy or vice versa. Interpret BMI with caution in highly muscular adults as it may be a less accurate measure of adiposity in this group. However, BMI is more commonly used than WC because of the convenience in measurement. Certain other ratios such as waist-to-hip ratio (WHR) and waist-to-height ratio have also been used to define obesity.

Obesity is multifactorial trait depending on both exogenous and endogenous factors such as ethnicity and genetic factors. Hence, definition of obesity varies according to the population studied and criteria for both BMI and WCs are lower for Asian-Indians compared to the Caucasian subsets (**Table 1**). Modified criteria of BMI classification for Asian Indians was found to have high sensitivity (67%) in predicting and diagnosing hypertension as compared to the WHO criteria (55%) or resembled sensitivity estimate obtained through direct body fat percentage estimation (69%). The reason for lowering cutoffs for defining obesity in Indian population is because Indians have higher risk for development of obesity-related noncommunicable diseases (NCDs) at lower BMI levels compared to several other races.

Additionally, obesity may be defined based on the abnormal regional fat distribution, especially VA. VA more accurately predicts the occurrence of metabolic

TABLE 1 Parameters used for defining obesity in people with different ethnicities.		
	Caucasian	**South Asians/ Indians**
BMI (overweight)	25–30	23–27.5
BMI (obesity)	>30	>27.5
Waist circumference (male)	102 cm	90 cm
Waist circumference (female)	88 cm	80 cm

complications including diabetes, hypertension, or atherosclerotic CVE. A strong correlation has been found between VA and WHR ($r = 0.936$, $p < 0.05$) in either gender, though the correlation between WC and BMI with visceral fat area (VFA) for males ($r = 0.739$, $r = 0.758$) and females ($r = 0.774$, $r = 0.605$) is relatively modest. WHR and WC are useful surrogate for assessing VA in clinical and epidemiological settings. More accurate measure of VA may be obtained by noninvasive modalities including bioimpedance analyzer, dual-energy X-ray absorptiometry (DXA), computed tomography (CT) or magnetic resonance imaging (MRI). But these modalities are restricted for research settings considering their expensive and labor-intensive nature.

METABOLIC SYNDROME

The clinical significance of obesity has been summed in a common definition known as MetS to correlate with cardiovascular outcomes. Abdominal obesity (AO) is considered as the single-most important risk factor for MetS and predisposition metabolic diseases including diabetes mellitus (DM). Therefore, the presence of AO assessed by either as WC [National Cholesterol Education Program's Adult Treatment Panel III (NCEP-ATPIII)] or WHR (the WHO criteria) is the mandatory criterion for the definition of MetS. There are various definitions of MetS but the most widely recognized definition is by the NCEP ATPIII that considers the presence of three out of five following factors in an individual: AO, high triglycerides, low high-density lipoprotein cholesterol (HDL-C), hypertension, and hyperglycemia.

- Raised triglycerides: ≥150 mg/dL (1.7 mmol/L) or history of specific treatment for this lipid abnormality
- *Reduced HDL-C*: <40 mg/dL (1.03 mmol/L) in males and <50 mg/dL (1.29 mmol/L) in females or history of specific treatment for this lipid abnormality
- *Raised blood pressure*: Systolic BP ≥ 130 mm Hg or diastolic BP ≥ 85 mm Hg or on treatment for previously diagnosed hypertension
- *Raised fasting plasma glucose (FPG)*: ≥100 mg/dL or previously diagnosed type 2 diabetes mellitus (T2DM)

Additional components include presence of NAFLD. About 25–30% of urban Indian population has the MetS. Fat deposition is also seen in ectopic tissues such as liver, pancreas, dorsocervical region and under the chin ("double chin") and this is strongly associated with the MetS.

OBESITY IN SOUTH ASIAN AND INDIANS

High prevalence of AO is characteristic of South Asians, even at BMI levels < 25 and is seen at a young age. Asian Indians have greater total, truncal, intra-abdominal and subcutaneous (SC) adipose tissue at similar BMI as compared to white Caucasians. WC is a surrogate of AO. As higher morbidities are seen at lower level of WC in Asian Indians, cutoffs for diagnosis of AO have been advocated as 90 and 80 cm, as opposed to international cutoffs of 102 and 88 cm for men and women, respectively.

EPIDEMIOLOGY

The prevalence of obesity in India is increasing with increasing urbanization and mechanization. The 2017 National Nutrition Monitoring Bureau prevalence estimates suggested overweight/obesity in 34% and 44% in males and females, respectively according to international cutoffs. However, if Asian-Indian cutoff (BMI value of > 23 kg/m^2) are taken in consideration, the prevalence of obesity/overweight shoots to 52% and 59%, respectively. In a recent study from rural Indian population, the prevalence of overweight and obesity was found to be 49.62% using modified criteria for the Asian Indians (BMI ≥ 23 kg/m^2) but 34.62% according to the WHO criteria (BMI ≥ 25 kg/m^2). Furthermore, obesity is more prevalent in women compared to men and is increasing in children and adolescents.

Regional adiposity, particularly AO, is pertinent for the prediction of chronic metabolic complications in addition to the generalized obesity (GO). Prevalence of both AO and GO is high in India. In a recent ICMR-INDIAB (Indian Council of Medical Research–India Diabetes) survey with samples from three states and one union territory, the extrapolation of data to the whole country revealed that 135, 153, and 107 million individuals will have GO, AO, and combined obesity (CO), respectively.

The main contributors to the rise of obesity in India include increased adoption of sedentary lifestyle and consumption of energy-dense and added sugar foods. In the ICMR-INDIAB study, female gender, hypertension, diabetes, higher socioeconomic status, physical inactivity, and urban residence were significantly associated with GO, AO, and CO on multiple logistic regression analysis.

ETIOLOGY AND RISK FACTORS

Most cases of obesity are due to imbalance between caloric intake and expenditure coupled with a sedentary lifestyle. However, there are various endogenous disorders causing obesity independent of calorie intake as shown in **Box 1**.

- *Familial*: Obesity commonly runs in families. This is because of shared genetics and environmental factors (e.g., excess food intake and sedentary lifestyle).
- Endocrine causes of obesity include Cushing syndrome, hypogonadism, hypothyroidism, and growth hormone deficiency.
- Monogenic causes are caused by a single-gene mutation, primarily located in the leptin-melanocortin

BOX 1	Various causes of endogenous obesity.
• **Monogenic disorders including gene mutations in:**	
◦ *Leptin, leptin receptor*	
◦ *POMC, MC4R*	
◦ AgRP	
◦ *Fat, Tub*	
◦ *PCSK1*, and *BDNF*	
◦ *TrkB, Sim1, SH2B1*	
◦ *FTO*	
• **Endocrine causes:**	
◦ Cushing's syndrome, hypothyroidism, insulinoma, post-craniopharyngioma hypothalamic disorders	
• **Syndromic obesity:**	
◦ Prader–Willi syndrome	
◦ Laurence–Moon–Biedl, Ahlstrom, Cohen, Carpenter	

pathway, e.g., congenital leptin deficiency, leptin receptor deficiency, proopiomelanocortin (*POMC*) gene mutations.

- *Syndromic obesity*: It causes severe obesity associated with other phenotypes such as neurodevelopmental abnormalities, and other organ system abnormalities. Obesity in these individuals is evident in childhood.
- *Polygenic obesity*: It is caused by cumulative contribution of many genes whose effect is amplified in a "weight gain promoting" environment. *MC4R, PCSK1, POMC,* and *BDNF* genes have been implicated in polygenic as well as monogenic forms of obesity.
- Psychosocial factors: Social factors (socioeconomic status, ethnicity etc.) and psychological factors (stress, depression) may lead to obesity. Psychologically directed specific eating disorders include binge eating and night eating syndrome.
- Other factors include medications.

HEALTH IMPLICATIONS

Obesity is commonly associated with abnormal metabolic function contributing to various s NCDs including T2DM, dyslipidemia, hypertension, coronary heart disease (CHD), NAFLD, and several cancers as elaborated in **Box 2**. In general, these comorbidities are more prevalent in Indians at a relatively lower BMI levels than other ethnicities.

DIAGNOSTIC APPROACH

CLINICAL EXAMINATION

Weight and height are essential for physical examination. Weight should be measured on a calibrated balance scale and height by standard stadiometer to obtain BMI. WC is obtained at midway of lower intercostal margin and superior margin of iliac crest. WHR is calculated by dividing WC (cm) by height (cm). Truncal SC adipose tissue can be measured by subscapular and supra-iliac skinfold thickness obtained by a caliper.

Patients should be examined for physical characteristics of obesity including acanthosis nigricans, excess dorso-cervical fat deposition, xanthelasma, arcus, hepatomegaly, hernia, and varicose veins.

BOX 2	Pathological consequences of obesity.
• Metabolic syndrome	
• Insulin resistance and type 2 diabetes mellitus	
• Dyslipidemia	
• Hypertension	
• Acute coronary syndrome, congestive heart failure, cerebral ischemic events	
• NAFLD	
• Hypogonadism (MOSH), subfertility, infertility	
• Polycystic ovarian syndrome	
• Osteoarthritis	
• Hyperuricemia and gout	
• Obstructive sleep apnea, obesity hypoventilation syndrome	
• Gall stone disease	
• Malignancy (higher risk of deaths)	
◦ *Males*: Esophagus, colon, rectum, pancreas, liver, and prostate	
◦ *Female*: Breast, cervix, endometrium, ovaries, gallbladder, and bile ducts	
◦ *Wither gender*: Renal, multiple myeloma, non-Hodgkins lymphoma	
• Venous stasis, varicose veins	

(MOSH: male obesity secondary hypogonadism; NAFLD: nonalcoholic fatty liver disease)

EVALUATION FOR COMORBID CONDITIONS

Investigations are often required to assess associated complications or to rule out secondary causes of obesity.

- 75-gram oral glucose tolerance test and glycated hemoglobin (HbA1c) for diagnosis of prediabetes and diabetes.
- Fasting lipid panel for dyslipidemia
- Serum uric acid for hyperuricemia
- Liver function tests for NAFLD
- Ultrasound of abdomen for assessment of NAFLD and polycystic ovarian disease
- Electrocardiogram and echocardiogram for assessment of left ventricular hypertrophy and CHD.
- Polysomnography (PSG) for obstructive sleep apnea.
- Thyroid function test for hypothyroidism
- Serum cortisol and other hormonal tests for Cushing's syndrome, growth hormone deficiency etc.

THERAPEUTIC APPROACH

GOAL OF THERAPY

The primary goal of treatment is to prevent obesity related comorbidities and decrease the risk of the development of future complications. The intensity of treatment is also determined by the number of coexisting comorbidities.

After determining the degree of overweight or obesity, discuss the implications of the individual's weight by addressing:

- Concerns and presenting symptoms
- Underlying causes of being overweight or obese
- Lifestyle (diet and physical activity)
- Eating behaviors
- Psychosocial distress and psychological problems
- Environmental, social, and family factors
- Comorbidities (e.g., T2DM, hypertension, cardiovascular disease, osteoarthritis, dyslipidemia, and sleep apnea)
- Risk factors assessed using lipid profile
- Blood pressure
- Glycemic management
- Person's willingness and motivation to change lifestyle
- Potential of weight loss to improve health

BEHAVIORAL INTERVENTIONS

Behavioral intervention is a broad term that includes dietary habits, exercise patterns, and food shopping habits of the individuals. The strategies for behavioral interventions include:

- Self-monitoring of behavior and progress
- Setting of goal
- Impulse and stimulus control for binge eating
- Slowing rate of eating
- Ensuring social support for problem-solving
- Assertiveness and cognitive restructuring (modifying thoughts)
- Reinforcement of changes for relapse prevention and strategies for dealing with weight regain

The initial weight loss can be sustained for as long as 10 years with appropriate behavioral modification and reinforcement as shown in LOOK AHEAD (Action for Health in Diabetes) trial.

PHYSICAL ACTIVITY

Encourage adults to increase their level of physical activity even if they do not lose weight because of the other health benefits it can bring (e.g., reduced risk of T2DM and cardiovascular disease).

- Encourage to build up to the recommended activity levels for weight maintenance, using a managed approach with agreed goals.
- Encourage adults to do at least 30 minutes of moderate- or greater-intensity physical activity on 5 or more days a week. The activity can be in one session or several sessions lasting 10 minutes or more.
- Most people may need to do 45–60 minutes of moderate-intensity activity a day. Few individuals may need to do 60–90 minutes of activity a day to avoid regaining weight, particularly if they do not reduce their energy intake.
- Recommend types of physical activity, including activities that can be incorporated into everyday life, such as brisk walking, gardening, or cycling.
- Supervised exercise programs to promote other activities, such as swimming, aiming to walk a certain number of steps each day, or stair climbing are advisable.
- Current physical fitness and individual ability are to be considered before prescribing physical activity.
- Encourage people to reduce the sedentary time, i.e., the amount of time spent inactive, such as watching television, using a computer, or playing video games.

DIETARY INTERVENTIONS

The main requirement of a dietary approach to weight loss is that total energy intake should be less than energy expenditure. Diets that have a 600 kcal/day deficit (i.e., they contain 600 kcal less than the person needs to stay the same weight) or that reduce calories by lowering the fat content (low-fat diets) may be offered for sustainable weight loss. Restricting fat in the diet without decrease in total calorie content may also not serve the purpose of weight loss. Very low-calorie diets (VLCD, 800 kcal/day or less) has been used to manage obesity with significant weight loss and metabolic benefits. But the sustainability of VLCD is questionable and is less likely to be nutritionally complete. Only consider VLCD as part of a multicomponent weight management strategy, for people who are obese and who have a clinically assessed need to rapidly lose weight, for example, people who need joint replacement surgery or who are seeking fertility services.

The diet should be nutritionally complete, so that diet could be followed for a minimum of 12 weeks (continuously or intermittently) to observe its effects. Encourage people to eat a balanced diet in the long term, consistent with other healthy eating advice.

PHARMACOLOGICAL INTERVENTIONS

Consider pharmacological treatment only after dietary, exercise, and behavioral approaches have been started and the person is not able to reach their target weight loss or have reached a plateau on dietary, activity, and behavioral changes. Most medications available to treat obesity are associated with only modest weight loss and rebound weight regain after cessation of therapy. The potential benefits and limitations of pharmacotherapy need to be discussed with the person, including the mode of action, adverse effects, and monitoring requirements, and the potential impact on the person's motivation. Various pharmacological agents used for weight loss are elaborated in **Table 2**. Presently, five antiobesity drugs have been approved by the US Food and Drug Administration (FDA) for long-term use with variable weight-lowering potential. Weight loss is found to be maximum with phentermine/topiramate > liraglutide 3.0 mg > naltrexone/bupropion > lorcaserin = orlistat. However, the use of many of these agents is restricted

TABLE 2 Pharmacological therapies for weight loss.

Drug class and name	Mechanism of action	Dose and route	Weight loss efficacy
Phentermine	Sympathomimetic	15–37.5 mg, oral, thrice a day	5%
Orlistat	Inhibit pancreatic Lipase	120 mg three times/day before meals	2–3%
Liraglutide	GLP-1 analog	3.0 mg daily subcutaneous	4–6%
Phentermine–topiramate extended release	Sympathomimetic/appetite suppressant	3.75/23 mg, once daily, oral	6–9%
Lorcaserin	Selective 5HT2c agonist	10 mg twice a day, oral	2–4%
Naltrexone/Bupropion	Mu-opioid receptor antagonist/ norepinephrine-dopamine reuptake inhibitor	32/360 mg, oral	5–6%
Gliflozins	SGLT-2 inhibitors	10/25 mg	2–3%

(GLP-1: glucagon-like peptide-1; SGLT-2: sodium-glucose cotransporter-2)

because of significant side effects including increased CVE with lorcaserin, increased neuropsychiatric adverse events with phentermine/topiramate, increased blood pressure with naltrexone. Some other investigational agents include leptin analog (metreleptin), glucagon-like peptide-1/ glucose-dependent insulinotropic polypeptide (GLP-1/ GIP) receptor dual agonists, neuropeptide-Y inhibitor, ghrelin antagonist, cannabinoid type-1 receptor antagonists and melanocortin receptor-4 agonist. Presently, orlistat and liraglutide are the only drugs approved for weight loss in India.

Orlistat: Orlistat inhibits pancreatic lipase and reduces enteric absorption of fatty acids. It is given in doses of 120 mg three times a day before major meals. Meta-analysis has shown that only 50% of patients have meaningful weight loss with orlistat. The average weight loss at the end of 1 year is 5 kg and most patients have weight loss in first 3 months of therapy. Continue orlistat therapy beyond 3 months only if the person has lost at least 5% of their initial body weight since starting drug treatment. Make the decision to use drug treatment for longer than 12 months (usually for weight maintenance) after discussing potential benefits and limitations with the person. The common side effect of orlistat is fatty diarrhea that limits compliance. The coprescribing of orlistat with other drugs aimed at weight reduction is not recommended.

Liraglutide: Liraglutide is a GLP-1 analog which has 97% homology with the native GLP-1. It predominantly induces satiety by acting on hypothalamic centers and delays gastric emptying causing prandial fullness. It is approved by the FDA for inducing weight loss in people with BMI >30 kg/m^2 or > 27.5 kg/m^2 in those with comorbidities. It is given as a once daily injection SC at a dose of 3.0 mg daily (compared with up to 1.8 mg daily for treatment of diabetes). Absolute weight loss reported with liraglutide 3.0 mg is up to 5.9 kg over 56 weeks. The significant side effects include nausea occurring in one third of patients and vomiting.

SURGICAL INTERVENTIONS

Bariatric surgery is the predominant and most reliable treatment option for people with obesity particularly for those with comorbidities of pre-existing diabetes, hypertension, dyslipidemia, NAFLD, cardiovascular diseases, sleep apnea, cancers, and pulmonary complications. The weight loss with bariatric surgery is substantial depending upon the type of surgery and sustained for prolonged years. Weight loss has been shown to sustain for up to 16 years after surgery, unlike the weight regain often occurs between 6 and 24 months following behavioral and pharmacologic treatments. The present recommendations for bariatric surgery are:

- BMI > 40 kg/m^2, or between 35 kg/m^2 and 40 kg/m^2 in the presence of significant disease such as T2DM or hypertension that could be improved if they lose weight.
- The modified cutoffs for Indians are BMI > 37.5 without presence of any obesity-related comorbidities or BMI > 32.5 with the presence of T2DM/any obesity-related comorbidities.
- All appropriate nonsurgical measures have been tried but the person has not achieved or maintained adequate, clinically beneficial weight loss.
- The person is generally fit for anesthesia and surgery.
- The person commits to the need for long-term follow-up.

Four surgical procedures are performed for obesity therapy including gastric banding, SG, RYBG, and biliopancreatic diversion (BPD). SG and RYBG are the two most performed procedures. Currently more than 0.3 million bariatric surgeries are performed annually in USA because of their significant metabolic benefits. Bariatric surgery usually produces weight loss that ranges between 50% and 75% of excess body weight and weight loss is maintained longer than that observed following nonsurgical treatment of obesity.

Approximately 80% of gastric bypass patients experience a 60–80% excess weight loss in the first year, with longer-term stabilization at 50–60% loss of excess body weight. The purported mechanisms for weight loss with bariatric surgery include early satiety, malabsorption, and increase in satiety hormones (GLP-1, GIP, cholecystokinin, peptide YY), decrease ghrelin, vagal interruption, and alteration in gut microbiota. The weight loss with bariatric surgery is associated with remission of diabetes in 40–70% of patients. Bariatric surgery is associated with remission of other comorbidities as well including sustained remission of hypertension in 70–90%, NAFLD in 50–80% of obese individuals. It has been noticed that bariatric surgery was associated with a reduced rate of all-cause mortality [pooled odds ratio (POR) 0.62, 95% confidence interval (CI) 0.55–0.69, $p < 0.001$], cardiovascular mortality (POR 0.50, 95% CI 0.35–0.71, $p < 0.001$) or cancer 0.47 (95% CI, 0.36–0.63, $p < 0.001$).

The treating team should discuss the potential benefits, the longer-term implications of surgery, associated risks, complications, and perioperative mortality before contemplating bariatric surgery.

CONCLUSION

Obesity is a complex, multifactorial disorder that contributes to significant morbidity and mortality. BMI is used as an index of obesity, though regional adiposity, particularly visceral obesity closely correlated with adverse metabolic consequences. Evaluation of obese individuals for the cause of obesity and obesity-associated comorbid conditions is essential. Interventions for obesity should include dietary therapy, increasing physical activity, and reinforcement for sustained weight loss. Lack of benefits with lifestyle interventions may prompt pharmacological therapy but have limited efficacy. Bariatric surgery, though invasive, is a reliable option for weight loss and remission of comorbid conditions including diabetes in morbid obese individuals.

RECOMMENDED READINGS

1. World Health Organization (WHO). (2012). World Health Statistics 2012. [Online] Available from https://www.who.int/gho/publications/world_health_statistics/EN_WHS2012_Full.pdf.
2. Verma M, Rajput M, Kishore K, Kathirvel S. Asian BMI criteria are better than WHO criteria in predicting Hypertension: A cross-sectional study from rural India. J Family Med Prim Care. 2019;8(6):2095-100.
3. Pradeepa R, Anjana RM, Joshi SR, Bhansali A, Deepa M, Joshi PP, et al. Prevalence of generalized & abdominal obesity in urban & rural India–the ICMR-INDIAB Study (Phase-I) [ICMR- NDIAB-3]. Indian J Med Res. 2015;142(2):139-50.
4. Gadekar T, Dudeja P, Basu I, Vashisht S, Mukherji S. Correlation of visceral body fat with waist-hip ratio, waist circumference and body mass index in healthy adults: A cross sectional study. Med J Armed Forces India. 2020;76(1):41-6.
5. Ahirwar R, Mondal PR. Prevalence of obesity in India: A systematic review. Diabetes Metab Syndr. 2019;13(1):318-21.
6. Look AHEAD Research Group. Wing RR, Bolin P, Brancati FL, Bray GA, Clark JM, Coday M, et al. Cardiovascular effects of intensive lifestyle intervention in type 2 diabetes. N Engl J Med. 2013;369(2):145-54.
7. Davies MJ, Bergenstal R, Bode B, Kushner RF, Lewin A, Skjøth TV, et al; NN8022-1922 Study Group. Efficacy of liraglutide for weight loss among patients with type 2 diabetes: The SCALE Diabetes Randomized Clinical Trial. JAMA. 2015;314(7):687-99.
8. Sjöström L, Lindroos AK, Peltonen M, Torgerson J, Bouchard C, Carlsson B, et al. Lifestyle, diabetes, and cardiovascular risk factors 10 years after bariatric surgery. N Engl J Med. 2004;351:2683-93.
9. Christou NV, Sampalis JS, Liberman M, Look D, Auger S, McLean APH, et al. Surgery decreases long-term mortality, morbidity, and health care use in morbidly obese patients. Ann Surg. 2004;240(3):416-24.
10. Wiggins T, Guidozzi N, Welbourn R, Ahmed AR, Markar SR. Association of bariatric surgery with all-cause mortality and incidence of obesity-related disease at a population level: A systematic review and meta-analysis. PLoS Med. 2020;17(7):e1003206.
11. Cardoso L, Rodrigues D, Gomes L, Carrilho F. Short- and long-term mortality after bariatric surgery: A systematic review and meta-analysis. Diabetes Obes Metab. 2017;19(9):1223-32.

CHAPTER 118 Endocrine Tumors and Malignancies

Suneel Mattoo, Roma Pradhan, Amit Agarwal

ABSTRACT

Each and every endocrine organ can undergo tumorigenesis. Tumors of the thyroid glands are not uncommon and include differentiated thyroid cancers (DTCs) and medullary thyroid carcinomas (CAs). Papillary thyroid carcinoma (PTC) is the most common type of DTC followed by follicular thyroid carcinoma (FTC). Parathyroid adenomas result in primary hyperparathyroidism (PHPT), however, parathyroid carcinomas are very rare and usually portend a grave prognosis. Adrenocortical neoplasms include adenoma and carcinomas. Both can result in cortisol and/or androgen hypersecretion. Neoplasms of the adrenal medulla include pheochromocytomas, which are usually benign but can rarely be malignant. Pheochromocytomas can be sporadic or occur as a part of syndromes, notably, multiple endocrine neoplasia type 2 (MEN2) or von Hippel–Lindau (VHL). Lastly, neuroendocrine tumors (NETs) of the pancreas and the rest of the gastrointestinal tract are often encountered in routine clinical practice. NETs of the pancreas can be either nonfunctional or associated with hormone hypersecretion, namely, insulinomas, gastrinomas, among others. Pancreatic NETs are often associated with multiple endocrine neoplasia type 1 (MEN1).

The E-chapter has many other tables and figures. Those who are interested in the topic in greater detail can refer to the E-chapter which has all the extra tables and figures.

"Faith is the bird that sings when the dawn is still dark"

—Rabindranath Tagore

INTRODUCTION

Endocrine tumors are a unique group of neoplasms which have an enormous impact on the patient's life disproportionate to their actual size. They tend to be functional most of the times and this has a tremendous impact on the normal physiology of the patient, but once surgically removed there is rapid return to normal and the results are extremely gratifying. They are elusive to diagnosis, elusive to localize, and elusive to find at surgery. They are also heterogeneous group of tumors ranging from the good ones like the papillary microcarcinoma to the ugly ones like the anaplastic and adrenal cancer. However, once surgically removed the patients are frequently cured and lead near normal lives and even in cases of advanced functional carcinomas significant palliation can be achieved by debulking leading to improvement in quality of life. Because of complexity in their diagnosis and treatment they are best treated in specialized endocrine units.

THYROID TUMORS AND MALIGNANCIES

Thyroid gland is present in the cervical region and is enclosed by pretracheal fascia. It is bound to cricoid cartilage and upper trachea by suspensory ligament of Berry. The isthmus lies against 2nd to 4th tracheal rings. The gland develops from the median downgrowth from the floor between first and second pharyngeal pouches.

It is suppled by superior thyroid artery (anterior and posterior branches), which is a branch of external carotid artery and inferior thyroid artery (ITA) which is a branch of thyrocervical trunk.

The lymphatics drain chiefly into middle and deep cervical lymph nodes (LNs) (levels 3 and 4). Subcapsular lymphatics however, drain into pretracheal and prelaryngeal LNs which then drain into lower deep cervical and mediastinal LNs.

External branch of superior laryngeal nerve (nerve of Galli-Curci) runs close to superior thyroid vessels and supplies cricothyroid muscle which is a tensor of vocal cord. This nerve must be preserved during ligation of superior thyroid vessels as it can lead to dampening of high notes which can be particularly devastating in professional singers, public speakers, and teachers.

CLINICAL FEATURES

The various clinical features and their significance is shown in the table below.

Neck swelling:

Duration/progression	
Short duration and rapid growth	• Likely malignant (e.g., carcinomas) • The rate of growth of anaplastic carcinomas is much faster when compared to DTCs
Long duration and slow growth	• Likely benign [e.g., benign multinodular goiter (MNG)] • Rapid growth of a nodule in a lump of long duration can indicate malignant transformation

Pressure symptoms:

Pressure symptoms	Cause
Dyspnea	• Tracheal compression in large goiters. Initially occurs in recumbent position and is relieved by lying on the sides • Tracheal infiltration with luminal invasion in malignancies • Cardiac failure in secondary thyrotoxicosis
Dysphagia	• Retrotracheal extension leading to compression of esophagus between trachea and vertebral column • Relatively uncommon because esophagus is a muscular and readily displaced tubular structure
Hoarseness of voice	• Compression of recurrent laryngeal nerve (RLN) in a benign goiter • Infiltration of RLN in malignancy

Toxic features:

Toxic features	Probable etiology
Mainly central nervous system (CNS) symptoms (e.g., tremors, sweating, excitability, heat intolerance, irritability, and prominent eyes)	Primary thyrotoxicosis (Graves' disease)
Mainly cyclic vomiting syndrome, cardiovascular symptoms (e.g., palpitations, chest pains, and dyspnea)	Secondary thyrotoxicosis (e.g., toxic MNG and FTC)

Important note: Follicular thyroid cancers and their metastatic lesions can be functional.

Classical features on clinical examination (Fig. 1):

Finding	Probable diagnosis
• Butterfly-shaped thyroid swelling • Bosselated surface • Variegated consistency • Mobile with deglutition • No cervical lymphadenopathy • Carotid artery pulsations pushed posteriorly	Benign thyroid swelling, e.g., MNG
• Solitary thyroid swelling • Firm to hard • Cervical lymphadenopathy • Fixed to straps/larynx/prevertebral fascia • Absent ipsilateral carotid artery pulsation (Berry sign positive suggestive of encasement of carotid artery)	Malignant thyroid swelling

CLASSIFICATION

Tumors within the thyroid gland can arise from follicular cells, C cells, and other mesenchymal cells. Those arising from the follicular cells form the vast majority and can range from benign to malignant. Other tumors of thyroid gland include medullary thyroid cancer (MTC), squamous cancer, mucoepidermoid cancer, paragangliomas (PGLs), mesenchymal tumors, hematolymphoid tumors, germ cell tumors etc.

A group of borderline thyroid tumors has been introduced for the first time by the WHO in 2017.

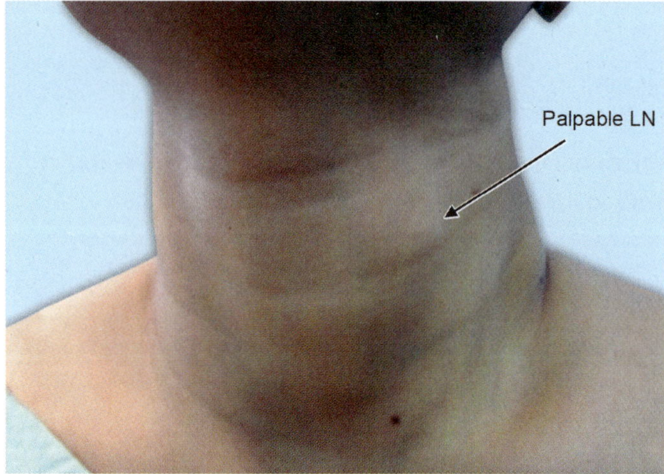

FIGURE 1: Patient of papillary thyroid carcinoma (PTC) presenting with goiter and lymph node (LN) enlargement

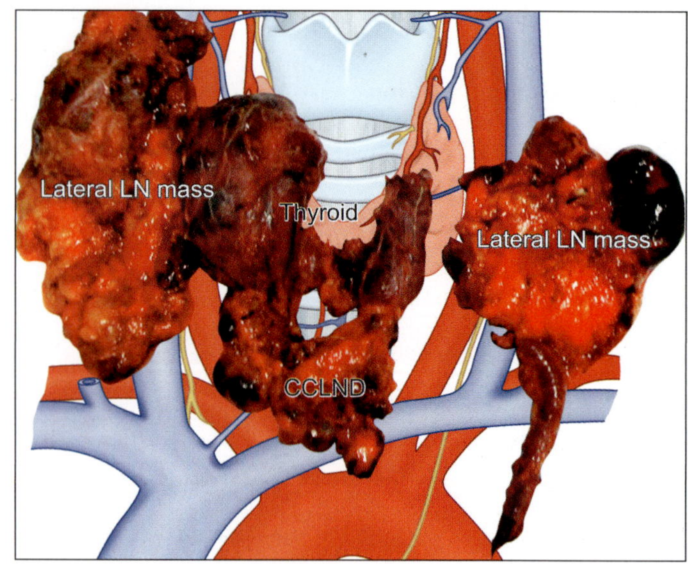

FIGURE 2: Specimen of total thyroidectomy of papillary thyroid carcinoma (PTC) treated with central compartment and bilateral modified radical neck dissection; note the black lymph nodes characteristic of papillary thyroid cancer

DIAGNOSIS AND MANAGEMENT

High-resolution ultrasonography (USG) of neck (7.5–15 MHz linear array transducer) with color Doppler is used to evaluate thyroid lesions. Thyroid Imaging Reporting and Data system (TI-RADS) is widely used to determine the risk of malignancy and need for cytologic examination. American College of Radiology (ACR) TI-RADS is the most widely used system.

An adequate FNA sample needs to have at least six groups of well-visualized follicular cells with at least 10 cells on a single slide. Cytomorphological features are then categorized according to the 2017 Bethesda System for Reporting Thyroid Cytopathology.

Papillary thyroid cancer (PTC): This is the most common thyroid cancer and may present as an incidentally discovered palpable or nonpalpable thyroid nodule which is highly suspicious/positive for malignancy on USG and fine-needle aspiration cytology (FNAC) (most common presentation), or reported to be DTC on a lobectomy specimen done for a Bethesda category 2, 3, 4 or 4 lesion, or as a thyroid incidentaloma on a positron emission tomography (PET) scan done for unrelated reason or detected on aspiration of a deep cervical LN with no palpable lesion in thyroid. After a confirmed diagnosis the treatment consists of surgery (**Fig. 2**), radioactive iodine (RAI) therapy and thyroid-stimulating hormone (TSH) suppression. The pathological diagnosis of classical PTC is relatively straight forward. The stoma has a papillary architecture and the characteristic nuclear changes of PTC include nuclear enlargement and overlap, nuclear elongation, irregular nuclear contours, nuclear pseudoinclusions or prominent longitudinal grooves, empty appearance of the nucleoplasm described as optically clear or ground glass nuclei. Psammoma bodies (lamellated calcifications) occur in about 50% cases. Multifocal diseases may be present in 20–40% cases. It carries an excellent prognosis with almost 95% survival.

Follicular thyroid cancer (FTC): It differs from PTC in all aspects. Usually presents with a solitary thyroid nodule but since FTC spreads hematogenously, distant metastases (DM) at presentation (M1) may be seen in a quarter of patients, thus patients may present with either a girdle bone mass like sternal mass, skull bone mets, or long bones metastases or even soft tissue metastases like eye/scalp. Cervical LN metastases are much less common seen only in 2–8%. Unlike PTC, FTC cannot be diagnosed by FNAC because the distinction between FTC (which shows capsular and/or vascular invasion) and benign FA (which does not show invasion) requires pathological examination of tumor capsule after thyroidectomy. On cytology all these lesions will either be categorized as Bethesda class III (rate of malignancy being 5–15%) or class IV (rate of malignancy being 15–30%). Thus a diagnosis of FTC is rarely confirmed prior to surgery—usually the patients with the Bethesda category III or IV cytology result would have undergone hemithyroidectomy with the pathology report of FTC. Surgical treatment could be either a hemithyroidectomy is considered sufficient if histopathological examination (HPE) is minimally invasive follicular thyroid cancer (MIFTC) with:

- Only CI with no VI
- <45 years old
- Tumor <4 cm
- No lymph node metastasis (LNM) and no DM

All others should undergo completion thyroidectomy. In patients presenting with thyroid nodule/goiter along with distant bone metastases, total thyroidectomy is the procedure of choice. Unlike the classical PTC, where the histopathological diagnosis is straightforward, the pathological diagnosis of FTC is rather difficult because of the need of examination of multiple sections/whole of the capsule; lack of standardized definition of types of FTC; and because of significant inter- or intraobserver variations. The WHO divided FTC into three main pathological categories:

1. *Minimally invasive*: Tumor with only CI
2. *Encapsulated angioinvasive*: Without reference to number of blood vessel
3. *Widely invasive*: Gross invasion

Radioactive iodine for FTC is generally administered to treat or discover DM and not to treat local recurrence or persistent local disease.

Following factors have been identified as independent predictors of recurrence, survival and DM: Older age, large tumor size, advanced stage, angioinvasion, DM, ETE, and presence of TERT mutations. In fact, follicular thyroid cancer histotype itself is thought to be an independent predictor of poorer survival.

Multiple metastases are best treated by RAI and sometimes with external beam radiation therapy (EBRT); multiple RAI doses can be given every 6 months along with suppressive thyroxine therapy. Spinal metastatic disease and spinal cord compression are major causes of morbidity and mortality. The treatment of metastatic disease of spine requires surgical decompression, reconstruction, and stabilization of spine in addition to EBRT. Patients with multiple brain metastases can be treated with EBRT or gamma knife. For single, demonstrable resectable metastasis, in long bones or brain, surgical resection should be considered. Recurrence rates in FTC vary from 3% to 40%. Local recurrences (thyroid bed/LNM) are rare in FTC while DM are more common (lungs, bones, brain, and soft tissues).

Hürthle cell carcinoma: It is a variant of FTC and its biological behavior is similar to FTC. They are primarily composed of Hürthle cells (also known as oncocytic or oxyphilic cell) which are large cells with increased granular cytoplasm due to increased mitochondria, along with large, hyperchromatic nuclei with increased cytoplasmic/nuclear ratio. On histopathology capsular and vascular invasion is necessary for diagnosis of hepatocellular carcinoma (HCC). However, LN metastases and soft tissue DM are more common than FTC. Unlike FTC, upfront total thyroidectomy is more acceptable for Hürthle cell neoplasm. Two studies concluded that total thyroidectomy was the only independent factor for improved cancer specific survival. Unfortunately, HCC is much less likely to be RAI avid. In HCC, tyrosine kinase inhibitors (TKIs) are best approach to systemic radioactive iodine refractory (RAIR) progressive disease.

Medullary thyroid cancer (MTC): It arises from parafollicular cells, the "C cells". It accounts for 5–10% of all thyroid malignancies. Three unique features of this thyroid malignancy are: (1) It is hereditary in 25% as part of MEN2A and MEN2B familial syndromes; (2) It secretes calcitonin which can be measured to make the diagnosis as well as used postoperatively as a very specific and sensitive tumor marker; (3) It metastasizes frequently to central and lateral LN of the neck (50%). Treatment is total thyroidectomy with LN compartmental dissection. 10-year survival is excellent (100%) in stage 1. Metastatic disease is treated by 2 TKIs approved by the Food and Drug Administration (FDA): Vandetanib and cabozantinib.

Poorly differentiated thyroid cancer: Poorly differentiated thyroid cancer (PDTC) can occur de novo or as a result of progression from DTC and it occupies an intermediate position between DTC and ATC. PDTC generally presents at an older age (median age 60 years) and unlike DTC, PDTC tends to present with locally invasive extrathyroidal disease in almost 50% cases. Also, DM are much more frequent in PDTC, occurring in up to 85% of cases when compared to 30% of cases in DTC. Distinguishing pathological features include presence of necrosis and mitosis [>3/10 high-power field (HPF)]. Most PDTC are now classified according to Turin criteria. Unlike DTC, treatment of PDTC has not been standardized due to heterogeneity of inclusion criteria. Surgery is the treatment of choice for PDTC. Total thyroidectomy and clearance of all gross disease can achieve satisfactory locoregional control (5-year locoregional control in up to 80% of PDTC patients. In addition, central and/or lateral neck dissection should be performed if there is clinical or radiological evidence of enlarged LNs. Regarding adjuvant treatment, when compared to DTC, PDTC does not usually respond as well. Radioiodine (RAI) avidity of PDTC is variable and role of postoperative EBRT in PDTC is equally controversial. PDTC is the most common cause for disease-specific mortality (DSM) in fatal nonanaplastic follicular cell-derived thyroid carcinomas. PDTC shows a more aggressive course with a higher propensity for local recurrence and DM to lungs and bone.

Anaplastic thyroid cancer (ATC) (Fig. 3): These are very aggressive thyroid cancers with median survival of 6 months. Majority present with a rapidly growing thyroid mass which is fixed on examination, dysphagia, dyspnea, vocal cord palsy, and neck pain. 50% present with DM. All anaplastic carcinoma are staged as Stage IV. So in majority upfront surgery is not an option and any radical

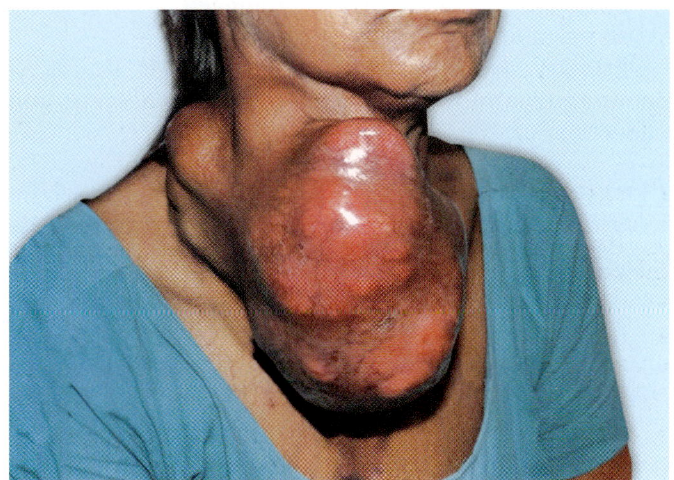

FIGURE 3: Anaplastic thyroid cancer.

morbid surgery is discouraged and they are usually put on chemotherapy or TKIs.

PARATHYROID TUMORS AND MALIGNANCIES

Most humans have four parathyroid glands. Superior parathyroid glands develop from the fourth branchial pouch and are located on the posteromedial aspect of thyroid gland near the tracheoesophageal groove. Majority of them are located in a circumscribed area 2 cm in diameter, about 1 cm above the intersection of RLN and ITA. Inferior parathyroid glands develop from the third branchial pouch and are more widely distributed from the posterior aspect of the thyroid lobe to the superior mediastinum along the path of descent of thymus.

The average weight and size of a parathyroid gland is 35–40 mg (range: 10–70 mg) and 5 mm × 3 mm × 1 mm, respectively. They are maroon, faintly globular or oblong, and softer than surrounding thyroid and LNs. Both superior and inferior glands are chiefly supplied by the branches of ITA.

TYPES

An inappropriately high parathyroid hormone (PTH) level for a particular calcium level is considered as hyperparathyroidism (HPT). It is of three types:

1. **Primary hyperparathyroidism:** It is a biochemical syndrome characterized by inappropriately high PTH due to increased secretion of PTH from one or more parathyroid glands. In outpatients, it is the most frequent cause of hypercalcemia. About 10% are familial and are inherited as autosomal dominated disease (three common familial HPTs: Familial isolated HPT (FIHPT), MEN1/MEN2A, or HPT-Jaw tumor syndrome.
2. **Secondary hyperparathyroidism (SPTH):** Excessive production of PTH secondary to a chronic abnormal stimulus such as chronic renal failure, vitamin D deficiency, and malabsorption syndromes.
3. **Tertiary hyperparathyroidism:** Autonomous hypersecretion of PTH causing hypercalcemia often seen in chronic secondary HPT (prolonged compensatory stimulation.

Primary hyperparathyroidism: PHPT is the most common type of HPT managed by endocrinologist and endocrine surgeons.

CLINICAL SYMPTOMS

The classically described symptom complex of PHPT includes:

- Painful bones (osteitis fibrosa cystica) (**Fig. 4**)
- Renal stones
- Abdominal groans (calcium-induced hypergastrinemia or pancreatitis)
- Psychiatric moans (hypercalcemia-induced psychiatric disease including depression, anxiety, and psychosis)
- Fatigue overtones

DIAGNOSIS

Hyperparathyroidism is a biochemical diagnosis. We need a set of investigations to diagnose PHPT and also to rule out causes of secondary HPT.

Traditionally biochemical diagnosis was made by elevated total calcium and intact PTH levels, however presently it is important to ask for an ionized calcium as it is unaffected by other factors like hypoalbuminemia. About 24-hour urine calcium levels are done to rule out benign idiopathic hypocalciuric hypercalcemia as the management is medical in such cases. Vitamin D and creatinine done to rule out secondary HPT.

Localizing investigations: Localizing investigations like US and sestamibi scans are done to plan the surgical procedure and not for making a diagnosis or to decide if surgery is needed or not which is a clinical decision.

The preoperative imaging commonly used is one anatomic and one functional imaging. The goal of preoperative imaging for HPT is to identify the location of abnormal parathyroid tissue as precisely as possible. Accurate preoperative imaging techniques such as technetium (99mTc) sestamibi scan and US can reduce unnecessary search and enable minimal invasive surgery. 99mTc sestamibi scan is the imaging of choice with sensitivity ranging from 54% to 88%. The high resolution US has sensitivity ranging from 59% to 89%.

The results of two imaging can be either concordant or discordant.

Concordant imaging means identifying same gland on both US and sestamibi scan. Nonidentification of any gland on both is called negative localization. Discordant imaging is when there is difference in the gland localized on both imaging. It can be either discordant for side (left or right) or gland position (superior or inferior gland) or for both side and position.

Investigations for end-organ effect: Before planning patient for surgery, it is important to document the end-organ effect especially on bones, kidney, and heart.

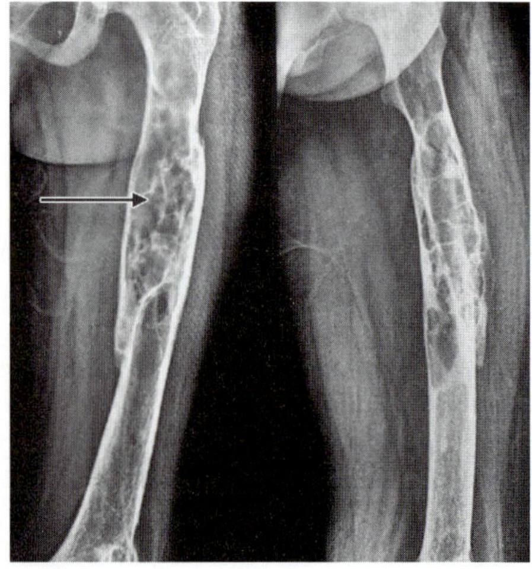

FIGURE 4: Brown tumor of femur: *Cystic, osteolytic, expansile thin* walled lesion.

Skeletal survey will reveal multiple brown tumors thus in such case it is advisable for proper handling of the patient while shifting or transferring them, 3 site dual-energy X-ray absorptiometry (DEXA) would reveal severe osteoporosis thus forewarning the possibility of hungry bone syndrome.

The role of FNAC in parathyroid lesions is limited as a diagnostic modality; however, it may have been unknowingly done in parathyroid lesions which are thought to be as thyroid lesions. The pathologist should be aware of the characteristics of the aspirate such as vascular proliferation and intracytoplasmic fat vacuoles which are highly suggestive of parathyroid origin.

MANAGEMENT

Surgery is the only cure for symptomatic patients and also for asymptomatic patients (**Flowchart 1**).

Surgical:

Surgical approach: The surgical approaches used in parathyroid surgery are BNE, unilateral neck exploration (UNE), and focused or limited parathyroidectomy (**Table 1**).

Bilateral neck exploration is the gold standard and includes visualization of all four glands and removal of the offending gland. If any of the glands is not seen then we have to search at embryological places.

Unilateral neck exploration is visualizing the glands on one side. Focused or limited parathyroidectomy is removal of the offending gland without visualization or search for other glands.

Focused or limited parathyroidectomy can be performed by various incisions that are either small incision right over the offending gland or conventional incision. Focused parathyroidectomy is attempted after one has concordant imaging on preoperative evaluation. In our series, 57 underwent focused parathyroidectomy out of 75 patients with concordant imaging. There were various reasons like concomitant PTC, intraoperative suspicion of carcinoma, and reoperation for patient who did not underwent focused approach with concordant imaging.

Intraoperative parathyroid hormone (IOPTH) is the most commonly used adjunct with focused parathyroidectomy. Most criteria of IOPTH require a PTH decline of ≥50% within 10 minutes after excision of the gland during surgery for primary PHPT (Miami criteria). A number of other criteria are mentioned in literature such as the Vienna criteria, 5 minute criteria, Halle criteria, and the residual criteria by Libutti et al. Because of cost constraints in India where IOPTH is used only in selected centers as routine adjunct; therefore, a method to reduce time and financial burden was suggested in our study. Two modifications can help in bringing down the cost of IOPTH. One way could be to reduce the number of samples needed to define cure. The second modification that could be made is the use of central laboratory for quick results.

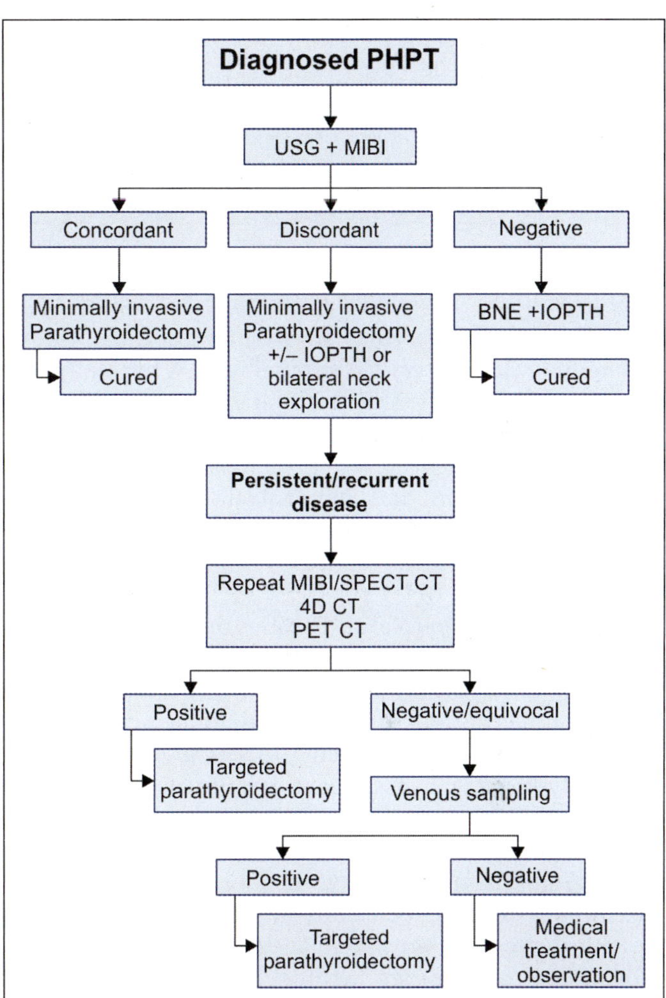

FLOWCHART 1: Managment of primary and recurrent primary hyperparathyroidism (PHPT).

TABLE 1 Extent of surgery in various pathologies of hyperparathyroidism.

Diagnosis	Treatment
Adenoma (e.g., sporadic and MEN2A)	• Focused single gland excision/minimally invasive parathyroidectomy
Hyperplasia (e.g. SHPT, THPT, and MEN syndromes)	Bilateral neck exploration (BNE) with: • Subtotal parathyroidectomy without autotransplantation • Total parathyroidectomy without autotransplantation • Total parathyroidectomy with autotransplantation
Carcinoma	• En bloc excision of parathyroid carcinoma with surrounding invaded structures • Radioresistant and chemoresistant

TABLE 2 Various drugs used in the management of hypercalcemia.

Class	Examples	Comments
Calcimimetics	Cinacalcet (Sensipar), evocalcet, and etelcalcetide	• Type 2 allosteric modulators of calcium-sensing receptor (CaSR) • Reduce serum calcium and PTH both • No effect on stabilizing bone mineral density (BMD) • Infrequent side effects, e.g., nausea and vomiting
Bisphosphonates	Zoledronic acid, alendronate, risedronate, and ibandronate	• Inhibit osteoclastic bone resorption • Slower onset and longer duration of action • Oral bisphosphonates have no effect on reducing calcium/PTH • Used to treat mainly severe bone disease • Intravenous (IV) drugs used to treat hypercalcemia in severe PHPT
Calcitonin	Salmon and human	• Inhibits osteoclastic bone resorption and promotes calciuresis • Rapid hypocalcemic action (in 2 hours) • Effect lasts for a week
Diuresis	Saline diuresis Loop diuretics	• Reserved in hypercalcemic crisis • Both together can lower serum calcium by 1.5–2 mg/dL in 24 hours

Histopathology: Parathyroid glands have chief cells, oxyphil cells, fibrovascular stroma, and adipose tissue. The median parenchyma to stromal ratio is normally 50% (40–70%). Tumors identified in parathyroid glands have varying composition of these primary elements apart from other distinguishing features. It is important to distinguish between adenoma and hyperplasia as the surgical management differs with the disease and the encountered pathology.

A vast majority of lesions (>95%) leading to PHPT are adenomas and hyperplasia. Parathyroid carcinomas are a cause of PHPT in only 0.5–2% cases. They are highly aggressive and typically presents between 45 and 59 years of age and has a slight male preponderance in contrast to adenoma which occurs mostly in females (3:1). 15% of seemingly sporadic cancers have germline CDC73/HRPT2 mutation and hence, genetic testing is recommended in all patients.

In comparison to parathyroid adenomas, parathyroid carcinomas tend to be relatively large and bulky with variable degrees of fibrosis and irregular borders. Common morphological findings include broad fibrous bands, necrosis, and solid growth pattern. The presence of increased mitotic activity, atypical mitoses, and nuclear atypia should raise the suspicion for an underlying malignancy.

Medical (Table 2):

Indications:

- Severe hypercalcemia in PHPT and parathyroid cancer
- Failure of surgical treatment of PHPT/when parathyroidectomy is contraindicated
- Uremic SHPT patients on dialysis

ADRENAL TUMORS, PARAGANGLIA AND MALIGNANCIES

Adrenal glands are paired glands in the perinephric fascia on the upper pole of each kidney. The right adrenal is pyramidal and located anterolateral to the right crus. The left adrenal is crescent shaped and related to spleen tail of pancreas and left crus of diaphragm. The glands are supplied by superior, middle, and inferior suprarenal arteries which are branches of inferior phrenic, abdominal aorta, and renal arteries, respectively. A single wide, short vein drains right adrenal gland into inferior vena cava and on the left; it is longer and drains into left renal vein.

Normal adrenal gland consists of two parts:

1. *Cortex*: It is made up of three layers; outermost is zona glomerulosa which secretes aldosterone, middle is zona fasciculata which secretes cortisol, and innermost is zona reticularis which secretes androgens.
2. *Medulla:* Secretes catecholamines including epinephrine (predominant), norepinephrine, and dopamine.

The hormonal hypersecretion corresponds to the region of the gland where the tumor arises (**Table 3**).

TABLE 3 2017 WHO classification of tumors of adrenal gland and paraganglia.

Tumors of adrenal cortex	Tumors of adrenal medulla and paraganglia
Cortical carcinoma	Pheochromocytoma
Cortical adenoma	Head and neck PGL
Sex cord stroma tumors	Sympathetic PGL
Adenomatoid tumors	Neuroblastic tumor of adrenal gland
Mesenchymal and stromal tumors: Myelolipoma and Schwannoma	Composite pheochromocytoma
Hematological tumors	Composite PGL
Secondary tumors	

ADRENAL INCIDENTALOMAS

- These are adrenal masses <1 cm in size detected on imaging done for reasons wherein adrenal pathology is not suspected initially.
- Up to 10% secrete excess hormones (cortisol—6.4%, catecholamines—3.1%, and aldosterone—0.6%)
- Risk of malignancy increases with size (**Table 4**)
- *Features suggestive of malignancy*: Abrupt onset, rapid increase in size, pyrexia, androgenic/feminizing tumors size >4 cm, irregular borders, heterogenous mass, infiltration into surrounding structures, elevated dehydroepiandrosterone (DHEA), and urinary ketosteroids.
- All adrenal incidentalomas should undergo testing for functional assessment as well as imaging (**Table 5**).

TABLE 4 Relation of size with risk of malignancy.

Size	Risk of malignancy
<4 cm	2%
4–6 cm	10%
>6 cm	25%
>8 cm	47%

Wash out studies on contrast-enhanced computed tomography (CECT) can help to predict malignancy as malignant tumors show washout less than 40%.

MANAGEMENT

- *Observation and follow-up*: For nonfunctional masses of size <4 cm with no pressure symptom or suspicion of malignancy
- *Laparoscopic adrenalectomy*: Preferred in all functional masses as well as nonfunctional symptomatic masses <6 cm in diameter with no suspicion of malignancy
- *Open adrenalectomy*: Preferred in masses >6 cm in diameter with high suspicion of malignancy

PANCREATIC ENDOCRINE TUMORS AND MALIGNANCIES

The pancreas is a retroperitoneal organ located in the epigastrium and upper left quadrants of abdomen. It is 15–20 cm long and extends along L1-2 vertebrae. It has both exocrine and endocrine parts. The exocrine parts has compound acinar gland, and the endocrine part has islets of Langerhans which has cells of different types (**Table 6**).

TABLE 5 Functional evaluation.

To rule out	Tests	Indication
Subclinical Cushing syndrome	Overnight 1 mg dexamethasone suppression test	All cases
Subclinical pheochromocytoma	24 hours urine fractionated (nor)metanephrines/plasma (nor) metanephrines	All cases
Subclinical hyperaldosteronism	Plasma aldo/plasma renin activity (PRA) ratio	• Hypertension (HTN) • Hypokalemia

TABLE 6 Distribution of different secretory cells in pancreas.

Islet cell	Location	Peptide	Physiological role
Alpha (10%)	Body and tail	• Glucagon • Peptide YY	Inhibit insulin and glucagon secretion
Beta (70%)	Throughout	• Insulin • Amylin	• Glucose uptake into cells • Inhibit insulin secretion • Increase insulin resistance • Decrease glucagon release
Delta (5%)	Throughout	• Somatostatin • VIP (D2 cells)	• Inhibit secretion of insulin, glucagon, gastrin, secretin, VIP, CCK, and motilin • Inhibits secretion of bile, pancreatic, and gastric juice • Inhibits gastrointestinal motility • Peripheral and splanchnic vasodilation • Smooth muscle relaxation • Inhibits gastrin-stimulated gastric acid secretion
F (15%)	Uncinate process	Pancreatic polypeptide	• Inhibits secretion of bile, pancreatic juice, and insulin • Inhibits gastrointestinal motility

INSULINOMA

- Insulin-producing tumor of pancreas
- *Incidence*: 4 per one million patient years
- F > M
- *Mean age of surgery*: 50 years (12–80)
- Benign and usually <2 cm
- Associated with MEN1 in 1–10% patients

Signs and symptoms:

- *Neuroglycopenic symptoms*: Apathy, confusion, dizziness, clouded sensorium, behavioral changes, and in severe cases stroke, convulsions, coma, and death
- *Gastrointestinal symptoms*: Hunger, nausea, and vomiting. Hunger leads to obesity in many cases.
- *Cardiovascular symptoms*: Episodic palpitation, pallor, chest pain, and tachycardia

> *Points to remember:*
> - Insulinoma leads to fasting hypoglycemia.
> - Signs and symptoms can mimic neurologic/psychiatric diseases.

Diagnosis:

Classical diagnosis by Whipple's triad:
- Signs and symptoms of hypoglycemia during fasting/exertion
- Blood sugar >45 mg/dL at the time of symptoms
- Relief of symptoms by administration of oral or IV glucose

Modern biochemical diagnosis:
- Fasting plasma glucose < 45–50 mg/dL
- Elevated insulin > 6 µ/mL by IRMA
- C-peptide > 200 pmol/L
- Negative screening levels for oral hypoglycemia agents—sulfonylureas and meglitinides
- Low beta hydroxybutyrate ≤2.7 mmol/L

Surgical management:

- Various localization modalities are available to localize the tumor pre-operatively.
- *Sporadic insulinoma*: Enucleation if present in head or body; distal pancreatectomy if present in tail of pancreas
- *Associated with MEN1*: Subtotal pancreatectomy + enucleation of lesions in head/Whipple's procedure
- *Malignant insulinoma*: Pancreatic resection with lymph nodal dissection

The other pancreatic neuroendocrine tumors are shown in **Table 7**.

Medical management:

Indications:
- Failed surgical management
- Unresectable tumor
- Metastatic tumor

Drugs:
- *Diazoxide*: 50–300 mg/day
  - Side effects: Hypotension, hirsutism, peripheral edema, nausea, and vomiting
- *Somatostatin analogs*:
  - Used in patients who cannot tolerate or are refractory to diazoxide
  - Octreotide: 100–500 µg IV/SC TDS
  - Long-term depot octreotide (Sandostatin LAR 30 mg/4 weeks IM) or lanreotide (Somatuline Autogel 120 mg/4 weeks deep SC)
- Mechanistic target of rapamycin (mTOR) inhibitor: Everolimus (10 mg/day)

MULTIPLE ENDOCRINE NEOPLASIAS

Multiple endocrine neoplasia refers to a group of autosomal dominant disorders with generally high penetrance that lead to the development of a wide spectrum of endocrine and nonendocrine manifestations (**Table 8**).

TABLE 7 Other pancreatic neuroendocrine tumors.

Tumor	Clinical syndromes	Malignancy (%)	MEN1 (%)
Gastrinoma	Zollinger–Ellison syndrome	60–90	25
Glucagonoma	Rash (necrolytic migratory erythema), diabetes, cachexia, and thrombophlebitis	70	3
Somatostatinoma	Steatorrhea, diabetes, and gallstone	40	1
VIPoma	Secretory diarrhea (Verner–Morrison syndrome)	40	1
GRFoma	Acromegaly	30	33
Corticotropin-producing tumor	Cushing's syndrome	100	-
Parathyroid hormone-related protein (PTHrP)-producing tumor	Hypercalcemia	Majority	-
Nonfunctioning tumors or PPoma	None	70–92	30

TABLE 8 Various clinical and genetic features of MEN syndromes.

Feature	MEN1	MEN2A	MEN2B
Eponyms	Wermer syndrome	Sipple syndrome	Wagenmann–Froboese syndrome
Prevalence	1 in 35,000	1 in 40,000	1 in 1,000,000
Gene responsible	MEN1 (11q13)	RET (10q11) Codons 634 (most common), 609, 618, 611, 631 etc.	RET (10q11) codon 918, 883
Age of presentation	20–40 years (Usually PHPT)	<35 years (usually MTC)	Infancy to early adulthood
Major clinical features	3Ps • PHPT (>95%) • Pancreatic/duodenal NETs (50–75%) • Pituitary tumors (30–55%)	• MTC (70–95%) • Pheochromocytoma (50%) • PHPT 13–30%)	• MTC (85%) • Pheochromocytoma (50%)
Other manifestations	• Adrenal cortical tumors • Foregut carcinoids • Nonmedullary thyroid neoplasms • Lipomas • Facial angiofibromas • Hypomelanotic macules • Gingival papules • Collagenomas	• Hirschsprung's disease • Cutaneous lichen amyloidosis	• Intestinal/mucosal ganglioneuromatosis • Marfanoid habitus • Conjunctival/mucosal neuromas • Thickened corneal nerves • Enlarged/bumpy lips • Skeletal abnormalities: Pes cavus, pes excavates, and scoliosis

RECOMMENDED READINGS

1. Silverberg SJ, Walker MD, Bilezikian JP. Asymptomatic primary hyperparathyroidism. J Clin Densitom. 2013; 16(1): 14-21.
2. Pradhan R, Gupta S, Agarwal A. Focused Parathyroidectomy Using Accurate Preoperative Imaging and Intraoperative PTH: Tertiary Care Experience. Indian J Endocrinol Metab. 2019;23(3):347-52.
3. Libutti SK, Alexander HR, Bartlett DL, Sampson ML, Ruddel ME, Skarulis M, et al. Kinetic analysis of the rapid intraoperative parathyroid hormone assay in patients during operation for hyperparathyroidism. Surgery. 1999;126:1145-50.
4. Riss P, Kaczirek K, Heinz G, Bieglmayer C, Niederle B. A "defined baseline" in PTH monitoring increases surgical success in patients with multiple gland disease. Surgery. 2007;142:398-404.
5. Riss P, Dunkler D, Selberherr A, Brammen L, Heidtmann J, Scheuba C. Evaluating a shortened interpretation criterion for intraoperative parathyroid hormone monitoring in patients with primary hyperparathyroidism: 5-minutes criterion in primary hyperparathyroidism and intraoperative algorithm. Head Neck. 2018;40(12):2664-9.
6. Udelsman R, Donovan PI, Sokoll LJ. One hundred consecutive minimally invasive parathyroid explorations. Ann Surg. 2000;232:331-9.
7. Agarwal A, Pradhan R, Kumari N, Krishnani N, Shukla P, Gupta SK, et al. Molecular Characteristics of Large Parathyroid Adenomas. World J Surg. 2016;40(3): 607-14.
8. Kumari N, Chaudhary N, Pradhan R, Agarwal A, Krishnani N. Role of Histological Criteria and Immunohistochemical Markers in Predicting Risk of Malignancy in Parathyroid Neoplasms. Endocr Pathol. 2016;27(2):87-96.
9. Pradhan R, Agarwal A, Gupta SK. PHPT Masquerading as Rickets in Children and Presenting with Rare Skeletal Manifestations: Report of Three Cases and Review of Literature. Indian J Endocrinol Metab. 2018;22(5):705-9.
10. Kumari N, Chaudhary N, Pradhan R, Agarwal A, Krishnani N. Role of Histological Criteria and Immunohistochemical Markers in Predicting Risk of Malignancy in Parathyroid Neoplasms. Endocr Pathol. 2016;27(2):87-96.
11. Singh DN, Gupta SK, Kumari N, Krishnani N, Chand G, Mishra A, et al. Primary hyperparathyroidism presenting as hypercalcemic crisis: Twenty-year experience. Indian J Endocrinol Metab. 2015;19(1):100-5.
12. Singh DN, Gupta SK, Chand G, Mishra A, Agarwal G, Verma AK, et al. Intra-operative parathyroid hormone kinetics and influencing factors with high baseline PTH: a prospective study. Clin Endocrinol (Oxf). 2013;78(6):935-41.

CHAPTER 119

Diabetes Mellitus: Diagnosis, Classification, and Pathophysiology

Anshita Aggarwal, Sri Venkata Madhu, Sanjay K Bhadada

ABSTRACT

Diabetes mellitus (DM) has been growing at pandemic proportions all over the world, with India being one of the leaders. The rapid increase in the prevalence of obesity and metabolic syndrome have lead to this steep rise which seems to be relentless. The classification of diabetes has broadened over the years with addition of certain types such as latent autoimmune diabetes in adults (LADA) and maturity onset diabetes of the young (MODY) which have distinct pathophysiology and clinical features compared to type 1 diabetes mellitus (T1DM) or type 2 diabetes mellitus (T2DM). The clinical picture of T2DM has also evolved over the years with many children or adolescents also presenting with it. Similarly, obesity and metabolic syndrome are now commonly observed even in T1DM, which was classically believed to be lacking features of insulin resistance. Different international [American Diabetes Association (ADA)] and national (Research Society for the Study of Diabetes in India) organizations have provided detailed guidelines for the diagnosis of diabetes. Apart from the glycemic cut-offs, auto-antibody assessment, and genetic workup may also help in the diagnosis and correct classification of diabetes.

"If someone had said to me, "What's your No. 1 health problem?" I would have said heart disease and then diabetes. And what doctors tell me now is that I can transpose them and say diabetes first"

—Larry King

INTRODUCTION

The term "Diabetes mellitus" is derived from the Greek word "diabetes" meaning siphon-to pass through and the Latin word "mellitus" meaning honeyed or sweet. This simplistic nomenclature, however, belies the complex pathophysiology and the wide spectrum of the disease. It is associated with significant morbidity and mortality, and is a great economic burden to the individual and the nation alike. DM has been growing at pandemic proportions the world over. India has the dubious distinction of being one of the major contributors to the global burden of diabetes. As per the data by the International Diabetes Federation guidelines, in the year 2017, India had the second-largest populace of 73 million diabetic patients, after China. Unfortunately, this figure is expected to double by the year 2045.

Diabetes has been traditionally classified broadly as T1DM and T2DM. However, in the current times, the lines between the different types of diabetes have blurred. For instance, with an increase in obesity and metabolic syndrome in children and adolescents, the incidence of T2DM has increased significantly in this age group. Autoimmune diabetes, which had been described classically in the younger age groups, is now known to occur in the older age groups as well, and presents in a latent and indolent form called as "LADA". The different types of diabetes have some overlapping features, making diagnosis challenging. The current classification of DM has been tabulated in **Table 1**.

The salient features of the various major types of diabetes have been described subsequently.

TYPE 2 DIABETES MELLITUS

DIAGNOSIS

The ADA has provided clear-cut criteria for the diagnosis of diabetes which have been accepted worldwide. In a patient without classic symptoms of hyperglycemia, the diagnosis requires two abnormal test results from the same sample or from two separate test samples. If using two separate test samples, it is recommended that the second test, which may either be a repeat of the initial test or a different test, be performed without delay. If a patient undergoes two different tests, and has discordant results, then the test result that is above the diagnostic cut point should be repeated, keeping in mind the possibility of A1c assay interference.

The diagnosis is made on the basis of the confirmed test. Few points should be kept in mind while running the samples. For instance, it is critical that samples for plasma glucose be spun and separated immediately after they are drawn. For results that are at the margins of the diagnostic threshold, the tests should be repeated after 3–6 months. In the Chennai Urban Rural Epidemiology Study (CURES), it was demonstrated that there was 88.0% sensitivity and 87.9% specificity for detection of diabetes when glycated hemoglobin (HbA1c) cut-off point is 6.1% (based on 2 h

TABLE 1 Classification of diabetes.

Type of diabetes mellitus	Etiology	Salient Features
Type 1 diabetes mellitus	β-cell destruction (mostly immune-mediated)	• Absolute insulin deficiency • Onset most commonly in childhood or early adulthood
Type 2 diabetes mellitus	Insulin resistance, and β-cell dysfunction	• Most common • Commonly associated with overweight and obesity
Hybrid forms of diabetes		
Slowly evolving, immune-mediated diabetes in adults **OR** Latent autoimmune diabetes in adults **(LADA)**	Slow, immune-mediated β-cell destruction	• Positive anti-GAD auto-antibodies • Good glycemic control with oral antidiabetic agents for at least 6 months after diagnosis • Onset in adulthood
Ketosis-prone type 2 diabetes mellitus		• Presents with ketosis and insulin deficiency • Later does not require insulin • Not immune-mediated
Other specific types of diabetes		
Monogenic diabetes: • Monogenic defects of β-cell function **OR** Maturity-onset diabetes of young **(MODY)**	Caused by specific genetic mutations	• Has several clinical manifestations depending on the type of mutation • Some occurring in the neonatal period, others by early adulthood
• Monogenic defects in insulin action	Caused by specific genetic mutations	• Has features of severe insulin resistance without obesity • Diabetes develops when β-cells do not compensate for insulin resistance
Diseases of the exocrine pancreas leading to secondary diabetes	Conditions such as trauma, inflammation or tumor which can affect the pancreas	• Most of the cases require insulin due to β-cell destruction • Concomitant involvement of the alpha cells (i.e., glucagon deficiency) results in reduced frequency of acute complications such as diabetic ketoacidosis (DKA)
Endocrine-disorders leading to secondary diabetes	Multiple endocrine-diseases can lead to diabetes due to varied causes such as insulin resistance, interference with postreceptor insulin signaling etc. These include: • Cushing's syndrome • Acromegaly • Pheochromocytoma	• Features vary depending on the disease involved
Other types such as drug-induced, and infection-related	Such as with glucocorticoid use, in the treatment of HIV/AIDS, or after organ transplantation	
Unclassified	Used to describe diabetes that does not clearly fit into other categories. This category should be used temporarily when there is not a clear diagnostic category especially close to the time of diagnosis	
Gestational diabetes mellitus	Diabetes diagnosed in the second or third trimester of pregnancy that was not clearly overt diabetes prior to gestation	

(Anti-GAD: antiglutamic acid decarboxylase)

postload plasma glucose) and 93.3% sensitivity and 92.3% specificity when HbA1c cut-off point is 6.4% [when diabetes was defined as fasting plasma glucose (FPG ≥ 7.0 mmol/L)] (**Box 1**).

PATHOPHYSIOLOGY

Type 2 diabetes mellitus is the most common type of diabetes, comprising >90% of cases of diabetes. Its hallmarks are insulin resistance, defective insulin secretion by

BOX 1 Diagnostic criteria of T2DM.
FPG > 126 mg/dL (7.0 mmol/L). (Fasting is defined as no caloric intake for at least 8 hours)
OR
2-hour PG > 200 mg/dL (11.1 mmol/L) during OGTT. The test should be performed as described by WHO, using a glucose load containing the equivalent of 75 g anhydrous glucose dissolved in water
OR
A1c > 6.5% (48 mmol/mol). The test should be performed in a laboratory using a method that is NGSP certified and standardized to the DCCT assay
OR
In a patient with classic symptoms of hyperglycemia or hyperglycemic crisis, a random plasma glucose > 200 mg/dL (11.1 mmol/L)

(DCCT: Diabetes Control and Complications Trial; NGSP: National Glycohemoglobin Standardization Program)

the pancreatic β-cells, and inadequate compensatory response by the β-cells leading to hyperglycemia. The risk of acquiring T2DM is determined by an interplay between genetic factors and the environment. Patients with T2DM are characteristically obese, with predominantly centripetal obesity. Obesity is associated with ectopic fat distribution in the liver, skeletal muscle, and peripancreatic area. Also, it is associated with production of various biologic products such as tumor necrosis factor-alpha (TNF-α), resistin etc., which contribute to insulin resistance. These adipocyte products also create a proinflammatory state, characterized by an increase in interleukin-6 and C-reactive protein. The precise mechanism for insulin resistance remains elusive. Studies have shown that insulin receptor levels and tyrosine kinase activity are reduced in the skeletal muscle of diabetic patients. However, these are more likely to be due to hyperinsulinemia rather than causing it. It is likely that the "postreceptor" defects in insulin mediated phosphorylation/dephosphorylation play a pivotal role in insulin resistance. These defects include:

- Phosphatidylinositol-3-kinase signaling defect leading to reduced translocation of glucose transporter type 4 (GLUT4) to the plasma membrane.
- Reduced insulin-mediated mitochondrial adenosine triphosphate (ATP) production due to lipid accumulation in the skeletal myocytes.
- Generation of reactive oxygen species in the skeletal myocytes.

The hepatic insulin resistance is reflected in the increased hepatic gluconeogenesis and increased very-low-density lipoprotein (VLDL) and triglyceride accumulation in the liver, leading to hepatic steatosis.

TYPE 1 DIABETES MELLITUS

DIAGNOSIS

The diagnostic criteria for T1DM are same as the aforementioned ones for T2DM. However, since dysglycemia can progress rapidly in patients with T1DM, HbA1c is less sensitive for diagnosis than fasting or post prandial blood glucose measurements. Children with T1DM usually present with osmotic symptoms such as polyuria and polydipsia, and nearly one-third present with diabetic ketoacidosis. Though traditionally described as childhood onset, it can occur in any age-group. There are no specific symptoms that can differentiate between T1DM and T2DM, low serum C-peptide levels can serve as markers of severe endogenous insulin deficiency. Over 90% of people with newly diagnosed T1DM have measurable antibodies against specific β-cell proteins, including insulin, glutamate decarboxylase, islet antigen 2, zinc transporter 8, and tetraspanin-7.

PATHOPHYSIOLOGY

Type 1 diabetes mellitus is a polygenic disease with a strong human leukocyte antigen (HLA)-association. Nearly half of the cases are associated with two HLA class 2 haplotypes involved in antigen presentation, HLA DRB1*0301-DQA1*0501-DQ*B10201 (DR3) and HLA DRB1*0401-DQA1*0301-DQB1*0301 (DR4-DQ8). T1DM is results from an interaction between genetic, environmental, and immunologic factors that culminate into pancreatic β-cell destruction and insulinopenia. This autoimmune β-cell destruction is triggered by an infectious or environmental stimulus. This leads to a gradual decline in the β-cell mass and progressive impairment of insulin secretion. The rate of decline is variable with some individuals progressing rapidly while others have a more indolent course. By the time diabetes is diagnosed, >80% of the β-cells have been lost. The ultimate trigger for the transition to frank diabetes may be an event associated with increased insulin requirement, such as infection, or puberty.

After the initial clinical presentation of T1DM, a "honeymoon phase" may follow, wherein there is a drastic decrease in the requirement of insulin. However, after this transient phase, the insulin production by the residual β-cells wanes off, and the individual becomes completely insulinopenic.

LATENT AUTOIMMUNE DIABETES OF ADULTS

A proportion of patients with adult-onset autoimmune diabetes do not require insulin-therapy at the time of diagnosis and are clinically similar to patients with T2DM. Earlier these patients were classified as T2DM, but now it is known that they have autoimmune diabetes that has an older age of onset and slower destruction of pancreatic β-cells, as evidenced by a more gradual decline in C-peptide levels.

The diagnosis of LADA requires the fulfilment of the following criteria:

- Adult age of onset (>30 years)
- Presence of any islet cell autoantibody; and
- Absence of insulin requirement for at least 6 months after diagnosis.

Glutamic acid decarboxylase (GAD) autoantibody is the most sensitive marker in both adult-onset T1DM and LADA.

MATURITY ONSET DIABETES OF THE YOUNG

Maturity onset diabetes of the young is a monogenic and nonautoimmune form of DM. The genetic defects in MODY impact the insulin production, resulting in hyperglycemia. Generally, these individuals lack features of insulin resistance and also lack pancreatic autoantibodies. The phenotypic features may vary depending on the gene involved. Certain mutations may have slightly raised blood glucose throughout their lifetime with minimal or no symptoms. They are usually picked up during routine screening and have a lower risk of diabetic complications. Certain other mutation types may require treatment with insulin or sulfonylureas. Although both T2DM and MODY can have a family history, such inheritance is autosomal dominant in MODY, thereby meaning that, it does not skip any generation. **Table 2** summarizes the different subtypes of MODY depending on the gene involved.

The diagnostic criteria for MODY are as follows: (a) Presence of overt diabetes in at least three consecutive generations with autosomal dominant mode of inheritance, (b) at least one family member diagnosed with diabetes before the age of 25, (c) absence of ß-cell autoantibodies, and (d) relatively preserved endogenous insulin secretion with a serum C-peptide level of >0.6 ng/mL. These diagnostic criteria can help to discriminate MODY from T1DM and T2DM. Nevertheless, distinguishing MODY from T1DM or T2DM at presentation is often challenging.

GESTATIONAL DIABETES MELLITUS

It deserves special mention as it can have important implications for the mother and the fetus alike. Gestational diabetes mellitus (GDM) is often indicative of underlying β-cell dysfunction, which confers marked increased risk

TABLE 2 Different subtypes of MODY.

Type of MODY	Gene involved	Pathophysiology
MODY 1	*HNF4A*/transcription factor	Progressive β-cell dysfunction, leading to macrosomia and hyperinsulinemic hypoglycemia
MODY 2	*GCK*/glycolytic enzyme	Disrupts glucose sensing leading to hyperglycemia
MODY 3	*HNF1A*/transcription factor	Causes gradual β-cell dysfunction, leading to reduced insulin production and progressive hyperglycemia
MODY 4	*IPFI/PDX1*/transcription factor	Causes pancreatic agenesis, β-cell developmental errors, and defective insulin secretion
MODY 5	HNFIB/transcription factor	Results in dysfunctional pancreatic embryonic development, the formation of kidney cyst, and suppresses cytokine signaling
MODY 6	*NEURODI*/transcription factor	Impairs pancreatic morphogenesis and β-cell differentiation
MODY 7	*KLFII*/transcription factor	Disrupts the activation of some insulin promoters. It also suppresses the expression of certain free radical scavengers such as catalase and superoxide dismutase, disrupting pancreatic β-cell function
MODY 8	Carboxyl-ester lipase	Alters C-terminal sequencing. It can also disrupt exocrine and endocrine functioning of pancreas
MODY 9	*PAX4*/transcription factor	Truncates embryonic β-cell development, inhibiting β-cell differentiation
MODY 10	*INS*/insulin synthesis	Causes molecular defects in the β-cell and increases endoplasmic reticulum (ER) stress, resulting in the synthesis of structurally altered (pre) proinsulin molecules and low insulin biosynthesis
MODY 11	BLK/B-cell receptor signaling and development	Suppresses MIN6 B-cells, disrupting β-cell functions
MODY 12	*ABCC8*/regulates insulin secretion	Causes congenital hyperinsulinism, adversely affecting the biogenesis and insulin trafficking of K_{ATP} channels
MODY 13	*KCNJII*/regulates insulin secretion	Causes congenital hyperinsulinism, adversely affecting the biogenesis and insulin trafficking of K_{ATP} channels
MODY 14	*APPL1*/regulates cell proliferation, and cellular signaling pathways	Starts off the β-cell structural abnormality and gradual death, leading to developmental delay. It can also suppress the insulin-uptake regulatory role of AKT2

(MODY: maturity onset diabetes of the young)

BOX 2 Diagnostic criteria for GDM.

One-step strategy

Perform a 75-g OGTT, with plasma glucose measurement when patient is fasting and at 1 and 2 hours, at 24–28 weeks of gestation in women not previously diagnosed with diabetes

The OGTT should be performed in the morning after an overnight fast of at least 8 hours

The diagnosis of GDM is made when any of the following plasma glucose values are met or exceeded:

- Fasting: 92 mg/dL (5.1 mmol/L)
- 1 hour: 180 mg/dL (10.0 mmol/L)
- 2 hours: 153 mg/dL (8.5 mmol/L)

Two-step strategy

Step 1: Perform a 50-g GLT (nonfasting), with plasma glucose measurement at 1 hour, at 24–28 weeks of gestation in women not previously diagnosed with diabetes

If the plasma glucose level measured 1 hour after the load is ≥130, 135, or 140 mg/dL (7.2, 7.5, or 7.8 mmol/L, respectively), proceed to a 100-g OGTT

Step 2: The 100-g OGTT should be performed when the patient is fasting

The diagnosis of GDM is made when at least two of the following four plasma glucose levels (measured fasting and at 1, 2, and 3 hours during OGTT) are met or exceeded (Carpenter-Coustan criteria):

- Fasting: 95 mg/dL (5.3 mmol/L)
- 1 hour: 180 mg/dL (10.0 mmol/L)
- 2 hours: 155 mg/dL (8.6 mmol/L)
- 3 hours: 140 mg/dL (7.8 mmol/L)

(GDM: gestational diabetes mellitus; OGTT: oral glucose tolerance test)

for later development of diabetes, generally but not always T2DM, in the mother after delivery. **Box 2** and **Table 3** summarize the guidelines for diagnosis of GDM.

Women found to have diabetes by the standard diagnostic criteria used outside of pregnancy should be classified as having diabetes complicating pregnancy (most often T2DM, rarely T1DM or monogenic diabetes) and managed accordingly. Women who meet the lower glycemic criteria for GDM should be diagnosed with that condition and managed accordingly. Other women should be rescreened for GDM between 24 and 28 weeks of gestation.

TABLE 3 Diagnostic criteria for GDM as given by DIPSI.

Criteria	In pregnancy	Outside pregnancy
2 hours ≥ 200 mg/dL	Diabetes mellitus	Diabetes mellitus
2 hours ≥ 140 mg/dL	GDM	IGT (impaired glucose tolerance)
2 hours ≥ 120 mg/dL	DGGT	

(DGGT: decreased gestational glucose tolerance; DIPSI: Diabetes in Pregnancy Study Group India; GDM: gestational diabetes mellitus)

DIPSI (Diabetes in Pregnancy Study Group India) has recommended a single step procedure irrespective of the last meal for the screening of GDM. A 2-hour plasma glucose after 75 g of anhydrous glucose if ≥140 mg/dL is taken as GDM.

RECOMMENDED READINGS

1. American Diabetes Association. Glycemic Targets: Standards of Medical Care in Diabetes–2021. Diabetes Care. 2021;44(Suppl 1):S73-84.
2. Chawla R, Madhu SV, Makkar BM, Ghosh S, Saboo B, Kalra S. RSSDI-ESI Clinical Practice Recommendations for the Management of Type 2 Diabetes Mellitus 2020. Indian J Endocrinol Metab. 2020;24(1):1-122.
3. Skyler JS, Bakris GL, Bonifacio E, Darsow T, Eckel RH, Groop L, et al. Differentiation of Diabetes by Pathophysiology, Natural History, and Prognosis. Diabetes. 2017;66(2):241-55.
4. Yahaya TO, Ufuoma SB. Genetics and Pathophysiology of Maturity-onset Diabetes of the Young (MODY): a review of current trends. Oman Med J. 2020;35(3):e126.
5. Jang KM. Maturity-onset diabetes of the young: update and perspectives on diagnosis and treatment. Yeungnam Univ J Med. 2020;37(1):13-21.
6. Galicia-Garcia U, Benito-Vicente A, Jebari S, Larrea-Sebal A, Siddiqi H, Uribe KB, et al. Pathophysiology of Type 2 Diabetes Mellitus. Int J Mol Sci. 2020;21(17):6275.
7. Deepa M, Pradeepa R, Rema M, Mohan A, Deepa R, Shanthirani S, et al. The Chennai Urban Rural Epidemiology Study (CURES)--study design and methodology (urban component) (CURES-1). J Assoc Physicians India. 2003;51:863-70.
8. Stenström G, Gottsäter A, Bakhtadze E, Berger B, Sundkvist G. Latent autoimmune diabetes in adults: definition, prevalence, β-cell function, and treatment. Diabetes. 2005;54(Suppl 2):S68-72.
9. Rani PR, Begum J. Screening and Diagnosis of Gestational Diabetes Mellitus, Where Do We Stand. J Clin Diagn Res. 2016;10(4):QE01-4.

CHAPTER
120
Complications of Diabetes

Rakesh K Sahay, Manisha Sahay

ABSTRACT

Microvascular complications of diabetes commonly involve target organs, such as the retina, kidney, and peripheral nerves. Diabetes is the most common cause of end-stage renal disease (ESRD) and one of the most frequent factors contributing to blindness and foot-related complications as a result of neuropathy. Most individuals with diabetes remain undiagnosed for a long time and can therefore present with complications of diabetes at the time of detection of diabetes. The biggest benefit in terms of reduction in progression of microangiopathy is by glycemic optimization.

Diabetic nephropathy (DN) is reported in approximately 40% of type 2 diabetes mellitus (T2DM) and 30% of type 1 diabetes mellitus (T1DM). Both albuminuric and nonalbuminuric phenotypes can be seen. Though albuminuric phenotype can be easily diagnosed and monitored by urine estimation, newer biomarkers such as transferrin, type IV collagen, laminin, podocalyxin, neutrophil gelatinase-associated lipocalin (NGAL), kidney injury molecule-1 (KIM-1), N-acetyl-β-D-glucosaminidase (NAG), and cystatin C can aid in early detection of nonalbuminuric kidney disease.

Diabetic retinopathy (DR) is regarded as the sine-qua-non of diabetes as it best correlates with the degree and duration of hyperglycemia. Detailed retinal examination is mandatory for all diabetic patients for early detection of DR as it can be present even at time of diagnosis of T2DM.

Diabetic neuropathy is one of the most common complications of diabetes, affecting >50% of patients with diabetes. It is clinically heterogeneous and can be present even in the prediabetes stage. However, routine evaluation even using simple bedside tests such as the tuning fork and monofilament can help diagnose it. Autonomic neuropathy assessment should be a part of the evaluation as it can have disastrous consequences, if undiagnosed.

"You can live with diabetes. It's not the worst thing to have, but you have to manage yourself and have some self-control"

—Tony Rock

INTRODUCTION

India is home to more than 70 million people with diabetes. The major problems in patients with diabetes are due to its complications namely the microvascular and macrovascular complications. The microvascular complications—retinopathy, neuropathy, and nephropathy—are related to the duration and severity of hyperglycemia and are often contributing to significant morbidity while the major mortality in patients with diabetes is due to the macrovascular complications namely the cardiovascular, cerebrovascular, or peripheral vascular disease. Most individuals with diabetes remain undiagnosed for a long time and can therefore present with complications of diabetes at the time of detection of diabetes.

MICROVASCULAR COMPLICATION

DIABETIC NEPHROPATHY

Diabetic nephropathy is a microvascular complication of diabetes mellitus and leading cause of chronic kidney disease (CKD) throughout the world. The natural history of diabetic kidney disease (DKD) includes glomerular hyperfiltration, progressive albuminuria, declining glomerular filtration rate (GFR), and ultimately, ESRD. Though ESRD is long-term consequence of DN, most of individuals succumb to infections and atherosclerotic heart disease long before initiation of renal replacement therapy.

Diabetic nephropathy was reported in approximately 40% of T2DM and 30% of T1DM. With the improvement in management of DM the prevalence of classic DN has come down in T1DM but not in T2DM which is attributed to its increased prevalence, obesity, and ageing population. Though optimal glycemic, blood pressure, and lipid control and the use of renin-angiotensin-aldosterone system (RAAS) inhibitors are proven to be beneficial, even more effective therapies are needed for even better outcomes. Hence, early diagnosis is very essential to deliver appropriate therapy to prevent the occurrence and progression of the disease, for reducing morbidity and mortality.

RISK FACTORS

Diabetic nephropathy is a result of complex interplay between genetic and environmental factors. The major risk factors are susceptibility factors (age, sex, race/ethnicity, and family history), initiation factors (hyperglycemia), and progression factors (e.g., hypertension, dietary factors, nonalcoholic fatty liver disease, and obesity). Epigenetic alterations secondary to hyperglycemia contribute to the progression of the disease. Genetic factors related to DN are not clearly understood and studies for identification of genetic loci are ongoing with GWAS candidate gene approaches.

PATHOGENESIS

Though multiple factors play a role in the pathogenesis of DN, hyperglycemia is a prime culprit that triggers and sustains the molecular signaling pathways in a genetically susceptible individual. Hyperglycemia triggers metabolic injury mediated by increased advanced glycation end products (AGE), polyol pathway, and protein kinase C activation in both the glomerular and interstitial cells.

Hyperglycemia activates the diverse downstream intracellular signaling pathways leading to RAAS activation and inflammatory cytokine production. RAAS activation results in enhanced production of increased production of aII and upregulation of angiotensin receptors 1 (AT1R) in leading to potentiation of glomerular hypertension. Hyperglycemia results in generation of reactive oxygen species (ROS), inflammatory mediators [nuclear factor (NF)-kβ, toll-like receptor (TLR)], growth factors [vascular endothelial growth factor (VEGF) and connective tissue growth factor], transforming growth factor beta (TGF-β), and proinflammatory and profibrotic cytokines causing structural and functional renal injury.

Hyperglycemia is also reported to upregulate sodium-glucose cotransporter-2 (SGLT-2) channels in proximal tubule resulting in loss of tubuloglomerular feedback and glomerular hypertension. SGLT-2 inhibitor restores the tubuloglomerular feedback.

Hyperglycemia leads to increased expression of connective tissue growth factor (CCN2) in the kidney which causes proliferation of fibroblasts, expansion of extracellular matrix, and causes renal fibrosis. DKD is associated with upregulation of dipeptidyl peptidase-4 (DPP-4) in the kidney and DPP4-phosphorylated beta-1 integrin complex promotes fibrogenesis by activating both vascular endothelial growth factor receptor (VEGFR1) and TGF-β.

Fibroblast growth factor 23 (FGF23) is an independent predictor for progression of DN and its levels are higher in the DM patients. It is phosphaturic hormone which suppresses 1-alpha hydroxylase resulting in decreased calcitriol synthesis and enhances the renin activity.

Growing data suggests the role of elevated FGF23 and deficient alpha klotho in the pathogenesis of DN.

PATHOLOGY

Glomeruli: Thickening of glomerular basement membrane, mesangial expansion due to accumulation of matrix, causing diffuse mesangial sclerosis, the hallmark lesion of DN. The distinctive nodular accumulations of mesangial matrix are known as Kimmelstiel-Wilson nodules.

Kimmelstiel-Wilson nodules, capsular drops, fibrin caps, and other exudative lesions are specific to DN however not pathognomic.

Tubules: Tubular basement thickening, accumulation of glycogen in cells of pars recta, and tubular atrophy (Armanni-Ebstein change).

Afferent and efferent arteriolar hyalinosis in blood vessels and fibrosis of the interstitium.

NATURAL HISTORY

Though Mogensen described distinct phases of DN in T1DM, natural history of nephropathy in T2DM is similar to T1DM with the exception that microalbuminuria or proteinuria may be present at diagnosis, because onset of diabetes may go undetected for many years and the relationship of microalbuminuria to T2DM duration is not precisely known.

Stage 1: It is seen at diagnosis of T1DM and is considered as stage of hyerperfusion and hyperfiltration. Glomerular hyperfiltration is an independent risk factor for DN.

Stage 2: A stage of clinical quiescence associated with thickening of basement membrane and mesangial expansion. GFR is normal or may be higher. Patients with upper limit of normoalbuminuria and structural changes of diabetic glomerulosclerosis have a higher chance of developing microalbuminuria. Nocturnal nondipping on 24 hour ambulatory blood pressure (BP) monitoring may be an early sign of DN, which precedes the development of stage 3.

Stage 3: Incipient nephropathy stage, characterized by persistent microalbuminuria. It starts 5–10 years after the onset of T1DM. GFR remains normal or may show decline. Persistent microalbuminuria is an independent predictor of future cardiovascular risk, and progression to macroalbuminuria is associated with arterial hypertension and decrease in GFR.

Stage 4: It is a stage of overt proteinuria which usually manifests 10–20 years after the onset of T1DM and if not managed appropriately, GFR decline progresses rapidly at mean annual rate of 10–12 mL/min/1.73 m^2. At this stage diabetes-associated chronic vascular complications are noted in most patients.

Stage 5: Progression to ESRD occurs 5–15 years after the onset of proteinuria.

Table 1 lists the current categories of diabetic kidney disease based on eGFR.

DIAGNOSIS

Diabetic nephropathy diagnosis is based on clinical features, urine albumin secretion (UAE), and assessment of estimated GFR (eGFR).

Albuminuria: First clinical indicator of DN is albuminuria. It is measured in the following ways (**Table 2**):

- 24-hour urine collection
- Timed overnight urine albumin excretion (UAE)
- Urine albumin–creatinine ratio (UACR)

TABLE 1	GFR categories (mL/min/1.73 m²) for staging.	
G1	Normal or high	≥90
G2	Mildly decreased	60–89
G3a	Mildly to moderately decreased	45–59
G3b	Moderately to severely decreased	30–44
G4	Severely decreased	15–29
G5	Kidney failure	<15

TABLE 2 Definition of abnormal albumin excretion.

Category	24 hour collection (mg/24 h)	Timed collection (µg/min)	Spot collection (UACR mg/g)
Normal	<30	<20	<30
Microalbuminuria	30–300	20–200	30–300
Overt albuminuria	>300	>200	>300
KDIGO 2020	A1 (normal to mildly increased)	A2 (moderately increased)	A3 (severely increased)

(KDIGO: Kidney Disease: Improving Global Outcomes; UACR: urine albumin–creatinine ratio)

Recent guidelines recommend the use of UACR as it is performed easily on spot urine sample.

Persistent albuminuria is considered when at least two of three measurements of urine ACR examined within 3–6 months are abnormal.

Estimated glomerular filtration rate: Estimated GFR is considered as the better index of renal function. Regular equations like Modification of Diet in Renal Disease (MDRD) and the Chronic Kidney Disease Epidemiology (CKD-EPI) collaboration equation use serum creatinine (SCr) for estimation of the GFRs.

Cystatin C, a cysteine protease inhibitor, is filtered freely by the glomerulus and absorbed in the proximal tubule, and considered to be a reliable marker of renal function.

As it is not widely available in routine practice, most guidelines use SCr-based eGFR for diagnosing and monitoring DKD.

Early diagnosis with new biomarkers: Significant glomerular damage has already occurred by the time albuminuria is evident and decline in renal function is not always associated with increased albuminuria so new biomarkers of glomerular, tubular injury, inflammation, and oxidative stress are being investigated.

Albumin accounts for minor fraction of total urinary protein and becomes unreliable in the presence of normoalbuminuria so nonalbumin proteinuria (NAP) may be considered as a marker for early detection of DN.

Urinary NAP:

- Glomerular biomarkers include—transferrin, immunoglobulin G, ceruloplasmin, type IV collagen, laminin, podocalyxin, and VEGF.
- Tubular biomarkers include—NGAL, alpha 1 microglobulin, KIM-1, NAG, cystatin C, angiotensinogen, and liver-type fatty acid-binding protein.
- Inflammatory markers include—tumor necrosis factor-alpha (TNF-α) and orosomucoid.

Though small studies showed promise of multiple biomarkers in early diagnosis of DN, larger longitudinal trials are required to validate their clinical use in day-to-day practice.

TREATMENT

The disease progresses over many years and multiple factors are known to modulate the course. Approved interventions target hypertension, glycemic control, dyslipidemia, smoking, dietary protein intake, hyperuricemia, hyperphosphatemia, and metabolic acidosis. Other therapies yet to be approved will be discussed in detail.

Smoking: Smoking is one of prime factors for progression of kidney disease. So it is compulsion to quit smoking as studies showed progressive risk of microalbuminria, macroalbuminuria, and ESRD to be higher in smokers compared to nonsmokers.

Nutritional management: Reduction in salt intake reported to reduce BP and UAE in T2DM. Salt paradox was reported in T1DM (low salt intake in the setting of hyperglycemia resulted in increased glomerular hyperfiltration). It is also reported that both higher and lower urinary sodium levels are associated with reduced survival and highest risk of progression of ESRD reported with low urinary sodium levels.

The 2013 KDOQI (Kidney Disease Outcomes Quality Initiative) clinical practice guidelines on diabetes and CKD endorsed the role of appropriate protein nutrition in DKD.

For CKD stages 1 and 2, recommended daily protein intake is 0.8 g/kg and 0.6–0.8 g/kg is allowed in stages 3 and 4.

Optimization of glycemic control: Intensive glycemic control mitigated the progression of DKD at every stage from normoalbuminuria to microalbuminuria or microalbuminuria to overt proteinuria.

The target hemoglobin A1c (HbA1c) of 7.0% is recommended to prevent or delay progression of DKD and target HbA1c beyond 7.0% is indicated in individuals with comorbidities, limited life expectancy, and risk of hypoglycemia.

The Diabetes Control and Complications Trial (DCCT) in T1DM and long-term follow-up Epidemiology of Diabetes Interventions and Complications (EDIC) study showed the beneficial effect of intensive glycemic control. Similarly the Kumamoto Study, the United Kingdom Prospective Diabetes Study (UKPDS), and the Veterans Affairs Cooperative Study on glycemic control and complications in T2 Diabetes Feasibility Trial. The follow-up studies of UKPDS also demonstrated that initial intensive glycemic control persisted beyond glycemic benefits, which was due to metabolic memory or legacy effect.

The more recent ADVANCE (Action in Diabetes and Vascular Disease: Preterax and Diamicron Modified Release Controlled Evaluation), ACCORD (Action to Control Cardiovascular Risk in Diabetes), and VADT (Veterans Affairs Diabetes Trials) did not show great benefits of intensive glycemic control on creatinine-based estimates of GFR and increased risk of hypoglycemia by 1.5 to 3-fold hence lowering of HbA1c beyond 7% is not recommended. Stricter glycemic control is associated with increased risk of hypoglycemia in more advanced stages of DN with excess mortality as observed in ADVANCE and ACCORD.

The glycemic targets should be individualized aiming to strike a balance between the risk of hypoglycemia and clear benefit of renoprotection.

Antidiabetic agents metformin, thiazolidinediones (TZDs), glucagon-like peptide-1 (GLP-1) agonists, DPP-4 inhibitors, and SGLT-2 inhibitors were reported to have renoprotective benefits beyond glycemic control.

Metformin: Metformin activates adenosine monophosphate kinase (AMPK) pathway which leads to inhibition of intracellular downstream signaling pathways of inflammation like mammalian target of rapamycin (mTOR) pathway and also protects podocytes from hyperglycemia-induced apoptosis.

United States Food and Drug Administration (FDA) suggests stoppage of metformin in men with a serum creatinine (SCr) of 1.5 mg/dL or in women with a SCr of 1.4 mg/dL.

The British National Formulary and the Japanese Society of Nephrology recently proposed that use of metformin to be reassessed when GFR is 45 mL/min/1.73 m^2 and stopped when 30 mL/min/1.73 m^2.

Sulfonylureas: Progression of DN results in decreased clearances of the sulfonylureas or their active metabolites, requiring a decrease in dose of drug to prevent episodes of hypoglycemia. First-generation sulfonylureas (tolbutamide and chlorpropamide) are completely avoided as elimination of the drug and its metabolites is through kidneys resulting in increased half-lives in the setting of kidney disease increasing the risk of hypoglycemia.

Among second-generation sulfonylureas (e.g., glipizide, glyburide, and glimepiride), glipizide is the preferred agent as due to lack of active metabolites and risk of hypoglycemia in minimal in patients with CKD. Gliclazide also has been recommended by the KDOQI guidelines as not requiring change in dosage with declining eGFR. However caution is required with eGFR below 30 mL/min.

Thiazolidinediones: The TZDs (pioglitazone and rosiglitazone) are metabolized by the liver, and are preferably avoided in CKD as they may worsen the edema.

Though experimental studies showed renoprotective benefits of TZDs, post-hoc analysis of the PROactive (Prospective Pioglitazone Clinical Trial in Macrovascular Events) study results did not show any change in eGFR compared to placebo.

Safety concerns of TZDs like fluid retention, osteoporosis, and congestive cardiac failure make them less likely as option in management of hyperglycemia.

Meglitinide analogs: Though increased risk of hypoglycemia was not demonstrated with progressive fall in GFR, when GFR is <30 mL/min/1.73 m^2 it is important to start therapy with a 0.5 mg dose of repaglinide or 60 mg dose of nateglinide with each meal and cautiously titrate the dose upward.

Alpha-glucosidase inhibitors (AGIs; acarbose, miglitol, and voglibose): Use of acarbose and miglitol is not recommended in patients with eGFR of <25 mL/h/1.73 m^2.

Glucagon-like peptide-1 receptor agonists: Gut-derived GLP-1 is the incretin hormone reported to have renoprotective benefits independent of glycemic control.

Liraglutide in LEADER (Liraglutide Effect and Action in Diabetes: Evaluation of Cardiovascular Outcome Results) trial reported lower incidence of nephropathy [new onset albuminuria, doubling of SCr and creatinine clearance <45 mL/min/1.73m^2, need for renal replacement therapy (RRT), and death from renal causes].

Among T2DM patient with moderate to severe CKD dulaglutide in AWARD-7 showed reduced decline in eGFR compared to glargine though glycemic control achieved was similar among both the groups.

Semaglutide in SUSTAIN-6 showed that the rates of new or worsening nephropathy were lower in the semaglutide group, however, retinopathy complications were higher.

The probable mechanisms involved are reduction in the levels of renal NADPH (reduced nicotinamide adenine dinucleotide phosphate) oxidase, ROS generation, UAE, and mesangial expansion.

Dipeptidyl peptidase-4 inhibitors: Small studies reported renal benefits of sitagliptin and vildagliptin, future trials adequately powered and designed are needed. Sitagliptin in TECOS (Trial Evaluating Cardiovascular Outcomes with Sitagliptin) trial did not show clinically significant outcomes related to cardiovascular or CKD outcomes, irrespective of baseline eGFR.

SAVOR-TIMI with saxaglitin comparing with placebo showed reduction in UAE without effect in eGFR independent of glycemic control. Pooled analysis of four clinical studies of T2DM patients randomized to receive either linagliptin or placebo showed 32% reduction in UAE in linagliptin compared to placebo.

CARMELINA showed that renal outcomes (time to first occurrence of death due to renal failure, ESRD, or sustained

40% or higher decrease in eGFR from baseline) occurred at lower rate in linagliptin arm compared to the placebo arm.

Sodium-glucose cotransporter-2 inhibitors: Sodium-glucose transporter inhibition promotes tubuloglomerular feedback which results in generation of adenosine causing afferent arteriole vasoconstriction reducing intraglomerular pressure. SGLT-2 inhibitors demonstrated favorable outcome in delaying the progression of DN.

Empagliflozin in EMPA-REG trial and canagliflozin in CANVAS program showed significantly better renal outcomes in T2DM.

Canagliflozin in CREDENCE showed that relative risk reduction of the primary outcome [composite of end-stage kidney disease (dialysis, transplantation, or a sustained estimated GFR of <15 mL/min/1.73 m^2), a doubling of the SCr level, or death from renal or cardiovascular causes] was 30% in the canagliflozin group than in the placebo group.

Insulin: Intensified insulin therapy resulted in a reduction of nephropathy over conventional therapy from 25% to only 9%. Insulin can be used at any stage of DN, but with dose titration as per ambient glycemia.

Blood pressure control: Hypertension is an independent modifiable risk factor for the onset and progression of DN. In both diabetic and nondiabetic adults with CKD with an UAE <30 mg/24 h and whose office BP is persistently >140 mm Hg systolic or >90 mm Hg diastolic recommendation is to use antihypertensives to maintain a BP that is consistently <140 mm Hg systolic and <90 mm Hg diastolic. If UAE is >30 mg/24 h BP should be consistently maintained <130 mm Hg systolic and <80 mm Hg diastolic.

Glomerular hypertension plays a key role in the pathogenesis of DN even in normotensive diabetic animals, indicating that effectively managing systemic BP without reduction in intraglomerular pressure may not be enough to prevent glomerular injury.

Renin–angiotensin–aldosterone system blockers [angiotensin-converting enzyme (ACE) inhibitor and angiotensin receptor blocker (ARBs)] are known to reduce both systemic and glomerular hypertension and have a dose-dependent action in reducing proteinuria.

Pronounced RAAS blockade using ACE inhibitor and ARBs together showed increased adverse events and hyperkalemia. Similarly, usage of direct renin inhibitor aliskiren along with combination of ACE inhibitor/ARB has been contraindicated following the adverse outcomes noted in ATTITUDE trial.

Though RAAS blockers are used as first-line therapy for hypertension in patients with diabetes, marked reduction in the development of DN is less likely. National Kidney Foundation Kidney Disease Outcomes Quality Initiative recommend usage of ACE inhibitor and ARBs is suggested in normotensive diabetic patients with microalbuminuria who are at risk for development of DKD in the future.

Nondihydropyridine calcium channel blockers (diltiazem or verapamil) are a better choice, if albuminuria persists along with uncontrolled BP on ACE inhibitor/ARB monotherapy.

Aldosterone receptor antagonists—spironolactone, eplerenone, and finrenone—are reported to have renoprotective effects but combination with RAS inhibition found greater risk of hyperkalemia.

Finrenone in Mineralocorticoid Receptor Antagonist Tolerability Study–Diabetic Nephropathy (ARTS-DN) study showed dose-dependent reduction of albuminuria.

Lipid-lowering therapy: The renoprotective effects of statins with statistically significant results are lacking in T1DM and T2DM patients with micro- and macroalbuminuria. AURORA trial showed that statin therapies reduced the risk of major atherosclerotic events, in all stages of CKD 1–4 or postrenal transplant patients, but not in patients on maintenance hemodialysis. Use of ezetimibe along with statin is also recommended to achieve better reduction of LDL-C with lower doses of statins due to risk of myopathy on high-dose statins.

Hyperuricemia: Serum uric acid (UA) is a strong and independent predictor for the increased UAE and overt proteinuria in T1DM patients. Allopurinol and febuxostat showed significant reduction in UAE and eGFR decline among T2DM patients.

Phosphate management: Impaired excretion of phosphorous from failing kidney results in hyperphosphatemia. Renal elimination of phosphate is dependent on FGF23. Sevelamer carbonate, an oral noncalcium phosphate binder having marked anti-inflammatory properties, showed significant reduction in FGF23 levels, markers of inflammation, and oxidative stress.

Dietary restriction of phosphate and sevelamer together significantly reduced the overall mortality and progression to renal replacement therapy among T2DM CKD patients.

CONCLUSION

Diabetic nephropathy is the one of the most common complications of diabetes and throughout the world it is becoming the most common cause of ESRD. In patients with diabetes, an annual screening of albuminuria and SCr (eGFR) is recommended. Early detection of eGFR decline and albuminuria would allow interventions to decrease the rate of eGFR decline and prolong the time for the onset of ESRD. It is important to identify naïve and modifiable risk factors which allow us to recognize subjects at high risk for development of early DN. Several clinical trials reported the importance of strict glycemic control and BP management in reducing the incidence and progression of DN. Though currently approved therapeutic interventions may only delay the progression of DN, newer therapeutic modalities are needed for prevention of DN.

DIABETIC RETINOPATHY

Diabetic retinopathy is one of the leading causes of preventable blindness in India and worldwide. Annual retinal examinations are mandatory for all diabetic patients for early detection of DR as it can be asymptomatic and its development and progression can be prevented by control of the risk factors and visual loss can be prevented by laser photocoagulation at an appropriate stage. Early Treatment Diabetic Retinopathy Study (ETDRS) has shown that argon laser photocoagulation treatment is beneficial in reducing the risk of visual loss from clinically significant diabetic macular edema (DME) and proliferative diabetic retinopathy (PDR). Newer technology like optical coherence tomography (OCT) and newer treatment options like intravitreal steroids and antiangiogenic agents have offered new hope to the diabetic patients with severe vision impairment.

The overall prevalence of DR was 17.6% in the Chennai Urban Rural Epidemiology Study (CURES), among the known diabetic subjects it was 20.8% and 5.1% in the newly detected diabetic subjects. The prevalence of PDR was 0.9% and that of DME, 5%. In the CURES study, male gender (p = 0.041), duration of diabetes (p < 0.0001), glycated hemoglobin (HbA1c; p < 0.0001), macroalbuminuria (p = 0.0002), and insulin therapy (p = 0.0001) were significantly associated with severity of DR. In the Sankara Nethralaya Diabetic Retinopathy Epidemiology and Molecular Genetics Study, prevalence of DR was 18.0% while in Aravind Eye Study it was 10.5%. The overall studies from India confirm the lower prevalence of DR in Indians compared to other ethnic groups.

CLINICAL EVALUATION

Detailed retinal examination is mandatory for all diabetic patients for early detection of DR. The details of ocular evaluation in patients with diabetes are depicted in **Tables 3** and **4** gives details about the assessment for diabetic macular edema.

- Direct ophthalmoscopy produces high magnification (15 Å~) and is very useful in identifying microaneurysms, retinal hemorrhages, hard exudates, cotton wool spots, and new vessels.
- Indirect ophthalmoscopy aids to assess the periphery of the fundus.
- Slit lamp biomicroscopy with contact lens is very helpful to assess DME. It is important to detect DME in the assessment of DR as this is the most frequent cause of decreased vision from retinopathy.

INVESTIGATIONS

The useful investigations are retinal color photography, fundus fluorescein angiography (FFA), OCT, and B-scan.

TABLE 4 International disease severity scale for diabetic macular edema by Wilkinson.

Absent	No retinal thickening or hard exudates in posterior pole
Present	• **Mild DME:** Some retinal thickening or hard exudates in posterior pole but distant from the macula • **Moderate DME:** Retinal thickening or hard exudates approaching the center of the macula but not involving the center • **Severe DME:** Retinal thickening or hard exudates involving the center of macula

(DME: diabetic macular edema)

TABLE 3 Stages of diabetic retinopathy.

Stage	Description	Findings on ophthalmoscopy
Mild NPDR	Small areas of balloon-like swelling in the retina's tiny blood vessels, called microaneurysms, occur at this earliest stage of the disease. These microaneurysms may leak fluid into the retina	Microaneurysms only
Moderate NPDR	As the disease progresses, blood vessels that nourish the retina may swell and distort. They may also lose their ability to transport blood. Both conditions cause characteristic changes to the appearance of the retina and may contribute to DME	More than just microaneurysms but less than severe NPDR
Severe NPDR	Many more blood vessels are blocked, depriving blood supply to areas of the retina. These areas secrete growth factors that signal the retina to grow new blood vessels	• More than 20 intraretinal hemorrhages in each of the four quadrants • Definite venous beading in two or more quadrants • Prominent intraretinal microvascular abnormalities in one or more quadrant and • No signs of proliferative retinopathy
PDR	At this advanced stage, growth factors secreted by the retina trigger the proliferation of new blood vessels, which grow along the inside surface of the retina and into the vitreous gel, the fluid that fills the eye. The new blood vessels are fragile, which makes them more likely to leak and bleed. Accompanying scar tissue can contract and cause retinal detachment—the pulling away of the retina from underlying tissue, like wallpaper peeling away from a wall. Retinal detachment can lead to permanent vision loss	• Neovascularization • Vitreous or preretinal hemorrhage

(DME: diabetic macular edema; NPDR: nonproliferative diabetic retinopathy; PDR: proliferative diabetic retinopathy)

Source: Adapted from https://nei.nih.gov/health/diabetic/retinopathy

Retinal color photography: It is useful to document retinal lesions. It is more reproducible than clinical examination and useful in research studies. It helps to document not only progression of DR, but also the response of treatment.

Fundus fluorescein angiography: It involves the photographic surveillance of fluorescein passing through the retinal and choroidal circulations on intravenous (IV) injection of 5 mL of 10% fluorescein dye into a peripheral vein and serial angiogram pictures at different phases are taken using digital retinal camera.

Fundus fluorescein angiography is indicated in patients with DR, clinically significant macular edema (CSME) to assess areas of leakage and also for macular ischemia (where laser has to be avoided), and in those with unexplained sudden visual loss. In severe nonproliferative diabetic retinopathy (NPDR), it helps to assess risk of developing PDR.

Optical coherence tomography: It is a noninvasive, noncontact imaging system which provides high-resolution cross sectional images of retina and optic nerve. OCT uses light instead of sound waves.

It is indicated:

- To quantify the retinal thickness in the different areas of the macula
- To identify cystic spaces in the macula
- Identify macular holes, neurosensory detachment, and vitreomacular traction
- Helps to assess the response of treatment like laser and intravitreal injections
- Helps in analysis of optic nerve head and retinal nerve fiber layer.

Even in absence of foveal center edema, a center point thickness between 225 µm and 299 µm on OCT scan, is called as subclinical DME. A significant number of eyes with subclinical DME will progress to more definite thickening or predict the need for treatment for DME within 2 years after its identification.

More recently a "spectral domain OCT" with a better scan rate of at least 20,000 axial scans per second, an improved axial resolution of 5 µm, has been introduced and this has improved visualization of different retinal layers and interpretation of various macular diseases.

B-scan ultrasound: It is the other modality which helps to assess the presence of vitreous hemorrhage and retinal detachment in diabetic patients with opaque media.

TREATMENT

Absent or mild NPDR: Patient with mild NPDR require individualized counseling as this stage is reversible and appropriate medical care will prevent sight-threatening complications.

- Strict control of blood glucose, blood pressure, and lipids should be emphasized.
- Yearly retinal examination is mandatory and specialized investigation like FFA is not required.

Moderate nonproliferative diabetic retinopathy without macular edema:

- Patients at this stage of DR should have a repeat examination within 6–12 months, because disease progression is common.
- Digital retinal color photography should be taken to document the lesions and to assess the condition on follow-up.
- Fundus fluorescein angiography and laser are not required.

Severe nonproliferative diabetic retinopathy:

- There is high risk of progression to sight-threatening PDR.
- Panretinal photocoagulation (PRP) should be considered in severe NPDR, especially in patients with impending cataract surgery, pregnancy, or poor access to healthcare facilities.
- Fundus fluorescein angiography can help to assess the extent of retinal ischemia and decide on laser treatment.

Laser photocoagulation for sight-threatening diabetic retinopathy:

Indications: Laser photocoagulation is indicated for PDR, CSME, neovascular glaucoma, and associated retinal disorders like ischemic retinal vein occlusion. Eyes with severe ischemia have high risk of anterior segment neovascularization and should be considered for PRP.

Type of laser:

- The slit-lamp biomicroscope, the laser indirect ophthalmoscope, and the endolaser probe are the three types of laser delivery systems commonly used in DR.
- Argon green and Nd:YAG (neodymium-doped yttrium aluminum garnet) are commonly used lasers for DR.

Principle of laser: Lasers produce a photocoagulative tissue effect by transforming light energy into thermal energy, which produces the desired tissue effect in the photocoagulated tissue or, sometimes, in neighboring tissues by thermal conduction.

In macular edema, the destruction of photoreceptors by the laser increases the availability of oxygen to the inner retinal layers thereby relieving hypoxia. Additionally the proliferation of the retinal pigmented epithelium induced by laser photocoagulation can produce cytokines to antagonize the permeabilizing effects of VEGF.

Laser photocoagulation in proliferative retinopathy causes regression of abnormal new vessels due to destruction of ischemic zones thus eliminating the source of angiogenic stimulus.

Diabetic macular edema: Fundus fluorescein angiography is performed to assess the extent of leakage and any associated signs of macular ischemia.

Focal and grid photocoagulation are used for the treatment of DME. Focal photocoagulation applies light, small-sized burns to leaking microaneurysms in the macula (outside the foveal avascular zone). The laser burns should be located 500 and 300 µm from center of fovea.

TABLE 5 Comparison of different anti-VEGF therapies for intravitreal injection.

	Ranibizumab	Bevacizumab	Aflibercept
Target	All VEGF-A isoforms	All VEGF-A isoforms	All VEGF-A isoforms. VEGF-B and PDGF
Molecular characteristics	Fab fragment (no Fc)	Full length monoclonal antibody (Fc containing)	Fusion protein (Fc containing)
Molecular weight	48 kDa	149 kDa	115 kDa
Formulation/ Administration	Intravitreal injection from a single use vial or prefilled syringe	Manufactured for IV use not licensed for intraocular use	Intravitreal injection from a single use vial
Intravitreal elimination (half-life)	• 2.88 days (rabbit eye) • 9 days (human eye)	• 4.32 days (rabbit eye) • 8.25 days (human eye)	• 4.79 days (rabbit eye) • Unknown (human eye)
Systemic elimination (half-life)	~2 h	20 days	5–6 days

(IV: intravenous; PDGF: platelet-derived growth factor; VEGF: vascular endothelial growth factor)

The ETDRS demonstrated that photocoagulation reduced the risk of moderate vision loss, especially for those eyes with macular edema that involved or threatened the center of the macula. Laser photocoagulation resulted in moderate visual gain and decrease in the amount of retinal thickening.

Grid photocoagulation applies a grid or pattern of burns (mimicking PRP but using smaller burns) to the areas of macular edema arising from diffuse capillary leakage shown on fluorescein angiography. They should be applied to areas located >500 µm from center of fovea and 500 µm from the temporal margin of optic disk. They should be one burn width apart. A follow-up is needed 2–3 months after laser.

Diabetic macular edema should be treated before PRP for PDR and also before cataract surgery because of potential progression DME and retinopathy after surgery. Even if treatment for macular edema is deferred, when center of macula is not involved or not threatened, patient should be observed closely for progression (3–4 months).

Proliferative diabetic retinopathy: PRP should be performed for virtually all eyes with high-risk proliferative retinopathy. Laser photocoagulation can be either total or sectorial. The goal of PRP is regression of new vessels in the retina, which can otherwise bleed causing vitreous/ preretinal hemorrhage or result in fibrous proliferation (tractional RD).

Anti-VEGF injections: VEGF is a key mediator in the development of both macular edema and PDR. Anti-VEGF injections have become the treatment of choice for DME and also have an important role to play in the management of PDR. Intravitreal injections of these agents are done periodically. The procedure is done under topical anesthesia using a 30G needle. A comparison of the three different agents available is shown in **Table 5**.

SCREENING FOR RETINOPATHY

The gold standard for the detection and classification of DR is stereoscopic color fundus photographs in seven standard fields, as defined by the ETDRS group. But it is a cumbersome procedure which is time-consuming and requires skilled photographer. American Academy of Ophthalmology guidelines states that seven field stereoscopic fundus photography is not an ideal screening technique, but it can serve as the standard with which to compare other screening technologies.

Adults and children above 10 years of age with T1DM should have an initial dilated examination by an ophthalmologist within 5 years of the onset of diabetes. While for T2DM may be present for years before the diagnosis, up to 20% of patients with T2DM have retinopathy at the time of diagnosis.

The eye should have an initial dilated examination by an ophthalmologist at the time of their diagnosis. Screening of DR is routinely done with the help of direct ophthalmoscope by the ophthalmologist in the clinic scenario. When access to specialist is not available, other modes of screening have to be considered. In these settings, remote interpretation of film-based or digital photographs of the retina may be employed. Digital retinal photography can be taken by either using mydriatic or nonmydriatic retinal camera.

CONCLUSION

Screening for DR is very important for early detection to prevent the progression to more advanced sight losing forms of eye involvement. The availability of nonmydriatic fundus cameras has made screening for DR more accessible to every diabetic clinic. **Box 1** summarizes the current recommendations from the RSSDI-ESI on screening and management of diabetic retinopathy.

DIABETIC NEUROPATHY

Diabetic neuropathy is one of the most common complications of diabetes and at any point of time would be affecting >50% of persons with diabetes. It is strongly associated with the duration and extent of hyperglycemia and therefore increases significantly with longer duration and poor control of diabetes. The diabetic neuropathies are a heterogeneous group of disorders with diverse clinical manifestations. The early recognition and appropriate

BOX 1	RSSDI-ESI recommendations for diabetic retinopathy.

- **Documentation** of formal history of vision and visual acuity either by recording it on sheet or electronic medical record (EMR) should be made mandatory first at the time of diagnosis and then periodically
- Ensure that examination of the eyes of people with T2DM is performed around the time of diagnosis and then routinely every 1–2 years as part of a formal recall process
- Measure and document visual acuity, corrected with glasses or pinhole
- Record ocular pressure and assess the condition of the iris and lens
- **Assess retinopathy:** Using retinal photography through dilated pupils, performed by an appropriately trained health-care professional, or
- Through examination by an ophthalmologist
- Discuss the reasons for eye examination with the person with diabetes
- **Counseling** must include components on smoking, diet, alternative medicines, exercise, and appropriate choice of drugs for BP and lipids
- Counsel women who are planning pregnancy on the risk of progression of retinopathy during pregnancy, especially if there is preexisting retinopathy
- Ensure regular follow-up throughout pregnancy and up to 1 year postpartum
- Use tropicamide to dilate pupils, unless contraindicated (rule out history of glaucoma), after discussing the implications and obtaining agreement of the person with diabetes
- **Classify the findings** of eye examination to stratify the review required as: Routine review, earlier review, or referral to an ophthalmologist (if not making the examination)
- The following **frequency of screening** is suggested:
    - 1–2 years, if no retinopathy, depending on clinical situation
    - 12 months, if minimal unchanged retinopathy
    - 2–4 months, after any active ophthalmic intervention
    - 3–6 months, if worsening since last examination
    - More often during pregnancy
- The following situations require **specialist referral**:
    - The same day: Sudden loss of vision
        - Evidence of retinal detachment
    - Within 1 week:
        - Evidence of preretinal and/or vitreous hemorrhage
        - New vessel formation or rubeosis iridis
        - Inability to see or assess disk or fovea
        - Raised ocular pressure
    - Within 1–2 months:
        - Advanced retinal lesions (4:2:1 rule)
        - Microaneurysms or retinal hemorrhages in four quadrants
        - Venous beading in two quadrants
        - IRMAs in one quadrant

Continued...

Continued...

        - Unexplained deterioration of visual acuity
        - Macular edema
        - Unexplained retinal findings
        - Cataract
        - Inability to visualize fundus
- **Stepped approach** should be adapted to manage hyperglycemia, as intensive glycemic control can cause transient (early) worsening of symptoms and even lead to cotton wool spots
- GLP-1 agonists may initially worsen diabetic retinopathy, and hence must be used with caution
- Advice that good control of blood glucose, BP and blood lipids, and cessation of smoking can help to reduce the risk of development or worsening of eye complications
- Advice that DR is not a contraindication for use of aspirin, if this is indicated for prevention of CVD
- Advise that tests of intraocular pressure should be done periodically
- Explain guarded prognosis about regaining vision after intraocular lens (IOL) surgery in mature/hypermature cataract because of poor assessment of retina in the presence of mature cataract
- Discourage use of alternative medicines as they can cause further complications

(BP: blood pressure; CVD: cardiovascular disease; DR: diabetic retinopathy; GLP-1: glucagon-like peptide-1; IRMAs: intraretinal microvascular abnormalities; RSSDI-ESI: Research Society for the Study of Diabetes in India-Endocrine Society of India; T2DM: type 2 diabetes mellitus)

management of neuropathy in the patient with diabetes is important.

Diabetic neuropathy is defined as the presence of peripheral nerve dysfunction in a diabetic patients in the absence of other causes. Hence, it is a diagnosis of exclusion. The classification of diabetic neuropathy is shown in **Box 2**. The risk factors for the developement of diabetic neuropathy are listed in **Box 3**.

In T1DM, distal polyneuropathy typically becomes symptomatic after many years of chronic prolonged hyperglycemia, whereas in T2DM, it may be apparent after only a few years of known poor glycemic control or even at diagnosis.

SYMPTOMS

These include the following:

- Sensory—negative or positive, diffuse or focal; usually insidious in onset and showing a stocking-and-glove distribution in the distal extremities
- Motor—distal, proximal, or more focal weakness, mostly occurring along with sensory neuropathy (sensorimotor neuropathy)
- Autonomic—neuropathy that may involve the cardiovascular, gastrointestinal, and genitourinary systems and the sweat glands with typical manifestations

BOX 2	Classification of diabetic neuropathies.
• **Generalized symmetrical polyneuropathies:**	
◦ Distal sensory or sensorimotor polyneuropathy	
◦ Small-fiber neuropathy	
◦ Autonomic neuropathy	
◦ Large-fiber sensory neuropathy	
• **Focal and asymmetrical neuropathies:**	
◦ Cranial neuropathy (single or multiple)	
◦ Truncal neuropathy (thoracic radiculopathy)	
◦ Limb mononeuropathy (single or multiple)	
◦ Proximal motor neuropathy (lumbosacral radiculoplexopathy, amyotrophy)	
• **Combinations:**	
◦ Polyradiculoneuropathy	
◦ Diabetic neuropathic cachexia	

BOX 3	Risk factors for diabetic neuropathy.
• Poor glycemic control	
• Duration of diabetes	
• Advancing age	
• Male sex	
• Alcohol consumption	
• Hypertension	
• Hyperlipidemia	
• Tobacco use	
• Aldose reductase gene hyperactivity	
• Angiotensin-converting enzyme genotypes	
• Presence of other diabetic complications like retinopathy or nephropathy	

Physical examination should include the following assessments:

- Peripheral neuropathy testing—gross light touch and pinprick sensation; vibratory sense; deep tendon reflexes; strength testing and muscle atrophy; dorsal pedal and posterior tibial pulses; skin assessment; Tinel testing; and cranial nerve testing (**Box 4**).
- Autonomic neuropathy testing—simple bedside screening to assess supine and upright BP and heart rate, with measurement of sinus arrhythmia ratio, can be supplemented with objective evaluation of cardiovascular, adrenergic, and sudomotor function in a specialized autonomic laboratory (**Box 4**).

The tests to rule out other causes of neuropathy are given in **Box 5**.

MANAGEMENT

The most important step in the management of any diabetic neuropathy is strict glycemic control. The DCCT and UKPDS trials have shown that meticulous control of blood sugar not only decreases the risk of developing neuropathy but also slows the progression in established neuropathy. Measures aimed at improvement of lipid and BP indices, and the avoidance of cigarette smoking and excess alcohol consumption, are recommended for the prevention of other complications of diabetes though there are no clear prevention studies involving these. **Box 6** summarizes the various measures that can be adopted to prevent the developement and progression of diabetic neuropathy.

BOX 4	Diagnostic tests used for diagnosis of diabetic neuropathy.
• Light touch sensation	
• Thermal thresholds	
• Vibration perception thresholds	
• Electromyography—nerve conduction velocity	
• Autonomic testing	
• Punch biopsy of skin and immunohistochemical staining	
• Quantitative sensory testing	
• Corneal confocal microscopy to assess nerve fiber density	

BOX 5	Screening blood tests for exclusion of other disorders.
• Complete blood cell count to check for anemia	
• Complete metabolic panel (electrolytes and liver function panel)	
• Vitamin B12 and folate levels	
• Thyroid function tests	
• Erythrocyte sedimentation rate	
• C-reactive protein	
• Serum protein electrophoresis with immunofixation electrophoresis	
• Antinuclear antibody	
• Anti-SSA and SSB antibodies	
• Rheumatoid factor	
• Paraneoplastic antibodies where indicated	
• Genetic screens where indicated	

(SS: Sjögren's syndrome)

BOX 6	Measures for prevention of progression of neuropathy.
• Glycemic control	
• Blood pressure control	
• Cessation of smoking	
• Cessation of alcohol intake	
• Regular exercises	
• Foot care	

Treatment options: In view of the multifactorial nature of the pathogenesis, multiple treatment options may be needed to provide optimum relief to a patient of diabetic neuropathy. The different pharmacological agents that have been used with variable results are listed below.

Aldose reductase inhibitors reduce the flux of glucose through the polyol pathway, inhibiting tissue accumulation of sorbitol and fructose and preventing reduction of redox potentials. Alrestatin, the first ARI studied, was shown to improve sensory impairment scores in one study while it did not show similar benefit in other studies. Patient selection may have complicated interpretation of these trials because more severe neuropathy may be irreversible. Sorbinil, another widely studied ARI, generated more promising clinical effects. In a double-blind crossover trial, treatment with sorbinil resulted in a small but significant improvement in both motor and sensory conduction velocities compared with placebo but long-term studies are lacking. Tolrestat showed significant improvement in autonomic function tests as well as in vibration perception, while epalrestat has shown efficacy in preventing the progression of diabetic neuropathy and retinopathy.

Intravenous immunoglobulin:

- *Gamma-linolenic acid*: It preserves the prostaglandin E2 and is believed to increase the nerve blood flow.
- *Aminoguanidine*: It is an inhibitor of AGEs formation, trials in animals has shown improved nerve conduction (NC) in diabetic neuropathy.
- *Alpha-lipoic acid*: It is a derivative of octanoic acid, acts as a thiol, is normally present in the food, and is also synthesized by the liver. When used parenterally, it acts as a replenishing and redox-modulating agent.
- *Capsaicin*: An alkaloid found in red pepper depletes the tissue of substance P: a mediator of pain. It is best used for localized pain syndromes.
- *Protein kinase C inhibitors*: Protein kinase C has been implicated in the pathogenesis of microvascular complications. An inhibitor (LY333531), now named ruboxistaurin, has shown promise in preliminary studies and more extensive studies are going on.
- *Frequent rhythmic electrical modulation system*: Transcutaneous frequency-modulated electromagnetic neural stimulation [frequency rhythmic electrical modulation system (FREMS)] is a safe treatment for symptomatic diabetic neuropathy with transient but immediate reduction in pain but without any change in NC velocity (NCV).
- Angiotensin-converting enzyme inhibitors
- Calcium channel blockers
- Nerve growth factors
- Gangliosides
- Continuous insulin infusions

Treatment of autonomic neuropathy: Management of diabetic autonomic neuropathy is summarized in **Table 6**. Attention to strict glycemic control can alleviate autonomic neuropathy to some extent. Different studies have found benefits of ACE inhibitors, spironolactone, ARIs, beta-blockers, and anticholinergic drugs in various forms of autonomic neuropathy. Multifactorial intervention often helps in alleviating diabetic autonomic neuropathy.

Management of entrapment neuropathies: Medical management consists of rest, placement of a splint, and anti-inflammatory medication. Carbamazepine is particularly useful for the pain in this condition. Surgical treatment is indicated when conservative methods fail, e.g., sectioning of the volar carpal ligament of Carpal tunnel syndrome. Reassurance and physical therapies have an important role to play.

TABLE 6 Treatment options for diabetic autonomic neuropathy.

Dysfunction	Treatment options
Diabetic gastroparesis	Frequent small meals; prokinetic drugs, e.g., cisapride, domperidone, metoclopramide, erythromycin, rarely surgery
Diabetic constipation	Stimulant laxatives, e.g., senna and dulcolax
Diabetic diarrhea	Loperamide, codeine, tetracyclines, and erythromycin
Neuropathic bladder	Manual pressure, Crede's method, intermittent self-catheterization, and antibiotics for infection
Erectile dysfunction	Sex therapy, psychotherapy, counseling; drugs: Yohimbine, sildenafil, vardenafil, tadalafil; intracavernosal injection of vasoactive agents, e.g., alprostadil, phentolamine, papaverine, and vacuum tumescence devices
Vaginal dryness	Vaginal lubricants
Sudomotor dysfunction	Emollients and skin lubricants, scopolamine, glycopyrrolate, botulinum toxin, and vasodilators
Postural hypotension	Head end elevation, gradual rising from the bed, pressure stockings; fludrocortisone (up to 1 mg/day), midodrine (2.5–10 mg/day)

BOX 7 Treatment options for management of painful neuropathy.

- Stabilization of glycemic control (preferably with the use of insulin)
- **First-line treatment with antidepressants:**
  - Tricyclic antidepressants—amitriptyline and desipramine
  - SNRI, SSRI—duloxetine, venlafaxine
- **Second-line treatment with antiepileptic drugs:**
  - Gabapentin, carbamazepine, pregabalin, and topiramate
- **Third-line treatment with opioid and opioid-like drugs:**
  - Tramadol and tapentadol
- Referral to a pain clinic

(SNRI: serotonin and norepinephrine reuptake inhibitors; SSRI: selective serotonin reuptake inhibitor)

Management of painful neuropathies: Management of the painful neuropathies is often very challenging. The various agents used for management of pain are listed in **Box 7**. The response to these agents is highly variable. There is no single correct approach to the management of any given patient, with painful neuropathy. Often it requires patience on the part of the patients and physicians who must try a variety of different medications on a trial and error basis until a satisfactory regimen is established.

CONCLUSION

It is very important for all doctors, especially primary care physicians to look for and recognize diabetic neuropathy. Early diagnosis with clinical tests or simple inexpensive methods, such as monofilament tests, can go a long way in preventing the limb-threatening and life-threatening consequences of neuropathy.

MACROVASCULAR COMPLICATIONS

Macrovascular complications of diabetes include coronary heart disease, cardiomyopathy, arrhythmias and sudden death, cerebrovascular disease and peripheral artery disease. Cardiovascular disease is the primary cause of death in most of the diabetic patients. Unlike microvascular complications which are related to the duration and severity of hyperglycemia, the macrovascular complications are also related to the insulin resistance, obesity, hypertension, dyslipidemia and can present even at the onset of diabetes or even before the individual develops diabetes. Hence it is important to know about the cardiovascular complications and screen for and treat them appropriately.

RECOMMENDED READINGS

1. Textbook of Diabetes, Fifth Edition. Edited by R. Holt, C. Cockram, A. Flyvbjerg and B. Goldstein. Published John Wiley & Sons, 2017.
2. Faselis C, Katsimardou A, Imprialos K, Deligkaris P, Kallistratos M, Dimitriadis K. Microvascular Complications of Type 2 Diabetes Mellitus. Curr Vasc Pharmacol. 2020;18:117-24.
3. Acute and Chronic Complications of Diabetes - Endocrinology and Metabolism Clinics of North America 2013;42(4):721-970.
4. Diabetic Complications Clinical Aspects in Joslin's Diabetes Mellitus, 14th Edition, Kahn CR, Weir GC ed Publ. Lippincott William & Wilkins, Section VIII Pages 885-1143.

CHAPTER 121

Diabetes Mellitus: Management

Subhankar Chowdhury, Partha Pratim Chakraborty

ABSTRACT

Comprehensive care in patients with diabetes mellitus (DM) not only involves successful management of hyperglycemia, but control of hypertension (HTN) and dyslipidemia, effective treatment of underlying vascular complications and associated comorbidities as well. Atherosclerotic cardiovascular disease (ASCVD) is the leading cause of mortality in patients with DM; hence, control of underlying cardiovascular (CV) risk factors is of utmost importance.

Management algorithm starts with an effort to identify the type of diabetes, particularly in youths, as all patients with type 1 diabetes mellitus (T1DM), and majority of patients with pancreatic diabetes require insulin from the very beginning. Type 2 diabetes mellitus (T2DM), on the other hand, is treated either with oral agents or noninsulin injectable molecules or insulin preparations depending on symptoms, clinical characteristics, prevailing glycemic status, on-going treatment, and underlying comorbidities.

All patients with DM should adopt a healthy dietary habit and engage in regular physical activities. Randomized controlled trials (RCTs), published in recent past, have documented the effectiveness of certain class of molecules like glucagon-like peptide-1 receptor agonists (GLP-1 RAs) and sodium-glucose cotransporter-2 (SGLT-2) inhibitors in preventing major adverse CV events, progression of nephropathy, and reducing hospitalization with heart failure (HF) in patients with T2DM. All current guidelines, therefore, recommend these agents as the preferred second-line therapy after metformin.

Glycemic targets have long been centered on fasting and postmeal glucose and glycated hemoglobin (HbA1c); however, the importance of reducing glycemic variability (GV) and avoidance of hypoglycemia has been highlighted in recent times. Blood glucose, blood pressure (BP), and lipid targets need to be individualized.

Regular follow-up is essential and patients with DM should be screened periodically for micro- and macrovascular complications of diabetes.

"The way to deal with the devil of obesity and diabetes is literally one day at a time"

—Stephen Furst

INTRODUCTION

Diabetes mellitus (DM) is a chronic multisystem disease; hence successful management of DM requires multidisciplinary approach, in addition to diabetes self-management education (DSME) and support. Long-standing uncontrolled hyperglycemia is associated with micro (nephropathy, retinopathy, and neuropathy) and macrovascular [cerebrovascular disease, coronary artery disease (CAD), and peripheral arterial disease (PAD)] complications of diabetes, while acute perturbation in diabetes care in patients with significant endogenous insulin deficiency may result in life-threatening hyperglycemia, diabetic ketoacidosis (DKA), or hyperosmolar hyperglycemic state (HHS). Hypoglycemia is another acute complication, actually of treatment of diabetes, which is more often encountered in patients with underlying target organ damage (TOD), or poor β-cell reserve, being treated with insulin secretagogues or exogenous insulin. Such metabolic and vascular complications of DM may be prevented or delayed with effective management of hyperglycemia and associated comorbidities, like hypertension (HTN) and dyslipidemia.

DM is broadly classified into four categories—(1) T1DM, (2) T2DM, (3) specific type of diabetes due to "other causes," and (4) gestational DM (GDM). Diseases, included in the "other causes" are monogenic causes of β-cell secretory defect [neonatal diabetes, maturity onset diabetes of the young (MODY)], monogenic causes of insulin resistance (IR) (including lipodystrophies), disorders of the exocrine pancreas [pancreatitis, fibrocalculous pancreatic diabetes (FCPD), cystic fibrosis-related diabetes (CFRD)], endocrinopathies (Cushing's syndrome and acromegaly), drug/chemical-induced diabetes [glucocorticoid, antiretroviral therapy, and new onset diabetes after transplant (NODAT)], viral infections (including SARS-CoV-2), immune-mediated diabetes, and diabetes-associated with different syndromes.

INITIAL EVALUATION

The first step in evaluation of a patient with DM, particularly in a young individual, is to identify the type of DM, if possible. Family history of DM in first and second-degree relatives, prior history of DKA, history of GDM in mother (in children), menstrual irregularities in adolescents and adult women, history of GDM in previous pregnancy (in adult women), history of pain abdomen, and oily stool should always be sought for. Clinical examination should focus on body mass index (BMI), waist circumference (WC) in those with normal BMI, presence of acanthosis nigricans (nape of neck, axillae, groins), and hepatomegaly. Diagnosis is achieved in a majority of patients from the mode of clinical presentation, supplemented by detailed history, thorough clinical examination, and a handful of investigations (**Figs. 1** and **2**).

Onset of DM before 6 months of life in an infant without acanthosis nigricans suggests neonatal diabetes. New onset osmotic symptoms in a nonobese child without family history of DM, particularly when associated with DKA is typical of T1DM. However, with increasing prevalence of childhood obesity, T2DM is also seen in children. Family history of DM in first-degree relative, presence of obesity, and acanthosis nigricans in any adult individual with diabetes points toward T2DM. Presence of DM in at least three successive generations, either in paternal or maternal side, in a nonobese youth without IR increases the likelihood of MODY. No/minimal antihyperglycemic response to noninsulin agents from beginning, particularly when associated with pain abdomen or oily stool indicates pancreatic diabetes (also known as type 3c DM), while insulin dependence following initial response (≈6 months) to oral agents suggests possible latent autoimmune diabetes in adult (LADA) or latent autoimmune diabetes in the young (LADY).

The next step is to evaluate for diabetes-related complications and potential comorbid conditions. All

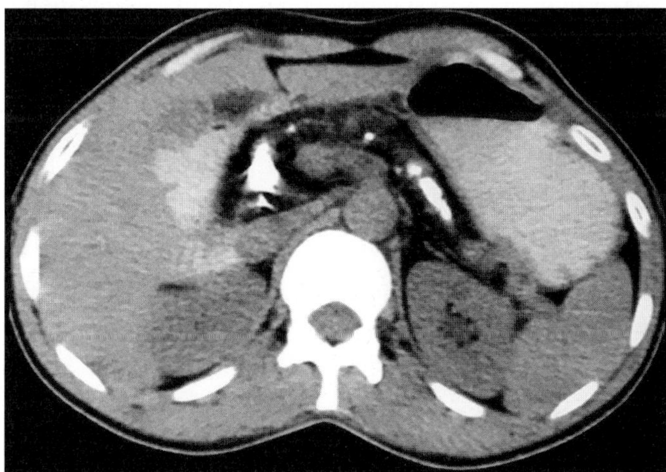

FIGURE 1: CT scan of abdomen showing calcifications along the main pancreatic duct in a patient with insulin requiring diabetes, suggesting FCPD.

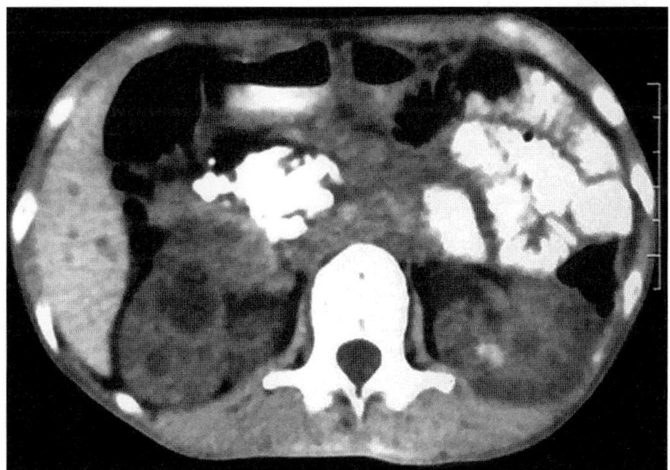

FIGURE 2: Bilateral renal cysts on CT scan in a young patient with diabetes. The patient finally was diagnosed to have MODY 5 or RCAD (renal cyst and diabetes).

TABLE 1 Summary of investigations performed during initial evaluation of patients with diabetes.

Parameters	Comments
CBC	Part of routine investigation. May reveal iron deficiency or vitamin B12 deficiency
HbA1c	Helps to decide on antihyperglycemic agent(s) in T2DM
Creatinine	Calculate eGFR by CKD-EPI or MDRD equation in adults and by bedside Schwartz equation in children (<18 years). Choice of therapy partly depends on eGFR
Urine ACR*	Done on spot sample, preferably in morning
Lipid profile*	Combination of low HDL-c and high TG suggests insulin resistance, while high HDL-C points toward insulin deficiency
LFT*	Elevated transaminases suggest NAFLD
USG/CT scan whole abdomen	Pancreatic and renal morphology may be helpful to classify diabetes (**Figs. 1** and **2**). Helps to identify NAFLD
Pancreatic autoantibodies	Includes anti-GAD antibody, anti-IA2 antibody, and anti-insulin antibody#. Confirms autoimmune T1DM or LADY/LADA; negative test does not rule out autoimmune diabetes
TSH	In T1DM
Total IgA and IgA anti-tTG antibody	In T1DM
c-peptide*	Stimulated c-peptide is preferred over fasting c-peptide. Performed in young onset diabetes, when diagnosis is uncertain

*To be performed once satisfactory glycemic control is achieved

#Anti-insulin antibody should always be sent before starting insulin therapy

(CKD-EPI: Chronic Kidney Disease Epidemiology Collaboration); GAD: glutamic acid decarboxylase; IA-2: islet antigen-2; Ig: immunoglobulin; LADY: latent autoimmune diabetes in the young; LADA: latent autoimmune diabetes in adult; MDRD: Modification of Diet in Renal Disease; tTG: tissue transglutaminase)

adults with DM should also be subjected to comprehensive foot examination (including evaluation of footwear), dilated direct fundoscopy, dental examination, and orthostatic BP measurement. Foot examination includes inspection for ulcer, callous, deformity, and infection; measurement of ankle-brachial pressure index (ABPI); evaluation for loss of protective sensation (LOPS) by determining temperature, pinprick, or vibration sensation and 10-g monofilament test.

Investigations, recommended during initial visit, have been summarized in **Table 1**.

TREATMENT

Comprehensive diabetes care encompasses control of hyperglycemia, HTN, and dyslipidemia along with effective management of underlying complications of DM, if any, and associated comorbidities. Focus should be on known CV risk factors for prevention of ASCVD, when appropriate. These objectives are achieved with a combination of pharmacologic and nonpharmacologic approaches.

LIFESTYLE MODIFICATION

Medical nutrition therapy (MNT) and physical activity are essential components of diabetes management. For all patients with overweight/obesity, lifestyle modification (LSM) to achieve and maintain a minimum weight loss of 5% is recommended. "Ideal" macronutrient composition is debatable, and there is no "best" diet that has to be followed universally. Meal plan should better be individualized and patients may be counseled to adhere to the Mediterranean or Dietary Approach to Stop Hypertension (DASH)-style eating pattern if possible. For an average Indian, carbohydrate, fat, and protein should contribute to roughly 50–60%, <30%, and 15% of total daily calorie intake (TDCI), respectively. Foods with low glycemic index (GI) and low glycemic load (GL) should be preferred; for an example, brown rice (GI: 68) may be preferred over white rice (GI: 73). Patients, particularly those on intensive insulin regimes, should be familiar with carbohydrate counting. Reduction of saturated fat (<10% of TDCI) and trans-fat, increase of dietary ω-3 fatty acids, viscous fiber (25–40 g/day), and plant stanols/sterols intake are beneficial. They should also be advised for smoking cessation, reducing dietary sodium (<2,300 mg/day, equivalent to <5,000 mg/day of salt), increasing potassium intake, and moderation of alcohol consumption.

Children and adolescents with DM should engage in at least 60 min/day of moderate or vigorous intensity aerobic exercise. Adults should spend at least 150 min/week for similar activities, spread over at least 3 days a week. In addition, resistance exercise needs to be performed on at least 3 days/week. Prolonged sitting should be avoided, and be interrupted every 30 minutes.

PHARMACOLOGICAL MANAGEMENT

T2DM: Management of T2DM depends on several factors like duration of disease, symptoms, associated comorbidities, findings on clinical examination (BMI, acanthosis nigricans), and prevalent glycemic status. Majority of patients with "garden variety" of T2DM are treated with oral antidiabetic agents (OADs), and the indications of insulin therapy in T2DM have been listed in **Box 1**.

All major guidelines across the globe recommend *treatment initiation with LSM, metformin* (if not contraindicated) with/without other agent(s) depending on glycated hemoglobin (HbA1c) at presentation. For an example, if the baseline HbA1c is between 7.5% and 9%, patients may be put on dual oral therapy, and when HbA1c is above 9%, triple therapy may be considered. The mean HbA1c reduction with the available agents when used as monotherapy is summarized in **Table 2**. However, higher the baseline HbA1c more is the percentage reduction.

BOX 1 Indications of insulin therapy in patients with T2DM.

- Secondary OAD failure (HbA1c above target despite combination therapy at optimal dose for at least 3 months)
- HbA1c > 9–10% with osmotic symptoms and loss of muscle mass
- Hyperglycemic crisis (hyperosmolar hyperglycemic state and diabetic ketoacidosis)
- Patients hospitalized with critical illnesses (acute coronary syndrome and cerebrovascular accident)
- Hospitalized patients on nil-per-os or on parenteral nutrition
- Patients with systemic infection (with/without sepsis)*
- Selected patients with organ failure (chronic kidney disease, chronic liver disease, and congestive heart failure) when one or more OADs are contraindicated
- Patients contemplating pregnancy or patients with pregnancy (though there is growing trend to use metformin as first-line drug therapy in gestational diabetes mellitus)
- Selected patients undergoing surgery
- Selected patients on systemic glucocorticoid therapy

*Tuberculosis per se is not an indication for insulin treatment

(OAD: oral antidiabetic drug)

In addition, combining two agents are likely to exert a synergistic effect on HbA1c.

Choice of the second agent after metformin depends on the following factors—high risk or established ASCVD, chronic kidney disease (CKD) or HF, compelling need to minimize hypoglycemia, compelling need to minimize weight gain or promote weight loss, cost, safety, tolerability, and patient preference (**Table 2**). The American Diabetes Association (ADA) suggests using GLP-1 RA or SGLT-2 inhibitor in patients with ASCVD, CKD, or HF irrespective of baseline HbA1c.

The 2019 European Society of Cardiology/European Association for the Study of Diabetes (ESC/EASD) guideline, however, recommends SGLT-2 inhibitor or GLP-1 RA as first-line therapy over metformin in patients with established ASCVD, or at very high/high CV risk to reduce CV events.

To summarize, in patients with established ASCVD or who are at high risk of ASCVD [age ≥ 55 years, left ventricular hypertrophy (LVH) or coronary, carotid, or lower-extremity arterial stenosis > 50%], the preferred second-line agent is either a GLP-1 RA or SGLT-2 inhibitor with proven CV benefit (**Table 3**). SGLT-2 inhibitor use is associated with reduction in HF and CV death in patients with or without DM and left ventricular ejection fraction (LVEF) ≤ 40% (DAPA-HF and EMPEROR-reduced trials), hence, preferred in such patients. Patients with albuminuria or CKD should also be offered SGLT-2 inhibitor upfront, and if that is not tolerated or contraindicated, GLP-1 RA. Patients with estimated glomerular filtration rate (eGFR) of <60 mL/min/1.73 m^2 are at increased risk of CV events irrespective of albuminuria; in absence of albuminuria, any one of these two agents should be used according to the eGFR. Agents associated with no/minimal hypoglycemia are preferred in elderly patients and in patients at high risk of hypoglycemia (**Table 2**). GLP-1 RA and SGLT-2 inhibitor are associated with weight loss, hence preferred in overweight or obese patients.

In low-income countries, cost of therapy needs to be considered as well, and sulfonylureas (SUs) and pioglitazone, being relatively cheaper, are often used in India. The Endocrine Society of India (ESI) and the

TABLE 2 Average HbA1c reduction with different blood-glucose lowering agents, when used as monotherapy. Change in body weight and risk of hypoglycemia are also shown.

Agent	Reduction in HbA1c (%)	Effect on weight	Risk of hypoglycemia
Insulin	No ceiling effect	Gain	High
Metformin	1–2	Neutral/Loss	Low/Absent
Sulfonylureas	1–2	Gain	High
GLP1RAs	1–1.5	Loss	Low/Absent
Thiazolidinediones	1–1.5	Gain	Low/Absent
SGLT-2 inhibitors	0.5–1.5*	Loss	Low/Absent
DPP-4 inhibitors	0.5–1.5*	Neutral/Loss	Low/Absent
Meglitinides	0.5–1.5	Gain	High
AGIs	0.5–1*	Neutral	Absent

* HbA1c reduction with SGLT-2 inhibitor and DPP-4 inhibitor use in most of the studies is around 0.5–0.9%. For AGI, reduction is around 0.5–0.8%.

TABLE 3 Summary of all the cardiovascular outcome trials (CVOTs) with different glucose-lowering agents.

Agent	Name of the study	Inclusion criteria	Comparator	Primary outcome	Nonfatal MI	Nonfatal stroke	CV death
DPP4Is							
Alogliptin	EXAMINE	Recent ACS	Placebo	N	N	N	N
Saxagliptin	SAVOR-TIMI 53	Established ASCVD or multiple risk factors	Placebo	N	N	N	N
Sitagliptin	TECOS	Established ASCVD	Placebo	N	–	–	N
Linagliptin	CARMELINA	Established ASCVD and elevated UACR	Placebo	N	N	N	N
Linagliptin	CAROLINA	Established ASCVD or multiple risk factors	Glimepiride	N	N	N	N
SGLT-2 inhibitors							
Empagliflozin	EMPA-REG OUTCOME#	Established ASCVD	Placebo	S	N	N	S
Canagliflozin	CANVAS	Established ASCVD or multiple risk factors	Placebo	S	N	N	N
Dapagliflozin	DECLARE-TIMI 58	Multiple risk factors or established ASCVD	Placebo	S*	N	N	N
Ertugliflozin	VERTIS CV	Established ASCVD	Placebo	N	N	N	N
GLP-1 RAs							
Liraglutide	LEADER#	Established ASCVD or multiple risk factors	Placebo	S	N	N	S
Semaglutide (injection)	SUSTAIN-6	Established ASCVD or multiple risk factors	Placebo	S	N	S	N
Semaglutide (oral)	PIONEER 6#	Established ASCVD or multiple risk factors	Placebo	N	N	N	S
Lixisenatide	ELIXA	ACS within 180 days	Placebo	N	N	N	N
Exenatide (extended release)	EXSCEL#	With or without ASCVD	Placebo	N	N	N	N
Albiglutide	HARMONY OUTCOMES	Established ASCVD	Placebo	S	S	N	N
Dulaglutide	REWIND	Established ASCVD or multiple risk factors	Placebo	S	N	S	N
Insulins							
Glargine	ORIGIN	Established ASCVD or CV risk factors	Placebo	N	–	–	N
Degludec	DEVOTE	Established ASCVD or risk factors	Glargine	N	N	N	N

* Significant reduction in composite of CV death or HHF; not in MACE

Reduction in "death from any cause" was noted

(**N:** neutral; **I:** inferior; **S:** superior)

Research Society for the Study of Diabetes in India (RSSDI) recommend these agents over others to reduce the cost of therapy in certain patients. Moreover, World Health Organization (WHO) strongly recommends SU as a second-line agent in patients with inadequate response or intolerance to metformin in low-resource settings. In India, some of the DPP4Is (vildagliptin, teneligliptin, evogliptin, and alogliptin) and SGLT-2 inhibitors (remogliflozin and dapagliflozin) are relatively inexpensive, and may be used in appropriate patients.

If HbA1c target is not achieved after about 3 months, another appropriate agent, from a different class should be added. In patients with uncontrolled hyperglycemia, particularly when three or four OADs have already been used in optimal dosage, injectable therapies are to be considered. Though GLP-1 RAs are recommended over insulin by ADA, insulin is widely used in India in such circumstances. If the difference between fasting and postprandial glucose concentrations is <100 mg/dL, initiation with long-acting basal insulin at bedtime is preferred (0.1–0.2 IU/kg or 10 U), and if the difference is >100 mg/dL, two shots of premixed insulin preparations (BIAsp 30:70, lispro mix 25:75, lispro mix 50:50, biphasic human 30:70, and biphasic human 50:50) or coformulations (IDegAsp) are often effective. One shot of premixed insulin preparations or coformulations may also be used in place of basal insulin during initiation. Subsequent intensification of insulin regime depends on glycemic status of the patient.

Type 1 diabetes mellitus: Insulin is the "fact of life" in patients with T1DM. Due to absolute deficiency of endogenous insulin, such patients must have "round-the-clock" insulin coverage either with multiple subcutaneous insulin injection (MSI) in the form of basal-bolus therapy or continuous subcutaneous insulin infusion (CSII) with insulin pump. Majority of them need at least four shots, prandial insulin before each meal (breakfast, lunch, and dinner) and one shot of long-acting insulin at any time of the day, preferably after evening. An additional shot of prandial insulin is required in some, if the predinner glucose values are consistently high. In rare instances, patients with T1DM may have satisfactory glycemic control with two shots of premixed insulin formulations.

Insulin analogs are preferred over conventional human insulin preparations in T1DM due to better pharmacokinetic properties of the latter, which is associated with better postprandial coverage and less hypoglycemia (overall, nocturnal, and severe). Such a benefit, however, if present at all, is likely to be minimal. Human short-acting insulin (regular insulin) and intermediate-acting insulin [neutral protamine Hagedorn insulin (NPH)], being cheaper, are widely used in resource-restricted settings. To reduce the number of daily pricks, regular and NPH insulin are at times mixed in the same syringe immediately before administration, in the so-called "split-mix" regime. The approval statuses of different insulin analogs have been summarized in **Table 4**. Insulin preparations, approved in pregnancy are human insulin (regular and NPH), lispro, aspart, and detemir. Insulin glargine has also been found to be safe in pregnancy, and though not an approved agent, can be used off-label.

In addition to insulin deficiency secondary to autoimmune destruction of the pancreatic β-cells, IR and postprandial hyperglucagonemia have also been described in T1D, and, may be potential adjunctive targets for intervention in addition to insulin therapy. IR in T1DM is secondary to the disease per se, underlying genetic predisposition, sedentary lifestyle, and over-insulinization following insulin therapy. Puberty, increasing age, and intercurrent illnesses also contribute to IR in T1DM. While IR is often encountered in obese T1DM patients, the disease itself is likely to have a component of systemic IR; poor glycemic control is associated with hepatic IR, while skeletal muscle glucose utilization is reported to be lower even in those with well-controlled diabetes.

Metformin has been tried in overweight/obese adolescents (T1D Exchange Clinic Network Metformin RCT Study) and adults (≥40 years) with T1DM (REMOVAL study), but failed to provide additional long-term antihyperglycemic benefit. However, metformin use is likely to be associated with reduction in total daily dose of insulin, reduction in adiposity, and improvement in CV risk parameters. Sotagliflozin, an oral inhibitor of SGLT-1 and SGLT-2, has recently been tried with insulin in T1DM (Tandem 3 study). Use of this agent is associated with higher proportion of patients with satisfactory glycemic control without severe hypoglycemia, albeit at higher risk of DKA. So far only two noninsulin agents have been approved by regulatory agencies to be used exclusively in adults with T1DM as *adjuncts (not in lieu of)* to insulin.

Pramlintide is approved by United States Food and Drug Administration (USFDA) in addition to mealtime insulin if desired glycemic control is not achieved despite optimal insulin therapy. European Commission, but not USFDA, has approved sotagliflozin, for patients with a BMI of 27 kg/m^2 or more. However, metformin and α-glucosidase inhibitors

TABLE 4 Current approval status of available insulin analogs.

Insulin analog	Approval status
Rapid/Ultrarapid-acting insulin analogs	
Aspart	Children ≥ 2 years and adults
FiAsp	Children ≥ 2 years and adults
Lispro	Children ≥ 3 years and adults
Lispro-aabc	Adults
Glulisine	Children ≥ 4 years and adults
Long-acting insulin analogs	
Degludec (U-100, U-200)	Children ≥ 1 years and adults
Detemir	Children ≥ 2 years and adults
U-100 glargine	Children ≥ 6 years and adults
U-300 glargine	Children ≥6 years and adults
Icodec	Not yet approved

TABLE 5	HbA1c target in majority of nonpregnant patients with diabetes.
ADA-2021	≤7%
AACE/ACE-2020	≤6.5%
IDF-2017	≤7%
Canadian Diabetes Association	≤7%
RSSDI-ESI 2020	≤7%
NICE-2019	≤6.5%

(ADA: American Diabetes Association; AACE/ACE: American Association of Clinical Endocrinologists and American College of Endocrinology; IDF: International Diabetes Federation; RSSDI-ESI: Research Society for the Study of Diabetes in India and Endocrine Society of India; NICE: National Institute for Health and Care Excellence)

are often used off-label in T1DM, particularly in patients with clinical features of IR and postsnack hyperglycemia, respectively.

Other types of DM: Management of GDM has been covered in the chapter entitled "Endocrine Disorders in Pregnancy". Choice of antihyperglycemic agents in other forms of DM depends on the type of the disease. For an example, insulin is the treatment of choice in majority of patients with pancreatic diabetes, while insulin sensitizers with/without insulin secretagogues are used in lipodystrophies.

GLYCEMIC TARGETS

The glycemic targets are broadly classified into two groups:

Efficacy-oriented goals: *Fasting glucose, postmeal glucose, HbA1c* (**Table 5**) Glycemic targets need to be individualized based upon patient and disease-related factors, and reassessed over time. ADA recommends preprandial capillary plasma glucose of 80–130 mg/dL and peak postprandial capillary plasma glucose of <180 mg/dL for majority of non-pregnant adults with diabetes. Glucometers though measure capillary whole blood glucose, most of the available instruments provide plasma equivalent values; hence postprandial capillary glucose measurements are ≈20% higher than venous plasma glucose. The authors recommend fasting plasma glucose (FPG) of 90–110 mg/dL and postmeal plasma glucose (2 hours after beginning of meal) of 140–160 mg/dL in majority of patients outside pregnancy.

HbA1c reflects average glycemic status over approximately 3 months, i.e., average life span of the red blood cells; however, almost 50% of the HbA1c value reflects contribution of the preceding 1 month and about 75% of the total HbA1c is attributed to the glycemic status of the preceding 2 months. HbA1c should preferably be tested in National Glycohemoglobin Standardization Program (NGSP)-certified assays at the time of diagnosis and then every 3–6 months depending on overall glycemic status of the patients. Though HbA1c is the gold standard for glycemic monitoring and has a robust predictive value for diabetes complications, alterations in hemoglobin metabolism can interfere with its reliability. Glycated albumin, fructosamine (total glycated proteins), and 1,5-anhydroglucitol are alternative markers of average glycemia in such conditions.

Majority of the non-pregnant adults with diabetes should achieve an HbA1c goal of <7% without significant hypoglycemia. However, a more stringent goal of <6–6.5% may be set in highly motivated relatively younger subjects with short duration of diabetes, no comorbidities, absence of established vascular complications, and long-life expectancy who have access to resources and support systems, if that can be achieved without clinically significant hypoglycemia. On the contrary, an HbA1c target of 8–8.5% is sufficient in elderly individuals with long-standing diabetes, limited life expectancy, associated comorbidities, established vascular complications, and those at high risk of hypoglycemia with/without hypoglycemia unawareness. An HbA1c of <7% is also appropriate for many children with diabetes, while less stringent goal (<7.5%) is preferred in children with hypoglycemia unawareness, who are unable to communicate for symptoms of hypoglycemia, those being treated with human insulins and/or do not perform self-monitoring of blood glucose (SMBG) or have access to continuous glucose monitoring (CGM). In addition, a target of <8% is suitable for children with a history of severe hypoglycemia, while those with T1DM during their honeymoon phase should have a more stringent HbA1c goal of <6.5%. It is important to note that insulin requirement is significantly reduced during honeymoon phase of T1DM (may be even 2–3 U/day); however, insulin should never be completely withdrawn during this time.

Glycemic variability (GV): There is growing interest in and some evidence for glycemic variability (GV) as another target of glycemic control. HbA1c fails to identify GV and episodes of hypoglycemia, two clinically relevant conditions in patients with severe insulin deficiency. SMBG and/or CGM are effective supplements to HbA1c in such cases. CGM data provides with the following three measures—interquartile range (IQR), standard deviation (SD) around the mean and coefficient of variation (CV). One way to measure GV is % CV, and the target being ≤ 36%; though lower targets (<33%) provide additional protection against hypoglycemia in patients treated with SUs or insulins. Time in range (TIR) has recently been put forward as a useful metric of glycemic control as it correlates with the risk of microvascular complications. In addition, time below range (TBR) and time above range (TAR) direct reevaluation of treatment regimen. A strong correlation between TIR and HbA1c has been found with 70% TIR corresponds to an HbA1c of 7%. Recommended target TIR values have been summarized in **Table 6**.

Daily frequent monitoring of capillary blood glucose (CBG): In the form of SMBG by glucometer or CGM, is an essential component of management in all patients treated either with MSI or CSII and in those with recurrent hypoglycemia. Ambulatory glucose profile (AGP), which is CGM metrics derived from CGM use over the preceding 2 weeks is often used now-a-days to evaluate TIR. Though SMBG up to 6–10 time points everyday have been

TABLE 6 CGM-based targets in different populations with diabetes.

Glucose value	Time spent			
	T1DM* and T2DM	Elderly patients/high-risk patients with T1DM or T2DM	Pregnant patient with T1DM#	Pregnant patient with T2DM or GDM$
>250 mg/dL	<5%	<10%		
>180 mg/dL	<25%	<50%		
>140 mg/dL			<25%	<5%
70–180 mg/dL	>70%	>50%		
63–140 mg/dL			>70%	>95%
<70 mg/dL	<4%	<1%		
<63 mg/dL			<4%	<4%
<54 mg/dL	<1%		<1%	<1%

*TIR target is ≈ 60% in patients younger than 25 years of age and HbA1c goal of 7.5%.

#Limited evidence

$Very sparse data:
>250 mg/dL: level 2 hyperglycemia; 181–250 mg/dL: level 1 hyperglycemia; 54–69 mg/dL: level 1 hypoglycemia; <54 mg/dL: level 2 hypoglycemia

advocated, particularly in children and adolescents, the authors of this chapter suggest SMBG monitoring at fasting, 2-hour postbreakfast, 2-hour postlunch, predinner, 2-hour postdinner, 3:00 am, and during symptoms suggestive of hypoglycemia. In addition, SMBG is recommended immediately before exercise and driving. In low-income groups, the frequency of SMBG may be further reduced in patients with satisfactory glycemic control.

Self-monitoring of blood glucose is not mandatory in patients on OADs. However, SMBG is often advised in those who experience frequent episodes of hypoglycemia or in situations, where HbA1c does not correlate with laboratory glucose values.

MANAGEMENT IN DIABETES WITH COMPLICATIONS

Cardiovascular disease and risk management: Atherosclerotic cardiovascular disease is the leading cause of morbidity and mortality in individuals with DM. These individuals are also at higher risk of HF, both with preserved EF or reduced EF. The 10-year risk of a first ASCVD event needs to be calculated. A number of risk calculators like Framingham Risk score-Coronary heart disease (FRS-CHD), Framingham Risk Score-Cardiovascular Disease (FRS-CVD), QRISK2, Joint British Society risk calculator 3 (JBS3), American College of Cardiology/American Heart Association (ACC/AHA), ASCVD, and WHO risk charts are available. Though the various risk calculators may not be accurate in Indians, FRS-CVD appears to be the most useful for CVD risk assessment. ADA recommends using the ACC/AHA risk calculator to stratify ASCVD risk.

Blood pressure control: Patients with confirmed office-based BP of ≥140/90 mm of Hg should be put on antihypertensive medication; it is prudent to start with two agents if BP is ≥160/100 mm of Hg. Angiotensin-converting enzyme inhibitors (ACEIs) and/or angiotensin receptor blockers (ARBs) are preferred in hypertensive patients with CAD and/or albuminuria. However, control of BP is more important than the choice of agent. A combination of ACEI and ARB should be avoided. BP targets need to be individualized in patients with diabetes and HTN; those with established ASCVD or 10-year risk of ≥15%, should target BP of <130/80 mm of Hg, while those at lower risk preferably have BP of <140/90 mm of Hg. Patients should be encouraged for home BP self-monitoring and 24-hour ambulatory BP monitoring.

Lipid management: The indications of statin therapy have been summarized in **Table 7**.

If recommended dose of statin is not tolerated, maximally tolerated statin dose should be used. If maximally tolerated statin dose fails to reduce low-density lipoprotein cholesterol (LDL-C) by the desired amount, ezetimibe may be used. Very high-risk patients with established ASCVD should achieve a LDL-C goal of <70 mg/dL, and if that is not achieved with maximally tolerated dose of statin, ezetimibe or proprotein convertase subtilisin/kexin type 9 (PCSK9) inhibitor may be considered. Once LDL-C goal is reached, the next target is nonhigh-density lipoprotein cholesterol (HDL-C), and the target being 30 mg/dL higher than the LDL-C target. Triglyceride (TG) is to be targeted next, and treatment of hyperTG is not required unless the baseline TG is >1,000 mg/dL, which greatly increases the risk of pancreatitis. Uncontrolled hyperglycemia (with/without insulin deficiency), obesity, and alcohol intake are the common causes of secondary hyperTG and serum TG often normalizes with lowering of plasma glucose (with/without insulin therapy). Icosapent ethyl may be added to statin therapy in patients with established ASCVD or those with multiple risk factors having elevated TG (135–499 mg/dL) and controlled LDL-C. Combination of statin and fibrate or niacin may provide additional benefit; however, combination therapy is associated with increased adverse effects. Combination of statin and fibrate may be considered in selected male patients at high risk of CV events with TG ≥ 204 mg/dL and HDL-C ≤ 34 mg/dL. Saroglitazar, a dual peroxisome proliferator-activated receptors (PPAR) α and γ agonist, is approved by Drug Controller General of India (DCGI) for the treatment of hypertriglyceridemia and diabetic dyslipidemia in India. The drug is also approved by DCGI in the treatment of T2DM as add on therapy with metformin.

Antiplatelet therapy: Aspirin therapy (75–150 mg/day) for secondary prevention is recommended in all patients. Low-dose aspirin for primary prevention is recommended in men and women aged ≥50 years with DM and at least one of the following risk factors—family history of premature ASCVD, HTN, dyslipidemia, smoking, and CKD/albuminuria. Clopidogrel should be used in documented aspirin allergy.

Diabetic nephropathy: To reduce the risk or slow the progression of CKD, patients should have satisfactory glycemic control and optimal BP control. Renin-angiotensin-aldosterone system (RAAS) blockade with either ACEI or ARB should be added in patients with albuminuria with/without HTN. SGLT-2 inhibitors and GLP-1 RAs have been associated with reduced risk of incident or worsening nephropathy. Dose adjustments of certain medications are needed when eGFR falls below 60 mL/min/1.73 m^2, and with further decline in renal function some of the agents need to be avoided (**Table 8**).

Diabetic retinopathy: Glycemic control, BP control, and lipid parameters need to be optimized to reduce the risk or slow the progression of diabetic retinopathy. Patients with severe nonproliferative diabetic retinopathy and proliferative diabetic retinopathy need to be treated with intravitreal antivascular endothelial growth factor (VEGF) and/or panretinal laser photocoagulation to reduce the risk of vision loss. Patients with diabetic macular edema are treated with anti-VEGF therapy with or without grid laser.

TABLE 7 Indication and dose of statin in diabetes.

High intensity statin (lowers LDL-C by ≥50%)	• Rosuvastatin: 20–40 mg • Atorvastatin: 40–80 mg	• Established ASCVD irrespective of age (secondary prevention) • 40–75 years of age and ASCVD risk ≥20% (primary prevention) • 50–70 years of age with multiple risk factors (primary prevention)
Moderate intensity statin (lowers LDL-C by 30–49%)	• Rosuvastatin: 5–10 mg • Atorvastatin: 10–20 mg • Simvastatin: 20–40 mg • Pravastatin: 40–80 mg • Lovastatin: 40 mg • Fluvastatin (extended release): 80 mg • Pitavastatin: 1–4 mg	• 40–75 years of age without ASCVD (primary prevention) • 20–39 years of age with multiple risk factors (primary prevention)

(ASCVD: atherosclerotic cardiovascular disease; LDL-C: low-density lipoprotein cholesterol)

TABLE 8 Use of different classes of noninsulin glucose lowering agents in CKD.

Agents	eGFR (mL/min/1.73 m^2)	Comments
Metformin	<30	Contraindicated
	30–45	Should not be initiated. Maximum dose to be reduced to 1 g/day in current users
	45–60	Maximum daily dose 2 g/day; monitor eGFR 3–6 monthly
	>60	Maximum daily dose 2 g/day; monitor eGFR yearly
Metformin should be temporarily discontinued at the time or before iodinated contrast administration in patients with eGFR 30–60 mL/min/1.73 m^2		
	SGLT-2 inhibitors	
Canagliflozin	<30	Should not be used
	30–45	Should not be initiated
Empagliflozin	<45	Should not be used
Dapagliflozin	<45	Should not be used
Ertugliflozin	<30	Should not be used
	30–60	Should not be initiated
EMPA-REG OUTCOME included participants with eGFR up to 30 and DAPA-CKD included patients with eGFR up to 25 and demonstrated benefit in subgroups with low eGFR. More frequent monitoring of renal function is required in patients having eGFR of <60 and being treated with any SGLT-2 inhibitor		

Continued...

Continued...

Agents	eGFR (mL/min/1.73 m²)	Comments
		GLP-1 RA
Liraglutide	<30	May be used, but there is paucity of data
Exenatide	>50	No dose adjustment is required
	30–50	Dose escalation from 5 to 10 µg conservatively
	<30	Not recommended
Lixisenatide	<30	Not recommended
Dulaglutide	<30	Not recommended
Albiglutide	<30	Not recommended
		DPP-4 inhibitors
Teneligliptin		No dose adjustment
Linagliptin		No dose adjustment
Evogliptin		No dose adjustment
Sitagliptin	<30	Maximum dose 25 mg/day
	30–50	Maximum dose 50 mg/day
	>50	No dose adjustment
Vildagliptin	<30	May be used with caution; maximum dose 50 mg/day
	30–50	Maximum dose 50 mg/day
	>50	No dose adjustment
Saxagliptin	>50	No dose adjustment
	<50	Maximum dose 2.5 mg/day
Saxagliptin is dialyzable. Dose to be repeated post hemodialysis		
Pioglitazone		No dose adjustment, caution needed in coexistent HF
		AGIs
All agents	Serum creatinine > 2 mg/dL	Not recommended

Diabetic neuropathy: Types of neuropathy encountered in patients with DM are distal symmetric peripheral neuropathy (small fiber and large fiber), autonomic neuropathy, and asymmetric neuropathy (cranial neuropathy, entrapment neuropathy, and plexopathy). Symptoms and signs of autonomic neuropathy should be assessed in patients with established microvascular complications. While satisfactory glycemic control prevents or delays the development of neuropathy in T1DM, it only helps to slow the progression of neuropathy in T2DM. Pregabalin, gabapentin, and duloxetine are recommended as initial pharmacologic treatments for painful diabetic neuropathy. Tricyclic antidepressant, however, is more effective than these agents to reduce diabetic neuropathic pain.

Other comorbidities: Other comorbidities, often associated with DM, are infections, obesity, obstructive sleep apnea (OSA), nonalcoholic fatty liver disease (NAFLD), periodontal diseases, psychiatric disorders ("diabetes distress," anxiety, depression, and disordered eating behavior) cognitive impairment, hypogonadism, pancreatitis, fractures, and cancers. Patients should be screened for these comorbidities and treated accordingly.

IMMUNIZATION SCHEDULE

Patients with diabetes should be provided Centers for Disease Control and Prevention (CDC) recommended immunization protocol according to their ages. Adults should receive influenza vaccine yearly. Patients aged between 19 years and 64 years should receive only one dose of pneumococcal polysaccharide vaccine (PPSV23), and those aged ≥ 65 years should receive one dose of PPSV23 and one dose of pneumococcal conjugate vaccine (PCV 13) at least a year apart. If the latter group had been vaccinated with PPSV23 before 65 years of age, the second dose of PPSV23 needs to be given at least 5 years after the previous dose. They should also receive hepatitis B, human papilloma virus (HPV), tetanus, diphtheria, pertussis (TDAP), and zoster (in ≥50 years) vaccines.

FOLLOW-UP

At every visit, patients should be enquired about symptoms of hypoglycemia along with frequency and time of such episodes. Body weight, BP, and insulin injection sites should be checked at every follow-up visit. FPG and postprandial plasma glucose (PPPG)/SMBG/AGP are checked at every visit, HbA1c every 3–6 months and serum creatinine, lipid profile, liver function test (LFT), urine albumin-to-creatinine ratio (ACR) should be tested annually. However, creatinine should be checked every 6 months in patients with stage 3b CKD, every 3 months in stage 4 CKD and every month in stage 5 CKD. Urine ACR needs to be monitored twice a year, if UACR is >300 mg/g of creatinine. Fundus, dental, and comprehensive foot examinations are undertaken annually. Fundus examination may be performed once every 2 years, if the initial findings are normal. In patients with T1DM, annual evaluation for complications should start when the disease duration is at least 5 years or from the time of puberty. All patients with DM should be followed up for the rest of their lives.

RECOMMENDED READINGS

1. Chawla R, Madhu SV, Makkar BM, Ghosh S, Saboo B, Kalra S, et al. RSSDI-ESI Clinical Practice Recommendations for the Management of Type 2 Diabetes Mellitus 2020. Indian J Endocrinol Metab. 2020;24(1):1-122.
2. American Diabetes Association. 9. Pharmacologic Approaches to Glycemic Treatment: Standards of Medical Care in Diabetes-2021. Diabetes Care. 2021;44(Suppl 1):S111-24.
3. Cosentino F, Grant PJ, Aboyans V, Bailey CJ, Ceriello A, ESC Scientific Document Group, et al. 2019 ESC Guidelines on diabetes, pre-diabetes, and cardiovascular diseases developed in collaboration with the EASD. Eur Heart J. 2020;41(2):255-323.
4. McMurray JJV, Solomon SD, Inzucchi SE, Køber L, Kosiborod MN, DAPA-HF Trial Committees and Investigators, et al. Dapagliflozin in patients with heart failure and reduced ejection fraction. N Engl J Med. 2019;381(21):1995-2008.
5. Packer M, Anker SD, Butler J, Filippatos G, Pocock SJ, EMPEROR-Reduced Trial Investigators, et al. Cardiovascular and renal outcomes with empagliflozin in heart failure. N Engl J Med. 2020;383(15):1413-24.
6. Scirica BM, Bhatt DL, Braunwald E, Steg PG, Davidson J, SAVOR-TIMI 53 Steering Committee and Investigators, et al. Saxagliptin and cardiovascular outcomes in patients with type 2 diabetes mellitus. N Engl J Med. 2013;369(14):1317-26.
7. Rosenstock J, Perkovic V, Johansen OE, Cooper ME, Kahn SE, CARMELINA Investigators, et al. Effect of linagliptin vs placebo on major cardiovascular events in adults with type 2 diabetes and high cardiovascular and renal risk: The CARMELINA Randomized Clinical Trial. JAMA. 2019;321(1):69-79.
8. Rosenstock J, Kahn SE, Johansen OE, Zinman B, Espeland MA, CAROLINA Investigators, et al. Effect of linagliptin vs glimepiride on major adverse cardiovascular outcomes in patients with type 2 diabetes: The CAROLINA Randomized Clinical Trial. JAMA. 2019;322(12):1155-66.
9. Zinman B, Wanner C, Lachin JM, Fitchett D, Bluhmki E, EMPA-REG OUTCOME Investigators, et al. Empagliflozin, cardiovascular outcomes, and mortality in type 2 diabetes. N Engl J Med. 2015;373(22):2117-28.
10. Neal B, Perkovic V, Mahaffey KW, de Zeeuw D, Fulcher G, CANVAS Program Collaborative Group, et al. Canagliflozin and cardiovascular and renal events in type 2 diabetes. N Engl J Med. 2017;377(7):644-57.
11. Wiviott SD, Raz I, Bonaca MP, Mosenzon O, Kato ET, DECLARE–TIMI 58 Investigators, et al. Dapagliflozin and cardiovascular outcomes in type 2 diabetes. N Engl J Med. 2019;380(4):347-57.
12. Cannon CP, Pratley R, Dagogo-Jack S, Mancuso J, Huyck S, VERTIS CV Investigators, et al. Cardiovascular outcomes with ertugliflozin in type 2 diabetes. N Engl J Med. 2020;383(15):1425-35.
13. Marso SP, Daniels GH, Brown-Frandsen K, Kristensen P, LEADER Steering Committee, LEADER Trial Investigators, et al. Liraglutide and cardiovascular outcomes in type 2 diabetes. N Engl J Med. 2016;375(4):311-22.
14. Marso SP, Bain SC, Consoli A, Eliaschewitz FG, Jódar E, SUSTAIN-6 Investigators, et al. Semaglutide and cardiovascular outcomes in patients with type 2 diabetes. N Engl J Med. 2016;375(19):1834-44.
15. Husain M, Birkenfeld AL, Donsmark M, Dungan K, Eliaschewitz FG, PIONEER 6 Investigators, et al. Oral semaglutide and cardiovascular outcomes in patients with type 2 diabetes. N Engl J Med. 2019;381(9):841-51.
16. Gerstein HC, Colhoun HM, Dagenais GR, Diaz R, Lakshmanan M, REWIND Investigators, et al. Dulaglutide and cardiovascular outcomes in type 2 diabetes (REWIND): A Double-Blind, Randomised Placebo-Controlled Trial. Lancet. 2019;394(10193):121-30.
17. Kovil R, Chawla M, Rajput R, Singh AK, Sinha B, Ghosal S, et al. Consensus on insulin dose and titration algorithms in ambulatory care of type 2 diabetes in India. J Assoc Physicians India. 2017;65(2):17-30.
18. Garg SK, Henry RR, Banks P, Buse JB, Davies MJ, Fulcher GR, et al. Effects of sotagliflozin added to insulin in patients with type 1 diabetes. N Engl J Med. 2017;377(24):2337-48.
19. Battelino T, Danne T, Bergenstal RM, Amiel SA, Beck R, Biester T, et al. Clinical targets for continuous glucose monitoring data interpretation: Recommendations From the International Consensus on Time in Range. Diabetes Care. 2019;42(8):1593-603.
20. Garg N, Muduli SK, Kapoor A, Tewari S, Kumar S, Khanna R, et al. Comparison of different cardiovascular risk score calculators for cardiovascular risk prediction and guideline recommended statin uses. Indian Heart J. 2017;69(4):458-63.

CHAPTER

122 Calcium and Phosphate Homeostasis

MK Garg, Madhukar Mittal

ABSTRACT

Calcium and phosphorus play important extracellular and intracellular physiological function in the human body. In adults, the normal reference ranges for serum total calcium are 2.2–2.6 mmol/L (8.7–10.2 mg/dL), for ionized whole blood calcium are 1.12–1.32 mmol/L (4.5–5.3 mg/dL), and for serum inorganic phosphorus are 0.81–1.4 mmol/L (2.5–4.3 mg/dL). It is important to maintain plasma calcium and phosphorus in normal physiological range which is regulated by mechanisms involving the gastrointestinal tract (GIT), kidneys, skin, parathyroid glands and bone through regulatory and sensing mechanisms.

Our endeavor is to help the reader to understand the various physiological pathways of calcium and phosphate homeostasis. Calcium homeostasis is maintained by active (transcellular and vitamin D dependent) and passive (paracellular and vitamin D independent) intestinal calcium absorption, which is kept static over wide range of calcium intake and serum 25(OH)D levels by local intestinal adaptation hypothetically called "intestinal calcistat". The renal excretion of calcium is about 2–4% of filtered load and rest is reabsorbed passively by proximal renal tubule and loop of Henle by paracellular pathway against electrochemical gradient and actively by distal convoluted tubule through channel called TRPV5.

The intestinal absorption of phosphorus happens via paracellular (passive and concentration dependent) or transcellular (active and sodium-phosphate type IIb cotransporters dependent) pathways. The renal phosphate reabsorption occurs in proximal renal tubular cells through renal sodium phosphate transporters (NaPi2a). A number of these transporters are dependent on various hormones, e.g., parathyroid hormone (PTH), fibroblast growth factor-23 (FGF-23), and calcitriol. Calcium-phosphorus homeostasis during pregnancy, and in the fetal and neonatal period is also briefly discussed.

"Provided one has the correct amount of vitamin, mineral and nutritional input, the body can overcome disease"

—Linus Pauling

HISTORICAL PERSPECTIVE

The Earth's crust is formed mainly by silicon, iron, calcium, magnesium, sulfates, and phosphates. All these minerals are utilized by nature to create body composition imparting various functions according to their properties. Calcium and phosphates are used to form body skeleton in addition to various functions. The Latin word "calx or calcis" which means "lime" denotes calcium oxide (CaO) which was the material obtained by heating limestone and has been used for centuries to make plaster and mortar. Though known from 1st century as lime, the element calcium was isolated by Sir Humphrey Davy in 1808 by electrolysis of its oxide. The biological significance of calcium was reported by Sydney Ringer in 1883 in an experiment where calcium was required in the bathing solution for frog heart to continue beating.

The word phosphorus is used in Greek mythology for planet Venus and is derived from the Greek words (φῶς = light, φέρω = carry) meaning "light-bearer." Elemental yellow phosphorus was isolated by the Hamburg merchant Hennig Brandt in 1669 by heating the residue of evaporated urine. Initially, production of phosphorus was done secretly till it was discovered that bone is made up of calcium phosphate and from then onward, phosphorus became more widely available.

INTRODUCTION

Besides the four organic basic elements (H, C, N, and O), the quantity elements (Na, Mg, K, Ca, P, S, and Cl) and essential trace elements (Mn, Fe, Co, Ni, Cu, Zn, Mo, Se, and I) play various important roles in the human body. Calcium is required for important cellular functions such as cell signaling, neuromuscular transmission, blood coagulation, as enzymatic cofactor, and for membrane and cytoskeletal functions. Phosphorus is ubiquitous and participates in cellular signaling, energy metabolism, nucleic acid synthesis, and membrane stabilization.

It is important to maintain plasma calcium and phosphorus in normal physiological range which is regulated by mechanisms involving GIT, kidneys, and bone. Critical organs (skeleton, parathyroids, skin, GIT, and kidneys) along with a number of hormones, including PTH, vitamin D, and calcitonin play a role in balancing the levels of the bone minerals—calcium and phosphorus through various regulatory and sensing mechanisms like calcium-sensing receptor (CaSR). Regulation of phosphate via FGF23, Klotho, and others has opened a new area of knowledge in phosphate pathways.

The goal of this chapter is to help the reader to understand the physiology of calcium and phosphate homeostasis especially in relation to bone mineral metabolism so that the clinician is able to better delineate the altered physiology seen in common clinical disorders that involve this homeostatic system.

BODY CALCIUM AND PHOSPHORUS

The total amount of *calcium in human body ranges from 1,000 to 1,200 g*. Approximately, 99% of body calcium stays in the skeleton as calcium hydroxyapatite [$Ca_{10}(PO_4)_6(OH)_2$]; rest 1% is present in the extracellular fluid (ECF) and intracellular fluid (ICF). Around 1% of skeletal calcium is freely exchangeable with calcium in the ECF compartment.

An *average adult human contains about 700 g of phosphorus*, about 85–90% in bones and teeth, and the remainder in soft tissues and ECFs. Phosphorus plays a major role in the structural framework of deoxyribonucleic acid (DNA) and ribonucleic acid (RNA). Phosphate as part of adenosine triphosphate (ATP) transports cellular energy necessary for every cellular process and helps in phosphorylation, which is a key regulatory event within cells. Phospholipids are the main structural components of all cellular membranes.

INTESTINAL REGULATION

CALCIUM

Recommended daily allowance (RDA) for calcium ranges from 600 to 1,300 mg according to age and gender. Although there is a great variability, the average daily diet contains about 1,000 mg of calcium and only about half of this undergoes net absorption. The *main sources of calcium* are dairy products such as milk, curd, and cheese. Other foods such as grains, legumes, fruits, and vegetables also contribute to calcium intake (**Table 1**, National Institute of Nutrition, Hyderabad, at fitjog.com).

Calcium homeostasis (**Figs. 1 A** and **B**) is maintained by the regulation of intestinal calcium absorption. Calcium is absorbed (75–90%) both actively and passively. It is actively absorbed in duodenum through transcellular process which is vitamin D dependent, whereas passive absorption occurs throughout intestine by paracellular process which is dependent on concentration of calcium in intestinal tract.

Transcellular transport occurs primarily in the duodenum where calcium enters intestinal cells through apical calcium channel—transient receptor potential cation channel, vanilloid family member 6 or TRPV6, expression of which is controlled by active vitamin D and calcium itself probably through CaSR. Further movement of calcium onward to the basolateral membrane is dependent on the calcium-binding protein, calbindin [also $1,25(OH)_2D_3$ dependent]. The actions of plasma membrane Ca-ATPase or Ca^{2+} pump (PMCA1b) and the Na^+/Ca^{2+} exchanger (NCX1) lead to efflux of calcium from the intestinal epithelium. The paracellular uptake is dependent on luminal—serosal electrochemical gradients and involves passive diffusion of calcium between mucosal cells (**Fig. 2**).

Total fraction of calcium absorbed from total intake can vary from 20 to 80%. Among this, 10–20% is contributed by passive diffusion (paracellular) and rest by active transport (transcellular). This suggests that calcium absorption can be kept static over wide range of calcium intake and serum 25(OH)D levels by local intestinal adaptation hypothetically called "intestinal calcistat (**Fig. 3**)." Calcium absorption is increased by increased calcium intake, vitamin D stores, intraluminal pH, protein, lactulose, and bile salts, whereas absorption is decreased by vitamin D deficiency, phosphorous, dietary fiber, excessive fat, and dietary constituents like phytates and oxalates.

Calcium-sensing receptors (blue) are located on intestinal cell brush border. Calcium (red with blue border) in intestinal lumen activates CaSRs, which modifies vitamin D system and calcium absorption.

- *Under condition of low calcium intake (arbitrarily ~250 mg)*: Assuming total body calcium requirement of ~200 mg, 80% of this calcium should be absorbed (maximal fractional calcium absorption has been

TABLE 1 Various sources of calcium (mg/100 g).

Dairy and poultry (mg/100 g)		Grains (mg/100 g)		Vegetables (mg/100 g)	
Milk powder	1,370	Ragi	344	Cauliflower	626
Cheese	790	Kidney beans	260	Yam leaves	460
Condensed milk	650	Soybean	240	Fenugreek	396
Milk buffalo	210	Sprouted beans	202	Coriander	190
Milk cow	120	Bengal gram	202	Carrot	80
Milk goat	170	Red gram	184	Spinach	73
Milk human	28	Green gram	124	Lady finger	66
Curd	150	Peas	76	Onion	60
Mutton	150	Lentil	69	French beans	60
Egg	60	Millet	42	Sweet potato	46

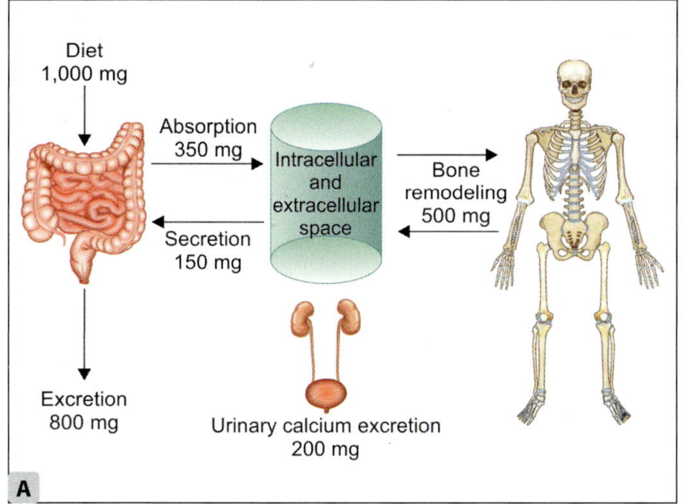

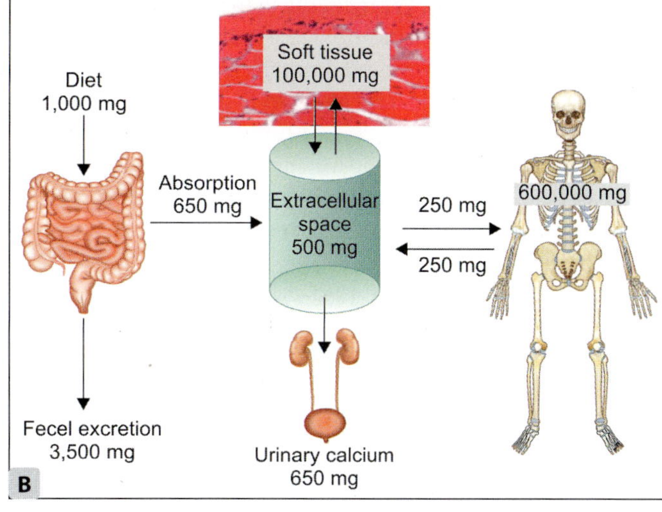

FIGURES 1 A & B: (A) Calcium and (B) phosphorus homeostasis.

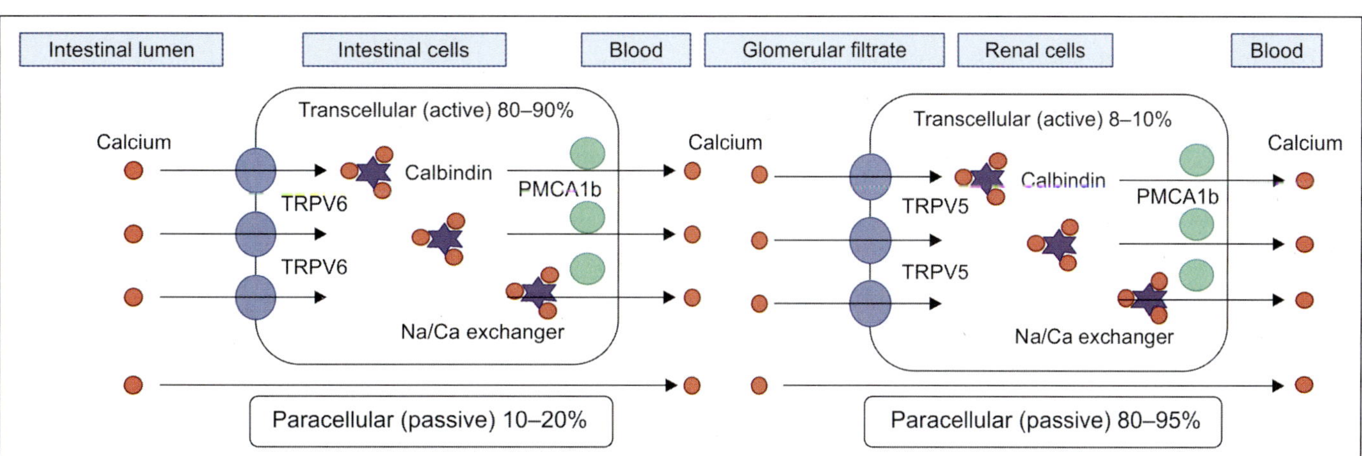

FIGURE 2: Mechanism of calcium absorption and excretion.

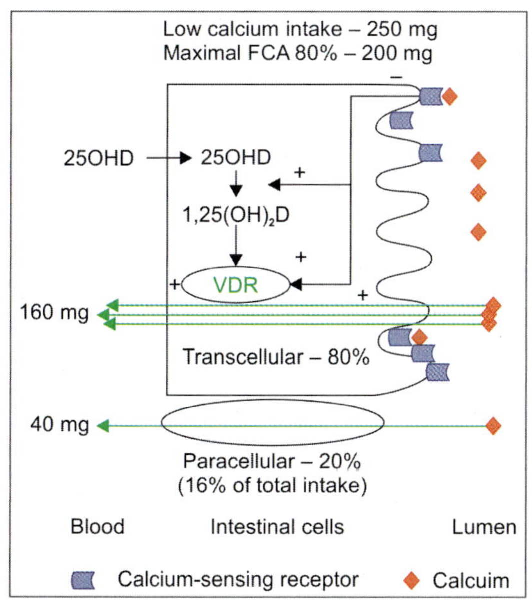

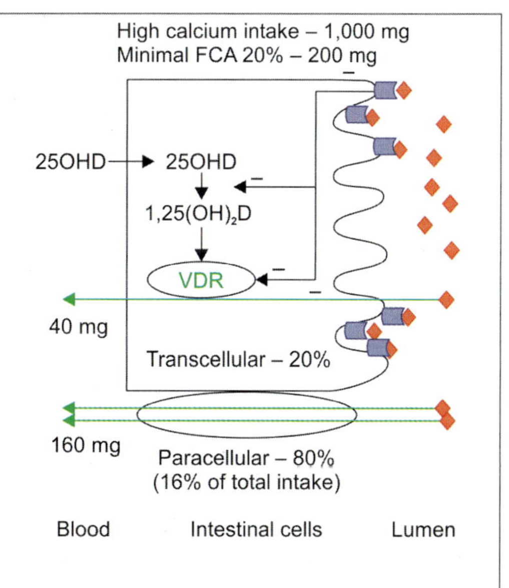

FIGURE 3: Interaction between calcium, calcium-sensing receptor (CaSR), and vitamin D system in intestine.

reported as ~80%). With decrease in occupancy of CaSR, the inhibition on vitamin D system will be removed. This will lead to enhanced active transport of calcium (80%, ~160 mg) which is vitamin D dependent, and rest by passive diffusion (20%, ~40 mg). Passive diffusion is vitamin D independent and it is calcium dependent. Passive diffusion contributes to about 10–20% of total calcium intake. Here, we have depicted it as 16% of total calcium intake.

- *Under the condition of high calcium intake (arbitrarily ~1,000 mg)*: Assuming total body calcium requirement of ~200 mg, and 16% of total calcium intake (160 mg) will be absorbed by passive diffusion. Hence, only 40 mg is required to be absorbed by active transport. This decrease in active transport will be mediated by dampening effect of activated CaSR on vitamin D system due to high occupancy of CaSRs by calcium (Reproduced with permission of authors).

Calcium flux between body compartments: Plasma calcium is present in three distinct fractions. About 10% of calcium is present complexed with anions such as citrate, bicarbonate, sulfate, lactate, and phosphate. About 40% calcium is bound to proteins, primarily albumin (nondiffusible) and around 50% circulates in free form as biologically active ionized calcium.

Conditions which result in decreased serum albumin levels will affect the total serum calcium levels. For every 1 g/dL decrease in serum albumin below normal (hypoalbuminemia), a correction factor of 0.2 mmol/L (0.8 mg/dL) needs to be added to get a true value of corrected total serum calcium. Ionized calcium concentrations, however, remain unaffected and may be preferable in such situations.

Alterations in systemic pH can lead to changes in the protein-bound fraction of calcium. A low pH can result in decreased protein binding leading to increase in ionized calcium. For every 0.1 decrease in serum pH, the ionized calcium may rise by 0.05 mmol/L (0.2 mg/dL). These approximations have been overtaken in clinical practice, with easy availability of reliable measurement methods for the biologically active ionized serum calcium fraction.

PHOSPHORUS

The current RDA for phosphorus for an adult is 700 mg/day. An adult with healthy diet consumes ~700–2,000 mg/day (average 1 g/day) of phosphorus, of which 60–80% is absorbed by intestine and the rest is directly excreted into the stool. *The main food sources* for phosphorus are the same as those containing protein such as cereals, milk, and meat. As a rule, if a diet has sufficient protein and calcium, the amount of phosphorus is probably sufficient.

Similar to absorption process of calcium, the intestinal absorption of phosphorus happens via paracellular (passive) or transcellular (active) pathways. The transcellular absorption occurs through the sodium-phosphate type IIb cotransporters (primarily NaPi-IIb), which is upregulated by 1,25$(OH)_2$D3 and the paracellular absorption is dependent on concentration gradient of phosphorus across the intestinal lumen and is nonsaturable.

RENAL REGULATION

The kidney plays an indispensable role in maintaining calcium and phosphorus homeostasis. Filtration, reabsorption, and excretion of these ions take place in the kidneys to maintain their serum concentrations and total body content.

CALCIUM

Losses of calcium occur through urine, faeces (predominantly unabsorbed calcium), perspiration, and cell sloughing (minor losses) and maternal losses (across the placenta to developing fetus in pregnancy and via breast milk for lactation in postpartum period). Endogenous fecal excretion related to bile acid and pancreatic enzymes is relatively constant and is about 100–200 mg/day. About 10,000 mg of calcium is filtered through glomerulus, whereas total excreted amount is equal to intestinal calcium absorption ~200–400 mg. Hence, total renal excretion is about 2–4% of filtered load and rest is reabsorbed.

Mechanism of renal reabsorption is just opposite to the intestinal absorption. About 80–95% is reabsorbed in proximal convoluted tubule (PCT) and loop of Henle through passive diffusion by paracellular pathway against electrochemical gradient. Only about 8–10% is reabsorbed by active transcellular through TRPV5, calbindin, and basolateral Ca-ATPase in distal convoluted tubule. This active pathway is controlled and affected by PTH, activated vitamin D, and calcium. Calcium transport in thick ascending limb of loop of Henle is also influenced by the CaSR, which is localized in the basolateral membrane. The calcium channel TRPV5 is the likely major isoform in distal convoluted tubule and the connecting tubule. This is also the rate limiting step, mirroring intestinal calcium absorption steps. The activity, movement, and endosomal recycling of the channel TRPV5 are regulated by a number of factors such as intracellular Ca^{2+} concentration, Klotho, tissue Kallikrein factor, pH, and estrogen. Klotho stimulates TRPV5 activity and thus increases calcium uptake by increasing the apical membrane concentration of the channels. Renal reabsorption of calcium is decreased by excessive sodium, phosphates, hypermagnesemia, acidosis and loop diuretics, and cyclosporin whereas it is increased by hypophosphatemia and thiazide diuretics (**Fig. 2**).

Normal calcium excretion and urinary calcium creatinine ratio (U_{Ca}/U_{Cr}) cutoff values to define hypercalciuria vary in different age groups and by region. Hypercalciuria has been defined as daily urinary excretion of >4 mg calcium/kg body weight if a child is over 2 years age. The most accepted method of evaluating normal calcium excretion is by collecting urine for 24 hours. Urinary calcium excretion of <200 mg calcium/L is considered normal. However, 24-hour urine collection in children and adolescents is cumbersome and inadequate compared to estimating by spot U_{Ca}/U_{Cr} ratio, which is easier and more practical. Hypercalciuria is defined as U_{Ca}/U_{Cr} ratio values above the 95th percentile, which is usually <0.21 in adults and is <0.13 in North Indian children and adolescents.

PHOSPHORUS

The concentration of phosphate in serum is controlled by renal reabsorption. This is usually quantified as tubular reabsorption of phosphorus and expressed as renal phosphate threshold [renal tubular reabsorption of phosphate to glomerular filtration rate ($TmPO_4$/GFR)]. Within the nephron, approximately 85% of phosphate reabsorption occurs within the PCT by an energy-dependent process that requires sodium.

The amount of phosphate reabsorbed from the filtrate is determined by abundance of cotransporters in the apical membrane of proximal tubule cells. There are three renal sodium phosphate cotransporters—(1) NaPi2a, (2) NapPi2c, and (3) PiT-2, positioned in the apical brush border membrane of PCT. Thus, hormones or dietary factors that alter phosphate reabsorption in the kidney do so by changing numbers of the sodium phosphate cotransporters in PCT. NaPi2a is responsible for majority (~70%) of renal regulation of phosphate transport.

Parathyroid hormone causes decreased renal reabsorption of phosphate (phosphaturia) by decreasing the abundance of NaPi2a, NaPi2c, and PiT-2 in PCT border membrane. In response to PTH, NaPi2a is removed rapidly (within minutes), whereas the decrease in apical membrane abundance of NaPi2c and PiT-2 takes hours.

Fibroblast growth factor-23 is produced by osteoblasts in response to increase in serum phosphates. To exert its physiologic effects on PCT, FGF23 requires the presence of a cofactor, Klotho, which is produced in kidney and activates FGF receptor-1. FGF23 reduces expression and activity of the sodium-phosphate cotransporters in renal proximal tubule and is also thought to decrease the activity of intestinal sodium-phosphate cotransporter. FGF23 also reduces serum levels of calcitriol by decreasing renal expression of 1α-hydroxylase, which is the rate-limiting step in calcitriol synthesis, and increasing the renal expression of 24-hydroxylase, which is required for calcitriol degradation (**Flowchart 1**). In addition, FGF23 suppresses PTH synthesis. Other phosphatonins namely secreted frizzled-related protein 4 (sFRP-4), matrix extracellular phosphoglycoprotein, sodium-hydrogen exchanger regulatory factor (NHERF1), and FGF7 have also been discovered and their actions are similar leading to a decrease in phosphorus uptake by renal proximal tubule cells.

The $TmPO_4$/GFR is usually estimated by a nomogram from measurements of serum and urinary phosphorus and creatinine.

$$TmPO_4 = TRP \times Sp \text{ (Normal} = 2.5\text{–}4.2 \text{ mg/dL)}$$

[TRP = 1-(Up × SCr/UCr × Sp) where Up = urinary phosphates, SCr = serum creatinine, UCr = urinary creatinine, and Sp = serum phosphates (normally >80%)]

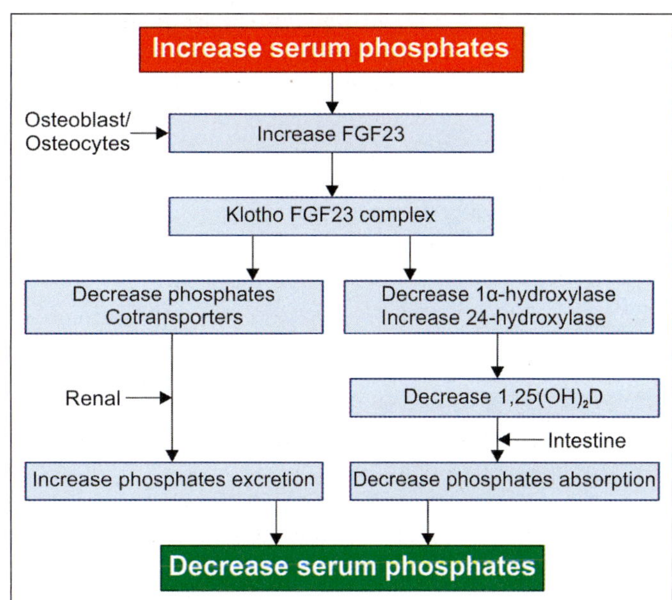

FLOWCHART 1: Fibroblast growth factor 23 (FGF23) and phosphate homeostasis.

HOMEOSTASIS MAINTENANCE

Normal levels of serum total calcium, ionized calcium and phosphates in Indian children and adolescents are 2.54–2.70 mmol/L in boys and 2.52–2.72 mmol/L in girls, 1.13–1.15 mmol/L in boys and 1.13–1.14 mmol/L in girls, 1.25–1.50 mmol/L in boys and 1.24–1.55 mmol/L in girls, respectively.

In adults, the normal reference ranges for serum total calcium are 2.2–2.6 mmol/L (8.7–10.2 mg/dL), for ionized whole blood calcium are 1.12–1.32 mmol/L (4.5–5.3 mg/dL), and for serum inorganic phosphorus are 0.81–1.4 mmol/L (2.5–4.3 mg/dL).

It is the coordinated action of hormonal regulators affecting intestinal absorption, renal tubular reabsorption, and bone resorption of these minerals which is the key to maintaining calcium and phosphorus homeostasis and thus preventing various endocrine diseases of the bone (**Table 2**). These organ systems are under the influence of various calcium regulatory hormones, including PTH, $1,25(OH)_2D3$, and calcitonin, which acting in harmony provide a further level of regulation.

Parathyroid hormone stimulates the renal 1α-hydroxylase which converts 25(OH)D to active $1,25(OH)_2D$ stimulating intestinal absorption of calcium through transcriptional regulation of TRPV6. Essential to process of calcium homeostasis is the G-protein-coupled Ca^{2+}-sensing receptors which are localized on the surface of parathyroid cells. The CaSR "senses" the ionized calcium levels based on which PTH release is regulated. With the lowering of serum calcium, the CaSR stimulates release of preformed and stored PTH which in turn leads to mobilization of calcium from the bone. PTH also directly increases renal tubular calcium reabsorption ($1,25(OH)_2D$-independent action) through TRPV5. All these actions have a cascading

TABLE 2 Calcium and phosphorus homeostasis.

Mineral	Calcium	Phosphorus
Total body content (g)	1,000–1,200	700
Skeletal distrubution (%)	99	85
Serum level (mg/dL)	2.2–2.6 mmol/L (8.7–10.2 mg/dL)	0.81–1.4 mmol/L (2.5–4.3 mg/dL)
Extraskeletal role	• Cell signaling • Neuromuscular transmission • Blood coagulation • Enzymatic cofactor • Membrane and cytoskeletal functions	• Cellular signaling • Energy metabolism (ATP) • Nucleic acid synthesis (DNA, RNA) • Regulation of intermediary metabolism (phosphorylation) • Membrane stabilzation (phospholipids)
Average daily intake (mg)	700–900	700–2,000
GI absorption (%)	30–35	40–80
Net absorption (%)	20	40–80
Major factors affectin serum levels	• Plasma proteins • Systemic pH • Major hormonal factors ◦ PTH ◦ 1,25(OH)D ◦ Calcitonin	• FGF23/Klotho • PTH • Kidney function • 125(OH)D (indirect)

(ATP: adenosine triphosphate; DNA: deoxyribonucleic acid; FGF23: fibroblast growth factor-23; RNA: ribonucleic acid; PTH: parathyroid hormone)

effect of restoring serum calcium back to the appropriate normal levels. The reverse processes happen in the case of increased ionized calcium levels which are again sensed by CaSR leading to inhibition of PTH secretion in such a scenario.

The CaSRs are also found in the thyroid parafollicular C cells and have been shown to regulate the release of calcitonin. Calcitonin acts by inhibiting osteoclastic activity and thereby inhibits Ca^{2+} release from bone into the circulation. The extent to which calcitonin plays a role in human calcium homeostasis is still not clear, although it is used pharmacologically to treat acute hypercalcemia of malignancy, painful metastasis in bone and Paget's disease. Calcitonin may also play a protective role in pregnancy and lactation by preventing excessive bone resorption.

From being not a true vitamin, vitamin D is becoming a true vitamin (mandatory nutritional supplementation being required) with increasing avoidance of sun exposure by the general population. After synthesis in skin following sun exposure (limited in elderly, the institutionalized, and those living in northern climates), the alternative source of vitamin D is dietary (egg yolk, fish oils etc.). Vitamin D exerts its action through formation of $1,25(OH)_2D$ (active form). Vitamin D plays a role in active calcium absorption through the transcellular pathway (definite, saturable). The extensively studied transcellular pathway involves stepwise entry of calcium into enterocyte (rate limiting), transport across the cell, and extrusion across basolateral membrane. It may also be involved in paracellular pathways by induction of formation of paracellular channels between neighboring cells via the expression of claudin-2 and claudin-12, contributing to intestinal calcium absorption. $1,25(OH)_2D$ has been shown to promote the intestinal phosphate absorption to some extent and to induce the expression of the phosphaturic FGF23.

Calcium and phosphorus in skeleton: The stores of the minerals calcium and phosphorous in the skeleton serve as a pool or bank from which they can be mobilized in times of need to maintain systemic mineral homeostasis. The osteoid matrix of bone is comprised of a mineral component (hydroxyapatite crystals) and an organic protein component (type 1 collagen). Although trabecular bone comprises only 20% of the skeleton, it has a larger surface area and is metabolically more active with remodeling rate of 20–30% per year. To maintain homeostasis, the minerals from bone may get depleted at cost of skeletal strength in certain pathological conditions.

HOMEOSTASIS IN PREGNANCY

Physiological changes in pregnancy also affect the Ca-P homeostasis. With an increase in vascular volume and a decrease in albumin levels, maternal total serum calcium levels decrease during pregnancy, with a nadir at 28–32 weeks. However, the albumin-adjusted total calcium and the ionized calcium concentrations actually are at low normal range. The urinary calcium excretion rate increases in parallel with an increase in GFR. The intestinal calcium absorption also undergoes a twofold increase.

Approximately 30 g of calcium is transferred from the mother to the fetus and most of this transfer occurs during the third trimester.

Parathyroid hormone-related protein (PTHrP) levels increase during pregnancy with the main sources being placenta and breasts. It is also expressed in uterus, amnion, umbilical cord, lactating breast, and fetal parathyroid glands. PTHrP is likely to be playing a role in calcium transport in these two places. PTH levels are within the normal range as for nonpregnant state.

There is a rise in the biologically active free fraction of 1,25$(OH)_2$D due to both increased synthesis by maternal renal 1α-hydroxylase activity and secretion by the placenta. This may be partly a reason for doubling of intestinal calcium absorption. There is a twofold increase in 1,25$(OH)_2$D concentrations in maternal circulation due to estrogen-induced rise in vitamin D–binding globulin although the 25-OHD levels remain unchanged.

FETAL AND NEONATAL HOMEOSTASIS

In utero, the fetus is in a high-calcium environment regulated by PTHrP and calcitonin. There is active transport via placenta of calcium from mother to the fetus. Concentrations of total calcium (2.75–3 mmol/L in third trimester), ionized calcium, and phosphate are higher in fetal circulation as compared to maternal circulation, emphasizing active transport of calcium across the placenta against a concentration gradient. This transferred calcium to the fetus is almost completely involved in mineralization of the fetal skeleton.

About 24 hours postdelivery, plasma calcium concentration falls, to a low of 9 mg/dL (2.3 mmol/L), and ionized calcium concentration to about 4.8 mg/dL (1.2 mmol/L) with removal of placenta.

The relatively low PTH concentrations (which are also minimally responsive to hypocalcemia) and high calcitonin concentrations lead to a period of 2–3 days of transient neonatal hypocalcemia. Calcitonin concentrations remain high for several days in the early neonatal period and are slightly lower in cord blood (~2000 ng/L). In fact, this rapid adjustment required in the neonatal period on moving from a high-calcium environment regulated by PTHrP and calcitonin to a low-calcium environment regulated by PTH and vitamin D, predisposes to transient hypocalcemia.

Stimulation of PTH secretion and inhibition of calcitonin secretion gradually increases the serum calcium concentrations in the neonate. The transitional mechanism from PTHrP to PTH secretion in neonatal parathyroid glands is still not clear.

CONCLUSION

The control of calcium and phosphorus homeostasis within normal range is crucial in the maintenance of normal physiological functions. Evolution of complex, integrated mechanisms helps to keep their serum concentrations within the narrow physiologic range. Disturbance in any of these regulatory mechanisms leads to significant alterations in calcium and phosphorus levels manifesting as pathological endocrine diseases. Transient alterations are seen in pregnancy and during transition from intrauterine to neonatal life.

RECOMMENDED READINGS

1. Taylor JG, Bushinsky DA. Calcium and phosphorus homeostasis. Blood Purif. 2009;27(4):387-94.
2. Blaine J, Chonchol M, Levi M. Renal control of calcium, phosphate, and magnesium homeostasis. Clin J Am Soc Nephrol. 2015;10(7):1257-72.
3. Bring FR, Leder BZ. Regulation of calcium and phosphate homeostasis. In: Degroot LJ, Jameson JL (Eds). Endocrinology, Volume 2, 5th edition. Philadelphia: Elsevier Saunders; 2006. pp. 1465-98.
4. Garg MK, Mahalle N. Calcium Supplementation: Why, Which, and How? Indian J Endocrinol Metab. 2019;23:387-90.
5. Garg MK, Mahalle N. Calcium absorption, clinical and subclinical vitamin D deficiency. Can a hypothesis of "Intestinal calcistat" hypothesis explain it all? Med Hypotheses. 2013;81:253-8.
6. Garg MK, Kalra S, Mahalle N. The Intestinal Calcistat: Determinant of clinical vitamin D deficiency. Indian J Endocr Metab. 2013;17:780-83.
7. Marwaha RK, Garg MK, Dang N, Mithal A, Narang A, Chadha A. et al. Reference range of random urinary calcium creatinine ratio in North Indian children and adolescents. Ann Pediatr Endocrinol Metab. 2019;24:34-40.
8. Marwaha RK, Khadgawat R, Tandon N, Kanwar R, Narang A, Sastry A, et al. Reference intervals of serum calcium, ionized calcium, phosphate and alkaline phosphatase in healthy Indian school children and adolescents. Clin Biochem. 2010;43(15):1216-9.
9. Jameson JL. Harrison's Principles of Internal Medicine. United States: McGraw-Hill Education; 2018.

CHAPTER
123

Parathyroid Disorders

Sanjay K Bhadada, Ravinder Goswami, Rimesh Pal

ABSTRACT

Parathyroid gland is the last organ identified in the human body. Parathyroid gland secretes a hormone called parathyroid hormone (PTH). Excess production of PTH leads to a condition called hyperparathyroidism while decreased or absent secretion of PTH is called hypoparathyroidism.

Excessive secretion of PTH in presence of hypercalcemia is defined as primary hyperparathyroidism (PHPT). PHPT is the second most common endocrine disorder. PHPT is an asymptomatic disease in the Western population while in India, PHPT is often symptomatic. Common symptoms of PHPT are related to bone and renal manifestations. The treatment of choice of PHPT is surgical resection of the abnormal parathyroid gland. Patients of PHPT require lifelong follow-up even after curative parathyroidectomy.

The deficiency or ineffectiveness of PTH is called hypoparathyroidism and pseudohypoparathyroidism, respectively. Common symptoms of hypoparathyroidism are tingling, numbness, carpal, and pedal spasm. Severe hypocalcemia due to hypoparathyroidism can present as laryngeal spasm and seizures. The treatment of choice for hypoparathyroidism is calcium supplementation with active vitamin D. Patients suffering from hypoparathyroidism also require lifelong follow-up and treatment. Knowledge about parathyroid disorders among physicians and general population is limited. Hypoparathyroidism and PHPT both have good prognosis, but need lifelong follow-up and treatment.

"These chemical messengers or 'hormones' as we might call them..."

—Ernest Starling

PARATHYROID DISORDERS

Parathyroid glands are the last organ discovered in the human body. Parathyroid glands are located parallel to the thyroid gland, hence named parathyroid glands. Parathyroid glands are four to five in number (two superior and two inferior) and weight of a single parathyroid gland is 40–50 mg. Parathyroid glands arise from the third and fourth branchial pouches. Parathyroid glands are composed of two types of cells: (1) chief (clear cytoplasm) and (2) oxyphil (eosinophilic granular cytoplasm) cells. Both types of cells from the parathyroid gland secrete PTH. PTH is a heat-labile peptide consists of 1–84 amino acids. PTH has circulating half-life of 3–4 minutes and liver and kidney metabolize it.

Normal range of PTH is 10–65 pg/mL. PTH has ultradian secretion, peaks in early morning, nadir in late afternoon, and small peak occurs in late afternoon. However, PTH secretion is closely linked to serum calcium, phosphate, and active vitamin D levels. The main function of PTH is to maintain serum calcium through three peripheral organs namely: (1) bone, (2) kidney, and (3) intestine.

Abnormally excess secretion of parathyroid gland is termed as hyperparathyroidism. However, deficiency or infectiveness of PTH is termed as hypoparathyroidism. Hyperparathyroidism is classified as primary, secondary, and tertiary hyperparathyroidism. Details of various types of hyperparathyroidism are described in **Table 1**. PHPT is more frequently seen in women (2–3:1). PHPT is considered a disease of postmenopausal women but in India, the mean age of presentation is 40 years. However, all age groups are affected with PHPT.

PRIMARY HYPERPARATHYROIDISM

Primary hyperparathyroidism is most frequently caused by a parathyroid adenoma (85–90%) followed by parathyroid hyperplasia (5–10%) and carcinoma (1%). Candidate genes implicated in the pathogenesis of sporadic PHPT are calcium-sensing receptor (CaSR), vitamin D receptor, and cyclin D1.

In sporadic parathyroid adenoma, CaSR is underexpressed. Due to the underexpression of the CaSR, calcium is not sensed by the parathyroid gland; to maintain serum calcium, parathyroid gland continues to secrete PTH and results in hypercalcemia with high PTH. Cyclin D1 is an oncogene and it is overexpressed in parathyroid adenoma. In sporadic PHPT, role of epigenetics is also documented. Various types of genetic mutations cause familial PHPT.

CLINICAL PRESENTATION

Primary hyperparathyroidism is clinically characterized by the pentad of PHPT namely bones, stones, abdominal pains, psychic moans, and fatigue overtones. Less common presentations of PHPT are pancreatitis, cholelithiasis,

TABLE 1 Etiological classification of hyperparathyroidism.

Primary hyperparathyroidism (high PTH and high calcium)	Secondary hyperparathyroidism (high PTH and low calcium)	Tertiary hyperparathyroidism (high PTH and high calcium)
• Parathyroid adenoma • Parathyroid hyperplasia • Parathyroid carcinoma • Chronic lithium therapy • MEN1 • MEN2A	• Vitamin D deficiency • Renal failure	• Renal failure

TABLE 2 Symptoms and signs of primary hyperparathyroidism (PHPT).

Symptoms related to hypercalcemia	Symptoms related to parathyroid hormone excess
• Anorexia and nausea • Constipation • Polyuria and polydipsia • Bone pain and fractures • Renal stone disease • Pancreatitis • Neuropsychiatric symptoms	• Muscle weakness • Anemia • Hypertension • Impaired glucose tolerance • Neuropsychiatric symptoms • Pruritus

rickets—osteomalacia, hypertension, arthralgia, arthritis, epulis, and deformities. These symptoms are caused by hypercalcemia and elevated PTH that are detailed in **Table 2**. In India, PHPT is mainly symptomatic; however, in the Western world, PHPT is predominantly asymptomatic and detected during routine biochemical screening. In India, asymptomatic PHPT is also on the rise.

Skeletal manifestations: Skelton is one of the most common sites involved in PHPT. Cortical bone (long bones) is more frequently and severely involved as compared to cancellous bone (vertebrae). The overt skeletal disease of PHPT is evident on conventional X-rays. The spectrum of bone symptoms varies from bone pains to osteitis fibrosa cystica (OFC) and pathological fractures (**Figs. 1 A** to **G**). The most sensitive and specific finding of bone involvement in PHPT is subperiosteal resorption of cortical bone. Physical examination is generally unremarkable, except for palpable brown tumor and skeletal deformities. Long bone fractures are commonly seen due to thinning of the cortex; however, vertebrae are affected in severe PHPT in the form of osteoporosis, codfish vertebrae, and occasionally vertebral fracture. Various radiological manifestations are depicted in **Figures 1 A** to **G**.

Bone mineral density is frequently and more severely reduced in symptomatic PHPT. Following parathyroidectomy, bone mineral density shows a rapid, remarkable, and striking recovery, often with >100% gains above baseline values over a period of months to years. In contrast to this, the average increase in bone mineral density in asymptomatic PHPT following parathyroidectomy is in the order of 15%. In spite of the spectacular rise in bone mineral density, the recovery of cortical bone density may be incomplete as compared to cancellous bone. Common dental changes of HPT are loose teeth, loss of teeth, and epulis.

Renal manifestations: Kidneys are one of the most common target organs involved in PHPT. In India, the incidence of the renal disease varies from 30 to 60% in different series. Hypercalciuria is seen in 30–40% of PHPT patients. Hypercalciuria is responsible for stone disease in the urinary tract. Hypercalciuria is proportional to the severity of hypercalcemia. Elevation in serum calcium is mainly caused by PTH-mediated bone resorption. Enhanced production of 1,25-dihydroxyvitamin D [$1,25(OH)_2D$] in PHPT also contributes to absorptive hypercalcemia and, in turn, results in hypercalciuria.

Another renal manifestation of PHPT is the diffuse deposition of calcium phosphate complexes in renal parenchyma known as nephrocalcinosis. The frequency of nephrocalcinosis in PHPT varies from 15 to 20%. Delayed diagnosis can cause recurrent renal colics, hydroureteronephrosis, and deranged renal functions in patients of symptomatic PHPT. The risk of renal stone disease in patients of PHPT remains high even after curative parathyroidectomy, compared to the general population.

Even in the absence of any other cause, PHPT may be associated with a reduction in creatinine clearance. Chronic hypercalcemia can also compromise the renal concentrating ability, resulting in polydipsia and polyuria. Various lithiases associated with PHPT are depicted in **Figures 2 A** to **F**.

Gastrointestinal manifestations: Gastrointestinal manifestations of PHPT are nausea, constipation, dyspepsia (peptic ulcer disease), pancreatitis and pancreatic pseudocyst, and gallstone disease. Nausea and constipation are related to hypercalcemia.

A high prevalence of gallstone disease is documented in symptomatic PHPT patients compared to the general population and asymptomatic PHPT patients. Animal studies showed increased biliary ionized calcium concentration with hypercalcemia and hence, favoring lithiatic milieu and one study has found that PTH is a smooth muscle relaxant, resulting in the lazy gallbladder. Both these factors can result in cholelithiasis in PHPT.

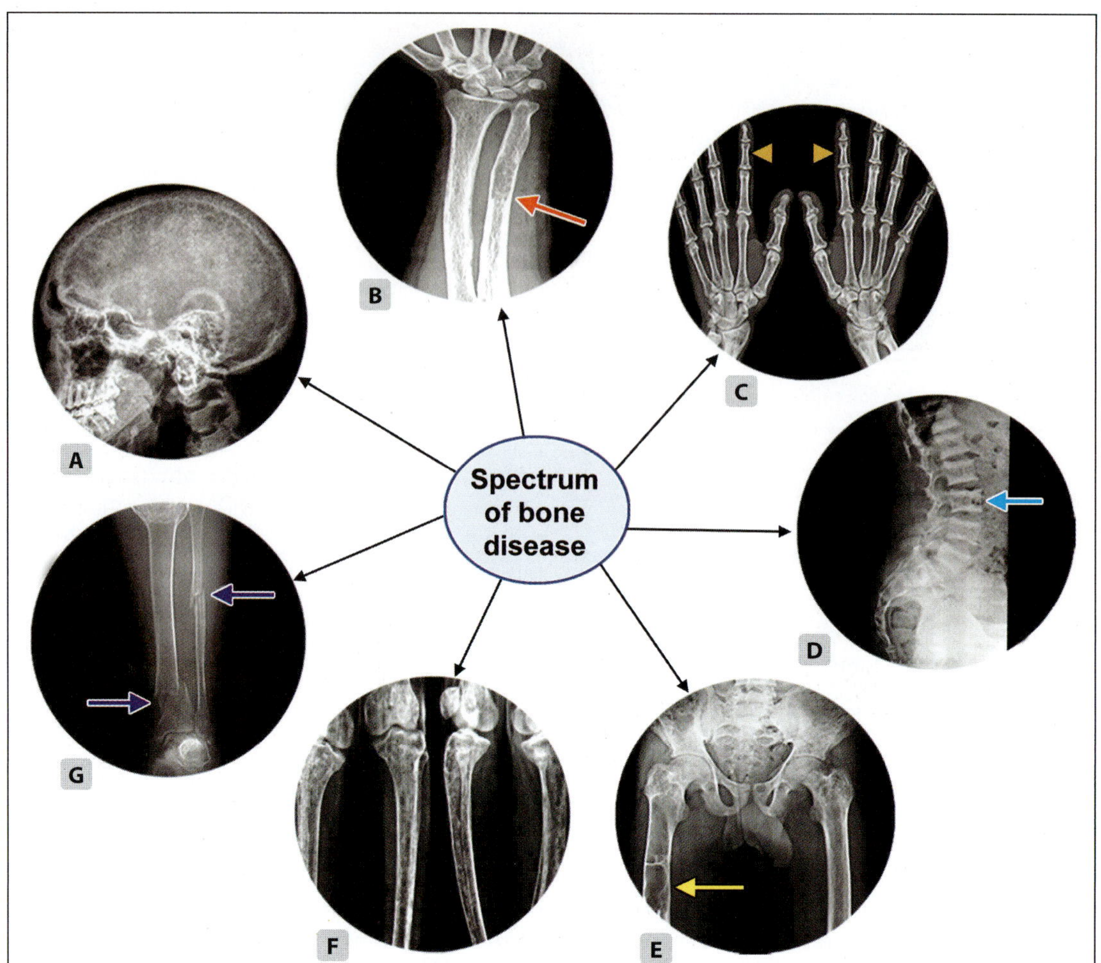

FIGURES 1 A to G: **(A)** Plain radiographs of patients with primary hyperparathyroidism showing salt-and-pepper appearance of skull; **(B)** Lytic lesion in the left ulna (marked in red arrow) suggestive of osteitis fibrosa cystica; **(C)** Subperiosteal bone resorption of the middle phalanges (marked in orange arrowheads); **(D)** Rugger-Jersey spine with anterior compression of the third lumbar vertebrae (marked in cyan arrow); **(E)** Lytic lesion involving the proximal shaft of right femur (marked in yellow arrow); **(F)** Multiple lytic lesions and diffuse osteopenia involving both the tibia; and **(G)** Fragility fractures involving the left tibia and fibula (marked in blue arrows).

Although an association between pancreatitis and hyperparathyroidism exists, the basis for it is not well known. In the West, pancreatitis is not considered as a complication of PHPT because hypercalcemia is very mild and of short duration. In developing countries, pancreatitis is reported in 10–20% of patients. In the author's series ($n = 225$), the prevalence of pancreatitis in PHPT is around 30%. Pancreatitis is often recurrent and associated with pancreatic calcification usually in the parenchyma and less commonly in the ducts. The presence of other features of PHPT (skeletal and renal) also helps to differentiate PHPT-related pancreatitis from other causes of pancreatitis.

Hematological manifestations: Hematological manifestations are common in symptomatic PHPT. Anemia is the most common (30–40%) hematological manifestation. This high prevalence of anemia in symptomatic PHPT is multifactorial and includes PTH-induced marrow fibrosis mediated by the effect of increased cytokines [interleukin (IL) and tumor necrosis factor-α (TNF-α)] and decreased erythropoietin levels. Anemia and marrow fibrosis both improve after curative parathyroidectomy. Less commonly, thrombocytopenia is seen possibly due to marrow fibrosis as well.

Miscellaneous manifestations: Primary hyperparathyroidism is a systemic disease; can affect any organ system of body and can have varied presentations such as arthralgia, arthritis, pseudogout, band keratopathy, skin necrosis, and left ventricular hypertrophy.

BIOCHEMICAL CHANGES

Primary hyperparathyroidism is biochemically characterized by persistently elevated PTH in the presence of hypercalcemia and hypophosphatemia. PHPT is the most common cause of hypercalcemia in the outpatient setting and differential diagnosis of hypercalcemia is depicted in **Table 3**.

TREATMENT

Treatment of choice for PHPT is surgical resection of abnormal parathyroid gland. While waiting for surgery,

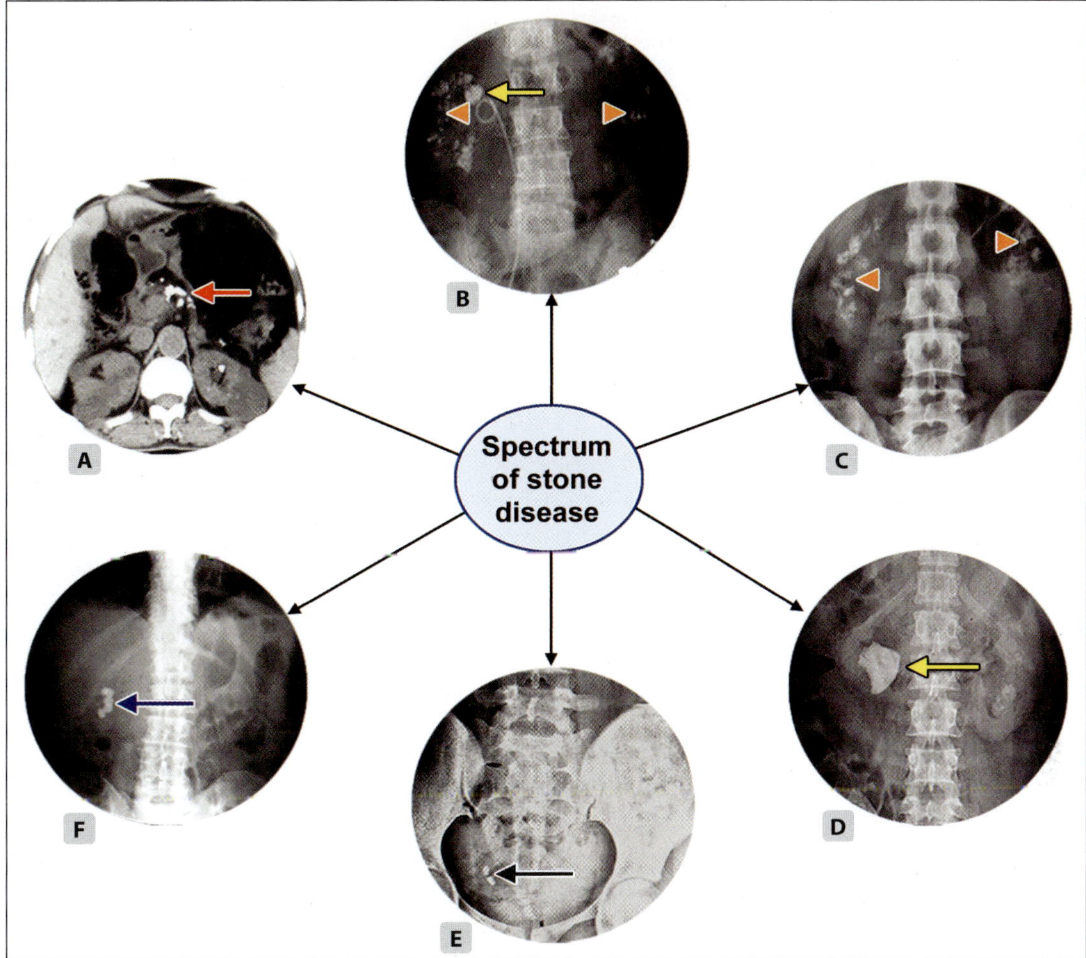

FIGURES 2 A to F: **(A)** Noncontrast computed tomography of the abdomen of a patient with primary hyperparathyroidism showing pancreatic calcifications (marked in red arrow); **(B and C)** Plain radiographs of patients with primary hyperparathyroidism showing bilateral nephrocalcinosis (marked in orange arrowheads) and right-sided nephrolithiasis (marked in yellow arrow); **(D)** Right-sided staghorn calculus (marked in yellow arrow); **(E)** Bladder calculus (marked in black arrow); and **(F)** Gallstones (marked in blue arrow).

moderate (serum calcium > 12–14 mg/dL) to severe hypercalcemia (>14 mg/dL) requires treatment.

Management of hypercalcemia (hypercalcemic crisis):

- *Hydration with increased salt intake and forced diuresis*: Many hypercalcemic patients are dehydrated because of vomiting and/or hypercalcemia-induced polyuria. The first principle of treatment is to restore normal hydration. Calcium levels start decreasing within hours.

  Under life-threatening circumstances, up to 4–6 L of isotonic saline plus furosemide in doses up to 100 mg every 1–2 hours may be required. Careful monitoring of central venous pressure and serum electrolytes is recommended.
- *Antiresorptive therapies such as intravenous bisphosphonates and subcutaneous denosumab*: Intravenous infusion of zoledronate (4–5 mg) over half an hour reduces serum calcium levels over 24–48 hours. Flu-like reactions are common with zoledronate infusion. Rarely, these drugs can precipitate renal dysfunction—proper hydration is essential. One also needs to be alert to the development of hypocalcemia, which can occur several days after the infusion. Zoledronate should be avoided in patients with glomerular filtration rate (GFR) below 45 mL/min/1.73 m^2 and contraindicated in GFR below 30 mL/min/1.73 m^2. Hypercalcemia with GFR below 30 mL/min/1.73 m^2 can be treated with denosumab (60–120 mg, single dose), calcitonin (200 IU twice a day for few days), or hemodialysis.

Preoperative localization of hyperfunctioning parathyroid tissue: The aim for locating abnormal parathyroid gland before surgery is that the glands can be abnormal in location and more than one gland may be active. Ultrasonography is often used as the first modality to localize abnormal parathyroid gland(s). Ultrasonography is a widely available and cost-effective technique. Additionally, it has reasonably good sensitivity and specificity (60–80%). 99mTc-sestamibi scintigraphy is often complementary to ultrasonography. It has better sensitivity and specificity compared to ultrasonography (80–90%). However, it is not widely available. Various other modalities are also used when ultrasonography and sestamibi scan failed to localize or show discordant results. In that case, choline

TABLE 3 Differential diagnosis for hypercalcemia.

Etiology	Serum PTH	Serum calcium	Serum PO_4	Urinary calcium	Remarks	Treatment
PHPT	↑↑	↑	↓	↑	RSD/GSD pathological fracture	Parathyroid surgery/ Calcimimetics
FHH	↑	(Mild)↑	N	↓	Elevated Mg	Calcimimetics
Granulomatous disorder	↓	↑↑	↑	↑	1,25(OH)$_2$ Vitamin D elevated	Glucocorticoids equivalent to 100 mg of hydrocortisone/day
Lithium	↑	↑	—	—	History of lithium intake	Stop lithium
Thiazide	↓	↑	—	↓	History of thiazide	Stop thiazide
Vitamin D intoxication	↓	↑	↑	↑	Elevated vitamin D levels (>150 ng/mL)	Glucocorticoids equivalent to 100 mg of hydrocortisone/day
Malignancy	↓	↑↑	N/↓	↑	Short history and elevated PTH-related peptide	Glucocorticoids equivalent to 100 mg of hydrocortisone/ day. Intravenous bisphosphonates/ subcutaneous denosumab

(FHH: familial hypocalciuric hypercalcemia; PTH: parathyroid hormone; PHPT: primary hyperparathyroidism)

and methionine positron emission tomography (PET)-CT (nearly 100% sensitivity and specificity), four-dimensional (4D)-CT, and MRI can be used for localization in selected patients.

Management of symptomatic primary hyperparathyroidism: All symptomatic PHPT patients need resection of abnormal parathyroid gland(s). In case of nonlocalization of parathyroid gland(s), patients not willing to undergo surgery or not fit for surgery can be managed medically. Medical management consists of bisphosphonates and calcimimetic agent such as cinacalcet (30–180 mg in divided doses).

Management of asymptomatic primary hyperparathyroidism: The National Institutes of Health (NIH) defines asymptomatic hyperparathyroidism as documented (presumptive) hyperparathyroidism without signs or symptoms attributable to the disease.

The need and indications for parathyroid surgery in asymptomatic PHPT are debatable because surgery does cause improvement in bone mineral density, left ventricular function, and decreases the risk of fracture and cardiovascular mortality. However, there is a lack of disease progression in most asymptomatic patients. The NIH sponsored a consensus development conference in 1990 and updated in 2002.

Asymptomatic patients should be monitored regularly as given below and parathyroidectomy can always be done when indicated.

- Serum calcium biannually
- Serum creatinine annually
- Bone density annually (lumbar spine, hip, and forearm)

PROGNOSIS

Asymptomatic PHPT is hardly associated with increased mortality, but symptomatic PHPT is associated with increased mortality and morbidity. Common causes of mortality in symptomatic PHPT are renal failure, respiratory exhaustion secondary to flail chest, pancreatitis, and sepsis (multiple fractures and bedsores). Persistent abnormalities after curative parathyroidectomy are bony deformities, low bone mineral density, renal dysfunction, and at times, diabetes secondary to pancreatitis.

HYPOPARATHYROIDISM

Hypoparathyroidism is a heterogeneous group of disorders characterized by inappropriate low or ineffective PTH secretion, leading to low serum calcium and increased inorganic phosphorus concentration. **Box 1** shows the common causes of hypoparathyroidism. Most common cause is postsurgical. This is followed by patients in whom it is difficult to assign any etiology based on syndromic etiologies. Disorders related to ineffective PTH action are labeled as PTH resistance syndrome or pseudohypoparathyroidism.

PREVALENCE OF THE DISEASE

Hypoparathyroidism is characterized as a rare disorder. There is limited information on the prevalence of the disorder. However, recent estimate indicates that overall prevalence of hypoparathyroidism is 22–37 cases per 100,000 persons. Idiopathic hypoparathyroidism (IH) is even rarer. Only 47 cases of IH were reported in the national registry of Denmark during 1977–2012. In a typical tertiary

BOX 1	Causes of hypoparathyroidism.
• Postsurgical	
• Idiopathic	
• **Autoimmune:** APECED and CaSR autoantibodies	
• **Genetic:** Nonsyndromic due to mutation of *PTH, CaSR, SOX3,* and *GNA11*	
• **Syndromic:** DiGeorge syndrome, Kenny–Caffey syndrome, Sanjad–Sakati syndrome, and GATA3	
• Irradiation, drugs, and infiltrative disorders	
• Severe hypomagnesemia	

(APECED: autoimmune polyendocrinopathy-candidiasis-ectodermal dystrophy; CaSR: calcium-sensing receptor; PTH: parathyroid hormone)

care center in India, on an average, 10–12 cases of IH are seen every year.

ETIOPATHOGENESIS

Causes of hypoparathyroidism are enumerated in **Box 1**.

Postsurgical hypoparathyroidism: Thyroid and parathyroid surgery or radical neck dissection can lead to postsurgical hypoparathyroidism which can be transient in 10–15% or permanent which persists for >6 months in up to 1–4%. Transient hypoparathyroidism after surgery for hyperparathyroidism occurs due to the suppression of normal parathyroid glands. Hypocalcemia due to hypoparathyroidism (low serum PTH) after surgery needs to be differentiated from hungry bone syndrome by its high serum PTH value. The risk factors for postsurgical hypoparathyroidism are total thyroidectomy, female gender, Graves' disease, recurrent goiter, and bilateral central ligation of the inferior thyroid artery. The degree of hypoparathyroidism may be more profound after treatment of laryngeal cancer with surgery combined with radiotherapy than with surgery alone. A chronic state of "decreased parathyroid reserve" may exist in some patients who manifest hypocalcemia only when mineral homeostasis is stressed further by other factors such as pregnancy, lactation, or illness.

Sporadic idiopathic hypoparathyroidism: This is the most common type of hypoparathyroidism encountered in our endocrine clinics. It is also called as nonfamilial, sporadic idiopathic hypoparathyroidism, or isolated. It is possibly a combination of various etiologies including autoimmune as indicated by CaSR antibodies in 10–12% and genetic with mutation in parathyroid transcription factor such as GCMB in another 10%. The disease has class I human leukocyte antigen (HLA) predisposition, indicating role of CD8-mediated damage to the parathyroid gland. Prevalence of coexistent disorders such as type 1 diabetes mellitus, autoimmune thyroiditis, and celiac disease is rare in them.

In the West, hypoparathyroidism commonly occurs as part of autoimmune polyendocrinopathy-candidiasis-ectodermal dystrophy (APECED) syndrome in association with autoimmune adrenal insufficiency and mutation in autoimmune regulator (*AIRE*) gene is expressed in thymus, lymph node, and fetal liver. APECED syndrome seems to be rare in India.

Genetic—hypoparathyroidism:

Nonsyndromic: Hypoparathyroidism has also been reported in families with autosomal dominant, autosomal recessive, and X-linked recessive inheritances. Mutations in the signal peptide region of the preproparathyroid hormone gene as well as in various domains of the CaSR have been reported in the familial form of hypoparathyroidism. Nonfamilial/*de novo PTH* gene mutation was observed in only one of the 160 patients with IH in India. Several mutations in the *CaSR* gene leading to its constitutive activation and decrease *PTH* gene synthesis and secretion and hypocalcemia have been recognized. Similar activation mutation of the CaSR would lead to a situation where renal tubules sense normal calcium excretion as excessive and normal reabsorption of calcium in the renal tubules is decreased. Thus, patients with mutation in the CaSR would, thus, demonstrate hypercalciuria and are prone to renal stones. Other nonsyndromic causes of hypoparathyroidism include *GCMB* mutation, *SOX3*, and *GNA11* mutation.

Syndromic: DiGeorge syndrome occurs because of abnormal development of 3rd and 4th branchial pouches, which give rise to the parathyroid glands. This syndrome has an eponym CATCH 22: *C*ardiac defects, *A*bnormal facies, *T*hymic hypoplasia/aplasia, *C*left palate, *H*ypocalcemia, and *22*q microdeletion. There are associated T-cell abnormalities leading to predisposition for infections and early mortality. Other syndrome associated with hypoparathyroidism includes mitochondrial dysfunction: Kearns–Sayre syndrome (KSS), characterized by progressive external ophthalmoplegia, pigmentary retinopathy before the age of 20 years, heart block, and cardiomyopathy. The MELAS syndrome comprising *M*itochondrial myopathy, *E*ncepalopathy, *L*actic *A*cidosis, and *S*troke-like episodes. Both KSS and MELAS syndrome are associated with hypoparathyroidism, insulin-dependent diabetes mellitus, and varying degrees of proximal muscle weakness.

Hypoparathyroidism occurs in 50% cases of patients with Kenny–Caffey syndrome characterized by short stature, otosclerosis and cortical thickening of long bones, delayed closure of anterior fontanel, and ophthalmic abnormalities. Recently, Kenny–Caffey syndrome and a related Sanjad–Sakati syndrome have been found to be associated with mutation of tubulin-specific chaperone E (TBCE). The TBCE encodes a chaperone protein required for folding of alpha-tubulin subunits and formation of alpha-beta-tubulin heterodimers. Usually, these syndromes are seen in countries in the Middle East.

Irradiation, drugs, and infiltrative disorders of parathyroid: External radiation or internal radiation, i.e., ^{131}I for Graves' disease, is a rare cause of hypocalcemia. Up to 58% incidence of diminished parathyroid reserve have been reported after high doses of ^{131}I in previous thyroid operation, external radiation, or Hashimoto's disease. Parathyroid glands are typically resistant to damage by toxic agents. Parathyroid tissue is resistant to most chemotherapeutic or cytotoxic agents except asparaginase that causes parathyroid necrosis and amifostine which causes reversible inhibition of PTH secretion. Pantoprazole has also been linked to transient hypoparathyroidism in occasionally, possibly related to associated hypomagnesemia. Most common toxic agent affecting parathyroid gland is alcohol, which is contributed further by associated hypomagnesemia.

Idiopathic hemochromatosis and chronic iron transfusion therapy are often associated with significant deposition of iron in the parathyroid glands. Decreased parathyroid reserve may occur as a consequence of iron infiltration in thalassemia. Wilson disease, metastatic neoplasia, miliary tuberculosis, amyloidosis, and sarcoidosis are other disorders associated with hypoparathyroidism.

Transient neonatal and hypomagnesemia-related adult transient hypoparathyroidism: Neonatal hypocalcemia, a self-limited disorder in premature and low birth weight infants, is related to deficient PTH secretion from immature parathyroid glands. Infants born to mothers with hyperparathyroidism or other causes of hypercalcemia also demonstrate transient suppression of the parathyroid gland. Infants born to diabetic mother are more predisposed. Severe deficiency of serum magnesium leads to reversible decrease in PTH secretion as well as resistance.

Pseudohypoparathyroidism: The condition is characterized by PTH resistance leading to poor cyclic adenosine monophosphate (cAMP) response and phosphaturic response to PTH (type 1a–1) or only poor phosphaturia response with normal cAMP (type 2). The type 1a and type 1c have clinical features of Albright's hereditary osteodystrophy (AHO) syndrome as short stature, obesity, dental enamel abnormality, short fourth and fifth metacarpals and rounded face, and obesity. They may have subcutaneous calcification. The abnormality in type 1 disorder is mutation of either $G\alpha_s$ or its imprinting. Multiple hormone resistance including TSH and gonadotropin is a feature of type 1a and c but not of type 1b.

CLINICAL SYMPTOMS AND SIGNS

Clinical manifestations of hypoparathyroidism are because of hypocalcemia. Clinical features depend upon rapidity and magnitude of fall of serum calcium. If there is acute fall of serum calcium concentration, symptoms are prominent, whereas chronic hypocalcemia has only few symptoms. Symptoms are mainly because of heightened neuromuscular irritability. However, there is no threshold value at which symptoms occur in acute hypocalcemia.

Acute hypocalcemia: A low extracellular ionized calcium symptom is often exacerbated by hypokalemia and hypomagnesemia and is related to enhanced neuromuscular excitability, circumoral numbness, and paresthesia of distal extremities. Severe hypocalcemia is associated with muscle cramps, carpopedal spasms, laryngospasms, and seizures. Clinical signs of neuromuscular excitability associated with latent tetany include Chvostek's sign and Trousseau's sign. Hypocalcemia is also associated with nonspecific electrocardiographic (ECG) changes, raised intracranial pressure, and papilloedema. Prolongation of corrected QT interval on ECG indicates severe hypocalcemia.

Chronic hypocalcemia: Symptoms of chronic hypocalcemia include dry skin, coarse hair, brittle nails, dental enamel hypoplasia, and loss of adult teeth. Intracranial calcification, most commonly in basal ganglia, can occur in all forms of hypoparathyroidism. Occasionally, basal ganglia calcification is associated with clinical features of extrapyramidal syndrome such as Parkinsonism, chorea, and increased prevalence of dyskinetic reaction to phenothiazine. Subcapsular cataracts are common in hypoparathyroidism and best seen with slit-lamp examination. Capsular calcification recurs even after cataract surgery and may need laser treatment. Patients with long-standing hypoparathyroidism have increased bone density and its effect on bone strength including fragility is under investigation.

INVESTIGATIONS AND DIAGNOSIS

The biochemical hallmarks are hypocalcemia, hyperphosphatemia, and inappropriately low PTH. Serum calcium levels may be as low as 5.0 mg/dL, whereas serum phosphorus levels may be >10 mg/dL especially in a growing child. Usually, serum alkaline phosphatase is normal. However, with coexistent vitamin D deficiency, serum alkaline phosphatase may be high. Serum $1,25(OH)_2D$ is usually low. The 24 hours urinary calcium excretion is typically decreased in hypoparathyroidism, but increased in those with activating mutation in the CaSRs. Nephrogenous cAMP excretion is low and fractional excretion of phosphorus is increased.

TREATMENT

Acute management: Slow intravenous injection of 10% calcium gluconate (10–30 mL) is given over a 10-minute period followed by continuous infusion of calcium using a solution of 5% dextrose with 100 mL of 10% calcium gluconate (930 mL of elemental calcium) given over 4–5 hours. Once the patient is stabilized, a plan is made to supplement oral treatment.

Chronic management: Vitamin D metabolite and calcium are mainstay of treatment. Because of variability in the intestinal calcium absorption, it is necessary to supplement 1–2 g of elemental calcium daily. Calcium is administrated in the divided doses with meals to minimize epigastric bloating and irritation. Vitamin D therapy is concomitantly used along with calcium. Vitamin D preparations such as ergocalciferol (vitamin D2) and cholecalciferol (vitamin D3) were widely used in the past due to their low cost. The duration of action of vitamin D2/D3 is prolonged due to its wide distribution in the body fat and currently is best avoided, these might not be good, should hypercalcemia occur due to drug overdose. Vitamin D analogs (1-alfa-hydroxylated analogs), i.e., alfacalcidol and calcitriol, are the drugs of choice. Both are equally effective but weight by weight the dose of alfacalcidol is double than that of calcitriol. However, currently cost advantage is with alfacalcidol in the management of hypoparathyroidism. The dose requirement varies from patient to patient and most patients can maintain serum calcium with daily dose of 1.5–1 μg of alfacalcidol. It is necessary to measure serum calcium, phosphorus, and urinary calcium excretion at periodic interval of 3–6 months. Goal is to maintain serum calcium between 8 and 9.0 mg/dL and 24-hour urinary calcium excretion below 100 mg/day in order to decrease the risk of nephrolithiasis. In patients with persistent hypocalcemia, despite hypercalciuria, hydrochlorothiazide in the dose of 12.5 mg daily can reduce urinary calcium excretion. Approximately, 40% of the patients can be managed by only alfacalcidol or calcitriol without oral calcium supplementation. Role of restricting dietary phosphate is limited in view of its presence mainly in diary product.

Treatment of different types of hypoparathyroidism is usually same. However, the dose requirement is minimum with pseudohypoparathyroidism, followed by idiopathic and highest in cases with postsurgical where all the glands have been removed.

Hypoparathyroidism and pregnancy: Usually, pregnant women with hypoparathyroidism are advised to continue the calcium and vitamin D therapy in the dose being taken in the prepregnancy period. Dose of calcitriol may be higher in the second half of the gestation. Occasionally, pregnant patient with hypoparathyroidism may require dose reduction due to alpha-hydroxylation in the placenta and release of parathyroid hormone-related protein (PTHrP) from breast tissue.

Parathyroid hormone (1-84) therapy: Parathyroid hormone (1-84) recombinant hormone therapy in dose of 50–100 μg/day by subcutaneous route has been approved in USA and European countries. However, currently approval is only as an adjunct to patients on conventional therapy with persisting symptoms. Its long-term advantage or disadvantages over the conventional therapy are under investigation.

RECOMMENDED READINGS

1. Bhadada SK, Bhansali A, Ahuluwalia J, Chanukya GV, Behera A, Dutta P. Anaemia and marrow fibrosis in patients with primary hyperparathyroidism before and after curative parathyroidectomy. Clin Endocrinol (Oxf). 2009;70(4):527 32.
2. Bhansali A, Masoodi SR, Bhadada S, Mittal BR, Behra A, Singh P. Ultrasonography in detection of single and multiple abnormal parathyroid glands in primary hyperparathyroidism: comparison with radionuclide scintigraphy and surgery. Clin Endocrinol (Oxf). 2006;65(5):340-5.
3. Varshney S, Bhadada SK, Saikia UN, Sachdeva N, Behera A, Arya AK, et al. Simultaneous expression analysis of vitamin D receptor, calcium-sensing receptor, cyclin D1, and PTH in symptomatic primary hyperparathyroidism in Asian Indians. Eur J Endocrinol. 2013;169(1):109-16.
4. Bhadada SK, Arya AK, Mukhopadhyay S, Khadgawat R, Sukumar S, Lodha S, et al. Primary hyperparathyroidism: insights from the Indian PHPT registry. J Bone Miner Metab. 2018;36(2):238-45.
5. Rao DS, Bhadada SK, Parfitt AM. Parathyroid growth: normal and abnormal. In: Bilezikian JP, Marcus R, Levine MA, Marcocci C, Silverbeg SJ, Potts J (Eds). The Parathyroids, 3rd edition. United States: Academic Press; 2014. pp. 255-72.
6. Gafni RI, Collins MT. Hypoparathyroidism. N Engl J Med. 2019;380(18):1738-47.
7. Shoback D. Clinical practice. Hypoparathyroidism. N Engl J Med. 2008;359(4):391-403.
8. Saha S, Goswami R. Auditing the Efficacy and Safety of Alfacalcidol and Calcium Therapy in Idiopathic Hypoparathyroidism. J Clin Endocrinol Metab. 2019;104(4):1325-35.
9. Goswami R, Brown EM, Kochupillai N, Gupta N, Rani R, Kifor O, et al. Prevalence of calcium sensing receptor autoantibodies in patients with sporadic idiopathic hypoparathyroidism. Eur J Endocrinol. 2004;150(1):9-18.
10. Tomar N, Gupta N, Goswami R. Calcium-sensing receptor autoantibodies and idiopathic hypoparathyroidism. J Clin Endocrinol Metab. 2013;98(9):3884-91.
11. Goswami R, Sharma R, Sreenivas V, Gupta N, Ganapathy A, Das S. Prevalence and progression of basal ganglia calcification and its pathogenic mechanism in patients with idiopathic hypoparathyroidism. Clin Endocrinol (Oxf). 2012;77(2):200-6.
12. Saha S, Gantyala SP, Aggarwal S, Sreenivas V, Tandon R, Goswami R. Long-term outcome of cataract surgery in patients with idiopathic hypoparathyroidism and its relationship with their calcemic status. J Bone Miner Metab. 2017;35(4):405-11.
13. Saha S, Kandasamy D, Sharma R, Bal C, Sreenivas V, Goswami R. Nephrocalcinosis, Renal Dysfunction, and Calculi in Patients With Primary Hypoparathyroidism on Long-Term Conventional Therapy. J Clin Endocrinol Metab. 2020;105(4):dgz319.
14. Tay YD, Tabacco G, Cusano NE, Williams J, Omeragic B, Majeed R, et al. Therapy of Hypoparathyroidism With rhPTH(1-84): A Prospective, 8-Year Investigation of Efficacy and Safety. J Clin Endocrinol Metab. 2019;104(11):5601-10.

CHAPTER 124 Diagnosis and Management of Osteoporosis

Sanjay K Bhadada, Sushil Gupta, Rekha Singh

ABSTRACT

Osteoporosis is a major public health problem, affecting nearly 30% of postmenopausal women. Osteoporosis increases the risk of new fragility fractures. Fragility fractures, in turn, contribute significantly to morbidity and increased mortality. However, early diagnosis and timely initiation of treatment can reduce the risk of incident fragility fractures in patients with osteoporosis. The diagnosis of osteoporosis is primary based on the measurement of bone mineral density (BMD) using dual-energy X-ray absorptiometry (DXA). BMD-derived T-scores measured at the lumbar spine, hip, and forearm are recommended for the diagnosis of osteoporosis ($T \le -2.5$) and osteopenia ($-2.5 < T < -1.0$) in postmenopausal women and in men aged 50 years and older.

The management of osteoporosis entails a treatment regimen consisting of a combination of nonpharmacologic and pharmacologic interventions. Nonpharmacologic interventions include calcium and vitamin D supplementation, weight-bearing exercise, muscle strengthening, and fall prevention. Pharmacological options include antiresorptive and osteoanabolic therapies. Antiresorptive therapies primary target bone resorption, while osteoanabolic therapies predominantly promote new bone formation. Antiresorptive therapies include bisphosphonates (BPs), denosumab, and estrogen/selective estrogen receptor modulators, while osteoanabolic therapies include teriparatide, abaloparatide, and romosozumab. Regular follow-up of patients is essential to ensure adherence and response to therapy.

"Osteoporosis and thinning bones is a major but unappreciated public health problem"

—Mariam Nelson

INTRODUCTION

Osteoporosis is a condition characterized by low bone mass and microarchitectural deterioration of bone tissue, with a consequent increase in bone fragility and susceptibility to fracture. Osteoporosis increases the risk of incident fragility fractures. Fragility fractures are major health concerns that contribute significantly to morbidity and increased mortality. As the population worldwide is aging, a significant increase in the incidence of osteoporosis is expected. Approximately, 30% of all postmenopausal women have osteoporosis in the United States and Europe. One in three women over age 50 years will experience osteoporotic fractures, as will one in five men over age 50 years. Despite marked advances in diagnosis and treatment for osteoporosis, very few patients receive appropriate treatment, even after a fragility fracture.

India is home to more than 1.3 billion people, with approximately 230 million Indians over 50 years. Most data on the prevalence of osteoporosis among women in India come from studies conducted in small groups spread across the country and estimates from 2015 have suggested that 20% of the 230 million Indian women over age 50 years have osteoporosis. Prevalence of osteoporosis ranging from 8 to 62% in Indian women of different age groups has been reported in several studies. The prevalence of osteoporosis in men older than 50 years is also variable, ranging from 8.5 to 24.6%.

DIAGNOSIS OF OSTEOPOROSIS

CLINICAL DIAGNOSIS

Any patient presenting with a fragility fracture should be suspected of having underlying osteoporosis. Fragility fractures are fractures that result from mechanical forces that would not ordinarily result in fracture, known as low-level (or "low-energy") trauma. The World Health Organization (WHO) has quantified this as forces equivalent to a fall from a standing height or less. However, vertebral fractures often go undiagnosed, as they remain clinically silent or present with nonspecific backache. Nonetheless, historical height loss of >4 cm in postmenopausal women raises the possibility of asymptomatic vertebral fractures and should be investigated for the presence of underlying osteoporosis.

MEASUREMENT OF BONE MINERAL DENSITY BY DUAL-ENERGY X-RAY ABSORPTIOMETRY

Diagnosis of osteoporosis based on the measurement of BMD using DXA has become the standard of practice. First introduced in the late 1980s, DXA scanners measure the attenuation through the body of two X-ray beams with different photon energies. DXA scans are two-dimensional projection images; hence, provide a measurement of areal BMD (in g/cm^2). A DXA scan is a set of point-by-point measurements of areal BMD across the chosen anatomical site. An edge detection software is used to find the bone outline and the pixels inside the bone edges are summed to find the bone area (in cm^2). The areal BMD report on the scan printout is the average areal BMD measurement within the bone area. The scan printout also provides the measurement of bone mineral content (BMC) obtained by multiplying the areal BMD with the bone area. The BMC is equal to the total mass of hydroxyapatite accrued within the selected bone area.

The use of DXA entails exposure to ionizing radiation; however, the radiation dose for a spine and hip examination is in the range of 1–10 μSv, a figure that is less than or comparable to the daily dose from natural background radiation (~7 μSv/day).

Fragility fracture risk: Fundamental to the clinical use of BMD measurements is their ability to predict fracture risk. When baseline BMD values are used to divide patients into quartiles, an inverse association is observed between fracture risk and BMD. The relationship between areal BMD and fracture incidence is best described by a gradient-of-risk model in which the risk increases progressively as BMD decreases following an approximately exponential relationship. The gradient-of-risk is described by the relative risk (RR), the increased risk of fracture for each standard deviation (SD) decreases in areal BMD. Results from meta-analysis have shown that RR values between 1.5 and 2.5, indicating that the ability of areal BMD measurement to predict fragility fracture, is comparable to the use of blood pressure to predict stroke and serum cholesterol to predict myocardial infarction. Not all types of fractures are equally well predicted by areal BMD measurements, which are best at predicting fractures at sites such as the hip, spine, forearm, humerus, and pelvis and are relatively ineffective for predicting fractures of the face, ankles, feet, and toes.

Scan sites: Dual-energy X-ray absorptiometry is primarily used to scan the central skeleton to measure BMD of the spine and hip. At the spine, DXA measurements are typically acquired at the lumbar spine extending from the first to the fourth lumbar vertebrae (L1-L4). Apart from the commonly acquired posteroanterior scans, lateral scans of L1-L4 can be acquired. Lateral spine DXA selectively measures the trabecular-rich vertebral bodies without the contributions of the cortical-rich posterior elements of the spine and is less affected by spinal degenerative disease than posteroanterior DXA.

Many DXA scanners can also measure forearm BMD at the radius (33% radius, also called 1/3 radius). Usually, the nondominant forearm is preferred. This is useful as an alternative site in circumstances when it is not possible to obtain a valid measurement at the spine or hip. This includes patients with bilateral hip replacement, elderly patients with severe degenerative disease in the spine, and patients whose weight exceeds the safety limit for the scanner. Forearm scans are also used to investigate patients with hyperparathyroidism by measuring cortical bone at the 33% radius site.

Areal BMD measurements across the whole skeleton can be performed using total body scans. These are usually interpreted after excluding the head from the scan analysis. They are useful in younger children with a growing skeleton in whom the adult hip scan may not be appropriate.

T-scores and Z-scores: The WHO recommends the use of T-scores at the spine, hip, and forearm for the diagnosis of osteoporosis and osteopenia in postmenopausal women and in men aged 50 years and older. T-scores are calculated by taking the difference between a patient's measured BMD and the mean BMD in healthy young adults (matched for gender and ethnicity and expressing the difference relative to young adult population SD):

T-score = (Measured BMD – Young adult mean BMD)/ Young adult population SD

The recommended T-score cut-offs have been summarized in **Table 1**.

Manufactures' scan printouts also report Z-scores which are similar to T-scores except that instead of comparing the patient's BMD with the young adult mean, it is compared with the mean BMD for a healthy subject matched for age, gender, and ethnicity.

Z-score = (Measured BMD – Age-matched mean BMD)/ Age-matched population SD

For premenopausal women and men younger than 50 years, Z-scores rather than T-scores are preferred for DXA scan interpretation. A Z-score ≤–2.0 is defined as low bone mass or below the expected range for age. Notably, the classical diagnosis of osteoporosis or osteopenia should not be based on Z-scores.

Controversies with regard to T-score and Z-score measurements: For the calculation of T-scores and Z-scores, whether the reference population should be matched for ethnicity is a matter of debate. Most of the data on fracture/BMD relationship has been derived using young Caucasian women as the reference population. The International Society for Clinical Densitometry (ISCD) and the WHO recommend the use of Caucasian female database as a reference. Although BMD reference data has been established for the Indian population by the Indian Council of Medical Research (ICMR) and several other institutions, the same are not routinely used for generating T-scores and Z-scores. Hitherto, for all practical purposes, the Caucasian

TABLE 1 The World Health Organization (WHO) definition of osteoporosis and osteopenia.

Terminology	T-score definition
Normal	T ≥ –1.0 (at all sites)
Osteopenia	–2.5 < T < –1.0 (at one or more sites)
Osteoporosis	T ≤ –2.5 (at one or more sites)
Severe osteoporosis	T ≤ –2.5 (at one or more sites) in the presence of one or more fragility fractures

female database derived from the National Health and Nutrition Examination Survey (NHANES) III is also used as the India's reference population.

The use of gender-specific reference population is also a matter of controversy. Data have accumulated that incident fracture risk at the same DXA-measured femoral neck BMD is very similar between men and women. As a result, the International Osteoporosis Foundation has recommended the use of young female reference data to derive femoral neck T-scores in men, a position previously endorsed by the ISCD. A uniform Caucasian (nonrace adjusted) female reference database should be used to calculate T-scores for men of all ethnic groups.

Indications: The National Osteoporosis Foundation (NOF) recommends BMD measurements in the following patients:

- Women aged 65 years and older and men aged 70 years and older, regardless of clinical risk factors
- Younger postmenopausal women and women in menopausal transition with clinical risk factors for fracture
- Men aged 50–69 years with clinical risk factors for fracture

In addition, BMD measurement by DXA can be recommended in other circumstances as outlined in **Box 1**.

Since data indicates that osteoporotic fractures occur at an earlier age in Indians than in the West, the Indian Society for Bone and Mineral Research (ISBMR) recommends screening at an earlier age in Indians starting at 60 years and 65 years in postmenopausal women and men, respectively.

Limitations: The limitations of DXA are given in **Box 2**.

Causes of overestimation or underestimation: Multiple conditions can lead to false overestimation or underestimation of BMD measured using DXA. The list of such conditions has been summarized in **Table 2**.

For spine scans, it is important to check that the correct vertebrae have been selected for analysis. Instead of L1-L4, scan analysis is sometimes erroneously performed for T12-L3 or L2-L5. Sometimes, source of confusion is patients with abnormal vertebral segmentation (sacralization of lumbar vertebra or lumbarization of sacral vertebra). In patients with fractures involving the L1-L4 lumbar vertebrae, the affected vertebral segment would lead to erroneously overall high BMD; hence, the final BMD should be interpreted after exclusion of the BMD of the affected vertebra. In patients who have recently had an investigation with barium-contrast medium, it may be necessary to wait up to a month for it to clear. For patients who have recently had a radionuclide scan with technetium-99m, it may be necessary to wait for 48 hours for it to decay.

Interpretation using fracture risk assessment tool: As it has been mentioned, BMD strongly correlates with fracture risk. Thus, the lower the BMD, the greater the chances of fragility fractures; nevertheless, most fractures occur in individuals with a BMD T-score that does not meet the conventional definition for osteoporosis (–2.5 or lower). The paradox is partly explained by the fact that multiple clinical risk factors (such as age, sex, and previous fractures) are independently associated with fracture risk. Thus, a new approach to DXA scan interpretation based on using femoral neck BMD combined with information on clinical risk factors (**Box 3**) to estimate patients' 10-year probability of a fracture at the hip or one of the major osteoporotic sites (defined as the hip, spine, forearm, or humerus) was introduced by the WHO and is designed for use in women

BOX 1 Additional indications for BMD measurement.

- Adults with a fragility fracture
- Adults with a disease or condition associated with low bone mass or bone loss
- Adults taking medications associated with low bone mass or bone loss
- Anyone being considered for pharmacologic therapy

Source: Adapted from the National Osteoporosis Foundation and the International Society for Clinical Densitometry recommendations.

BOX 2 Limitations of dual-energy X-ray absorptiometry.

- Two-dimensional measurement affected by bone size and shape
- Measurement errors caused by heterogeneity in soft-tissue composition
- Discordant BMD findings between different measurement sites in the same individual
- Degenerative disease affects spine BMD in older adults
- BMD measurements for fracture and nonfracture populations overlap
- Cannot differentiate low bone density resulting from osteoporosis or osteomalacia

TABLE 2 Conditions associated with overestimation or underestimation of BMD.

Overestimation of BMD	Underestimation of BMD
• Spinal degenerative disease (osteophytes) • Vertebral fracture • Extraneous calcification (aortic calcification) • Overlying metals (clips, coins, and navel ring) • Other overlying objects (buttons and wallets) • Sclerotic metastasis • Ankylosing spondylitis with paravertebral ossification • Exposure to strontium-containing medications	• Laminectomy • Lytic metastasis • Barium-contrast medium in bowel • Recent radionuclide examination

BOX 3 Risk factors included in FRAX®-WHO fracture risk algorithm.

- Age
- Gender
- Weight and height
- Previous history of low trauma fracture in adult life
- Parental history of hip fracture
- Current smoking habit
- Current or past use of oral glucocorticoids for >3 months at a dose of prednisolone of 5 mg daily or more (or equivalent doses of other glucocorticoids)
- Rheumatoid arthritis
- Secondary osteoporosis*
- Alcohol intake ≥ 3 units/day
- Femoral neck areal bone mineral density

* These include type 1 (insulin-dependent) diabetes mellitus, osteogenesis imperfecta in adults, untreated long-standing hyperthyroidism, hypogonadism or premature menopause (<45 years), chronic malnutrition or malabsorption, and chronic liver disease.

(FRAX: Fracture Risk Assessment Tool; WHO: World Health Organization)

and men aged 40–90 years. The Fracture Risk Assessment Tool (FRAX)-WHO is readily available for online use and has also been incorporated into manufacturers' DXA scan printouts. As it has been described later in the text, the 10-year probability of fracture risk derived using FRAX can be used to make treatment decisions.

The FRAX has been adapted for multiple ethnicities. Derivation of Indian-specific FRAX is based on the fracture risk in individuals living in Singapore and, therefore, may not be fully applicable in the native Indian population. The Indian-specific FRAX may underestimate the fracture risk in the native population.

Patients with diabetes mellitus [both type 1 diabetes mellitus (T1DM) and type 2 diabetes mellitus (T2DM)] are at a high risk of fragility fractures. While patients with T1DM tend to have low BMD, patients with T2DM often have either normal or slightly increased BMD compared to healthy subjects. Thus, measurement of BMD and T-scores might be fallacious in patients with T2DM. Similarly, FRAX may underestimate the 10-year probability of hip and major osteoporotic fractures in patients with T2DM and thereby inadvertently delay the initiation of appropriate therapy. Hence, while using FRAX in patients with T2DM, any of the three corrections have to be applied:

1. Reduce the T-score estimated by the DXA scanner by –0.5
2. Increase the age of the patient by 10 years
3. Select the option "rheumatoid arthritis"

BIOCHEMICAL INVESTIGATIONS

Biochemical investigations should be directed at identifying the underlying cause of osteoporosis. In all patients

TABLE 3 Biochemical investigations for cause of osteoporosis.

Mandatory tests in all	Tests in suspected secondary osteoporosis
• Complete blood count • Total calcium • Inorganic phosphate • Total alkaline phosphatase • Kidney function test • Liver function test • 25-hydroxyvitamin D • Intact parathyroid hormone • TSH	• Erythrocyte sedimentation rate and serum electrophoresis for suspected multiple myeloma • IgA tissue-transglutaminase antibody (IgA-tTg) in suspected celiac disease • Serum testosterone (in men) and estradiol (in women) in suspected hypogonadism • Overnight dexamethasone suppression test in suspected Cushing's syndrome • Fasting blood glucose, post-prandial blood glucose, and glycated hemoglobin in a known or suspected case of diabetes mellitus

(IgA: immunoglobulin A; TSH: thyroid-stimulating hormone)

with osteoporosis, prior to initiation of pharmacotherapy, a basic biochemical and hormonal profile that includes serum calcium, phosphorous, total alkaline phosphatase, creatinine, 25-hydroxyvitamin D, and intact parathyroid hormone (iPTH) would be desirable. Besides, in patients with secondary osteoporosis, detailed blood investigations should be pursued based on clinical suspicion (**Table 3**).

BONE TURNOVER MARKERS

Bone turnover markers (BTMs) are dynamic parameters that reflect short-term, acute changes in bone remodeling status that are not measured by BMD and are complementary to BMD measurement. BTMs include markers of bone formation and markers of bone resorption. However, BTMs have no role in the diagnosis of osteoporosis. Although BTMs are not routinely used to diagnose osteoporosis, they are increasingly used in the follow-up of patients who are on antiosteoporotic treatments. Hence, wherever available, patients contemplating antiosteoporotic therapy can get a baseline BTM level estimated prior to initiation of therapy for subsequent comparison during follow-up.

MANAGEMENT OF OSTEOPOROSIS

A treatment regimen consisting of both nonpharmacologic and pharmacologic interventions should be used to decrease the risk of incident fractures in patients with osteoporosis. Nonpharmacologic interventions include calcium and vitamin D supplementation, weight-bearing exercise, muscle strengthening, and fall prevention.

Patients should be counseled to maintain adequate dietary intake of calcium with a total intake (including diet plus supplement, if needed) of at least 1,000 mg/day for women ≥50 years. Serum 25-hydroxyvitamin D should be maintained at ≥20 ng/mL in all patients with osteoporosis, although a level of 30–40 ng/mL would be desirable. Daily maintenance therapy at a dose of 1,000–2,000 International Units (IUs) is typically required to maintain an optimal serum 25-hydroxyvitamin D level. Higher doses of vitamin D may be necessary in the presence of certain risk factors (e.g., obesity, malabsorption, older individuals).

Fall prevention is an integral part of comprehensive osteoporosis care. Important points that need to be reiterated to patients with osteoporosis include use of low-heeled shoes with rubber soles for more solid footing, avoiding walking on slippery floors/sidewalks, using hand rails while walking up or downstairs, keeping rooms, bathrooms, and stairs well-lit, securing in-room carpets, and installing grab bars on the bathrooms walls.

OSTEOPOROSIS PHARMACOTHERAPY

Indications for initiation: Based on the NOF 2010 guidelines, postmenopausal women and men aged 50 years and above presenting with the following should be considered for treatment:

- A hip or vertebral (clinical or morphometric) fracture
- T-score ≤ –2.5 at the femoral neck or lumbar spine after appropriate evaluation to exclude secondary causes
- Low BMD (–2.5 < T-score < –1.0 at the femoral neck or lumbar spine) and a 10-year probability of a hip fracture ≥3% or a 10-year probability of a major osteoporotic fracture ≥20% based on the FRAX®-WHO fracture risk algorithm.

However, as with the T-scores and Z-scores, the aforementioned FRAX cut-offs for initiating osteoporosis treatment are based on the white Caucasian population. Based on limited data available from India, it has been proposed that the FRAX thresholds might be lower for the Asian-Indian population. Data from community-dwelling rural South Indian postmenopausal women have shown that FRAX cut-offs predicting hip fractures and major osteoporotic fractures were 2.5% and 9%, respectively. However, more evidence is needed to support that treatment initiation based on these criteria truly results in absolute fracture risk reduction. Till conclusive data is available, it is prudent to use the standard Caucasian cut-offs even in the Indian setting.

Pharmacotherapy options: Osteoporosis pharmacotherapy can be broadly classified into antiresorptive therapy and osteoanabolic therapy. Antiresorptive therapies primarily target bone resorption, while osteoanabolic therapies predominantly promote new bone formation. The hitherto available antiresorptive and osteoanabolic therapies have been summarized in **Table 4**.

Bisphosphonates: Bisphosphonates are the most widely prescribed pharmacologic agent for the treatment of osteoporosis. They are synthetic analogs of inorganic pyrophosphate. BPs may be administered orally (alendronate, risedronate, ibandronate) or parenterally (ibandronate, pamidronate, zoledronate). Oral BPs are administered either daily, weekly, or monthly, while zoledronate, the most widely used intravenous BP, is usually administered once a year for the management of primary osteoporosis.

TABLE 4 Antiresorptive and osteoanabolic drugs used for the treatment of osteoporosis.

Antiresorptive therapies	Osteoanabolic therapies
• Bisphosphonates • Denosumab • Estrogen/selective estrogen receptor modulators • Calcitonin • Cathepsin K inhibitors*	• Recombinant human parathyroid hormone (teriparatide) • Abaloparatide* • Romosozumab*

* Not yet available in India.

The intestinal absorption of BPs is poor (<1%) and decreases further in the presence of food, calcium, or other minerals that bind them. Hence, oral BPs should be administered in the fasting state 30–60 minutes before meals with water. The absorbed dose of BP tends to concentrate in the skeleton, especially at sites of active remodeling. At the bone surface, BPs inhibit bone resorption and are subsequently embedded in the bone where they remain for long and are eliminated slowly from the skeleton, thereby explaining the slow speed of reversal of the effect of BPs on bone following cessation of treatment.

At the cellular level, BPs inhibit the activity of osteoclasts. BPs bound to bone hydroxyapatite that are released in the acidic environment of the resorption lacunae under the osteoclasts and are taken up by them. In osteoclasts, BPs lead to inhibition of the enzyme farnesyl pyrophosphate synthase (FPPS), an enzyme of the mevalonate biosynthetic pathway. The enzyme is responsible for the formation of isoprenoid metabolites required for the prenylation of small GTPases that are important for cytoskeletal integrity and function of osteoclasts. Thereby, BPs induce changes in the cytoskeleton that ultimately culminates in osteoclast apoptosis. This, in turn, leads to a decrease in bone resorption, which is followed by a slower decrease in bone formation, due to coupling of the two processes. A new steady state at a lower rate of bone turnover is reached 3–6 months after the initiation of BP treatment.

Bisphosphonates tend to increase BMD by approximately 5–7% with the BMD rise at the trabecular bone (lumbar spine) being more marked than at the cortical bone (femoral neck) over 2–3 years. The rise in BMD is associated with a reduction in the risk of incident vertebral fractures by approximately 35–65%, nonvertebral fractures by 20–30%, and hip fractures by 40–50%. In the landmark HORIZON (Health Outcomes and Reduced Incidence with Zoledronic Acid Once Yearly) trial, the use of the most potent BP, zoledronate, administered at a dose of 5 mg once yearly in postmenopausal women, reduced the incidence of vertebral fractures by 70%, hip fractures by 41%, and nonvertebral fractures by 25% after 3 years as compared to placebo.

TABLE 5 Adverse effects associated with bisphosphonate (BP).

Adverse effects	Possible means of prevention
Atypical femoral fracture resulting from severe suppression of bone turnover	Temporary cessation after 3–5 years of BP use (drug holiday)
Osteonecrosis of jaw	• Ensuring proper oral hygiene prior to and during BP use • Avoiding dental manipulation while on BP therapy (for oral BP) or at least 3 months before and after injectable BP use
Esophagitis (oral BP)	• Avoid oral BP use in patients with known esophageal disease (e.g., achalasia, stricture, Barrett's esophagus, severe reflux, and scleroderma) • Avoid lying in recumbent position for 30 minutes after an oral dose of BP • Switch from oral to intravenous BP
Hypocalcemia and/or hypophosphatemia	• Ensure vitamin D sufficiency prior to BP administration • Avoid intravenous BPs in patients with severe renal impairment [estimated glomerular filtration rate (eGFR) < 30–35 mL/min/1.73 m^2]
Atrial fibrillation with IV zoledronic acid	May avoid zoledronic acid use in elderly patients with underlying cardiac disease
Flu-like syndrome	
Iritis/uveitis	

The adverse effects associated with the use of BPs along with possible means to prevent them have been summarized in **Table 5**.

Denosumab: Denosumab is a fully human immunoglobulin G2 (IgG2) antibody that binds to the receptor activator of nuclear factor-kappa B ligand (RANKL) with very high affinity and high specificity. Thus, denosumab functions like osteoprotegerin (OPG) to reduce bone resorption by inhibiting the activity of RANKL. The drug is recommended for use at a dose of 60 mg and to be administered subcutaneously twice a year at 6-monthly intervals. After dosing with 60 mg of denosumab, bone resorption marker, serum C-terminal cross-linking telopeptide of type I collagen (CTX) reached a nadir at about 1 month, then gradually increased during the 6 months between doses. Similarly, markers of bone formation decreased after 2–3 months of treatment and gradually increased thereafter between doses.

The FREEDOM (Fracture Reduction Evaluation of Denosumab in Osteoporosis Every 6 Months) trial, performed in healthy postmenopausal women with osteoporosis, had shown that the drug administered at a dose of 60 mg every 6 months for 3 years had reduced the risk of new morphometric vertebral fractures by 68%. Similarly, denosumab led to a RR reduction of 40% and 20% for hip fractures and nonvertebral fractures, respectively. Compared to placebo, denosumab use was associated with an increase in BMD of 9.2% at the lumbar spine and 6.0% at the total hip over 3 years. Besides, denosumab was effective in increasing bone density and decreasing the incidence of vertebral fracture in women of the FREEDOM trial across the spectrum of baseline renal function. Thus, denosumab can be safely used even in patients with severe renal impairment.

Discontinuation of denosumab leads to an increase in bone remodeling with indices of bone turnover returning to baseline within 3 months of not taking a dose (9 months from the last dose). Thereafter, resorption and formation markers rise above the baseline over the next several months and then return to baseline levels within 24 months after stopping treatment. Gains in BMD achieved on therapy are lost within the 1st year off treatment. This rebound increase in bone remodeling in patients who inadvertently miss a schedule dose of denosumab predisposes them to a high risk of vertebral fractures. Thus, denosumab doses should be administered strictly at an interval of 6 months without any delay between subsequent doses. Besides, patients contemplating stoppage of denosumab therapy should follow the last dose of denosumab by a longer-acting antiresorptive such as zoledronic acid.

Like BPs, denosumab use has rarely led to atypical femoral fractures resulting from oversuppression of bone turnover. Occasional cases of osteonecrosis of jaw have been reported with denosumab as well, mostly in patients with skeletal-related malignancies receiving more frequent doses of denosumab. Besides, skin infections at the site of injections have been reported with denosumab. Lastly, denosumab use in patients with severe renal impairment can lead to hypocalcemia.

Estrogens or selective estrogen receptor modulators: The Women's Health Initiative (WHI) confirmed the value of estrogen administration (with or without a progestin) in the treatment of osteoporosis and reduction of risk for hip and other clinical fractures. However, the presumed extraskeletal benefits were not confirmed and the effect on BMD and fracture reduction disappeared within a year of discontinuation of estrogen (loss of BMD of approximately 5% in the 1st year after stopping). Thus, it appears that estrogen has protective effects on the skeleton only for as long as it is taken. However, women who take estrogen and then stop should be no worse off compared with women who have never taken estrogen at all.

Following the results of the WHI, estrogen treatment is recommended for relief of menopausal symptoms, but in the lowest dose and for the shortest time necessary. Most women are not sufficiently symptomatic at menopause to require estrogen therapy and the most who require estrogen will be able to stop after a few years. However, a minority will require estrogen long-term. For those women, estrogen may be sufficient for preventing and/or treatment of osteoporosis.

Thus, while estrogen is indicated for overcoming menopausal symptoms, bone effects may be considered a side benefit. Raloxifene, an estrogen agonist/antagonist, has a limited role for prevention and treatment of osteoporosis and for reducing the risk of breast cancer.

Calcitonin: Osteoclasts express receptors for calcitonin and respond to calcitonin with a rapid decline in resorptive capacity. As a pharmacologic agent, human, eel, and salmon calcitonin have all been tried, but synthetic salmon calcitonin has been the major product in clinical use. In women with osteoporosis who were at least 5 years postmenopausal, nasal spray salmon calcitonin at a dose of 200 IU/day was shown to reduce the risk of vertebral fractures. Changes in BMD and BTMs were minimal.

Although not included in the approved indications for calcitonin, studies suggest a possible analgesic effect, possibly mediated through an increase in circulating and central nervous system endorphins, which may be clinically useful in patients with acute painful vertebral fractures.

Recombinant human parathyroid hormone (teriparatide): Recombinant human parathyroid hormone (also know as rhPTH or teriparatide) is approved for use as an osteoanabolic agent for the management of osteoporosis. Teriparatide, administered subcutaneously at a dose of 20 μg/day, stimulates bone formation. This is in contrast to what is seen in primary hyperparathyroidism, a state of chronic endogenous PTH excess, where there is loss of BMD. The reason for this discrepancy is not fully elucidated.

Administration of teriparatide first stimulates bone formation within 1 month of therapy followed by a delayed increase in bone resorption markers, as the two processes are coupled. This difference in the rise of bone markers produces what has been termed the anabolic window, a period when bone formation is greater than bone resorption. The "anabolic window" lasts for 18–24 months following initiation of teriparatide therapy after which bone resorption equals bone formation and thereafter both the processes decline. This forms the basis for recommending teriparatide therapy for a period of 18–24 months following treatment initiation.

The beneficial effects of teriparatide on bone qualities are seen predominantly in the cancellous skeleton. At the cortical site (forearm), PTH does not typically increase bone density and there may be a small decline in BMD in association with an increase in cortical porosity. However, this does not translate into decreased bone strength because porosity only occurs in the inner one-third of bone, where mechanical effect is minimal. Other salutary effects of teriparatide occurring at cortical bone are periosteal apposition, increased cortical area, cortical thickness, and cross-sectional area. Treatment with teriparatide leads to bone strength increase for different loading conditions of about 30%.

As a monotherapy, teriparatide at a dose of 20 μg/day has been shown to increase lumbar spine BMD by 9.7% and femoral neck BMD by 3% over a median treatment period of 19 months. Accordingly, teriparatide reduces the risk of new vertebral fractures and nonvertebral fractures by 65% and 53%, respectively. Despite a small reduction in radius BMD, teriparatide also reduced the risk of incident forearm fractures.

In spite of such encouraging results, the routine use of teriparatide in Indian scenario is challenging, notably, because of the exorbitant price and the daily subcutaneous mode of administration that compromises patient compliance. Hence, teriparatide therapy should be reserved for the following patients:

- Patients with fragility fractures of the vertebrae (clinical or morphometric)
- Patients with other osteoporosis-related fractures with BMD in the osteoporosis range
- Patients with very low BMD (T-score < –3.0) even in the absence of fractures

Teriparatide therapy should also be recommended for individuals who have been on prior antiresorptive therapy and who have had a suboptimal response to treatment, defined as incident fractures or active bone loss during therapy, or who have persistent osteoporosis, despite therapy. Teriparatide should be avoided in individuals who might be at a high risk of osteosarcoma, such as those with a history of Paget's disease of bone, bone radiation, and unexplained elevation in alkaline phosphatase. Furthermore, people with metastatic bone cancer, primary bone cancer, multiple myeloma, primary hyperparathyroidism, unexplained hypophosphatemia, and hypercalcemia should not receive teriparatide.

Transient increase in serum calcium within 6 hours after subcutaneous administration of teriparatide is common; however, sustained increase (confirmed with at least one subsequent measurement) is seen in only about 3% of the patients. Animal studies have shown that administration of high-dose teriparatide to rodents is associated with osteosarcoma, dependent on dose and duration of administration. In patients with endogenous hyperparathyroidism or parathyroid carcinoma, there is no evidence of an increased risk of osteosarcoma.

Recent findings from a 15-year US postmarketing surveillance study showed that the incidence of osteosarcoma associated with teriparatide use during the 15-year surveillance period was no different than would be expected based on the background incidence rate of osteosarcoma. It was earlier believed that teriparatide administration in patients with open epiphyses (children, adolescents) would predispose them to a higher risk of osteosarcoma; however, the drug is nowadays safely used in young patients with hypoparathyroidism. Other possible adverse effects of teriparatide are dizziness, leg cramps, redness and irritation at injection sites, headache, nausea, arthralgia, myalgias, lethargy, and weakness.

Other pharmacologic agents: Cathepsin K inhibitors are a new class of antiresorptive drugs. However, considering the potential safety concerns with the use of cathepsin K inhibitors that include dermatologic (morphea-like skin lesions and systemic sclerosis), serious respiratory infections, skeletal (delayed fracture union, osteonecrosis of the jaw, atypical femoral fractures), and major adverse cardiovascular events, this drug class is not approved for use in clinical practice.

Abaloparatide: It is a 34-amino acid peptide with 76% homology with parathyroid hormone-related protein (PTHrP) (1–34) and 41% homology to PTH (1–34). Abaloparatide is a potent and selective activator of the PTHR1 signaling pathway. Abaloparatide is differentiated from teriparatide based on its affinity and greater selectivity for the G protein-dependent (RG) [rather than the G protein-independent (R0)] receptor conformation of PTHR1. This selectivity potentially produces a more transient stimulation of osteoblast cyclic adenosine monophosphate (cAMP) compared with PTH, resulting in less of an effect on bone resorption and less hypercalcemia.

A phase III study conducted in postmenopausal women with low BMD with or without prevalent fracture (ACTIVE trial) demonstrated that abaloparatide, 80 µg/day, subcutaneously reduced the incidence of new vertebral, nonvertebral, major osteoporotic, and clinical fractures by 86%, 43%, 70%, and 43%, respectively, compared with placebo.

Romosozumab: It is a humanized monoclonal antibody directed against the osteocyte-derived glycoprotein sclerostin. In normal physiology, sclerostin acts as an antagonist of the bone Wnt/β-catenin pathway. The Wnt/β-catenin pathway is essential for osteoblast differentiation and function. Thus, romosozumab, by blocking sclerostin, increases osteoblast differentiation, function and promotes bone formation. The drug is administered as subcutaneous injection at a dose of 210 mg once monthly. Of all the available pharmacologic agents, the gain in BMD is maximum with romosozumab. Available phase III clinical trials with romosozumab include the FRAME (Fracture Study in Postmenopausal Women with Osteoporosis), the ARCH (Active-Controlled Fracture Study in Postmenopausal Women with Osteoporosis at High Risk), and the BRIDGE study. Following 12 months of therapy, the risk of incident vertebral fractures is reduced by 37–73%, clinical fractures by 28–36%, and nonvertebral fractures by 26%. Adverse effects associated with the use of romosozumab include injection site reactions and occasionally, hypocalcemia, atypical femoral fractures, osteonecrosis of jaw, and serious cardiovascular events.

FOLLOW-UP OF PATIENTS

Follow-up of patients with osteoporosis is of paramount importance to assess treatment adherence and to monitor the response to therapy.

Clinical: At each visit, a brief history with an emphasis on assessing new incident fractures, new-onset/worsening of kyphosis/scoliosis, new-onset or worsening of back pain, and perceptible height loss should be elicited. A history of falls is a predictor of future falls and hence should be specifically queried. Patients should also be asked about the possible side effects of pharmacologic therapy, notably persistent thigh pain (suggestive of atypical femoral fractures) and jaw pain (suggestive of osteonecrosis of jaw).

Physical evaluation: A short physical examination focusing on the patient's height should be undertaken. Other characteristics to assess include spinal tenderness, kyphosis, decreased spacing between lower ribs and pelvis, and oral hygiene. Patients on antiresorptive therapy with poor dentition may be referred to a dental physician for a detailed oral evaluation.

Biochemical: Although no consensus exists, serum 25-hydroxyvitamin D may be estimated at 6-month intervals for the initial two to three visits, and thereafter annually, to ensure vitamin D sufficiency while on treatment and target a serum 25-hydroxyvitamin D >20 ng/mL (ideal 30–40 ng/mL).

Radiological: A new radiograph of the spine may be ordered at annual follow-up for all patients, particularly for patients complaining of new-onset or worsening back pain/kyphosis to rule out any incident vertebral fractures. In addition, patients on BP therapy complaining of thigh pain should undergo a radiograph of the upper femur to rule out cortical beaking, the precursor of atypical femoral fracture. Similarly, patients on antiresorptive therapy with suspected osteonecrosis of the jaw should undergo a computed tomography of the jaw to rule out the same.

Bone mineral density: Treatments for osteoporosis increase BMD, but only modestly. Evidence to support the use of BMD to monitor the treatment response is weak, but suggests that BMD can be used for this purpose. The latest Endocrine Society Guidelines suggest monitoring BMD by DXA at the spine and hip every 1–3 years to assess treatment response. It has been suggested that serial BMD measurements in treated patients may identify individuals who do not adhere to treatment or have a secondary cause for bone loss. An increase in BMD with treatment above the least significant change (LSC) is reassuring and is associated with a greater reduction in fracture risk than a stable BMD. Usually, changes in lumbar spine BMD are more robust, while those at the hip are less dramatic, irrespective of the treatment modality used. A stable BMD on treatment is also an acceptable endpoint; however, a loss of BMD beyond the LSC (usually 5% in the lumbar spine, 4% in the total hip, and 5% in the femoral neck) over 2 years suggests treatment failure. In addition, having two or more fractures, especially vertebral fractures, while on therapy, also constitute treatment failure. In such a case, low compliance, improper dosing, vitamin D deficiency, celiac disease, multiple myeloma, concurrent glucocorticoid use, and endocrinopathies (e.g., primary hyperparathyroidism, Cushing's syndrome, thyrotoxicosis, and unrecognized hypophosphatemic states) should be considered.

Assessing changes in BMD on serial follow-up measurements require careful attention to detail. Using the same scanner and a well-trained technologist who is aware of the pitfalls of bone densitometry can mitigate these problems.

BONE TURNOVER MARKERS

Bone turnover markers are dynamic parameters that can reflect short-term/acute changes in bone that are often missed by BMD. Hence, BTMs reflect the therapeutic responses to antiosteoporosis therapies much earlier than BMD and, therefore, can be used in clinical practice, especially to monitor compliance and adherence to treatment. The absolute values or the degree of change from baseline for BTMs can be used; considering the ethnic variations in BTMs and the preanalytical variables involved in their measurement, using the degree of change rather than absolute values is more reasonable. Of the commercially available BTMs, the International Osteoporosis Foundation (IOF) and the International Federation of Clinical Chemistry and Laboratory Medicine (IFCC) recommend using serum type I collagen C-telopeptide (CTX) and serum procollagen type I N-terminal propeptide (PINP). CTX and/or PINP can be used to evaluate patient adherence and drug responses to antiresorptive agents, with measurements suggested at baseline, 3, 6, and 12 months after starting treatment. Similarly, PINP can be used to evaluate patient adherence and drug responses to anabolic agents, with measurements at baseline, 1–3 months, 6 months, and 12 months after starting anabolic treatment. A decrease in CTX by at least 30% or by at least 100 ng/L from the pretreatment value is expected in a patient on antiresorptive therapy. For PINP, a threshold of >20% or >10 μg/L from baseline is considered to be significant.

CONCLUSION

Osteoporosis is a major public health problem. Osteoporosis increases the risk of fragility fractures with subsequent morbidity and mortality. Assessment of BMD using DXA is most commonly used for the diagnosis of osteoporosis. Treatment of osteoporosis should be individualized. Maintaining optimum serum 25-hydroxyvitamin D levels is essential, which, in most cases, would require regular vitamin D supplementation. Pharmacotherapy involves use of antiresorptive or osteoanabolic medications. Regular follow-up is essential to ensure adherence and response to therapy.

ACKNOWLEDGMENT

We are thankful to Dr Rimesh Pal, Department of Endocrinology, Post Graduate Institute of Medical Education and Research, Chandigarh for helping us prepare this chapter.

RECOMMENDED READINGS

1. Kanis JA, Johnell O, Oden A, Sernbo I, Redlund-Johnell I, Dawson A, et al. Long-Term Risk of Osteoporotic Fracture in Malmö. Osteoporos Int. 2000;11:669-74.
2. Khadilkar A, Mandlik RM. Epidemiology and treatment of osteoporosis in women: an Indian perspective. Int J Womens Health. 2015;7:841-50.
3. Aggarwal A, Pal R, Bhadada SK, Ram S, Garg A, Bhansali A, et al. Bone mineral density in healthy adult Indian population: the Chandigarh Urban Bone Epidemiological Study (CUBES). Arch Osteoporos. 2021;16:17.
4. Bilezikian JP, Bouillon R, Clemens T, Compston J, Bauer DC, Ebeling PR, et al. Primer on the Metabolic Bone Diseases and Disorders of Mineral Metabolism, 9th edition. United States: John Wiley & Sons, Inc.; 2021.
5. Pasco JA, Seeman E, Henry MJ, Merriman EN, Nicholson GC, Kotowicz MA. The population burden of fractures originates in women with osteopenia, not osteoporosis. Osteoporos Int. 2006;17:1404-9.
6. Compston JE, McClung MR, Leslie WD. Osteoporosis. Lancet. 2019;393:364-76.
7. Pal R, Aggarwal A, Sachdeva N, Ram S, Garg A, Bhansali A, et al. Age- and sex-specific concentrations of bone remodeling markers in healthy Indian adults with and without vitamin D deficiency. Arch Osteoporos. 2021;16:10.
8. Rajan R, Paul J, Cherian KE, Asha HS, Kapoor N, Paul TV. FRAX® with or without BMD and TBS predicts fragility fractures in community-dwelling rural southern Indian postmenopausal women. Arch Osteoporos. 2020;15:82.
9. Gilsenan A, Midkiff K, Harris D, Kellier-Steele N, McSorley D, Andrews EB. Teriparatide Did Not Increase Adult Osteosarcoma Incidence in a 15-Year US Postmarketing Surveillance Study. J Bone Miner Res. 2021;36:244-51.
10. Eastell R, Rosen CJ, Black DM, Cheung AM, Murad MH, Shoback D. Pharmacological Management of Osteoporosis in Postmenopausal Women: An Endocrine Society* Clinical Practice Guideline. J Clin Endocrinol Metab. 2019;104:1595-622.

CHAPTER

125 Endocrine Disorders in Pregnancy

Soham Mukherjee, Sanjay K Bhadada

ABSTRACT

During pregnancy, placenta acts as an endocrine organ and secretes several hormones which affect almost each and every endocrine organ system in the mother. The endocrine changes that occur during pregnancy are adaptive so that the developing fetus could be nurtured well. The hormonal changes that take place in pregnancy alter the manifestations of common endocrine diseases. The evaluation strategies and diagnostic criteria for various hormonal disorders are also different from those in nonpregnant state. Regarding the management, safety of the developing fetus should be given due consideration as well. Here we discuss some of the commonly encountered important endocrine disorders including gestational diabetes, hypo- and hyperthyroidism, primary hyperparathyroidism (PHPT), and pheochromocytoma during pregnancy.

"There is such a special sweetness in being able to participate in creation"

—Pamela S Nadav

GESTATIONAL DIABETES

INTRODUCTION

- Gestational diabetes mellitus (GDM) is classically defined as "onset or recognition of diabetes or impaired glucose tolerance occurred during pregnancy."
- The Hyperglycemia and Adverse Pregnancy Outcome (HAPO) study has shown that maternal hyperglycemia was independently associated with adverse perinatal outcomes such as increased birth weight and cord blood c-peptide level and higher rates of primary cesarean delivery and clinically recognized neonatal hypoglycemia.
- Evidences also suggest that treating even mild GDM can reduce adverse pregnancy outcomes.
- In addition, women who developed GDM are at increased risk of type 2 diabetes mellitus (T2DM) in future.
- All these underscore the importance of identifying this entity at the earliest followed by prompt initiation of treatment.

DIAGNOSTIC CRITERIA

- Diagnosis for GDM can be established by following either of the two approaches namely one step or two step strategies (**Table 1**).
- The one step approach is recommended by IADPSG (International Association of Diabetes and Pregnancy Study Groups) and is based on HAPO study. While the two step approach is based on older O'Sullivan–Mahan criteria (with Carpenter and Coustan interpretation).
- Diabetes in Pregnancy Study Group India (DIPSI) proposed separate criteria to diagnose GDM. In this protocol, 75 g anhydrous glucose dissolved in 250–300 mL of water to be ingested by the pregnant woman irrespective of the last meal, followed by plasma glucose estimation after 2 hours. A 2-hour plasma glucose level ≥140 mg/dL is considered to be diagnostic of GDM. A 2-hour plasma glucose value of ≥200 mg/dL is considered as diabetes mellitus

TABLE 1 Screening and diagnosis of gestational diabetes mellitus (GDM).

One step strategy	Two step strategy
• To perform in pregnant women not previously diagnosed with diabetes at 24–28 weeks of gestation • To perform a 75 g OGTT (oral glucose tolerance test) in the morning, after an overnight fast of at least 8 hours • Plasma glucose measurement at fasting, 1 and 2 hours • The diagnosis of GDM is made when any of the cutoff value is either met or exceeded ◦ *Fasting*: ≥92 mg/dL ◦ *1 hour*: ≥180 mg/dL ◦ *2 hours*: ≥153 mg/dL	**Step 1:** • To perform a 50 g GLT (glucose load test, nonfasting), with measurement of plasma glucose at 1 hour, at 24–28 weeks of gestation in women not previously diagnosed with diabetes • If the plasma glucose level measured 1 hour after the load is ≥135 mg/dL, proceed to step 2 **Step 2:** • A 100 g OGTT should be performed in fasting state • Plasma glucose measurement at fasting, 1, 2, and 3 hours • The diagnosis of GDM is made when any two of the cutoff values are either met or exceeded ◦ *Fasting*: ≥95 mg/dL ◦ *1 hour*: ≥180 mg/dL ◦ *2 hours*: ≥155 mg/dL ◦ *3 hours*: ≥140 mg/dL

TABLE 2 Gestational diabetes mellitus (GDM)—potential consequences in the offsprings.

Fetal period	Neonatal period	Childhood	Adult
• Congenital malformations • Stillbirth and birth asphyxia • Preterm delivery • Macrosomia	• Large for gestational age • Birth injury • Hypoglycemia • Respiratory distress syndrome • Polycythemia • Hyperbilirubinemia • Hypocalcemia	• Neurodevelopmental impairments • Obesity and insulin resistance • Impaired glucose tolerance	• Obesity insulin resistance impaired glucose tolerance • Type 2 diabetes mellitus

and ≥120 mg/ dL as decreased gestational glucose tolerance (DGGT). Although, convenient and patient friendly, DIPSI criteria have been criticized for its low sensitivity.

- At the initial prenatal visit, pregnant women having risk factors should be screened for T2DM using standard diagnosis criteria (used outside of pregnancy).
  - Women who are diagnosed to have diabetes with these criteria are classified as having diabetes complicating pregnancy.
  - Pregnant women who are meeting the lower glycemic diagnostic criteria for GDM are classified to have that condition only and to be managed accordingly.
  - Rest of the women who have absolutely normal glycemic profile at initial prenatal visit should be screened again for GDM between weeks 24 and 28.

OUTCOME IN OFFSPRING

- Congenital malformation usually develops if the fetus gets exposed to very high level of maternal hyperglycemia during the period of organogenesis, i.e., in the first trimester and may be observed if the mother already has pregestational diabetes during conception and is unlikely if she develops diabetes at second trimester. The risk usually steeply increases with a glycated hemoglobin (HbA1c) > 9.5–10%.
- Gestational diabetes may be associated with various short-term as well as long-term adverse outcomes which have been depicted in **Table 2**.
- Maternal hyperglycemia results in increased transplacental transfer of glucose into fetal circulation which leads to enhanced insulin release and fetal hyperinsulinemia. Excess insulin, being an anabolic hormone, leads to macrosomia and related complications. The increase birth weight is mainly contributed by rise in fat mass rather than lean body mass.
- There is a state of relative hypoxia in the fetus which may lead to still birth or birth asphyxia. This also induces erythropoietin secretion which may result in polycythemia and hyperbilirubinemia.
- Hyperinsulinemia in the fetus also may alter surfactant synthesis and lead to respiratory distress syndrome.

TREATMENT

Medical nutrition therapy:

- About 80–90% of GDM patients can be managed by medical nutrition therapy (MNT) alone.
- These patients are advised to eat three small to moderate-sized meals and two or three snacks and bedtime snack.
- The diet should be balanced, consisting of carbohydrates (whole-grain), protein, and unsaturated fats. Pregnant women are advised to eat less carbohydrate at breakfast as compared to that in lunch or dinner. They should preferably consume diet having low glycemic index.

Moderate-intensity aerobic exercise: For duration of 30 minutes per day for at least 5 days per week or a minimum of 150 minutes over the course of the week is recommended.

Pharmacologic therapy: To be started, if glycemic targets are not achieved with lifestyle modification alone within 1 week.

Insulin:

- Considered as first-line pharmacologic therapy
- It does not cross the placenta to a significant extent.
- Fasting and postprandial hyperglycemias are usually treated with basal and prandial insulin, respectively.
- Among basal insulin neutral protamine Hagedorn (NPH) and detemir, and among prandial insulin regular, lispro and aspart insulin have acceptable efficacy and safety profile. However, none of the human insulin preparations currently available for clinical use have been shown to cross the placenta.
- Insulin dose varies widely from patient to patient and may need titration on weekly basis or more frequently based on self-monitoring of blood glucose.

Metformin:

- It freely crosses the placenta.
- Metformin use was associated with lower prandial glucose excursions, reduced maternal weight gain, and decreased incidence of pregnancy-induced hypertension.
- However, it was shown to be linked with greater risk of preterm delivery.

- Although short-term effects on neurodevelopmental outcomes were reassuring, the possible long-term developmental and metabolic consequences on the offspring need to be explored in future.
- Couple of studies reported that children who were exposed to metformin in intrauterine period were found to have higher weight at 4 and 9 years of age.
- Up to 50% of the women treated with metformin for GDM still required add on insulin therapy to achieve target blood glucose level.

MONITORING

Self-monitoring of blood glucose:

- Blood glucose control worsens progressively during second and third trimester as insulin resistance increases with gradual rising level of diabetogenic hormones released from placenta over the course of gestation.
- Home monitoring of capillary blood glucose is essential to achieve the glycemic target (**Table 3**) by addition of antidiabetic agents as well as titration of insulin doses, if required.
- Gestational diabetes mellitus patients are advised to monitor capillary fasting and postprandial (1 or 2 hours after meals) blood glucose level as well as selective monitoring of prelunch and predinner blood glucose values to guide insulin dose adjustments.
- These patients usually need to submit weekly glucose update for optimum glycemic control.
- Changes in the therapeutic regimen are advised when 20–25% of glucose values at a particular point of time (i.e., fasting or after a particular meal) are above the glycemic target, despite compliance to the existing regimen, or if there is hypoglycemic episodes.

Glycated hemoglobin:

- It is more relevant for preexisting diabetes complicating pregnancy.
- Glycated hemoglobin target should be < 6%, if this can be achieved without any unwanted risk of hypoglycemia; otherwise it can be maintained at <7%.

FOLLOW-UP AFTER DELIVERY

- There is dramatic reduction in insulin resistance immediately after delivery.
- Insulin requirements should be reevaluated and adjusted accordingly.
- Women with recent history of GDM should be screened for diabetes mellitus with 75 g oral glucose tolerance test using nonpregnancy diagnostic criteria 4–12 weeks after delivery.

TABLE 3 Glycemic targets.

Blood glucose parameters	Values
Fasting blood glucose and	<95 mg/dL
1 hour postprandial blood glucose or	<140 mg/dL
2 hours postprandial blood glucose	<120 mg/dL

- Women having history of GDM should receive lifelong screening for diabetes mellitus every 3 yearly.

THYROID DISORDERS

- Pregnancy has profound effect on thyroid gland structure and function.
- In pregnancy, thyroid gland increases by 10–40% in size.
- Plasma level of thyroxine-binding globulin (TBG) and total thyroxine (T4) increases by 6–8 weeks of gestation and remain elevated up to delivery.
- Rise in circulating human chorionic gonadotropin (hCG) level in pregnancy induces T4 production by its action on thyroid-stimulating hormone (TSH) receptor due to its structural similarity with TSH and hence, there is decline in TSH level.
- Thyroid-stimulating hormone reference interval decreases by 0.1–0.2 mU/L and 0.5–1 mU/L for lower and upper normal limit, respectively in pregnancy. When available, trimester-specific reference intervals derived from local population data should be used.
- In the absence of local population data, the lower limit of reference range of TSH may be decreased by approximately 0.4 mU/L and upper limit can be reduced by about 0.5 mU/L in the first trimester. This should be applied from 7th to 12th week of gestation and to be followed by gradual increase in the second and third trimesters toward the nonpregnant reference range.
- Serum free T4 (FT4) estimation by the indirect analog immunoassays can be influenced by pregnancy; however, when used, assay method and trimester-specific reference intervals need to be considered.
- Total T4 (TT4) measurement with a pregnancy-adjusted reference interval may be used instead of FT4.
- Serum TT4 level starts to increase (due to rise in TBG level) from 7th week of gestation reaching peak at 16th week to attain 50% above the prepregnancy level which is then sustained throughout the pregnancy. Therefore, after week 16 of gestation the upper limit of normal reference range is 1.5 times the upper nonpregnant reference range. In between, weeks 7 and 16 of gestation, upper reference range of TT4 can be calculated by increasing the nonpregnant upper reference limit by 5% per week, beginning from week 7.

HYPOTHYROIDISM

- In pregnant women, hypothyroidism is characterized by elevation of serum TSH level above the upper limit of the pregnancy-specific reference interval.
- In the absence of trimester-specific TSH reference range, derived from local or similar population during pregnancy, an upper reference limit of approximately 4.0 mU/L may be used.
- Overt maternal hypothyroidism during pregnancy has been found to be associated with increased risk of miscarriage, preterm delivery, low birth weight baby, and lower IQ in the offspring.
- Most of the studies on subclinical hypothyroidism also reported a higher risk of adverse pregnancy outcomes.

- While overt hypothyroidism in pregnancy invariably needs to be treated, for subclinical hypothyroidism, indication for levothyroxine (LT4) therapy is selective and provided in the **Flowchart 1**.
- It is advisable to maintain a TSH in the lower half of the reference range (trimester specific). Maternal TSH may be targeted to <2.5 mU/L when trimester-specific reference range of the given population is not available.
- Pregnant patients with hypothyroidism should be monitored with serum TSH at 4 weekly interval till midgestation and then at around 30th week.
- Hypothyroid women receiving LT4 therapy, if become pregnant, should increase their LT4 dose by 20–30%. They have to inform their healthcare provider urgently for further testing and evaluation.
- After delivery, LT4 dose needs to be reduced to that in the preconception phase and additional testing to be performed at about 6 weeks postpartum.
- After delivery, LT4 therapy may be stopped in women when it was initiated during pregnancy and the dose is ≤50 μg/day. In such case, serum TSH should be re-evaluated at 6 weeks postpartum.

THYROTOXICOSIS

- Thyrotoxicosis is characterized by a suppressed serum TSH less than the lower limit of the reference range. In places, where local pregnancy and trimester-specific data are not available, 0.06 mU/L, 0.3 mU/L, and 0.3 mU/L may be considered as the lower limit of TSH reference interval in the first, second, and third trimester of pregnancy.
- When a low or suppressed TSH is detected in the first trimester, apart from a detail history and clinical examination, serum FT4 or TT4 should be measured. Estimation of total triiodothyronine (TT3) and TSH receptor antibody (TRAb) may be helpful in determining the etiology.
- Radionuclide or radioiodine scan is contraindicated in pregnancy and should be avoided.

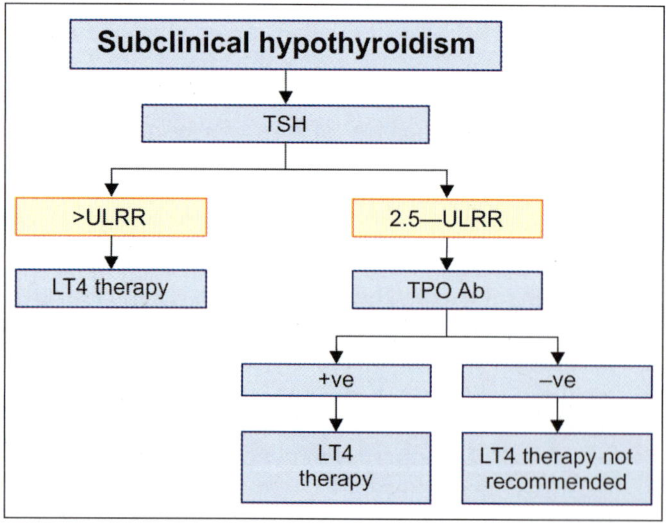

[TPO Ab: thyroid peroxidase antibody; ULRR: upper limit of the reference range (pregnancy and trimester specific); in absence of local population data it may be taken as 4 mU/L]

FLOWCHART 1: Indication of LT4 therapy in pregnant women with subclinical hypothyroidism.

Etiology:

- Graves' disease (GD) is the most common cause of hyperthyroidism in females of childbearing age. The frequency is 0.4–1.0% of women before pregnancy and about 0.2% during pregnancy.
- Toxic multinodular goiter and toxic adenoma are the less common causes of hyperthyroidism during pregnancy. Subacute thyroiditis, another etiology of thyrotoxicosis is less frequently observed in pregnancy.
- Gestational transient thyrotoxicosis is an important cause of hyperthyroxinemia in pregnancy and is limited to the first half of gestation. Often associated with hyperemesis gravidarum, this condition is characterized by elevated FT4 and suppressed TSH resulting from excessive hCG-induced stimulation of TSH receptor (specificity spill over).
- In early gestation, the differential diagnosis of hyperthyroidism in the majority of cases is between gestational transient thyrotoxicosis and GD. Although, they share common clinical manifestations, a detail history and physical examination may differentiate between the two (**Table 4**).
- If alternate etiologies for thyrotoxicosis are considered, TRAb measurement is useful. Thyroid ultrasound should be done if either thyroid nodules are suspected based on clinical examination or TRAb is negative.

Management: Gestational transient thyrotoxicosis should be treated with supportive therapy including correction of dehydration and hospitalization, if required. Although β-blockers may be considered, antithyroid drugs (ATDs) should be avoided.

Graves' disease:

- Uncontrolled overt thyrotoxicosis may lead to adverse perinatal outcomes including miscarriage, preeclampsia, preterm delivery, low birth weight baby, thyroid storm, and congestive heart failure in the mother.
- Thionamides including methimazole (MMI), carbimazole (CM), and propylthiouracil (PTU) are the mainstay of treatment. Initial doses of different ATDs are enlisted in **Table 5**.
- In a woman with GD, who recently conceives, and is euthyroid on a low dose of (ATD (i.e., MMI ≤ 5–10 mg/day), discontinuation of ATD may be considered due to their teratogenic potential. Maternal thyroid function test should be performed 1–2 weeks after ATD discontinuation and if the patient is found to be clinically and biochemically euthyroid then the test interval can be prolonged to 2–4 weeks.
- In all the other cases, pregnant patients of GD need ATD.
- In the first 16 weeks of gestation, PTU is recommended rather than MMI due to increased risk of severe form of birth defect associated with use of the latter. Pregnant women who are already on MMI or CM and need to be

TABLE 4 Gestational transient thyrotoxicosis versus Graves' disease.

Parameters	Gestational transient thyrotoxicosis	Graves' disease
Prior history of thyroid disease	Usually absent	Often present
Symptoms of emesis	Present	Usually absent
Goiter	Absent	Usually present
Orbitopathy	Absent	May be present
Disease progression	Self-limited mild disease	Persistent disease with varying severity

TABLE 5 Initial doses of ATDs during pregnancy.

ATD	Initial dose	Typical dose in an average patient	Frequency
MMI	5 30 mg/day	10–20 mg/day	Once daily*
CM	10–40 mg/day		Once daily*
PTU	100–600 mg/day	200–400 mg/day	Split into two or three daily doses
Equivalent anti thyroid potency			
• Therapeutic potency (antithyroid) ratio of MMI to PTU is at least 15:1 • 10 mg of CM is rapidly metabolized in human body to 6 mg of MMI (approximately)			

*In rare and severe cases of hyperthyroidism, twice daily dosing may be required.

(ATD: antithyroid drug; CM: carbimazole; MMI: methimazole; PTU: propylthiouracil)

continued on ATD should be switched to equivalent dose of PTU as soon as possible.

- After 16th week, if ATD is needed to be continued then either a switch from PTU to MMI/CM or continuation PTU beyond 16th week may be considered in absence of evidence of clear risk versus benefit of one approach over other, at present.
- Thyroid-stimulating hormone and FT4/TT4 should be monitored at about 4 weekly intervals during pregnancy.
- Lowest effective dose of ATD should be administered targeting maternal FT4/TT4 level at the upper limit or slightly above the reference interval.
- β-blockers (e.g., propranolol 10–40 mg 6–8 hourly) may be used to control adrenergic symptoms for a short duration (usually 2–6 weeks). However, when used for prolonged period may be associated with intrauterine growth retardation, fetal bradycardia, and neonatal hypoglycemia.
- Thyroidectomy during pregnancy may be required for unusual scenarios. Second trimester is the optimal time for thyroidectomy, if required at all. If maternal TRAb level is >3 times the upper limit of reference interval, the fetus needs to be monitored for development of fetal hyperthyroidism during the entire pregnancy, even when the mother remains euthyroid, postsurgery.
- The TRAb measurement is indicated in patients with GD on ATD at first trimester when pregnancy is confirmed. Then to be repeated at second trimester at week 18–22, if still she is on ATD. In the third trimester (week 30–34) again TRAb testing is needed if TRAb level was elevated in second trimester or the mother is still on ATD. This is required to evaluate the need for neonatal and postnatal monitoring.
- Further, if the pregnant patient had received a definitive therapy for GD (surgery or radioiodine) in past, maternal serum TRAb estimation should be performed during early pregnancy. Repeat testing is required at weeks 18–22, if maternal TRAb level was elevated in early gestation.
- If the pregnant woman has uncontrolled hyperthyroidism in the second half of pregnancy or has high TRAb concentration (>3 times the upper limit of normal), fetal surveillance with ultrasound for fetal growth, heart rate, amniotic fluid volume, and appearance of fetal goiter is mandatory.
- Screening for hypothyroidism in newborns should be carried out by blood spot analysis at 2–5 days after delivery.

Hyperthyroidism caused by autonomous nodules:

- If hyperthyroidism caused by autonomous nodules is treated with ATD, a low dose should be used with a target to maintain maternal serum FT4/TT4 level at the upper limit or slightly above the upper limit of reference range.
- The fetus must be monitored carefully for goiter and sign of hypothyroidism during second half of gestation.
- If sign of fetal hypothyroidism still develops, maternal surgery aiming at removal of the autonomous nodule need to be considered.

PRIMARY HYPERPARATHYROIDISM

DIAGNOSIS

- Diagnosis of PHPT in pregnancy is challenging.
- In a woman during normal pregnancy changes in calcium homeostasis result in relatively lower level of serum total calcium.
- Factors responsible for relatively lower total calcium level in pregnancy include—hemodilution, hypoalbuminemia, transplacental calcium transport to the fetus, and hypercalciuria resulting from an increased glomerular filtration rate. Besides, estrogen may also inhibit parathyroid hormone (PTH)-induced bone resorption.
- In the pregnancy, even serum total calcium at the upper normal level needs to be considered important.

- Most of the pregnant patients of PHPT are either asymptomatic or may have mild nonspecific symptoms which are similar to symptoms associated with normal pregnancy.
- A high index of suspicion for PHPT should be kept for women who have excessive pregnancy-associated symptoms.
- The ^{99m}technetium sestamibi scintigraphy, the gold standard imaging technology for PHPT, is contra-indicated during pregnancy. Neck ultrasonography is the safest modality in pregnancy and has a sensitivity of approximately 70%.

MATERNAL AND FETAL COMPLICATIONS

- Primary hyperparathyroidism may be associated with serious maternal and fetal complications.
- Maternal complications include renal stone disease, bone disease, pancreatitis, muscle weakness, hyperemesis gravidarum, preeclampsia-eclampsia, and altered sensorium. Hypercalcemic crisis, a life-threatening complication of PHPT, is characterized by nausea, vomiting, tremulousness, dehydration, and altered mental status and may progress to renal failure, coma, or even death.
- A very high rate of fetal complications (80%) has been noted in pregnant women with untreated PHPT.
- These fetal complications may encompass intrauterine growth restriction, neonatal tetany, or even neonatal death.
- Maternal hypercalcemia leads to transplacental excessive calcium flux into fetal circulation which results in fetal parathyroid gland suppression through negative feedback mechanism. Although this type of neonatal hypoparathyroidism is usually transient, it may lead to a fatal neonatal tetany, if remains unrecognized or untreated.

TREATMENT

Conservative management is preferred in mild and asymptomatic cases; however, surgery should be considered in more severe cases.

Medical therapy:

- Immediate hospitalization is necessary when pregnant patients have severe hypercalcemia or have significant manifestations including pancreatitis, hyperemesis gravidarum, altered mental status, arrhythmia, or any other life-threatening complications.
- These patients are usually dehydrated and require aggressive intravenous fluid resuscitation.
- The medical management options to normalize serum calcium level in pregnant PHPT patients are enlisted in **Table 6**.

Surgical therapy:

- This is the most definite treatment option for PHPT.
- Second trimester is the most appropriate time of surgery, if at all required due to severity of the disease.
- During this period, organogenesis is completed and the risk of anesthesia-induced preterm delivery is minimum.

PHEOCHROMOCYTOMA

Pheochromocytoma is extremely rare in pregnant women with an approximate frequency of 0.007%. However, it may be associated with very high rate of maternal and fetal mortality (up to 40–50%) if left untreated.

SYMPTOMS

- Hypertension is the most common presenting manifestation of pheochromocytoma and is noted in >80% of patients. Period of hypotension may also be observed in about 50% of patients.
- Pheochromocytoma-associated manifestations may worsen with progression of pregnancy. This may be related to increase in pressure on the pheochromocytoma resulting from progressive abdominal distension, uterine contractions, or fetal movements. Further, estrogens may act as a growth factor for the tumor per se.
- Pheochromocytoma needs to be differentiated from pregnancy-related hypertension (**Table 7**).

DIAGNOSIS

- Measurement of plasma and/or 24-hour urine metanephrine and normetanephrine concentrations is the most useful test similar to nonpregnant individuals. Mild elevation in the level might reflect a false positive result due to inherent limitations of these tests or issues with sample collection. Use of medications including labetalol or methyldopa may lead to false positive yields.
- After the biochemical diagnosis is made tumor localization should be done by either ultrasonography or magnetic resonance imagining (MRI). MRI without gadolinium has high accuracy in detecting pheochromocytoma in pregnancy. Metaiodobenzylguanidine (MIBG) scan should be avoided during pregnancy.
- A disease causing mutation is commonl found approximately in 30% of patients with pheochromocytoma diagnosed during pregnancy. Hence, after the diagnosis is confirmed, genetic counseling should be seriously considered during follow-up.

MANAGEMENT

- The tumor should be removed either in the second trimester before 24 weeks of pregnancy or after delivery.
- Preoperative preparation is required for optimal outcome. Pretreatment with α-blocker for at least 10–14 days before surgery improves the perioperative outcome.
- In pregnant patient, target blood pressure for pheochromocytoma is not known. However, for nonpregnant patients, the target is <130/80 mm Hg in sitting posture with systolic blood pressure > 90 mm Hg during standing. In pregnant women having chronic hyper-

TABLE 6 Medications in pregnant PHPT patients.

Drug name	Status in pregnancy	Mechanism of action	Comments
Calcitonin	• Category B • Does not cross placenta	Inhibits osteoclast function directly	• Acute lowering of serum calcium • Continuous use associated with tachyphylaxis
Cinacalcet	• Category C • Animal studies have reported that it crosses placenta • Embryonal or fetal toxicity or harmful effects with respect to pregnancy have not been observed	• Calcimimetic • Activates calcium-sensing receptor (CaSR) • Decreases PTH secretion • Decreases renal calcium reabsorption	• Delayed onset of action • For the rapid correction of severe hypercalcemia, monotherapy is not sufficient and should be combined with calcitonin
Bisphosphonates	• Category C • Crosses the placenta • Animal studies have shown that it interferes with endochondral bone development	Inhibit osteoclastic bone resorption	Should only be reserved in emergency condition as a short term measure for stabilization of severe and life-threatening hypercalcemic state before surgery
Furosemide	Category C	Inhibits renal tubular calcium reabsorption and promote calciuresis	Monitor serum electrolytes closely
Oral phosphates	Category C	• Promotes precipitation of calcium phosphate complexes (insoluble) in bone and soft tissues • Inhibition of osteoclastic activity • Reduction of intestinal calcium absorption	• Hypokalemia and diarrhea are the common side effects • It may cause intra- and extravascular calcium phosphate deposits which may lead to severe organ failure

(PHPT: primary hyperparathyroidism; PTH: parathyroid hormone)

TABLE 7 Pheochromocytoma versus pregnancy-related hypertension.

Parameters	Pheochromocytoma	Pregnancy-related hypertension
Onset	May present with hypertension at any time during pregnancy	Usually develops after 20 weeks of gestation
Characteristics	Often paroxysmal	Sustained hypertension
Hypotension	May be present	Absent
Associated features	Headache, palpitations, perspiration, hyperglycemia, or cardiomyopathy	Edema and proteinuria
Phenotypical features	Café-au-lait macules, freckles, or fibromas may suggest syndromic pheochromocytoma	Usually absent

tension without end-organ damage, a target blood pressure of <150/100 mm Hg along with diastolic blood pressure of >80 mm Hg should be maintained. When end-organ damage is present, the target is reduced to <140/90 mm Hg.

- Phenoxybenzamine (10–40 mg twice a day) and doxazosin (4–16 mg twice a day) are most commonly used α-blockers
- Phenoxybenzamine when used may lead to neonatal hypotension and respiratory depression as it can cross the placenta (category C drug).
- Doxazosin has also been used to treat pheochromocytoma during pregnancy, and is associated with lesser episodes of postoperative hypotension.
- Although doxazosin is also a category C drug and may cross placenta, neonatal outcome is relatively better without any report of neonatal hypotension and respiratory depression.
- β-blockers should be added to the regimen to counteract α-blockade-induced tachycardia. β-blockers may lead to intrauterine growth retardation and their use should be restricted to a short period of time during pregnancy.
- When hypertension is not controlled by α-blocker, calcium channel blocker (category C drug) can be added.
- Labetalol, a combined α- and β-blocker should not be used as a single therapeutic agent in pheochromocytoma due to its relatively weak α-blockade property and may

TABLE 8 Diagnostic criteria and treatment of Cushing disease, acromegaly, and prolactinoma during pregnancy.

Disease	Screening test	Treatment option
Cushing disease	• UFC: >4 times the upper limit of normal reference interval (nonpregnant) • Late-night salivary cortisol: ≥3–4 times above the upper limit of normal reference interval (nonpregnant) • Dexamethasone suppression test yields false positive result and not recommended	• Surgical resection: In second trimester—when pituitary adenoma or adrenal adenoma has been clearly localized • Metyrapone: Every 6–8 hourly dosing
Acromegaly	• Definite diagnosis should be postponed until postpartum period due to lack of normative data during pregnancy (if possible) • A high serum IGF-1 level before midgestation or higher GH levels > 1 μg/L by highly specific assays for pituitary GH during third trimester are suggestive	• Stop long-acting somatostatin receptor ligand (SRL) formulations and pegvisomant about 2 months before attempting for conception • If required, short-acting octreotide may be used until conception • Medical therapy for acromegaly should be withheld during pregnancy and only restricted use is advisable for headache and tumor control • Pregnant patients with macroadenomas should have serial visual field testing • GH-IGF-1 levels should not be monitored during pregnancy
Prolactinoma	• Hyperprolactinemia renders the women infertile • Usually, female patients of prolactinoma conceive when their hyperprolactinemia gets corrected on dopamine agonist therapy • During normal pregnancy serum prolactin concentration increases about 10-fold and may reach up to 150–300 μg/L by term • Serum prolactin estimation during pregnancy for monitoring purpose is not useful	• As soon as the patient identifies herself to be pregnant, she should discontinue dopamine agonist • In patients with macroadenomas which is either invasive or abutting the optic chiasma, who conceive on dopamine agonist therapy and do not have any prior history of surgery or radiotherapy, dopaminergic therapy may be continued in such cases throughout the pregnancy • Routine use of pituitary MRI in pregnant patients with intrasellar macroadenomas or microadenomas is not advisable • Pituitary MRI is only required when there is clinical evidence for tumor growth (e.g., visual field compromise) • Surgical resection before attempting pregnancy should be considered in women with macroprolactinomas who either do not have tumor shrinkage on medical management or develop drug intolerance • Formal visual field testing followed by pituitary MRI without gadolinium is advisable in pregnant patients with prolactinomas who develop severe headaches or visual field changes • Bromocriptine therapy should be initiated if there is symptomatic growth of the tumor during pregnancy

(IGF: insulin-like growth factor; UFC: urinary free cortisol)

precipitate paroxysmal hypertension. Methyldopa may also worsen the hypertension in pheochromocytoma and should be avoided.

- Restoration of intravascular volume is also important; and few days prior to surgery, intravenous fluids can be started and patients should receive a salt-rich diet.
- Commonly prescribed drugs (e.g., corticosteroids, opioids such as morphine and pethidine, metoclopramide, anesthetics such as thiopental, ephedrine, and ketamine, and muscle relaxants like mivacurium) which may precipitate pheochromocytoma crisis should be avoided.

PITUITARY DISORDERS

Some of the important issues relating to the diagnosis and management of pituitary disorders including Cushing disease, acromegaly and prolactinoma have been depicted in **Table 8**.

CONCLUSION

Pregnancy presents a unique challenge for the endocrinologist. Diagnosis of the common endocrine disorders is challenging and often confused with the exaggerated manifestations of normal pregnancy. The diagnostic criteria are also different from those in nonpregnant state. Some of the routinely performed radiological imaging and nuclear scintigraphy required to establish the diagnosis of various endocrine diseases are not safe at all in pregnancy and are contraindicated. Management is more complicated as we need to care for two lives simultaneously.

RECOMMENDED READINGS

1. HAPO Study Cooperative Research Group, Metzger BE, Lowe LP, Dyer AR, Trimble ER, Chaovarindr U, Coustan DR, et al. Hyperglycemia and adverse pregnancy outcomes. New Eng J Med. 2008;358:1991-2002.
2. Szmuilowicz ED, Josefson JL, Metzger BE. Gestational diabetes mellitus. Endocrinol Metab Clin North Am. 2019;48:479-93.
3. American Diabetes Association. 14. Management of Diabetes in Pregnancy: Standards of Medical Care in Diabetes—2020. Diabetes Care. 2020;43(Suppl 1): S183-92.
4. Metzger BE. Diabetes mellitus and pregnancy. In: Jameson JL, De Groot LJ, de Kretser DM, Giudice LC, Grossman AB, Melmed S, Potts, Jr JT, Weir GC (Eds). Endocrinology: adult and pediatric, Volume 1, 7th edition. Philadelphia: Elsevier; 2016. pp. 788-804.
5. Rani PR, Begum J. Screening and diagnosis of gestational diabetes mellitus, where do we stand. J Clin Diag Res. 2016;10:QE01-4.
6. Alexander EK, Pearce EN, Brent GA, Brown RS, Chen H, Dosiou C, et al. 2017 Guidelines of the American Thyroid Association for the diagnosis and management of thyroid disease during pregnancy and the postpartum. Thyroid. 2017;27:315-89.
7. Hollenberg A, Wiersinga WM. Hyperthyroid disorders. In: Melmed S, Auchus RJ, Goldfine AB, Koenig RJ, Rosen CJ (Eds). Williams Textbook of Endocrinology, 14th Edition. Philadelphia: Elsevier; 2020. pp. 364-403.
8. Leere JS, Vestergaard P. Calcium metabolic disorders in pregnancy: Primary hyperparathyroidism, pregnancy-induced osteoporosis, and vitamin D deficiency in pregnancy. Endocrinol Metab Clin N Am. 2019;48: 643-55.
9. Gokkaya N, Gungor A, Bilen A, Bilen H, Gviniashvili D, Karadeniz Y. Primary hyperparathyroidism in pregnancy: a case series and literature review. Gynecol Endocrinol. 2016;32:783-6.
10. Pal R, Bhadada SK, Gupta N, Behera A, Aggarwal N, Aggarwal A, et al. Primary hyperparathyroidism in pregnancy: observations from the Indian PHPT registry. J Endocrinol Inv. 2020.
11. van der Weerd K, van Noord C, Loeve M, Knapen MFCM, Visser W, De Herder WW, et al. Endocrinology in pregnancy: Pheochromocytoma in pregnancy: case series and review of literature. Eur J Endocrinol. 2017;177:R49-58.
12. Lenders JWM, Langton K, Langenhuijsen JF, Eisenhofer G. Pheochromocytoma and pregnancy. Endocrinol Metab Clin N Am. 2019;48:605-17.
13. Jung C, Ho JT, Torpy DJ, Rogers A, Doogue M, Lewis JG, et al. A longitudinal study of plasma and urinary cortisol in pregnancy and postpartum. J Clin Endocrinol Metab. 2011;96:1533-40.
14. Abucham J, Bronstein MD, Dias ML. Acromegaly and pregnancy: A contemporary review. Eur J Endocrinol. 2017;177:R1-12.
15. Katznelson L, Laws Jr ER, Melmed S, Molitch ME, Murad MH, Utz A, et al. Acromegaly: An endocrine society clinical practice guideline. J Clin Endocrinol Metab. 2014;99:3933-51.
16. Melmed S, Casanueva FF, Hoffman AR, Kleinberg DL, Montori VM, Schlechte JA, et al. Diagnosis and treatment of hyperprolactinemia: an Endocrine Society clinical practice guideline. J Clin Endocrinol Metab. 2011;96:273-88.

CHAPTER 126

Endocrine Disorders of Elderly

Surya K Singh, Vahid Bharmal

ABSTRACT

Physiological functions of body begin to decline with aging. With increased life expectancy consequent to better living, burden of age-related comorbidities and chronic illness will rise. Among various structural and functional changes, with aging, secretory patterns of hormones produced by hypothalamo-pituitary system and its sensitivity to negative feedback by end hormones change. Complex alterations of hormonal patterns with aging, inflammation, and altered metabolism lead to age-related chronic illness. Also, certain endocrine and metabolic disorders are more common as the age progresses, such as type 2 diabetes mellitus, hypothyroidism, and osteoporosis. In this chapter, an overview of physiological changes in endocrine system with aging and their implications in management of endocrine diseases of elderly have been described.

"Ageing is just another word for living"

—Cindy Joseph

DIABETES IN ELDERLY

Glucose homeostasis is under tight control of insulin, but gradually it is altered with increasing chronological age. Fasting and 2-hour after 75 g oral glucose load, glucose concentrations gradually increase with age in normal healthy elderly individuals. Elderly individuals have disordered insulin secretion with reduction in both amplitude and reduced frequency of ultradian pulses, which become less effective in suppressing hepatic glucose output. There is also gradual decrease in glucose disposal by muscle due to decrease in insulin action attributable to changing ratio of fat to lean muscle mass.

Although there is a continuum of risk of the development of diabetes, the risk reaches plateau or even declines after the age of 85 years. Prevalence of diabetes is 33% and of prediabetes is nearly 50% in the US population aged 65 years or older. Prevalence of diabetes in elderly in India varies in rural and urban areas. In urban area, prevalence varies from 3.33 to 30% in various studies.

CLINICAL PRESENTATION

Osmotic symptoms are rarely present in elderly population as renal threshold of glucose increases with age and thirst is impaired with aging. Symptoms are generally nonspecific such as confusion, delayed healing of ulcer and boils, and urinary incontinence. Several unique syndromes occur in elderly patients with diabetes such as diabetic neuropathic cachexia, diabetic amyotrophy, malignant otitis externa, and spontaneously resolving diabetic bullae on feet.

Risk of microvascular complications is also increased and risk of macrovascular events is doubled in elderly patients with diabetes compared with controls (**Fig. 1**). Risk of severe and fatal hypoglycemia increases with use of oral hypoglycemic agents and insulin in elderly patients with type 2 diabetes mellitus. Increased risk of hypoglycemia in elderly is related to reduced response of counterregulatory hormone especially glucagon and reduced awareness of autonomic warning symptoms.

DIAGNOSIS

Fasting plasma glucose and glycated hemoglobin (HbA1c) are recommended to diagnose diabetes or prediabetes in patients with aged 65 years or old. If fasting plasma glucose or HbA1c suggestive of prediabetes, glucose tolerance test is advisable. In high-risk patients with obesity, first-degree relative having diabetes, history of cardiovascular disease (CVD), hypertension (>140/90 mm Hg or on therapy for hypertension), high-density lipoprotein (HDL) cholesterol level <35 mg/dL (0.90 mmol/L) and/or a triglyceride level >250 mg/dL (2.82 mmol/L), sleep apnea or physical inactivity, and ethnic susceptibility glucose tolerance test are indicated for diagnosis of diabetes mellitus.

Diagnosis of diabetes is based on the American Diabetes Association (ADA) criteria: symptoms of diabetes plus a casual (any time of day without regard to time since last meal) plasma glucose value of >200 mg/dL (the classic symptoms of diabetes include fatigue, polyuria, polydipsia, and unexplained weight loss); a fasting plasma glucose value of >126 mg/dL (fasting is defined as no caloric intake for at least 8 hours); or a plasma glucose value in the 2-hour sample of the oral glucose tolerance test (OGTT) of >200 mg/dL (**Table 1**).

MANAGEMENT

Glycemic target: Glycemic target should be individualized depending on age and comorbidities of patient. Target fasting blood glucose (FBG) is 90–130 mg/dL and HbA1c <7.5% can be applied to patients with good health with few coexisting illness and intact cognitive function and functional status. Patient with poor health with multiple comorbidities and cognitive and functional impairment should have liberal glycemic targets of FBG 100–180 mg/dL and HbA1c <8.5%. Similarly, blood pressure goal should be <140/90 mm Hg in patients with good health and

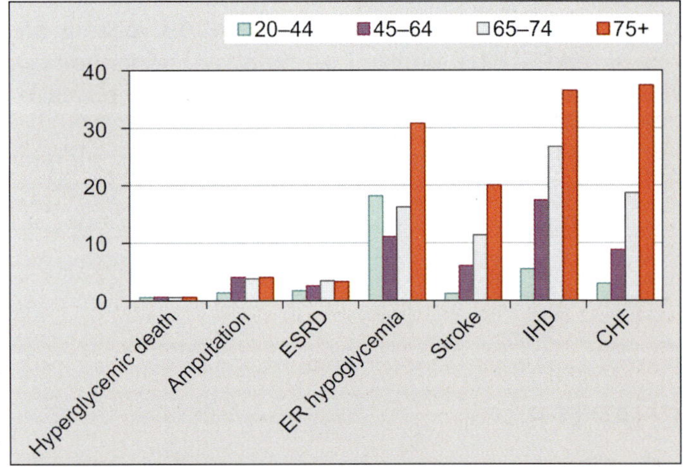

(ER: emergency room)

FIGURE 1: Incidence (per 1,000) of major diabetes complications according to age among adults with diabetes, 2009.

Source: Reproduced from Centers for Disease Control and Prevention (CDC). (2019). Diabetes Data and Statistics.

TABLE 1 Criteria for diagnosis of diabetes.

Fasting plasma glucose	≥126 mg/dL	After no calorie intake at least 8 h
2-hour plasma glucose	≥200 mg/dL	2 hours after 75 g glucose
Random plasma glucose	≥200 mg/dL	Without oral glucose but with classical symptoms
Glycated hemoglobin (HbA1c)	≥6.5%	Measured in certified laboratory

TABLE 2 Treatment targets for older patients with diabetes.

Patients characteristics and overall health	HbA1c goal	Fasting blood glucose	BP goal
Generally healthy (zero to two comorbidities)	<7.5%	90–130 mg/dL	<140/90 mm Hg
Intermediate health (three or more comorbidities)	<8.0%	90–150 mg/dL	<140/90 mm Hg
Very poor health (end-stage medical condition)	<8.5%	100–180 mg/dL	<150/90 mm Hg

<150/90 mm Hg in patients with poor health (**Table 2**). Statins should be prescribed to patients with good health unless contraindicated, while likelihood of benefit should be considered for patients with poor health.

Lifestyle management: Diabetes in aging population is associated with sarcopenia and frailty, which also occurs due to inadequate nutrition intake. Optimal nutrition with adequate protein intake combined with exercise program (that includes aerobic activity and resistance training) is recommended in elderly to prevent sarcopenia.

Pharmacological therapy: Metformin is first-line agent for older adults with diabetes. Evidence has emerged that metformin also delays senescence by mobilizing endogenous progenitor cells and enhancing regenerative potential of cells. Dipeptidyl peptidase-4 (DPP-4) inhibitors along with metformin, if dual therapy is needed, are most appropriate, which have minimal risk of hypoglycemia. Short-acting sulfonylureas such as glipizide may be preferred, but glinides are safer than sulfonylureas. Thiazolidinediones should be used very cautiously in those with at-risk of congestive heart failure and at-risk for falls or fractures. Glucagon-like peptide-1 (GLP-1) receptor agonists have shown cardiovascular benefits, but they are injectable and can cause poor appetite, nausea, vomiting, and weight loss. Sodium-glucose cotransporter-2 (SGLT-2) inhibitors are not safe in frail elderly but in tolerant individuals they have cardiorenal advantages. If patient needs insulin therapy, once-daily basal insulin injection therapy is reasonable option in many older patients.

THYROID DISORDERS IN AGING

Normal aging is accompanied by rising thyroid-stimulating hormone (TSH). Bioactivity may also change with increasing age making TSH less effective or set point of TSH receptor may increase making receptor less functional. Free thyroxine (T4) concentration remains stable with increasing age, whereas free triiodothyronine (T3) concentrations decrease over the course of life span.

HYPOTHYROIDISM

Etiology: Hashimoto's thyroiditis is most prevalent etiology of hypothyroidism in elderly above 60 years. Other causes are listed in **Box 1**.

BOX 1 Etiology of hypothyroidism in elderly.

- Hashimoto's thyroiditis
- Postsurgical hypothyroidism
- Postablative hypothyroidism
- Secondary hypothyroidism
- External beam radiation
- Drug-induced hypothyroidism
- Infiltrative disorders of the thyroid gland

Clinical presentation: Symptoms and signs of overt hypothyroidism in elderly include fatigue, weakness, constipation, reduced appetite, hair loss, and dry skin. These symptoms can be attributed to aging and, therefore, diagnosis of overt hypothyroidism is often overlooked.

Diagnosis of subclinical hypothyroidism on the basis of symptoms is a challenge in elderly. In a community-based study of individuals aged 70–79 years, investigators showed that subclinical hypothyroidism was associated with increased walking speed and retention of physical function across a 2-year period compared with euthyroidism.

Long-term consequences: Overt thyroid failure affects cognition, well-being, and cardiovascular system. Subclinical hypothyroidism can be progressive, but serum TSH concentrations <10 mIU/L are usually reversible to within normal range. In large study of 422,242 individuals, progression from slightly increased serum TSH concentrations (5.5–10 mIU/L) to high concentrations (>10 mIU/L) was reported in 2.9% of cases over a 5-year period.

Cardiac effects: Although subclinical hypothyroidism is associated with increased risk of atherosclerosis in younger individual, not in elderly subjects older than 65 years, in fact, in 85-year-old healthy individuals, subclinical hypothyroidism was associated with lower all-cause and cardiovascular mortality.

Levothyroxine treatment: In older patients, levothyroxine requirements are lower than in younger patients. The American Thyroid Association recommends initiating lower doses of levothyroxine to avoid overtreatment and iatrogenic hyperthyroidism. A treatment algorithm for hypothyroidism in elderly is given in **Flowchart 1**.

HYPERTHYROIDISM

Etiology: Most common cause of hyperthyroidism in elderly is Graves' disease, but number of studies have found toxic nodular hyperthyroidism to be underlying etiology

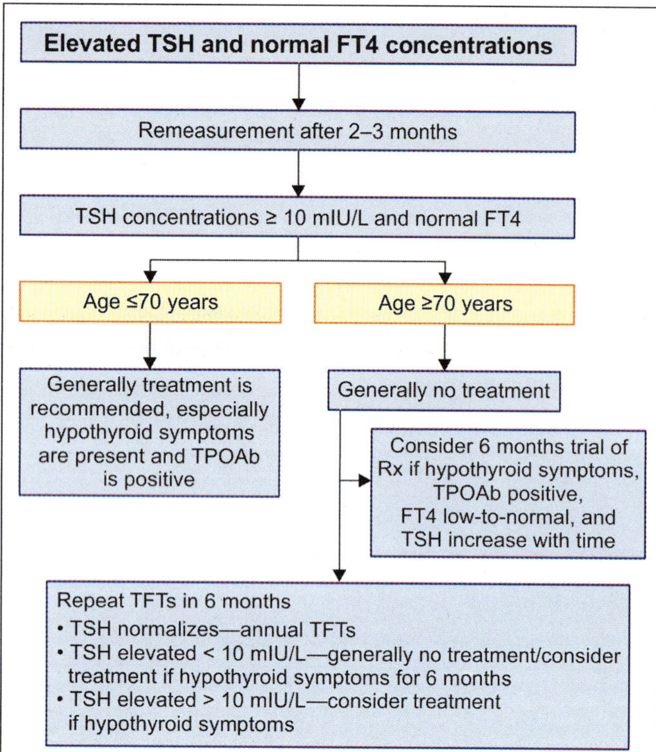

(TFTs: thyroid function tests; TPOAb: thyroid peroxidase antibody)

FLOWCHART 1: Treatment algorithm of hypothyroidism in elderly.

in 28–65% of individuals in elderly. Other causes include subacute thyroiditis, amiodarone-induced thyrotoxicosis, and thyrotoxicosis induced by iodine-containing contrast agents or drugs.

Subclinical hyperthyroidism can be due to exogenous levothyroxine intake or due to endogenous variant, which is caused by same etiologies that result in overt hyperthyroidism. Exogenous subclinical hyperthyroidism is more frequent than endogenous subclinical hyperthyroidism due to widespread use of levothyroxine to treat hypothyroidism and for suppressive therapy in patients with thyroid cancer.

Clinical presentation: Symptoms and signs of hyperthyroidism are less frequent in older patient than younger people. Patient can present as cardiac arrhythmias such as atrial fibrillation, weight loss (apathetic thyrotoxicosis), or heart failure.

Long-term consequences:

Cardiovascular consequences: Subclinical hyperthyroidism is also associated with increased risk of atrial fibrillation and increased risk of all-cause and cardiovascular mortality when serum TSH level is <0.1 mIU/L.

Skeletal consequences: Overt hyperthyroidism is associated with increased risk of osteoporotic hip fractures and spine fracture in women aged >65 years of age with baseline serum TSH <0.1 mIU/L compared with normal TSH concentration.

Dementia: Overt hyperthyroidism has been associated with impairment of concentration and changes in mood and perception. A meta-analysis of 11 prospective cohort studies reported an association of subclinical hyperthyroidism with increased risk of dementia.

Treatment: It depends on the etiology. For toxic nodular goiter, radioactive iodine is preferred. Surgery is alternative approach but course of antithyroid drugs should always be considered as rates of remission is higher in older subjects.

For subclinical hyperthyroidism, latest guidelines recommend treatment after diagnosis of underlying disorder based on the level of TSH suppression. When serum TSH is <0.1 mIU/L and confirmed after 3–6 months period, treatment is advised in individuals with hyperthyroid symptoms, all individuals with 65 years or more age, postmenopausal women not on bisphosphonates or estrogen, and patients with cardiac risk factors, heart disease, or osteoporosis. In serum TSH between 0.1 and 0.5 mIU/L, treatment should be considered only for individuals above 65 years or more age and in patients with cardiac disease, osteoporosis, and hyperthyroid symptoms.

THYROID NODULES AND CANCER

Thyroid nodules are more frequent in elderly and there is linear increase with age in both presence of nodules and absolute number of nodules per patient. Approximately, 50% of individuals aged 65 years have thyroid nodules by ultrasonography. Once identified, thyroid nodules should be evaluated by thyroid function tests, ultrasound, and fine-needle aspiration cytology. Differential diagnosis of thyroid nodularity includes benign and malignant nodules, multinodular goiter, autonomous functioning nodules, cysts, and inflammation or thyroiditis.

With advancing age, though prevalence of clinically relevant (>1 cm) nodules increases, however, risk of malignancy of such nodule decreases. In one of the study, it was demonstrated that nodular malignancy risk in youngest cohort is 14.8% at the time of diagnosis in comparison to 5.6% in oldest cohort.

Generally, peak occurrence of thyroid cancer is between 51 and 60 years. Most common thyroid cancer in elderly is papillary thyroid cancer. Anaplastic thyroid cancer was most common among poorly differentiated. Larger tumor size, advanced tumor, node and metastasis (TNM) stage, more widespread disease, and relative increase in the frequency of more aggressive histological subtypes are features of thyroid cancer in elderly. Advanced age is also risk factor for worse prognosis for thyroid cancer.

Treatment of differentiated thyroid cancer: Cornerstone of therapy for differentiated thyroid cancer is surgical resection, with radioiodine ablation and TSH suppression by thyroid hormone. Serum thyroglobulin and neck ultrasound are used for monitoring. Patients with progressive or metastatic disease may benefit from radioactive iodine ablation (RAIA), repeat surgery, or chemotherapy.

In elderly population, decision to pursue surgery and extent of surgery (total thyroidectomy vs. lobectomy) depends on associated comorbidities and life expectancy. Risk of surgical complications such as hypoparathyroidism, recurrent laryngeal nerve injury, and hematoma and wound infection may be higher in surgical population. Lobectomy may be considered in selected patients with low-risk disease having multiple comorbid conditions. Generally, patients with high and intermediate risk should be considered for RAIA with ^{131}I.

Thyroid-stimulating hormone suppression goal should be individualized in elderly patients. Patients with comorbid cardiac disease and/or osteoporosis with intermediate risk disease recurrence should be managed with TSH targets in the low, but not fully suppressed range to minimize adverse effects of therapy.

GROWTH HORMONE AND AGING

There is a progressive decline of growth hormone (GH) secretion by approximately 15% for every decade of life. There is marked reduction in GH amplitude with little change in frequency and loss of nocturnal sleep-related GH pulses. Growth hormone-binding protein (GHBP) also decreases from 60 years of age parallel to decrease in GH receptors with age. Circulating level of insulin-like growth factor-1 (IGF-1), main mediator of trophic effects of GH, also declines with age due to direct results of decrease in GH.

CLINICAL CONSEQUENCES

Age-related increase in body mass index, reduction in muscle mass and bone density, increase in total body fat, adverse changes in lipoprotein profile and decline in cognitive function, sarcopenic obesity, and frailty are consequences of age-related decline in GH secretion. Changes in the somatotropic axis are associated with increased survival, but no formal longevity studies have been performed in humans with dwarfism.

GROWTH HORMONE THERAPY

A large literature has led to a general consensus that GH replacement therapy can reverse many abnormalities in adult GH deficiency such as reduction of fat mass, increased lean body mass, improved exercise capacity and cardiac function, improved bone mineral density, and enhanced quality of life. This led to interest in administering GH or GH secretagogues in elderly population.

It was found that there was no positive effects of GH on muscle strength and muscle function. In contrast, when GH was administered in combination with resistance exercise training, significant positive effects on muscle mass and strength were observed.

Elderly peoples treated with GH are significantly more likely to develop adverse effects such as softtissue edema, arthralgias, carpal tunnel syndrome, gynecomastia, and hyperglycemia.

MENOPAUSE

Menopause is permanent cessation of menstruation resulting from loss of ovarian follicular function and diagnosed retrospectively after 12 months of amenorrhea. Average age of menopause is 51.4 years. The lengthening of cycle duration, missed periods, and prolonged intervals of amenorrhea signal onset of late menopausal transition, which end with near-total exhaustion of ovarian follicles and final menstrual period around the age of 51 years.

Hormonal changes throughout menopausal transition and menopause are characterized by increased luteinizing hormone (LH) and follicle-stimulating hormone (FSH) pulse amplitude. These changes are due to altered feedback resulting from ovarian decline in sex steroids inhibin A and B production.

PHYSIOLOGICAL CHANGES

In women 45–49 years of age, the incidence of cardiovascular disease is three times lower than men of same age. The Framingham study had shown that by age of 75–79 years, woman's risk of heart disease increases and equals to man's risk for age. Associations exist between low endogenous sex hormone-binding globulin (SHBG) and estradiol and elevated FSH with increased carotid-intima media thickness (CIMT) in perimenopausal women. Lipoprotein changes associated with menopause were increased low-density lipoprotein (LDL) and decreased cardioprotective HDL also contribute to increased cardiovascular risk. There is also increase in procoagulant factors such as plasminogen activator inhibitor-1 and factor 8, which cause procoagulant state.

Osteoporosis is major concern for postmenopausal women. At menopause, there is accelerated bone loss, 5% trabecular and 1.5% of the total bone mass is lost per year. In first 20 years after menopause, there is 50% reduction in trabecular bone and 30% reduction in cortical bone.

Vasomotor symptoms and hot flashes adversely affect quality of life. Hot flashes can occur in 85% of menopausal women. Mean [standard deviation (SD)] duration of vasomotor symptoms noted without HT was 5.2 (3.8) years. In past, hot flashes were thought to be related to withdrawal of estrogen, but there is no acute change in serum of estrogen and FSH. More recent work has found that activation of neurokinin 3 receptor in kisspeptin, neurokinin B, and dynorphin (KNDy) neurons can cause vasodilatation.

Loss of libido is a prevalent complaint in women of all ages and is present in approximately 9% of postmenopausal women. Causes for a menopause-related decline in sexual desire may be related to a drop in both estrogen and testosterone with decline in ovarian function and aging, respectively. After menopause, breast tissue is gradually replaced with increasing amounts of adipose tissue. Mammography becomes more effective for diagnosing breast cancer due to decrease in density.

MENOPAUSAL TREATMENT

Nonhormonal treatment:

Antidepressants: Selective serotonin reuptake inhibitors such as paroxetine have been found to reduce hot flashes. Long-acting paroxetine 7.5 mg is Food and Drug Administration (FDA) approved for treatment of hot flashes. Venlafaxine, serotonin norpeinephrine reuptake inhibitor, has also shown encouraging results in management of hot flashes. It has been used in dose of 37.5–150 mg/day.

Neurokinin B receptor inhibitors: In phase II trial, Oral NK3 receptor antagonist fezolinetant has showed 45% decrease in number of hot flashes per week compared with placebo. This drug is not associated with side effects of estrogens therapy.

Hormonal treatment:

Estrogens: Hormonal therapy with estrogen is the most effective therapy for bothersome menopausal symptoms. In addition, it acts as antiresorptive and also shown to reduce incidence of colon cancer by almost 40%. But the Women's Health Initiative (WHI) study had clearly shown increased risk of cardiovascular complications (coronary heart disease, stroke, and venous thromboembolism) and increased incidence of breast cancer. Subsequent reanalysis of data from WHI has led to interpretation that peri- and early postmenopausal women derive cardiovascular benefits from hormone replacement therapy (HRT) and estrogens are atheroprotective, if used in early phase of atherosclerosis development. So, current consensus is that HRT is usually prescribed for women 45–60 years of age who are experiencing moderate-to-severe vasomotor symptoms for maximum duration of 5 years having no contraindication to HRT (**Box 2**).

Estrogen therapy is available in various forms and routes. The efficacy of oral 17β-estradiol (1 mg daily), transdermal 17-β estradiol (0.05 mg daily), and conjugated estrogen (0.625 mg daily) is almost same with abolition of hot flashes in approximately 80% of women. Transdermal formulation has lower risk of venous thromboembolism, stroke, vaginal bleeding, and breast tenderness. Starting dose should be low (0.5 mg oral estradiol, 0.025 mg transdermal). Women with intact uterus need progestins.

BOX 2	Contraindications to hormone replacement therapy.
• History of stroke	
• History of breast cancer	
• History of venous thromboembolism	
• Coronary artery disease	
• Active liver disease	
• Unexplained vaginal bleeding	
• Thrombophilic state	
• Active gallbladder disease	

Selective estrogen receptor modulators: Selective estrogen receptor modulators (SERMs) have variable antiestrogenic and estrogenic actions in different tissues. Long-term treatment of menopausal patients with breast cancer with SERMs has prevented development of new breast cancer by 40% and number of cardiovascular incidents decreased by 70% and the age-related decrease in bone mineral density was also prevented.

Raloxifene causes increase in bone mineral density with significant reduction in vertebral fracture risk and neutral effects on incidence of cardiovascular events but higher incidence of stroke and venous thromboembolic events.

ANDROPAUSE

Men do not undergo equivalent of menopause. Testicular volume in men older than 75 years is decreased by 30% and number of Sertoli cells is reduced, reflected by increase in FSH concentrations and decrease in the ratio of serum inhibin B to FSH and decrease in fertility.

Normal serum testosterone circadian rhythmicity is blunted. Other male hormone concentrations such as dihydrotestosterone and androstenedione also decrease with age, but serum concentrations of estradiol do not decrease with aging.

CLINICAL CONSEQUENCES

No clinical consequences of decline in serum testosterone with age are known with certainty. Many epidemiological studies of older men have reported associations between low testosterone and health outcomes, but these associations are weak. Sexual dysfunction was observed at testosterone concentrations < 8 nmol/L. Decline in multiple domains of cognition such as verbal memory, visual memory, spatial abilities, and executive function is associated with decline in testosterone. In meta-analysis of epidemiological studies of community-dwelling men, low testosterone was associated with increased risk of all-cause and CVD death. In the Osteoporotic Fractures in Men (MrOS) study, odds of osteoporosis in men with testosterone was <200 ng/dL were 3.7-fold higher than in men with normal testosterone level.

Diagnostic criteria have been proposed for late-onset hypogonadism by Wu and colleagues from the European Male Aging Study (EMAS): Presence of three sexual symptoms (i.e., poor morning erections, decreased sexual interest, and erectile dysfunction) together with serum total testosterone levels <320 ng/dL and free testosterone levels <6.4 ng/dL.

TESTOSTERONE REPLACEMENT THERAPY

The Endocrine Society Clinical Practice guidelines for testosterone therapy suggested following recommendations:

- Testosterone therapy should be offered on individualized basis to older men who have symptoms and conditions suggestive of testosterone deficiency

- Testosterone therapy is not recommended in older men who have low testosterone in absence of symptoms and conditions suggestive of testosterone deficiency
- Testosterone therapy should not be initiated until further evaluation, if the patient has prostate nodule and prostate-specific antigen (PSA) >4 ng/mL or >3 ng/mL in men at increased risk of prostate cancer
- Monitoring is recommended with target value at low normal range for young men (300–400 ng/dL)
- Prostate-specific antigen and hematocrit should be measured every 3–6 months after initiation of testosterone treatment

RECOMMENDED READINGS

1. van den Beld AW, Lamberts SW. Endocrinology and aging. In: Melmed S, Koenig R, Rosen C, Auchus R, Goldfine A (Eds). Williams Textbook of Endocrinology, 14th edition. Philadelphia: Elsevier; 2019. pp. 1179-95.
2. van den Beld AW, Kaufman JM, Zillikens MC, Lamberts SWJ, Egan JM, van der Lely AJ. The physiology of endocrine systems with ageing. Lancet Diabetes Endocrinol. 2018;6:647-58.
3. Chaker L, Cappola AR, Mooijaart SP, Peeters RP. Clinical aspects of thyroid function during ageing. Lancet Diabetes Endocrinol. 2018;6:733-42.
4. Boelaert K. Thyroid dysfunction in the elderly. Nat Rev Endocrinol. 2013;9:194-204.
5. Meneilly GS, Tessier D. Diabetes in elderly adults. J Gerontol A Biol Sci Med Sci. 2001 Jan;56(1):M5-13.
6. Sesti G, Incalzi RA, Bonora E, Consoli A, Giaccari A, Maggi S, et al. Management of diabetes in older adults. Nutr Metab Cardiovasc Dis. 2018;28:206-18.
7. Ross DS, Burch HB, Cooper DS, Greenlee MC, Laurberg P, Maia AL, et al. 2016 American Thyroid Association Guidelines for Diagnosis and Management of Hyperthyroidism and Other Causes of Thyrotoxicosis. Thyroid. 2016;26:1343-421.
8. Bhasin S, Brito JP, Cunningham GR, Hayes FJ, Hodis HN, Matsumoto AM, et al. Testosterone Therapy in Men with Hypogonadism: An Endocrine Society Clinical Practice Guideline. J Clin Endocrinol Metab. 2018;103:1715-44.
9. Garcia JM, Marriam GR, Kargi AY. (2019). Growth Hormone in Aging. [online] Available from https://www.ncbi.nlm.nih.gov/books/NBK279163/.
10. Lechner MG, Hershman J. (2018). Thyroid Nodules and Cancer in Older Adults. [online] Available from https://www.ncbi.nlm.nih.gov/books/NBK278969/.
11. Roeca C, Al-Safi Z, Santoro N, Feingold KR, Anawalt B, Boyce A, et al. (2018). The Postmenopausal Woman. [online] Available from https://pubmed.ncbi.nlm.nih.gov/25905354/.

CHAPTER 127

COVID-19 and Endocrine Disorders

Sanjay K Bhadada, Rimesh Pal

ABSTRACT

The novel coronavirus disease (COVID-19), caused by the severe acute respiratory syndrome coronavirus 2 (SARS-CoV-2), primarily affects the lungs. However, the angiotensin-converting enzyme 2 (ACE2), the enzyme that acts as a receptor for SARS-CoV-2, is widely expressed in the human body including various endocrine organ systems. As a result, these endocrine organs might be affected either by direct viral intrusion or via the indirect effect of cytokines induced by the virus in the host. Although clinical evidence with regard to endocrine involvement in COVID-19 is limited and more data are expected to emerge as the pandemic wages, observations can be extrapolated from the SARS outbreak in 2003.

Hypothalamo-pituitary, thyroid, pancreatic β-cell, and testicular involvements have been reported in SARS. Considering the marked similarity in the genomic sequences of the SARS-CoV and the SARS-CoV-2, involvement of endocrine organs might be speculated in COVID-19 as well. Hitherto, thyroid involvement in the form of subacute thyroiditis, thyrotoxicosis, and hypothyroidism has all been reported in COVID-19. Besides, patients with COVID-19 have been shown to mount an adequate and robust cortisol response although occasional cases of primary adrenal insufficiency secondary to bilateral adrenal hemorrhagic infarction have been reported. In addition, although hyperglycemia in hospitalized patients with COVID-19 is not unknown and often multifactorial, cases of new-onset diabetes mellitus after COVID-19 have also been described. Lastly, male gonadal involvement in the form of primary testicular damage and hypocalcemia secondary to altered calcium metabolism have also been reported in association with COVID-19.

"True wisdom comes to each of us when we realize how little we understand about life, ourselves, and the world around us"

—Socrates

INTRODUCTION

The novel COVID-19 has affected over 57 million cases and inflicted >1.3 million casualties worldwide. The disease primarily affects the lungs, leading to pneumonia, often complicated by an inflammatory cytokine storm. Besides, the causative SARS-CoV-2 also affects the heart, kidneys, vascular endothelium, neural pathways, and the pancreas. Similarly, COVID-19 has been reported to affect multiple endocrine organs. Besides, there are various speculations of involvement of other endocrine systems, most of which are based on observations from the original SARS outbreak in 2003. Most of the speculations are fueled by the fact that ACE2, which acts as a receptor for the novel SARS-CoV-2, is expressed on multiple endocrine tissues.

This chapter outlines the endocrinological implications of COVID-19 that have been summarized in **Table 1**.

HYPOTHALAMO-PITUITARY AXIS

Involvement of the hypothalamo-pituitary axis could result from *direct or indirect injury*. Direct injury may relate to the ACE2 receptor-mediated SARS-CoV-2 infection of neuronal cells causing cell edema and necrosis. In fact, ACE2 expression has been demonstrated in the hypothalamus. The indirect effects on the HPA are mediated by cytokines, namely, interleukin-1 (IL-1), IL-6, and tumor necrosis factor-alpha (TNF-α) that can alter the hypothalamo-pituitary axis. Also, inflammation may result in damage to the pituitary and hypothalamus resulting in hypophysitis.

Biochemical evidence of hypothalamo-pituitary axis involvement in SARS was first reported by Leow et al. Of 61 SARS patients examined at 3 months postrecovery and thereafter annually, 24 patients (40%) showed signs of central hypocortisolism, majority of which resolved within a year. A small percentage of patients also had central hypothyroidism and low dehydroepiandrosterone sulfate. The authors had proposed the possibility of a reversible hypophysitis or a direct hypothalamic damage that could have led to a state of transient hypothalamo-pituitary dysfunction. Similar involvement of the hypothalamo-pituitary axis in COVID-19 might be speculated; in fact, it has been hypothesized that *post-COVID fatigue syndrome* could be attributed to secondary hypocortisolism. To lend support, hypothalamic and pituitary involvement has been demonstrated on imaging in COVID-19 patients presenting with ophthalmoparesis. Thus, it would be prudent to measure serum cortisol 12 weeks after recovery from COVID-19, especially those complaining of marked fatigue and lassitude. Any biochemical evidence of secondary hypocortisolism should be substantiated by sellar imaging to rule out the possibility of an underlying hypophysitis.

An autopsy report by Wei et al. demonstrated an increased expression of prolactin (PRL), follicle-stimulating hormone (FSH), and luteinizing hormone (LH), and a reduced expression of growth hormone (GH), thyroid-stimulating hormone (TSH), and adrenocorticotropic hormone (ACTH) in the anterior pituitary cells of five SARS patients compared to controls. These observations were supported by the serum levels of the corresponding hormones. Similarly, in COVID-19, two studies have shown low TSH, triiodothyronine (T3), and/or thyroxine (T4) suggesting a possible central mechanism mediated by

TABLE 1 Possible effects of COVID-19 on the endocrine organ systems.

Endocrine organ system involved	Possible pathogenic mechanisms	Clinical implications
Hypothalamo-pituitary axis	• Direct injury by SARS-CoV-2 to the hypothalamus and/or pituitary • Indirect immune-mediated injury to the hypothalamus and/or pituitary	• Secondary hypocortisolism and/or hypothyroidism • May contribute to post-COVID fatigue syndrome
Thyroid gland	• Direct injury by SARS-CoV-2 to the thyroid gland • Indirect immune-mediated injury to the thyroid gland	Atypical subacute thyroiditis
Adrenal glands	• Direct injury by SARS-CoV-2 to the adrenal glands • Bilateral adrenal hemorrhagic infarction • Anti-ACTH antibodies • Downregulation of ACE2	• Hypocortisolism • Hypokalemia
Islets of Langerhans	Direct injury by SARS-CoV-2 to the pancreatic β-cells	New-onset diabetes mellitus
Male gonadal system	Direct injury by SARS-CoV-2 to the testis	Primary hypogonadism
Bone mineral metabolism	Utilization of calcium for viral entry and replication	Hypocalcemia

cytokines. In another report, levels of LH were found to be elevated in patients with COVID-19.

Elevated IL-6, as reported in COVID-19 patients, is also known to suppress insulin-like growth factor-1 (IGF-1). Reduced IGF-1 has been speculated as a possible risk factor for autism in infants born to pregnant mothers with COVID-19; nevertheless, low IGF-1 has not yet been demonstrated in COVID-19 patients.

THYROID GLAND

A study performed during the SARS outbreak had reported lower levels of serum T3 and T4 in patients with SARS compared with controls. The low T3/T4 levels could be due to considerable destruction of the thyroid follicular cells that was demonstrated in SARS patients on autopsy studies. Data about COVID-19 are forthcoming. *Multiple cases of subacute thyroiditis* after COVID-19 have been reported. Another recent report by Muller et al. has highlighted the prevalence of atypical subacute thyroiditis in COVID-19 patients receiving high-intensity care. Of the 8 patients who were followed, 2 developed hypothyroidism and 6 had suppressed TSH suggesting long-term effects of COVID-19 on thyroid functions. They were negative for thyroid antibodies. A cell-mediated immune mechanism was proposed by the authors to explain these findings. Of 287 hospitalized patients with COVID-19, 58 patients (20.2%) had thyrotoxicosis, 15 (5.2%) had hypothyroidism, and 214 (74.6%) had normal thyroid function.

On the contrary, Huang et al. reported low normal T3, T4, and TSH in COVID-19 patients without clinically apparent hypothyroidism. In 50 patients with laboratory-confirmed COVID-19 without a history of thyroid disease who underwent thyroid function testing during their course of COVID-19 infection, TSH lower than the normal range was present in 56% (28/50) of the patients. The levels of TSH and serum total T3 of the patients with COVID-19 were significantly lower than those of the healthy control group and non-COVID-19 pneumonia patients. The degree of the decrease in TSH and T3 levels was positively correlated with disease severity.

Considering the commonality of thyroid involvement, it would be wise to measure thyroid function tests in COVID-19 patients, especially those with severe and critical disease. Patients with subacute thyroiditis with concomitant thyrotoxic symptoms should be managed conservatively with beta-blockers and/or glucocorticoids. Similarly, COVID-19 patients with low T3, T4, and TSH concordant with sick-euthyroid syndrome would require thyroxine supplementation only when serum T4 < 4 μg/dL as per standard protocol.

Involvement of thyroid gland in COVID-19 is supported by the fact that ACE2 is expressed in the thyroid follicular cells. Notably, lymphocytic infiltration has also been reported in the interstitium of thyroid tissue in three patients with COVID-19 on autopsy.

ADRENAL GLANDS

Autopsy studies on SARS patients had demonstrated *adrenal necrosis, vasculitis, and adrenal infiltration* with monocytes and lymphocytes. In addition, viral antigens and genomic sequence of SARS-CoV were demonstrated in the adrenal glands, which may reflect the direct cytopathic effect of the virus. Similarly, viral invasion of the adrenocortical cells by SARS-CoV-2 is not unlikely as ACE2 is also expressed on the adrenal glands. Occasional cases of acute adrenal infarction and primary adrenal insufficiency secondary to bilateral adrenal hemorrhages have been reported in COVID-19 patients.

One of the primary immunoinvasive strategies employed by the SARS-CoV, like influenza virus, is to knock down the host's cortisol stress response. To achieve the same, SARS-CoV expresses certain amino acid sequences that act as molecular mimics of the host ACTH. The first 24 amino acids of ACTH ($ACTH_{1-24}$) are highly conserved between different mammalian species while $ACTH_{25-39}$ represents the less conserved region. Six amino acids at position 26, 29, 31, 33, 37, and 39 represent the antigenically important positions for mammalian ACTH. SARS (and influenza virus) contain many permutations of amino acid sequences with homology to these ACTH key residues. Antibodies produced by the host to counteract the virus, in turn, would unknowingly destroy the host ACTH, thereby blunting the cortisol rise. The same mechanism might be operational in COVID-19; this would imply a high prevalence of relative adrenal insufficiency or critical illness-related corticosteroid insufficiency. However critical illness-related corticosteroid insufficiency is uncommon in the setting of COVID-19.

A recent report by Tan et al. has shown that COVID-19 patients could mount a robust and appropriate adrenal response; COVID-19 patients had higher serum cortisol compared to non-COVID-19 patients although disease severity was not matched between the two groups making head-to-head comparison biased. Besides, baseline serum cortisol was found to be a reliable predictor of mortality in COVID-19 with doubling of serum cortisol being associated with a 42% increase in mortality after adjusting for age, comorbidities, and other laboratory tests. Median survival was significantly lower in patients with cortisol concentrations of >744 nmol/L in the cohort. Conspicuously, however, the analysis did not include disease severity. A multivariate analysis performed after adjusting for disease severity might have been reflective of the true potential of cortisol in predicting clinical outcomes in COVID-19 patients.

The landmark RECOVERY trial had shown that low-dose dexamethasone was associated with significant benefits in critically ill COVID-19 patients. The trial had demonstrated that the drug reduced the risk of mortality by 17% in ventilated COVID-19 patients. However, the beneficial effects of dexamethasone in critically ill COVID-19 patients are unlikely to be due to adrenal insufficiency and possibly relate to the anti-inflammatory effect of glucocorticoids. Hence, routine measurement of serum cortisol to guide glucocorticoid therapy even in critically ill patients with COVID-19 is not rewarding and hence, not indicated. Endocrine implications of exogenous glucocorticoid use in COVID-19 patients include risk for long-term suppression of the hypothalamo-pituitary-adrenal axis, infections, and dysglycemia.

Apart from alteration in serum cortisol, perturbation in the renin–angiotensin–aldosterone axis has also been reported in COVID-19. Severe COVID-19 has been associated with hypokalemia; a biochemical abnormality that has been attributed to the downregulation of ACE2. In normal physiology, ACE2 breaks down angiotensin-II and to a little extent, angiotensin-I to smaller peptides. The downregulation of ACE2 following SARS-CoV-2 intrusion results in decreased degradation of angiotensin-II, increased aldosterone secretion, and subsequent increased urinary potassium loss, culminating in hypokalemia.

ISLETS OF LANGERHANS

Diabetes mellitus increases the risk of severe disease, acute respiratory distress syndrome (ARDS), and mortality in patients with COVID-19. There exists a two-way interaction between diabetes mellitus and COVID-19; while diabetes mellitus increases the chances of poor prognosis in patients with COVID-19, the hyperinflammatory state associated with COVID-19 tends to worsen dysglycemia in patients with diabetes mellitus.

Besides, there are speculations regarding *pancreatic β-cell damage by the SARS-CoV-2*. ACE2 is expressed in the pancreas with its mRNA expression being higher in the pancreas than in the lungs. The ACE2 expression is seen both on the exocrine pancreas and the endocrine islets. Accordingly, Yang et al. had reported that glucocorticoid-naïve patients with SARS had significantly higher fasting plasma glucose levels as compared to patients with non-SARS pneumonia. In another study, SARS-CoV-mediated damage of the pancreatic β-cells was proposed as the plausible mechanism behind the development of "acute diabetes" in patients with SARS. In fact, immunohistochemistry and in-situ hybridization have identified SARS-CoV in the pancreas of patients who died of SARS.

Clinical evidence about COVID-19 is limited but forthcoming. COVID-19 has been reported to cause *exocrine pancreatic injury* of varying severity. Wang et al. had reported pancreatic damage in 17% of 52 COVID-19 patients biochemically manifesting as elevated serum amylase or lipase levels. McNabb-Baltar et al. also found isolated hyperlipasemia in COVID-19 patients.

Just like the exocrine pancreas, *damage to the endocrine pancreas* has been reported in COVID-19. SARS-CoV-2 infection has been reported to trigger type 1 diabetes mellitus with/without diabetic ketoacidosis suggesting either direct beta-cell cytotoxicity or an immune-mediated reaction. Autoantibody-negative insulin-dependent diabetes mellitus has also been reported after SARS-CoV-2 infection. However, hyperglycemia developing in the setting of COVID-19 could be a transient phenomenon precipitated by stress, cytokine storm, hypokalemia, glucocorticoids, and other drugs like lopinavir/ritonavir, interferon-β, and remdesivir.

Persistence of hyperglycemia even after recovery would point toward the possibility of a new-onset diabetes mellitus triggered by the preceding COVID-19 infection. Hence, it would be prudent to advice every COVID-19 patient with in-hospital hyperglycemia to repeat a fasting blood glucose and postprandial blood glucose at 6 weeks along with a glycated hemoglobin (HbA1c) at 12 weeks after discharge. A global database (CoviDIAB Project) has been established to collect information on patients with COVID-19 and high blood glucose.

THE GONADS

Human testes express ACE2, involving the Leydig cells, Sertoli cells, and spermatogonia. While the expression of ACE2 is markedly high in testicular cells, the expression of ACE2 in ovarian cells is relatively low, reflecting an increased sensitivity of the male gonadal system to SARS-CoV-mediated dysfunction. Accordingly, autopsy samples of the testis from SARS victims showed evidence of orchitis.

Data regarding involvement of the male gonadal system in COVID-19 are also available. A study in 81 Chinese men with COVID-19 showed that serum total testosterone (T) was lower (although not statistically significant), while serum LH was significantly higher as compared to 100 age-matched healthy men. Serum T:LH ratio was also significantly lower in COVID-19 patients and was negatively associated with disease severity. Another German study had documented that both levels of LH and FSH were elevated along with decreased levels of testosterone and dihydrotestosterone in critically ill male patients with COVID-19. Similarly, decreased total and free testosterone with increased LH levels were reported in severe COVID-19 cases and were significantly correlated with increased plasma lactate dehydrogenase, ferritin, elevated neutrophil levels, and reduced lymphocyte count. Elevated serum LH in men with COVID-19 hints toward a primary Leydig cell damage.

Testicular damage could be mediated directly by COVID-19 or could be a result of the florid immune response. In fact, testicular tissues of patients infected with SARS-CoV-2 showed the presence of inflammatory infiltrates in the seminiferous tubules, immunoglobulin G (IgG) deposition in the seminiferous epithelium, and degenerated germ cells, Leydig cells, and Sertoli cells, which suggest that the inflammatory responses might be playing a significant role in the testicular damage induced by COVID-19. Considering the magnitude of the pandemic and the fact that a large proportion of patients are young and are presently in their reproductive age, testicular function in young men recovering from COVID-19 perhaps needs to

TABLE 2 Endocrine investigations that could be considered in hospitalized and recovered patients of COVID-19.

Endocrine organ system	Investigations in hospitalized patients with COVID-19	Investigations in recovered patients with COVID-19
Hypothalamo-pituitary axis	None	Serum cortisol, TFT at 12 weeks
Thyroid gland	TFT	TFT at 12 weeks
Adrenal glands	None	Serum cortisol at 12 weeks
Islets of Langerhans	FPG, PPG, HbA1c	• FPG, PPG at 6 weeks* • FPG, PPG, HbA1c at 12 weeks*
Male gonadal system	None	LH, FSH, testosterone at 12 weeks
Bone mineral metabolism	Serum calcium, phosphate, 25-hydroxyvitamin D	None

*To be considered only in patients who have had in-hospital hyperglycemia.

be monitored periodically. A morning sample of serum T, LH, and FSH performed at 12 weeks after recovery would be adequate with seminal analysis being ordered only when hormonal profile is deranged. Certain questions like how frequently and how long one needs to monitor remain still unanswered.

Several data suggest that COVID-19 severity and case fatality is more in males than in females. The gender disparity is explained by abundance of estradiol present in females. Interestingly, estrogen can interfere with glycan-glycan and glycan-protein interactions between human ACE2 and SARS-CoV-2 spike protein and can block host cell entry of the virus. Besides, high levels of 17β-estradiol and progesterone can synergize to reduce the level of proinflammatory cytokines, enhance anti-inflammatory response and immune tolerance and induce the production of antibodies by B-lymphocytes. Hormonal treatments with estradiol and progesterone in patients diagnosed with COVID-19 could alleviate the cytokine storm by increasing the levels of antibodies.

BONE-MINERAL METABOLISM

Multiple hematological and biochemical parameters have emerged as potential biomarkers to predict severe disease and mortality in COVID-19. One such biochemical biomarker is hypocalcemia. Hypocalcemia is associated with severe disease, organ failure, increased likelihood of hospitalization, admission to the intensive care unit, need for mechanical ventilation, and death in COVID-19.

Hypocalcemia in COVID-19 could be a direct effect of SARS-CoV-2 or could result from an imbalance in parathyroid hormone (PTH) and/or 25-hydroxyvitamin D. In general, calcium is required for virus structure formation, entry, replication, and virion release. In vitro and animal studies with SARS-CoV (responsible for the SARS outbreak in 2003) had shown that the viral E gene encodes a small transmembrane protein that functions as a calcium ion channel.

It was also demonstrated that alteration in calcium homeostasis within the host cell could lead to the activation of inflammatory pathways resulting in lung cell damage. Considering the remarkable similarity between SARS-CoV-2 and SARS-CoV genomes, the same mechanism may be operational in COVID-19 as well. Besides, elevated levels of unbound and unsaturated fatty acids have been reported in COVID-19 patients. Unsaturated fatty acids can bind calcium, causing hypocalcemia. An alternate explanation could be a reduction in renal 1α-hydroxylase activity in patients with COVID-19. ACE2, the receptor for the SARS-CoV-2, is expressed in the proximal renal tubule, the predominant site of expression of renal 1α-hydroxylase. The impaired renal 1α-hydroxylase activity would reduce calcitriol production that could explain both hypocalcemia and hypophosphatemia.

Table 2 summarizes the proposed endocrinological investigations that could be contemplated in hospitalized and recovered patients with COVID-19.

CONCLUSION

Coronavirus disease is associated with multiple endocrine abnormalities predominantly involving the thyroid, the pancreatic β-cells, and the male gonad. However, as the pandemic wages on, more robust clinical evidence of involvement of other endocrine organs are expected to emerge. Nevertheless, physicians managing COVID-19 patients need to be aware of the endocrine implications of the disease, especially while dealing with COVID-19 survivors.

RECOMMENDED READINGS

1. Pal R, Banerjee M. COVID-19 and the endocrine system: exploring the unexplored. J Endocrinol Invest. 2020;43:1027-31.
2. Leow MK-S, Kwek DS-K, Ng AW-K, Ong K-C, Kaw GJ-L, Lee LS-U. Hypocortisolism in survivors of severe acute respiratory syndrome (SARS). Clin Endocrinol (Oxf). 2005;63:197-202.
3. Pal R. COVID-19, hypothalamo-pituitary-adrenal axis and clinical implications. Endocrine. 2020;68: 251-2.

4. Garg MK, Gopalakrishnan M, Yadav P, Misra S. Endocrine involvement in COVID-19: Mechanisms, clinical features, and implications for care. Indian J Endocrinol Metab. 2020;24:381-6.
5. Brancatella A, Ricci D, Viola N, Sgrò D, Santini F, Latrofa F. Subacute Thyroiditis After SARS-COV-2 Infection. J Clin Endocrinol Metab. 2020;105:2367-70.
6. Muller I, Cannavaro D, Dazzi D, Covelli D, Mantovani G, Muscatello A, et al. SARS-CoV-2-related atypical thyroiditis. Lancet Diabetes Endocrinol. 2020;8:739-41.
7. Tan T, Khoo B, Mills EG, Phylactou M, Patel B, Eng PC, et al. Cortisol concentrations and mortality from COVID-19 - Authors' reply. Lancet Diabetes Endocrinol. 2020;8:809-10.
8. Pal R, Banerjee M, Bhadada SK. Cortisol concentrations and mortality from COVID-19. Lancet Diabetes Endocrinol. 2020;8:809.
9. Pal R, Bhansali A. COVID-19, diabetes mellitus and ACE2: The conundrum. Diabetes Res Clin Pract. 2020;162:108132.
10. Pal R, Bhadada SK. COVID-19 and diabetes mellitus: An unholy interaction of two pandemics. Diabetes Metab Syndr. 2020;14:513-7.
11. Rubino F, Amiel SA, Zimmet P, Alberti G, Bornstein S, Eckel RH, et al. New-Onset Diabetes in Covid-19. N Engl J Med. 2020;383:789-90.
12. Di Filippo L, Formenti AM, Giustina A. Hypocalcemia: the quest for the cause of a major biochemical feature of COVID-19. Endocrine. 2020;70:463-4.

MULTIPLE CHOICE QUESTIONS

To access the multiple choice questions of this Section online, kindly scan the QR code.

CHAPTER 128

Clinical Approach to Gastrointestinal Diseases

Anuraag Jena, Anupam Kumar Singh, Rakesh Kochhar

ABSTRACT

Gastrointestinal (GI) diseases are quite common and affect the GI tract from mouth to anus. Common symptoms of GI diseases, alone or in combination, may point toward a specific organ as the source of manifestations. General and systemic examination provides further clues and help in evaluation of the etiology. History and examination are often adequate to make a disposition in patients with minor complaints while other cases require further testing and evaluation based on clinical findings. Basic blood workup is required in all the major GI disorder while specific investigations should be ordered for suspected etiology based on clinical evaluation of the patient. Advanced GI tools not only help in diagnosis of specific GI disorders, but also provide an opportunity for a therapeutic intervention during the same session. Management of GI disorders is a combined approach and requires a dedicated team of gastroenterologists, physicians, surgeons, radiologists, pathologists, nurses, and dieticians.

"Certainly it is by their signs and symptoms, that internal diseases are revealed to the physician"

—Elisha Bartlett

INTRODUCTION

Gastrointestinal (GI) diseases are commonly encountered disorders in clinical practice. The management of GI diseases involves a combined approach by gastroenterologists, physicians, surgeons, radiologists, pathologists, nurses, and dieticians. Advances in investigations and therapeutics have revolutionized the management of GI disorders. However, the basic approach to GI disorders remains clinical which is crucial for better patient evaluation and management.

CLASSIFICATION

Gastrointestinal diseases can result from any abnormality from mouth to anal canal as well as abnormalities outside GI tract. They can be classified on the basic of pathophysiological alterations in basic structure and function of GI system (**Table 1**). The disease can involve one or multiple organs with varied clinical symptoms.

SYMPTOMS

The most common symptoms of GI diseases include abdominal pain, nausea, vomiting, GI bleeding, jaundice, dysphagia, constipation, and diarrhea. There can be a combination of one or more symptoms at presentation. Symptoms often point towards the specific disease or organ involved (**Table 2**).

TABLE 1 Classification of gastrointestinal (GI) diseases.

Defect	Diseases
Impaired digestion	• Acute gastroenteritis • Lactase deficiency • Small intestinal bacterial overgrowth • Inflammatory bowel disease • Malabsorption syndromes • Celiac disease • Tropical sprue
Altered gut transit	• Gastroparesis • Achalasia • Intestinal obstruction • Intestinal pseudo-obstruction
Altered secretion	• Laxative abuse • Diabetic diarrhea • Small intestinal bacterial overgrowth • Pernicious anemia • Zollinger–Ellison syndrome • Bile acid induced diarrhea • Colonic villous adenoma
Immune dysfunction	• Celiac disease • Inflammatory bowel disease • Eosinophilic gastroenteritis

Continued...

Continued...

Defect	Diseases
Altered blood flow	• Intestinal ischemia • Radiation enteritis
Neoplastic transformation	• Esophageal cancer • Gastric cancer • Colon cancer • Gall bladder cancer • Pancreatic cancer • Hepatocellular cancer • Anal cancer
Genetic defects	• Cystic fibrosis • Familial adenomatous polyposis
Functional disorders	• Functional dyspepsia • Functional heart burn • Irritable bowel syndrome

TABLE 2 Common causes of gastrointestinal (GI) symptoms.

Symptoms	Disease
Pain abdomen	• Peptic ulcer disease • Esophagitis • Acute biliary disease • Pancreatitis • Appendicitis • Diverticulitis • Inflammatory bowel disease • Abdominal compartment syndrome • Intestinal obstruction • Mesenteric ischemia
Nausea/Vomiting	• Enteric infections • Appendicitis • Drug induced • Motility disorders • Pregnancy • Neurological disorders • Endocrine disorders • Connective tissue disorders • Post surgery
GI bleeding	• Esophageal varices • Peptic ulcer disease • Esophagitis • Mallory–Weiss syndrome • Portal hypertensive gastropathy • Inflammatory bowel disease • Hemorrhoids • Diverticular bleed • Dieulafoy's lesion • Other vascular lesions

Continued...

Continued...

Symptoms	Disease
Jaundice	• Viral hepatitis • Bile duct stones • Hemolytic disorders • Carcinoma gallbladder • Carcinoma head of pancreas • Periampullary tumors • Cholangiocarcinoma • Recurrent pyogenic cholangitis • Choledochal cyst • Bile duct stricture
Dysphagia	• Esophageal motility disorders • Carcinoma esophagus • Esophageal web • Corrosive stricture • Neurological causes • Connective tissue disorders • Eosinophilic esophagitis
Constipation	• Motility disorders • Irritable bowel syndrome • Drug induced • Abdomen tuberculosis • Colon carcinoma • Neurological causes • Endocrine disorders • GI lymphoma • Electrolyte disorders • Porphyria
Diarrhea	• Irritable bowel syndrome • Infections • Inflammatory bowel disease • Drug induced • Celiac disease • Microscopic colitis • Food allergy • Endocrine disorders • Bile acid diarrhea • Post surgery

Abdominal pain: Abdominal pain can be acute lasting for several days, subacute lasting from several days to 6 months, or chronic lasting for more than 6 months. Abdominal pain can be visceral, somatic-parietal, or referred pain. Evaluation of acute abdominal pain requires proper history and physical examination. The characteristics, site, nature, intensity as well as radiation of abdominal pain can give clue to the diagnosis (**Table 3**). Referred pain is classically felt in areas remote from the affected organ. Subdiaphragmatic hematoma or splenic rupture can present as shoulder pain (Kehr's sign). Aggravating as well as relieving factors also give information regarding the etiology of pain. The

TABLE 3 Comparison of types of abdominal pain.

Cause	Onset	Site	Character	Type	Radiation	Intensity
Pancreatitis	Acute	Epigastrium	Localized	Boring	Back	Severe
Cholecystitis	Acute	Right upper quadrant and epigastrium	Localized	Constricting	Scapula	Moderate-to-severe
Appendicitis	Gradual	Periumbilical early and late lower quadrant	Diffuse early and later localized	Aching	None	Moderate-to-severe
GI obstruction	Gradual	Periumbilical area	Diffuse	Cramping and crescendo-decrescendo	None	Moderate-to-severe
Diverticulitis	Gradual	Left lower quadrant	Localized	Aching	None	Moderate-to-severe
Perforated peptic ulcer	Sudden	Epigastrium	Localized early and diffuse later	Burning	None	Severe
Mesenteric ischemia	Sudden	Periumbilical	Diffuse	Agonizing	None	Moderate-to-severe

relationship of the pain to change in position, meals, stress, and movements can help in diagnosis. Patients of peritonitis will be motionless while a patient of renal colic would be restless to find a comfortable position. Pain of duodenal ulcer is alleviated by food intake while gastric ulcer pain or pain of mesenteric ischemia worsens with food intake. History of chronic painkillers abuse will point towards peptic ulcer disease. Associated symptoms along with abdominal pain also give clue to the diagnosis. Bilious vomiting points to proximal small intestinal obstruction while feculent vomiting will suggest distal colonic obstruction.

Nausea and vomiting: Nausea is an unpleasant subjective sensation of impending vomiting. Vomiting is the act of forceful expulsion of gastric or intestinal contents through mouth. Retching is spasmodic and abortive respiratory movements against a closed glottis. Regurgitation is effortless reflux of gastric contents into esophagus or mouth. Mechanical obstruction of upper gut as well disorders of propulsion can cause nausea and vomiting. The duration, frequency, severity, characteristics as well as associated symptoms are essential for evaluation of etiology. The relation of vomiting to food intake is decisive to locate the site of obstruction. Drug history is crucial in all patients of undiagnosed vomiting. Early morning vomiting with secondary amenorrhea will suggest pregnancy. Vomiting along with distention, tenderness, and obstipation will suggest obstruction. Heart burn along with nausea will suggest gastroesophageal reflex disease. Headache and projectile vomiting will point towards nervous system causes. The patient can also present with complications of recurrent vomitings with fluid depletion and electrolyte abnormalities.

GI bleed: Acute upper GI bleed can present as hematemesis and/or melena. Hematemesis is vomit of blood or coffee ground like material while melena is black tarry stool. Melena results when at least 50–100 mL blood gets degraded into hematin by intestinal bacteria over several hours. Lower GI bleed can present as bright red or maroon colored stools. Sometimes a massive upper GI bleed can present as fresh bleeding per rectum but slow bleeding from right ascending colon can present as melena. Chronic GI bleeding can present as iron deficiency anemia. Occult bleeding denotes no clinically visible blood. Obscure GI bleeding is diagnosed when the site of bleed cannot be localized after endoscopy, colonoscopy, and enteroscopy. Severe GI bleeding is defined as bleeding accompanied with hypotension, drop in hemoglobin by 2 g/dL, or transfusion of at least 2 units of packed red blood cells (RBCs). History can give clue to the suspected site of GI bleed (**Table 4**). Clear nasogastric tube does not always rule out upper GI bleed.

Jaundice: It is an important symptom in GI and liver disorders. It is discussed in detail in the chapter *"Approach to Management of Jaundice: Obstructive Jaundice/Hepatitis"*.

Dysphagia: Dysphagia is the sensation of food being obstructed in its passage from mouth to stomach. The most important aspect of approach to dysphagia is differentiation of oropharyngeal from esophageal dysphagia. Oropharyngeal or transfer dysphagia is inability to transfer the food bolus from hypopharynx to esophagus across upper esophageal sphincter. Oropharyngeal dysphagia occurs immediately after food intake. Such patients can have associated features such as dysarthria, nasal speech, and nasal regurgitation. The causes of oropharyngeal dysphagia include neuromuscular causes such as Parkinson's disease and structural causes like Zenker's diverticulum. Swallowing difficulty associated with gurgling sound is associated with Zenker's diverticulum. Patient with esophageal dysphagia should be enquired about the type of food, nature of progression, and associated symptoms (**Flowchart 1**). Odynophagia is painful swallowing seen in caustic ingestion, infective esophagitis, and pill-induced esophagitis. Globus sensation is feeling of a lump in the throat unrelated to swallowing. Hiccups are due to contraction of diaphragm along with closed glottis.

Constipation: It is defined as per Rome IV criteria. It includes at least 25% defecations for past 3 months, with onset at

TABLE 4 Site of bleed localization from history.

Site of bleeding	History
Esophageal ulcers	• Heart burn and odynophagia • Traumatic nasogastric tube insertion • Pill ingestion
Esophageal carcinoma	• Dysphagia with significant weight loss • History of Barrett's esophagus • Chronic smoker
Mallory–Weiss tear	• Alcohol binge • Vomiting
Cameron lesions	Large hiatal hernia
Peptic ulcer	• *Helicobacter pylori* infection • NSAID abuse
Gastric cancer	• Early satiety • Significant weight loss
Gastric angiodysplasia	• Aortic stenosis • Chronic kidney disease • Scleroderma
Meckel's diverticulum	Unexplained GI bleed in <40 years age
Ampulla of Vater	Recent endoscopic sphincterotomy
Bile ducts	Recent liver biopsy
Small intestine ulcers	• Crohn's disease • NSAID induced
Ischemic colitis	• Previous cardiac comorbidities
Colonic cancer	• Recent altered bowel habits • Significant weight loss • Family history of malignancy
Ulcerative colitis	• Bloody diarrhea with rectal symptoms of tenesmus and urgency • Family history of IBD
Crohn's disease	• Bloody diarrhea • Chronic abdominal pain • Associated fistula • Family history of IBD
Hemorrhoids	Dripping blood sometimes without mixed with stool
Anal fissure	• Anal pain • Severe constipation
Radiation enteritis	• History of radiation therapy for malignancy

least 6 months prior and associated with any two of the following: straining, lumpy hard stools, sense of incomplete evacuation, sense of anorectal blockage, manual maneuvers for evacuation, and less than three spontaneous bowel movements per week. Risk factors include female gender, old age, low physical activity, low socioeconomic status, and drugs. A detailed history of duration of symptoms, frequency, and associated symptoms like distention should be enquired. In history, always rule out alarm features such as blood in stool, significant unintentional loss of weight or appetite, and family history of malignancy. A dietary history should also be asked for fluid and fiber intake. Obstetric and surgery history are important. A per rectal examination is paramount in evaluation of constipation.

Diarrhea: It is defined as passage of loose or watery stools typically three or more bowel movements per day with stool weight >200 g/day. The duration of acute diarrhea is <14 days while chronic diarrhea is duration of diarrhea >4 weeks. Any diarrhea lasting >14 days but <4 weeks is called persistent diarrhea. Diarrhea can be classified depending on stool characteristics (watery, fatty, or inflammatory), volume (large or small volume), and pathophysiology (secretory, osmotic, or complex). The important point to note in history of diarrhea is the presence of fecal incontinence, associated systemic diseases, drug history, and aggravating, and alleviating factors. Presence of alarm symptoms such as unintentional weight loss and rectal bleeding should be enquired. Excessive flatus and bloating suggests carbohydrate malabsorption. Nocturnal diarrhea denotes organic rather than functional diarrhea. Urgency and incontinence signify a rectal disorder. Dietary history is also important in history of patients with diarrhea. A detailed physical examination is necessary to pin point etiology of diarrhea (**Table 5**).

DIAGNOSTIC TOOLS

Laboratory: Baseline biochemical investigations should be obtained in all cases while specific investigations should be ordered based on clinical suspicion. Anemia is a common manifestation of many diseases and the type of anemia helps in identifying the etiology. Iron deficiency anemia will point towards blood loss, hook worm infestation, or malnutrition while vitamin B12 deficiency will suggest ileal disease or gastric resection. While evaluating GI disorders, other important investigations include thyroid profile, fasting glucose, anti-tissue transglutaminase (tTG), and fecal calprotectin. Anti-tTG [immunoglobulin A (IgA)-tTG] and anti-deamidated gliadin peptide (IgA-DGP) will be elevated in celiac disease. Serum gastrin and gastric acid quantification are tested when Zollinger–Ellison syndrome is suspected.

When ascites is present, its analysis is of paramount importance to identify the causes of ascites which include chronic liver disease, infections, and malignancy. Stool samples are tested for RBCs, pus cells, organisms, and antigens of *Giardia* or *Helicobacter pylori*. Fecal fat quantification is important for the evaluation of malabsorption. Fecal calprotectin is tested to quantify the intestinal inflammation while fecal elastase is advised for ruling out pancreatic insufficiency. Urine samples are tested for carcinoid, copper estimation, toxic screen, and porphyria. Urinary D-xylose test is used for assessment of proximal small intestinal mucosal functions

Endoscopy: Endoscopy is a crucial component in the evaluation of various GI symptoms. It not only helps in the diagnosis but also aids in therapeutics in the management (**Table 6**).

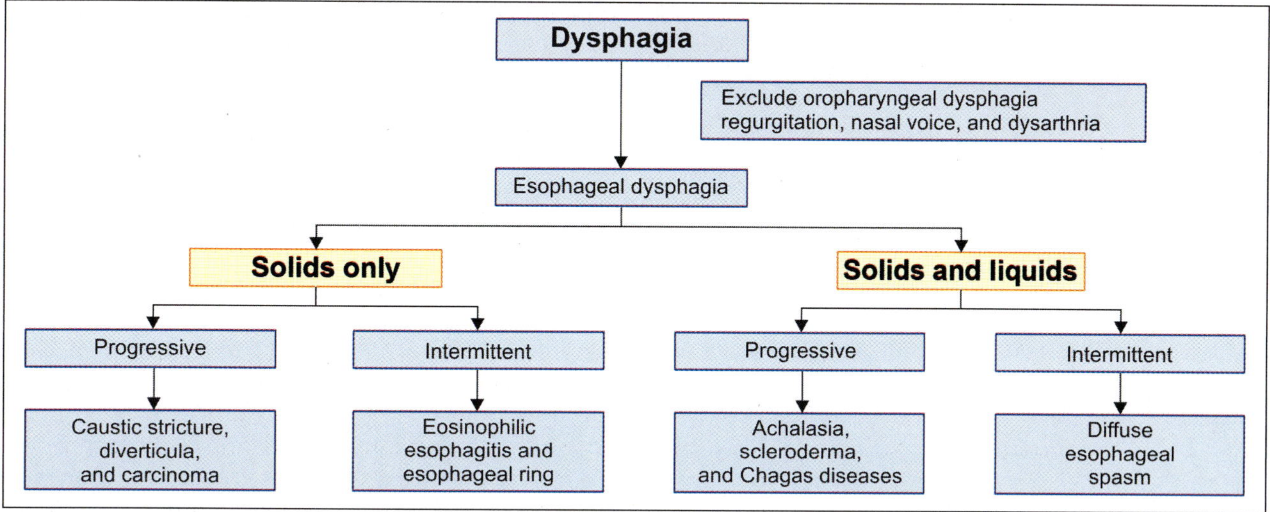

FLOWCHART 1: Approach to dysphagia.

TABLE 5 Physical examination in diarrhea.

Finding	Disease
Hyperpigmentation	Addison disease
Migratory necrotizing erythema	Glucagonoma
Flushing, right heart murmurs, and wheezing	Carcinoid
Tremors and lid lag	Hyperthyroid
Dermatitis herpetiformis	Celiac disease
Oculomasticatory myorhythmia	Whipple disease
Pinch purpura and macroglossia	Amyloidosis
Arthritis	IBD and whipple
Muscle wasting and edema	Malnutrition
Abdominal bruit	Chronic mesenteric ischemia
Lymphadenopathy	AIDS, lymphoma, and malignancy

(IBD: Inflammatory bowel disease)

Radiology: Radiological examination of the esophagus, small intestine, and large intestine using barium contrast can provide detailed information for suspected malabsorption. Barium studies delineate the mucosa from esophagus to rectum. Abdominal X-ray can aid in diagnosis of intestinal obstruction (multiple air fluid levels), intestinal perforation (air under diaphragm), chronic calcific pancreatitis (calcification in pancreas), acute pancreatitis (sentinel loop sign and colon cut off sign), intestinal volvulus (coffee bean sign), carcinoma colon (apple core sign), and intestinal ischemia (thumb printing).

Ultrasound and CT abdomen are useful for diagnosis of mass lesions, collections, vascular involvement, and lymphadenopathy. Magnetic resonance cholangiopancreatography (MRCP) helps to delineate the biliary tree and pancreatic duct using heavily T2-weighted sequences. CT and MR enterography provide better mucosal characteristics in diseases like inflammatory bowel disease. They help in better assessment of mucosal enhancement,

TABLE 6 Role of various modalities in gastrointestinal (GI) disease.

Investigation	Nature of investigation	GI disorders
Endoscopy	Diagnostic and therapeutic	• Dysphagia • GI bleed • Gastric outlet obstruction • Anemia evaluation • Malabsorption • Foreign body • Refractory dyspepsia
Colonoscopy	Diagnostic and therapeutic	• GI bleed • Cancer screen • Chronic diarrhea • Polypectomy • Anemia evaluation • Colonic obstruction • Inflammatory bowel disease
Endoscopic ultrasound (EUS)	Diagnostic and therapeutic	• Cancer staging • Drain pseudocyst • Biopsy/fine-needle aspirate • Submucosal mass evaluation • Anal continuity
Endoscopic retrograde cholangiopancreatography (ERCP)	Therapeutic	• Cholangitis • Biliary and pancreatic stricture management • Common bile duct (CBD) stone clearance • Pancreatic duct disruption • Chronic calcific pancreatitis • Bile leaks • Biliary parasites

Continued...

Continued...

Investigation	Nature of investigation	GI disorders
Capsule endoscopy	Diagnostic	• Obscure GI bleed • Crohn's disease
Enteroscopy	Diagnostic and therapeutic	• Small bowel bleed • Small bowel mass • Crohn's disease
Cholangio-scopy	Diagnostic and therapeutic	• Cholangitis • Large CBD stones • Hemobilia evaluation • Migrated stents • Indeterminate biliary strictures • Staging of biliary malignancy

mural thickening, and mesenteric vasculature. CT and MR angiography help delineate the vascular structures better for diagnosis of diseases such as pulmonary embolism and intestinal ischemia. Positron emission tomography can help distinguish malignancy from benign GI diseases. Scintigraphy evaluates both structural abnormalities as well as help in analysis of transit studies. RBC scan can be utilized for detection of GI bleed.

Histopathology: Mucosal biopsies obtained during endoscopy help in diagnosis of inflammatory, infectious, and malignant GI diseases. Ultrasound or CT or endoscopic ultrasound (EUS) guided biopsies and fine-needle aspiration can aid in diagnosis of underlying diseases. Liver biopsy is the gold standard for diagnosis of several liver disorders. It is used for diagnosis as well as for prognosis of the liver diseases. Liver biopsy can be performed by following routes: percutaneous, transjugular, and laparoscopic.

Functional testing: Testing for pancreatic function tests can help diagnose pancreatic insufficiency. Esophageal manometry is used for diagnosis of esophageal motility diseases like achalasia. Wireless motility capsule is used to measure contractility of stomach, small intestine, and colon. Anorectal manometry is used for evaluation of constipation, defecatory disorders, and fecal incontinence.

Breath tests: Urea breath test is used for the diagnosis of *H. pylori* infection. Hydrogen breath tests are utilized for carbohydrate malabsorption and small intestinal bacterial growth. They can also help in measurement of orocecal transit time. Octanoic breath test is used for study of delayed gastric emptying. Triglyceride breath test is used to diagnose pancreatic insufficiency.

DIFFERENTIATION

FUNCTIONAL VERSUS ORGANIC BOWEL DISEASE

Functional bowel disorders are very much prevalent in the society and include functional heartburn, functional dyspepsia, irritable bowel syndrome etc. It is important to differentiate functional bowel disorders from organic disorders to prevent unnecessary misuse of investigations and to avoid finical burden. Organic disorders on the other hand require further evaluation and treatment. Often initial history and examination provide clues toward the diagnosis of functional disorders (**Table 7**). Patients with functional disorders are often young or middle aged females with nonspecific symptoms and without alarming symptoms (old age, weight loss, hematemesis, or melena). Patients with functional disorders can have associated depression and frequently seek medical consultation for nonspecific symptoms. Blood and imaging investigations are often normal in the patients with functional bowel disorders.

INTESTINAL TUBERCULOSIS VERSUS CROHN'S DISEASE

Tuberculosis is common in India and other endemic countries. It is clinically important to differentiate intestinal tuberculosis from the Crohn's disease. Clinical features of abdominal pain, recurrent partial intestinal obstruction, fever, anorexia, weight loss, chronic diarrhea, hematochezia, and perianal involvement are seen in both the disorders. However, most of the studies report longer duration of disease, diarrhea, hematochezia, perianal disease, and

TABLE 7 Differentiation between functional and organic bowel disorder.

Features	Functional bowel disorder	Organic bowel disorder
Age	Young and middle age	More common in elderly, can also affect young patients
Gender	More common in females	Affect both the sex
Associated psychiatric symptoms	Yes	Rare
Frequent change of physicians	Yes	No
Symptoms	Nonspecific symptoms, more during day time	Occurs irrespective of time
Anorexia	Uncommon	Common
Weight loss	Uncommon	Common
Laboratory parameters	Normal	May be abnormal

TABLE 8 Differentiation features of intestinal tuberculosis and Crohn's disease.

Features	Intestinal tuberculosis	Crohn's disease
Favors Crohn's disease		
Duration of disease	Short (<2 years)	Long (>2 years)
Diarrhea	Less common (16–57%)	More common (43–85%)
Hematochezia	Less common (7–20%)	More common (24–68%)
Perianal disease	Less common (0–8%)	More common (16–32%)
Extraintestinal manifestations	Less common (2–13%)	More common (11–45%)
Favors intestinal tuberculosis		
Fever	More common (20–43%)	Less common (23–30%)
Night sweats	More common (7–31%)	Less common (1–20%)
Ascites	More common	Less common
Common in both		
Constipation	Common in both (60–80%)	
Abdominal pain	Common in both (60–90%)	
Intestinal obstruction	Common in both (10–55%)	

extraintestinal manifestations as being more common in Crohn's disease than intestinal tuberculosis (**Table 8**). Presence of fever, night sweats, lung involvement, and ascites favor a diagnosis of intestinal tuberculosis. However, none of the features is exclusive for either disease and alone cannot diagnose Crohn's disease or intestinal tuberculosis.

Endoscopic involvement of left-sided colon, presence of longitudinal ulcers, aphthous ulcers, cobblestoning, and skip lesions are more common in Crohn's disease while presence of transverse ulcers and patulous ileocecal valve favor a diagnosis of intestinal tuberculosis. Other features such as pseudopolyps, strictures, and nodularity can be seen in both the diseases.

TREATMENT

The management of various GI diseases depends on the etiology of symptoms. A multimodality approach is often needed for treatment.

Nutrition: Dietary modifications like gluten-free diet for celiac disease, lactose free diet for lactase deficiency, carbohydrate restrictions for dumping syndrome, liquid meals for delayed gastric emptying, low fermentable oligo-di-monosaccharides and polyols (FODMAP) diet for irritable bowel syndrome, and medium-chain triglycerides rich diet for severe ileal disease. Enteral nutrition is beneficial early in the course of acute pancreatitis through nasogastric or nasojejunal route. Parenteral nutrition is advised when patients cannot tolerate enteral nutrition.

Pharmacotherapy: Acid suppressants such as proton pump inhibitors and histamine receptor antagonists are used to treat peptic ulcer disease. Antidiarrheal agents include anticholinergics, antispasmodic, tricyclic agents, bile acid sequestrants, and serotonin antagonists. Bulk forming laxatives, osmotic laxatives, stimulant laxatives, and stool softeners are used to treat constipation. For abdominal pain, antispasmodics, antidepressants, and opiates are used as pain relief agents. Prokinetic agents are used in delayed emptying and pseudo-obstruction. Antiemetics such as serotonin antagonists, antimuscarinic, antihistaminics, and neurokinin-1 antagonists are used to suppress vomiting. Antibiotics are used to treat *H. pylori*, gastroenteritis, diverticulitis, small intestinal bacterial overgrowth, and liver abscess. Proton pump inhibitors and vasoconstrictors such as terlipressin and octreotide are used in management of GI bleed. Octreotide analogs are used for treatment of hypersecretory states. 5-aminosalicylic acid, steroids, immune-suppressants, and biological are used in management of inflammatory bowel disease. Pancreatic enzyme replacement therapy is used in treatment of pancreatic insufficiency. Chemoradiotherapy is used for the management of GI malignancies.

Interventional therapy: Nasogastric tube helps in decompression of upper gut in intestinal obstruction. Enemas help decompress in fecal impaction. Flatus tube decompresses distal colonic pseudo-obstruction.

There are various treatment modalities through endoscopy. Endoscopy is utilized for insertion of feeding tubes. Percutaneous endoscopic gastrostomy tube placement can help in nutrition in neurological diseases. Polypectomy, mucosal resection, submucosal dissection, dilatation of strictures, and placement of metal stents across strictures are some of the commonly used procedures done through endoscopy. Injection with sclerosing agents is used in bleeding ulcers and vascular malformations. Band ligation is used for esophageal varices while glue injection is indicated for gastric varices. Hemorrhoids are treated with sclerotherapy or banding. Radiofrequency ablation is used for Barrett's esophagus and in malignant biliary strictures. Endoscopic retrograde cholangiopancreatography (ERCP) is used for drainage of biliary system in cholangitis. ERCP is also indicated for pain relief in chronic pancreatitis not responding to medical management. EUS-guided drainage of pseudocyst, drainage of pancreatic duct, biliary drainage, hepaticojejunostomy, hepaticogastrostomy, and choledochoduodenostomy are various therapeutic modalities for management of GI diseases. EUS-guided coil insertion can be effective for gastric varices. Per oral endoscopic myotomy is the preferred modality for achalasia.

Radiological interventions also aid in management of GI diseases. Angioembolization is used to control bleeding through vessel leaks. Pigtail catheter drainage is an effective option for drainage of fluid collections in abdomen in acute necrotizing pancreatitis. Per-cutaneous transhepatic cholangiography helps to relieve biliary obstruction in cholangitis. Transjugular intrahepatic portosystemic shunts are used for treatment of variceal bleed and refractory ascites.

Surgery: Surgery is necessary for ulcer related complications such as bleeding, obstruction, and perforation. For medically unresponsive ulcerative colitis, Crohn's disease, diverticulitis, and appendicitis, surgery is the rescue option for management. Minimally invasive necrosectomy, video-assisted retroperitoneal debridement, and open necrosectomy are surgical options for necrotizing pancreatitis. Feeding jejunostomy can serve for nutrition in malnourished patients.

RECOMMENDED READINGS

1. Almario CV, Ballal ML, Chey WD, Nordstrom C, Khanna D, Spiegel BMR. Burden of Gastrointestinal Symptoms in the United States: Results of a Nationally Representative Survey of Over 71,000 Americans. Am J Gastroenterol. 2018;113(11):1701-10.
2. Mealie CA, Ali R, Manthey DE. Abdominal Exam. Treasure Island (FL): StatPearls Publishing; 2021.
3. Kim BS, Li BT, Engel A. Diagnosis of gastrointestinal bleeding: A practical guide for clinicians. World J Gastrointest Pathophysiol. 2014;5(4):467-78.
4. Gondal B, Aronsohn A. A Systematic Approach to Patients with Jaundice. Semin Intervent Radiol. 2016;33(4):253-8.
5. Philpott H, Garg M, Tomic D, Balasubramanian S, Sweis R. Dysphagia: Thinking outside the box. World J Gastroenterol. 2017;23(38):6942-51.
6. Pare P. The approach to diagnosis and treatment of chronic constipation: suggestions for a general practitioner. Can J Gastroenterol. 2011;25 Suppl B(Suppl B):36B-40B.
7. Sweetser S. Evaluating the patient with diarrhea: a case-based approach. Mayo Clin Proc. 2012;87(6):596-602.
8. Nguyen VX, Le Nguyen VT, Nguyen CC. Appropriate use of endoscopy in the diagnosis and treatment of gastrointestinal diseases: up-to-date indications for primary care providers. Int J Gen Med. 2010;3:345-57.
9. Lankarani KB. Diet and the Gut. Middle East J Dig Dis. 2016;8(3):161-5.
10. Ray DM, Srinivasan I, Tang SJ, Vilmann AS, Vilmann P, McCowan TC, et al. Complementary roles of interventional radiology and therapeutic endoscopy in gastroenterology. World J Radiol. 2017;9(3):97-111.

CHAPTER

129

Esophageal Disorders

Shobna Bhatia, Arshdeep Singh

ABSTRACT

Esophagus is a conduit for transportation of food from oral cavity to the stomach. Structural and functional disorders of esophagus are among the most common disorders in general medical as well as in gastroenterology practice. The common symptoms of esophageal disorders include dysphagia, odynophagia, heartburn, regurgitation, and pain. The esophageal disorders can broadly be divided into structural disorders, motility disorders, gastroesophageal reflux disease (GERD), infections, corrosive injuries, and tumors. Esophageal webs, rings, diverticula, and hiatus hernia are the commonly encountered structural disorders. With increasing awareness and access to high-resolution esophageal manometry, greater number of patients with motility disorders are being diagnosed.

Achalasia cardia is a common primary esophageal motility disorder that presents with dysphagia. Peroral endoscopic myotomy (POEM) has changed the therapeutic landscape for achalasia cardia and has emerged as an important therapy. GERD, caused due to loss of functional integrity of the lower esophageal sphincter (LES), is arguably the most commonly reported symptom in clinics that requires long-term therapy with proton pump inhibitors (PPIs). Corrosive injuries to esophageal mucosa, when complicated by strictures and malignancy, are associated with poor quality of life. Eosinophilic, infective, and pill esophagitis are not uncommon. This chapter provides an overview of the approach to common esophageal disorders.

"In all chaos there is a cosmos, in all disorder a secret order"

—Carl Jung

INTRODUCTION

The esophagus is a muscular tube starting at the upper esophageal sphincter (UES) and ends at the LES, and is a conduit for transit of food from mouth to the stomach. In normal circumstances, the passage of food through the esophagus is not sensed by an individual.

SYMPTOMS

The major symptoms of esophageal diseases are heartburn, regurgitation, chest pain, dysphagia, and odynophagia.

Heartburn (pyrosis) is defined as retrosternal burning pain or discomfort, is usually worse after meals, and relieved by antacids or acid-inhibiting drugs. Stress, fear, or anxiety can worsen symptoms of heartburn.

Regurgitation is described as effortless appearance of gastric content (acid, bile) into the esophagus. Bending, belching, or maneuvers that increase intra-abdominal pressures can provoke regurgitation. The regurgitation of sour content is associated with GERD. Regurgitation of bland content may occur when acid secretion has been inhibited by drugs, or when an obstruction exists in the lower esophagus.

Dysphagia, or difficulty in swallowing, is a sensation of obstruction to the passage of food through the mouth, pharynx, or esophagus. Oropharyngeal dysphagia is characterized by inability to initiate swallow, and occurs due to neuromuscular or structural abnormalities of mouth, hypopharynx, or upper esophagus. Esophageal dysphagia results from either mechanical obstruction to transit of food (webs, Schatzki ring, and benign or malignant stricture) or motor abnormalities like achalasia cardia. The dysphagia in mechanical obstruction usually starts for solid food and may be progressive; the severity varies with the degree of luminal narrowing, type of food bolus, and presence of associated esophagitis. On the other hand, dysphagia due to esophageal motor disorders may be equal to solids and liquids, and is usually slowly progressive (achalasia cardia) or intermittent (less specific motility disorder). It may be relieved by maneuvers which increase intraesophageal pressure such as Valsalva maneuver. Nonobstructive dysphagia occurs in patients with reflux disease who have esophageal inflammation associated with a motility disorder (**Flowcharts 1** and **2**).

Odynophagia or painful swallowing is due to mucosal inflammation due to infections [candidiasis, herpes, cytomegalovirus (CMV), and Epstein–Barr virus], corrosive intake, pill esophagitis, and radiation esophagitis (**Flowchart 3**).

Chest pain of esophageal origin is described as squeezing or burning substernal sensation, is often similar to cardiac angina; it is therefore imperative that a cardiac cause be ruled out when the symptom occurs for the first time. In most cases, noncardiac chest pain (NCCP) is associated with other esophageal symptoms, and may last for few hours, is related to meals and relieved by antacids.

Water brash is reflex salivary hypersecretion that occurs in response to gastroesophageal reflux (GER). It should not be confused with regurgitation. Globus sensation is a feeling of food stuck at pharyngeal level, but occurs between meal times.

Besides these symptoms, indications of organic disease including malignancy are gastrointestinal bleeding, involuntary weight loss, and anemia.

INVESTIGATIONS

Investigations of esophageal diseases include endoscopy, imaging studies, and manometry. The choice of investigation depends on the symptom complex that the patient presents with. For instance, barium swallow is useful for evaluation of dysphagia, endoscopy is the investigation of choice for mucosal diseases, and esophageal manometry is

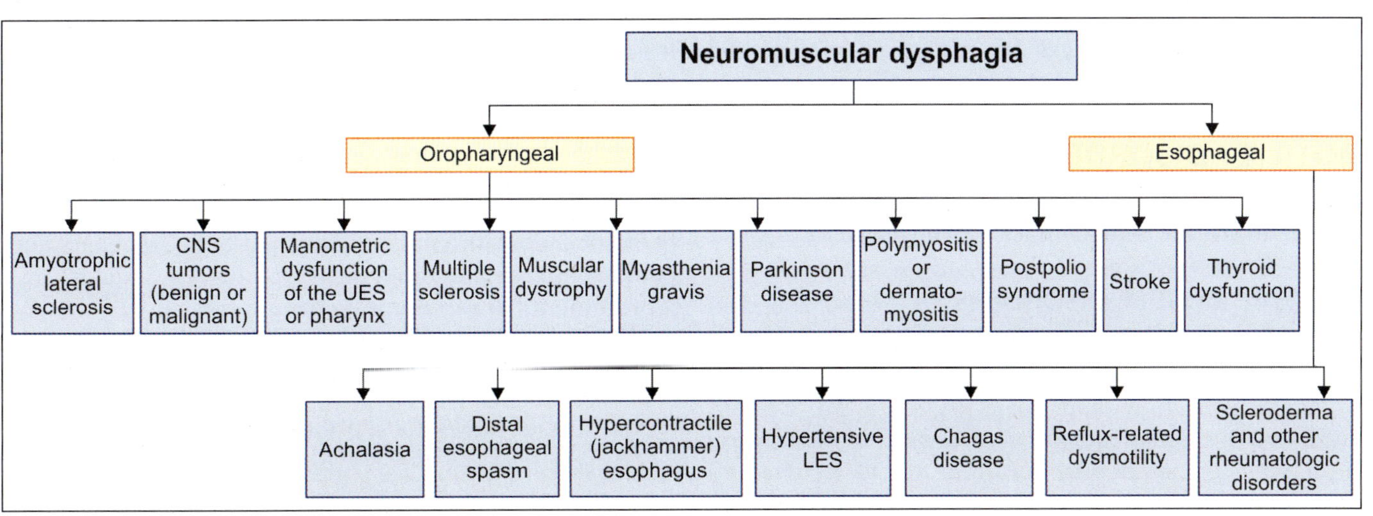

(LES: lower esophageal sphincter; UES: upper esophageal sphincter)

FLOWCHART 1: Causes of neuromuscular dysphagia.

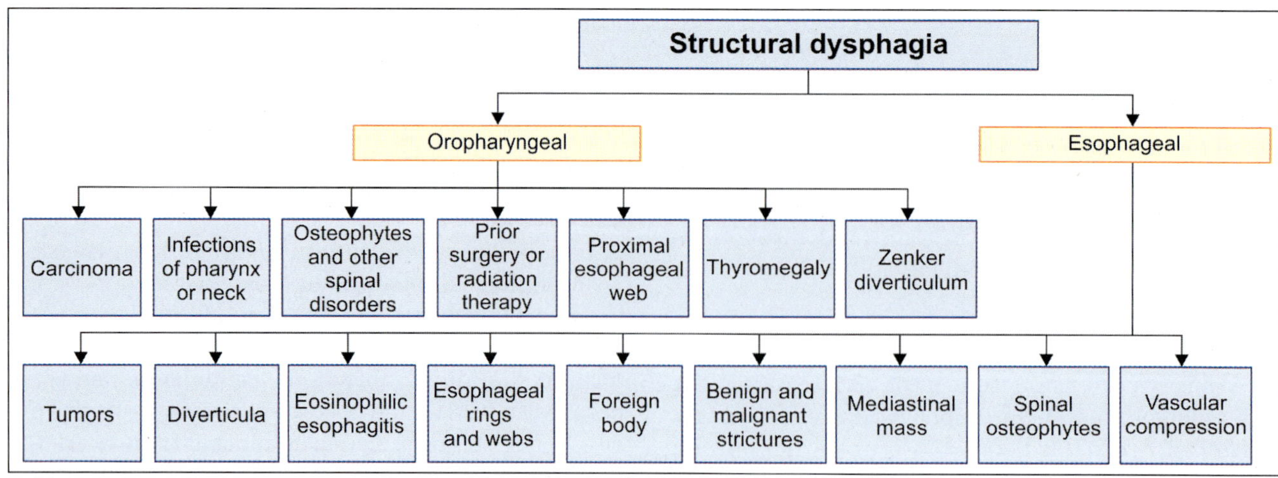

FLOWCHART 2: **Causes of structural dysphagia.**

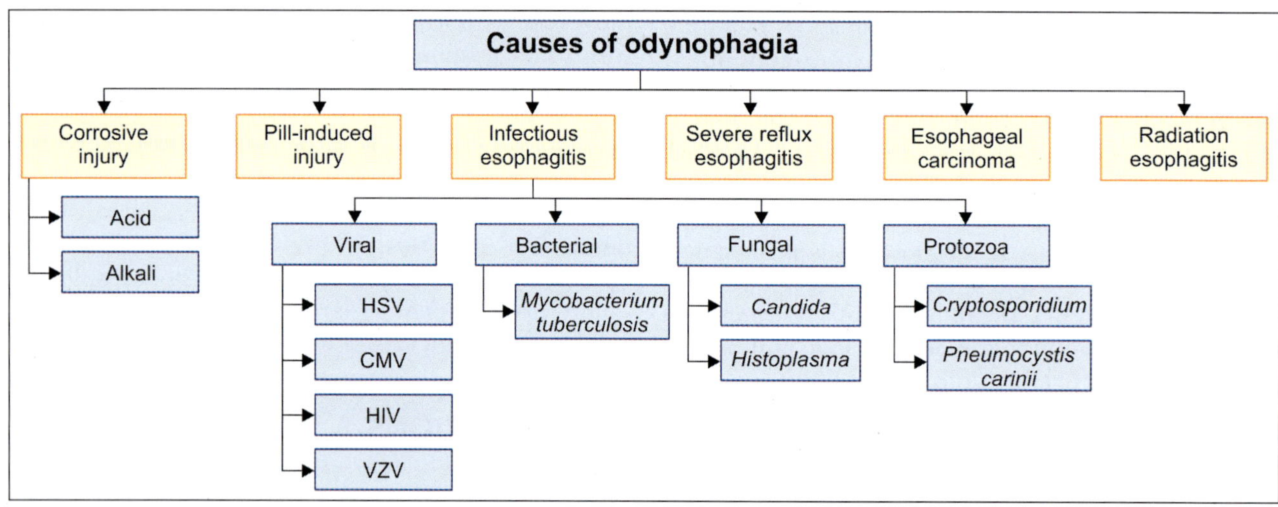

(CMV: cytomegalovirus; HSV: herpes simplex virus; VZV: varicella-zoster virus)

FLOWCHART 3: **Causes of odynophagia.**

useful when a motility disorder is suspected. Investigations like computed tomography (CT) scan and endoscopic ultrasound are useful when transmural pathologies or extraesophageal pathologies are suspected (mediastinal lymph nodes, invasion of tumors into aorta).

MOTILITY DISORDERS OF ESOPHAGUS

The motility disorders of esophagus can involve either skeletal muscles or smooth muscles (**Flowchart 4**).

SKELETAL MUSCLE DISORDERS

Pharyngeal paralysis may occur following neuromuscular diseases. It is characterized by transfer dysphagia, laryngeal aspiration, and nasal regurgitation. Barium swallow with cineradiography may reveal poor contraction of pharyngeal constrictors, barium in the valleculae and pyriform sinuses, and nasal and tracheal aspiration.

Patients who have pharyngeal paralysis due to myasthenia gravis or polymyositis respond to treatment of the primary disease. In patients with a cerebrovascular accident, the extent of impairment of swallowing and its subsequent recovery depend on the type and extent of lesion. The main aim of treatment is to improve swallowing and maintain nutrition. Swallowing exercises may help; however, in severe cases, a feeding gastrostomy may be required.

Cricopharyngeal achalasia is a disorder of unknown cause, and occurs due to failed relaxation of the UES and can be associated with Zenker's diverticulum. Dysphagia and choking are the predominant symptoms. On radiography, a prominent bar representing the contracted UES may be seen. Cricopharyngeal myotomy may be helpful in selected cases.

SMOOTH MUSCLE DISORDERS

Achalasia cardia: Achalasia cardia is a motor disorder of the esophageal smooth muscle in which the esophageal body is aperistaltic, the LES may be hypertensive, and does not relax completely with swallowing.

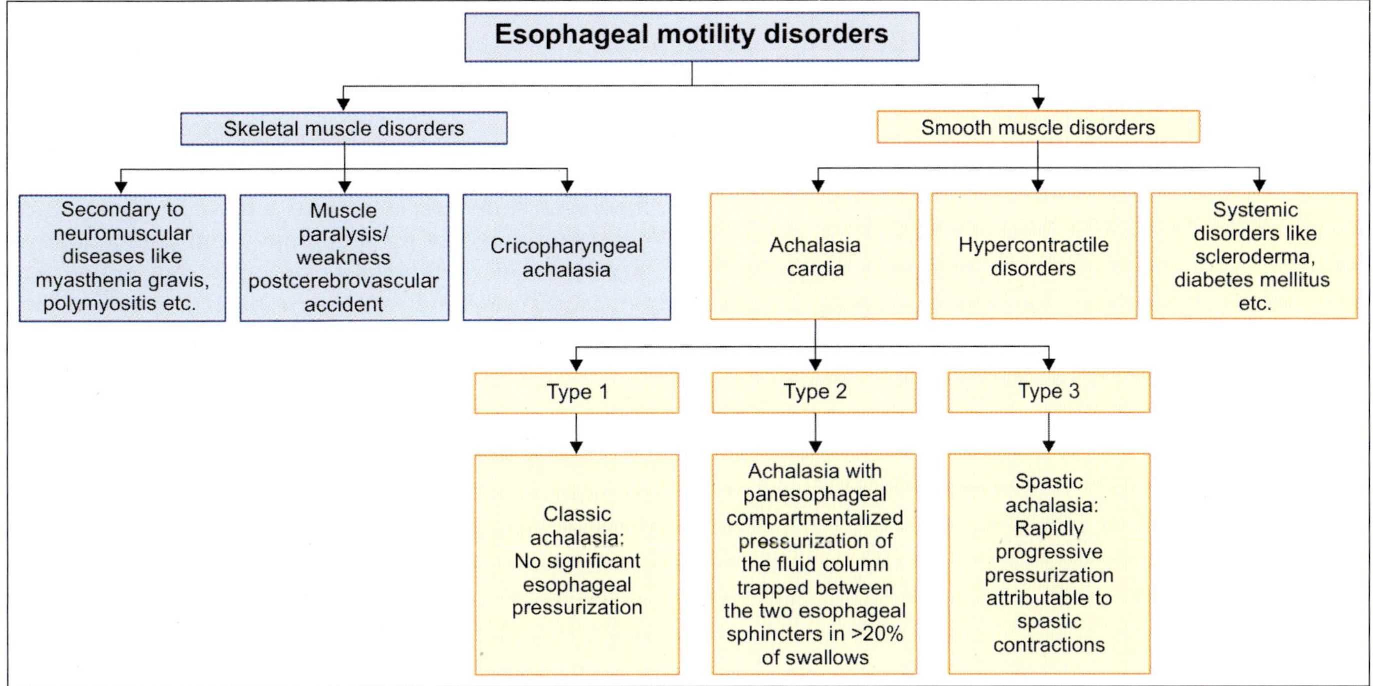

FLOWCHART 4: Esophageal motility disorders.

The underlying abnormality is defective innervation of the smooth muscle of the esophageal body and the LES. Classic achalasia shows a marked reduction in myenteric neurons. Secondary achalasia may be caused by gastric carcinoma infiltrating the esophagus, lymphoma, Chagas disease, neuropathic chronic intestinal pseudo-obstruction syndrome, irradiation, and certain toxins and drugs.

Nonprogressive or slowly progressive dysphagia, intermittent chest pain, and bland regurgitation are the main symptoms of achalasia. Dysphagia occurs with both liquids and solids. Various maneuvers like the Valsalva maneuver, may help passage of the bolus into the stomach. Regurgitation and pulmonary aspiration occur because of retention of large volumes of saliva and ingested food in the esophagus.

Barium swallow shows esophageal dilatation and a persistent beak-like narrowing, representing the nonrelaxing LES. In long-standing achalasia, sigmoid esophagus configuration due to severe dilation of the esophagus can be seen.

Endoscopic findings may range from normal endoscopy to tortuous dilated sigmoid esophagus with retained food and secretions. Endoscopy is helpful in excluding the causes of secondary achalasia, particularly gastric fundal carcinoma.

Esophageal manometry is the most sensitive and specific diagnostic test that shows the defining feature of distal body aperistalsis, and incomplete or absent swallow-induced relaxation of LES. On the basis of high-resolution esophageal manometry findings, achalasia is classified into three variants: type 1—Classic achalasia: No significant esophageal pressurization; type 2—Achalasia with panesophageal compartmentalized pressurization of the fluid column trapped between the two esophageal sphincters in >20% of swallows; and type 3—Spastic achalasia: Rapidly progressive pressurization attributable to spastic contractions. Type 2 achalasia patients respond best to therapy; type 3 achalasia does not respond well, and type 1 has intermediate response to any form of treatment.

The goal of *therapy* is to relieve symptoms by reducing the LES pressure; once the outflow obstruction is relieved food passes through with the help of gravity. Medical treatment using nitrates and calcium-channel antagonists such as nifedipine has been used with some success; these need to be administered sublingually 15–30 minutes prior to a meal. The best available nonsurgical therapies are endoscopy-assisted balloon dilatation of the LES, and POEM. Endoscopic injection of botulinum toxin into the LES is effective in the short term. Laparoscopic Heller's extramucosal myotomy of the LES in which the circular muscle layer is incised, is equally effective. Reflux esophagitis and peptic stricture may develop after successful treatment of achalasia; this complication is more frequent after POEM than with balloon dilation. During surgery, fundoplication is done to prevent GER.

Spastic disorders of distal esophagus other than achalasia: Hypercontractile disorders are a spectrum of disorders like diffuse esophageal spasm, jackhammer esophagus, nonspecific spastic disorders, and hypertensive LES. These are differentiated on the basis of high-resolution manometry findings. Patients present with history of chest pain, occasional dysphagia, and rarely regurgitation. Pain is often similar to angina, may occur at rest or after swallowing, and may radiate to the back or neck. These disorders are associated with other functional bowel disorders, and patients may have anxiety, depression, and other psychological abnormalities. Chronic opioid use causes loss of inhibitory signals involved in control of esophageal motility, resulting in spastic disorders of the esophagus; manometric findings may occasionally mimic achalasia cardia.

Diffuse esophageal spasm is characterized by normally relaxing LES with spasm in >20% of swallows nonperistaltic responses of normal amplitude after 30% or more of swallows with a normally relaxing LES. Barium swallow may reveal intermittent areas of esophageal spasm that produce an appearance of a corkscrew esophagus.

Management includes first ruling out ischemic heart disease; smooth muscle relaxants like nitrates and calcium channel blockers are beneficial in a few cases. Antidepressants like imipramine, trazodone, and sertraline have been found to be useful in some patients with NCCP.

Systemic diseases like scleroderma and diabetes mellitus cause motor disorders of the esophagus. Scleroderma esophagus is associated with atrophy of the esophageal smooth muscle, and patients present with severe GERD and its complications. Diabetes mellitus, when complicated by autonomic neuropathy, may be associated with asymptomatic esophageal dysmotility.

GASTROESOPHAGEAL REFLUX DISEASE

Gastroesophageal reflux is defined as backward flow of gastric contents into the esophagus, resulting in heartburn and/or sour regurgitation. The prevalence of GERD symptoms in India ranges from 8% to 12% of the population; the prevalence is lower than that in Western countries probably due to higher prevalence of *Helicobacter pylori* infection, lower body mass index, low fat consumption in diet, and genetic diversity.

PATHOPHYSIOLOGY

Functional integrity of gastroesophageal junction is maintained by baseline LES pressure, extrinsic compression of the LES by the crural diaphragm, the intra-abdominal location of the LES, integrity of the phrenoesophageal ligament, and maintenance of the acute angle of His. Disruption of any of these factors can result in GER.

Transient LES relaxation is one of the most important causes for GERD; it is stimulated by gastric distension due to food or gas. It is mediated via vagovagal reflex pathway in response to activation of stretch receptors in the stomach.

Hiatus hernia breaches the antireflux barrier by displacing the LES from the crural diaphragm. Hiatus hernia is seen in >50% of patients with reflux esophagitis, and is associated with higher degree of reflux.

Impaired esophageal motor function resulting in inadequate volume clearance occurs in esophagitis; peristaltic dysfunction increases with increasing severity of esophagitis.

The quantity of gastric acid secretion is not increased in GERD patients. However, there is a pocket of acid in the distal esophagus, especially when a hiatal hernia is present, which escapes the buffering action of food; hence the predilection for esophagitis at this location.

CLINICAL FEATURES

The symptom complex of GERD has been divided into esophageal and extraesophageal manifestations. Typical reflux symptoms are heartburn and sour regurgitation. These symptoms are present alone or in combination in >90% of patients. Reflux chest pain can be indistinguishable from pain of ischemic heart disease, but is usually associated with other symptoms of GERD.

Dysphagia in a patient with GERD could be an indicator of peptic stricture or development of malignancy. Dysphagia may also occur because of reflux esophagitis and motor functional abnormalities. Barrett's esophagus is an endoscopic diagnosis confirmed on histology showing specialized intestinal metaplasia. There are no symptoms which herald the development of Barrett's esophagus. Increasing age, male gender, long duration of GERD symptoms, obesity, and smoking are risk factors for Barrett's esophagus. Adenocarcinoma may develop in patients with Barrett's esophagus especially high-grade dysplasia.

Extraesophageal syndromes are classified as those with established associations and those with proposed associations. Established associations include reflux cough, reflux laryngitis, reflux asthma, and reflux dental erosions (**Fig. 1**). These syndromes usually occur with the concomitant manifestation of typical reflux esophageal symptoms and rarely in their absence. They have been found to respond to treatment of GERD. GERD is also seen in pregnancy, Zollinger–Ellison syndrome, scleroderma, prolonged nasogastric intubation, and after surgery involving the gastroesophageal junction (Heller myotomy for achalasia and laparoscopic gastric banding for obesity).

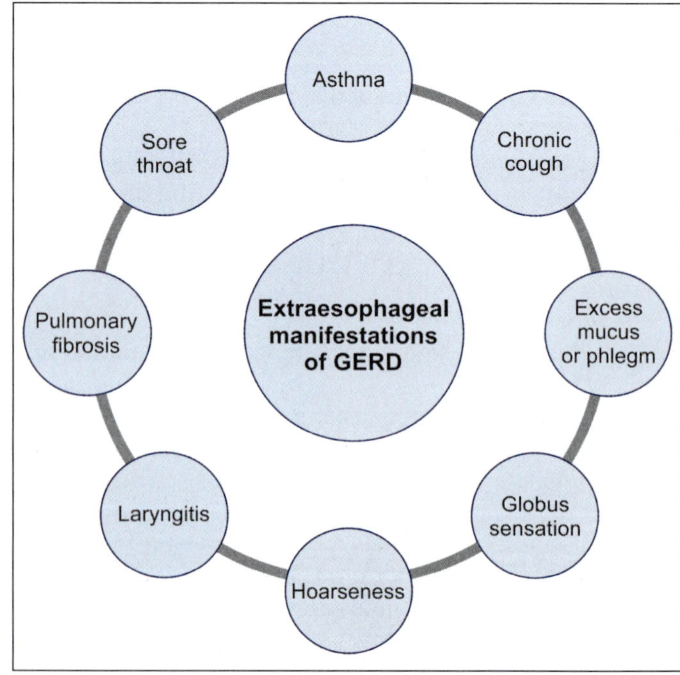

FIGURE 1: Extraesophageal manifestations of gastroesophageal reflux disease (GERD).

INVESTIGATIONS

The diagnosis of GERD is made on the basis of clinical history and confirmed by response to acid-suppressing medications. Diagnostic testing is done to avoid misdiagnosis of other conditions, to identify severity of esophagitis, complications of GERD, and to evaluate the reason for failure of standard therapy.

Endoscopy is done to assess presence of esophagitis; esophagitis is graded using the Los Angeles grading system in which Grade A and B are indications of mild damage, and grades C and D indicate severe esophagitis. Less than 50% of patients with GERD have endoscopic features of esophagitis. Peptic stricture seen in <5% of GERD patients manifests as troublesome mechanical dysphagia.

If endoscopy is normal, the patient should be treated empirically as GERD, and further investigated if symptoms do not resolve. Manometry is useful in detecting peristaltic dysfunction and decrease in LES pressure, as also to diagnose achalasia cardia (which presents with regurgitation and maybe misdiagnosed as GERD). Investigations to demonstrate esophageal acid exposure are ambulatory catheter-based pH-metry or wireless capsule pH-metry, and impedance-pH monitoring.

THERAPY

The aim of treatment is to alleviate symptoms, heal esophagitis, and prevent complications.

Treatment usually begins with *dietary and lifestyle modifications*. The patient should be asked to avoid food items that increase reflux (fatty or fried food, caffeinated drinks, chocolate, and mint) and decrease intake of acidic foods (citrus fruits, spicy food, carbonated drinks, tomatoes, and onions). Lifestyle modifications include weight reduction in those who are obese, elevation of the head end of the bed, and avoiding eating within 2–3 hours of bedtime in those with nighttime symptoms.

Empirical *initial management* with acid reduction is the accepted approach in patients with uncomplicated heartburn. Acid reduction helps in healing of esophagitis and relief from symptoms. PPIs are more effective than H2 receptor antagonists (H2RAs) in treating esophagitis and ameliorating symptoms. PPIs (e.g., omeprazole, lansoprazole, pantoprazole, rabeprazole, esomeprazole, and ilaprazole) are all equally effective in standard doses. There does not appear to be any additional benefit of higher dosage/twice daily dosing of PPIs or adding a H2RA, except in cases of severe esophagitis.

Maintenance therapy is usually necessary as GERD is a chronic disease. The lowest possible dose of PPI or H2RA should be titrated for symptom control. In patients with extraesophageal symptoms, maintenance therapy is indicated only to control esophageal symptoms. Long-term PPI therapy is potentially safe though there is a theoretical risk of hypergastrinemia, vitamin B12 and iron deficiency, pneumonia, *Clostridium difficile* colitis, and hip fractures.

Antireflux surgery (laparoscopic fundoplication) and long-term PPIs have equal efficacy for control of esophageal reflux symptoms. Surgery should be offered when an individual is intolerant to PPIs, or when a patient has troublesome sour regurgitation. The potential side-effects of antireflux surgery include excessive flatulence, inability to belch, and dysphagia.

INFECTIOUS ESOPHAGITIS

Infectious esophagitis can be due to viral, bacterial, and fungal causes. With an increase in the number of patients with immunocompromised states, there has been an increased frequency of esophageal infections.

Infections of the esophagus present with acute dysphagia, odynophagia, and chest pain. In patients with severe ulceration of the mucosa, bleeding may occur; this is usually self-limiting and small in quantity.

VIRAL

Herpes simplex virus (HSV) type 1 or 2 may cause esophagitis in immunocompromised individuals. Systemic manifestations like nausea, vomiting, and fever may be present. On endoscopy, the esophageal mucosa has 1–3 mm vesicles and small, discrete, punched-out lesions, which may proceed to confluent ulcers and diffuse erosive esophagitis. Biopsy or cytology may show ballooning degeneration, ground-glass change in nuclei with eosinophilic inclusions (Cowdry type A), and giant cell formation. Treatment consists of 14–21 day course of acyclovir (400 mg orally 5 times a day). In severe odynophagia, initial treatment with acyclovir 250 mg/m^2 intravenous 8 hourly and as the patient improves, oral therapy may be started with 200–400 mg acyclovir 5 times a day. Symptoms usually resolve within a week.

Varicella-zoster virus occasionally produces esophagitis in children with chicken pox and in adults with herpes zoster. The esophageal lesions are similar to those of HSV, and necrotizing esophagitis may occur in a severely compromised patient. Biopsy from the edge of the ulcer shows findings similar to those of HSV, and differentiation requires culture studies. Acyclovir, in doses higher than for HSV, is required for treatment.

Cytomegalovirus infection occurs only in immunocompromised host. Endoscopy shows serpiginous ulcers which are large and deep with surrounding normal mucosa. In distal esophagus, the ulcers may coalesce. Biopsy should be taken from the center of the ulcer and reveals intranuclear and small cytoplasmic inclusions in fibroblasts and endothelial cells of blood vessels. Early diagnosis may be made by immunohistochemistry using monoclonal antibodies to CMV. Ganciclovir (5 mg/kg every 12 hourly) is the treatment of choice. Valganciclovir or foscarnet can also be used. Complete healing may take a few weeks to months and treatment should be continued until then.

Human immunodeficiency virus causes esophagitis during seroconversion and during inversion of T-cell helper:suppressor ratio. The esophagitis is self-limiting. Steroids may help in this condition.

BACTERIAL

Primary tuberculosis of the esophagus is rare. Tuberculosis affects the esophagus by contiguous spread from the lung or mediastinal lymph nodes. Patients may have an ulcerated lesion with stricture, or have dysphagia due to extrinsic compression from mediastinal lymph nodes.

FUNGAL

Candidiasis of the esophagus occurs in immunodeficiency disorders like diabetes mellitus, chronic renal failure, alcoholism, and acquired immunodeficiency syndrome (AIDS). Individuals receiving steroids or immunosuppressive chemotherapy for malignancy, and those with underlying esophageal diseases that cause stasis of food (achalasia or scleroderma) may also develop candidiasis.

Candida is present in the nonpathogenic form in the oral flora in normal individuals. Patients who develop esophagitis may be asymptomatic, or may have odynophagia and dysphagia. Rarely, bleeding may occur, and the deep ulcers may perforate or may form a stricture. Systemic invasion from esophageal candidiasis is also reported.

Oral candidiasis, if present, suggests the diagnosis by its white flakes appearance. Endoscopy reveals raised white pseudomembranous plaques with mucosal erythema. In severe cases, confluent linear and nodular plaques with underlying ulcerations may be present. A smear taken from these plaques may reveal hyphae. Treatment in mild cases is with 10–20 mL of oral nystatin (100,000 units/mL) 6 hourly, or oral clotrimazole (10 mg 6 hourly), or fluconazole 100 mg/day for 7 days. If symptoms persist, endoscopic biopsy and culture are recommended. If antifungal resistance is demonstrated, caspofungin may be effective.

PROTOZOAL

Protozoal esophagitis is very rare. However, patients with AIDS may develop esophagitis due to *Cryptosporidium* or *Pneumocystis carinii.*

CORROSIVE INJURY

Corrosive is any substance which causes tissue injury upon contact. Caustic injury of the esophagus occurs following accidental or suicidal ingestion of strong alkali (e.g., sodium hydroxide) or acid (hydrochloric and sulfuric acid). Most corrosives are available as over-the-counter drain cleaners, dish washing detergents, bleaches, battery fluids, button batteries, nail polish removers etc.

Alkali ingestion provokes liquefaction or saponification necrosis of the esophageal wall and thrombosis of blood vessels. Acids cause superficial necrosis due to coagulative necrosis which limits its penetration into deeper layers of esophageal, and also it is ingested in small quantity due to offensive smell and taste. Severity of tissue injury depends upon factors like substance pH, physical state (solids adhere to mucosa and cause more damage), quantity, tissue contact time, and concentration. There is an acute inflammatory response with mucosal necrosis, followed by sloughing of necrotic tissue and ulceration over 4–15 days. Risk of perforation is maximum up to 7 days. After 3–4 weeks, cicatrization begins. Significant esophageal strictures develop when there is circumferential damage.

In the esophagus, corrosives pool at the postcricoid area, level of the aortic arch, tracheal bifurcation, and LES. These are common locations for strictures. In severe cases, there may be perforation into the mediastinum or pleural cavity or development of a tracheoesophageal fistula.

Symptoms include burning pain in the mouth and throat, odynophagia, excessive salivation, stridor, hoarseness, dysphagia, and chest pain. There may be edema and ulceration of the lips, tongue, and pharynx. Airway obstruction from severe epiglottic and laryngeal edema may occur. As the acute inflammatory reaction subsides, odynophagia and dysphagia decrease; with the development of esophageal stricture, dysphagia gradually returns, usually within 1–3 months after the ingestion. Mortality rate is of 1%, usually due to mediastinitis or peritonitis resulting in multiorgan failure.

The aim of *therapy* in the acute phase is resuscitation and supportive care. Clinical features do not correlate with severity of damage. X-ray or CT scan of chest and abdomen is done to check for perforation, pneumomediastinum or pneumoperitoneum. If there is evidence of perforation, patient may need surgery. Flexible endoscopy should be done at the earliest or up to 96 hours of corrosive ingestion, after ruling out a perforation and is the best way to assess the severity of mucosal damage. Patients who have minimal injury can be started on oral liquids by 48 hours and can be discharged early. In patients with advanced damage, a nasojejunal tube can be placed during endoscopy; this serves as a route for maintaining nutrition. Measures which have shown to be of no use or are harmful are administration of activated charcoal, pH neutralization or dilution, by inducing emesis, and intravenous steroids. Antibiotic therapy is required only if secondary infection is present.

Stricture of the esophagus is the major long-term complication. Caustic strictures are often extensive and multiple. They respond to repeated dilatation, and the frequency of dilatation may decrease over time. Self-expandable plastic stents can be placed at the site of stricture for 6–8 weeks, with good results. Esophageal resection with colon or gastric tube replacement may be necessary in cases of extensive damage.

PILL-INDUCED ESOPHAGEAL INJURY

Pill-induced esophageal injury results from damage due to ingestion of certain medications which cause injury by either production of caustic solution, hyperosmolar solution, or direct drug damage. Drugs commonly implicated are tetracycline, doxycycline, potassium chloride, nonsteroidal anti-inflammatory drugs, alendronate, ferrous sulfate, theophylline, and quinidine. The injury is more common if inadequate water is taken with the medication, or the patient lies down immediately after taking a pill. The most common location of pill-induced esophagitis is the mid-esophagus at the crossing of aorta or carina. Symptoms include severe sudden onset chest pain, odynophagia, and dysphagia. Endoscopy may reveal an ulcer, diffuse esophagitis, or pseudomembrane at the site of damage. Withdrawal of the offending medication, viscous lignocaine solution, adequate hydration, and use of PPIs to reduce acid exposure results in healing of the lesion. Rarely there can be perforation, esophagorespiratory fistula, or a chronic stricture at the site of the ulcer.

EOSINOPHILIC ESOPHAGITIS

Eosinophilic esophagitis (EoE) is characterized by eosinophilic infiltration of the esophageal mucosa. Almost 80% of children and 40–60% of adults have history of food/environmental allergies.

Patients may present with dysphagia, recurrent food impaction, and heartburn. Often, they are treated as GERD and do not respond adequately to therapy.

Endoscopic findings include esophageal rings (felinization or trachealization), raised white specks, longitudinal furrows, whitish exudates, and strictures. Multiple (>5) biopsies from different levels of the esophagus should be taken. The pathognomonic feature of EoE is eosinophilic infiltration of 15 eosinophils/HPF (high power field) in the esophageal mucosa; other features are eosinophilic microabscesses.

Drugs used for treatment include corticosteroids to control the inflammation. Topical preparation of fluticasone propionate (440–500 mg/day) should be given orally twice daily for 6 weeks; swallowed budesonide mixed with sucralose and beclomethasone has also been used. Symptoms recur in 50% of patients when treatment is stopped and can be managed with reintroduction of same therapy or, use of steroid-sparing drugs like azathioprine. Systemic steroids (prednisolone) are used as second-line treatment in severe cases and in patients who do not respond to topical steroids. Endoscopic dilatation of strictures should preferably be limited to patients after a trial of medical therapy, because of the risk of perforation. Dietary therapy by eliminating foods like dairy, peanuts, soy, fish, eggs, wheat, and other foods identified by allergic testing has been found to be successful in 70% of children with EoE.

HIATUS HERNIA

Herniation through the esophageal hiatus occurs in two forms: (1) axial or sliding type; and (2) paraesophageal or rolling type.

In sliding hernia, both the distal esophagus and a varying portion of the stomach are situated above the diaphragm. The size of the sliding hernia alone does not predict the presence or severity of symptoms; larger, long-standing hernias are more likely to be associated with symptomatic GER.

In the less common paraesophageal or rolling hernia, the lower esophagus and the esophagogastric junction retain their position below the diaphragm, while a portion of the proximal stomach protrudes into the thorax alongside the esophagus. With positive intra-abdominal pressure exerting an upward push, this hernia tends to enlarge progressively. The typical paraesophageal hernia is rarely associated with GER; however, it can get incarcerated and strangulation or bleeding may occur.

The management of symptomatic sliding hiatus hernia is similar to that of GERD. Paraesophageal hernia needs surgical correction to avoid complications.

ESOPHAGEAL WEBS, RINGS, AND DIVERTICULA

Esophageal webs usually occur in the upper esophagus, but may occur in the mid or lower esophagus as well. They are thin horizontal membranes of stratified squamous epithelium, usually protrude from the anterior wall. A syndrome of cervical esophageal web, anemia, and platynychia, which occurs mainly in middle-aged women, is called the Paterson–Kelly or Plummer–Vinson syndrome.

Esophageal rings are found near the LES. They are of two types. Type A is a muscular ring, 4–5 mm thick and is the hypertrophied upper portion of LES. Type B ring, or Schatzki ring, is a mucosal ring at the squamocolumnar junction; its upper surface is squamous epithelium and undersurface is columnar. It is usually associated with GERD.

Rings and webs present with intermittent, mild dysphagia to solid food. Treatment consists of breaking the web or ring by dilatation. The underlying disorder like anemia or GER needs appropriate treatment.

Diverticula are outpouchings of the esophageal wall from an area of muscular weakness. Zenker's diverticulum occurs due to weakness in the posterior hypopharynx; patients present with dysphagia and regurgitation. Treatment consists of cricopharyngeal myotomy. Epiphrenic diverticula occur in the distal esophagus and are associated with esophageal motility disorders.

RECOMMENDED READINGS

1. Mittal R, Vaezi MF. Esophageal Motility Disorders and Gastroesophageal Reflux Disease. N Engl J Med. 2020;383(20):1961-72.
2. Jawaid S, Draganov PV, Yang D. Esophageal POEM: the new standard of care. Transl Gastroenterol Hepatol. 2020;5:47.
3. Jung HK, Hong SJ, Lee OY, Pandolfino J, Park H, Miwa H, et al. 2019 Seoul Consensus on Esophageal Achalasia Guidelines. J Neurogastroenterol Motil. 2020;26(2):180-203.
4. Maret-Ouda J, Markar SR, Lagergren J. Gastroesophageal Reflux Disease: A Review. JAMA. 2020;324(24):2536-47.
5. Young A, Kumar MA, Thota PN. GERD: A practical approach. Cleve Clin J Med. 2020;87(4):223-30.
6. Hoffman RS, Burns MM, Gosselin S. Ingestion of Caustic Substances. N Engl J Med. 2020;382(18):1739-48.
7. Katzka DA. Eosinophilic Esophagitis. Ann Intern Med. 2020;172(9):ITC65-ITC80.
8. Malfertheiner P, Kandulski A, Venerito M. Proton-pump inhibitors: understanding the complications and risks. Nat Rev Gastroenterol Hepatol. 2017;14(12):697-710.

CHAPTER

130 Dyspepsia and Peptic Ulcer Disease

Amit Kumar Dutta

ABSTRACT

Dyspepsia is a common clinical condition, which includes multiple symptoms such as epigastric pain, epigastric burning sensation, bloating, and early satiety. In majority of patients, symptoms arise without an underlying organic pathology and are considered functional. However, in some patients, an underlying organic pathology may be present. Considering the prevalent nature of symptoms, an understanding of the clinical and etiological factors as well as role of investigations is essential for optimum management of patient. Older individuals and those with alarm symptoms require endoscopy while younger patients without alarm symptoms do not need this test. Treatment is aimed at providing symptom relief and treating any underlying cause, if present.

Peptic ulcer disease is an important cause of organic dyspepsia. The chief etiological agents include *Helicobacter pylori* infection, nonsteroidal anti-inflammatory drugs (NSAIDs) and aspirin. The main symptom is pain in upper abdomen. Some patients may present with complications such as bleeding, perforation, or gastric outlet obstruction. Diagnosis is usually made during upper gastrointestinal endoscopy. Treatment includes acid-suppressant medications to heal the ulcer and eradication of *H. pylori* infection, if present. This chapter discusses the evaluation and management of patients with dyspepsia and peptic ulcer disease.

"No matter how dark things seem to be or actually are, raise your sights and see the possibilities – always see them, for they're always there"

—Norman Vincent Peale

DYSPEPSIA

INTRODUCTION

The word "dyspepsia" is derived from the Greek language and means bad or difficult digestion. In clinical practice, dyspepsia includes a variety of symptoms originating from the stomach and duodenum. This includes epigastric pain or burning sensation, bloating, belching, early satiety, nausea etc. It is one of the most common gastrointestinal conditions seen in clinical practice. Multiple etiological factors can lead to dyspeptic symptoms, although in about two-thirds of cases, no cause is identified. Due to the heterogeneous nature of this condition, in terms of type and severity of symptoms as well as causative factors, a systematic approach is essential for appropriate evaluation and management.

EPIDEMIOLOGY AND ETIOLOGICAL FACTORS

Globally, the prevalence of dyspeptic symptoms varies from 15–35%. In India, the prevalence is estimated to be around 25–30% and is more common in urban than rural population. There is no consistent gender predilection, although in some population, females are more commonly affected. The disease affects all age groups and the peak incidence is noted during fourth to sixth decade of life. The nature and severity of symptoms vary and about 15–30% of individuals with dyspepsia seek medical care. Based on the evaluation of symptoms and underlying etiological factor, dyspepsia has been grouped under the following subtypes:

- **Uninvestigated dyspepsia:** Patients in whom evaluation of etiology has not been done.
- **Functional dyspepsia:** Patients where no causative factor is identified during evaluation.
- **Organic dyspepsia:** Patients where an underlying cause is identified during evaluation.

Among patients who undergo evaluation of symptoms, no cause is found in about 70% cases (functional dyspepsia). Hence the proportion of patients with organic cause of dyspepsia is much lower compared to the functional group. The list of conditions associated with dyspeptic symptoms is large (**Box 1**) and among them peptic ulcer disease and erosive esophagitis are common while gastric/esophageal malignancy is noted in <1% cases. *H. pylori* infection is also recognized as a cause of dyspepsia but this occurs in <10% of patients with this infection. Earlier, this was grouped under functional dyspepsia but currently it has been reclassified as a separate entity called "*H. pylori*-associated dyspepsia" and is considered distinct from functional dyspepsia.

Investigations do not reveal any visible abnormality in stomach, duodenum, or other organs in upper abdomen on endoscopy and imaging in functional dyspepsia. However, a number of physiological abnormalities have been identified in a subgroup of these patients. This includes abnormal gastric accommodation and motility, visceral hyper-

BOX 1	Causes of organic dyspepsia.
• Peptic ulcer disease	
• Gastroesophageal reflux disease	
• Drugs (NSAID, aspirin, potassium supplements, iron supplements, alendronate, SSRI, antibiotics, steroids, digitalis, theophylline etc.)	
• Ethanol intake	
• Other infections (cytomegalovirus, tuberculosis, *Giardia*, *Strongyloides*, fungal infection)	
• Inflammatory disorders (Crohn's disease, Sarcoidosis)	
• Systemic and metabolic disorders: Hypothyroidism, Type 2 diabetes mellitus, heart failure, chronic kidney disease	
• Gastric dysmotility (Gastroparesis)	
• Pregnancy	
• Pancreatic, liver, and biliary diseases	
• Dietary factors	
• Upper gastrointestinal tract malignancy	

(SSRI: selective serotonin reuptake inhibitor)

sensitivity, abnormal processing of signals in central nervous system and duodenal inflammation. Other functional gastrointestinal disorders may coexist with functional dyspepsia. Gastroesophageal reflux symptoms are present in about 30% of patients with functional dyspepsia while 15% have symptoms of irritable bowel syndrome.

CLINICAL FEATURES

The four main symptoms of dyspepsia are: (1) Epigastric pain, (2) epigastric burning sensation, (3) bloating, and (4) early satiety. Patients may report any combination of these symptoms and severity may vary. Based on the dominant type of symptoms, functional dyspepsia is categorized into two groups: (1) Postprandial distress syndrome—patients with early satiety and/or bloating as the chief symptom, (2) epigastric pain syndrome—patients with epigastric pain and/or epigastric burning sensation as the chief symptom. This classification may have some benefits in making therapeutic decisions although overlap of the symptoms from the two groups is frequently noted. Other symptoms, which may be present in patients with dyspepsia, include belching, nausea, heartburn, and regurgitation. Heartburn is usually associated with gastroesophageal reflux but around 25% of patients with dyspepsia may have this symptom although it is not the predominant symptom. Some patients may have coexisting psychiatric symptoms such as anxiety or depression.

Clinical evaluation should include detailed assessment of the above symptoms including their duration, relationship to meals, dietary triggers, severity, and progression. As a number of conditions are associated with dyspepsia (**Box 1**), the presence of coexisting illnesses, medications, smoking and alcohol consumption and past abdominal surgery should be ascertained. In addition, it is essential to look for alarm symptoms such as dysphagia, vomiting, weight loss, feeling of mass in abdomen and gastrointestinal bleed. Alarm symptoms may be suggestive of an underlying organic cause and warrant a thorough investigation instead of empirical treatment. A family history of significant gastrointestinal illness, especially upper gastrointestinal malignancy, should be obtained.

As two-thirds of the patients with dyspepsia have no organic disease, physical examination is often normal. However, physical examination is an important aspect of clinical evaluation. They may provide a clue to an underlying organic cause. This includes pallor, icterus, edema, features of nutritional deficiency, and peripheral signs of malignancy such as acanthosis nigricans, thrombophlebitis, and enlarged supraclavicular lymph node. Abdominal examination may reveal a mass lesion, ascites, or organomegaly in patients with organic lesions.

INVESTIGATIONS AND DIAGNOSIS

The diagnosis of dyspepsia is based mainly on symptoms. Recommended investigations include blood tests for hemoglobin, renal function, glucose level and thyroid function and stool test for parasites. Tests for *H. pylori* are also recommended in the Western countries and in Asian countries with high prevalence of gastric cancer. However, based on the data from randomized controlled trials in India, the benefit of *H. pylori* eradication for dyspepsia is unclear and is not routinely recommended.

Further investigations are required to look for an underlying cause in a subgroup of patients and include upper gastrointestinal (UGI) endoscopy and imaging of abdomen. This depends on the age of patient, presence of alarm features, and failure to respond to empirical therapy.

- *Patients <40 years of age*: The key benefit of endoscopy is in detecting an underlying organic lesion especially malignancy as a cause of dyspepsia. In Western countries, the risk of malignancy is very low in patients <55 years of age and hence endoscopy is not recommended if they do not have alarm features. However, in India about 15% of upper gastrointestinal malignancy occurs in patients between 40 and 55 years of age and therefore a cutoff of 40 years is more appropriate. Therefore, among Indian patients who are <40 years of age and do not have alarm features, UGI endoscopy is not essential.
- *Patients ≥40 years of age*: UGI endoscopy is recommended in patients ≥40 years of age with dyspepsia to exclude malignancy.
- *Patients with alarm features*: Alarm features include weight loss, gastrointestinal bleeding, dysphagia, vomiting, pallor/anemia, peripheral signs of malignancy, mass in abdomen, ascites, and organomegaly. All patients with alarm features should undergo UGI endoscopy, irrespective of their age. In addition, patients with family history of gastric malignancy should also undergo UGI endoscopy.
- *Persistent symptoms*: Patients in whom the symptoms persist, despite empirical therapy, may also require further evaluation like UGI endoscopy to look for an underlying organic cause.

BOX 2 ROME IV criteria for functional dyspepsia.

- *At least one of the following symptoms, which is bothersome*:
  - (i) Postprandial fullness
  - (ii) Early satiety
  - (iii) Epigastric pain
  - (iv) Epigastric burning sensation
- No organic cause of symptoms on evaluation
- The criteria should be fulfilled for at least 3 months and symptom onset should be at least 6 months before diagnosis
- **Subclassification:**
  - *Postprandial distress syndrome*: Patients who have symptom (i) and/or (ii) for at least 3 days per week
  - *Epigastric pain syndrome*: Patients who have symptom (iii) and/or (iv) for at least 1 day per week

Source: Stanghellini V, Chan FK, Hasler WL, Malagelada JR, Suzuki H, Tack J, et al. Gastroduodenal Disorders. Gastroenterology. 2016;150(6):1380-92.

In addition to UGI endoscopy, imaging of abdomen may also be required to assess for other conditions associated with dyspepsia. This includes pancreatic disorders, gallbladder and biliary disorders, liver disorders etc. An ultrasound of abdomen is often sufficient but occasionally a higher imaging like computed tomography may be required in patients with alarm features such as anemia, weight loss, and mass lesion.

The investigations mentioned above are aimed at identifying an organic cause of dyspepsia. When no organic cause is found, dyspepsia is considered functional. The diagnostic criteria for functional dyspepsia recommended by the ROME committee are frequently used. The most recent of these criteria were published in 2016 (ROME IV criteria, **Box 2**). However, these may not be strictly applicable in all patients and clinical judgment is important, especially with regards to duration of symptoms. These criteria are more helpful in clinical research to ensure uniformity of included subjects. With regards to the subtypes of dyspepsia, an overlap of the two subtypes is more common in India followed by postprandial distress syndrome and epigastric pain syndrome.

MANAGEMENT

The management of dyspepsia involves a multipronged approach and includes pharmacological and nonpharmacological interventions. It depends on the nature and severity of symptoms.

Gastric acid suppressants: This includes proton-pump inhibitors (PPIs) and histamine 2 receptor antagonists (H2RAs). They are generally the first-line therapy for dyspeptic symptoms. PPIs have better efficacy than H2RAs. The duration of therapy should generally be limited to 8–12 weeks. Further use of these agents should be tailored according to recurrence of symptoms. Long-term use of PPIs has been associated with adverse effects such as vitamin B12 deficiency, bacterial overgrowth, osteoporosis, and renal dysfunction. Although the absolute risk of these adverse effects is low, caution should be exercised when prescribing them for longer duration.

Prokinetic agents: These include drugs such as domperidone and itopride. They are less effective than acid suppressants and are seldom used as monotherapy. They may be useful as an adjunctive therapy, in addition to PPI, in patients with postprandial distress subtype of functional dyspepsia.

Drugs affecting gastric accommodation: Impaired gastric accommodation has been identified in up to 40% patients with functional dyspepsia. Drugs such as buspirone and acotiamide improve gastric accommodation and have shown benefit in relieving symptoms although data is limited.

Antidepressants: In patients not responding to acid suppressants and those with coexisting symptoms of depression, antidepressants may be used. Tricyclic antidepressants such as amitriptyline and tetracyclic antidepressants such as mirtazapine have been shown to be effective in management of dyspepsia. In addition to drugs, psychotherapy has also been used in treating dyspeptic symptoms.

***H. pylori* eradication therapy:** As discussed earlier, this is not recommended as a first-line therapy in Indian patients with dyspepsia due to the lack of evidence showing benefit. However, patients not responding to acid suppressants or in those with frequent and recurrent symptoms, this may be an option.

Diet and lifestyle measures: Strong evidence for specific dietary measures in treating dyspepsia is lacking. However, they may be beneficial in some patients. Dietary measures include avoiding food triggering symptoms and eating small and frequent meals in patients with postprandial distress syndrome. Eating balanced diet, regular meal timings, avoiding lying down for 2–3 hours after meals, regular exercise, and avoiding smoking are some of the measures to promote a healthy lifestyle and may help in dealing with the negative perception of symptoms.

Complementary and alternative therapy: Products such as STW5 and menthacarin have shown some benefit in relieving dyspeptic symptoms, although experience with these agents is limited.

Treatment of underlying organic cause: In patients with organic cause of dyspepsia, treating the underlying cause is important in addition to the symptomatic therapy discussed in the earlier text. This includes treating the underlying conditions such as peptic ulcer disease, erosive esophagitis, pancreaticobiliary disorders, diabetes mellitus, and neoplastic lesions. In addition, drugs causing dyspeptic symptoms should be avoided if feasible.

PROGNOSIS

Functional dyspepsia may not affect survival but may have a significant impact on the quality of life. Hence appropriate management is important. The response rate in placebo arm of drug trials varies from 30 to 40% and therefore in addition to drug therapy, paying attention to patient's symptoms, empathizing with the patient, acknowledging the presence of symptoms and reassurance about their benign nature may go a long way in improving the outcome of treatment. After diagnosis and initial therapy, about 20% patients have persistent symptoms, 30% have recurrent symptoms and the rest experience long-term relief from symptoms. Therefore, follow-up after initiation of therapy is an integral part of management.

PEPTIC ULCER DISEASE

INTRODUCTION

Peptic ulcer disease (PUD) denotes a break in gastric or duodenal mucosa, which is greater than 5 mm in diameter and extends at least up to muscularis mucosa. A lesion, which is smaller in size and more superficial, is called erosion. Duodenum is more commonly affected than stomach; although, in the past two decades, the ratio of duodenal ulcer (DU) to gastric ulcer (GU) is declining. PUD may also develop in ectopic gastric mucosa in Meckel's diverticulum or esophageal inlet.

The incidence of PUD is estimated to be around 0.1–0.3% and is more common in males. Majority of the patients are in the fourth to sixth decade of life, although any age group may be affected. PUD is noted in about 5–6% of patients with dyspepsia and is an important cause of organic dyspepsia.

ETIOPATHOGENESIS

The mucosa of stomach and duodenum are exposed to acidic secretions in the lumen. There are multiple defense mechanisms, which protect the mucosal surface including mucus coating on the surface, epithelial lining, and vascular supply. Prostaglandins and nitric oxide play an important role in maintaining mucosal barrier function. Multiple factors may lead to impairment of barrier function and result in PUD. This includes extrinsic factors, host genetic factors, and immune response. Two most common causes of PUD are infection with *H. pylori* and NSAIDs.

Infection with *H. pylori* is the most common cause of PUD. *H. pylori* is a gram-negative spiral bacterium and is present in more than half of the world's population. In India, the prevalence is estimated to be around 60–75%. Despite the infection being common, only a small proportion (<10%) of individuals develop significant illness. This may be due to variations in strain and pathogenic property of bacteria. The diseases cause by *H. pylori* include PUD, gastric cancer, and gastric mucosa-associated lymphoid tissue (MALT) lymphoma. Other conditions associated with this infection include iron deficiency anemia, idiopathic thrombocytopenic purpura, and vitamin B12 deficiency, although the association is weak. In addition, *H. pylori* infection is also associated with dyspeptic symptoms without causing PUD (*H. pylori*-associated dyspepsia). Infection leads to chronic inflammation in gastric mucosa (**Fig. 1 A**) and may progress in some individuals to atrophic gastritis and intestinal metaplasia and subsequently gastric cancer. The bacteria can be detected on hematoxylin and eosin (H&E) staining but special stains such as modified Giemsa stain make them easier to identify (**Fig. 1 B**). Overall, *H. pylori* leads to PUD by causing chronic inflammation, disrupting mucosal barrier function and affecting acid secretion. **Figure 2** shows the histopathology image of chronic gastric ulcer.

Nonsteroidal anti-inflammatory drugs and aspirin are the next most common cause of PUD. They inhibit prostaglandin secretion, which are important for maintaining mucosal barrier function. Other risk factors for PUD include smoking, older age, previous history of PUD, comorbid conditions such as chronic liver disease, chronic kidney disease and chronic obstructive pulmonary disease. Steroids, antiplatelet drugs, and anticoagulants may potentiate the effect of other factors in causing PUD. Patient with critical illnesses such as burns, head injury,

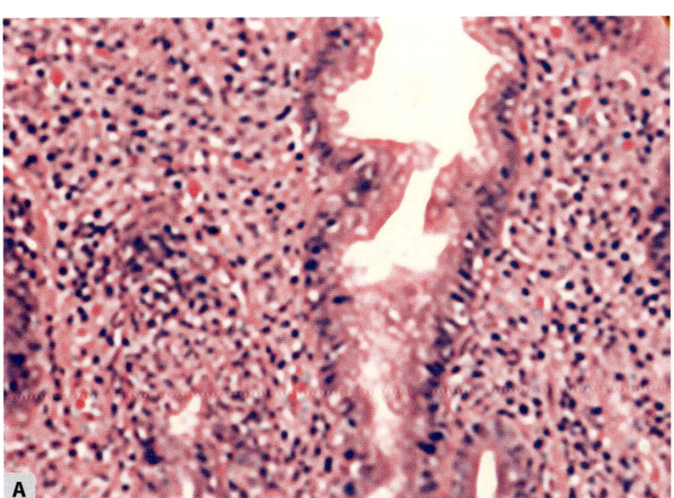

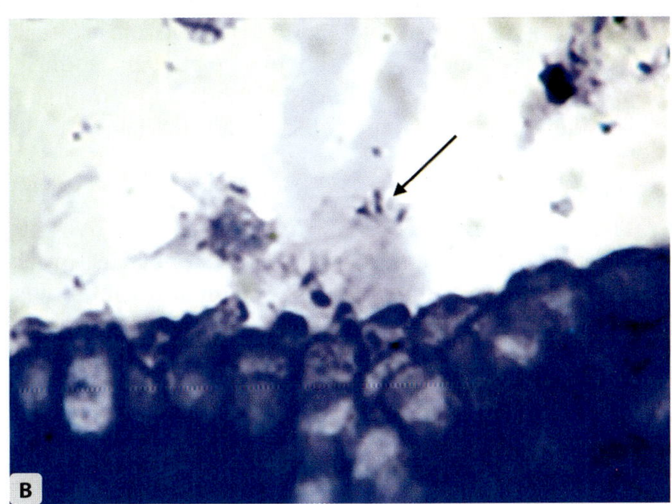

(H&E: hematoxylin and eosin)

FIGURES 1 A & B: Histopathology: **(A)** Chronic gastritis with severe foveolitis due to *Helicobacter pylori* infection (H&E stain); **(B)** Modified Giemsa stain showing *H. pylori* (arrow) above the gastric surface epithelium.

Courtesy: Dr Anna Pulimood, Professor, Department of Gastrointestinal Sciences, CMC Hospital, Vellore.

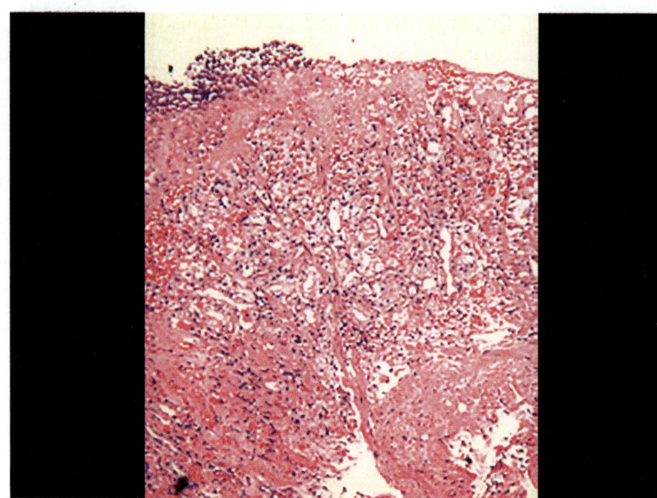

(H&E: hematoxylin and eosin)

FIGURE 2: Histopathology of chronic gastric ulcer (H&E stain).

Courtesy: Dr Anna Pulimood, Professor, Department of Gastrointestinal Sciences, CMC Hospital, Vellore.

BOX 3	Causes of ulcer in stomach and duodenum.
• **Peptic ulcer disease** (*Helicobacter pylori* infection, NSAID, and aspirin)	
• **Drugs:** Bisphosphonate, potassium chloride, iron tablets, antiplatelet drugs etc.	
• **Malignancy** (adenocarcinoma, lymphoma, metastatic lesion)	
• **Inflammatory:** Crohn's disease, sarcoidosis, eosinophilic gastritis	
• **Infection:** Tuberculosis, CMV, HSV, syphilis	
• **Others:** Ischemia, post-radiation, corrosive ingestion, iatrogenic (postendoscopic resection of lesions)	
• **Idiopathic**	

and multiorgan failure are also at risk of developing ulcers in stomach. Contrary to popular belief, spices and chili have not been shown to be a risk factor for PUD. The role of stress is also controversial. In some patients, no etiology is found (idiopathic PUD). In addition to PUD, ulcers in stomach and duodenum may be due to other conditions (**Box 3**).

CLINICAL FEATURES

The symptoms are often nonspecific and overlap with functional dyspepsia. Pain or discomfort in upper abdomen, mainly in the epigastric region and sometimes in right upper quadrant of abdomen, is the chief symptom. Other symptoms include bloating, belching, heartburn, and nausea. The symptoms may be intermittent and present for several weeks to months. The classic symptoms of DU has been described as nocturnal epigastric pain, which occurs 2–3 hours after meals, awakens the patient, and is relieved by food. The pain of gastric ulcer classically occurs or worsens after food intake and anorexia and weight loss may be present in about 30–40% cases. In clinical practice, however, symptoms are not very useful in differentiating between gastric and duodenal ulcer. Presence of alarm features, as discussed earlier for dyspepsia, should be assessed to guide investigation. History of drug intake (NSAID, aspirin, antiplatelets, steroids, anticoagulants etc.), smoking, and coexisting illnesses should be obtained. In 20–30% patients, there may be no symptoms related to PUD and ulcers are detected during investigations (endoscopy and imaging) for other indications. Although clinical examination is usually normal in PUD, a proper general and systematic examination is essential.

Complications: Three important complications related to PUD are: (1) Bleeding, (2) perforation, and (3) gastric outlet obstruction.

This may be the initial presentation of PUD in a subgroup of patients, especially bleeding ulcer in patients taking NSAIDs. While patients with bleeding and perforation present acutely, symptoms of gastric outlet obstruction are usually chronic. The symptoms of bleeding ulcer are hematemesis and melena. Perforated ulcer causes acute-onset severe pain in upper abdomen with rigidity and guarding on clinical examination. Patients with gastric outlet obstruction complain of vomiting, which usually occurs 30–60 minutes after meals. Visible gastric peristalsis and succession splash may be noted on examination.

INVESTIGATIONS

The diagnostic test of choice for PUD is UGI endoscopy. The ulcer is directly visualized and its size, location, and number (in case of multiple ulcers) noted during examination (**Figs. 3 A** to **C**). In addition, gastric mucosal biopsy sample for testing for *H. pylori* infection is also obtained during endoscopy, *H. pylori* can be diagnosed by performing rapid urease test (RUT) on the biopsy specimen, which is simple, and results are obtained within 1–24 hours. The bacterial urease enzyme cleaves urea in the test kit and leads to change in pH, which is detected by a color change in patients with infection. Patients should not be on antibiotics or acid suppressants for about 2 weeks before the test.

Mucosal biopsy specimen from stomach may also be sent for histopathology to detect *H. pylori,* although this test is more expensive and takes more time than RUT. For duodenal ulcer, visualizing the ulcer and RUT is sufficient. In contrast, for gastric ulcer, biopsy should be taken from the margin of ulcer and sent for histopathology to exclude malignancy. Malignant gastric ulcers are more likely to have raised and irregular margin while benign ulcers have smooth edges and flat base. Duodenal ulcers are rarely malignant and hence routine biopsy from the ulcer margin is not recommended. In the past, PUD was usually diagnosed on barium meal study of stomach and duodenum but is seldom used currently with the widespread availability of endoscopy facilities. It may have a role in patients where endoscopy is contraindicated.

MANAGEMENT

The goals of therapy include healing of ulcer and prevention of recurrence.

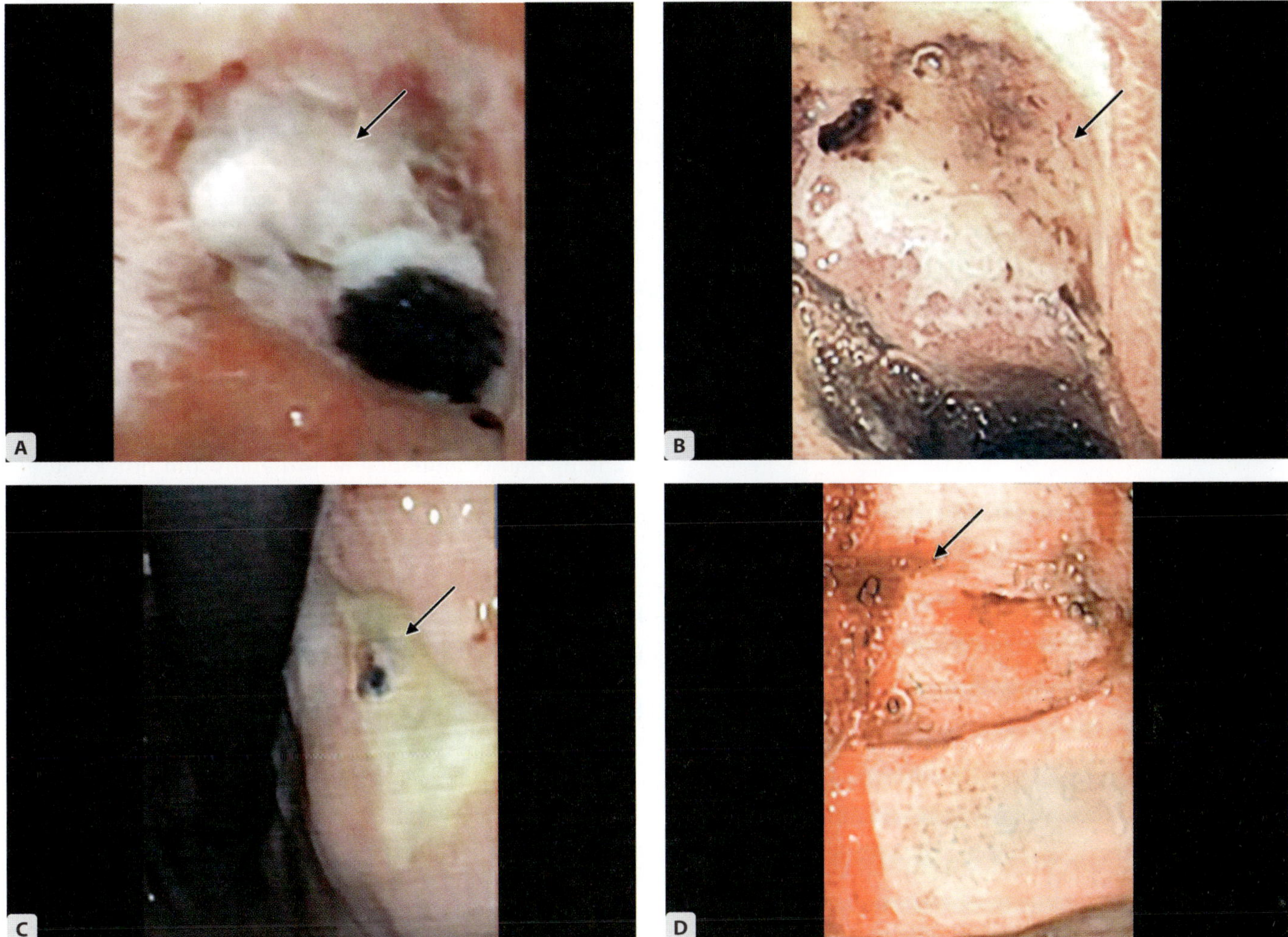

FIGURES 3 A to D: Endoscopy images: **(A)** Peptic ulcer in gastric antrum (arrow); **(B)** Peptic ulcer in duodenal bulb (arrow); **(C)** Peptic ulcer in body of stomach (arrow); **(D)** Peptic ulcer in antrum of stomach with active bleeding (arrow).

Courtesy: Dr Lalji Patel, Consultant, Department of Gastrointestinal Sciences, CMC Hospital, Vellore.

Ulcer healing: Acid-suppressant drugs are the cornerstones of therapy for healing of ulcers. Acid-suppressant drugs include PPIs and H2RAs. Among them, PPIs are the drugs of choice as they are more potent at suppressing gastric acid secretion and lead to faster healing of ulcers. Examples of PPIs include omeprazole, pantoprazole, lansoprazole, and rabeprazole (**Box 4**). There is no significant difference among them for efficacy of ulcer healing and any one of them may be prescribed. For DU, PPI therapy is recommended for 4 weeks and for GU therapy should be continued for 8 weeks. H2RAs are also effective in healing ulcers but are seldom used as first-choice drugs with the availability of PPIs. Examples of H2RAs include ranitidine, famotidine, and nizatidine. Other drugs such as sucralfate, misoprostol, and bismuth compounds have also shown efficacy in healing ulcers but are infrequently used as PPIs have much better efficacy. Antacids such as magnesium or aluminum compounds neutralize acid in lumen but do not suppress acid secretion and should not be used primarily for ulcer healing. They are often used as over-the-counter medication for relief of dyspeptic symptoms.

Prevention of recurrence: To prevent recurrence of PUD, the underlying cause should be evaluated and managed accordingly. *H. pylori* infection is the most frequent cause and all patients with PUD should be tested for *H. pylori* infection. In patients with infection, eradication therapy should be administered. The therapy includes a combination of antibiotic and acid suppressants and there are different regimens based on the drugs used (triple therapy, quadruple therapy, sequential therapy, concomitant therapy, and hybrid therapy). The duration of therapy is 2 weeks and clarithromycin-based triple therapy and bismuth-based quadruple therapy are the main regimens (**Box 5**). In areas with low prevalence of *H. pylori* resistance to clarithromycin (<15%), triple therapy containing this drug is used as first-line treatment. In areas with higher resistance, bismuth-based quadruple therapy is the preferred initial therapy.

BOX 4	Standard dose of proton-pump inhibitors in adults.
• Pantoprazole: 40 mg once daily	
• Esomeprazole: 40 mg once daily	
• Omeprazole: 20 mg once daily	
• Lansoprazole: 30 mg once daily	
• Rabeprazole: 20 mg once daily	

BOX 5	*Helicobacter pylori* eradication therapy regimen.
• **Clarithromycin-based triple therapy (duration 14 days):**	
◦ PPI twice daily (e.g., tablet pantoprazole 40 mg twice daily)	
◦ Tablet clarithromycin 500 mg twice daily	
◦ Capsule amoxycillin 1,000 mg twice daily	
• **Bismuth-based quadruple therapy (duration 14 days):**	
◦ PPI twice daily (e.g., tablet pantoprazole 40 mg twice daily)	
◦ Tablet bismuth subcitrate (120 mg) *or* bismuth subsalicylate (300 mg)—four times daily	
◦ Capsule tetracycline 500 mg four times daily	
◦ Tablet metronidazole 500 mg three times daily	

(PPI: proton-pump inhibitor)

The data on clarithromycin resistance from India is scanty and conflicting and hence either therapy is appropriate. Reports from India suggest a very high incidence of resistance of *H. pylori* to metronidazole and hence triple therapy based on metronidazole is not recommended. However, metronidazole may still be used as a component of bismuth-based quadruple therapy, as the efficacy is not significantly reduced.

Another important aspect of managing *H. pylori* infection is to test for success of eradication after therapy is completed. The efficacy of standard therapies in bacterial eradication ranges from 75 to 90%. Hence it is important to confirm eradication as persistent infection may lead to recurrent ulcer and its complications. For confirming *H. pylori* eradication, nonendoscopic test like urea breath test or stool antigen test is appropriate and should be done a month after therapy is completed. If infection is persistent, alternative therapeutic regimen may be used as second-line therapy. Failure of second-line therapy warrants culture to determine antibiotic sensitivity and decide on appropriate drugs but this test is generally not available as the organism is difficult to culture. Molecular tests may also detect antibiotic resistance but again, this is not freely available.

The next important etiological factors for PUD are NSAIDs and aspirin. These agents should be avoided if feasible, and if they need to be continued, then patient may require long-term PPI, especially if there is a history of PUD-related complication. Using COX-2 (cyclooxygenase-2) selective NSAIDs is another option as they have less effect on gastric mucosal prostaglandin secretion. In patients who smoke, smoking cessation is strongly recommended to promote healing of ulcer.

Management of complications: Patients with symptoms of gastrointestinal bleeding require resuscitation and stabilization followed by upper gastrointestinal endoscopy. Endoscopy has both diagnostic and therapeutic roles. Patients with active bleeding or visible vessel in ulcer base require therapy and >90% are successfully managed with endoscopic therapy (**Fig. 3 D**). When endoscopic therapy is not successful, radiological or surgical intervention should be considered. For perforation, urgent surgical intervention is recommended. Patients with gastric outlet obstruction should be initially managed with PPIs and *H. pylori* eradication therapy (if infection is present). They should be advised to take small-volume meals. This leads to improvement in symptoms in many patients and for those with persistent or recurrent symptoms, surgery may be considered.

Majority of the patients with PUD respond well to medical therapy and the risk of persistent or recurrent ulcer is low. Repeat endoscopy after 3 months is recommended in patients with GU to assess healing as some cases of GU may harbor malignancy. In patients with persistent or recurrent ulcers (GU or DU), one should look for persistent *H. pylori* infection, ongoing NSAID or aspirin intake, smoking and compliance with therapy and other causes of ulcers. In the past, surgery had an important role in managing PUD. This included vagotomy (truncal or highly selective) and drainage procedure. With the availability of PPI and eradication of *H. pylori* infection, the role of surgery has significantly diminished and is generally reserved for complications of PUD and refractory nonhealing ulcers.

RECOMMENDED READINGS

1. Stanghellini V, Chan FK, Hasler WL, Malagelada JR, Suzuki H, Tack J, et al. Gastroduodenal Disorders. Gastroenterology. 2016;150(6):1380-92.
2. Miwa H, Ghoshal UC, Fock KM, Gonlachanvit S, Gwee KA, Ang TL, et al. Asian consensus report on functional dyspepsia. J Gastroenterol Hepatol. 2012;27(4):626-41.
3. Talley NJ, Ford AC. Functional Dyspepsia. N Engl J Med. 2015;373(19):1853-63.
4. Sugano K, Tack J, Kuipers EJ, Graham DY, El-Omar EM, Miura S, et al. Kyoto global consensus report on *Helicobacter pylori* gastritis. Gut. 2015;64(9):1353-67.
5. Kuo YT, Liou JM, El-Omar EM, Wu JY, Leow AHR, Goh KL, et al. Primary antibiotic resistance in *Helicobacter pylori* in the Asia-Pacific region: a systematic review and meta-analysis. Lancet Gastroenterol Hepatol. 2017;2(10):707-15.
6. Malfertheiner P, Megraud F, O'Morain CA, Gisbert JP, Kuipers EJ, Axon AT, et al. Management of *Helicobacter pylori* infection—the Maastricht V/ Florence Consensus Report. Gut. 2017;66(1):6-30.
7. Lanas A, Chan FKL. Peptic ulcer disease. Lancet. 2017;390(10094):613-24.
8. Dutta AK, Chacko A, Balekuduru A, Sahu MK, Gangadharan SK. Time trends in epidemiology of peptic ulcer disease in India over two decades. Indian J Gastroenterol. 2012;31(3):111-5.
9. Ghoshal UC, Singh R, Chang FY, Hou X, Wong BC, Kachintorn U, et al. Epidemiology of uninvestigated and functional dyspepsia in Asia: facts and fiction. J Neurogastroenterol Motil. 2011;17(3):235-44.
10. Milosavljevic T, Kostic-Milosavljevic M, Jovanovic I, Krstic M. Complications of peptic ulcer disease. Dig Dis. 2011;29(5):491-3.

CHAPTER

131 Nonvariceal Upper Gastrointestinal Bleeding

Sanjay Khanna, Ajay Kumar

ABSTRACT

Nonvariceal upper gastrointestinal bleed (UGIB) is a medical emergency with about 65 per 100,000 patients requiring hospitalization. The most common cause remains a peptic ulcer bleed. The patients may present with hematemesis and/or melena and may have hemodynamic compromise depending on the severity of bleed. The patients should be triaged in the emergency itself, possibly by the Glasgow–Blatchford score and decision to whether patient needs ward or intensive care unit (ICU) admission needs to be taken.

Fluid resuscitation needs to be done along with intravenous proton pump inhibitor (PPI) treatment. Packed cells should be transfused to build hemoglobin to 8 g/dL. Fresh frozen plasma (FFP) needs to be transfused if international normalized ratio (INR) is more than 2 and platelet concentrate to be transfused if platelets are less than 50,000/mL. Early upper GI endoscopy (within 24 hours of admission) is done in majority of the patients after adequate resuscitation and endotherapy done as per etiology. Cardiac and renal comorbidities may increase the morbidity in these patients. Patients with acute UGIB, however, have a good outcome after proper resuscitation, drug treatment, and endotherapy.

"It is our attitude at the beginning of a difficult task which, more than anything else, will affect its successful outcome"

—William James

INTRODUCTION

The common manifestations of nonvariceal upper gastrointestinal bleed (UGIB) include hematemesis and/or melena. The primary assessment of patients with acute UGIB begins with history taking and evaluation of hemodynamic status, followed by the search for the underlying cause. The patient needs to be resuscitated, accordingly and thereafter, plan for the diagnostic studies, commonly endoscopy, may be initiated to localize and treat the cause.

ETIOLOGY

The annual incidence of hospitalization for acute UGIB is 65 per 100,000 individuals and is sixfold higher than lower GI bleed (LGIB). The incidence is higher in men than in women and increases with age. Peptic ulcer disease is still the most common cause of UGIB and is responsible for approximately 20–25% of all cases of UGIB. Gastric ulcers are becoming more common a cause of UGIB than duodenal ulcers due to decreasing incidence of *Helicobacter pylori* secondary to the test and treat policy. Dieulafoy's lesion, seen in about 6% population, is an aberrant arteriole usually in the proximal stomach and is an important and easily missed cause of UGIB (**Box 1**).

APPROACH

The initial evaluation of a patient with a suspected acute UGIB includes history, physical examination, and laboratory tests with aim to:

- Determine extent of blood loss
- Localize source of the bleed
- Identifying comorbidities, if any

If the source of bleeding is in upper GI tract, it generally presents as hematemesis, i.e., presence of blood or coffee ground material in vomitus, melena, or melenic stool observed on per rectal examination. The ligament of Treitz (duodenojejunal flexure) is the anatomical landmark that can be used to differentiate an UGIB and LGIB. Hematemesis usually occurs when the source is proximal to it, and if accompanied by tachycardia or hemoglobin <8 g/dL, is highly suggestive of an ongoing bleed. Melena mostly originates proximal to the ligament of Treitz (90%), though it may also originate from the small bowel or right colon and may be seen with as little as 50 mL of blood loss. Blood clots in the stool or hematochezia (red or maroon blood in the stool) generally point toward a pathology in

BOX 1 The common causes of upper gastrointestinal bleed (in descending order of frequency).

- Gastric and/or duodenal ulcers
- Severe or erosive gastritis/duodenitis
- Esophagogastric varices
- Portal hypertensive gastropathy
- Dieulafoy's lesion and angiodysplasias
- Mallory–Weiss syndrome
- Mass lesions (polyps/cancers)
- Gastric antral vascular ectasia (GAVE)

lower GI. However, it can occur with a massive UGIB, where it is typically associated with orthostatic hypotension.

PAST MEDICAL HISTORY

Information on any past history of bleed is crucial as in approximately 60% patients; there is recurrence of bleeding from the same site. Presence of comorbidities in acute UGIB can have an impact on management strategies.

Patients with coronary artery disease are more prone to manifest the adverse effects of falling hemoglobin.

- In patients with heart failure or renal disease, fluid resuscitation or blood transfusions should be carefully monitored to avoid volume overload.
- Management of bleeding can be particularly difficult in patients with coagulopathies, thrombocytopenia, or significant hepatic dysfunction
- There is a high risk of aspiration of GI contents into the lungs in patients suffering from neurological disorders like dementia and hepatic encephalopathy.

Medication history: A complete detailed history of medications is crucial. Use of NSAIDs is frequently associated with peptic ulcers. Antiplatelet drugs like clopidogrel and anticoagulants like heparin and warfarin are known to promote bleeding. Drug esophagitis can sometimes be the culprit behind the bleed.

SYMPTOM ASSESSMENT

Severe bleeding can lead to hypovolemia and hypotension, and cause symptoms like orthostatic dizziness, confusion, palpitations, and cold/clammy extremities.

A detailed symptomatology can point toward a specific etiology of GI bleeding. For example:

- Pain in upper abdomen is suggestive of peptic ulcer, while esophageal ulcer usually manifests as painful or difficult swallowing and gastroesophageal reflux. Emesis or retching just before hematemesis is seen in Mallory–Weiss tear. Bleeding due to esophageal varices or portal hypertensive gastropathy is often accompanied by jaundice or ascites. In the presence of symptoms like early satiety, involuntary weight loss, cachexia, and malignant etiology must be ruled out.

PHYSICAL EXAMINATION

Hypovolemic signs include:

- Resting tachycardia, when blood loss <15%.
- Orthostatic hypotension, when blood loss is at least 15%.
- Supine hypotension, when blood loss is ≥40%.

LABORATORY TESTS

Patients with acute UGIB should undergo a complete blood count, serum chemistries, liver tests, coagulation studies, and an electrocardiogram. Echocardiography should be done in the cardiac patients and the elderly. Excessive volume administration can lead to a falsely low hemoglobin value. Packed cell volume (PCV) may give a better idea of the severity of bleed; however, higher values may be seen in severe bleeds leading to hemoconcentration. The initial hemoglobin level is monitored every 2–8 hours, depending upon the severity of the bleed. Patients with acute upper GI bleeding typically have an elevated blood urea nitrogen (BUN)-to-creatinine ratio.

GENERAL MANAGEMENT

GENERAL SUPPORT

Patients should receive supplemental oxygen by nasal cannula and should receive nothing per mouth. Two large caliber (18 gauge or larger) peripheral intravenous catheters or a central venous line should be inserted. Elective endotracheal intubation in patients with ongoing hematemesis or altered respiratory or mental status may facilitate endoscopy and decrease the risk of aspiration.

NASOGASTRIC LAVAGE

Nasogastric tube (NGT) placement is controversial. It is usually preferred by the endoscopists, as fresh blood in aspirate is suggestive of ongoing bleeding and even in clinically stable patients, it suggests urgency. These patients might benefit from an early endoscopy. An NGT lavage can also be used to remove particulate matter, fresh blood, and clots from the stomach to facilitate endoscopy. Some people have reservations about it, thinking that it may cause retching and increase bleeding or it may not dislodge the clot if any. Also there is risk of aspiration in patients with altered sensorium. Thus, it is avoided in patients who are not cooperative or are delirious.

FLUID RESUSCITATION

Planning for endoscopy must be preceded with hemodynamic stabilization of the patient to avoid treatment related complications. Fluid resuscitation in active bleeding should preferably be done with crystalloids, initially and blood transfusion, if needed, after typing and cross matching. Patients at risk of fluid overload like those with coexisting cardiac and renal comorbidities require intensive monitoring. If the hemodynamics do not improve with initial efforts, use of vasopressors may be considered.

RISK STRATIFICATION

Various scoring systems like Blatchford score and the Rockall score have been proposed for risk stratification for recurrent or life-threatening hemorrhage. They can provide guidance regarding decision to manage the patient on an outpatient or inpatient basis, and endoscopy and discharge timings as well. The hemodynamically unstable patients or those with active bleeding should be closely monitored in ICUs. Electrocardiographic monitoring for all inpatients should be done.

Risk scores: The International Consensus Group recommends that all patients with upper GI bleeding at presentation undergo risk stratification using the Glasgow–Blatchford score as it does not take endoscopic data into account. The score ranges from 0 to 23. A score of 0 identifies low-risk patients who are at a very low risk for rebleeding or mortality who might be suitable for outpatient management, while scores of 6 or more are associated with a >50% risk of rebleeding and need an intervention (**Table 1**).

The Rockall score is based upon age, the presence of shock, comorbidity, diagnosis, and endoscopic stigmata of recent hemorrhage (**Table 2**).

BLOOD PRODUCT TRANSFUSION

ANEMIA

Patients with active bleeding and hypovolemia may require red blood cell transfusion despite an apparently normal hemoglobin, particularly if the patient remains hemodynamically unstable despite appropriate fluid resuscitation. Goal for most patients (including those with stable coronary artery disease) is maintaining hemoglobin at a level ≥8 g/dL and a level of ≥9 g/dL for patients with unstable coronary artery disease or in those with evidence of ongoing active bleeding. For patients with signs of active ischemia, maintaining the hemoglobin at ≥10 g/dL is appropriate.

Because packed red blood cells do not contain coagulation factors, transfusion of a unit of FFP should be given after every four units of packed red blood cells. It is particularly important to avoid over transfusion in patients especially with suspected variceal bleeding, as it can precipitate worsening of the bleeding.

THROMBOCYTOPENIA

Patients with active bleeding and a low platelet count (<50,000/μL) should be transfused with platelets. Upper endoscopy can be done in patients who are not actively bleeding even when platelet count is >20,000/μL.

COAGULOPATHY

Patients with a coagulopathy and a prolonged prothrombin time with an international normalized ratio (INR) >2.0 should generally be transfused with FFP.

Provided the patient is hemodynamically stable, urgent endoscopy can usually proceed simultaneously with transfusion. However, in patients with an INR ≥2.5,

TABLE 1 Glasgow–Blatchford score for risk stratification.

	GBS
Blood urea (mmol/L)	
<6.5	0
6.5–7.9	2
8–9.9	3
10–25	4
>25	6
Hemoglobin	
Men (g/L)	
>129	0
120–129	1
100–119	3
<100	6
Women (g/L)	
>119	0
100–119	1
<100	6
Systolic blood pressure (mm Hg)	
>109	0
100–109	1
90–99	2
<90	3
Other markers	
Pulse BPM ≥100	1
Melena	1
Syncope	2
Liver disease*	2
Heart failure*	2

*Based on past medical history, clinical, or laboratory evidence.

Note: Total score is obtained by adding the value of all items.

(BPM: beats per minute; GBS: Glasgow–Blatchford bleeding score)

Source: Adapted from Stanley AJ, Laine L. Management of acute upper gastrointestinal bleeding. BMJ. 2019;364:l536.

TABLE 2 Rockall score for risk stratification.

Rockall Scoring System				
Variable	**Score = 0**	**Score = 1**	**Score = 2**	**Score = 3**
Age (years)	<60	60–79	>80	
Comorbidity			Congestive heart failure, ischemic heart disease	Renal failure, liver disease, metastatic disease
Shock	No shock	Pulse >100 bpm	Systolic BP <100 mm Hg	
Source of bleeding	Mallory–Weiss tear	All other diagnoses: e.g., esophagitis, gastritis, peptic ulcer disease, varices	Malignancy	
Stigmata of recent bleeding	None		Adherent clot or spurting vessel	

***Note*: On a scale of 0–11, with 11 representing the highest risk.**

one should attempt to correct it prior to starting an endoscopy.

DRUG TREATMENT

Majority of patients with bleeding peptic ulcers will stop bleeding spontaneously and not rebleed during hospitalization but a subgroup of patients are at high risk for recurrent hemorrhage and require endoscopic therapy to decrease this risk. If endoscopic therapy fails, interventional angiography or surgery may be required.

Despite advances in pharmacologic and endoscopic therapy, mortality rates have not improved.

ACID SUPPRESSION

Treatment with a PPI leads to elevation of gastric pH levels above 4 which stabilizes blood clots and improves clinical outcomes.

Admitted patients with acute upper GI bleeding are treated with a PPI as a high-dose bolus (e.g., esomeprazole 80 mg) followed by a continuous infusion at a rate of 8 mg per hour for 72 hours and then at 40 mg twice a day. Oral formulations (e.g., esomeprazole 40 mg orally twice daily) are a reasonable alternative if intravenous (IV) formulations are not available. All PPIs work well. The goal of treatment in low-risk patients should be directed at healing the ulcers and eliminating precipitating factors such as *H. pylori* and nonsteroidal anti-inflammatory drugs. PPIs have also shown to reduce the need for endotherapy in these patients when started early, while awaiting endoscopy. Studies have compared PPIs with H2RA (H2 receptor blockers) in patients with UGIB and found H2RAs less effective than PPIs, because of inability to sustain gastric pH above 4.

High-dose oral PPIs in patients with high-risk stigmata of recent hemorrhage are continued for a total of 2 weeks and then changed to a once daily dose.

PROKINETICS

The goal of using a prokinetic agent such as erythromycin 3 mg/kg intravenously over 20–30 minutes may be given 30–90 minutes prior to endoscopy to improve gastric visualization at the time of endoscopy by clearing the stomach of blood, clots, and food residue. Parenteral erythromycin is not available in India, hence, prokinetics like injectable metoclopramide and levosulpiride are used with intent to clear the gastric contents prior to endoscopy.

OTHER MEDICATION

Vasoactive agents like terlipressin are not recommended for routine use in patients with acute nonvariceal upper GI bleeding. If cause of bleeding (variceal or nonvariceal) is not clear, and endoscopy is being delayed, then some patients may be helped by combining both the drugs together, i.e., terlipressin and PPI. Antibiotics also have no role except in those patients with aspiration. Tranexamic acid does not appear to be beneficial.

UPPER GASTROINTESTINAL ENDOSCOPY

Upper endoscopy is the diagnostic modality of choice for acute upper GI bleeding. Endoscopy has a high sensitivity and specificity for locating and identifying bleeding lesions in the upper GI tract. In addition, once a bleeding lesion has been identified, therapeutic endoscopy can achieve acute hemostasis and prevent recurrent bleeding in most patients.

TIMING OF ENDOSCOPY

Early endoscopy (within 24 hours) is recommended for most patients with acute upper GI bleeding but only after adequate resuscitation. Very early endoscopy (within 12 hours of presentation), however, is not associated with improved clinical outcomes and may lead to poorer outcomes in specific populations with upper GI bleeding. For patients with suspected variceal bleeding, endoscopy should be performed within 12 hours of presentation.

ANTICOAGULANTS AND ANTIPLATELETS

For most patients, endoscopy should not be delayed because of anticoagulant or antiplatelet agent use.

Wherever possible, anticoagulants and antiplatelet agents should be stopped in patients with upper GI bleeding. The decision to reverse anticoagulation depends on the associated risk of thrombosis against risk of continued bleeding, and should be patient centric. A cardiac consultation is warranted if patient started taking antiplatelets from the past 1 year, after undergoing vascular stent placement or has suffered from cardiac ailments.

The decision to restart these drugs also depends on thrombotic risk against risk of recurrent bleeding. Antiplatelets can be reintroduced if it is ascertained that the bleeding is controlled.

RISKS OF EARLY ENDOSCOPY

These include pulmonary aspiration, adverse reactions to medications used to achieve conscious sedation, GI perforation, and increasing bleeding while attempting therapeutic intervention. These risks are more for very early endoscopies as compared to those done within 12–24 hours of presentation as the patient gets more stable for the endoscopy by this time.

The risks versus benefits of upper endoscopy should be considered in high-risk patients. Complications (including ventricular tachycardia, respiratory arrest, and hypotension) occurred more often in patients who had a recent myocardial infarction (MI) and in patients who were very ill (APACHE II score > 16 or hypotension prior to endoscopy).

STIGMATA OF RECENT BLEEDING

Endoscopic findings in patients with bleeding peptic ulcers may be described using the Forrest classification. Findings include spurting hemorrhage (class Ia), oozing hemorrhage (class Ib), a nonbleeding visible vessel (class IIa), an adherent clot (class IIb), a flat pigmented spot (class IIc), and a clean ulcer base (class III). The endoscopic appearance helps determine which lesions require endoscopic therapy. Class IIc and class III have a low risk of rebleed and do not require endotherapy. Class Ia, Ib, and IIa ulcers are associated with increased risk of rebleeding (**Figs. 1 A to E**).

RISK STRATIFICATION FOR REBLEEDING

The decision to discharge a patient after endoscopy is governed by the following:

- If source of bleeding is localized or not
- If source is identified, is there any risk of recurrence or rebleeding. Variceal bleeding, active bleeding, bleeding from a Dieulafoy's lesion, or an ulcer bleeding with

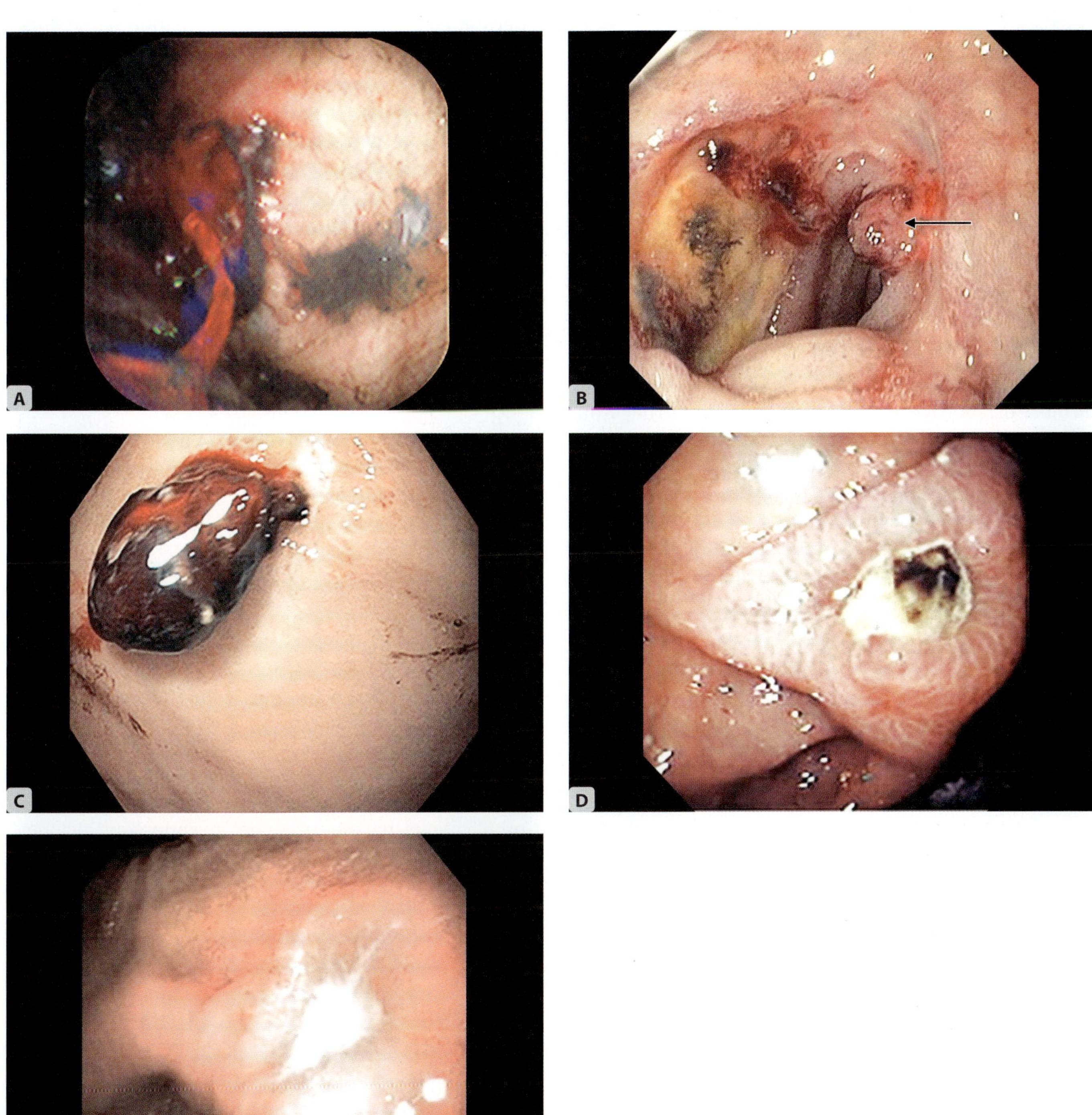

FIGURES 1 A to E: (A) Forrest Ia: spurting hemorrhage; **(B)** Forrest IIa: nonbleeding visible vessel; **(C)** Forrest IIb: adherent clot; **(D)** Forrest IIc: flat pigmented spot; **(E)** Forrest III: clean ulcer base.

high-risk stigmata is the high risk bleeding source. Also, clinical features suggestive of increased recurrence of recurrent bleeding should not be missed.

Apart from these, discharge can be considered, if patient:

- Has no comorbidities
- Is hemodynamically stable
- Has a normal hemoglobin level

The risk of rebleeding is high if the patient:

- Is hemodynamically unstable, suggested by systolic blood pressure <100 mm Hg, heart rate > 100 beats/minute
- Has hemoglobin <10 g/L
- Had active bleeding at the time of endoscopy
- Has ulcer of size >1–3 cm
- Has ulcer in the posterior duodenal bulb or high lesser gastric curvature
- Has BUN levels raised at 24 hours from the baseline.

The Rockall score is a useful score to predict rebleed in such patients. Most patients who have received endoscopic treatment for high-risk stigmata should be hospitalized for 72 hours to monitor for rebleeding, since most rebleeding occurs during this time.

ENDOSCOPIC THERAPY

Endoscopic therapy is indicated for the treatment of most ulcers with stigmata of recent hemorrhage that increases the risk of recurrent bleeding.

CHOICE OF ENDOSCOPIC TREATMENT

Several types of endoscopic treatment for bleeding peptic ulcers have been described, including injection therapy, thermal coagulation, hemostatic clips, fibrin sealant (or glue), argon plasma coagulation, and combination therapy (typically injection of epinephrine combined with another treatment modality).

Currently, most patients are treated with either thermal coagulation therapy or hemostatic clips, with or without the addition of injection therapy as shown by results from meta-analyses of randomized trials comparing different forms of treatment to control bleeding (**Table 3**).

Standard approaches to treatment include thermal coagulation and hemoclip placement. Both of these modalities can be combined with injection therapy, an approach known as combination therapy.

Injection therapy: Injection therapy should be used in conjunction with other forms of therapy, such as thermal coagulation or hemoclip placement and should not be used as monotherapy because it is associated with higher rates of recurrent bleeding than treatment with thermal coagulation, hemoclip placement, or combination therapy.

Injection therapy with dilute epinephrine results in local tamponade and vasospasm. Epinephrine diluted with saline to 1:10,000–1:20,000 is injected in 0.5–2.0 mL aliquots in four quadrants within 3 mm of the bleeding site. A potential advantage of epinephrine injection is that it is easy to administer, can help slow or stop bleeding.

TABLE 3 Available endoscopic modalities.

Modality	Agent	Effect
Injection	Epinephrine, saline	Local tamponade, vasoconstriction
Mechanical	Endoclips	Occlusion of vessels
Thermal	Heater probe, APC	Cauterization
Topical	Hemospray, endoclot	Hemostat

(APC: argon plasma coagulation)

Thermal coagulation: Thermal coagulation with contact probes achieves acute hemostasis and prevents recurrent bleeding by coaptive coagulation of the underlying artery in the ulcer base.

Hemoclips: The endoscopic application of hemoclips is an alternative to thermal coagulation. Once applied, the clips achieve hemostasis in a manner similar to surgical ligation.

Alternative approaches: Alternatives to standard endoscopic therapy include the use of tissue adhesives and agents that promote hemostasis, i.e., fibrin sealant and hemostatic nanopowder. These agents may provide a temporary benefit where other methods have been less effective and while awaiting a more definite therapy.

SECOND-LOOK ENDOSCOPY

Second-look endoscopy refers to performing a planned follow-up endoscopy, generally within 24 hours of the initial endoscopy. If there is active bleeding or a nonbleeding visible vessel, endoscopic therapy is performed. Routine second-look endoscopy for patients at high risk for rebleeding is associated with a decreased risk of rebleeding.

Situations that might warrant a second-look endoscopy include:

- If visualization during the initial endoscopy was limited by blood or debris.
- If there is concern on the part of the endoscopist that the prior endoscopic therapy was suboptimal.
- If there is recurrent bleeding.

TREATMENT-RELATED COMPLICATIONS

Complications that may occur before endoscopy include:

- Aspiration (especially in a sedated, combative, or encephalopathic patient)
- Hypoventilation (related to over sedation), or
- Hypotension (due to inadequate volume replacement or transfusions, in addition to sedation with opiates)

TREATMENT OF PERSISTENT AND RECURRENT BLEEDING

Although the majority of bleeding ulcers can be controlled endoscopically, some patients have persistent or recurrent bleeding. Patients with one episode of recurrent bleeding following initially successful endoscopic therapy are typically treated with a second attempt at endoscopic therapy. Surgery or angiography-guided intervention is indicated for patients who fail endoscopic therapy

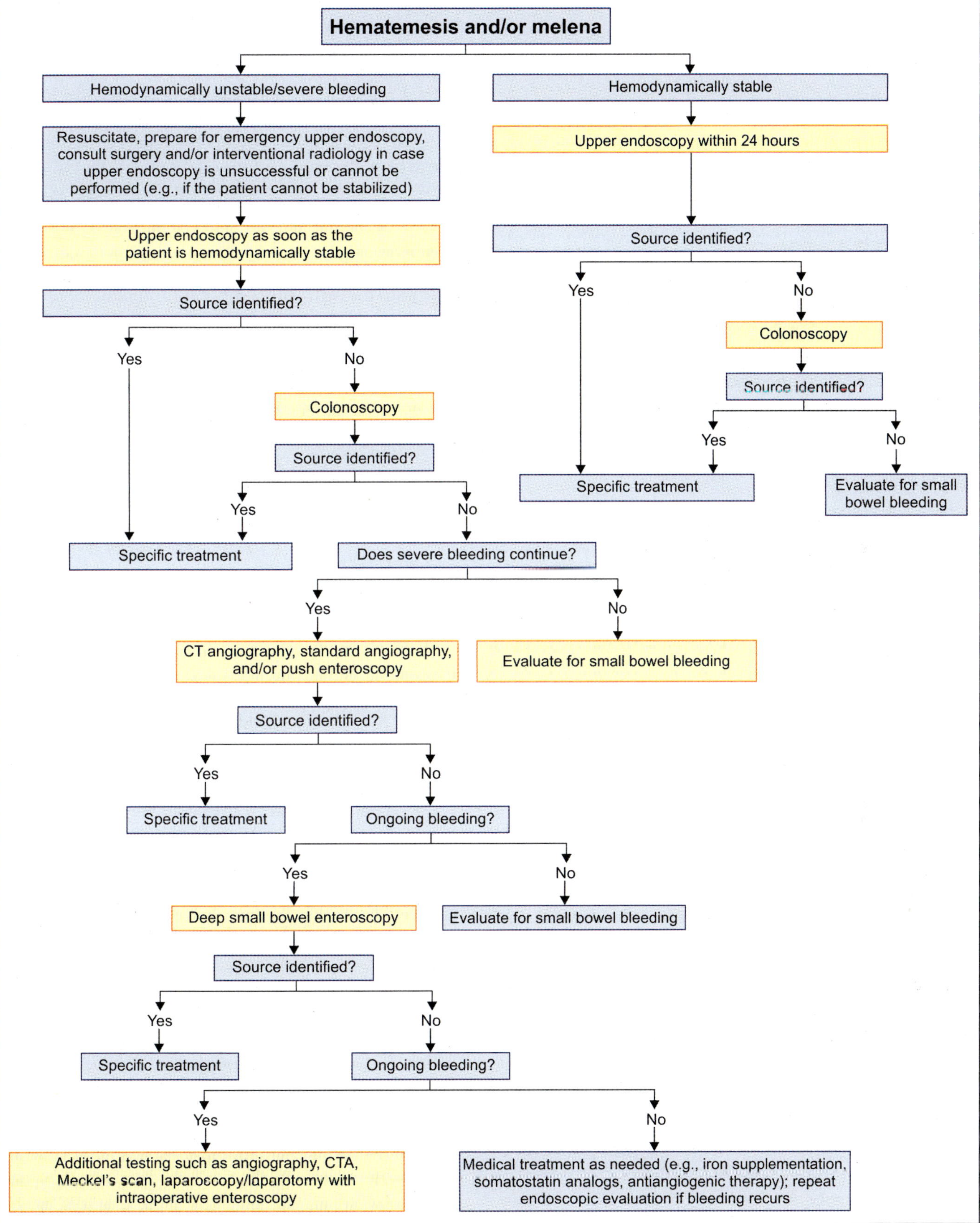

(CTA: computed tomography angiography)

FLOWCHART 1: Evaluation of suspected upper gastrointestinal bleeding.

(persistent bleeding or recurrent bleeding after two therapeutic endoscopies).

RISK FACTORS

They include ulcer location, the patient's presentation, the appearance of the ulcer at the time of endoscopy, size of the ulcer, and presence of comorbid illnesses.

Predictors of recurrent bleeding included active bleeding at endoscopy, large ulcers (>1–2 cm), posterior duodenal ulcers, and gastric ulcers on the lesser curvature. End-stage kidney disease also increases the risk of recurrent bleeding.

TEAM WORK

At times, when there is a possibility of failure of endoscopic therapy, high risk of recurrent bleeding or endoscopy-related complications, or there is a suspicion of an aortoenteric fistula, surgical or radiological intervention may be needed. It would be wise to alert a surgeon and an interventional radiologist in any case of severe acute bleed from upper GI.

INTERVENTIONAL ANGIOGRAPHY

To manage bleeding from persistent or recurrent peptic ulcer bleeding, angiography with transarterial embolization (TAE), being less invasive, can be a suitable alternative to surgery Success rates of 52–98% have been reported in patients with acute peptic ulcer bleeding, so far.

- Endoscopy is the first and the best procedure recommended for diagnostic and therapeutic purpose.
- In case, therapeutic endoscopy fails, we can consider surgery or transcatheter arteriography/intervention. Though both are equally effective, latter is preferred in patients with high risk for surgery.
- Although deranged coagulation factors disfavor the success of transcatheter arteriography/intervention, this technique is preferred for management bleeding into the biliary tree or pancreatic duct.
- Transarterial embolization has been associated with lower mortality and complication rates. Rebleeding was seen more commonly with TAE.

SURGERY

Traditionally, surgery was required for patients who failed endoscopic therapy, though many patients now undergo an attempt at interventional angiography prior to surgery.

Surgical treatments for peptic ulcer disease include oversewing of the artery with truncal vagotomy and pyloroplasty, antrectomy with gastrojejunostomy (Billroth II procedure), and highly selective vagotomy. Emergency surgery for bleeding peptic ulcer disease involves oversewing of the ulcer (to ligate the bleeding artery) plus truncal vagotomy (to decrease acid secretion) and pyloroplasty (for gastric drainage).

In addition to failure of endoscopic therapy, other indications for surgery for peptic ulcer hemorrhage include:

- Hemodynamic instability despite vigorous resuscitation (more than a three-unit transfusion)
- Shock associated with recurrent hemorrhage.

Given the less invasive nature of angiography, it is suggested that patients who have failed endoscopic therapy first undergo attempted angiography with TAE, and that surgery be reserved for those who fail angiographic therapy.

FOLLOW-UP

All patients with bleeding peptic ulcers need to be evaluated *H. pylori* and treated as appropriate. However, in the setting of a duodenal ulcer-related bleed treatment of *H. pylori* can be done even without testing for it (**Flowchart 1**).

RECOMMENDED READINGS

1. Barkun AN, Almadi M, Kuipers EJ, Laine L, Sung J, Tse F, et al. Management of nonvariceal upper gastrointestinal bleeding: guideline recommendations from the International Consensus Group. Ann Intern Med. 2019;171(11):805-22.
2. Stanley AJ, Laine L. Management of acute upper gastrointestinal bleeding. BMJ. 2019;364:1536.
3. Lau JY, Yu Y, Tang RS, Chan HC, Yip HC, Chan SM, et al. Timing of endoscopy for acute upper gastrointestinal bleeding. N Eng J Med. 2020;382(14):1299-308.
4. Sung JJ, Chiu PW, Chan FK, Lau JY, Goh KL, Ho LH, et al. Asia-Pacific working group consensus on non-variceal upper gastrointestinal bleeding: An update 2018. Gut. 2018;67(10):1757-68.
5. Samuel R, Bilal M, Tayyem O, Guturu P. Evaluation and management of Non-variceal upper gastrointestinal bleeding. Dis Mon. 2018;64(7):333-43.
6. Gralnek I, Dumonceau J, Kuipers E, Lanas A, Sanders D, Kurien M, et al. Diagnosis and management of nonvariceal upper gastrointestinal hemorrhage: European Society of Gastrointestinal Endoscopy (ESGE) Guideline. Endoscopy. 2015;47(10):a1-46.
7. Fujishiro M, Iguchi M, Kakushima N, Kato M, Sakata Y, Hoteya S, et al. Guidelines for endoscopic management of non-variceal upper gastrointestinal bleeding. Dig Endosc. 2016;28(4):363-78.
8. Siau K, Chapman W, Sharma N, Tripathi D, Iqbal T, Bhala N. Management of acute upper gastrointestinal bleeding: an update for the general physician. J R Coll Physicians Edinb. 2017;47(3):218-30.
9. Holster IL, Kuipers EJ. Management of acute nonvariceal upper gastrointestinal bleeding: current policies and future perspectives. World J Gastroenterol. 2012;18(11):1202-7.
10. Laine L, Jensen DM. Management of patients with ulcer bleeding. Am J Gastroenterol. 2012;107(3):345-60.

CHAPTER
132
Small Bowel Evaluation

Shivaraj Afzalpurkar, Usha Goenka, Mahesh K Goenka

ABSTRACT

Small intestine is a specialized tubular part of gastrointestinal (GI) tract in continuity with stomach proximally and large intestine distally with a length of 6–8 meters in adults. Small bowel diseases are important causes of morbidity and mortality. Appropriate diagnosis requires high index of clinical suspicion. Adequate evaluation is imperative for diagnosis and management of these diseases. History and physical examination will not only play an important role in suspecting small bowel disease but also choosing right investigation or procedure for further evaluation of small bowel. The various procedures which are available are broadly divided into endoscopic-based and radiologic techniques.

Direct visualization of small bowel mucosa is possible with endoscopic-based techniques including capsule endoscopy and device-assisted enteroscopy. Capsule endoscopy has revolutionized the diagnosis and treatment of small bowel diseases. It is the first-line modality to investigate small bowel bleeding and complementary to radiology for assessing inflammatory bowel disease and refractory celiac disease. Various other platforms available for evaluating small bowel are double-balloon enteroscopy (DBE), single-balloon enteroscopy (SBE), spiral enteroscopy (SE), and balloon-guided endoscopy (BGE). The motorized SE (power spiral) is the new addition to the armamentarium. Obtaining tissue for histological examination and performing therapeutic procedures are the additional benefits of these deep enteroscopy procedures.

The radiological investigations like computed tomography (CT) and magnetic resonance enterography (MRE) have gradually replaced barium-based studies. CT enterography (CTE) is a simple and effective method with high sensitivity in evaluating intestinal wall changes along with an additional information of associated extraintestinal and mesenteric alterations. However, due to absence of ionizing radiation, MRE is often preferred radiological imaging of small bowel.

"Happiness: a good bank, a good cook and a good digestion"

—JJ Rousseau

INTRODUCTION

Intestinal tract has several functions which include digestion, absorption, and transport of nutrients, synthesis of proteins required for absorption of fats and elimination of waste products. Small bowel diseases are major causes of morbidity and mortality. Appropriate diagnosis requires high index of clinical suspicion. There is significant advancement in the small bowel evaluation techniques in recent times which has helped us in early diagnosis and treatment of patients. Earlier we had nothing else but barium to evaluate small bowel. For endoscopist, it was considered to be out of bounds. In last two decades, significant progress has been made both in radiology and endoscopy.

ANATOMY OF SMALL INTESTINE

- It is a specialized tubular structure in continuity with stomach proximally and large intestine distally.
  - *Length*: 6–8 meters in adults
  - Divided into three parts: (1) Duodenum, (2) jejunum, and (3) ileum
    i. *Duodenum*: Shortest, widest, and most fixed part and 25 cm in length. It is shaped in the form of letter C and curved around the head of pancreas. Except its two ends, most part of it is retroperitoneal and fixed. It is divided into following parts.
       - *First (superior) part*: 5 cm
       - *Second (descending) part*: 7.5 cm
       - *Third (horizontal) part*: 10 cm
       - *Fourth (ascending) part*: 2.5 cm

    ii. *Jejunum*: Present in upper and left part of the abdomen
       - Walls are thicker and more vascular.
       - Lumen is often empty and more wide.
       - It has fewer solitary lymphatic follicles.
       - Payer's patches are absent.

    iii. *Ileum*: Present in right and lower part of abdomen
       - Walls are thinner and less vascular.
       - Lumen is often loaded and comparatively narrow.
       - It has more numerous solitary lymphatic follicles.
       - Payer's patches are present.
  - *Meckel's diverticulum*: It is the persistent proximal part of the vitellointestinal duct.
    - Present in 2% population
    - Has length of 2 inches

- Situated 2 feet proximal to ileocecal valve
- *Clinical importance*: It may cause intestinal obstruction. It may have small regions of gastric mucosa and the inflammation of which may produce symptoms similar to acute appendicitis.

- *Blood supply*:
  - Duodenum up to the opening of bile duct in the second part is supplied by superior pancreaticoduodenal artery (a branch of celiac artery) and below it is supplied by inferior pancreaticoduodenal artery (a branch of superior mesenteric artery).
  - Jejunum and ileum are supplied by branches of superior mesenteric artery.

OUTLINE OF EVALUATION

The method of evaluation from history and simple investigations to the endoscopic and radiological evaluation is shown in **Box 1**.

BOX 1	Method for evaluation of small bowel.
• **History and physical examination**	
• **Laboratory investigations**	
• **Endoscopic procedures**	
◦ Push enteroscopy	
◦ Small bowel capsule endoscopy (SBCE)	
◦ Device-assisted endoscopy	
– Single-balloon enteroscopy	
– Double-balloon enteroscopy	
– Spiral enteroscopy (manual and motorized)	
– Balloon-guided endoscopy	
– Intraoperative enteroscopy	
• **Radiologic procedures**	
◦ Conventional radiology	
– Barium meal follow-through (BMFT)	
– Enteroclysis	
◦ Ultrasonography (USG)	
◦ Computed tomography	
– Enterography	
– Enteroclysis	
– Angiography	
◦ Magnetic resonance imaging	
◦ Nuclear scans	

HISTORY AND PHYSICAL EXAMINATION

- *Small bowel diarrhea*: Patients give history of passing frequent large quantity of foul-smelling loose stools usually associated with periumbilical pain and steatorrhea.
- *Small bowel bleeding*: History of passing black tarry stools with characteristic smell (melena) and/or passing of red blood from rectum (hematochezia). It may be associated with pain abdomen, easy fatigability, lethargy, and dyspnea on exertion. Painless passage of large amount of blood-mixed stools is seen in vascular causes of bleeding.
- *Malabsorption*: The key points to help reaching the diagnosis of malabsorption:
  - History of stomach or small bowel resection
  - Excessive alcohol consumption
  - Receiving any drugs which can cause malabsorption
  - History of intake of food rich in poorly absorbable carbohydrates (sweeteners such as fructose or sorbitol)
  - History of organ transplantation or abdominal radiation
  - Preexisting diseases like chronic pancreatitis, Whipple disease, diabetes mellitus, thyrotoxicosis, biliary, or liver disease
  - History suggestive of extraintestinal manifestations of inflammatory bowel disease, celiac, or Whipple disease
- Drug history—regular intake of anticoagulants, antiplatelets, nonsteroidal anti-inflammatory drugs (NSAID), and history of drug allergy—is important in patients presenting with small bowel bleeding.
- *Analysis of problems*: The following history will help in detecting the small bowel disease:
  - *Excessive gas*: Carbohydrate malabsorption
  - *Unusually offensive stool and gas*: Protein malabsorption
  - *Intolerance to milk or milk products*: Lactose malabsorption
  - *Sudden onset proximal muscle weakness*: Potassium loss
  - *Carpopedal spasm*: Calcium/vitamin D malabsorption
  - *Weight loss despite good appetite*: Malabsorption of all nutrients
- *Examination*: General physical examination from head to toe gives clue in detection of underlying disease and also in assessing its severity. Dry mouth, pallor, tachycardia, and postural hypotension are signs of hypovolemia.
  - *Important physical signs*: Important physical signs suggesting underlying etiology are pigmented lips (Peutz–Jeghers syndrome), purpuric lesions of the skin (Henoch–Schonlein purpura), acanthosis nigricans (underlying GI malignancy), xanthomas of trunk, face or extremities (primary biliary cirrhosis), bronze-brown skin color mainly in sun-exposed sites (hemochromatosis), palpable mass in the right iliac fossa (intestinal tuberculosis), and perianal fissure/fistula (inflammatory bowel disease).

LABORATORY INVESTIGATIONS

Certain laboratory investigations (blood and stool) will not only act as simple screening tools for diagnosis of small bowel disorders but also help in choosing the definitive diagnostic modalities in confirming the diseases. **Table 1**

TABLE 1 Laboratory investigations.	
Blood investigation	**Comments**
Hematocrit	Decreased in vitamin B12, folic acid, and iron malabsorption, blood loss
White blood cells	Lymphopenia in lymphangiectasia, eosinophilia in parasitic infestation and eosinophilic gastroenteritis
Albumin	Hypoalbuminemia in protein losing enteropathy
Alkaline phosphatase	Elevated in vitamin D and calcium malabsorption
Cholesterol	Decreased in bile acid or fat malabsorption
Iron/Ferritin	Decreased in chronic blood loss and celiac disease. Elevated in inflammatory disease
Zinc	Decreased in extensive small intestinal mucosal disease.
Citrulline	Decreased in intestinal resection and extensive small bowel mucosal disease
Vitamin B12	Decreased in terminal ileal disease and small intestinal bacterial overgrowth
Beta carotene	Decreased in fat malabsorption
Stool investigation	**Comments**
Calprotectin	Elevated in inflammatory disease of intestine
Occult blood	Intestinal erosion, ulceration or tumor
Ova and parasites	Worm infestation

summarizes the commonly used laboratory investigations and their value in diagnosing small bowel diseases. **Flowchart 1** shows evaluation and approach to small bowel diarrhea.

ENDOSCOPIC PROCEDURES

Push enteroscopy:

- It is the long endoscope with standard diameter used to visualize the GI tract from esophagus to proximal jejunum.
- It can rapidly diagnose the bleeding source in the proximal jejunum (about 50–70 cm distal to pylorus).
- The main advantage of this procedure over device-assisted enteroscopy is shorter examination time. The major disadvantage, however, is unable to visualize the entire small bowel.
- Push enteroscopy plays an important role in early evaluation of small bowel lesions but has largely been replaced by device-assisted enteroscope.

Small bowel capsule endoscopy (SBCE):

- Capsule endoscopy has revolutionized the diagnosis and treatment of small bowel diseases.
- It is the first-line modality to investigate small bowel bleeding and complementary to radiology for investigating inflammatory bowel disease and refractory celiac disease.
- *Capsule endoscopy systems*:
  - *First-generation SBCE (PillCam SB1)*: It captures two images per second with 140° angle of view. It provides 8-hour battery life and eightfold magnification.
  - *Second-generation SBCE (PillCam SB2)*: Wider angle of view (156°) and has automatic light control with better optics.
  - *Third-generation SBCE (PillCam SB3)*: It has superior optics and frame rate is adaptive, i.e., it can capture up to six frames per second depending upon the speed of movement of capsule in the GI tract. This saves the battery when it travels slowly in the small bowel.
- *Indications and contraindications* of capsule endoscopy are listed in **Table 2**. **Figures 1 A** to **D** show images of various disorders on capsule endoscopy.
- European Society of Gastrointestinal Endoscopy (ESGE) recommends video capsule endoscopy (VCE) as first-line investigation in patients of small bowel bleeding (strong recommendation, moderate quality of evidence). It is also considered as investigation of choice for small bowel inflammatory conditions such as Crohn's disease.
- *Diagnostic yield*: The pooled diagnostic yield is about 62% for detection of small bowel lesions and the detection rate of small bowel bleed is approximately 60%. **Table 3** summarizes various Indian studies on SBCE in small bowel bleed.
- *Timing*:
  - *Small bowel bleed*: The diagnostic yield increases if it is done soon after the bleeding episode.
  - *Small bowel tumor*: Early use of SBCE is recommended in patients with obscure GI bleed and unexplained iron-deficiency anemia for the diagnosis of small bowel tumors.
- *Optimal bowel preparation*: There is no consensus for the optimal timing of bowel preparation prior to SBCE. The most commonly followed preparation method is administration of 2 liter polyethylene glycol (PEG)-based solution one day prior to SBCE. A 2-liter PEG solution is similar to 4-liter solution in terms of diagnostic yield.

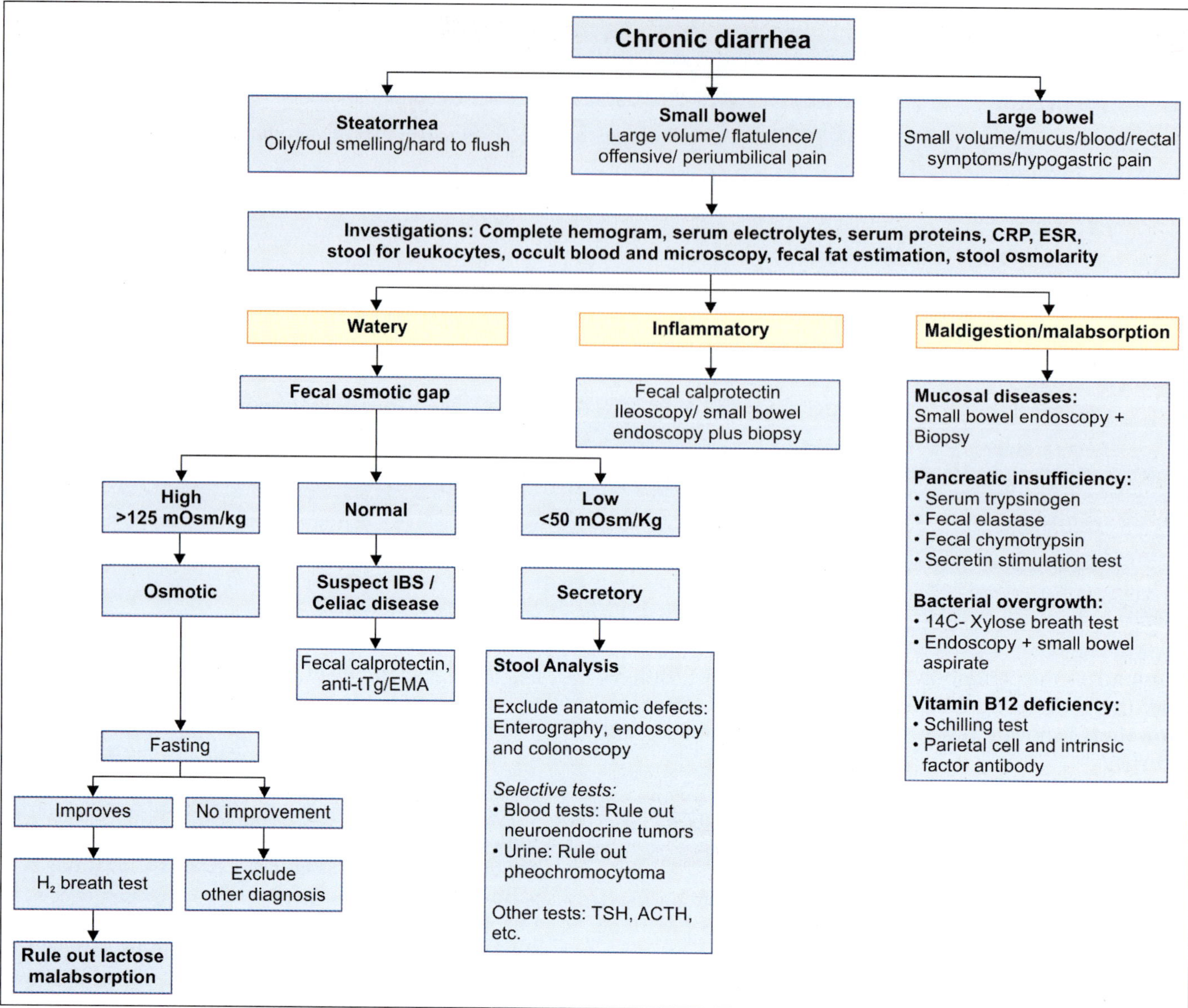

(EMA: endomysial antibody)

FLOWCHART 1: Approach to small bowel diarrhea.

TABLE 2 Indications and contraindications of small bowel capsule endoscopy (SBCE).

Indications	Contraindications
• Small bowel bleeding (occult or obscure)	• Absolute contraindications
• Small bowel tumors	• Evidence of bowel obstruction
• Crohn's disease	• Intestinal pseudoobstruction
• Celiac disease (if patient is unable to undergo conventional endoscopy)	• Relative contraindications
• Nonsteroidal anti-inflammatory drug-induced enteropathy	• Cardiac pacemakers
• Portal hypertensive enteropathy	• Pregnancy
• Inherited polyposis syndromes	• Dysphagia
• Chronic unexplained pain abdomen	• Extensive intestinal diverticulosis
	• Previous intestinal surgeries

- *Challenges and future directions*: New devices need to be developed in order to add the ability to provide therapy, inflation of air for better visualization of bowel, external control system to control the movement of the capsule, and additional systems attached to capsule for obtaining biopsy.

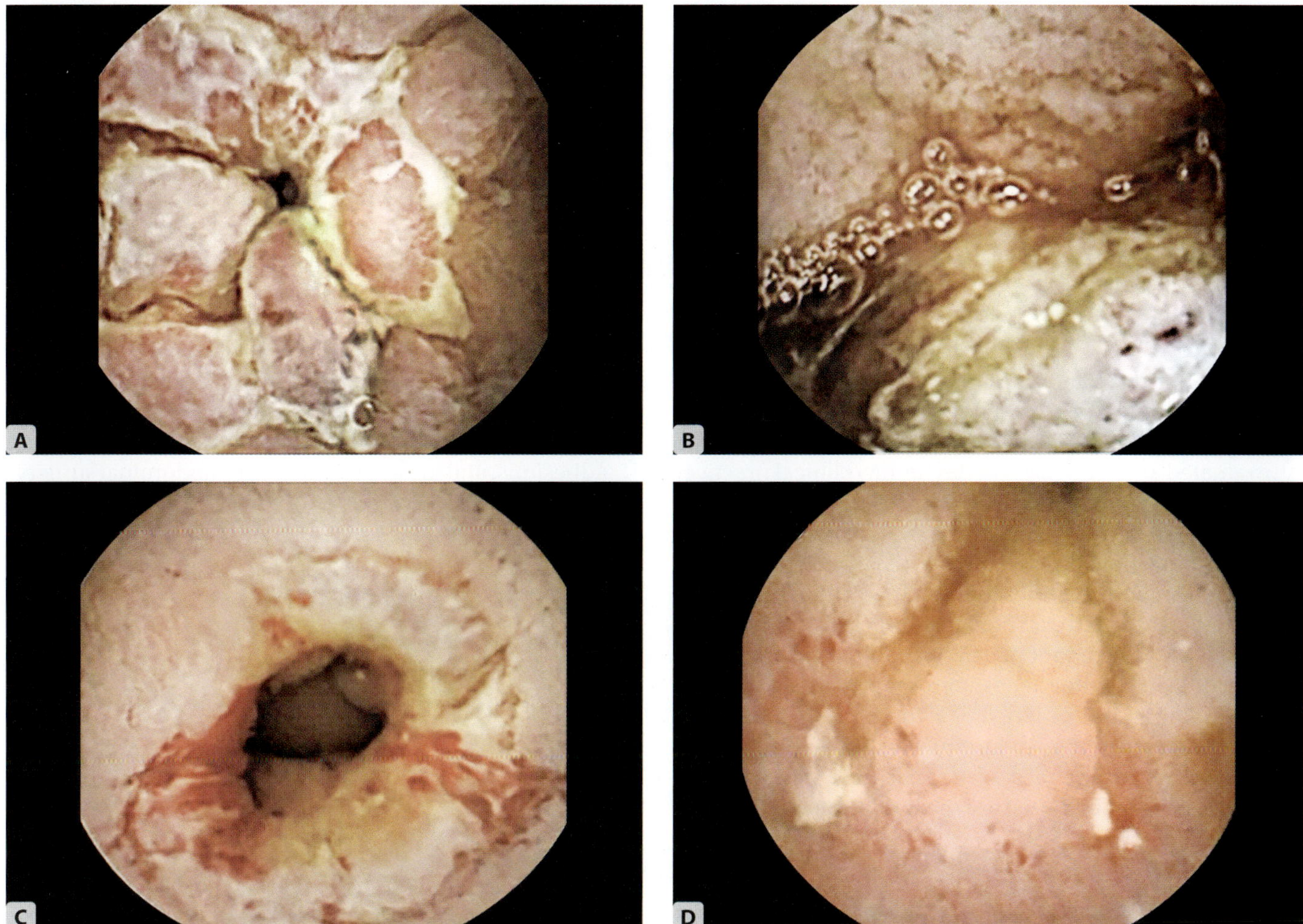

FIGURES 1 A to D: Capsule endoscopy images. (A) Cobblestone appearance characteristic of Crohn's disease; **(B)** an ileal tumor; **(C)** circumferential ulcer with narrowing and minor ongoing bleeding in a patient with Crohn's disease; and **(D)** small intestinal ulcers in a patient with tuberculosis.

Source: Goenka MK, Majumder S, Kumar S, Sethy PK, Goenka U. Single center experience of capsule endoscopy in patients with obscure gastrointestinal bleeding. World J Gastroenterol. 2011;17(6):774-8.

TABLE 3 Summary of Indian studies on SBCE in patients with occult small bowel bleed.

Author	Year	City	N	Yield	Most common lesion(s) identified
Gupta R et al.	2006	Hyderabad	154	27%	• Angiodysplasia (23%)
UC Ghoshal et al.	2011	Lucknow	86	82%	• Ulcers/Erosions (74%) • Tumors (22%)
Goenka MK et al.	2011	Kolkata	284	59%	• Ulcers/erosions (70.3%), • Tumors (18.8%)
Pandey V et al.	2016	Mumbai	68	75%	• NSAID-induced lesions (15%), • Angiodysplasias (14%)

Device-assisted enteroscopy:

- Various different platforms available for evaluating small bowel are DBE, SBE, SE, and BGE. The motorized SE (power spiral) is the new addition to the armamentarium.
- **Figures 2 A and B** show overview of SBE and DBE scope advancement techniques for diagnostic and therapeutic access into the small intestine.
- *Double-balloon enteroscopy*: It was first introduced in Japan by Yamamoto. It is the combination of flexible endoscope, an overtube, distal balloon mounted onto the endoscope and the proximal balloon mounted on the overtube tip. Both the balloons can be inflated and deflated independently and they help in anchoring the bowel while advancing the endoscope.
- *Single-balloon enteroscopy*: It uses one balloon which is attached to the tip of the overtube. While advancing the overtube, to maintain the scope in stable position, it uses "hook and suck technique" (angulation of the scope tip and suction) instead of balloon inflation.

- *Spiral enteroscopy*: It utilizes the principle of converting rotational energy into linear force. Here, instead of applying the pushing force the scope is advanced by active rotation of the instrumentation shaft. It uses the manually rotatable endo-ease overtube with the flexible spiral thread over its distal end for pleating the small intestine. It generally requires the assistance of second endoscopist for its appropriate use.
- *Balloon-guided endoscopy*: In this system, through the scope balloon is inserted in the working channel of endoscope. The scope is advanced by push-and-pull maneuver after anchoring the balloon in the small bowel. Main advantage of this system is it can be used as "on demand" enteroscope or can be added to any standard endoscope. However, this is not properly evaluated and is not used in day-to-day clinical practice.
- *Motorized spiral enteroscope (MSE)*: It has been introduced in 2015. It consists of a disposable, short, spiral, and flexible overtube with an electric motor embedded in the endoscope with a rotation coupler. This spiral overtube can be rotated clockwise or counter-clockwise using a foot pedal. Available data shows it is safe and effective for deep enteroscopy.
- Motorized spiral enteroscope therefore is the more advanced, emerging, and promising procedure with an advantage of deeper access of small intestine. However, availability and high cost are the limiting factor.

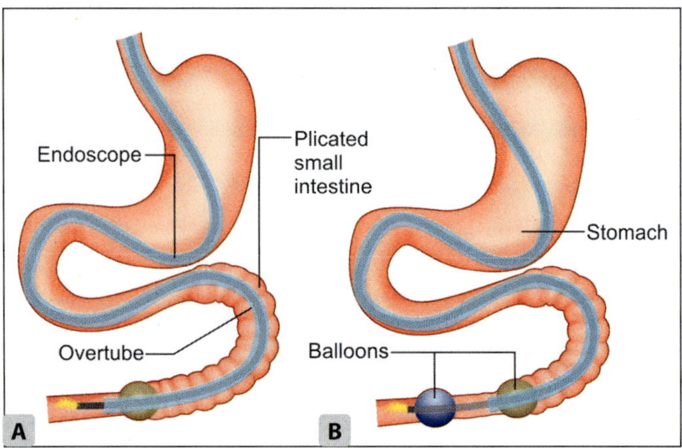

FIGURES 2 A & B: Comparison of **(A)** single-balloon and **(B)** double-balloon enteroscopy system.

Courtesy: Bowen LK, et al. Journal of the Mechanical Behaviour of Biomedical Materials. 2020 Nov 1;111.

- The diagnostic yield and safety profile of SBE, DBE, and SE are comparable and appear equivalent for routine clinical practice.
- Single-balloon enteroscopy appears to be least complicated procedure to perform. However, the rate of panenteroscopy is only about 20%. **Table 4** shows the rates of panenteroscopy achieved during SBE in the recently published studies.
- Overall adverse event rates of device-assisted enteroscopy for diagnostic procedures are 0.8% while for therapeutic interventions are up to 10%.
- *Intraoperative enteroscopy*: It is used only in certain situations like unstable patient, unsuccessful deep enteroscopy in patient with ongoing bleed or if deep enteroscopy cannot be performed without lysis of adhesions, and in patients with prior abdominal surgery.

Flowchart 2 shows the approach toward the patient with small bowel bleeding.

RADIOLOGIC PROCEDURES

Barium examination:

- Barium studies are readily available across the globe and are still the first-line investigation in many centers of India.
- It is a fluoroscopic technique which is easy to perform, relatively well tolerated, reproducible and gives high-resolution images of the small bowel.
- Barium meal follow through and barium meal small bowel enema are the two main techniques used. Small bowel enema involves placement of a tube beyond distal duodenum and then instilling barium through the tube.
- *Indications*: Obstruction, stricture, masses, diverticulosis, abnormal motility, extraluminal tethering, and fistulas.
- The detailed mucosal evaluation can be done using small bowel barium study.
- It has got limited role in assessment of extraluminal diseases and diagnosis of ileus or acute small intestinal obstruction. The yield is only 3–17% in suspected small bowel bleeding. Hence, barium studies should not be performed in the evaluation of obscure GI bleeding.

Ultrasonography:

- It is widely available and does not involve any radiation. However, the skill and experience of the operator determine the success of small bowel evaluation at USG.

TABLE 4 Panenteroscopy rates using single-balloon enteroscopy.

Author	Year	Study design	No. of procedures or cases	Rate of panenteroscopy
Goenka et al.	2020	Prospective	180	5/22 (22.72%)
Li et al.	2014	RCT	106	37/106 (34.9%)
Takano et al.	2011	RCT	14	0/14 (0%)
Domagk et al.	2011	RCT	65	7/65 (11%)
May et al.	2010	RCT	50	11/50 (22%)
Ramchandani et al.	2009	Case series	131	5/20 (25%)

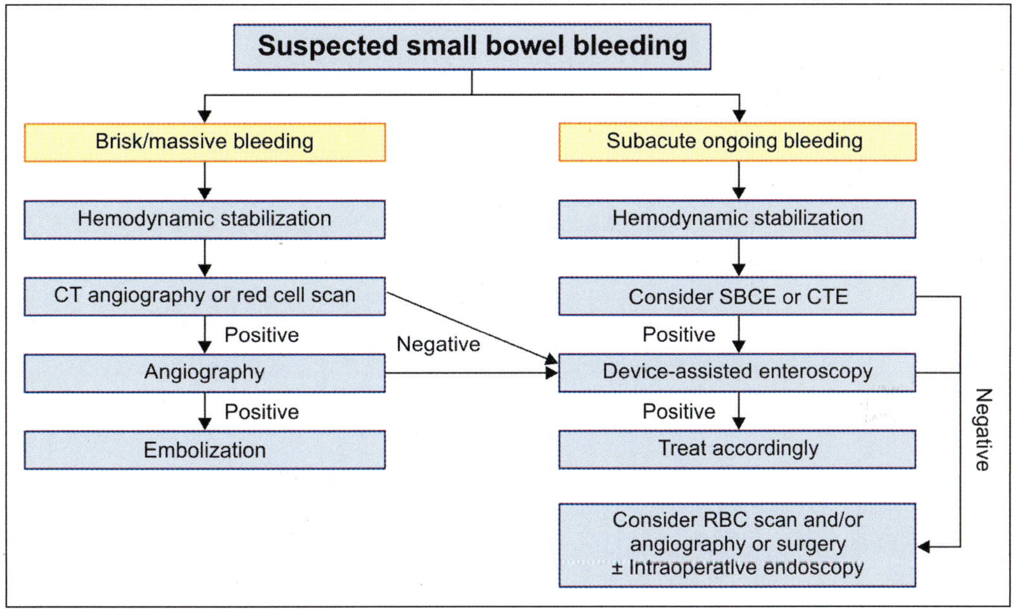

(CTE: CT enterography)

FLOWCHART 2: Approach toward the patient with small bowel bleeding.

- Most commonly used in diagnosis of Crohn's disease with reported sensitivity and specificity between 75–94% and 67–100%, respectively. It is more effective in evaluation of inflammatory bowel disease involving terminal ileum and less effective elsewhere in small intestine and colon.
- A unique advantage of USG is real-time imaging of the small bowel. This helps in assessing peristalsis (which is impaired in high-grade small bowel obstruction, enteritis, and ischemia), compressibility (which is lost in appendicitis, bowel malignancy, intussusception, and distended bowel in obstruction), and performing Valsalva maneuver (in diagnosing hernias of bowel, mesentery, and peritoneum).
- The major disadvantage is it is operator dependent and majority of the small bowel lesions are missed in inexperienced hands.

Computed tomography:

- Conventional CT using oral and intravenous contrast agents is used widely to investigate nonspecific abdominal pain and other symptoms related to small bowel.
- The performance of routine cross-sectional imaging of the abdomen can be increased by ingestion of large volumes of contrast (enterography) or by administration of contrast through nasoenteric tube (enteroclysis). **Flowchart 3** shows the approach toward the patient with intestinal obstruction.
- *Computed tomography enterography*:
  - It should be considered before SBCE in the setting of previously established inflammatory bowel disease, prior radiation therapy, past history of surgery of small bowel, and/or stenosis of small bowel.
  - A meta-analysis has shown that CTE has lower pooled yield in comparison to SBCE (40% vs. 53%). However, it has got improved detection of mural-based small bowel lesions.
  - If there is high suspicion of small bowel source of bleeding, CTE should be performed despite the performance of prior standard CT of the abdomen and negative SBCE (conditional recommendation, very low level of evidence).
  - Its noninvasive nature (in comparison to enteroclysis and device-assisted enteroscopy) and speed of investigation, it is the preferred technique for evaluation of small bowel.
- *Computed tomography enteroclysis*:
  - It has become a popular imaging technique for evaluation of small bowel disorder.
  - Here, the bowel is distended using a controlled infusion of enteral contrast at rate of 120–200 mL/min until up to 2,000 mL is delivered.
  - It has got multiplanar reformatting capability of cross-sectional imaging using enteral contrast.
  - The major limitation of CT enteroclysis is high radiation dose involved and poor toleration of high volume of enteral contrast material.
- *Computed tomography angiography (CTA)*:
  - It is used to detect active bleeding in patients with acute overt bleeding and can detect bleeding as slow as 0.3 mL/min with pooled sensitivity and specificity in detecting the source of acute GI bleeding is 89% and 85%, respectively.
  - It can also be used to triage the patients presenting with acute overt GI bleeding.
  - Conventional angiography should be performed in hemodynamically unstable patients presenting with acute overt GI bleeding. On the other hand, multiphasic CTA should be performed in hemodynamically stable patients for the identification of the site of bleeding, before planning a conventional angiography.
  - *Limitations*: The lesions can be detected only if the patient is bleeding at the time of scan. In elderly

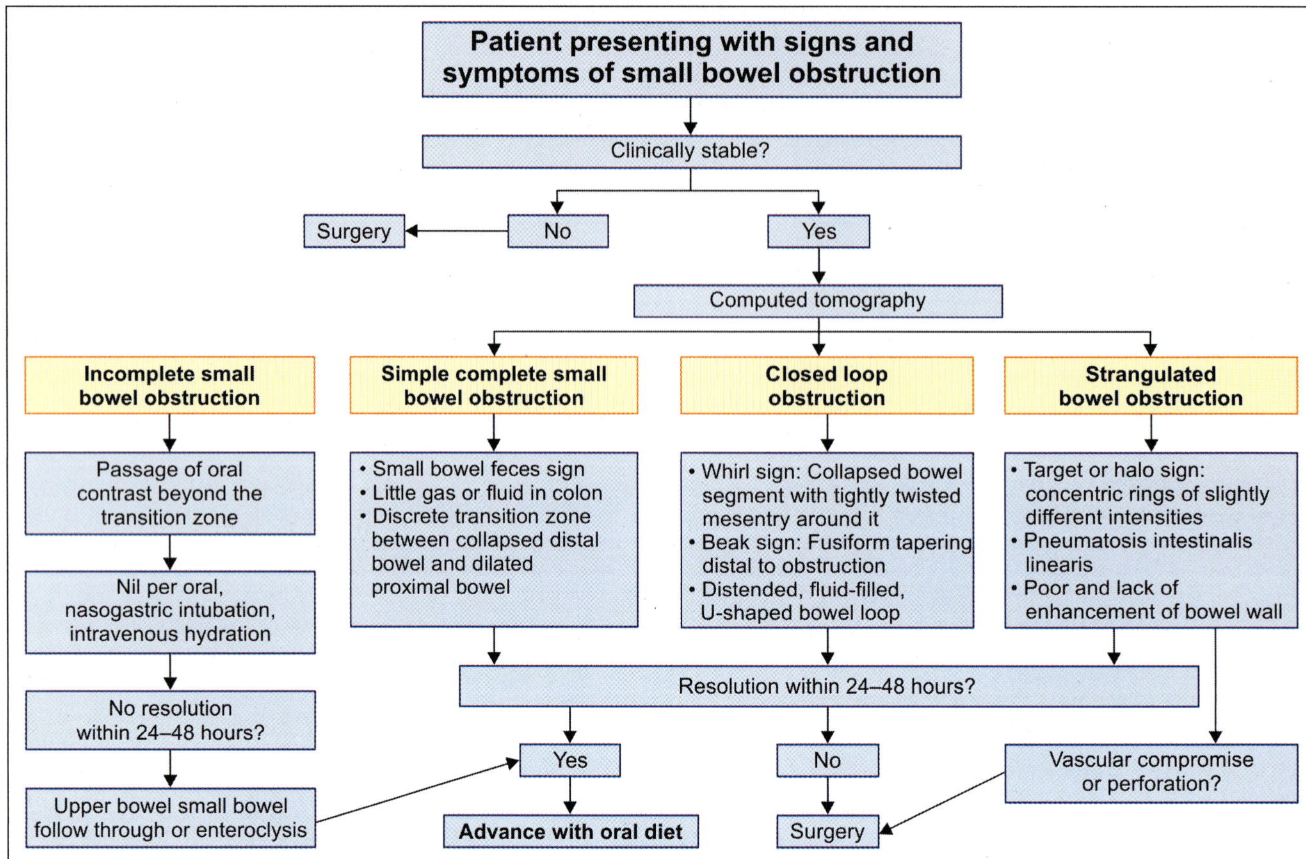

FLOWCHART 3: Approach toward the patient with intestinal obstruction.

patients, administration of contrast agent may increase the risk of renal impairment.

Magnetic resonance imaging:

- Magnetic resonance imaging (MRI) has important role in imaging of small bowel owing to its excellent soft tissue contrast, lack of ionizing radiation, and availability of new ultrafast breath-holding pulse sequences.
- Due to increased awareness of radiation exposure, globally MRI is becoming a preferred modality over CT.
- Similar to CT, MR enteroclysis (administration of contrast using nasojejunal tube) and MRE (using oral contrast) are two major techniques used to evaluate small bowel.
- Different pulse sequence techniques are available for imaging small bowel. These are—half-Fourier acquisition single-shot turbo spin echo (HASTE) techniques [single-shot fast spin echo (SSFSE) and single-shot turbo spin echo] and the balanced gradient echo [fast imaging employing steady-state acquisition, true fast imaging with steady-state precession (FISP), and balanced fast field echo] sequences.
- Half-Fourier acquisition single-shot turbo spin echo sequence is ideal for imaging small bowel due to lack of artifacts from peristalsis, however, the information of mesenteries is limited.
- Mural and extraintestinal complications are better diagnosed using true-FISP sequence.
- In patients with Crohn's disease, MR enteroclysis delineates superficial changes better than MRE. There is limited experience in using MRI in evaluating other small bowel diseases.

Scintigraphy:

- ^{99m}Tc-tagged red blood cell (RBC) scintigraphy can detect bleeding as slow as 0.2 mL/min.
- It helps in detection of delayed bleeding by performing delayed imaging.
- Wide range of diagnostic yields (26–87%), localization accuracy (19–100%), sensitivity (33–93%), and specificity (30–95%) has been reported in the literature. Due to these large variations, there is considerable controversy in using scintigraphy in diagnosing acute overt GI bleeding.
- *Limitations*: Inability to characterize the source of bleeding and difficulty to localize the foregut lesions are few of the limitations.
- The authors do not support the use of ^{99m}Tc-tagged RBC scintigraphy.
- Meckel scan (Technetium-99m pertechnetate scintigraphy) should be performed in younger patients with normal VCE and ongoing overt bleeding to detect Meckel diverticulum.

Evaluation of small bowel is challenging and requires high index of clinical suspicion. Small bowel diseases are important causes of morbidity and mortality. Adequate evaluation is imperative for diagnosis and management of these diseases. History and physical examination will not only play an important role in suspecting small bowel disease but also in choosing right investigation or procedure for further evaluation of small bowel. Significant progress has been made both in radiology and endoscopy in past few years which has eased the job of physician and the endoscopist to a great extent.

RECOMMENDED READINGS

1. Feldman M, Friedman LS, Brandt LJ. Sleisenger and Fordtran's gastrointestinal and liver disease E-book: pathophysiology, diagnosis, management. Netherlands: Elsevier Health Sciences; 2019.
2. Gerson LB, Fidler JL, Cave DR, Leighton JA. ACG clinical guideline: diagnosis and management of small bowel bleeding. Am J Gastroenterol. 2015;110(9):1265-87.
3. Yamada T, Alpers DH, Kalloo AN, Kaplowitz N, Owyang C, Powell DW. Textbook of gastroenterology. United States: John Wiley and Sons; 2015.
4. Schneider M, Höllerich J, Beyna T. Device-assisted enteroscopy: A review of available techniques and upcoming new technologies. World J Gastroenterol. 2019;25(27):3538.
5. Chaurasia BD. BD Chaurasia's Human Anatomy, Volume 2: Lower Limb, Abdomen and Pelvis. New Delhi: CBS Publishers & Distributors; 2013.
6. Laghi A, Hara AK. Small bowel disease. In: Laghi A, Hara AK (Eds). Diseases of the Abdomen and Pelvis 2018-2021: Diagnostic Imaging-IDKD Book. Germany: Springer; 2018. pp. 117.
7. Kopylov U, Seidman EG. Diagnostic modalities for the evaluation of small bowel disorders. Curr Opin Gastroenterol. 2015;31(2):111-7.
8. Hara AK, Leighton JA, Sharma VK, Heigh RI, Fleischer DE. Imaging of small bowel disease: comparison of capsule endoscopy, standard endoscopy, barium examination, and CT. Radiographics. 2005;25(3): 697-711.
9. Goenka MK, Majumder S, Kumar S, Sethy PK, Goenka U. Single center experience of capsule endoscopy in patients with obscure gastrointestinal bleeding. World J Gastroenterol. 2011;17(6):774-8.
10. Goenka MK, Afzalpurkar S, Rai VK, Agarwal R, Shah BB, Rodge GA, et al. Single-balloon enteroscopy in management of small-bowel disorders. Indian J Gastroenterol. 2020;39(6):550-6.

CHAPTER 133

Celiac Disease and Other Causes of Malabsorption

Ajit Sood, Vandana Midha, Arshdeep Singh

ABSTRACT

Malabsorption, a clinical syndrome resulting from a variety of infectious and noninfectious conditions, is characterized by malnutrition, diarrhea, and weight loss. Celiac disease (CeD) is a common cause of malabsorption both in developed and developing countries. The global prevalence of CeD is increasing. CeD develops in genetically susceptible [human leukocyte antigen (HLA) DQ2/DQ8 positive] individuals who elicit an aberrant immune response triggered by gluten ingestion. It has diverse clinical manifestations ranging from frank malabsorption to minimal intestinal/extraintestinal or asymptomatic presentations, necessitating high index of suspicion, especially in areas with high prevalence. The diagnosis of CeD is based on clinical features, serologic testing, and histologic evaluation. Gluten-free diet (GFD) forms the mainstay of treatment. However, lifelong adherence to GFD is a challenge and nondietary therapies are therefore being evaluated. This chapter discusses in detail the pathophysiology, clinical features, diagnosis, treatment, and complications of CeD. Other causes of malabsorption in India are reviewed in brief.

"Good health begins in the gut and plays a key role in natural immunity"

—Rick Rockhill

INTRODUCTION

Small intestine, due to its large surface area (attributable to numerous villi and microvilli) and presence of digestive enzymes on the mucosal surface, is the main site for uptake and absorption of dietary nutrients. Intact small intestinal mucosal surface, sufficient secretion of digestive enzymes, uninterrupted blood supply, normal intestinal motility, and healthy gut microbiota are prerequisites for normal absorptive functions. A defect in any of the components of this complex framework results in malabsorption.

Physiologically, there are three phases of absorption: luminal phase, mucosal phase, and transport phase. A defect in any of the three phases results in malabsorption. **Table 1** summarizes the pathophysiology of common causes of malabsorption.

The clinical syndrome of malabsorption is characterized by diarrhea, steatorrhea, malnutrition, weight loss, abdominal pain, and anemia. The etiology of malabsorption syndrome (MAS) is different in developed and developing world. While short bowel syndrome, Crohn's disease, chronic pancreatitis, celiac disease (CeD), and eosinophilic enteropathies remain the common causes of malabsorption in West; infections like giardiasis, strongyloidiasis, intestinal tuberculosis, parasitic infestations, tropical sprue, and bacterial overgrowth are exclusive to developing countries in the tropics. In an observational study from north India, tropical sprue (37%), CeD (19%), small intestinal bacterial overgrowth (10%), acquired immunodeficiency syndrome (5.4%), and giardiasis (5%) were the common causes of malabsorption in adults. Another study from south India found tropical sprue (41%), CeD (21%), acquired immunodeficiency syndrome (7.5%), giardiasis (5%), and intestinal tuberculosis (3%) as common causes of malabsorption. Yadav and colleagues analyzed the clinical,

TABLE 1 Common causes of malabsorption.

Phase	Pathophysiology	Example
Luminal phase	Abnormal anatomy of the absorptive surface	• Short bowel syndrome • Intestinal fistula • Mechanical obstruction (stricture/tumor/polyp/adhesions/peritoneal carcinomatosis) • Bariatric surgery
	Abnormal mucosal surface	• Celiac disease • Crohn's disease • Intestinal tuberculosis • Giardiasis • Tropical sprue • Whipple's disease • Amyloidosis • Radiation enteritis • Allergic and eosinophilic gastroenteritis • Neonatal enteropathies • Abetalipoproteinemia • Autoimmune enteropathy • Drugs (nonsteroidal anti-inflammatory drugs, opioid analgesics, mycophenolate mofetil, gold, and olmesartan)
	Deficiency of digestive enzymes	• Chronic pancreatic insufficiency • Cystic fibrosis • Inactivation of pancreatic enzymes in Zollinger–Ellison syndrome • Primary or secondary disaccharidase deficiency
	Deficiency of bile salts	• Ileal resection or dysfunction (increased loss) • Cirrhosis (decreased synthesis) • Chronic cholestasis (ineffective secretion) • Bacterial overgrowth (deconjugation) • Gastrectomy and bypass (rerouting)
Mucosal phase	Brush border enzyme deficiency	Lactase deficiency (primary, developmental, or secondary)
	Enterocyte dysfunction	• Celiac disease • Crohn's disease
Transport phase	Lymphatic obstruction	• Intestinal lymphangiectasia • Lymphoma • Abetalipoproteinemia • Waldenstrom macroglobulinemia • Tuberculosis • Whipple's disease • Filariasis • Resection of abdominal aortic aneurysm • Retroperitoneal lymph node dissection

endoscopic, and histological features of 94 consecutive patients with MAS and reported CeD (65%) and tropical sprue (22%) as the most common etiologies.

This chapter reviews the pathogenesis, clinical features, diagnosis, and management of CeD and other common causes of malabsorption in India.

CELIAC DISEASE

DEFINITION

CeD is a chronic small intestinal immune-mediated enteropathy caused by ingestion of gluten in genetically susceptible individuals. Gluten is the alcohol-soluble protein component of wheat, rye, and barley. Exposure to gluten in at-risk individuals (discussed below) results in a variable degree of damage to the intestinal mucosa resulting in MAS.

A combination of suggestive clinical manifestations, positive celiac serological tests, a supportive duodenal histology, and response to GFD is needed to make a diagnosis of CeD. On the basis of these parameters, multiple terminologies are used in relation to CeD. A multidisciplinary task force reached agreement on the definitions of terms used in clinical practice and research related to CeD. These definitions are called the "Oslo definitions" (**Table 2**). The use of terminologies like silent CeD, latent CeD, overt CeD, typical CeD, and atypical CeD is discouraged.

EPIDEMIOLOGY

The global prevalence of CeD is approximately 1% of the general population. In one of the first study from India, conducted by our group, the estimated prevalence of CeD among school children in north India was 1 in 310. A subsequent nationwide study reported 1.23%, 0.87%, and 0.1% age-adjusted seroprevalence of CeD in northern, northeastern, and southern India. Prevalence of CeD was 8.53/1,000 in northern, 4.66/1,000 in northeastern, and 0.11/1,000 in southern India. The difference in prevalence of CeD in different parts of India can be attributed to higher consumption of wheat (and therefore gluten) in northern India as prevalence of celiac compatible HLA haplotypes (discussed below) is similar in different parts of the country (38.1% in northern, 31.4% in north-eastern, and 36.4% in southern India). There are also racial and ethnic differences in the prevalence of CeD with highest prevalence in persons of Punjab ethnicity and lesser in non-Hispanic blacks. The prevalence of CeD is increasing worldwide owing to increased physician awareness and recognition of varied intestinal and extraintestinal presenting features of CeD.

ETIOPATHOGENESIS

GENETIC SUSCEPTIBILITY

Celiac disease has a strong genetic component as is evident from high rates of positive family history (in first-generation relatives) and high prevalence among monozygotic twins. HLAs DQ2 and DQ8 (heterodimeric proteins associated with CeD) play an important role in the causation of CeD. Almost all patients with CeD express either HLA DQ2 or DQ8. Expression of HLA DQ2 on the surface of antigen-presenting cells is seen in >90% of patients, while majority of the remainder are HLA DQ8 positive. In India, nearly one-third (30–35%) of general population expresses HLA DQ2 or DQ8, however the prevalence of CeD is only 1%; implying that though HLAs DQ2 and DQ8 are vital for predisposition to CeD, these alone are not sufficient and additional non-HLA associated genes are required to develop CeD. More than 100 such non-HLA associated genes have been identified till date, though their clinical relevance is not yet clear.

GLUTEN

Gluten refers to a family of proteins called prolamins and is composed of a complex group of alcohol-soluble gliadins and alcohol-insoluble glutenins that are resistant to proteolytic enzymes.

Gliadins are not completely digested by the intestinal enzymes and the partially digested peptides have the potential to trigger an immune response by entering the lamina propria of the small intestine via transcellular or paracellular routes. The partially digested gliadin peptides (GPs) bind to chemokine receptor CXCR3 on the apical membrane of enterocytes resulting in release of zonulin that via disintegration of intercellular tight junctions increases paracellular permeability. Once the tolerance to gluten is broken, GPs can translocate from intestinal lumen to lamina propria through the transcellular route also.

The GPs in the lamina propria are subjected to deamidation by resident tissue transglutaminase 2 (tTG2) to form deamidated gliadin. The deamidated gliadin is immunogenic and it is identified and presented by HLA DQ2/DQ8-positive antigen presenting cells to gluten-sensitized CD4+ T helper cells. The stimulated CD4+ T helper cells further increase the production and release of proinflammatory cytokines, keratinocyte growth factor,

TABLE 2 Oslo definitions of celiac disease (CeD) and related terms.

Terminology	Clinical symptoms of malabsorption or malabsorption syndrome	Extraintestinal manifestations	Response to gluten withdrawal	Serology	Histology
Asymptomatic CeD	–	–	–	+	+
Classical CeD	+	–	+	+	+
Nonclassical CeD	–	+	+	+	+
Potential CeD	+			+	–

and metalloproteases and activate B cells to produce immunoglobulin A (IgA), IgM, and IgG antibodies against tTG2, gliadin, and actin. The proinflammatory milieu in the lamina propria culminates in damage to enterocytes. The damaged enterocytes express CD71 on the apical membrane, which binds to IgA-gliadin complex and mediates its retrotranscytosis. The increased trafficking of gliadin into the lamina propria further compounds the immune-mediated enteropathy.

The GPs trigger the production of interleukin-15 (IL-15), IL-8, and interferon α; and also induce toll-like receptor 4 (TLR 4)-mediated release of proinflammatory cytokines (interferon γ and tumor necrosis factor α) thereby initiating the inflammatory cascade in lamina propria. IL-15 plays an important role in loss of oral tolerance to gluten, loss of immune regulation, increased lymphokine killer activity and epithelial cell destruction, and increased expansion and survival of an abnormal subset of $CD3^-$ intraepithelial lymphocytes in patients with refractory CeD.

Figure 1 summarizes the immune pathogenesis of CeD.

OTHER FACTORS

As discussed earlier, not all individuals carrying susceptible HLA DQ2/DQ8 alleles develop CeD, implying the role of environmental factors in the pathogenesis of CeD. Age of introduction and amount of gluten in the diet have been evaluated. However, no significant association between early introduction or higher quantity of gluten and CeD has been proven. The European guidelines however suggest to introduce gluten between the age of 4 and 12 months and consumption of large quantities should be avoided early after introduction. Elective cesarean section, and gastrointestinal and respiratory infections, have demonstrated association with subsequent development of CeD. However, these observations need validation.

CLINICAL FEATURES

Celiac disease, more common in females, can present at any age from infancy to senior adulthood. The average age of diagnosis is between the second and the fourth decades of life, with approximately 20% of cases diagnosed in those who are >60 years of age. The clinical presentation of CeD can be divided into classical/gastrointestinal and nonclassical/extraintestinal features. The classical presentation of CeD is usually characterized by diarrhea, steatorrhea, weight loss, failure to thrive, and nutritional deficiencies. The diarrhea in CeD is usually episodic and occurs during night or early morning. Diarrhea in CeD is multifactorial and commonly occurs due to a combination of increased osmotic load in colon due to malabsorption, cathartic action of fatty acids, increased luminal contents due to secretion of electrolytes in the lumen, impaired intraluminal digestion, and bile acid diarrhea. It is important to note that in CeD, weight loss occurs despite preserved appetite.

The nonclassical (constipation, bloating) or extra-intestinal (hematological, musculoskeletal, neurological,

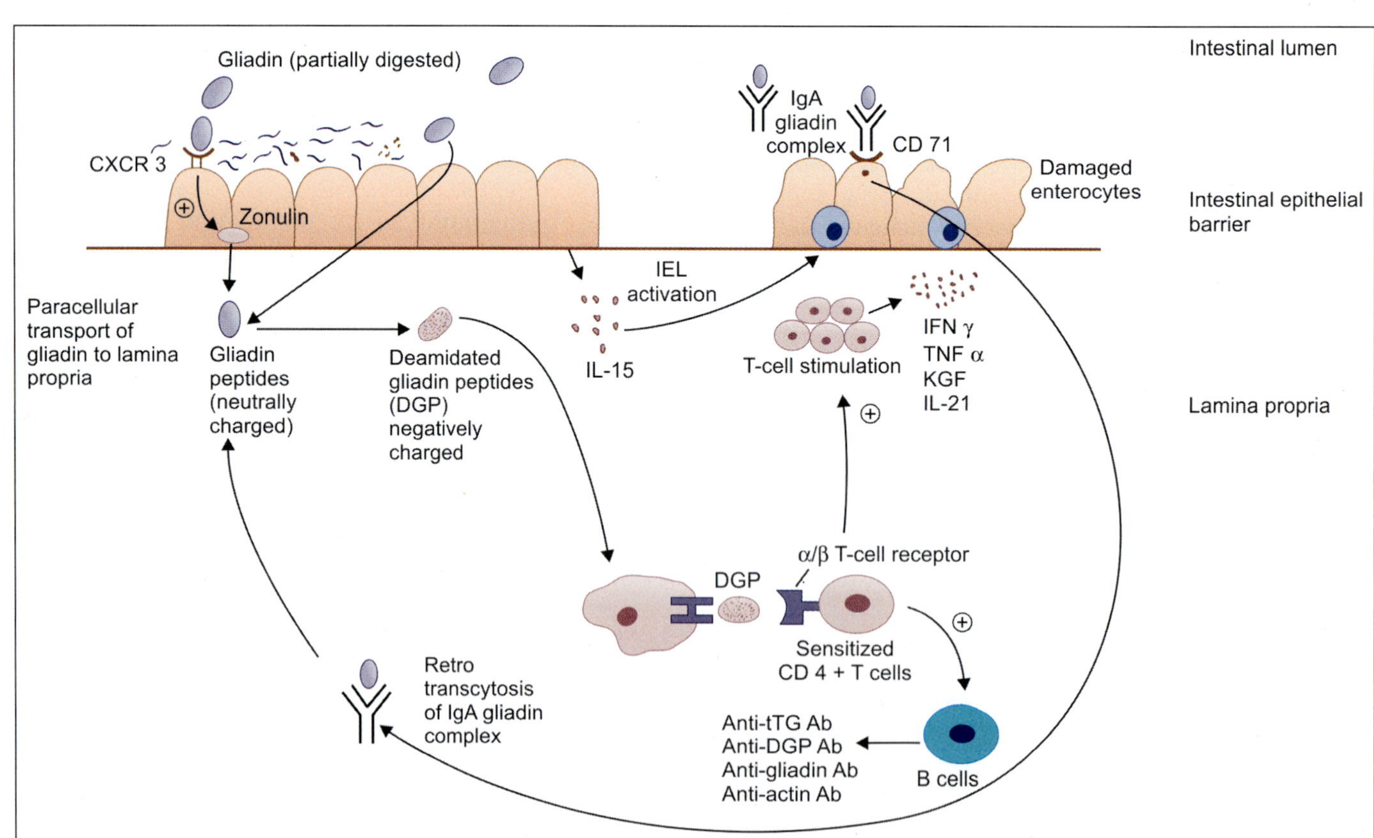

(DGP: deamidated gliadin peptide; IL: interleukin; IEL: intraepithelial lymphocytes; IFN: interferon; IL-21: interleukin-21; IgA: immunoglobulin A; KGF: keratinocyte growth factor; TNF: tumor necrosis factor; tTG: tissue transglutaminase)

FIGURE 1: Immune pathogenesis of celiac disease.

TABLE 3 **Extraintestinal manifestations of celiac disease.**

System	Clinical presentation	Remarks
Hematological	Anemia	• Iron deficiency • Folate deficiency
	Coagulopathy	
	Thrombocytosis	Secondary to hyposplenism, Howell–Jolly bodies seen
Musculoskeletal	Osteoporosis/osteopenia	• Malabsorption of calcium and vitamin D • Secondary hyperparathyroidism, that is refractory to gluten-free diet, may develop
	Muscle weakness	Presents as chronic fatigue
Neurological	Ataxia	Cerebellar atrophy, not reversible with gluten-free diet
	Peripheral neuropathy	Damage to posterior column (patchy demyelination) and peripheral nerves, not reversible with gluten-free diet
	Seizures	Complex partial seizures
	Headache	
Hepatic	Liver parenchymal damage, increased aminotransferases	
Dermatological	Dermatitis herpetiformis	• More common in males • Pruritic papulovesicular lesions commonly located on the extensor surfaces of elbows, knees, and buttocks • Only a minority of individuals have enteropathy • High risk of lymphoma
	Hyperkeratosis follicularis	
	Psoriasis	
	Alopecia areata	
	Chronic urticaria	
Oral cavity	• Dental enamel defects • Aphthous stomatitis • Angular cheilitis • Glossitis	
Psychiatric	• Depression • Anxiety • Increased suicidal tendencies	
Reproductive	Intrauterine growth retardation	Due to binding of anti tissue transglutaminase to trophoblast
	Recurrent abortions	
	Amenorrhea	
	Delayed menarche	Can be delayed up to 1 year
	Infertility	
	Oligozoospermia	Due to hypothalamic pituitary dysfunction and gonadal androgen resistance

hepatic, dermatological, and reproductive system) involvement is not uncommon (**Table 3**). The gastrointestinal symptoms dominate the clinical presentation in children, whereas extraintestinal manifestations may be common initial presentation in adults, with minimal or subclinical gastrointestinal manifestations.

Because of diverse clinical presentations, a high index of suspicion is required to diagnose CeD. A delay in diagnosis can lead to complications and poor quality of life. **Table 4** summarizes the National Institute for Health and Care Excellence (NICE) indications for testing for CeD.

DIAGNOSIS

The diagnosis of CeD is based on clinical features, serology, and histology.

It is important that patient is on gluten-containing diet at the time of serologic and histologic testing. If the suspected patient is on GFD with a questionable/unconfirmed diagnosis of CeD, a gluten challenge can be given to induce serologic or histologic changes. In gluten challenge, 3 g gluten is introduced in the diet of HLA DQ2/DQ8-positive patient and the patient is advised to continue it for 2 weeks. At the end of 2 weeks, if the patient is symptomatic, a

TABLE 4 NICE recommendations for testing for celiac disease (CeD).

Recommended testing for CeD	• Persistent unexplained abdominal or gastrointestinal symptoms • Impaired growth • Chronic fatigue • Unintentional weight loss • Severe or persistent oral ulcers • Unexplained iron, vitamin B12, or folate deficiency • Coexistent autoimmune diseases (type 1 diabetes mellitus, autoimmune thyroid disease, Sjögren's syndrome) • First-degree relatives of people with CeD • Dermatitis herpetiformis
Consider testing for CeD	• Metabolic bone disorders • Unexplained peripheral neuropathy/ataxia • Persistently increased hepatic aminotransferases of unknown etiology • Dental enamel defect • Unexplained infertility • Down syndrome • Turner syndrome

(NICE: National Institute for Health and Care Excellence)

TABLE 5 Serological tests for diagnosis of celiac disease.

	Sensitivity	Specificity	Remarks
Anti-tTG (IgA)	88–90%	98%	• Test of choice • False positive in other autoimmune diseases, liver disease, congestive heart failure and inflammatory bowel disease • False negative in children <2 years of age, mild enteropathy and IgA deficiency
Anti-EMA	90%	99%	• Immunofluorescence based, so needs expertise
Anti-DGP (IgA and IgG)	75–96%	98–100%	• IgG anti-DGP useful in IgA deficiency • IgG anti-DGP more accurate in children

(DGP: deamidated gliadin peptide; EMA: endomysial antibody; Ig: immunoglobulin; tTG: tissue transglutaminase)

duodenal biopsy is taken. If the patient is able to tolerate gluten at the end of 2 weeks, gluten challenge is continued for additional 6 weeks and serology is repeated at the end of challenge. A positive serology after 8 weeks indicates potential CeD. If the serology is negative at 8 weeks, a repeat serological testing is performed 2–6 weeks after the end of challenge and a second negative serological test rules out CeD.

Serology: The presence of antibodies against GPs and connective tissue proteins like tissue transglutaminase (tTG) is the hallmark of CeD (**Table 5**).

The sensitivity and specificity of current anti-tTG IgA assays used to detect CeD approach 90–95% and anti-tTG IgA is therefore the most commonly used serological test used for screening and diagnosing CeD because of its ease to use and objectivity in interpretation. Various enzyme-linked immunosorbent assay (ELISA) kits that measure anti-tTG IgA are available commercially. Because of the use of different substrates [guinea pig liver tTG (gpl-tTG) or erythrocyte tTG or recombinant human tTG (rHu-tTG)] in different kits, the results may vary from one kit to another. Additionally, the cutoff values for kits developed by different manufacturers are different, even if they all use same substrate. Therefore the cutoff values need to be adjusted via ROC plot analysis for the referral population.

The discrepancies between the ROC analysis-derived cut-off values and manufacturer-recommended cut-off values highlight the importance of revalidation of cutoff points by the testing laboratories. Anti-tTG (IgA) antibodies will not manifest in IgA-deficient patients. In such patients, measurement of serum IgA levels or performing both IgA and IgG-based tests, such as anti-deamidated gliadin peptide (DGP) (IgG and IgA), is recommended. As children below 2 years of age are likely to have subnormal levels of IgA, IgA anti-tTG test should be combined with (IgA and IgG) DGP when screening for CeD. If selective IgA deficiency is documented, IgG-based testing (IgG DGP and IgG tTG) should be performed. Anti endomysial antibody (anti EMA) IgA is the most specific serologic test. Despite high specificity, the use of anti-EMA in clinical practice is limited due to its semiquantitative nature and operator-dependent technique for testing. Anti-EMA may be used as a confirmatory test, particularly when anti-tTG has a low titer (<2 times the upper normal limit) or the results are equivocal.

Sequential testing (anti-tTG IgA followed by anti-EMA IgA in those who tested positive for anti-tTG IgA) has been employed for diagnosis of CeD in large epidemiological studies but its accuracy in clinical practice needs further evaluation. Antibodies against native gliadin (anti-gliadin antibodies, AGA) were previously used to diagnose CeD. However, they have wide variability in the diagnostic accuracy and are less sensitive and specific than anti-tTG and anti-DGP. Therefore their use as diagnostic tool for CeD is not recommended. Combining different antibody tests in commercially available panels increases the sensitivity of diagnosing CeD; however, this increased sensitivity comes at the expense of decreased specificity. The combination testing is therefore not performed routinely.

A positive serological test warrants histological examination to confirm the diagnosis of CeD. However in children with signs or symptoms suggestive of CD and high anti-tTG (IgA) titers (>10 times upper limit of normal);

a positive anti-EMA (done on a second serum sample) confirms the diagnosis and duodenal biopsy may not be required.

Apart from serological testing for celiac antibodies, there are certain molecules which can serve as a biomarker for enterocyte mass and function (citrulline, cytochrome P450 3A4), enterocyte injury (intestinal fatty acid-binding protein), and enterocyte regeneration (regenerating gene 1α). These noninvasive markers can predict enteropathy (villous atrophy) and are being tested as diagnostic tools in CeD.

Histology: A positive serological test is followed by an esophagogastroduodenoscopy to obtain duodenal biopsy. Endoscopy may show scalloped and grooved duodenal mucosa; however, these changes are not specific for CeD. A normal-looking mucosa also does not rule out CeD. The histological changes associated with CeD are patchy and therefore, multiple duodenal biopsies are required (at least two from duodenal bulb and four from different quadrants of second part of duodenum).

Additionally, interpretation of the biopsy from duodenal bulb alone is challenging due to presence of abundant Brunner's glands and inflammatory changes inflicted by gastric acid or pancreatic secretions. Therefore deeper biopsies from second or third part of duodenum are essential and biopsies from multiple sites need to be interpreted in totality. Orientation of biopsy fragments is important for correct classification of the disease severity. For this, a single biopsy should be obtained per pass and each biopsy fragment should be mounted separately on a piece of laboratory grade 1 filter paper.

The histopathologic examination of duodenal biopsies may reveal increased intraepithelial lymphocytes, crypt hyperplasia, and villous atrophy. The severity of mucosal damage is classified according to modified Marsh (Marsh-Oberhuber) classification. Recently, Corazza and Ensari classification systems have been proposed; however, modified Marsh (Marsh-Oberhuber) classification is most widely used in clinical practice. It is important to exclude other differentials that cause villous atrophy on duodenal histology (**Table 6**).

Genetic testing: Human leukocyte antigen-DQ2 and HLA-DQ8 testing is not routinely recommended. However in scenarios where there is discordance between serology and histology, or the patient is on self-imposed GFD with a questionable diagnosis, genetic testing may be considered. The absence of HLA-DQ2 and HLA-DQ8 almost always excludes CeD, with a negative predictive value of >99%.

SERONEGATIVE CELIAC DISEASE

A small subset of patients with CeD have seronegative villous atrophy. The seronegativity can be due to IgA deficiency, coexistent autoimmune conditions requiring immunosuppressives or deposition of anti-tTG antibodies in the small bowel mucosa rendering the antibodies unable to enter the circulation. Seronegative CeD requires careful diagnosis, with the presence of HLA-DQ2 or HLA-DQ8 and a response to a GFD after excluding other causes of

TABLE 6	Histologic differential diagnosis of celiac disease.
Infections	• Bacterial overgrowth • Peptic duodenitis (*Helicobacter pylori*) • Giardiasis • Tropical sprue
Immunodeficiency states	• Common variable immunodeficiency • Selective IgA deficiency • Severe combined immunodeficiency
Autoimmune conditions	• Autoimmune enteropathy • Collagenous and lymphocytic colitis • Crohn's disease
Miscellaneous	• Cow's milk protein allergy • Eosinophilic enteritis • Nonsteroidal anti-inflammatory drugs (NSAIDs)-induced enteropathy • Olmesartan-induced enteropathy • Graft versus host disease • Radiation enteritis • Intestinal lymphoma

seronegative villous atrophy (drugs like mycophenolate mofetil and olmesartan, common variable immune deficiency, Crohn's disease, tropical sprue, giardiasis, autoimmune enteropathy etc.).

Flowchart 1 summarizes the diagnostic approach to CeD.

TREATMENT

Gluten-free diet: Gluten-free diet (containing <20 parts per million of gluten) forms the mainstay of treatment of CeD. Gluten-containing cereals such as wheat, barley, and rye should be excluded from the diet. Consumption of rice, corn, and maize is permitted. Oats contain smaller proportion of prolamins and are not allowed initially; however, they may be consumed in small amounts later in the disease course. Caution is advised while consuming commercial oat products, candies, ice creams, soups, and sausages as these contain gluten. Beer also contains gluten, whereas wine and whisky are gluten free (**Table 7**). Inadvertent intake of gluten will result in persistence of symptoms and continuous immune-mediated injury. Improvement and resolution of symptoms with GFD typically occurs within days or weeks. At times, dyspepsia-like symptoms may appear or get aggravated when the patient is started on GFD. However, these are transient and regress gradually. Clinical recovery precedes serological and histological recovery. Simultaneous testing and replacement of deficient micronutrients (iron, folic acid, vitamin B12, and vitamin D) is vital to improve growth parameters and quality of life.

Glucocorticoids: Currently, the most common indication for the use of corticosteroids in CeD is the treatment of refractory symptoms. The second indication of glucocorticoids in CeD is in celiac crisis (a life-threatening condition characterized by severe diarrhea, dehydration, electrolyte disturbances, renal dysfunction, and shock). Patients with celiac crisis

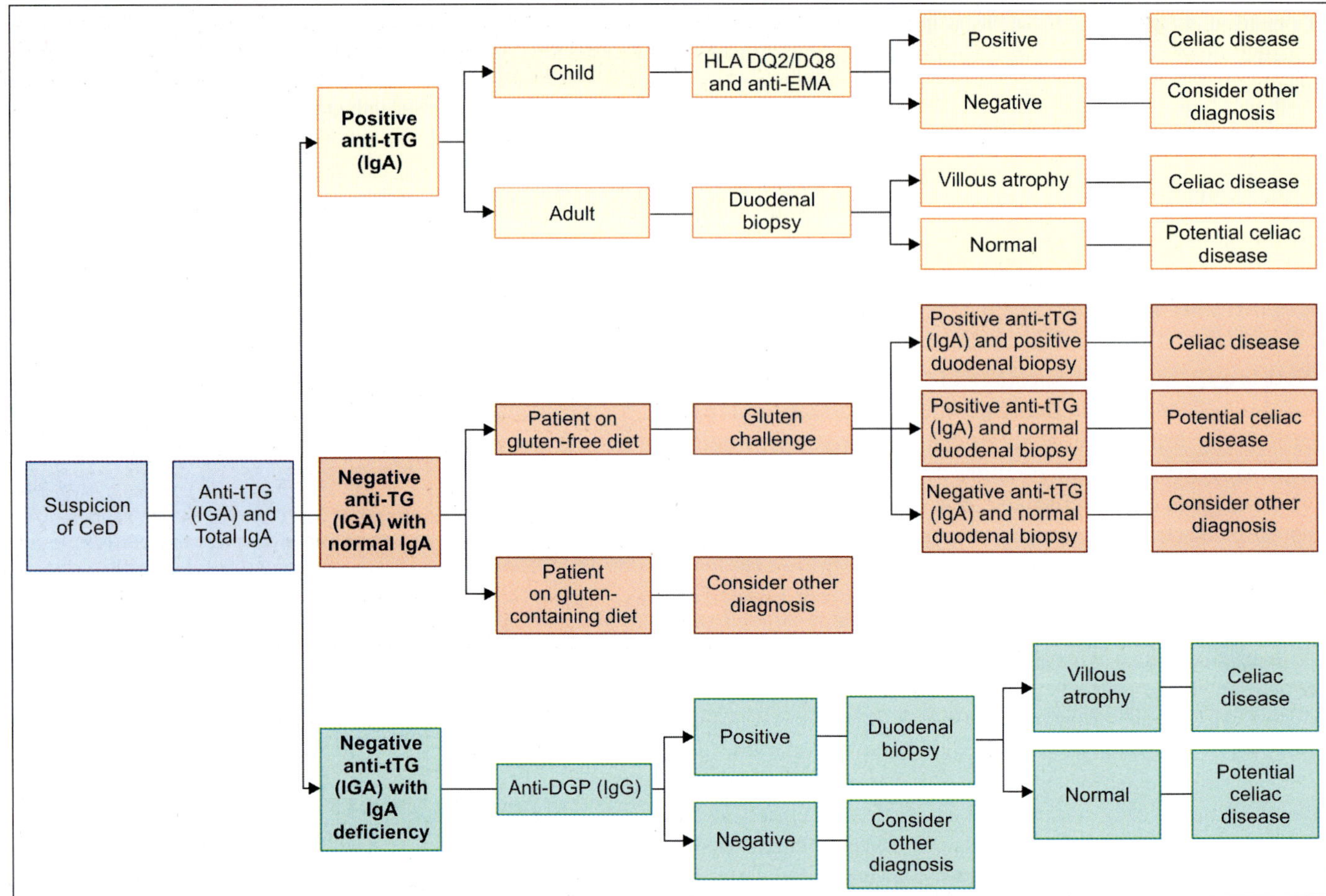

(DGP: deamidated gliadin peptide; EMA: endomysial antibodies; IgA: immunoglobulin A; tTG: tissue transglutaminase)

FLOWCHART 1: Diagnostic algorithm for celiac disease (CeD).

TABLE 7 List of allowed and restricted dietary items in celiac disease.

Allowed	Not allowed
• Corn • Buckwheat • Flax • Legume flours (bean, chickpea, lentils, and pea) • Millets, quinoa, rice • Rice flour, rice bran • Amaranth, sago • Sorghum flour • Tapioca, lentils • Dried peas, dried beans • Plain tofu • All fruits and vegetables • Meat • Fish, poultry, eggs • Butter, cream, margarine, lard, and vegetable oil • Milk, buttermilk • Plain yogurt • Cream cheese • Most ice cream, cakes, cookies, pastries made with allowed ingredients • Plain popcorn • Nuts, soy nuts • Potato chips • Taco (corn) chips • Tea, coffee • Homemade broth and soup	• Wheat bran • Wheat flour • Wheat starch • Durum flour • Graham flour • Barley • Rye • Canned or frozen meat, fish, poultry-containing hydrolyzed wheat protein • Contaminated oils • Baking powder, Brewer's yeast • Ice creams made from ingredients not allowed • Bread pudding • Ice cream cones and wafers • Chocolate bars with wafers and candies • Beer, ale, and lager • Malted beverages • Soups made from ingredients not allowed

TABLE 8 Nondietary therapies in celiac disease (CeD).

Mechanism	Approach	Remarks
Decreasing immunogenicity of gluten	Genetically modified gluten	Development of genetically engineered wheat with attenuated immunotoxicity while preserving its gastronomic or agronomic properties
	Intraluminal digestion of gluten	Gluten degrading enzymes (glutenases) that digest gliadin into peptides with nine or less amino acids
	Modified wheat gluten	Enzymatic predigestion or thermal modification of wheat gluten
Intraluminal sequestration of gliadin peptides	Polymeric binders	Bind gluten in the gut and preventing their breakdown/absorption, e.g., poly (hydroxyethyl methacrylate-co-styrene sulfonate) or P(HEMA-co-SS)
	Antigluten antibody	IgY antibody harvested from the yolk of eggs laid by hens that have been super immunized against gliadin
Prevention of uptake of gliadin peptides	CXCR3 antagonist, CD71 inhibitor, zonulin antagonist	Zonulin antagonist larazotide acetate, currently in phase-3 trials
Tissue transglutaminase inhibition	Tissue transglutaminase inhibitors	Currently in clinical trials, the inhibition of tTG-2 can result in cross-inhibition of other members of the transglutaminase family, several of which are indispensable for pathways like the coagulation cascade and the maintenance of epidermal integrity
	Silencing RNA-based therapy	Silencing RNA molecules target human tTG-2 and IL-15
Prevention of downstream immune activation	HLA blockers	Prevent the interaction of antigen presenting cells that process and present gluten to the T-cell receptor (TCR) of CD4+T helper cells
	Vaccine	Nexvax 2, targets HLA DQ2.5-epitope-TCR complex linking the antigen presenting cell to the gluten-reactive CD4+T cells, currently in phase-2 clinical trial
	Cathepsin inhibitor	Cathepsin S is important for the MHC II to function normally to present processed antigens to CD4+ cells, e.g., RG7625, RG7236
	Stem cell therapy	Case reports of using hematopoietic autologous stem cell transplant being successfully used to treat the enteropathy of CeD patients
	IL-15 antagonists	Humanized Mik-Beta-1 monoclonal antibody and AMG 714 have been developed to target IL-2/IL-15R beta (CD122)
	Immunosuppressants	Anti-TNF-α, anti-integrins, IL-10 blockers etc., are being investigated
Miscellaneous	Probiotics and prebiotics, low FODMAP diet, pancreatic enzyme supplements, helminth therapy using hookworms	Investigational
Identifying safe varieties of wheat	Testing old landraces of wheat	A pilot study used C273 wheat variety in patients with CeD and demonstrated that consumption of C273 wheat did not result in development of symptoms or evident changes in serology and histology at 28 weeks. However, variations in circulating inflammatory markers were noted

(RNA: ribonucleic acid; tTG: tissue transglutaminase; TNF: tumor necrosis factor; IL: interleukin; HLA: human leukocyte antigen; FODMAP: fermentable oligosaccharides, disaccharides, monosaccharides, and polyols; MHC: major histocompatibility complex)

who receive corticosteroids experience rapid clinical improvement within 2 weeks of treatment initiation and eventually maintain on GFD. Adjuvant treatment with corticosteroids has been reported to expedite clinical and histological recovery in patients with newly diagnosed CeD, though this is not a standard practice.

Nondietary therapies: Adherence to GFD is a challenge. The high cost, variability in information on the gluten-free status of food ingredients, peer pressure, and risks of inadvertent intake of gluten increase the disease-related burden on the patients. Attempts are therefore being made to look for effective and safe nondietary therapeutic alternatives. The nondietary therapies are summarized in **Table 8**.

COMPLICATIONS

A late diagnosis of CeD and nonadherence to GFD predispose to complications. The common complications of CeD are discussed below.

Hyposplenism: Hyposplenism can be functional or anatomical. It should be suspected in patients with thrombocytosis or Howell–Jolly bodies on peripheral smear. Hyposplenism is associated with development of encapsulated bacterial infections (i.e., *pneumococcus*, *Haemophilus influenzae*, *meningococcus*) and some physicians recommend vaccination against these infections.

Refractory celiac disease and intestinal lymphoma: It is characterized by persistence of clinical symptoms of malabsorption, weight loss, and diarrhea along with villous atrophy despite maintaining a strict GFD for at least 6–12 months. The adherence to GFD is confirmed by negative CeD serology. There are two subtypes of refractory CeD: type I and type II. Type I has a phenotypically normal CD3/CD8+ population of intraepithelial lymphocytes, whereas type II refractory CeD has an abnormal clonal proliferation of surface CD3–/intracytoplasmic CD3+ intraepithelial lymphocytes. Additionally there is monoclonal rearrangement of the gamma chain of the T-cell receptor. Type II refractory CeD is an aggressive disease and carries a poor prognosis. The increased mortality in type II refractory CeD is due to progression to intestinal lymphoma [enteropathy-associated T-cell lymphoma (EATL)]. Treatment of type I refractory CeD consists of immunosuppressants (glucocorticoids, azathioprine and methotrexate etc.). Type II refractory CeD requires chemotherapeutic agents such as cladribine, fludarabine, IL-15 antagonists, and JAK3 inhibitors. Once EATL develops, Scottish (ifosfamide, etoposide, epirubicin, methotrexate + autologous stem cell transplantation) or French (cyclophosphamide, doxorubicin, prednisone + autologous stem cell transplantation) regimes of chemotherapy are administered depending on CD30 negative (Scottish) or positive (French) status.

Ulcerative jejunoileitis: Ulcerative jejunoileitis is closely related to refractory CeD and presents with abdominal pain, diarrhea, weight loss, and malnutrition. Small intestinal lesions can result in gastrointestinal bleeding (ulcer), bowel obstruction (stricture) and perforation. Most of the patients progress to develop EATL.

Malignancy and mortality: Celiac disease is associated with an increased risk of malignancies of esophagus, small intestine (adenocarcinoma), colon, liver, pancreas, and ovary. Symptomatic but untreated CeD is associated with a modestly increased risk of mortality.

OTHER CAUSES OF MALABSORPTION

Celiac disease remains the most common cause of malabsorption in India. However, as discussed earlier, the clinical presentation of MAS is similar (diarrhea, steatorrhea, malnutrition, weight loss, abdominal pain, and anemia) no matter what the etiology is. The commonly encountered causes of MAS in India, other than CeD, are enumerated in **Tables 1** and **9**.

TABLE 9	Common causes of malabsorption in India (other than celiac disease)
Protein energy malnutrition	
Etiology	Starvation Metabolic stress
Pathogenesis	Protein or energy intake, or both, chronically fail to meet the body's requirements
Clinical Presentation	Weight loss, reduced muscle mass and strength, hypothermia, apathy, edema, immunodeficiency, thinning of skin, decreased metabolic rate, impaired wound healing, decubitus ulcers, fatigue
Diagnosis	• Physical examination • Anthropometry
Treatment	• Provision of adequate protein and energy • Mobilization and exercises as a component of nutritional rehabilitation • In critically ill, parenteral nutrition
Tropical sprue	
Etiology	• Primary malabsorption syndrome • Small intestinal bacterial overgrowth
Pathogenesis	Damage to stem cells in intestinal crypts leading to villus atrophy
Clinical Presentation	Diarrhea, steatorrhea, glossitis, cognitive defects, muscle wasting, weight loss, bone disease, hypomagnesemia leading to sprue coma
Diagnosis	No single test, diagnosis of exclusion; electron microscopy shows degenerating cells at the base of crypt
Treatment	• Correction of fluid and electrolyte abnormalities • Antibotics (tetracycline or doxycycline) for 3–6 months
Intestinal tuberculosis	
Etiology	*Mycobacterium tuberculosis*
Pathogenesis	• Through infected food or milk (primary intestinal tuberculosis) • Ingestion of infected sputum (secondary intestinal tuberculosis) • Hematogenous spread from distant tubercular focus • Contagious spread from infected adjacent foci • Spread through lymphatic channels
Clinical presentation	Fever, pain abdomen, diarrhea, borborygmi, vomiting, intestinal obstruction, ascites, loss of weight and loss of appetite

Continued...

Continued...

Intestinal tuberculosis	
Diagnosis	• Clinical history, history of contact • Mantoux test • Interferon gamma release assay (IGRA) • X-ray of chest, X-ray of abdomen, computed tomography or magnetic resonance imaging of abdomen, documentation of necrotic lymph nodes on imaging • Transverse ulcers on ileocolonoscopy, diseased ileo caecal valve • Confluent caseating granuloma containing acid fast bacilli and surrounded by a lymphoid cuff on histology
Treatment	• Anti-tubercular therapy • Endoscopic dilatation/surgery of refractory stricture
Crohn's disease	
Etiology	• Genetic predisposition • Dysregulated immune system • Gut microbial dysbiosis • Environmental influences (diet, pollution, gastrointestinal infections, antibiotic use, smoking etc.)
Pathogenesis	Dysregulated immune response
Clinical Presentation	• Diarrhea, fever, fatigue, abdominal pain and cramping, blood in stools, oral ulcers, loss of appetite, weight loss, fistula formation (perianal, entero-cutaneous, entero-enteric, entero-visceral) • Extra-intestinal manifestations (joint pains, scleritis, episcleritis, erythema nodosum, nephrolithiasis)
Diagnosis	• Clinical history, family history of Crohn's disease • Fecal calprotectin, C-reactive protein • Computed tomography enterography or magnetic resonance imaging enterography • Capsule endoscopy • Ileocolonoscopy showing aphthous ulcers or deep linear serpiginous ulcers, skip lesions, cobblestoning of mucosa • Multiple small non caseating non confluent granuloma
Treatment	• Nutritional therapy • Immunomodulators (azathioprine, 6-mercaptopurine, methotrexate) • Biologics (anti TNF agents, anti integrins, anti IL12/23) • Surgery
Giardiasis	
Etiology	*Giardia duodenalis* (also referred to as *Giardia lamblia* and *Giardia intestinalis*)
Pathogenesis	• Protozoa disrupt small intestine epithelial cell junctions and brush border enzymes • Increased intestinal permeability
Clinical Presentation	Asymptomatic or Abdominal pain, nausea, flatulence, and large volume watery, foul-smelling, greasy stools
Diagnosis	• Stool antigen detection assays and nucleic acid amplification tests (NAAT) • Difficult to detect with microscopy as the protozoa are only intermittently shed
Treatment	• Correction of fluid and electrolytes • Metronidazole 250–500 mg three times a day for 5–10 days
Strongyloidiasis	
Etiology	*Strongyloides stercoralis* or *Strongyloides fuelleborni*
Pathogenesis	• Direct contact of intact skin with contaminated soil results in inoculation of the larva • Larvae migrate to reach pulmonary circulation and then alveoli • Larvae are coughed up into the trachea and then swallowed into the gastrointestinal tract • Within the intestine, they mature and eggs are produced by females • Autoinfection can occur in immunocompromised hosts

Continued...

Continued...

Strongyloidiasis	
Clinical Presentation	• Pruritic edematous petechial rash at the site of penetration • ***Larva currens*** or ***migrans*** • Abdominal bloating, heartburn, constipation or diarrhea, reduced appetite • Chronic dry cough or wheezing, Low grade fever, • Weight loss • Hyper infection syndrome: Intestinal obstruction, peritonitis, pneumonitis, respiratory failure • Disseminated infection: Massive weight loss, meningitis, encephalitis, or SIADH
Diagnosis	• Microscopic examination of stool for larva • Serologic testing by Enzyme-linked Immunosorbent assay(ELISA) • Endoscopy and duodenal biopsy may reveal larva or signs of chronic inflammation • High serum IgE levels
Treatment	• Ivermectin (200 mg/kg for 2 consecutive days); repeat dosing is necessary after two weeks • Ivermectin is not recommended for body weight less than 15 kg • Albendazole and thiabendazole (25 mg/kg twice daily for 5 days, 400 mg maximum) are also effective

(IgE: immunoglobulin E; IL: interleukin; TNF: tumor necrosis factor; SIADH : Syndrome of inappropriate secretion of antidiuretic hormone)

RECOMMENDED READINGS

1. Sood A, Midha V, Sood N, Avasthi G, Sehgal A. Prevalence of celiac disease among school children in Punjab, North India. J Gastroenterol Hepatol. 2006;21(10):1622-5.
2. Singh P, Arora S, Singh A, Strand TA, Makharia GK. Prevalence of celiac disease in Asia: A systematic review and meta-analysis. J Gastroenterol Hepatol. 2016;31(6):1095-101.
3. Lindfors K, Ciacci C, Kurppa K, Lundin KEA, Makharia GK, Mearin ML, et al. Coeliac disease. Nat Rev Dis Primers. 2019;5(1):3.
4. Grover J, Chhuneja P, Midha V, Singh A, Mahajan R, Mehta V, et al. An open-label randomised pilot trial on safety of wheat variety C273 in patients with adult celiac disease. Therap Adv Gastroenterol. 2020;13:1756284820944089.
5. Makharia GK, Catassi C. Celiac Disease in Asia. Gastroenterol Clin North Am. 2019;48(1):101-13.
6. Mehtab W, Singh N, Malhotra A, Makharia GK. All that a physician should know about gluten-free diet. Indian J Gastroenterol. 2018;37(5):392-401.
7. Caio G, Volta U, Sapone A, Leffler DA, De Giorgio R, Catassi C, et al. Celiac disease: a comprehensive current review. 2019;17(1):142.
8. Krishnareddy S. The Microbiome in Celiac Disease. Gastroenterol Clin North Am. 2019;48(1):115-26.
9. Lebwohl B, Rubio-Tapia A. Epidemiology, Presentation, and Diagnosis of Celiac Disease. Gastroenterology. 2021;160(1):63-75.
10. Lindfors K, Ciacci C, Kurppa K, Lundin KEA, Makharia GK, Mearin ML, et al. Coeliac disease. Nat Rev Dis Primers. 2019;5(1):3.

CHAPTER 134

Intestinal Tuberculosis

Ashish Chauhan, Archita Makharia, Govind K Makharia

ABSTRACT

Extrapulmonary tuberculosis accounts for approximately 20% of patients having tuberculosis and 7–10% of them have abdominal tuberculosis. Amongst abdominal tuberculosis, intestinal tuberculosis is the most common. Ileocecum is the most common site involved in them, because of relative stasis and abundance of lymphatics in this region. Phenotypically, intestinal tuberculosis is of three types namely (1) Ulcerative, (2) Hypertrophic, and (3) Ulcerohypertrophic.

Symptoms of intestinal tuberculosis include abdominal pain, partial bowel obstruction, and constitutional symptoms such as fever, malaise, and weight loss. Pulmonary lesions, either healed or active, may be noted in 3–25% of subjects; hence, it may be worthwhile getting a contrast-enhanced computed tomography (CECT) chest along with computed tomography (CT) enterography. For evaluation of the lesions, colonoscopy for the large intestine and CT or magnetic resonance (MR) enterography for small intestine are the modalities of the choice. The histological characteristic lesions of intestinal tuberculosis are caseating granuloma, confluent granuloma, and large granuloma. Microbiological confirmation, while is the gold standard, their yield is not high.

The most important differential diagnosis of intestinal tuberculosis is Crohn's disease (CD). Both of the diseases can be distinguished in one-half to two-thirds of cases using clinical, endoscopic, histological, and radiological characteristics. The confirmed diagnosis of intestinal tuberculosis is based upon one of the three criteria namely, (1) demonstration of organism by culture or (2) demonstration of acid-fast bacilli (AFB) or (3) caseating granuloma. More often, the diagnosis of intestinal tuberculosis is confirmed with healing of lesions with a therapeutic trial of antitubercular therapy. Six months of treatment with antituberculosis drugs regimen is effective for intestinal tuberculosis. If patient is treated on a presumptive evidence, it is ideal to demonstrate the healing of the lesions after completion of the therapy.

"Science knows no country because science belongs to humanity, and is the torch which illuminates the world"

—Louis Pasteur

INTRODUCTION

Tuberculosis, from being a stigmatizing disease to a disease having complete cure, has been one of the examples of success stories of modern science. While being curable, this disease is still far from eradication because of both human factors and adaptation of the bacteria to survive in the challenging environment. Globally, tuberculosis is amongst the top 10 causes of death and the top infectious disease causing death. While, approximately one-fourth to one-third of the world's population is infected with *Mycobacterium tuberculosis*, only 10% of them, however, ever develop active disease.

India is amongst the countries with highest burden for tuberculosis in the world, in the year 2019 alone, 26.9 lakh patients had tuberculosis. Extrapulmonary tuberculosis accounts for approximately 20% of patients having tuberculosis and 7–10% of them have abdominal tuberculosis. Amongst those having abdominal tuberculosis, gastrointestinal (GI) tract, peritoneum, hepatobiliary system, spleen, ovaries, and pancreas may be affected. Of all, intestinal tuberculosis is the most common. We shall focus on intestinal tuberculosis in the following sections.

SITE OF INVOLVEMENT

While any part of the GI tract may be affected by *M. tuberculosis* infection, the most common site of involvement is ileocecum [ileum, ileocecal (IC) valve, and cecum]. Intestinal tuberculosis involves the ileocecum in up to three-fourths of the patients. Ileocecum is a favorable location for tuberculosis because of relative stasis, and abundance of lymphatics in this region. Other common sites of involvement in those having intestinal tuberculosis are the colon (decreasing frequency from ascending colon to the rectum), jejunum, stomach, duodenum, and esophagus. Isolated colonic involvement and gastroduodenal involvement are seen in 10% and 0.5–2.5% of the GI tuberculosis patients, respectively (**Box 1**).

PATHOGENESIS

Mycobacterial infection can develop primarily within the intestinal tract or from another focus elsewhere in the body. Tubercular bacilli can reach the GI tract by four routes including ingestion of *M. tuberculosis* bacilli either via infected milk or ingested sputum, transport by the way of infected bile, extension from the adjacent diseased organs or tissues such as peritoneum, and rarely via mycobacterial bacteremia. Intestinal involvement is probably related to the number and virulence of the bacilli and the nutritional status of the patient. In the

BOX 1 Investigations for intestinal tuberculosis.

- Hemogram:
  - High ESR
  - Anemia: Mostly normochromic, normocytic
  - Relative thrombocytosis
- Mantoux test:
  - Positive in 70% of patients in endemic regions
  - A negative Mantoux test does not rule out tuberculosis
- HIV serology
- Interferon gamma release assay
- Chest X-ray
- Specific investigations:
  - Colonoscopy and retrograde ileoscopy
  - CT enterography/MR enterography/BMFT
- Microbiological tests:
  - Culture for *M. tuberculosis*
  - AFB staining
  - AFB-PCR/GeneXpert
  - AFB-PCR/GeneXpert

(PCR: polymerase chain reaction)

initial stage of illness, the lesions caused by the disease are mostly superficial and does not result in luminal compromise and hence patients may not have any GI symptoms. With advancing disease, the lesions involve deeper layers of intestinal wall along with fibrogenesis and cicatrization associated with inflammation. Such events lead to ulceration and strictures in the intestine which can cause obstruction to the flow of luminal contents forward. The contraction of proximal segment in order to push the contents forward through the strictures results in colicky abdominal pain. Further compromise of the lumen can result in partial obstruction, which can be recognized by its symptoms such as colicky abdominal pain, bloating and distension of the abdomen, gurgling sounds, feeling of movement of ball of wind, vomiting, and obstipation (may be). Such episodes of intestinal colic occurred episodically and precipitated by GI infection or a fiber ball, but as the diseases further progress, the frequency and intensity of symptoms increase. Ultimately, patients develop partial intestinal obstruction and land in the emergency departments.

After effective treatment of intestinal tuberculosis, while inflammatory components subside, the fibrotic components may persist. Even with the complete microbiological cure, the existing strictures may not reverse completely and fibrotic strictures may persist. The distinction between fibrotic and active stricture is of paramount importance, as management for active disease is antitubercular therapy and for fibrotic stricture is either endoscopic dilatation or surgical resection.

PHENOTYPES

Traditionally, intestinal tuberculosis is described to be of three types such as (1) *Ulcerative*, (2) *Hypertrophic*, and (3) *Ulcerohypertrophic*. The ulcerative form of the disease is mainly due to deprivation of blood supply, because of endarteritis. In GI tuberculosis, ulcerogenesis is relatively slow, and an inflammatory wall develops ahead of the advancing ulcer and thus if perforation occurs, they remain contained. There is an accumulation of collagenous tissue during the process of ulcer healing that subsequently contracts and causes circumferential stricture of the intestinal lumen.

The diseased segment is moderately indurated and the serosa is studded with nodules. Mesenteric lymph nodes are usually enlarged. The mucosal surface may show single or multiple ulcers, and skip areas may be present with normal appearing mucosa between involved segments. The ulcers are characteristically transverse and circumferential, but may be round, stellate, or longitudinal. The ulcers are deep; however, they generally do not penetrate the muscularis propria. In the acute phase, there may be a functional stenosis of the involved segment because of the spasm of a segment of intestine. In the more chronic phase, circumferential strictures may develop. In hypertrophic form of the disease, there is a marked inflammatory fibroblastic reaction in the submucosa and subserosa of the involved segment, mostly ileocecum.

TABLE 1 Clinical symptomatology of pathological phenotypes of intestinal tuberculosis.

Pathological process	Symptoms
Ulceroconstrictive	Intestinal colic, abdominal distension, nausea, vomiting, constipation, and gastrointestinal bleed
Chronic inflammation	Fever, weakness, weight loss, and night sweats
Adjacent tissue involvement	Ascites, lymph node enlargement, and tubo-ovarian symptoms
Associated pulmonary tuberculosis	Chronic cough, expectoration, and hemoptysis

CLINICAL FEATURES

The symptoms in a patient with intestinal tuberculosis arise because of various pathological processes as described in **Table 1**. The symptoms of GI tuberculosis depend upon the site(s) of involvement of the GI tract and also on the type of lesions. IC area is the most common site of involvement in patients with intestinal tuberculosis, and mostly lesions are ulcerative or ulceroconstrictive. *Abdominal pain* is the most common manifestation and can occur because of a stricture of the intestinal lumen, mesenteric inflammation, or peritoneal involvement. While pain arising from the intestine is mostly colicky in nature, pain arising from the mesentery or the peritoneum is diffuse and may not have specific character. As disease advances with time, the severity and frequency of painful episodes increase and patient may develop partial intestinal obstruction (abdominal distension, gurgling in the abdomen, partial or complete cessation of flatus, and vomiting or movement of ball of wind in the abdomen) or even complete intestinal obstruction. *Diarrhea* is seen in 20–30% of patients and can be because of involvement of both the small and large intestine. Almost half of the patients with intestinal tuberculosis report having *constipation*. *Constitutional symptoms* in the form of fever, malaise, night sweats, anorexia, and weight loss are common in patients with intestinal tuberculosis.

Intestinal tuberculosis mostly is a localized disease, and diffuse mucosal involvement is uncommon and hence, frank mucosal malabsorption is less common in patients with intestinal tuberculosis. These patients can have *malabsorption* because of reasons such as (1) decrease in small intestinal mucosal surface, (2) lymphatic obstruction, (3) fistula formation, (4) deconjugation of bile salts secondary to bacterial overgrowth, and (5) decreased bile salt pool because of impaired active absorption in the distal ileum. While *lower GI bleeding* is seen in 10–15% of patients with intestinal tuberculosis, the bleeding from tubercular ulcers is rarely massive. A few patients may have active tuberculosis elsewhere, especially lungs.

One-half to two-thirds of patients have low-grade fever. Abdominal tenderness may be present in the right lower quadrant. A mass may be palpable in 10–20% of patients and is because of a conglomerate of adhered bowel loops, lymph nodes and sometimes, mesentery. Extensive fibroadhesive inflammation in the peritoneum can make the consistency of the abdominal wall doughy.

When to suspect intestinal tuberculosis?

Intestinal tuberculosis should always be suspected in all those patients who presents with recurrent intestinal colic with or without intestinal obstructive symptoms.

INVESTIGATIONS

The aims of the investigations in patients suspected to have intestinal tuberculosis are detection of the lesion(s), site and extent of the lesion(s), type of lesion, detection of any associated complication(s), histological diagnosis, microbiological confirmation, and detection of tuberculosis either active or healed elsewhere. In a patient suspected to have intestinal tuberculosis, hematological and biochemical investigations are nondiagnostic, they, however, should be done to estimate the effects of the disease and also as a baseline for monitoring the effects or complications of the therapy (**Box 1**).

Pulmonary lesions, either active or healed, on chest radiograph may be noted in 3–25% of subjects. In prospective data from our centre, 24% of patients with suspected intestinal tuberculosis had pulmonary lesions on contrast enhanced computed tomography (CECT) chest and addition of CECT chest to computed tomography (CT) enterography increased the sensitivity of intestinal tuberculosis diagnosis by 24–51%. Hence, in a patient with ulceroconstrictive disease of the intestine where intestinal tuberculosis is a differential diagnosis, it may be worthwhile getting a CECT chest along with CT enterography in the same setting. Abdominal X-ray during pain episodes may be helpful in documenting intestinal obstruction. All patients suspected to have intestinal tuberculosis should be screened for HIV infection as HIV infection may be the reason for reactivation of latent tuberculosis in that patient.

EVALUATION OF THE SITE OF THE DISEASE

Large intestine: Since ileocolonic is the most common site of involvement, which can be reached by an ileocolonoscopic examination, hence colonoscopy is amongst first-line investigation for patients suspected to have intestinal tuberculosis. Colonoscopic examination allows visualization of the lesions directly and biopsies can be taken from the lesions at the same time. Endoscopic findings seen most commonly in intestinal tuberculosis are ulcers, which are circumferential in orientation, strictures, pseudopolyps, nodularity, and patulous IC valve (**Fig. 1**). Ulcers in intestinal tuberculosis are transverse and may progress to become circumferential with surrounding inflamed areas. One of the most important differential diagnoses of the lesion mimicking intestinal tuberculosis is Crohn's disease (CD), described below. Presence of longitudinal ulcers, aphthous ulcers, skip lesions, and cobblestoning of the intestinal mucosa favors a diagnosis of CD.

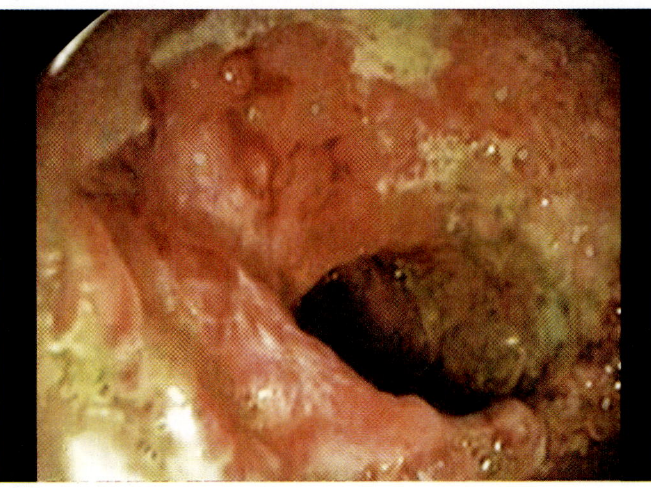

FIGURE 1: A colonoscopic picture in a patient with intestinal tuberculosis showing ulceration of the ileocecal valve.

After examination of the lesions during colonoscopy and retrograde ileoscopy or even enteroscopy, multiple mucosal biopsies should be obtained both for histological examination and microbiological tests.

Small intestine: Small intestine can be evaluated using endoscopic examination such as enteroscopy (single balloon, double balloon, or spirus enteroscopy) or capsule enteroscopy. Capsule enteroscopy should be avoided in all such patients where there is a possibility of intestinal stricture, such as tuberculosis. Facilities for enteroscopic examination are not available widely, technically demanding and one may not reach the site of the disease if the lesions are deep in the intestine.

Therefore, the first line of investigation for evaluation of small intestine in the intestinal inflammatory disorders is radiological evaluation including cross-sectional imaging such as CT and magnetic resonance (MR) enterography. Barium-based studies are now not preferred because they do not provide all the necessary information and they are much inferior to CT or MR enterography.

The foremost thing to remember is that luminal imaging should be done as enterography and positive contrast should not be given. Since the intestine remains collapsed, imaging of the luminal component of the intestine is not complete unless the intestine is distended. In CT enterography or MR enterography, intestinal lumen is distended using a negative contrast such as polyethylene glycol or mannitol which allows simultaneous cross-sectional imaging of the intestinal lumen, the intestinal wall, and the surrounding tissues. Therefore, CT enterography or MR enterography is preferable imaging techniques than CECT or MRI for imaging of the small intestine. CT enterography may show intestinal wall thickening (unifocal or multifocal), a stricture with proximal dilation of the intestine, and regional lymphadenopathy. The pattern of lymphadenopathy in tuberculosis may vary widely, including increased number of normal-sized nodes, mildly enlarged nodes to large confluent nodal masses. The involved lymph nodes are necrotic which typically

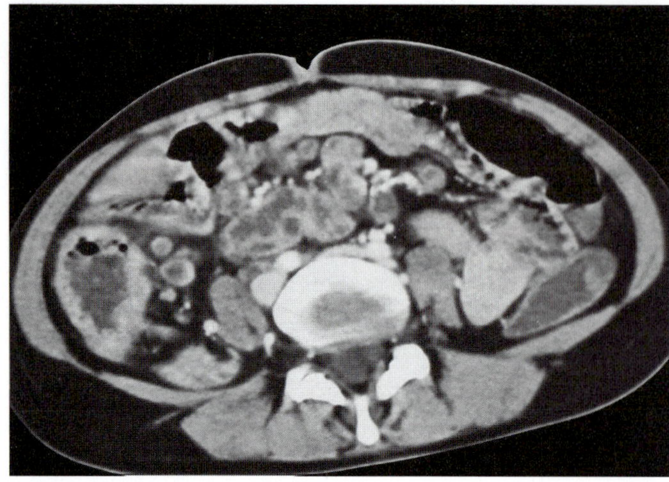

FIGURE 2: Contrast-enhanced computed tomography (CECT) showing enlarged mesenteric lymph nodes with central hypodensity and thickening of the cecum.

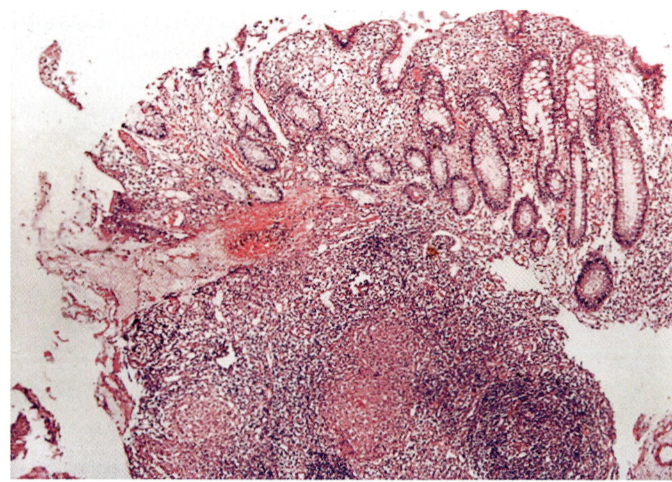

FIGURE 3: A photomicrograph showing caseating granuloma.

show hypodense center and peripheral enhancement in 40–70% cases; which reflects central necrosis (**Fig. 2**). A study from India has shown that features such as IC involvement, short segment involvement (≤3 cm), lymph nodes >1 cm, and necrotic lymph nodes, suggest intestinal tuberculosis, whereas left colonic involvement, long segment involvement, smaller lymph nodes, skip lesions, and comb sign suggest a diagnosis of CD.

EVALUATION OF MUCOSAL BIOPSIES

With the increasing use of endoscopic procedures to visualize the intestinal lumen and obtain targeted biopsies from diseased and normal areas, endoscopic mucosal biopsies have now mostly replaced the surgical biopsies for microscopic examination. Granulomas are found in only 50–80% of intestinal mucosal biopsies from patients with clinically confirmed tuberculosis. Caseation and AFB, the diagnostic features of tuberculosis, are found in only 18–33% of cases and in as low as 5% of cases, respectively. Other features suggestive of tuberculosis include confluent granulomas, a lymphoid cuff around granulomas, granulomas >400 μm in diameter, 5 or more granulomas in biopsies from one segment, granulomas located in the submucosa or in granulation tissue, often as palisaded epithelioid histiocytes, and disproportionate submucosal inflammation (**Fig. 3**).

In a recent meta-analysis of studies on histological features, three features specific for tuberculosis include caseation, confluent granuloma, and a lymphoid cuff around the granulomas.

MICROBIOLOGICAL TESTS

Isolation of *M. tuberculosis* using culture or by staining the smear is the most specific methods for the diagnosis of active tuberculosis, the sensitivity of both these techniques being really low. While culture can detect 10–100 bacilli per mL of the sample, *M. tuberculosis* can be cultured from 10 to 30% of mucosal biopsies in patients with colonic tuberculosis. A presumptive diagnosis of tuberculosis may be considered by detection of AFB on intestinal biopsies which have been reported with a variable frequency (25–36%) in patients with intestinal tuberculosis.

Polymerase chain reaction (PCR) using *M. tuberculosis* specific primer shows a positivity varying from 20 to 64%. Detection of *M. tuberculosis* by PCR has a fair sensitivity, but the results of a positive PCR should be interpreted cautiously. PCR may be reported positive because of contamination in laboratories. Passage of saprophytic mycobacteria may also test positive in colonic biopsies. In one study, in situ PCR for tuberculosis in mucosal biopsies was positive in six out of 20 intestinal tuberculosis patients.

DIAGNOSTIC CRITERIA

A definitive diagnosis of intestinal can be made based on the presence of any of the following three criteria:

1. Culture of tissue (colonic biopsy, lymph nodes) resulting in growth of *M. tuberculosis*
2. Histological demonstration of typical AFB
3. Histological evidence of necrotizing granuloma.

While a positive culture, demonstration of AFB on smear and histological evidence of a caseating granuloma are gold standard tests for the definitive diagnosis of tuberculosis, the sensitivity of the combination of the three or any one test is approximately 30–50%. In rest of the patients, the diagnosis is considered presumptive based on clinical, endoscopic, radiological, and histological evidence. The unequivocal response to antituberculosis therapy (ATT) for 6 months confirms the diagnosis of tuberculosis in these patients. It should be emphasized that adherence to treatment is extremely important in those with presumptive diagnosis of tuberculosis who are receiving antituberculous therapy empirically. Nonresponse to treatment may occur because of nonadherence of the treatment, an alternative diagnosis or multidrug-resistant tuberculosis.

DIFFERENTIAL DIAGNOSIS

The closest differential diagnosis of intestinal tuberculosis is CD. Both intestinal tuberculosis and CD are granulomatous diseases of the intestine. The clinical, morphological, and histological features of intestinal tuberculosis and CD are so similar that it becomes difficult to differentiate between these two entities. In geographical regions like Asia where both intestinal tuberculosis and CD are prevalent, differential diagnosis between the two may be challenging. In India, intestinal tuberculosis is common, but CD is also being increasingly reported from all over India. Natural history of CD is quite different from that of intestinal tuberculosis. While intestinal tuberculosis gets cured by appropriate antituberculous therapy; CD has a remitting/relapsing or persistent course and usually stays lifelong. Because of similarity in the clinical presentation and morphology of these two entities, at times such patients are treated empirically with antituberculous drugs.

The clinical, endoscopic, and histological features which can differentiate these two diseases as reported are summarized in **Table 2**. From this table, it is obvious that almost all the features are present in these two conditions and not many are diagnostic feature of one or another. However, with the use of a combination of these features, one is able to make a diagnosis of either tuberculosis or CD in almost half of the patients.

There are often situations where a differentiation between intestinal tuberculosis and CD remains unclear despite extensive investigation. Under these circumstances, both the Asia Pacific Association of Gastroenterology (APAGE) and Indian Society of Gastroenterology consensus on CD suggest a trial of antituberculosis treatment. This is based on the rationale that the treatment of tuberculosis is finite, whereas treatment for CD continues indefinitely. Also there is a risk in treating patients with corticosteroids, if there is a possibility that the diagnosis may actually be tuberculosis. Obviously, the decision to treat for one disease or the other would take into account other clinical considerations including the nature of presentation of the patient, whether acutely ill and requiring immediate definitive therapy or not. It would also be accompanied by a complete discussion with the patient of the possibilities and therapeutic alternatives.

In patients treated for intestinal tuberculosis, it is expected that there will be a complete resolution of the lesions, detectable by endoscopy or by imaging, following therapy. It is therefore appropriate to re-endoscope the patients who were treated empirically for intestinal tuberculosis and to establish complete mucosal healing at the end of 6 months.

Compounding the problem of differentiation between intestinal tuberculosis and CD and a therapeutic trial of antituberculous drugs to resolve the issue, a proportion of patients with CD also responds to antituberculous therapy at least symptomatically.

TREATMENT

Patients with intestinal strictures should be advised to take low-fiber diets. All these patients should undergo a nutritional assessment and nutritional deficiencies should be addressed.

All patients with tuberculosis should receive anti-tuberculous drugs. Patients with active tuberculosis

TABLE 2 Clinical, endoscopic, and histological differentiation between intestinal tuberculosis and Crohn's disease.

	Variables	Intestinal tuberculosis	Crohn's disease
Symptoms	Chronic diarrhea	20–40%	60–80%
	Blood in the stools	10–20%	50–70%
	Abdominal pain	90%	60–80%
	Constipation	50%	10–30%
	Partial intestinal obstruction	50–60%	20–30%
	Perianal disease	5%	30–80%
	Fever	40–70%	30%
	Loss of appetite	40–80%	40–60%
	Weight loss	60–90%	50–60%
	Extraintestinal manifestations	10%	20–50%
Involvement of intestine	Anal canal	<5%	15–50%
	Rectum	10–20%	40–60%
	Sigmoid colon	5–10%	10–50%
	Descending colon	5–10%	10–50%
	Ascending colon	40–60%	50–70%
	Ileocecal area	70–90%	60%
	Ileum	10–20%	20–40%

Continued...

	Variables	Intestinal tuberculosis	Crohn's disease
Endoscopic features	Aphthous ulcers	5–10%	30–50%
	Longitudinal ulcers	5%	20–30%
	Deep ulcers	50–70%	30–40%
	Nodularity	50%	20%
	Cobblestoning	None	15–20%
Histological features	Granuloma	30–60%	30%
	Necrosis in the granuloma	10–30%	None

should be treated with multiple agents to achieve bacterial clearance, to reduce the risk of transmission, and to prevent the emergence of drug resistance.

A 6-month-antituberculosis drugs regimen using a combination of rifampicin, isoniazid, ethambutol, and pyrazinamide for 2 months, followed by rifampicin, isoniazid, and ethambutol for 4 months, cures approximately 90% in human immunodeficiency virus–negative patients and is the globally accepted treatment for drug-susceptible, active tuberculosis. Since the treatment of tuberculosis is prolonged, adherence to treatment is a major problem in many parts of the world including India. In order to increase the rate of adherence to treatment and reduction in the duration of exposure of potentially toxic drugs, efforts are being made to decrease the duration of treatment. The duration of treatment for GI tuberculosis whether, 6 months or longer has remained to be a matter of debate. Furthermore, in spite of the recommended 6-month-treatment duration, many physicians treat such patients for longer than 6 months. In a recent Korean study including 90 patients with intestinal tuberculosis, Park, et al showed comparable efficacy (93.3% vs. 91.1%; $p = 1.00$) and recurrence rate (2.4% vs. 0%; $p = 1.00$) between 6-months and 9-months treatment. Overall, 6-month-treatment is as effective as 9-month-treatment. A small pilot study from the southern part of India has shown a comparable efficacy of antituberculous therapy administered for 6 months and 9 months using DOTs strategy. We also conducted a multicenter randomized controlled trial including 196 patients with abdominal tuberculosis using ATT using intermittent directly supervised therapy. The complete clinical response was equal in both in those who received 6 months or 9 months of treatment.

In summary, even 6 months of ATT is effective in patients with intestinal tuberculosis and efficacy is comparable to that achieved by a therapy delivered for 9 months.

FOLLOW-UP AND MONITORING

Patients receiving treatment for tuberculosis should be counseled regarding the adverse effects of drugs and should be evaluated clinically at least once a month for assessment of adherence and possible adverse effects of antituberculous drugs. Patients should be assessed from time to time for regression in their symptoms. While fever and constitutional symptoms start improving within weeks, they may take up to 8 weeks before any improvement is appreciated. As the inflammatory component of the intestinal lesions starts resolving, the luminal diameter starts getting better and thus the frequency and severity of abdominal pain improve. Patients should be monitored for the side effects of the drugs especially drug-induced hepatitis.

RECOMMENDED READINGS

1. Makharia GK, Srivastava S, Das P, Goswami P, Singh U, Tripathi M, et al. Clinical, endoscopic, and histological differentiations between Crohn's disease and intestinal tuberculosis. Am J Gastroenterol. 2010;105:642-51.
2. Kedia S, Das P, Madhusudhan KS, Dattagupta S, Sharma R, Sahni P, et al. Differentiating Crohn's disease from intestinal tuberculosis. World J Gastroenterol. 2019;25:418-32.
3. Limsrivilai J, Shreiner AB, Pongpaibul A, Laohapand C, Boonanuwat R, Pausawasdi N, et al. Meta-analytic Bayesian model for differentiating intestinal tuberculosis from Crohn's disease: Am J Gastroenterol. 2017;112:415-27.
4. Mehta V, Desai D, Abraham P, Rodrigues C. Making a positive diagnosis of intestinal tuberculosis with the aid of new biologic and histologic features: How far have we reached? Inflamm Intest Dis. 2019;3:155-60.
5. Epstein D, Watermeyer G, Kirsch R. Review article: the diagnosis and management of Crohn's disease in populations with high-risk rates for tuberculosis: Aliment Pharmacol Ther. 2007;25:1373-88.
6. Kedia S, Sharma R, Makharia GK, Ahuja V, Desai D, Kandasamy D, et al. Imaging of the small intestine in Crohn's disease: Joint position statement of the Indian Society of Gastroenterology and Indian Radiological and Imaging Association. Indian J Gastroenterol. 2017;36:487-508.
7. Pratap Mouli V, Munot K, Ananthakrishnan A, Kedia S, Addagalla S, Garg SK, et al. Endoscopic and clinical responses to anti-tubercular therapy can differentiate intestinal tuberculosis from Crohn's disease. Aliment Pharmacol Ther. 2017;45:27-36.
8. Ramakrishna BS, Makharia GK, Ahuja V, Ghoshal UC, Jayanthi V, Perakath B, et al. Indian Society of Gastroenterology Task Force on Inflammatory

Bowel Diseases. Indian Society of Gastroenterology consensus statements on Crohn's disease in India. Indian J Gastroenterol. 2015;34:3-22.

9. Ooi CJ, Hilmi I, Makharia GK, Gibson PR, Fock KM, Ahuja V, et al. Asia Pacific Association of Gastroenterology (APAGE) Working Group on Inflammatory Bowel Disease. The Asia Pacific Consensus Statements on Crohn's Disease Part 2: Management. J Gastroenterol Hepatol. 2016;31:56-68.

10. Makharia GK, Ghoshal UC, Ramakrishna BS, Agnihotri A, Ahuja V, Chowdhury SD, et al. Intermittent Directly Observed Therapy for abdominal tuberculosis: A multicenter randomized controlled trial comparing 6 months versus 9 months of therapy. Clin Infect Dis. 2015;61:750-7.

11. Jullien S, Jain S, Ryan H, Ahuja V. Six-month therapy for abdominal tuberculosis. Cochrane Database Syst Rev. 2016;11:CD012163.

CHAPTER

135

Irritable Bowel Syndrome

Uday C Ghoshal

ABSTRACT

Irritable bowel syndrome (IBS) is a common disorder in the community and in clinical practice. The diagnosis of IBS is based on symptom-based criteria such as Manning criteria and different version of the Rome criteria, absence of alarm features, and minimum investigations. Subtyping of IBS into constipation, diarrhea, mixed and alternating subtypes is important as the treatment of the condition is largely symptom based. However, in the recent times, pathophysiological basis of IBS and an attempt to target these pathophysiological factors therapeutically are evolving.

"Anything that affects the gut always affects the brain"

—C Major

INTRODUCTION

Irritable bowel syndrome (IBS) is a chronic (onset at least 6 months ago and symptoms present during the last 3 months) disorder of gut–brain interaction in which recurrent abdominal pain is associated with a change in bowel habits (altered stool form and/or passage), which are not explained by any organic cause detected on routine investigations (Rome IV criteria released in May, 2016). However, with highly sensitive investigations, many organic causes that could not have been picked up by routine investigations may be found. This challenges the concept of functional basis of this disorder in all the patients. These factors include gut dysbiosis and small intestinal bacterial overgrowth (SIBO), acute infection gastroenteritis, Corona virus disease-19 (COVID-19), altered gut motility and transit, gut inflammation and permeability alteration, dietary intolerance, visceral hypersensitivity, genetic factors, and psychological issues.

These data suggest that IBS is multidimensional in nature with several microorganic factors contributing to its pathogenesis. Patients with IBS have significant reduction in their quality of life. IBS is a common problem in the world as shown in several epidemiological studies including the Rome Foundation global epidemiology study published recently and is one of the most common disorders seen by gastroenterologists worldwide. There has been major paradigm shift in understanding of epidemiology, pathophysiology, diagnosis, and management of IBS in the last decade. This chapter will review some aspects of advances in diagnosis and treatment of this disorder.

DIAGNOSIS

Irritable bowel syndrome used to be considered as a diagnosis of exclusion earlier. However, Manning and Thompson, in a landmark publication in 1978, for the first time introduced the concept of positive diagnosis of IBS without the need of multiple unnecessary investigations to exclude organic diseases. The diagnostic criteria introduced by them is popularly known as the Manning criteria (**Box 1**).

Manning criteria brought in a paradigm shift in the diagnosis of IBS as the authors noted in their study that fulfilling four of the six criteria was associated with a diagnosis of functional disorder, currently called gut–brain interaction disorder, such as IBS on investigation mitigating the need

BOX 1 The Manning criteria.

- Onset of pain associated with more frequent bowel movements
- Onset of pain associated with more loose bowel movements
- Relief of pain with defecation
- Abdominal distension
- Sense of incomplete evacuation
- Passage of mucus

BOX 2 Rome IV criteria.

Recurrent abdominal pain, on average, at least 1 day per week in the last 3 months, associated with two or more of the following criteria:

- Related to defecation
- Associated with a change in frequency of stool
- Associated with a change in form (appearance) of stool

Criteria fulfilled for the last 3 months with symptom onset at least 6 months before diagnosis

to consider these disorders as "diagnosis of exclusion." It is important to note that in the study by Manning and Thompson, peptic ulcer, gastrointestinal malignancy, and stricture were excluded before the diagnosis of IBS was made. Hence, in reality, several other organic diseases such as lactose malabsorption, celiac disease, microscopic colitis, SIBO, fecal evacuation disorder, collagenous colitis, and microscopic colitis are not excluded even after Manning criteria are fulfilled. Manning criteria did not give due consideration for symptom duration and age of onset of the symptoms, even though organic disorders are well known to present with symptoms for a shorter duration at an older age; these are the other limitations of the Manning criteria.

Though the *Rome IV criteria* (**Box 2**) is the most recent iteration of the criteria laid down by the Rome Foundation (www.romecriteria.org) after the Rome I, II, and III criteria, it is somewhat less sensitive than the Rome III criteria to diagnose IBS anywhere in the world and in India in particular, possibly due to the facts that abdominal pain has been considered essential to diagnose IBS and symptom frequency threshold has been increased.

ALARM FEATURES

Before a diagnosis of IBS is made, it is important to elicit some features known as "red flags" while history-taking and physical examination. These include symptom onset at an age 45 years or older, blood in the stools, unintended weight loss, nocturnal symptoms, fever, a family history of colorectal cancer, presence of anemia, and abdominal mass. It is important to note that a patient with one or more of these alarm features may even be diagnosed having IBS provided appropriate investigations are undertaken to exclude organic diseases. Several conditions may mimic IBS at least in the early stages (**Box 3**); some of these conditions such as SIBO, food intolerance, and tropical sprue may even be hidden behind the diagnosis of IBS diagnosed by symptom-based criteria.

Several guidelines on investigating patients with possible IBS have been published. However, it is important to mention here that most clinical trials necessitate a definite diagnosis of IBS and hence recommend at least blood counts, erythrocyte sedimentation rate, C-reactive protein, and limited colonoscopic examination, and other investigations, as indicated.

BOX 3 Conditions that may mimic or underlie the diagnosis of irritable bowel syndrome.

- Celiac disease
- Tropical sprue
- Food intolerance including lactose intolerance
- Crohn disease
- Collagenous or microscopic colitis
- Small intestinal bacterial overgrowth
- Colonic diverticulosis
- Giardiasis

RECENT ADVANCES IN DIAGNOSIS

In recent time, there has been a paradigm shift in understanding of the pathogenesis of IBS. A microorganic basis of IBS has received considerable attention in the recent time. Several of these factors including gut microbiota dysbiosis, SIBO, low-grade gut inflammation, dietary malabsorption, abnormal gut transit, prior gastrointestinal infection and infestation, abnormal intestinal permeability, and neurohormonal dysregulation may have significant therapeutic implications. At least three studies, one from India, the other from China, and yet another from USA showed that the patients with IBS and SIBO respond more often with antibiotic treatment than those without SIBO. It is also important to understand that patients with less severe symptoms, those with considerable psychological comorbidity may not require such extensive investigations and specific treatment for a microorganic cause. Considering all these, the Rome IV algorithm brought a new dimension to management of IBS, the multidimensional clinical profile (MDCP) (**Box 4**).

Treatment of IBS is largely dependent on the subtype of the condition (**Fig. 1**), e.g., patients with diarrhea-predominant IBS (IBS-D) would not respond to drug used to treat patients with constipation-predominant IBS (IBS-C) and vice versa. Moreover, patients with mixed subtype of IBS (change in symptoms, e.g., constipation and diarrhea in days) and those with alternating subtype (change in weeks to months) may necessitate pathophysiology-directed

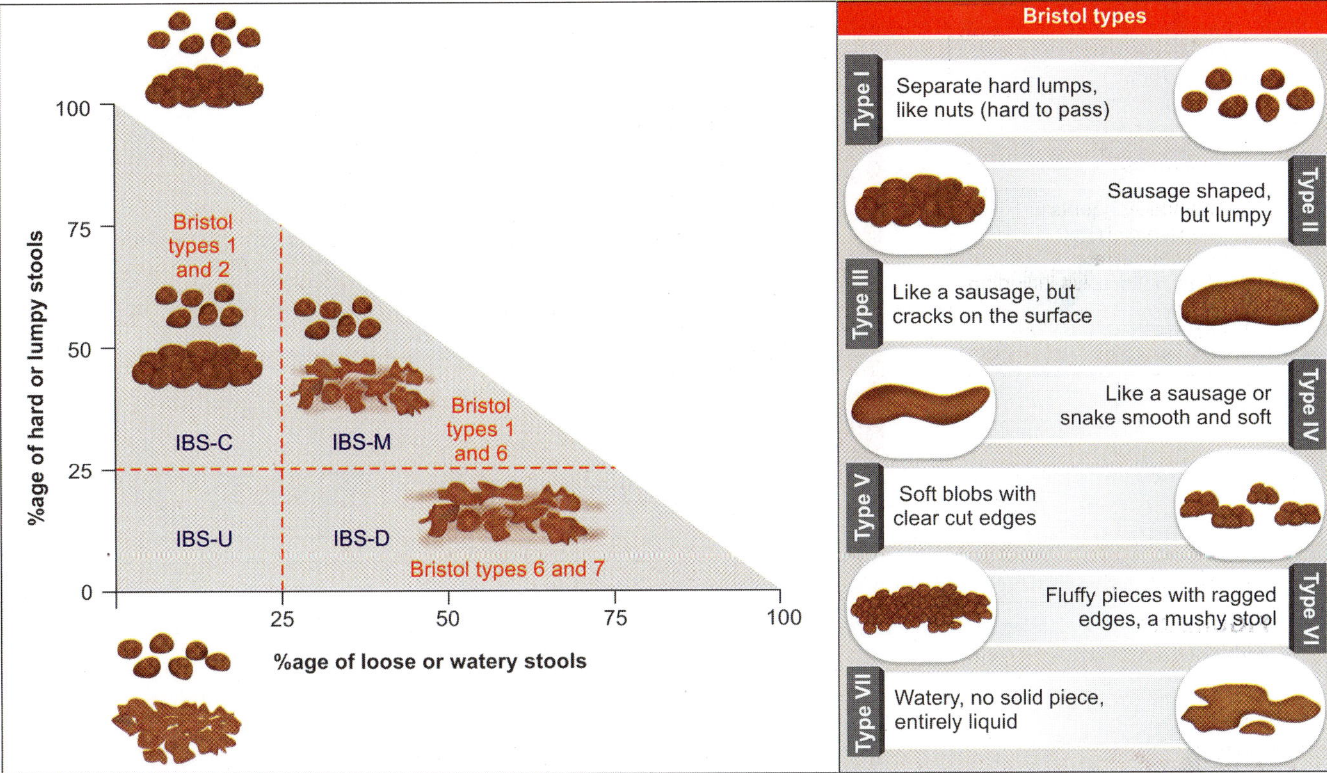

(IBS-C: constipation-predominant IBS; IBS-D: diarrhea-predominant IBS; IBS-M: IBS-mixed; IBS-U: IBS-unsubtyped)

FIGURE 1: Bristol stool types and method of subtyping of IBS according to the Rome IV system. IBS subtypes should be established according to stool consistency, using the Bristol stool form scale. Whether 25% of the stools are constipating types (type I and II) or 25% of the stools are diarrheal types (type VI or VII), determine IBS subtypes according to the Rome IV criteria. According to Asian and India data, type III stool is also considered as constipation-defining stool.

BOX 4	Multidimensional clinical profile (MDCP).

- Diagnosis based on Rome criteria
- Additional information that subclassifies the diagnosis leading to more specific treatment (e.g., diarrhea-predominant, constipation-predominant, pain-predominant, and overlapping)
- The personal impact of the disorder on the patient (severity)
- Physiological abnormalities or biomarkers
- Psychological influences of the disorder

treatment such as gut microbiota manipulators (e.g., rifaximin, probiotics).

Like any other disease, assessment of severity of IBS is another component MDCP, which is of considerable clinical implication. Self-reported severe IBS had more reduction in productivity and incurred higher expenditure than those with mild or moderate disease. Patients with severe IBS also had greater degree of impairment of health-related quality of life (HRQOL). Recent studies also showed patients with overlap functional gastrointestinal disorders (FGIDs) (e.g., IBS with functional dyspepsia) had more severe disease than those with a single condition. Obviously, patients with severe IBS would require more aggressive and multimodal management than those with mild disease. Several questionnaires are available for assessment of severity of IBS and impairment of QOL. However, there is lack of consensus on method of severity assessment of IBS symptoms and till date no single set of criteria is universally accepted. Some of the commonly used criteria for assessment of severity of IBS are listed in **Box 5**.

BOX 5	Severity assessment for irritable bowel syndrome (IBS).

- Functional Bowel Disorder Severity Index (FBDSI)
- IBS Symptom Severity Score (IBS-SSS)
- Health-related quality of life (IBS-QOL)
- Hospital Anxiety and Depression Scale (HADS)
- IBS 36

TREATMENT

Treatment of IBS may include several options including *lifestyle and dietary modifications, psychological management, relaxation techniques, and pharmacotherapy*. Even alternative and complementary therapy is also gaining popularity. The current model of single therapy to treat a disorder with multiple clinical manifestations and overlap with other FGIDs is being increasingly challenged in favor of combination treatment. It is often best to focus on the predominant symptom: Diarrhea (**Fig. 2**), constipation, or pain/gas/bloat and then treat accordingly (**Table 1**). Team

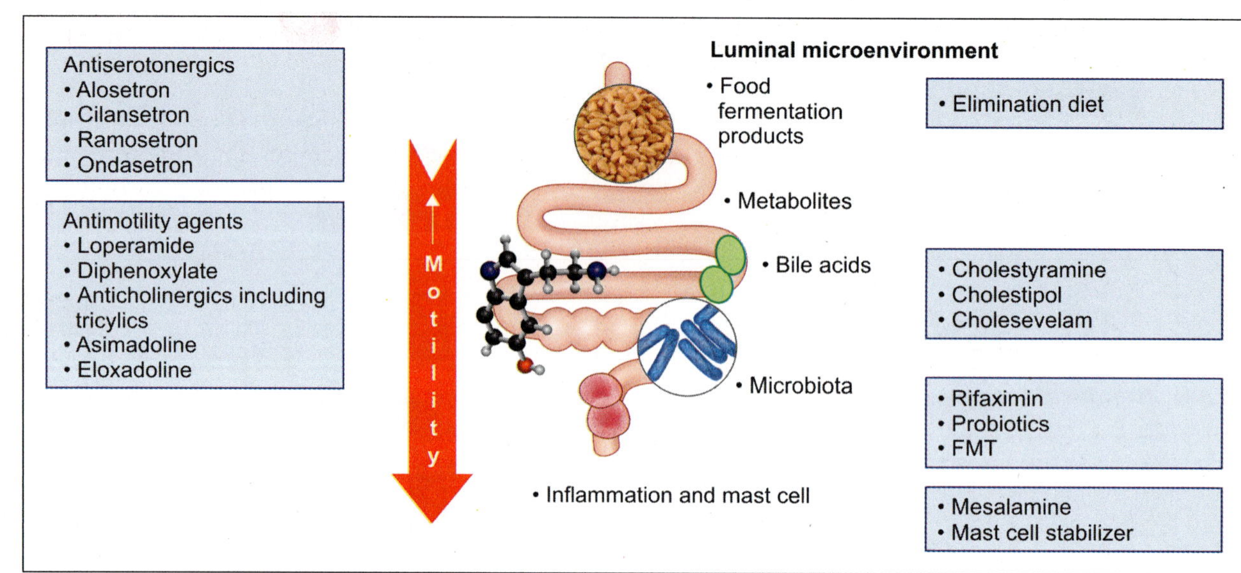

[FMT: fecal microbiota transplant (currently in experimental stage)]

FIGURE 2: Abnormalities in luminal microenvironment in diarrhea-predominant IBS that are used as therapeutic targets with different pharmacological agents.

TABLE 1 Current symptom based management of irritable bowel syndrome (IBS).

Symptom	First line	Second line
Constipation	• Fiber • Osmotic laxative including polyethylene glycol • Lactulose/Lactitol • Stool softner, e.g., docusate	• Bisacodyl • Sodium picosulfate • Tegaserod (withdrawn) • Lubiprostone • Linaclotide • Prucalopride (5-HT4 agonist) • Elobixibat (ileal bile acid transporter inhibitor)
Diarrhea	• Loperamide • Diphenoxylate	• Alosetron • Ramosetron • Ondansetron • Bile acid sequestrant (cholestyramine, colestipol) • Obeticholic acid • Rifaximin • Clonidine
Bloating	• Treat constipation	• Probiotic • Antibiotic (rifaximin)

Pain		• Antispasmodics
		• Anticholinergics
		• Mebeverine
		• Pinaverium
		• Otilonium bromide
		• Antidepressant
		  ◦ Tricyclic anti-depressants
		  ◦ Serotonin and serotonin nor-epinephrine reuptake inhibitors

approach to treat patients with FGIDs in general and IBS is particular is being found to be increasingly more effective than pharmacotherapy alone.

Many of the above-mentioned drugs underwent clinical trials in IBS, which showed variable response rates. Such variations in the response rates might be related to multiple factors including different inclusion criteria and regional, dietary, and cultural variations. It is also important to note that the placebo response rate is quite high among patients with IBS. Therefore, more trials are required for many of the therapies that claim on their efficacy in treatment of IBS.

Combinations of antispasmodic, laxative, and anti-diarrheal agents: The first-line treatment of IBS should include variable combinations of antispasmodic, laxative, and antidiarrheal agents. Antispasmodics are effective when pain is the predominant symptom. Antispasmodics include antimuscarinics, smooth-muscle relaxants, and anticholinergic agents. Anticholinergic agents may result in adverse effects such as dry mouth, dizziness, blurry vision, confusion, urinary retention, and constipation; hence, these agents should be carefully used in spite of their efficacy and low cost, particularly in the elderly patients. Bulking agents are quite commonly prescribed in patients with IBS-C, though the evidence for this drug in IBS is surprisingly scanty. These agents have also been shown to aggravate abdominal pain and bloating. Loperamide has the best quality of evidence for controlling diarrhea. Several serotonin agonists have been used in treatment of IBS-C and functional constipation (cisapride, tegaserod, and prucalopride). However, tegaserod and cisapride have been withdrawn from the market due to their cardiovascular adverse effects.

Psychotropic agents, now renamed as visceral neuro-modulators by the experts in the Rome IV Committee, are another group of drugs quite often used in the treatment of IBS. These drugs include tricyclic antidepressants, serotonin reuptake inhibitors (SSRIs), serotonin norepinephrine reuptake inhibitors (SNRIs). Interestingly, these work in IBS even in absence of psychiatric comorbidity suggesting their action peripherally in the enteric nervous system. These may alter pain perception, improve sleep, alter gut motility and secretion, and improve any associated psychological illness. Another unique approach of treating IBS is psychotherapy. Aims of psychotherapy include reframing maladaptive beliefs, reduction of over-responsiveness to stress, reduction of maladaptive psychological responsiveness, and modification of maladaptive behaviors. The specific content of the therapy is based on a biopsychosocial assessment of the patient's background and current difficulties. Hypnotherapy is one of the important tools in psychotherapy. The essence of hypnotherapy is to create a relaxing and calming environment and allowing the patient to refocus away from uncomfortable symptoms and toward a more pleasant perception of his or her current state. There is little evidence for efficacy of such an approach in IBS. Major drawback of hypnotherapy is a requirement of a well-trained mental health professional.

Rifaximin, a broad-spectrum nonabsorbable antibiotic, has been evaluated for treatment of IBS without constipation (Target 1 and Target 2 studies). Patients with IBS receiving rifaximin (550 mg thrice daily for 2 weeks) had a greater frequency of improvement (41%) compared to those on placebo (30%). However, in this study, treatment with rifaximin was administered to IBS patients without considering the fact that only 10–20% patients with IBS might have gut microbiota dysbiosis including SIBO and hence, are expected to respond to antibiotic treatment.

At least three studies, one from India, the other from China, and yet another from USA showed that the patients with IBS and SIBO responded more often with antibiotic treatment than those without SIBO. However, in spite of these limitations, this study is important as it brings a novel concept of treating a "functional disorder", which is now believed to result from altered gut microbiota, with antibiotic.

Dietary modifications: Recently, dietary modifications have become a cornerstone of therapy of patients with IBS. Several studies showed that some cereals (which contain complex carbohydrates) and dairy products are well known to aggravate IBS symptoms. In Asia including India, chilli and curry are the possible food triggers for symptoms in patients with IBS. Lactose malabsorption was as common in IBS and healthy controls but patients with IBS reported symptoms more commonly following the lactose load. Fructose malabsorption has also been reported to be commoner among IBS patients than healthy controls.

Recently, a new concept of dietary management of IBS by exclusion of fermentable olio-di-monosaccharides and polyols (FODMAP) has become quite popular. Dietary FODMAPs are not absorbed completely in the gut and their bacterial fermentation in the colon produces osmotically active metabolites and gases that induce gastrointestinal and systemic symptoms. Elimination of high FODMAP foods and encouragement to use low FODMAP diet may help in improving symptoms of IBS, particularly abdominal bloating (**Fig. 3**).

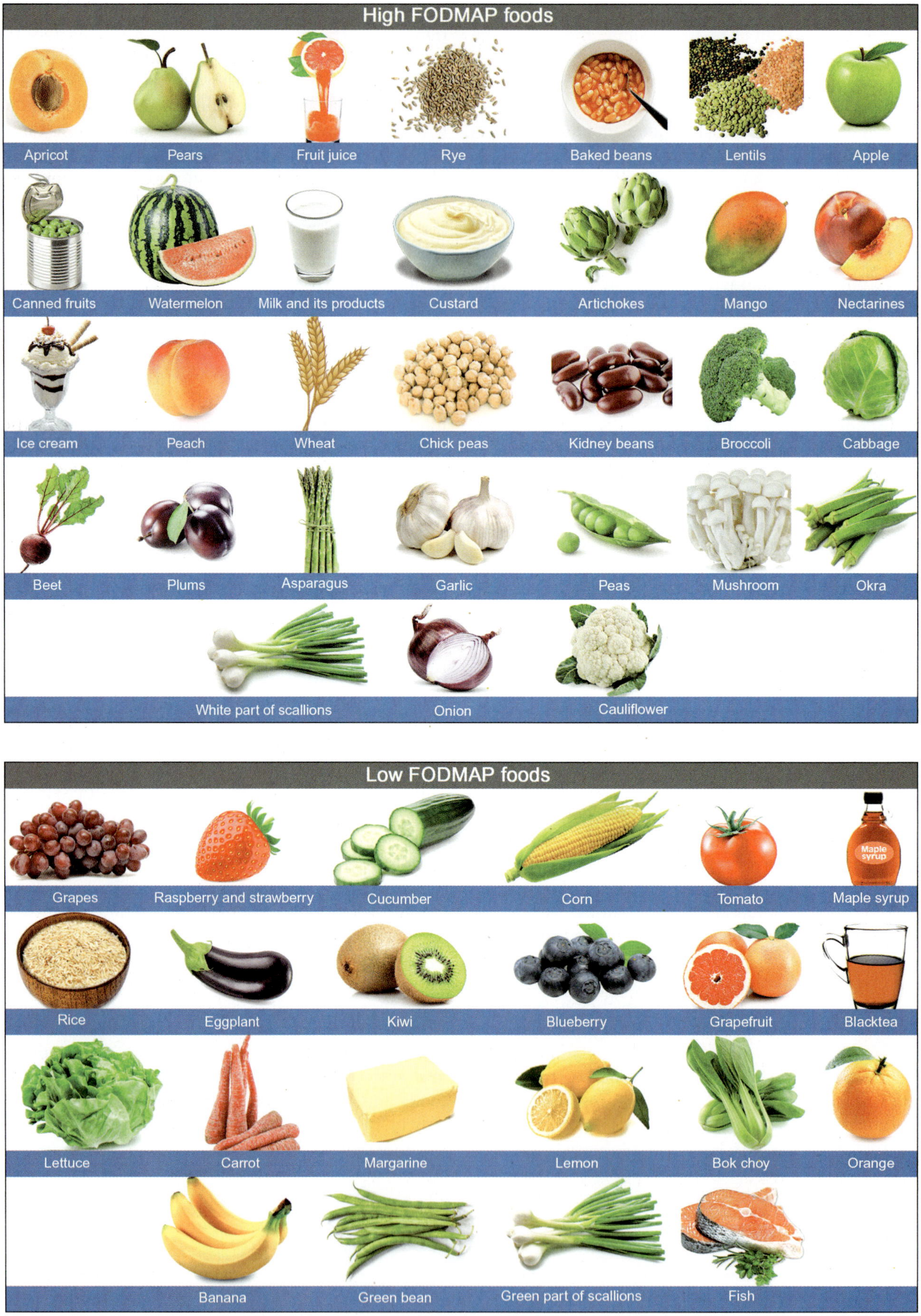

High FODMAP foods
Apricot
Pears
Fruit juice
Rye
Baked beans
Lentils
Apple
Canned fruits
Watermelon
Milk and its products
Custard
Artichokes
Mango
Nectarines
Ice cream
Peach
Wheat
Chick peas
Kidney beans
Broccoli
Cabbage
Beet
Plums
Asparagus
Garlic
Peas
Mushroom
Okra
White part of scallions
Onion
Cauliflower
Low FODMAP foods
Grapes
Raspberry and strawberry
Cucumber
Corn
Tomato
Maple syrup
Rice
Eggplant
Kiwi
Blueberry
Grapefruit
Blacktea
Lettuce
Carrot
Margarine
Lemon
Bok choy
Orange
Banana
Green bean
Green part of scallions
Fish

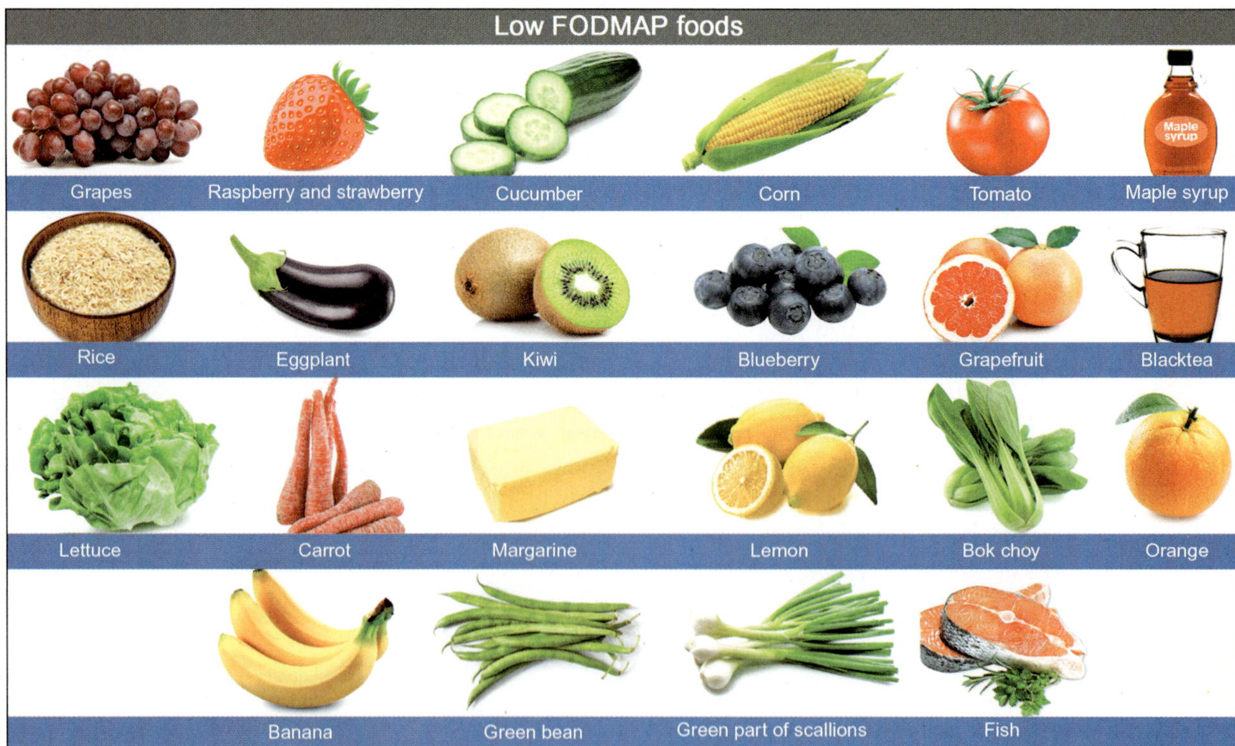

FIGURE 3: High and low Fermentable Oligo-, Di- and MonosAccharides and Polyols (FODMAP) foods.

RECOMMENDED READINGS

1. Mearin F, Lacy BE, Chang L, Chey WD, Lembo AJ, Simren M, et al. Bowel Disorders. Gastroenterology 2016;S0016-5085(16)00222-5.
2. Schmulson M, Ghoshal UC, Barbara G. Managing the inevitable surge of post-COVID-19 functional gastrointestinal disorders. Am J Gastroenterol. 2021;116(1):4-7.
3. Ghoshal UC. Marshall and Warren Lecture 2019: A paradigm shift in pathophysiological basis of irritable bowel syndrome and its implication on treatment. J Gastroenterol Hepatol. 2020;35(5):712-21.
4. Barbara G, Feinle-Bisset C, Ghoshal UC, Quigley EM, Santos J, Vanner S, et al. The intestinal micro-environment and functional gastrointestinal disorders. Gastroenterology. 2016;S0016-5085(16)00219-5.
5. Drossman DA, Camilleri M, Mayer EA, WhiteheadWE. AGA technical review on irritable bowel syndrome. Gastroenterology. 2002;123(6):2108-31.
6. Gwee KA, Lu CL, Ghoshal UC. Epidemiology of irritable bowel syndrome in Asia: something old, something new, something borrowed. J Gastroenterol Hepatol. 2009;24(10):1601-7.
7. Ghoshal UC, Abraham P, Bhatt C, Choudhuri G, Bhatia SJ, Shenoy KT, et al. Epidemiological and clinical profile of irritable bowel syndrome in India: report of the Indian Society of Gastroenterology Task Force. Indian J Gastroenterol. 2008;27(1):22-8.
8. Sperber AD, Bangdiwala SI, Drossman DA, Ghoshal UC, Simren M, Tack J, et al. Worldwide prevalence and burden of functional gastrointestinal disorders, results of Rome Foundation Global Study. Gastroenterology. 2021;160(1):99-114.e3.
9. Gwee KA, Bak YT, Ghoshal UC, Gonlachanvit S, Lee OY, Fock KM, et al. Asian consensus on irritable bowel syndrome. J Gastroenterol Hepatol. 2010;25(7):1189-205.
10. Drossman DA. Guidelines for use of the multi-dimensional clinical profile. Multi-dimensional clinical profile (MDCP) for the functional gastrointestinal disorders, 1st edition. North Carolina: Rome Foundation; 2015. pp. 7-14.
11. Gibson PR, Shepherd SJ. Evidence-based dietary management of functional gastrointestinal symptoms: The FODMAP approach. J Gastroenterol Hepatol. 2010;25(2):252-8.

CHAPTER

136

Inflammatory Bowel Disease

Sudheer K Vuyyuru, Saurabh Kedia, Vineet Ahuja

ABSTRACT

Inflammatory bowel diseases (IBDs) are a group of complex immune-mediated diseases [ulcerative colitis and Crohn's disease (UC and CD)] with variable clinical presentations and significant morbidity. IBD is predominantly seen in Western population, but recently there has been an epidemiological shift to East with increase in incidence in countries like India and other Asian countries. The clinical course is often complicated with requirement of multiple hospital admissions, and surgery. Diagnosis is made with the help of a combination of clinical, endoscopic, radiological, and histological features and there is no single diagnostic feature of IBD. In countries like India, where infectious conditions are much prevalent, diagnostic dilemma often arises in differentiating from diseases like intestinal tuberculosis (ITB) and infectious causes of diarrhea. Treatment strategy depends on disease phenotype, behavior, severity, and risk factors for aggressive disease. Timely decision-making is of prime importance. There are many therapies available in the therapeutic armamentarium and right choice at right time helps in better control of the disease. Recent technological advances provided better understanding of pathogenesis of IBD and newer drugs targeting various immune and microbial pathways are underway.

"Death sits in the bowels and bad digestion is the root of all evil"

—Hippocrates

INTRODUCTION

Inflammatory bowel diseases are a group of immune-mediated chronic inflammatory disorders predominantly comprising two major disorders namely UC and CD with estimated 6.8 million cases globally. UC and CD are phenotypically distinct disorders with differences

TABLE 1 Differentiating features between Crohn's disease and ulcerative colitis.

Feature	CD	UC
Clinical		
Presenting symptoms	Abdominal pain and diarrhea are the most common symptoms	Chronic diarrhea with hematochezia and rectal symptoms like urgency and tenesmus
Fever and weight loss	Common	Uncommon
Features of small bowel involvement	Malabsorption features seen	Not seen
Intestinal obstruction	Common in presence of stricturing disease	May occur in presence of colorectal cancer complicating ulcerative colitis
Perianal fistula	Seen in 20–30% of patients	Not seen
Endoscopic		
Ulcers	Aphthous ulcers, linear serpiginous ulcers seen with cobblestoning	Superficial ulcers are more common, but larger ulcers can be seen. Deep ulcers may indicate underlying CMV. Pseudopolyps are more common
Extent of involvement	Segmental involvement with skip areas	Continuous involvement
Upper gastrointestinal involvement	May be seen	Not seen
Ileal involvement	Often involved (approximately 75% of cases)	Not involved (except as backwash ileitis in pancolitis)
Rectum	Usually spared	Most commonly involved (can be spared, if patient on medical therapy and in children)
Histological		
Inflammation	Focal active inflammation	Diffuse inflammation
Transmural inflammation	All layers of intestine are involved	Inflammation is limited to lamina propria. Transmural inflammation can be seen in acute severe fulminant cases
Granulomas	Granulomas are present in 15–60% of patients	Granulomas are not seen (should not be confused with pericryptal microgranulomas)
Radiological		
Small bowel involvement	Common	Not seen
Creeping fat	Commonly seen	Not seen
Strictures	Common complication of CD. Strictures can be fibrotic or inflammatory	Strictures are rare, presence of which may raise suspicion for malignancy

(CD: Crohn's disease; UC: ulcerative colitis)

in immunopathogenesis, genetic predisposition and management, but in approximately 10% of cases, it is not possible to classify IBD based on clinical features as UC or CD which is then called as IBD-U (IBD-unclassified) (**Table 1**).

EPIDEMIOLOGY

Inflammatory bowel disease is traditionally considered as a Western disease with highest incidence and prevalence in Western Europe and North America. According to global burden of disease estimates of 195 countries, highest prevalence was noted in North America (422 per 100,000). Since the mid of 20th century, the incidence of IBD has steadily increased and now stabilized in Western world. In the last two decades, there has been significant increase in IBD incidence in newly industrialized countries like Japan, South Korea, China, and India. India is also witnessing increasing burden of IBD and faces unique problem of simultaneous existence of infectious diseases like ITB and noncommunicable diseases like IBD.

ETIOPATHOGENESIS

The etiopathogenesis has not been clear but appears to be multifactorial. It has been hypothesized that IBD occurs due to complex interaction of environmental and microbial factors in genetically susceptible individuals leading to aberrant immune response (**Fig. 1**).

GENETIC FACTORS

Familial aggregation of IBD is well known and twin studies have shown high concordance in monozygotic twins, more in CD than in UC. Genome-wide association studies (GWAS) have revealed association of over 240 genetic loci with IBD; among which, 37 are specific to CD and 32 are for UC. NOD2/CARD15 is the first gene shown to be strongly associated with CD. Other susceptibility genes include *ATG16L1, LRRK2, IRGM, Il23R, HLA, STAT3, JAK2,* and *MUC2* which are involved in bacterial sensing, innate immunity, and mucus layer production; autophagy and Th-17 pathway have been implicated in pathogenesis.

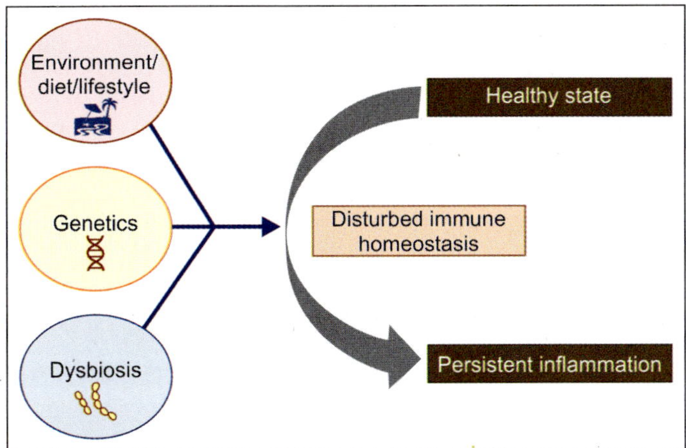

FIGURE 1: Pathogenesis of inflammatory bowel disease.

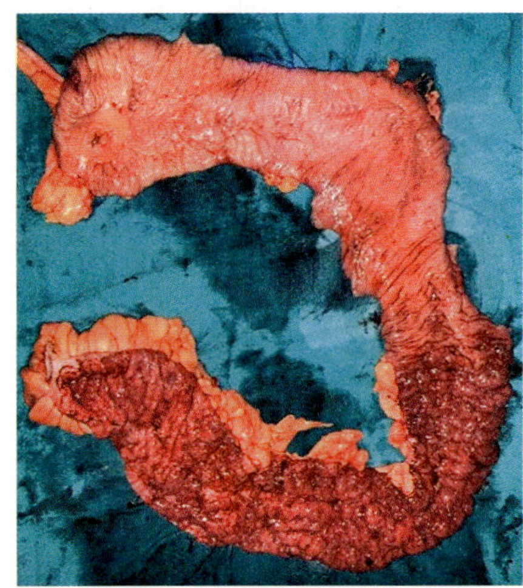

FIGURE 2: Resected surgical specimen showing clear macroscopic demarcation between involved and uninvolved segments.

ENVIRONMENTAL FACTORS

It has been shown that immigration from low-incidence countries to high-incidence countries results in increased risk especially for those who migrated in childhood, indicating role of environmental factors. Factors such as breastfeeding, living on farms, and childhood contact with animals have only inconsistently been identified as being protective for CD. Cigarette smoking has been found to be associated with CD, but protective for UC. Other factors including antibiotic exposure in childhood, low-fiber intake, high-saturated fat intake etc., have been associated with increased risk of CD.

GUT MICROBIOTA-RELATED FACTORS

Microbiota plays an important role in maintaining gut homeostasis. IBD has been shown to be associated with change in composition of microbiota referred to as dysbiosis. It is characterized by decreased microbial diversity and decline in the population of useful bacteria such as *Ruminococcus, Faecalibacterium prausnitzii, Lachnospiraceae,* and *Bifidobacteria* and increased population of pathogenic bacteria such as *Enterobacteriaceae*. However, there are many factors like age, drugs, diet, lifestyle, ethnicity, and environment which can influence microbiota and the causal role of microbial dysbiosis has not been proven yet.

ULCERATIVE COLITIS

CLINICAL FEATURES

Diarrhea and hematochezia are the most common clinical symptoms. Patients usually complain of urgency, tenesmus, nocturnal frequency, abdominal cramps, and fatigue. Up to 10–15% patients can present with severe disease at presentation. Disease starts in rectum and progresses proximally with clear macroscopic demarcation between involved and spared areas macroscopically (**Fig. 2**). Based on extent of involvement, UC is categorized into proctitis (E1 or confined to rectum), left-sided colitis (E2 or up to splenic flexure), and extensive colitis (E3 or beyond splenic flexure) (**Table 2**). About 30–60% patients have E2 disease at presentation, and 15–45% have E1 disease. In 20% cases, entire colon can be involved which is then referred to as pancolitis. Extraintestinal manifestations (EIM) occur in one-third of patients. Primary sclerosing cholangitis and pyoderma gangrenosum are more common in UC than in CD. Axial arthropathies or primary sclerosing cholangitis is independent of disease activity. Whereas, erythema nodosum and pauciarticular large joint arthritis (type 1) are associated with active intestinal disease (**Table 3**).

TABLE 2 Montreal classification of extent of ulcerative colitis.

Extent	Anatomy
E1—ulcerative proctitis	Involvement limited to the rectum (that is, proximal extent of inflammation is distal to the rectosigmoid junction)
E2—left-sided colitis	Involvement limited to a proportion of the colon distal to the splenic flexure
E3—extensive colitis	Involvement extends proximal to the splenic flexure

DIAGNOSIS

Endoscopy: Classic endoscopic findings in UC include erythema, loss of normal vascular pattern, granularity, erosions, friability, bleeding, and ulcerations (**Figs. 3 A to D**). The disease generally begins in the rectum, extending proximally in a continuous, circumferential pattern. Rectal sparing can be seen in patients on topical therapy. Ulcers can be superficial or deep especially when associated with cytomegalovirus (CMV) infection.

Histopathology: Inflammation in UC is confined to mucosa and inflammatory changes are diffuse with basal cell plasmacytosis, cryptitis, crypt abscess, architectural distortion, ulceration, and paneth cell metaplasia. Basal cell plasmacytosis is one of the early findings, and along with chronic crypt architectural changes, it helps in differentiating UC from acute self-limiting infectious colitis.

TABLE 3	Extraintestinal manifestations associated with IBD.
System involved	**Manifestations**
Ocular	• Anterior uveitis (or iritis) • Episcleritis • Keratopathy • Night blindness • Scleritis
Mucocutaneous	• Oral aphthous stomatitis • Oral granulomatous inflammation • Leukocytoclastic vasculitis • Sweet syndrome (neutrophilic dermatosis) • Cutaneous polyarteritis nodosa • Epidermolysis bullosa acquisita
Hepatobiliary	• Autoimmune hepatitis • Cholelithiasis • Hepatic amyloidosis • NAFLD • PSC • Pancreatitis
Cardiopulmonary	• Chronic obstructive pulmonary disorder • Bronchiectasis • Chronic bronchitis • Coronary artery disease • Cardiomyopathy • Pleuritis, pericarditis, and myocarditis
Musculoskeletal	• Ankylosing spondylitis • Sacroiliitis • Osteoporosis/Osteopenia • Sarcopenia • Arthralgia • Peripheral arthritis • Type 1: Pauciarticular • Type 2: Polyarticular
Hematologic	• Arterial thrombosis • Anemia • B12 deficiency • Iron deficiency • Venous thromboembolism
Renal	• Interstitial nephritis • Glomerulonephritis • Nephrolithiasis • Renal amyloidosis
Others	• Secondary amyloidosis

(PSC: primary sclerosing cholangitis)

Radiological imaging: Radiological imaging has limited role in UC. Plain X-ray is useful in acute severe colitis for detecting toxic megacolon (**Fig. 4**). Transverse colon diameter of >6 cm is considered as significant. Contrast enhanced computed tomography (CT) with enterography is indicated when there is diagnostic confusion between UC and CD so as to evaluate small bowel involvement.

MANAGEMENT

Many options are available in the therapeutic armamentarium for UC and choice of therapy depends on disease severity and extent. UC can be categorized into mild, moderate, and severe grades based on modified Truelove and Witts criteria, Mayo clinic score or Simple Clinical Colitis Activity Score (SCCAI), and endoscopic activity can be graded as per Baron Criteria or UCEIS (UC Endoscopic Index of Severity). An algorithm for management of UC has been shown in **Flowchart 1**.

Management of mild-to-moderate ulcerative colitis:

Induction therapy:

- For E1 disease, topical mesalamine (1 g) in the form of suppositories is recommended, but enema can also be used as an alternative.
- Mesalamine enema has better efficacy than steroid enema.
- Steroid enema is added in E1 disease, if there is no response to 5ASA suppository/enema. Subsequently, if required oral 5ASA can also be added.
- For E2 and E3 disease, oral mesalamines are recommended with minimum dose of 2.4 g/day along with topical mesalamines in the form of suppositories or enema.
- Combination of oral and topical therapy is better than oral therapy alone.
- Refractory cases to 5ASA are treated with oral steroids, immunomodulators, or biologics in a step-up manner.
- Oral steroids are given for not more than 12–16 weeks duration and started at a dose of 40 mg/day prednisolone followed by gradual taper at the rate of 5 mg/2 weeks.
- In case of steroid dependence, thioguanines (azathioprine or 6-mercaptopurine) are added as steroid-sparing therapy. If there is no response to steroids (steroid refractory), or in case of thioguanine failure/intolerance, biologics are recommended.
- Second-line therapy is in the form of antitumor necrosis factor (TNF) monoclonal antibodies (biologics) like infliximab and adalimumab (ADA).
- On failure of anti-TNF biologics, lymphocyte trafficking inhibitors like vedolizumab (VDZ) or oral small molecules which inhibit Janus kinase/signal transducers and activators of transcription (JAK/STAT) pathway like tofacitinib can be used.

Surgery in form of two or three-step procedures which entails subtotal colectomy followed by ileal pouch anal anastomosis (IPAA) is an attractive option in patients not responding to second-line therapy.

Maintenance of remission:

- For E1 disease, first line of therapy is topical therapy for maintenance.
- For E2 and E3 disease, maintenance therapy with oral mesalamine is recommended.
- Maintenance with immunomodulators (azathioprine/6-mercaptopurine) is recommended in case of steroid dependency or requirement for >1 steroid course per year.

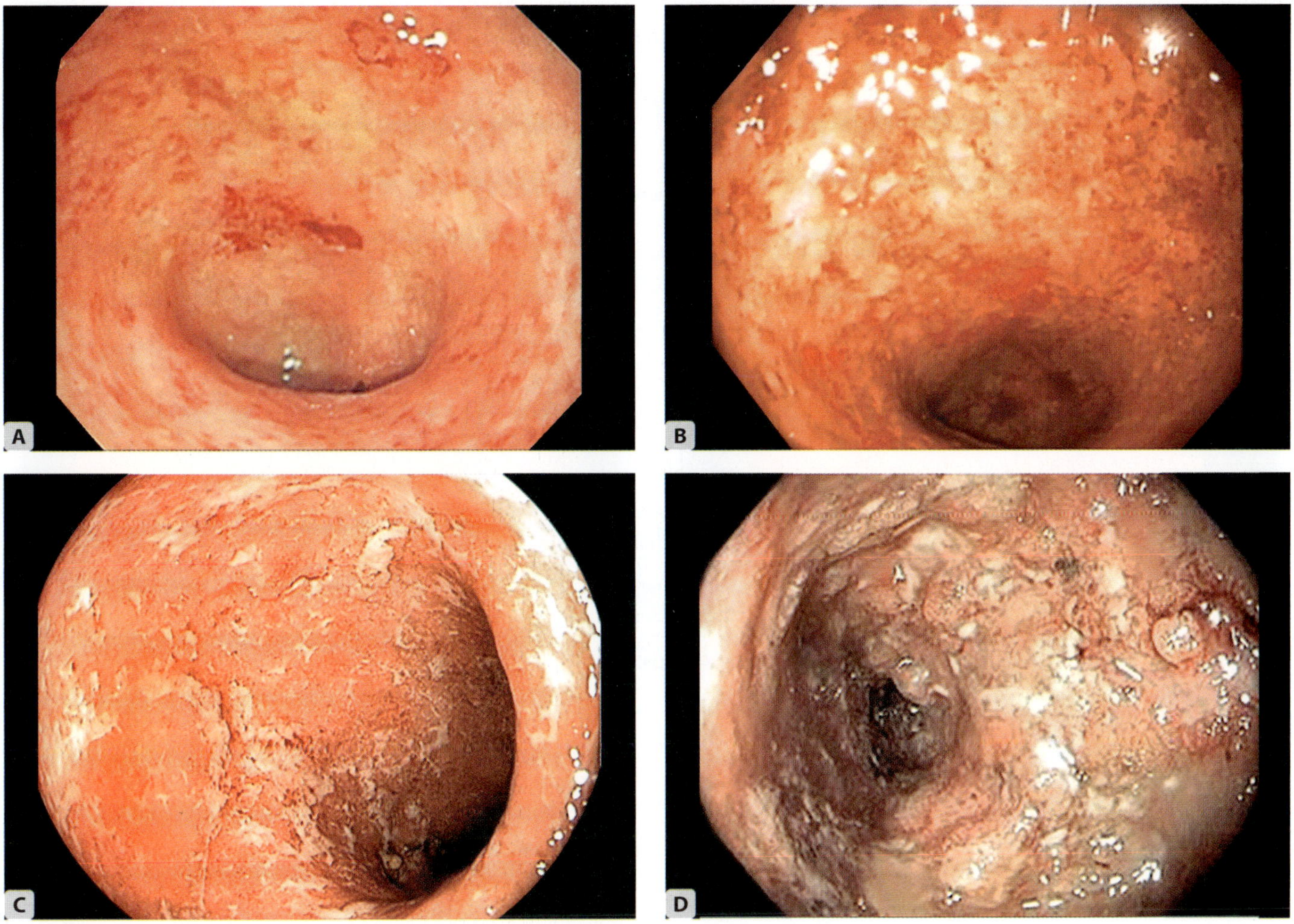

FIGURES 3 A to D: Endoscopic images showing features of ulcerative colitis: **(A)** Patchy loss of vascular pattern; **(B)** Complete loss of vascular pattern with mucosal bleeding; **(C)** Superficial ulceration; **(D)** Deep ulcers with pseudopolyps.

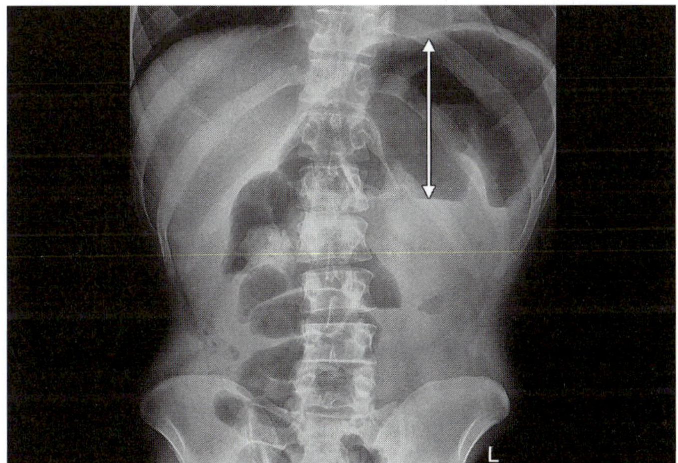

FIGURE 4: Plain X-ray abdomen showing dilated transverse colon suggestive of megacolon in a patient with acute severe ulcerative colitis.

- Steroid dependency is defined by relapse within 3 months of stopping steroids or inability to taper steroids below 10 mg/day.
- Those patients who achieved remission with biological therapy, maintenance with same therapy is recommended.

Management of acute severe ulcerative colitis:

- Acute severe UC (ASUC) is a life-threatening medical emergency which requires hospital admission and timely management.
- Acute severe UC is diagnosed by modified Truelove and Witts criteria (**Table 4**).
- Approximately 25% of patients will have one episode of ASUC during their lifetime.
- Patients should be managed with intensive monitoring of vital parameters, serum electrolytes, and underlying infections like *Clostridium difficile* and CMV should be rule out especially in patients with steroid dependence.
- A recent study from India showed that high mucosal CMV viral load > 2,000 copies/mg of tissue is associated with poor short-term outcomes in patients with ASUC. Hence, unprepared sigmoidoscopy should be done at admission and rectal biopsies must be taken to exclude CMV infection.

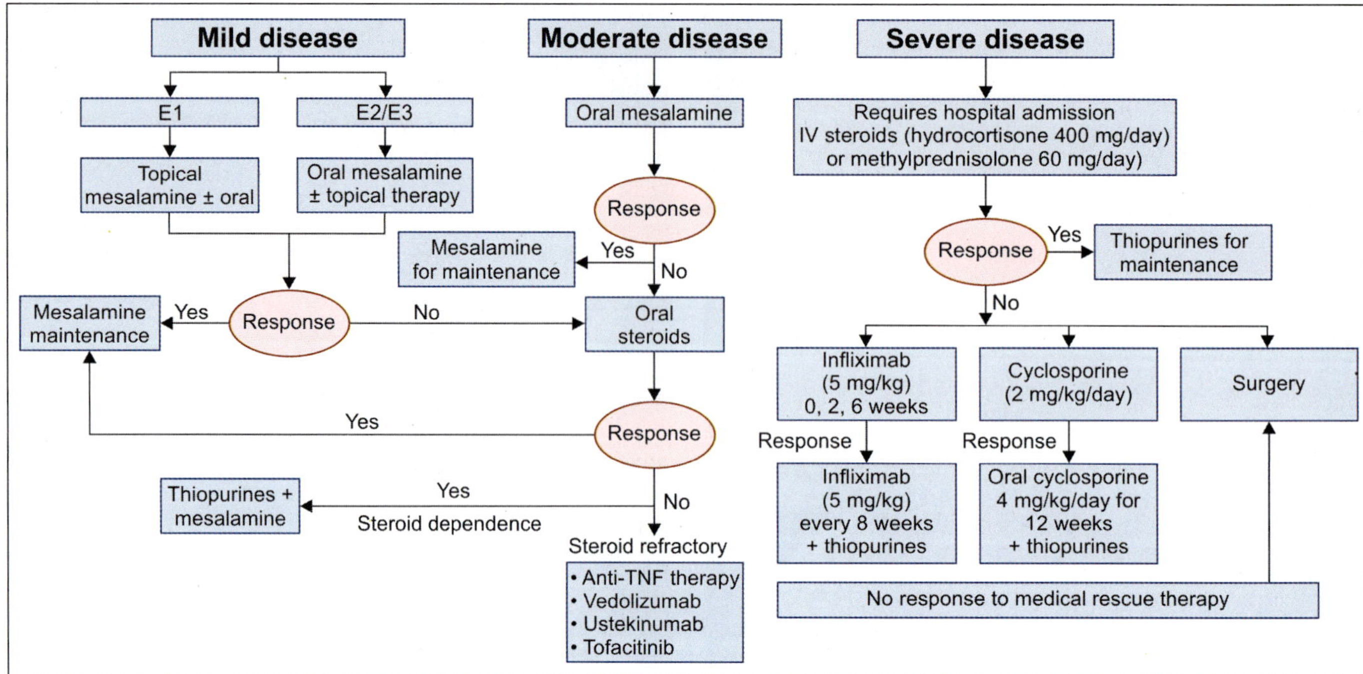

FLOWCHART 1: Algorithm for management of ulcerative colitis.

TABLE 4 Modified Truelove and Witts criteria.

Parameter	Mild	Moderate	Severe
Bloody stools per day	<4	4–6	≥6 and
Pulse (per min)	<90	≤90	>90 or
Temperature (°C)	<37.5	≤37.8	>37.8 or
Hemoglobin (g/dL)	>11.5	≥10.5	<10.5 or
ESR (mm/h)	<20	≤30	>30 or
CRP (mg/L)	Normal	≤30	>30

Severe disease is defined by ≥6 bloody stools with any one of the rest of the features.

- Abdominal X-ray should be done to rule out megacolon. Patients should be allowed to take oral nutrition except in cases of suspected toxic megacolon.
- Thromboprophylaxis with heparin must be provided to every patient.
- Intravenous (IV) steroids are first-line drugs of choice and antibiotics may be recommended if features of toxemia are present.
- Response is assessed on day 3 based on Oxford criteria.
- A recent study from India showed UCEIS score or >6 on day one along with fecal calprotectin >1,000 μg/g of stool (AIIMS index) showed better predictive ability than Oxford score.
- Two-thirds of cases respond to IV steroids and rest require some form of rescue therapy and those who respond to IV steroids are switched to oral steroids after 5–7 days of IV steroid therapy and also started on azathioprine at the time of discharge.
- Those patients who had partial response or no response are qualified for medical rescue therapy with either infliximab or cyclosporine, and there is no difference in efficacy or long-term colectomy rate between these two agents.
- Response is assessed between 4 and 7 days following medical rescue therapy.
- If there is no response, patient should be considered for colectomy.
- A recent randomized clinical trial (RCT) from India has shown the addition of exclusive enteral nutrition for 7 days to steroids was associated with increased steroid response rates to 85% which needs to be validated in further studies.

Other therapies:

- Vedolizumab targets $\alpha_4\beta_7$ integrin which prevents binding of lymphocytes to endothelium by blocking interaction of integrins with MAdCAM receptors.
- Vedolizumab acts in gut selective manner thereby it has less adverse events compared to other biologics.
- Recent head-to-head RCT showed better efficacy of VDZ compared with ADA in moderate to severe UC.
- Ustekinumab (anti-IL-12/23 inhibitor) and tofacitinib (Pan JAK inhibitor) are recommended as second-line drugs after anti-TNF failure in moderate to severe UC.
- Fecal microbial transplantation (FMT) has also been shown to be effective in inducing remission and maintaining it in mild-to-moderate UC. However, there is no uniform consensus on mode of delivery, dose, and frequency.

Surgery: 10–20% of patients with UC require colectomy during their lifetime. Indications for surgery include medically refractory disease, toxic megacolon, perforation, and colorectal carcinoma. Commonly performed surgery is restorative proctocolectomy with IPAA. Surgery offers permanent cure with good long-term quality of life. It is usually performed as two- or three-staged procedure with either laparoscopic or open approach. Pouch success rates are >90% at 20 years. Common complications include pouchitis (70% by 20 years), small bowel obstruction, anastomotic stricture, abscess, and fistula.

CROHN'S DISEASE

CLINICAL FEATURES

Crohn's disease may have a presentation either as inflammatory or stricturing or fistulizing phenotype. CD is a chronic inflammatory disease with progressive disease progression and often complicated by fistulae and strictures. Any part of intestine from mouth till anus can be involved. CD is a disease of young with peak onset between second and fourth decade, although a second peak has been described in sixth decade. Males and females are equally affected. Clinical features are heterogeneous and depend on location, severity of inflammation, and behavior of disease (**Table 5**). Abdominal pain and diarrhea are most common symptoms. Other symptoms include anorexia, fatigue, weight loss, symptoms of recurrent partial intestinal obstruction, perianal fistulae, and symptoms related to EIM. Most common site of involvement is terminal ileum. Approximately, one-third of cases involve terminal ileal region, one-third involve colonic region, one-third involve ileocolonic region, and isolated upper gastrointestinal involvement is not very common. Patients with strictures can present with intestinal obstruction and in severe cases with penetrating behavior, patients can present with perforation and diffuse peritonitis or abdominal lump or abscess which requires urgent surgical intervention. Fistula can form between two intra-abdominal organs or can open externally forming cutaneous fistulae.

TABLE 5 Montreal revision of Vienna classification of Crohn's disease.

Phenotypic character	Subclassification
Age at diagnosis	• A1 < 16 years • A2 between 17 and 40 years • A3 > 40 years
Location	• L1 ileal • L2 colonic • L3 ileocolonic • L4 isolated upper GI disease
Behavior	• B1 nonstricturing, nonpenetrating • B2 stricturing • B3 penetrating • P perianal disease modifier

- L4 is a modifier that can be added to L1–L3 when concomitant upper gastrointestinal (GI) disease is present. Upper GI involvement includes esophagus, stomach, duodenum, jejunum, and proximal ileum.
- "P" is added to B1–B3 when concomitant perianal disease is present.

DIAGNOSIS

Diagnosis is made by constellation of clinical, radiological, histopathological, and endoscopic features. Laboratory parameters include thrombocytosis, elevated erythrocyte sedimentation rate (ESR), C-reactive protein (CRP), and hypoalbuminemia. Anti-*Saccharomyces cerevisiae* antibody (ASCA) is observed in 60–70% of patients and is not useful as a diagnostic test.

Endoscopy: Mucosal changes range from mild erythema, erosions, and aphthous ulcers to deep serpiginous ulcers. Changes are segmental in nature and rectal sparing is often seen. Serpiginous ulcerations interspersed with nodular edematous mucosa produces the so-called cobblestone pattern (**Figs. 5 A** to **C**). Severe transmural inflammation causes luminal narrowing and internal opening of fistula sometimes can be appreciated in endoscopy. Diagnostic small bowel capsule endoscopy is reserved for cases in which endoscopic studies have been negative despite suggestive symptoms and imaging shows absence of small bowel stricture.

Histopathology: Crohn's disease is characterized by chronic focal, patchy, discontinuous, and transmural inflammation. Microscopic picture reveals architectural changes in the form of ulceration, cryptitis, crypt abscess, branching, hyperplasia, transmural lymphoid aggregates, and pyloric gland metaplasia. The histological hallmark of CD is the epithelioid granuloma, which is seen in only about 15% of mucosal biopsies but in up to 70% of cases in surgical specimens. The granulomas are not well formed, small and can be seen in extraintestinal tissues like skin and lymph nodes. Presence of granuloma is not a specific feature of CD. Granulomas can be found in other conditions like ITB, sarcoidosis, and vasculitis (**Table 6**). These granulomas should not be confused with pericryptal granulomas seen near ruptured crypt, which can be found even in UC.

Radiological imaging: Plain X-ray has limited role in CD. It can be useful in cases of perforation or obstruction. CT or magnetic resonance (MR) enterography (CTE/MRE) should be done at diagnosis to map out the disease extent and presence of complications such as strictures or fistulas, thereby providing information about disease behavior and CTE also helps in differentiating CD from its close mimicker, ITB. Important features that are commonly seen in CD are long segment thickening with stratified enhancement, Comb sign, multisegmental involvement (>4), increased visceral fat, fistulae, and strictures (**Figs. 6 A** to **C**). Advantage of MRE over CTE includes lack of exposure to ionizing radiation, better soft tissue resolution, and ability to differentiate inflammatory stricture from fibrotic stricture. Pelvic MRI is preferred modality for perianal fistula.

MANAGEMENT

Disease severity is commonly measured by CD activity Index (CDAI) (**Table 7**). Management of IBD has progressed from symptomatic relief to prevention of progression

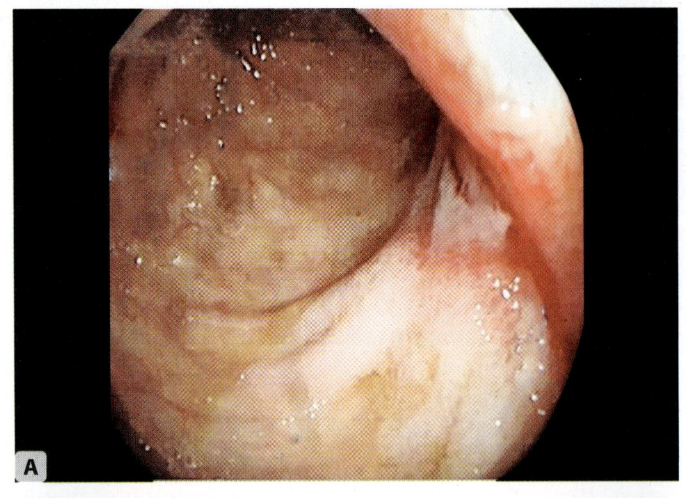

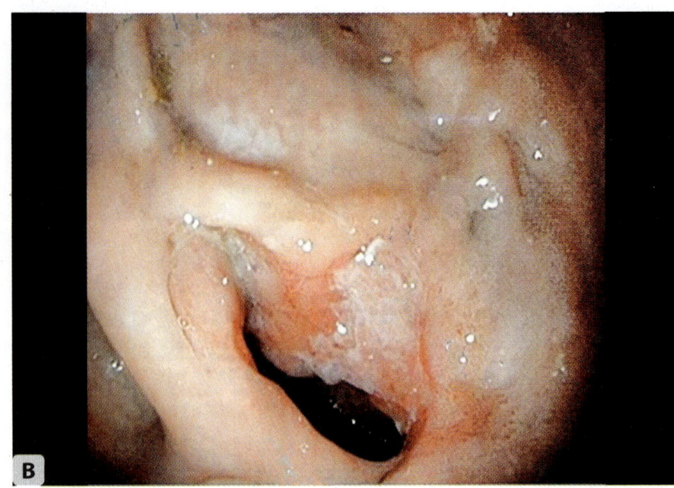

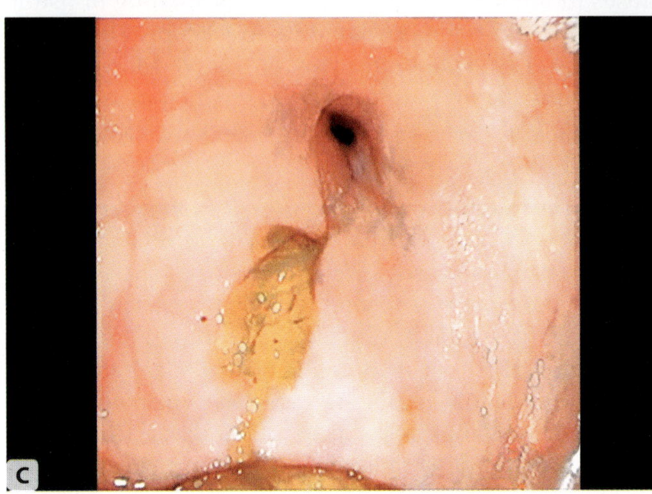

FIGURES 5 A to C: Endoscopic images. (A) Terminal ileal ulcer in a patient with Crohn's disease; **(B)** Longitudinal ulcer at anastomotic site in a patient with Crohn's disease; and **(C)** Ulcerated stricture in a patient with Crohn's disease.

TABLE 6 Differences between Crohn's disease and intestinal tuberculosis.

	Favoring Crohn's disease	Favoring ITB
Clinical features	• Chronic diarrhea • Hematochezia • Perianal disease • Longer duration of symptoms	• Ascites
EIM	• Peripheral arthropathy • Aphthous ulcers • Any/Multiple EIMs	• Pulmonary TB
Endoscopic features	• Left as well as right colonic involvement • Longitudinal ulcers • Aphthous ulcers • Cobblestoning	• Transverse ulcers • Ileocecal valve involvement
Histology (six to eight biopsies)	• Micrgranuloma	• Large caseating confluent granuloma
Radiology	• Long segment involvement • ≥3 segments involvement • Colonic involvement • Comb sign • Visceral fat: Subcutaneous fat ratio > 0.63 • Pseudosacculation	• Ileocecal involvement • Lymph node > 1 cm • Necrotic lymph node • <3 segment involvement • Short segment involvement
Others	• FOXP3 + CD4+ T-cell fraction in peripheral blood < 32.5%	

(EIM: extraintestinal manifestation)

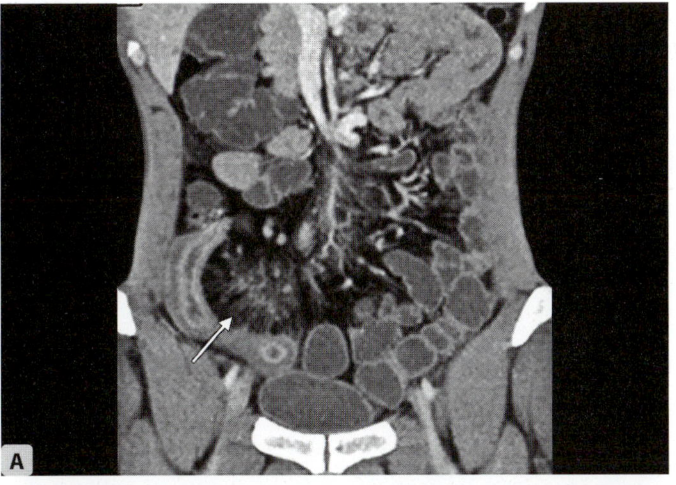
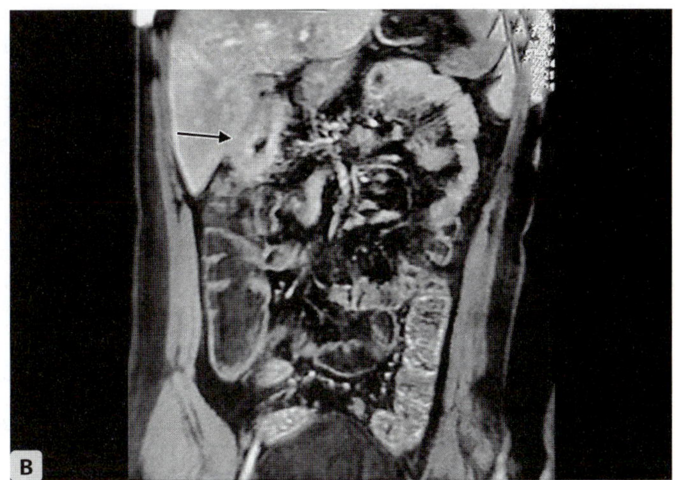
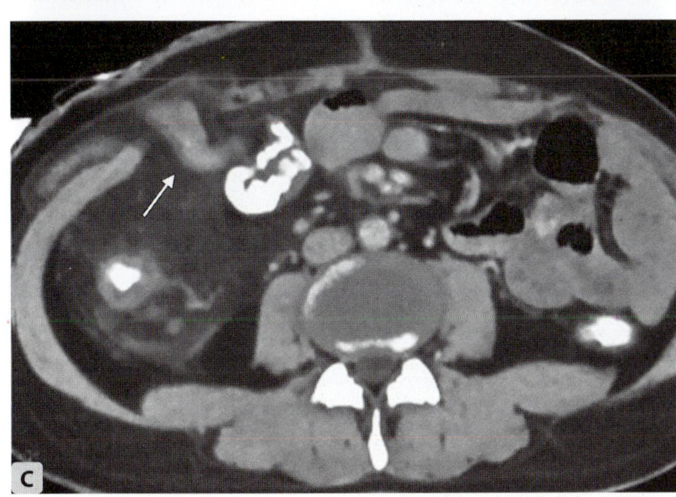

FIGURES 6 A to C: Radiologic images (CT enterography). (A) Long segment thickening with Comb sign in a patient with Crohn's disease (CD); **(B)** Stricture of hepatic flexure of colon in a patient with CD; and **(C)** Enterocutaneous fistula in a patient with CD.

TABLE 7 Crohn's disease activity index (CDAI).

S.no	Variable description	Multiplier
	Date	
1	No. of liquid or soft stools (each day for 7 days)	2
2	Abdominal pain, sum of 7 daily ratings (0 = none, 1 = mild, 2 = moderate, 3 = severe)	5
3	General well-being, sum of 7 daily ratings (0 = generally well, 1 = slightly under par, 2 = poor, 3 = very poor, 4 = terrible)	7
4	Number of listed complications [arthritis or arthralgia, iritis or uveitis, erythema nodosum or pyoderma gangrenosum or aphthous stomatitis, anal fissure or fistula or abscess, other fistula, fever over 37.8°C (100°F)]	20
5	Use of diphenoxylate or loperamide for diarrhea (0 = no, 1 = yes)	30
6	Abdominal mass (0 = no, 2 = questionable, 5 = definite)	10
7	Hematocrit [males, 47-Hct (%); females, 42-Hct (%)]	6
8	Body weight (1-weight/standard weight) × 100 (add or subtract according to sign)	1
	CDAI total score	

of disease. Treatment protocol includes either step-up approach (stepwise increase in immunosuppressive drugs) or top-down approach (most potent drugs are initiated first) depending on severity and behavior of the disease. The top-down approach (biologics) has been recommended only in the presence of high-risk features such as young age of onset, and presence of complications such as fistulae and strictures. Endoscopic healing of mucosal ulcers has been shown to be associated with less frequent surgeries, hospitalization, and morbidity. Early initiation of therapy (within 2 years of onset) has also been shown to be associated with less complications (**Flowchart 2** and **Table 8**).

Management of mild-to-moderate disease:

- Sulfasalazine can be used for induction of therapy in mild colonic CD, but mesalamines have not been shown to be effective.

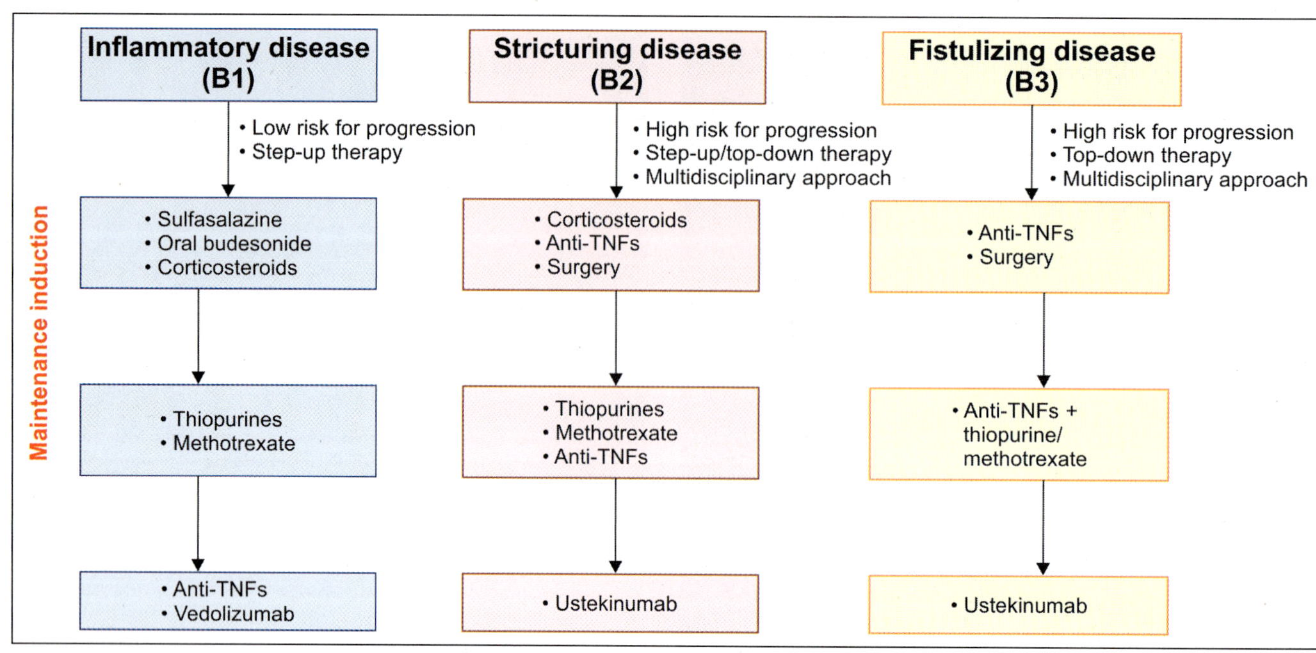

FLOWCHART 2: Algorithm for management of Crohn's disease.

TABLE 8 Different pharmacological therapies available for management of IBD.

Type of therapy	Mechanism of action	Dose	Induction/ Maintenance	Indication in UC	Indication in CD
5-ASA/ sulfasalazine	• Multiple mechanisms of action and act locally • Inhibit proinflammatory cytokines, leukotrienes, scavenge free radicals	• 2.4–4.8 mg/day • Once daily or split dosing	• Induction and maintenance	• Mild to moderate UC	• Colonic CD
Glucocorticoids	• Inhibit both innate and adaptive immune system nonspecifically	• Prednisolone 40 mg/day for not >12 weeks with gradual taper • IV hydrocortisone 400 mg/day	• Induction only	• Moderate to severe UC • Acute severe UC	• Moderate to severe CD
Thiopurines	• Inhibition of purine in lymphocytes	• AZA: 2–2.5 mg/kg/day • 6-MP: 1–1.5 mg/kg/day	• Maintenance only	• Steroid dependence • Following episode of ASUC • Following medical rescue therapy with cyclosporine	• Mild to moderate CD for maintaining remission • Combination therapy with anti-TNFs
Methotrexate	• Folate antimetabolite and inhibits DNA synthesis	• 25 mg/week SC for induction • 15 mg/week SC for maintenance	• Maintenance only	• Not recommended	• Mild to moderate CD for maintaining remission • Combination therapy with anti-TNFs
Cyclosporine	• Inhibit the action of calcineurin thereby inhibit production and release of interleukin II	• 2 mg/kg/day IV for induction followed by 4 mg/kg/day in BD dose for 3 months	• Induction	• Medical rescue therapy in ASUC	• Not recommended

Continued...

Continued...

Type of therapy	Mechanism of action	Dose	Induction/ Maintenance	Indication in UC	Indication in CD
Infliximab	• Blocks TNF-α	• 5 mg/kg per dose, IV at 0, 2, and 6 weeks followed by every 8 weeks	• Induction and maintenance	• Moderate to severe UC • Medical rescue therapy in ASUC	• Moderate to severe CD nonresponsive to steroids • Perianal fistulizing CD • Moderate to severe CD with high-risk features
Adalimumab	• Blocks TNF-α	• 160/80/40 mg SC every 2 weeks followed by 40 mg every 2 weeks	• Induction and maintenance	• Moderate to severe UC	• Moderate to severe CD nonresponsive to steroids • Perianal fistulizing CD • Moderate to severe CD with high-risk features
Vedolizumab	• Anti-α4β7 integrin antibody	• 300 mg IV at 0, 2, and 6 weeks followed by every 8 weeks	• Induction and maintenance	• As a second-line drug in moderate to severe UC	• As a second-line drug in moderate to severe CD
Tofacitinib	• JAK inhibitor	• 10 mg, oral tablet twice a day for 8 weeks followed by 5 mg twice a day	• Induction and maintenance	• As a second-line drug in moderate to severe UC after anti-TNF	• Not recommended
Ustekinumab	• Anti-IL-12/23 antibody		• Induction and maintenance	• As a second-line drug in moderate to severe UC after anti-TNF failure	• As a second-line drug in moderate to severe CD after anti-TNF failure
Fecal microbial transplantation	• Manipulating gut microbiota	• There is no standard dose	• Induction and maintenance	• No recommendation for use outside clinical trial setting	• No recommendation for use outside clinical trial setting

(ASUC: acute severe ulcerative colitis; AZA: azathioprine; JAK: Janus kinase)

- Oral budesonide can be used to induce remission in mild cases limited to ileum and ascending colon.
- In mild-to-moderate cases not responding to budesonide, oral prednisolone can be used for inducing remission.

Management of moderate-to-severe disease:
- Oral steroids are recommended in inducing remission in moderate-to-severe cases.
- Remission is maintained by immunomodulators (azathioprine/6-mercaptopurine or methotrexate).
- Steroid refractory cases are managed with anti-TNF agents (infliximab or ADA).
- Anti-TNF therapy (infliximab) is given in combination with azathioprine or methotrexate to prevent formation of antidrug antibodies.
- In countries like India with high-TB infection rate, chances of TB reactivation following anti-TNF therapy can be as high as 11%. Therefore, proper screening for TB infection should be performed before initiation and prophylaxis should be given. This should involve tests for latent TB (interferon gamma release assay and Mantoux test) and chest imaging (CT chest).
- Ustekinumab has been recommended as second-line agent after failure of anti-TNF therapy.

Surgery: Common indications for surgery in CD include the following:
- Perforation or abscess
- Acute intestinal obstruction due to stricture
- Predominantly fibrotic strictures, in which case stricturoplasty can be attempted
- In limited ileocolonic disease, laparoscopic resection has been shown to be equally efficacious to anti-TNF therapy.
- Complex perianal fistulae refractory to medical therapy—diversion stoma or rarely proctocolectomy can be done.

Other therapeutic options:
- Vedolizumab was shown to be effective in non-stricturing and nonfistulizing CD. However, it is less effective in patients who have already experienced anti-TNF therapy.
- Unlike in UC, JAK inhibitor—Tofacitinib has not been shown to be beneficial in CD.

- Anti-IL-12/23 drug ustekinumab is recommended as a second-line agent in CD following failure of anti-TNF therapy.
- Newer drugs targeting IL-12 and sphingosine-1-phosphate receptors are in development.

Principles of management of perianal fistula:

- Simple fistulas can be managed with antibiotics, followed by surgical drainage in the absence of active proctitis.
- Curative surgery without immunosuppression is rarely possible in complex fistula and aggressive surgery sometimes might lead to incontinence due to sphincter damage.
- Adequate drainage with seton is preferred along with a course of antibiotics.
- Anti-TNF therapy (infliximab) is preferred first-line agent with or without thiopurines in a complex fistula or fistula with active proctitis in the absence of significant collection.
- Local injection of mesenchymal stem cells is newer therapy with promising results.

CONCLUSION

Inflammatory bowel disease results from complex interaction of environmental and microbial factors in genetically predisposed individuals. There has been epidemiological shift with increasing incidence of UC and CD in India. In developing countries like India, conditions like acute infectious colitis and ITB pose diagnostic dilemma by mimicking IBD. Therapy of IBD is targeted toward immune pathways in the form of steroids, immunomodulators, and biological therapies. Surgery plays a major role in therapy of both UC and CD. There has been significant progress in understanding of pathophysiology, and many newer therapeutic modalities are underway.

RECOMMENDED READINGS

1. Ng SC, Shi HY, Hamidi N, Underwood FE, Tang W, Benchimol EI, et al. Worldwide incidence and prevalence of inflammatory bowel disease in the 21st century: a systematic review of population-based studies. Lancet. 2017;390(10114):2769-78.
2. Singh P, Ananthakrishnan A, Ahuja V. Pivot to Asia: inflammatory bowel disease burden. Intest Res. 2017;15(1):138-41.
3. Kedia S, Ahuja V. Epidemiology of Inflammatory Bowel Disease in India: The Great Shift East. Inflamm Intest Dis. 2017;2(2):102-15.
4. Ananthakrishnan AN. Environmental risk factors for inflammatory bowel diseases: A review. Dig Dis Sci. 2015;60(2):290-8.
5. Satsangi J, Silverberg MS, Vermeire S, Colombel J. The Montreal classification of inflammatory bowel disease: controversies, consensus, and implications. Gut. 2006;55(6):749-53.
6. Ordás I, Eckmann L, Talamini M, Baumgart DC, Sandborn WJ. Ulcerative colitis. Lancet. 2012;380(9853):1606-19.
7. Warren BF. Classic pathology of ulcerative and Crohn's colitis. J Clin Gastroenterol. 2004;38(5 Suppl 1):S33-5.
8. Harbord M, Eliakim R, Bettenworth D, Karmiris K, Katsanos K, Kopylov U, et al. Third European Evidence-based Consensus on Diagnosis and Management of Ulcerative Colitis. Part 2: Current Management. J Crohns Colitis. 2017;11(7):769-84.
9. Jain S, Namdeo D, Sahu P, Kedia S, Sahni P, Das P, et al. High mucosal cytomegalovirus DNA helps predict adverse short-term outcome in acute severe ulcerative colitis. Intest Res. 2020.
10. Jain S, Kedia S, Bopanna S, Sachdev V, Sahni P, Dash NR, et al. Faecal Calprotectin and UCEIS Predict Short-term Outcomes in Acute Severe Colitis: Prospective Cohort Study. J Crohns Colitis. 2017;11(11):1309-16.
11. Williams JG, Alam MF, Alrubaiy L, Arnott I, Clement C, Cohen D, et al. Infliximab versus ciclosporin for steroid-resistant acute severe ulcerative colitis (CONSTRUCT): a mixed methods, open-label, pragmatic randomised trial. Lancet Gastroenterol Hepatol. 2016;1(1):15-24.
12. Sands BE, Peyrin-Biroulet L, Loftus EV Jr, Danese S, Colombel JF, Törüner M, et al. Vedolizumab versus adalimumab for moderate-to-severe ulcerative colitis. N Eng J Med. 2019;381(13):1215-26.
13. Makharia GK, Sachdev V, Gupta R, Lal S, Pandey RM. Anti-Saccharomyces cerevisiae antibody does not differentiate between Crohn's disease and intestinal tuberculosis. Dig Dis Sci. 2007;52(1):33-9.
14. Pratap Mouli V, Munot K, Ananthakrishnan A, Kedia S, Addagalla S, Garg SK, et al. Endoscopic and clinical responses to anti-tubercular therapy can differentiate intestinal tuberculosis from Crohn's disease. Aliment Pharmacol Ther. 2017;45(1):27-36.
15. Kedia S, Sharma R, Makharia G, Ahuja V, Desai D, Kandasamy D, et al. Indian guidelines on imaging of the small intestine in Crohn's disease: A joint Indian Society of Gastroenterology and Indian Radiology and Imaging Association consensus statement. Indian J Radiol Imaging. 2019;29(2):111-32.
16. Agarwal A, Kedia S, Jain S, Gupta V, Bopanna S, Yadav DP, et al. High risk of tuberculosis during infliximab therapy despite tuberculosis screening in inflammatory bowel disease patients in India. Intest Res. 2018;16(4):588-98.
17. Ponsioen CY, de Groof EJ, Eshuis EJ, Gardenbroek TJ, Bossuyt PM, Hart A, et al. Laparoscopic ileocaecal resection versus infliximab for terminal ileitis in Crohn's disease: a randomised controlled, open-label, multicentre trial. Lancet Gastroenterol Hepatol. 2017;2(11):785-92.
18. Sands BE, Anderson FH, Bernstein CN, Chey WY, Feagan BG, Fedorak RN, et al. Infliximab maintenance therapy for fistulizing Crohn's disease. N Eng J Med. 2004;350(9):876-85.
19. Tandon R, Ahuja V. Chapter 1 : Clinical Manifestations. In: Tandon R, Ahuja V (Eds). Inflammatory Bowel Diseases. India: Macmillan Publishers; 2014. pp. 1-24.

CHAPTER
137
Lower GI Bleed

Pradev Inavolu, Mohan Ramchandani

ABSTRACT

Lower gastrointestinal (GI) bleed can present as frank bleeding such as hematochezia or melena (acute) or as iron deficiency (chronic). Conventionally bleeding beyond the ligament of Treitz is defined as lower GI bleed. Incidence of lower GI bleed is 20–80/10,000 population (Western world). In >80% of cases, the source of lower GI bleed is colon. The most common cause is diverticulosis in western population whereas hemorrhoidal/ulcer-related bleed is more common in Indians. Hence, colonoscopy is the most important investigation of choice in identification and management. Lower GI bleed is less acute and less common compared to upper GI (UGI) bleed. As there are no randomized clinical trials (RCTs) regarding resuscitation protocols for lower GI bleed, the same resuscitation protocol for UGI bleed is followed at present. Management of lower GI bleed is usually done with the help of endotherapy (hemoclipping/band ligation) and angioembolization (interventional radiology). Rarely, a surgery is required to tackle the bleeding. In 3–5% of cases, small intestine is the source of lower GI bleed where special investigations such as radionuclide RBC scan, capsule endoscopy, balloon-assisted enteroscopy, and novel motorized spiral enteroscopy are required in evaluation and management.

"Problems are solved from the inside out not the other way around"

—Vivian Amis

INTRODUCTION

Lower GI bleed was previously defined as bleeding in the GI tract beyond the ligament of Treitz. However, in recent times, due to the distinct nature of small bowel bleeds, bleeding from beyond the ligament of Treitz to the ileocecal valve is defined as middle GI bleed and from the ileocecal valve to the anorectum as lower GI bleed. Generally, the term lower GI bleeding signifies bleeding from the colon to the anorectum. It constitutes 20% of the total GI bleeds.

In 70–80% of cases, the source of lower GI bleed is colonic, and in 15–20% of cases the source of the bleed is upper GI (UGI) tract. A small percentage of bleeds are from the small bowel (1–10%), and the source is unknown in 3–5% of cases.

Classifications: Lower GI bleeds are classified as:

- **Acute lower GI bleed:** Presenting as hematochezia, diarrhea (with/without unstable vitals) or maroon stools or melena (50–100 mL of blood in the GI tract is required to cause melena).
- **Chronic lower GI bleed:** Presenting as clinically overt [melena/bleeding per rectum (PR)] or occult (iron deficiency anemia).
- **Severe GI bleeding** is defined as bleeding with orthostatic hypotension, shock, drop in hemoglobin >2 g/dL from the baseline, fall in hematocrit >6% from the baseline or needing >2 units of packed RBC transfusion.

EPIDEMIOLOGY

There is no data about the incidence of lower GI bleeds available from India. In the Western world, incidence of lower GI bleed is 20–80/10,000 population, the incidence increasing with age. The mortality due to lower GI bleed is around 2–3% and it increases to 18% when it occurs in hospitalized patients, mainly due to associated comorbidities. Risk factors for poor outcome are hypotension, tachycardia, ongoing hematochezia, age > 60 years, elevated creatinine (>1.7 mg/dL), and/or associated significant comorbidities.

In the Western world, diverticular bleed is the most common source of lower GI bleed, followed by hemorrhoids, anal fissure, and ulcer-related bleeding. In India, lower GI bleed is seen in a comparatively younger population. It is less common than UGI bleed. Anorectal source (hemorrhoids and fissure) is the most common cause of lower GI bleed. Acute self-limiting colitis (infective—*Shigella, Entamoeba, Salmonella*), ileocecal tuberculosis, irritable bowel disease (IBD), ulcers [solitary rectal ulcer syndrome (SRUS)/ stercoral)], colorectal cancers, diverticulosis etc., are the other causes of lower GI bleeding.

The spectrum of lower GI bleed in the earlier studies from India by MK Goenka et al. reported ulcer-related bleeding as most common cause of lower GI bleed but recent data reported from South India and Eastern India that around half of the lower GI bleeding was hemorrhoidal. The recent data from North India reported the most common cause of lower GI bleed to be polyp related (23.3%), followed by colitis (infections and nonspecific etiology), IBD, and malignancy. The spectrum of lower GI bleed in pediatric population as reported by SK Yachha et. al the most common cause was colitis (42%) followed by colorectal polyps.

APPROACH TO ACUTE LOWER GI BLEED

Diagnosis and management of acute lower GI bleed is given in **Flowchart 1**.

- **Age of presentation:**
  - Elderly: Colorectal cancer, diverticulitis, and ischemic colitis
  - Adults: Anorectal bleeds, infection, SRUS (**Fig. 1**), and IBD.
  - Pediatric: Rectal polyp (**Fig. 2**) and Meckel's diverticulitis

HISTORY

- History of fever: Infection and IBD
- Chronic history of altered bowel habit [IBD and tuberculosis (TB) (**Fig. 3**)].
- Chronic constipation [hemorrhoids (**Figs. 4** and **5**), SRUS, stercoral ulcers]
- Drug history [nonsteroidal anti-inflammatory drugs (NSAIDs), anticoagulants and antibiotics] and history of radiation exposure.
- Past history of subacute intestinal obstruction (SAIO) [Crohn's disease (**Fig. 6**)]
- Acute obstruction, surgeries in the past (anastomotic site ulcer)
- Recent interventional procedures: Iatrogenic (post polypectomy)
- History of cirrhosis (portal hypertension related): Varices (**Fig. 7**) and colopathy

CLINICAL ASSESSMENT

- Painless bleeding (diverticulosis, hemorrhoidal, SRUS, stercoral ulcers)/painful bleeding (anal fissure, IBD, infections)
- Character of bleed: Red/maroon (anorectal, diverticulosis), melena (colon cancer, ulcers/colitis, small bowel bleed, and UGI bleed), blood mixed with stool—(nonanorectal cause) blood seen separately from stool (hemorrhoidal or anal fissure related bleed)
- Presence of tenesmus: Rectal source

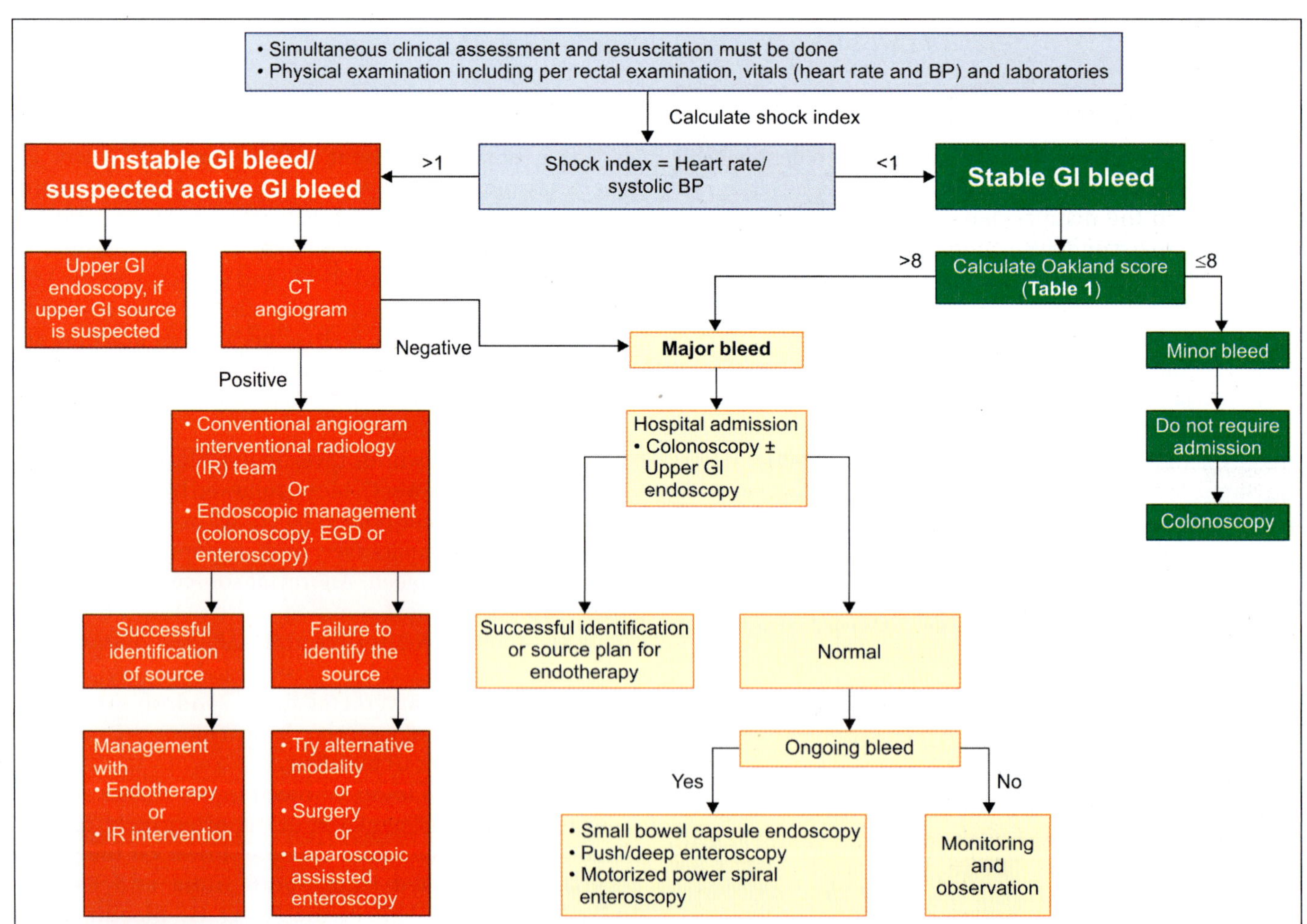

(EGD: esophago-gastro-duodenoscopy)

FLOWCHART 1: Evaluation of acute lower GI bleeding.

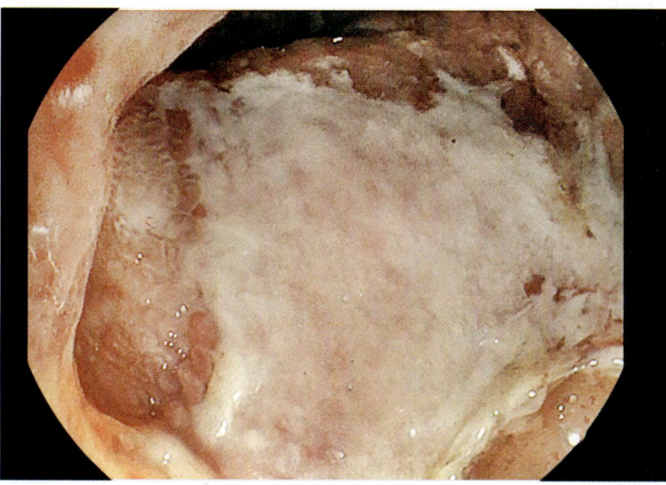

FIGURE 1: Large rectal ulcer in a patient with chronic constipation with a history of digital evacuation suggestive of solitary rectal ulcer syndrome.

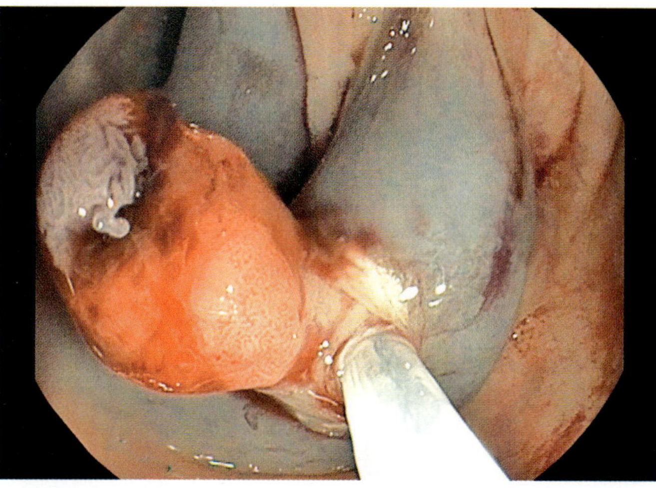

FIGURE 2: Snare polypectomy of bleeding rectal polyp (juvenile polyp) in a young child.

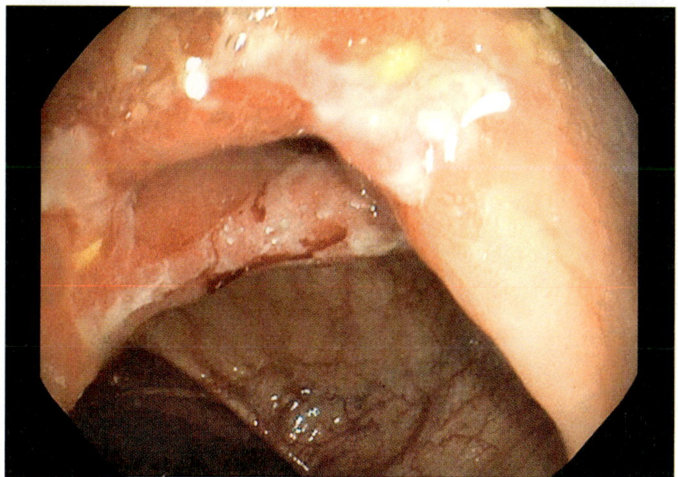

FIGURE 3: A 25-year-old patient presenting with episodes of pain abdomen, colonoscopy showed ileocecal ulceration causing narrowing of IC valve (ileocecal tuberculosis).

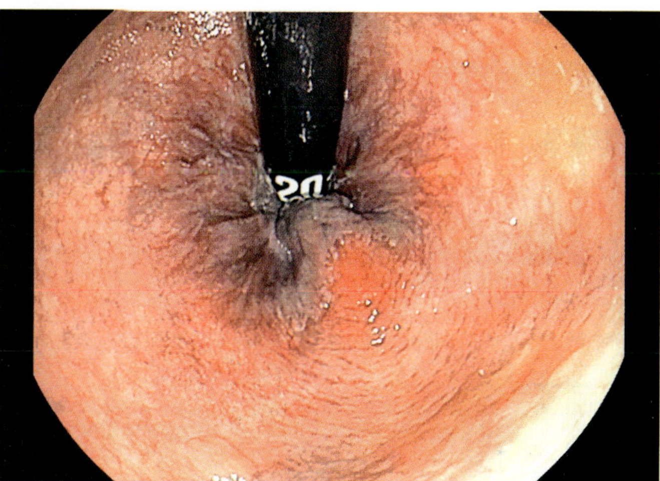

FIGURE 4: Retroflexion image (rectum) of a 45-year-old female with constipation and bleeding per rectum, showing internal hemorrhoids.

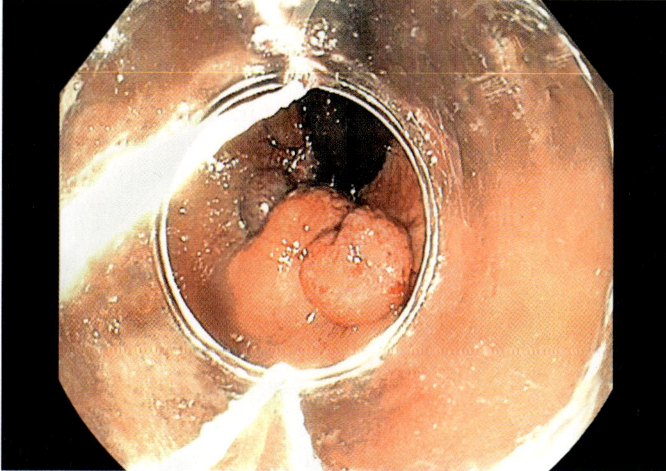

FIGURE 5: Management of bleeding hemorrhoids with the help of band ligation.

- Tachycardia, hypotension, shock—probably indicate UGI source of bleed
- Telangiectasia: Cardiac diseases, chronic liver disease, chronic kidney disease, malignancies, hereditary hemorrhagic telangiectasia (Osler–Weber–Rendu syndrome)
- Palpable lymph nodes: Malignancy or TB
- Lump or mass per abdomen: Malignancy, portal hypertension
- Tenderness: Infective/IBD

EVALUATION

Most of the lower GI bleeds are slow, intermittent, and do not require admission. Primary clinical management depends on the mode of presentation.

In a stable patient, apart from routine history-taking and investigations, a targeted history and clinical assessment

TABLE 1 Oakland score—calculated using various variables.

Predictor	Score
Age	
<40 years	0
40–69 years	1
>70 years	2
Gender	
Female	0
Male	1
Previous lower gastrointestinal (GI) admission	
No	0
Yes	1
Digital rectal examination	
No blood	0
Blood	1
Heart rate	
<70/min	0
70–89/min	1
90–109/min	2
>110/min	3
Systolic blood pressure	
<90 mm Hg	5
90–119 mm Hg	4
120–129 mm Hg	3
130–159 mm Hg	2
>160 mm Hg	1
Hemoglobin	
<7 g/dL	22
7–8.9 g/dL	17
9–10.9 g/dL	13
11–12.9 g/dL	8
13–15.9 g/dL	4
>16 g/dL	0

along with a digital rectal examination and proctoscopy is essential. Cardiovascular and respiratory assessment is of prime importance. Colonoscopy is the primary investigation of choice.

In an unstable patient:

- Resuscitation and management should be started simultaneously:
  - Two large wide-bore cannula/central venous line must be secured.
  - Fluid resuscitation must be started with crystalloid or plasma expanders.
  - Blood transfusion should be arranged for, if necessary: The trigger level of Hb is <7 g, target Hb being 7–9 g; in a cardiac comorbid individual, the trigger is <8 g and target 10 g

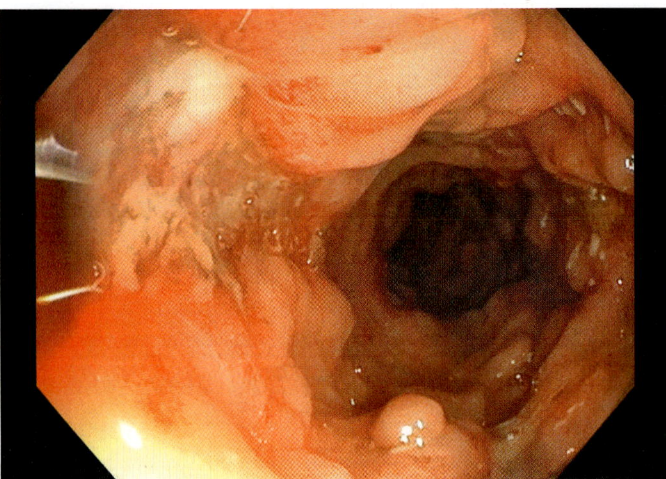

FIGURE 6: Longitudinal serpiginous ulcers in ileum suggestive of Crohn's disease.

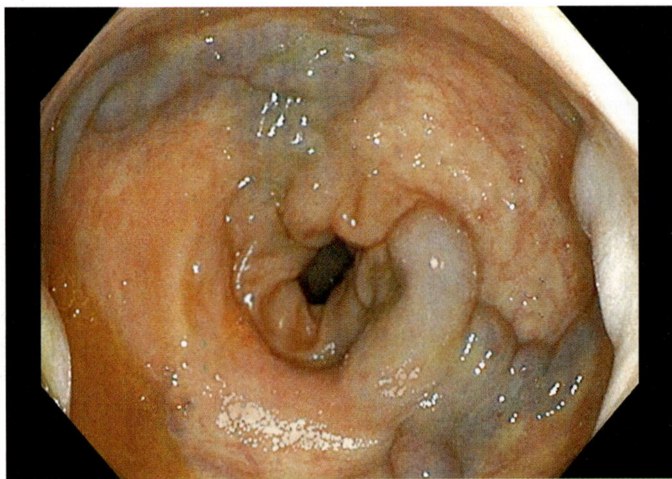

FIGURE 7: A 45-year-old chronic liver disease patient presenting with significant intermittent hematochezia, dilated tortuous ectopic veins noted in rectum—rectal varices.

Blood biochemistry: workup should be started—complete blood count (CBC), serum electrolytes, blood urea etc.

- History of drug intake:
  - Warfarin must be stopped at presentation. Reversal agent should be considered before endotherapy [prothrombin complex concentrate (PCC) and vitamin K] in a low thrombotic risk individual. It is restarted after 7 days of hemostasis. In a high-risk individual (prosthetic mitral value), AF with prosthetic value or MS (or <3 months of thrombotic event)—LMWH is started 48 hours after hemostasis.
  - Aspirin: If used for primary prophylaxis, it must be discontinued and in individuals using it for secondary prophylaxis. It should not be stopped as routine, if stopped it must be restarted immediately, after hemostasis is achieved.
- *Cardiovascular and respiratory* assessment is of prime importance.

Digital rectal examination must be done to look for active bleeding. Proctoscopy is useful in case of anorectal bleed.

- **Endoscopy:** Flexible sigmoidoscopy and colonoscopy are primary investigations of choice. Timing of colonoscopy—a randomized controlled trial on urgent (<12 h) versus elective (36–60 h) suggested no advantage of urgent over elective colonoscopy in diagnosis, treatment, length of hospital stay, morbidity, or need for blood transfusions.
- Colonoscopic bowel preparation is very important in patient with lower GI bleeding, poor mucosal visibility leads to difficulty in identification of the source of bleeding or sometime missing the lesion. Ryle tube placement for colon preparation (rapid purge—4–6 L), or if UGI bleed is suspected. About 11–15 % of lower GI bleeds actually have UGI source. History of peptic ulcer disease (PUD), portal hypertension, raised blood urea nitrogen (BUN)-creatinine ratio, and use of antiplatelet raises our suspicion towards UGI source.

TREATMENT

Endoscopic: Various endoscopic hemostasis methods are shown in **Table 2**.

- Injection of adrenaline/saline
- Heater/Gold probe
- Argon plasma coagulation (APC)
- Hemoclip applications

Interventional radiology: On identification of culprit vessel/vasculature on conventional angiogram, selective embolization can be done using micro coil, gelatin sponge, polyvinyl alcohol sponge, and N-butyl cyanoacrylate glue injection. The technical success of this therapy has been reported to be 93–100%.

Surgery: Emergency laparotomy for severe lower GI bleed is very uncommon. Surgery is the treatment option for Meckel diverticulosis bleed and small/large intestinal malignancies (**Table 2**).

TABLE 2 Causes of acute lower GI bleed and their evaluation and management.

Cause	Features and management
Hemorrhoidal bleed	• Presents as dripping of blood with bowel movement or hematochezia with normal bowel movement, usually mild intermittent, self-limiting but occasionally severe and presents as acute lower GI bleeding • *Treatment*: Band ligation (**Fig. 5**), sclerotherapy, laxative, lubricant rectal suppositories, warm sitz bath
Anal fissure	• Hematochezia with anal pain, usually mild bleed and rarely cause moderate-to-severe bleed • *Treatment*: Medical management- topical creams, calcium channel blocker (2% diltiazem), laxatives use, warm sitz bath
Stercoral ulcer	• Chronic constipation due to impaction manifests with disimpaction, most common site is rectosigmoid area; it is especially seen in the hospitalized elderly patients • *Treatment*: Laxative, sucralfate enema
SRUS	• Chronic constipation due to excessive straining, usually single (rarely multiple) ulcer. Seen commonly on the anterior wall of rectum • *Treatment*: Laxatives, biofeedback therapy, sucralfate enema
Diverticulosis	• Painless hematochezia or maroon stools without abdominal pain with prior history of diverticulosis, usually seen in 60–70-year-old individuals, right-sided diverticula are most likely to bleed (**Fig. 8**), usually resolve spontaneously • *Treatment*: Hemoclip application (**Fig. 9**), angioembolization, epinephrine injections, multipolar electrocautery, and band ligation (risk of perforation)
Angioectasia	• Usually presents with chronic blood loss and rarely severe bleed. Usually small (**Fig. 10**) (<5 mm), multiple and located in the right colon (cecum). Only 10 % of the angioectasia bleed. Advancing age (>60 years), renal insufficiency, prior irradiation, cardiovascular diseases (aortic valve disease), chronic liver disease, chronic kidney disease etc., are certain predisposing conditions for angioectasia • *Treatment*: ◦ For chronic (slow, intermittent bleeds)—iron therapy ◦ For acute lower GI bleed: Endotherapy—Argon plasma coagulation (APC) ◦ Diffuse disease: Estrogen progesterone therapy, octreotide, thalidomide
Ischemic colitis	• Abdominal pain with low-volume hematochezia with concurrent illness such as cardiovascular disease, past history of abdominal or vascular surgeries, vasculitis, clotting disorders • *Treatment*: Conservative medical treatment—anticoagulants (antiplatelet if arterial)
IBD	• Grossly bloody diarrhea usually seen in ulcerative colitis (**Fig. 11**); major hemorrhage is uncommon • *Treatment*: Mesalamine—oral, suppositories, enemas; steroids; immunosuppressants (azathioprine); biological agents—infliximab, adalimumab
Radiation proctitis	• It may occur many months or years after radiation exposure, especially seen in individuals who had radiation therapy for prostate cancer and pelvic tumors such as ovarian or cervical malignancies. Colonoscopy finding is usually mucosal telangiectasia as the source of GI bleed. Rarely, it causes severe bleeding • *Treatment*: Endotherapy—APC of the lesions

Continued...

Continued...

Infections	• *Campylobacter, Salmonella, Shigella, Escherichia coli*, CMV, *Clostridium difficile* (**Fig. 12**), parasitic infestations (**Figs. 13** and **14**) etc., are usually the common causes of bloody diarrhea (dysentery) • *Clinical presentation*: Fever, rash, arthralgia, eosinophilia, diarrhea, and travel history. In HIV, immunocompromised or immunosuppressed individuals, CMV infection, and lymphoma must be suspected • *Medical management*: Hydration, antibiotics based on causative organis
Neoplasia	• Intermittent bleeding or occult blood loss in elderly individuals, colorectal malignancy (**Fig. 15**) always is of high suspicion. Small bowel neoplasm is rare, but commonly seen in individuals with Crohn disease or celiac disease

(CMV: cytomegalovirus; SRUS: solitary rectal ulcer syndrome)

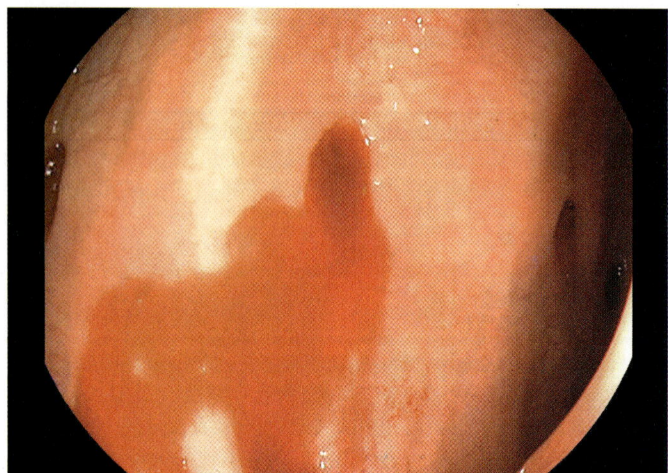

FIGURE 8: Elderly male presenting with acute lower gastro-intestinal (GI) bleed, colonoscopy showing diverticular bleed.

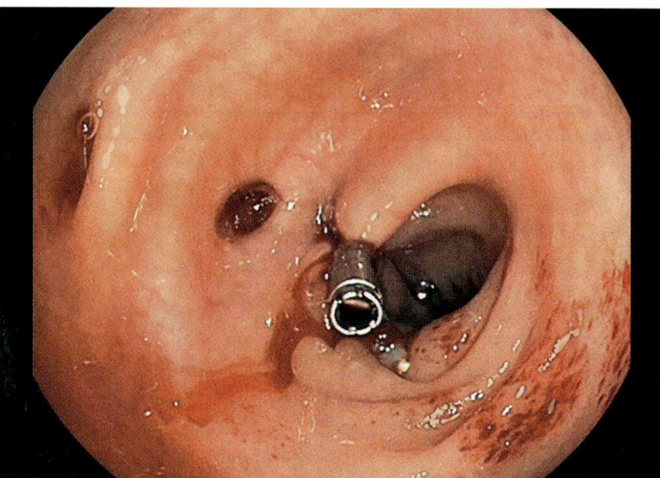

FIGURE 9: Diverticular bleed controlled with the help of hemoclips.

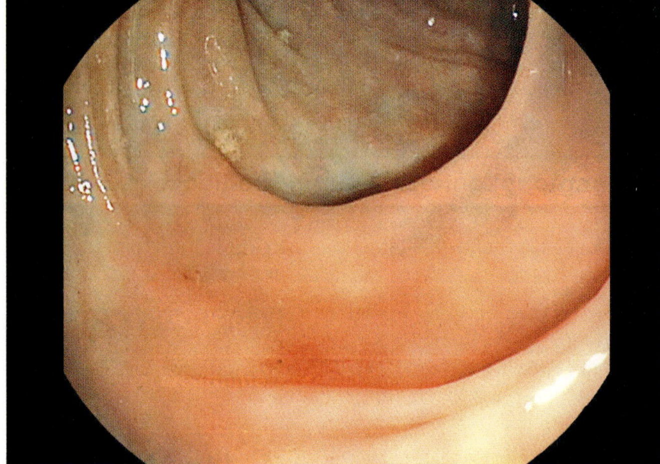

FIGURE 10: A colonoscopy image showing dilated prominent tortuous thin-walled vessel suggestive of angioectasia.

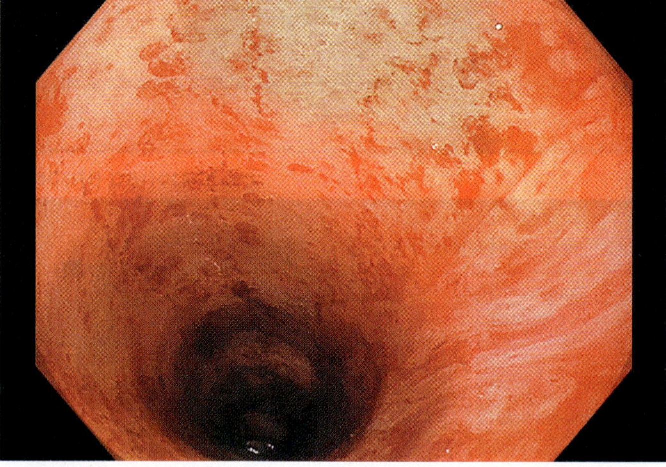

FIGURE 11: A 24-year-old female who is a known case of ulcerative colitis presented with increase stool frequency bloody stools. Colonoscopy shows active colitis with spontaneous bleeding, Mayo score—6/8.

OBSCURE GASTROINSTESTINAL BLEED

Obscure GI bleed is defined as GI bleeding of uncertain cause after a nondiagnostic UGI endoscopy, colonoscopy, and small bowel radiological imaging. Obscure GI bleed can be classified as overt and occult based on clinical presentation.

Obscure overt GI bleed refers to clinically apparent bleed (visible acute bleed) in the form of melena, maroon stools, or hematochezia in a patient with nondiagnostic UGI endoscopy, colonoscopy, and small bowel imaging.

Obscure occult GI bleed refers to clinically suspected bleeding without overt signs of bleeding usually presents with unexplained iron deficiency anemia or fatigue.

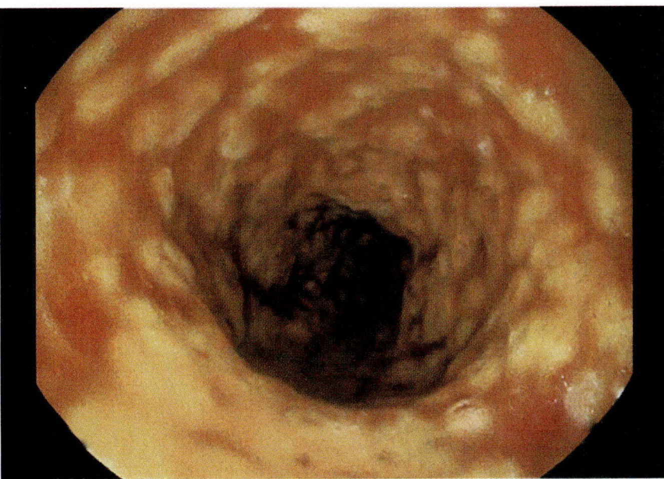

FIGURE 12: A 66-year-old women, recently hospitalized, (pneumonia) presented with bleeding per rectum—pseudomembranous colitis (*Clostridium difficile*).

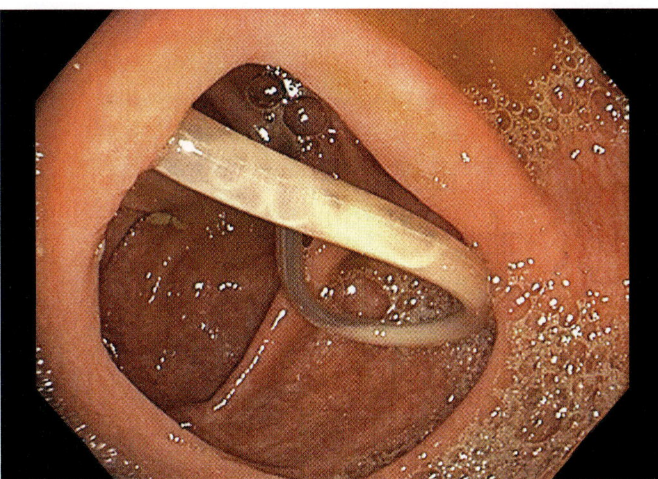

FIGURE 13: A 52-year-old male presenting with abdominal pain and iron deficiency anemia, colonoscopy—worm infestation (ascariasis).

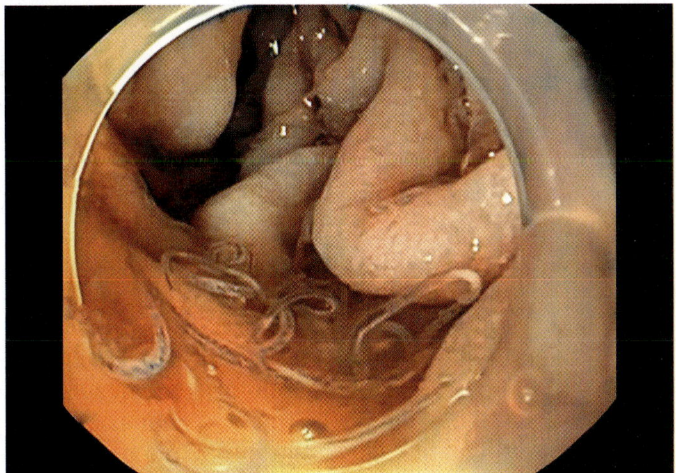

FIGURE 14: A 60-year-old male presenting with melena need multiple blood transfusion for the last 3 months, upper gastrointestinal (UGI) endoscopy, and colonoscopy were normal. Single balloon enteroscopy showed worm hyperinfestation all along the small intestine.

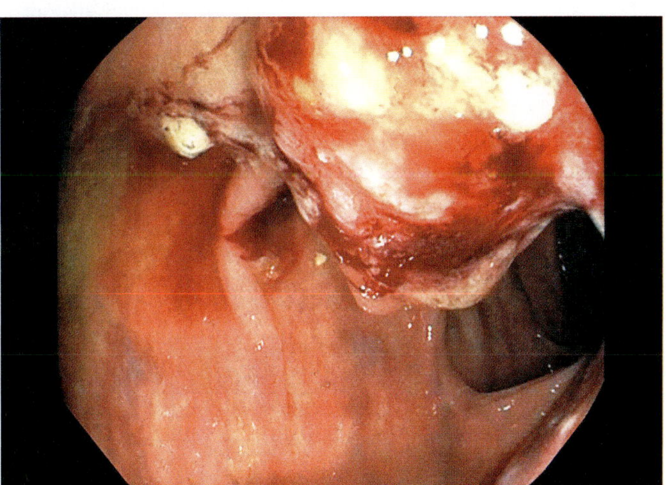

FIGURE 15: A 56-year-old male presenting with melena and anemia, colonoscopy revealed ulceroproliferative growth (colorectal carcinoma).

In 75% of cases, the source of bleed in obscure GI bleed is located in small intestine. In other cases, either the lesion was not recognized as a bleeding site on previous endoscopy (Cameroon lesion, angioectasia, internal hemorrhoid) or lesion was difficult to visualize (present of blood clot obscuring the visibility, in apparent varices in hypovolemic patient) or lesion was bleeding intermittently (Dieulafoy's lesion/angioectasia).

EVALUATION

Physical examination: Patient with obscure GI bleed might present with feature of anemia such as pallor, tachycardia, postural hypotension with hyperdynamic circulation or koilonychias or features of malignancy such as lymphadenopathy, palpable mass hepatosplenomegaly, or jaundice (**Flowcharts 2** and **3**).

INVESTIGATIONS

Fecal blood testing: Normal fecal blood loss is 0.5–1.5 mL/day. Fecal immune chemical test (FIT) is more sensitive when compared to guaiac preparation tests [fecal occult blood test (FOBT)]. The false positivity of FOBT is seen on taking peroxidase-containing foods (radish, turnip, cantaloupe, beans, sprouts, broccoli, and grapes or some medication such as sucralfate and cimetidine). The false-negative result of FOBT are noticed on use of ascorbic acid, antacids, heat, and pH-inhibiting substances. In large screening studies, it was found that 2–10% of patients with positive guaiac-positive stools have colorectal cancers.

Endoscopy: UGI endoscopy and colonoscopy must be done to rule out any missed lesions on initial endoscopy.

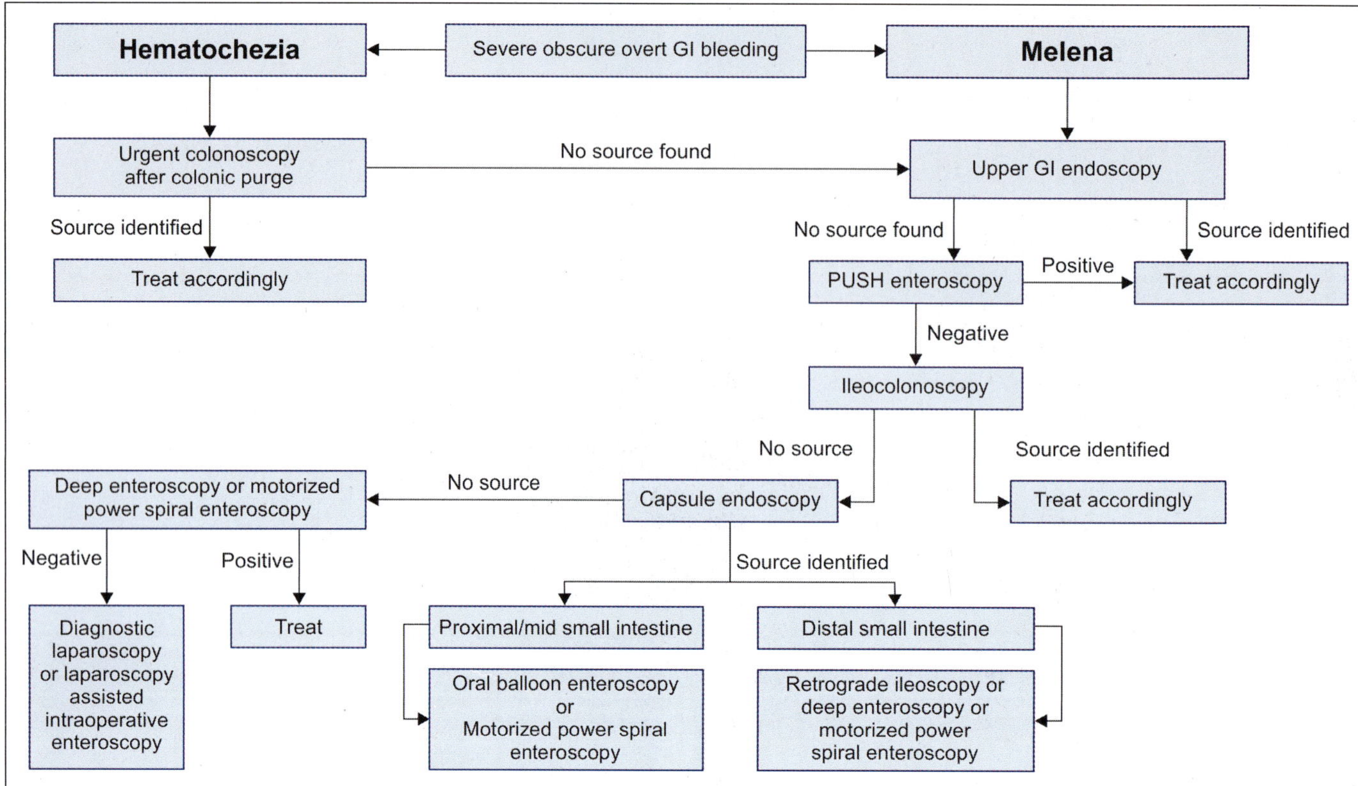

FLOWCHART 2: Evaluation of overt GI bleeding.

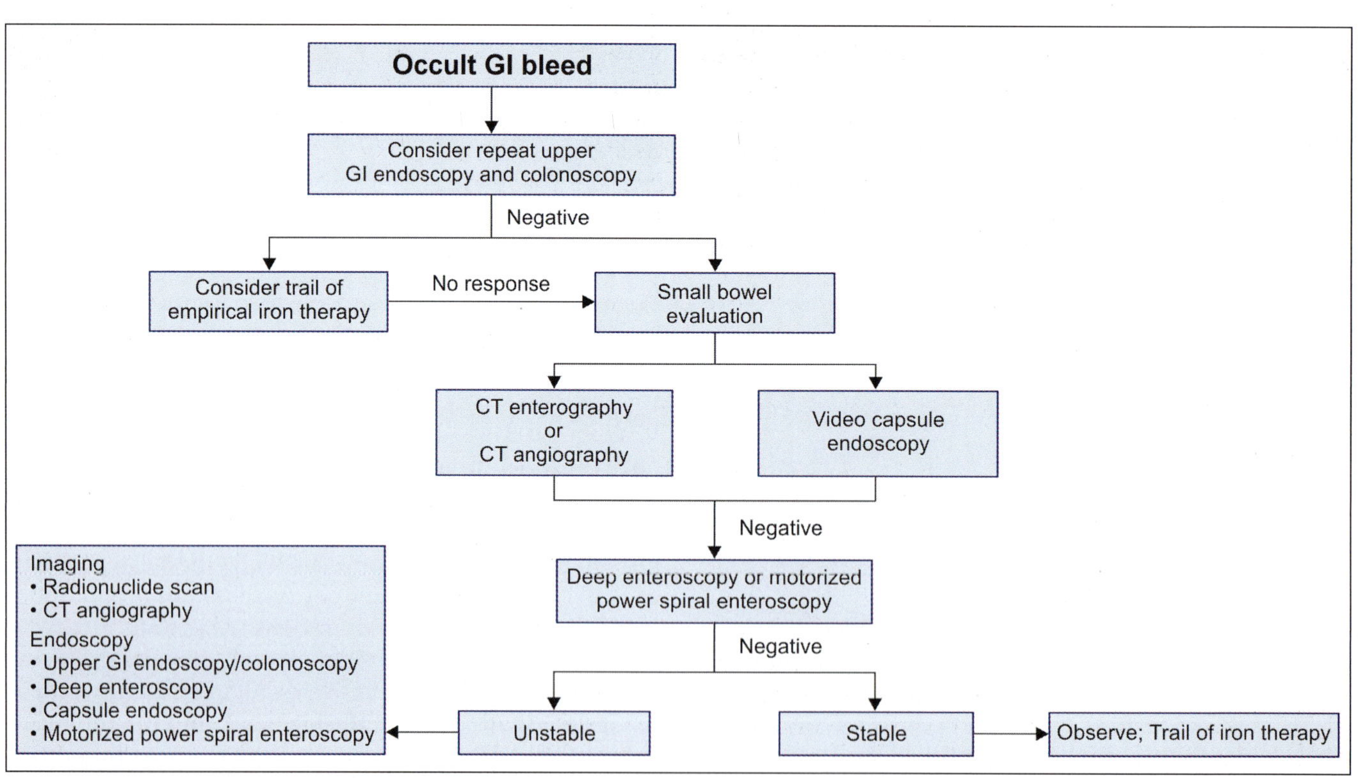

FLOWCHART 3: Evaluation of occult GI bleeding.

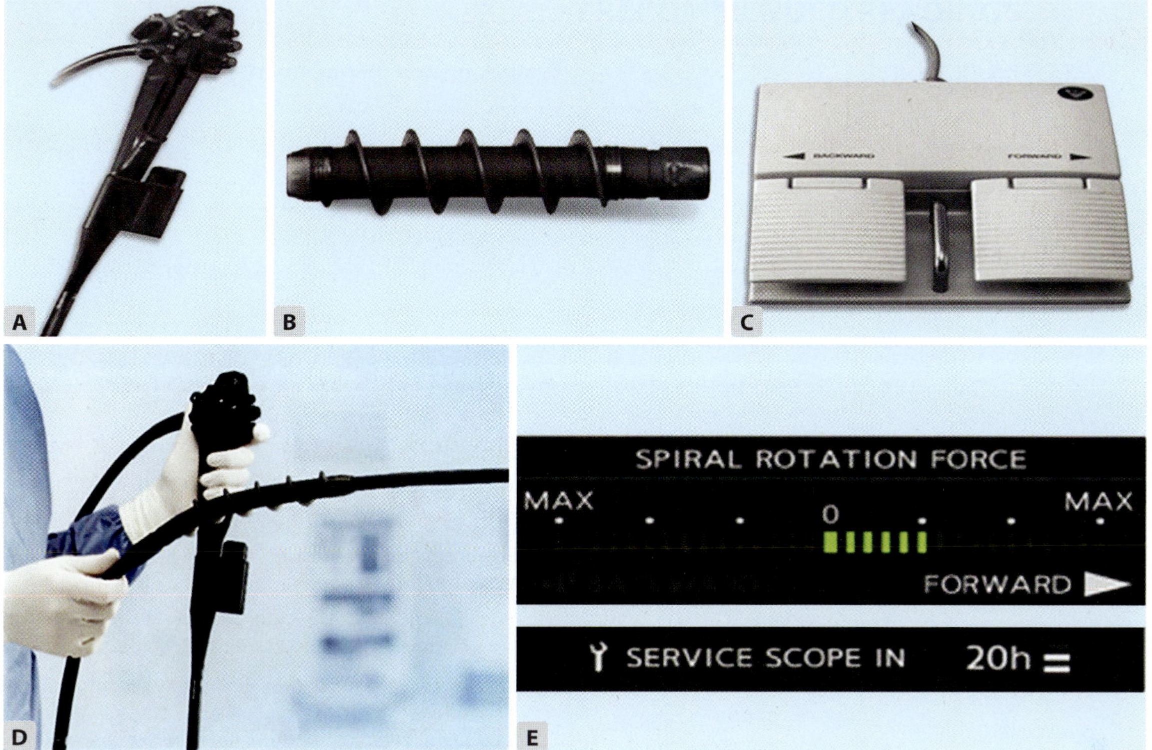

FIGURES 16 A to E: Novel motorized spiral enteroscope. **(A)** Integrated motor in the handle of the motorized spiral enteroscope; **(B)** spiral overtube; **(C)** Foot pad with switch pedal to operate the scope forward and backward; **(D)** Motorized spiral enteroscope; **(E)** Force gauge on control unit for visual indication of the rotational direction.

Capsule endoscopy has a diagnostic yield of 50–72% in obscure GI bleeds and is helpful in identifying the source of bleed. Its yield is better when done close to the bleeding episode (<48 h from the bleed: 87–91.9 % and >3 days after the bleed < 50%). The disadvantage of video capsule endoscopy is that therapeutics cannot be performed. Enteroscopy is a useful tool in diagnosis and is also helpful in performing therapeutic interventions. Push enteroscopy has a yield of around 50%. Double-balloon enteroscopy (DBE) reaches deeper depths of insertions when compared to single-balloon enteroscopy (SBE); randomized controlled studies comparing DBE versus SBE have shown the diagnostic yield for both the groups ranged from 40 to 60%, with an overall rate of adverse events including pancreatitis, bleeding, and perforation being 1.2–1.6%. Novel motorized spiral enteroscopy (**Figs. 16 A to E**) is a recent advancement in the small bowel evaluation. It has an integrated electric motor which is controlled with the help of a footswitch. The motor helps rotate a short spiral overtube segment present at one end of the scope to pleat and unpleat the small bowel over the scope. This new technology has increase the speed of performing the procedure, helped facilitate greater depth of insertion, and advantage of being a single-operator technique. In the recent literature published, it has been reported to have diagnostic yield of 74%. Intraoperative enteroscopy is very rarely done nowadays; it has a diagnostic yield of 70%.

Computed tomography (CT) enterography helps in identifying small bowel pathology such as strictures and neoplasms. CT angiography has sensitivity of 79–95% and specificity of 95–100%. Its sensitivity and specificity depends on velocity of bleed (0.5–1.0 mL/min) and is usually helpful in diagnosis of acute lower GI bleeding. Radionuclide scan is helpful if the bleeding rate is >0.1–0.5 mL/min. Meckel scanning is a radiolabeled scan where technetium compound accumulates in acid-producing mucosa present in the diverticulum.

Diagnostic laparoscopy is rarely performed for lower GI bleed due to the better diagnostic and therapeutic tools available recently.

DIFFERENTIAL DIAGNOSIS

The common causes of obscure GI bleeding in individuals younger than 40 years bleeding is more likely to be due to tumor, Meckel's diverticulum, or Crohn's disease. In individuals older than 40 years, angioectasia or an NSAIDs-induced ulcer are common causes. Other causes of obscure GI bleed are illustrated **Table 3**.

- *Inflammatory lesions*:
    - Acid peptic disease-related longitudinal erosions or ulcers noted in hiatus hernia
    - Inflammatory bowel disease—Crohn's disease
    - Celiac sprue
    - Meckel's diverticulum
    - Eosinophilic gastroenteritis
    - Radiation enteritis
    - Whipple's diseases
- *Infections*: With hookworm, *Mycobacterium tuberculosis*, amoeba, ascariasis etc.

TABLE 3	Cause of obscure GI bleed and their evaluation and management.	
Site	**Cause**	**Evaluation and management**
Proximal to ligament of Treitz	Cameron erosion	• 20–60 years, usually seen in individuals with large hiatus hernia • Treatment: Proton-pump inhibitors (PPIs) (double dose), antacids, and endotherapy if required (in case of active bleeding)
	NSAIDs enteropathy	• >20 years, history of use of NSAIDs in the past. It is reported that 8% of patient taking NSAIDs in the preceding 6 months presented with NSAID enteropathy • Treatment: Stopping NSAIDs use, COX2 inhibitors preferred instead, PPI therapy
	Dieulafoy lesion	• >40 years, intermittent large-volume bleeding • Treatment: Endotherapy or angioembolization
	Crohn's disease	• 20–60 years, history of multiple episodes of SAIO, family history of Crohn's disease, presence of extraintestinal manifestations • Treatment: Steroid—topical budesonide, steroid therapy; immunosuppressant, biologics
	Gastric antral vascular ectasia	• 20–60 years, associated with autoimmune disease or chronic liver disease • Treatment: APC, endoscopic band ligation
Small intestine	Angioectasia	• Younger than 40 years, usually intermittent occult bleeding. Frequent nose bleeds. Hereditary hemorrhagic telangiectasia (Osler–Weber–Rendu disease) • Treatment: APC, Hyde syndrome (aortic stenosis with intestinal angioectasia)—treated with valve replacement, von Willebrand disease: Desmopressin, replacement of relevant deficient factors
	Peutz–Jeghers syndrome	• Younger than 20 years at presentation, perioral pigmentation, obstructive symptoms due to intussusception • Treatment: Polypectomy or surgical resection, cancer surveillance
	Meckel's diverticulum	• 20–60 years, abdominal pain with lower GI bleed, 100 cm proximal to IC valve in location, 50% of them have gastric mucosa and may bleed. May present as unexplained bleeding (since childhood or in a young adult) • Treatment: Surgery
	Malignancy	• >50 years, present with weight loss and abdominal pain. Carcinoid, neuroendocrine tumors, gastrointestinal stroma tumor (GIST), lymphoma, metastatic lesions, leiomyoma, leiomyosarcoma, adenomatous polyps, juvenile polyps • Treatment: Surgery, chemotherapy, radiotherapy
	Pancreaticobiliary	Fundal variceal bleed after an episode of acute pancreatitis due to portal vein thrombosis
Colonic	Diverticulosis	>50 years, intermittent painless bleeding
	Malignancy	>50 years, weight loss, family history of malignancy
	Angioectasia	>40 years, intermittent painless bleeding
	Varices	20–60 years, associated CLD or EHPVO/NCPF
	Hemorrhoids	>40 years, painless bleeding per rectum

(COX: cyclooxygenase; EHPVO: extrahepatic portal vein obstruction; IC: ileocecal; NCPF: noncirrhotic portal fibrosis)

- *Vascular*: Portal hypertensive gastropathy, gastric vascular angioectasia, ectopic varices

MANAGEMENT

The management of obscure GI bleed depends on the cause. The plan and choices are given in **Table 3**.

RECOMMENDED READINGS

1. Feldman M, Friedman LS, Brandt LJ. Gastrointestinal Bleeding. Sleisenger and Fordtran's gastrointestinal and liver disease E-book: Pathophysiology, diagnosis, management, 11th edition. USA: Elsevier; 2020.
2. Oakland K, Chadwick G, East JE, Guy R, Humphries A, Jairath V, et al. Diagnosis and management of acute lower gastrointestinal bleeding: guidelines from the British Society of Gastroenterology. Gut. 2019;68(5):776-89.
3. Gralnek IM, Neeman Z, Strate LL. Acute lower gastrointestinal bleeding. N Engl J Med. 2017;376(11):1054-63.
4. Strate LL, Gralnek IM. ACG Clinical Guideline: Management of patients with acute lower gastrointestinal bleeding. Am J Gastroenterol. 2016;111(4):459-74.

CHAPTER
138
Acute Pancreatitis

Anshuman Elhence, Soumya Jagannath Mahapatra, Pramod Kumar Garg

ABSTRACT

Acute pancreatitis (AP) is an acute inflammatory disease of the pancreas presenting clinically as acute abdominal pain. In about 20% of patients, it may lead to pancreatic and/or peripancreatic fat necrosis. AP is generally mild but may be severe and associated with organ failure in up to 20% of patients leading to a high mortality. Gallstones and alcohol remain the most common etiologies responsible for nearly two-thirds of cases. Intracellular calcium overload and premature trypsinogen activation are key central pathogenic mechanisms in the initial phase of the inflammatory cascade. The diagnosis of AP is based on the presence of two of the following: Abdominal pain, serum level of amylase or lipase more than three times the upper normal limit, and imaging evidence of AP. Early prediction of severity is necessary for triage and hospitalized care for patients. Persistent systemic inflammatory response syndrome (SIRS) is an important clinical biomarker to predict severe AP and a high probability of developing organ failure.

Management of AP has evolved from being a surgeon's domain to a disease requiring multidisciplinary care with a critical role for the medical gastroenterologist, interventional radiologist, surgeon, and nutritionist. The "one size fits all" approach cannot be recommended for AP and the management needs to be tailored to each patient. Prompt and adequate care has been able to bring down the mortality of patients with AP, but still remains high in severe AP. Although no specific therapy is currently available, newer targeted therapy based on insights into the pathogenic processes are in development. Prevention of recurrence and management of long-term sequelae are equally important, but often neglected part of management.

"Patience is the key that connects efforts to success"

—Anonymous

INTRODUCTION

Acute pancreatitis is an acute inflammatory disease of the pancreas which constitutes one of the most common causes of hospitalization related to gastrointestinal diseases. AP may be associated with both local and systemic complications. In the majority of patients, it has a self-limiting mild course but in up to 20% of the patients it leads to severe systemic inflammation resulting in organ failure with a high mortality of up to 40%. Among the local complications, patients may develop acute fluid collections in and around the pancreas and/or necrosis.

Most patients with AP have acute interstitial (edematous) pancreatitis, but in around 20% of patients, the disease process leads to pancreatic necrosis and/or peripancreatic fat necrosis termed as acute necrotizing pancreatitis. Later in the course of disease, there is a tendency for the necrotic collections to develop infection, i.e., infected pancreatic necrosis (IPN) which may lead to sepsis. Following resolution of the inflammatory insult, there is a possibility of recurrence of AP and progression to chronic pancreatitis in a subset of patients as well as for long-term consequences such as endocrine and exocrine insufficiency.

In spite of rapidly accumulating information on the pathogenesis of AP, there is no specific therapeutic agent currently in use. Treatment often needs to be tailored to each patient specifically, but general principles of early management entail optimal fluid therapy, adequate analgesia, early enteral nutrition, and management of organ failures with supportive therapy in an intensive care unit (ICU). Later in the course beyond 2 weeks of illness, the management revolves around treating local complications particularly IPN.

ETIOLOGY

Gallstones are the most common cause of pancreatitis (40%) followed by alcohol (25%). Gallstone pancreatitis develops when a small stone passes down the common bile duct (CBD) and impacts at the ampulla of Vater leading to transient obstruction of both the bile and pancreatic ducts. This causes a rise in the intrapancreatic ductal pressure which leads to perturbation in the acinar cell physiology. Obstruction of the CBD leads to increased serum alanine aminotransferase (ALT) levels to more than three times the upper normal limit which is an important biomarker for biliary etiology of AP within 48 hours of onset of pain. Apart from gallstones, any transient ampullary obstruction might lead to pancreatitis through a similar mechanism, e.g., small ampullary tumors and intraductal papillary mucinous neoplasms

(IPMNs) trigger pancreatitis by a similar mechanism and must be considered among differentials in patients above 50 years of age presenting with apparently idiopathic pancreatitis. Similarly, passage of *Ascaris* worm through the ampulla should be considered in patients particularly from an endemic zone such as Kashmir. Post-endoscopic retrograde cholangiopancreatography (ERCP) pancreatitis (PEP) is a well-known complication in 5–7% of patients undergoing ERCP and occurs due to injury and edema causing obstruction at the ampulla of Vater.

Alcohol intake in amounts >60 g/day for at least 5 years predisposes to AP. Despite alcohol being a well-known risk factor for AP, <5% of people who drink significant amount of alcohol develop AP pointing to yet another cofactor, e.g., an underlying genetic predisposition in these patients. Alcohol has well-known adverse effects on pancreatic acinar and ductal cells that predispose to AP.

Metabolic risk factors such as hypertriglyceridemia (>1,000 mg/dL) and hypercalcemia also predispose to AP. Apart from these well-known risk factors, certain *pancreato-biliary anatomical variants* and abnormalities such as pancreas divisum, abnormal pancreato-biliary duct junction, choledochal cyst, and annular pancreas may also predispose to AP. *Blunt trauma to abdomen* during road traffic accidents predisposes to AP by injury to the proximal pancreatic body due to compression, e.g., between the steering wheel and vertebra. *Drugs* such as antiepileptics such as valproate, carbamazepine and anticancer drugs such as L-asparaginase and cytarabine are well known to cause AP. Other miscellaneous causes include *postviral pancreatitis* due to hepatitis viruses, corona viruses, and human immunodeficiency virus (HIV). Despite standard investigations, the etiology of pancreatitis may not be evident in 20–30% of patients and such patients are labeled as having idiopathic pancreatitis.

PATHOGENESIS

Studies on animal models of pancreatitis have shown that the key pathophysiologic events that trigger the cascade of AP are (1) a rise in intra-acinar calcium, (2) premature activation of pancreatic enzymes within the acinar cells, (3) impaired autophagy, and (4) mitochondrial dysfunction and failure to generate adenosine triphosphate (ATP) with consequent acinar cell death. Injured acinar cells release damage-associated molecular patterns (DAMPs) such as high-mobility group box protein-1 (HMGB1), and secrete cytokines such as monocyte chemoattractant protein-1 (MCP-1) and CXC chemokines which attract innate immune cells such as monocytes and neutrophils to the site of injury.

The DAMPs via their actions on pattern recognition receptors (PRRs), e.g., toll-like receptors (TLRs) lead to activation of NF-κβ pathway. The NF-κβ pathway is a transcription factor which further leads to secretion of cytokines such as interleukin-1 (IL-1), IL-6, and IL-18 and thus contribute to the inflammatory cascade and SIRS. Severe systemic inflammation and injury may cause distant organ dysfunction. The lipolysis of pancreatic and peripancreatic fat leads to release of unsaturated free fatty acids (FFAs) which might have a role in causing organ failure. The initial proinflammatory phase is followed by a compensatory anti-inflammatory response syndrome (CARS) which is characterized by an increase in anti-inflammatory cytokines such as transforming growth factor-β (TGF-β) and IL-10. During CARS, patients are predisposed to secondary infections particularly in the necrotic fluid collections.

These unique pathogenetic events lead to two distinct phases in the disease course of AP (**Fig. 1**), the early phase which is characterized by a sterile inflammatory response and a late phase with infectious complications that may cause sepsis.

CLINICAL PRESENTATION AND DIAGNOSIS

Patients with AP commonly present with acute-onset severe abdominal pain, particularly in the upper abdomen, that is frequently associated with nausea and vomiting. Pain may radiate to the back in about 50% of the patients. Patients with severe AP may also present with features of accompanying organ failure such as breathlessness, shock, and decreased urine output. A detailed systemic examination should be done to look for features of SIRS (tachycardia, tachypnea, and temperature). Abdominal examination may show tenderness, distension, and sometimes paralytic ileus. Periumbilical (Cullen's sign) and flank (Grey Turner's sign) discoloration are well known but uncommon findings of necrotizing pancreatitis. Later in the course, patients may present with symptoms arising from local complications predominantly fluid collections.

The diagnosis of AP should be made according to the *Revised Atlanta Classification (RAC)* if two of the following three criteria are met: (1) upper abdominal pain, (2) serum amylase or lipase more than three times the upper limit of normal, and (3) imaging evidence of AP. Usually, a cross-sectional imaging is not required for the diagnosis if clinical and biochemical criteria are met. A computed tomography (CT) scan is required in the beginning only in case of a diagnostic dilemma. It is generally done later during the course of disease to assess local complications such as necrosis and fluid collections.

PROGNOSTICATION AND PREDICTION OF SEVERITY

It is important to differentiate between "prediction of severity" early in the disease course and final severity of the disease. Prediction of severity is required primarily for triage and referral of patients likely to require intensive care. A "classification of severity" system is generally used for better understanding of disease course and protocolized management.

CLASSIFICATION OF SEVERITY

The most commonly used classification system for severity is the RAC (**Table 1**). According to RAC, AP is classified as mild if there are no accompanying local or

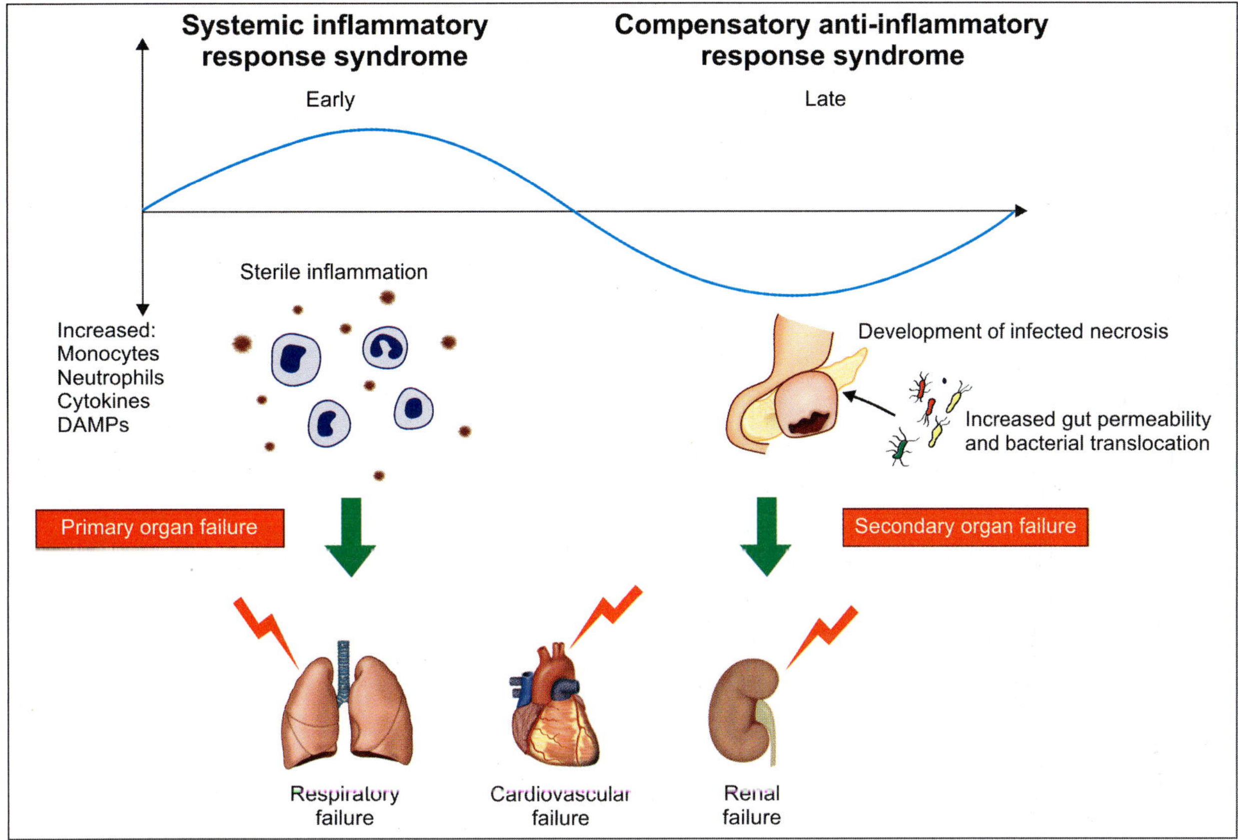

FIGURE 1: Clinical course of acute pancreatitis. Sterile inflammation and secondary infection phases, if severe may lead to primary and secondary organ failure respectively.

TABLE 1 Severity classification systems for acute pancreatitis.

Severity	Revised atlanta classification (RAC)	Determinant-based classification (DBC)
Mild	No local complications or organ failure	No local complications or organ failure
Moderate	Presence of local complications and/or transient (<48 hours) organ failure or exacerbation of previous illness	Sterile local complications (pancreatic/peripancreatic necrosis) and/or transient organ failure
Severe	Persistent organ failure	Infected necrosis or persistent organ failure
Critical	-	Infected necrosis and persistent organ failure

systemic complications. Moderately severe AP (MSAP) is characterized by transient organ failure (<48 hours) and/or local complications or exacerbation of pre-existing comorbid illness while severe AP is characterized by persistent (>48 hours) organ failure. The terminology for local complications of AP as suggested by RAC is depicted in **Figure 2**. Organ failure is defined according to modified Marshall criteria in RAC and a score of more than or equal to two qualifies as organ failure (**Table 2**).

PREDICTION OF SEVERITY

A number of single parameter laboratory tests such as hematocrit (>44%) at admission, C-reactive protein (>150 mg/L) within 48 hours of onset, and IL-6 (>130 IU/L) can be used to predict severity early in the course. In addition, multiparameter scores based on clinical and laboratory parameters such as Ranson score (>3), Imrie score (>3), acute physiology and chronic health evaluation II (APACHE II >8), and bedside index for severity in acute pancreatitis (BISAP >3) predict a severe course. Persistent SIRS beyond 48 hours has a high sensitivity of 85%, but a low positive predictive value for severe disease.

MANAGEMENT IN EARLY PHASE

FLUID THERAPY

Vomiting, decreased oral intake, and loss of fluid in third space contribute to fluid depletion in pancreatitis. The median fluid deficit in AP is estimated to be around 3–4 L in 24 hours depending on the severity of AP. Fluid

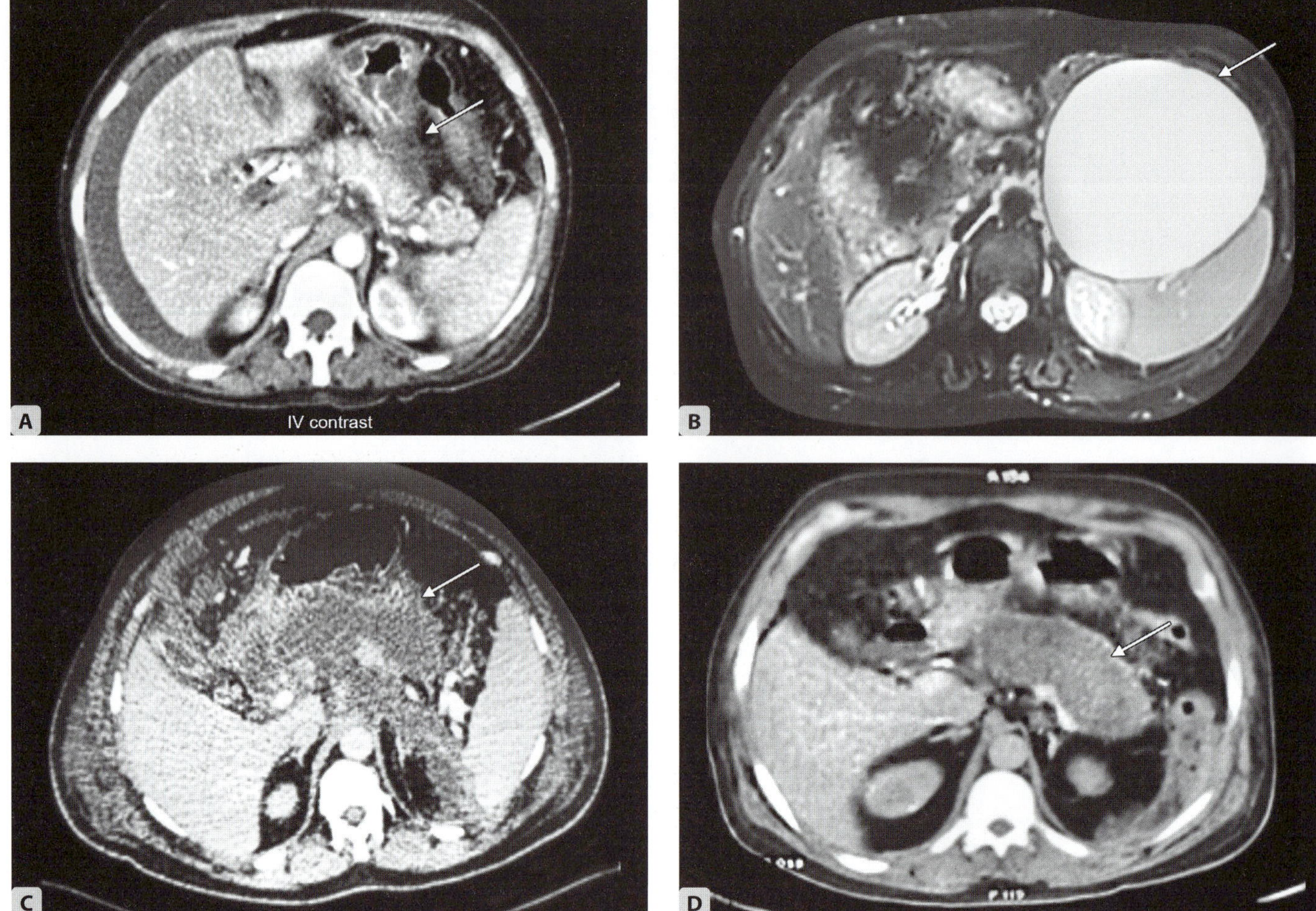

FIGURES 2 A to D: Local complications of acute pancreatitis as per the Revised Atlanta Classification. **(A)** Mild edematous pancreatitis with small acute fluid collection (arrow); **(B)** Pseudocyst with well defined wall but no necrotic debris (arrow); **(C)** Acute necrotic collection with heterogenous density (arrow); **(D)** Walled off necrosis with defined wall and heterogenous density (arrow).

TABLE 2 Modified Marshall scoring for organ failure in acute pancreatitis.

Organ system	Score				
	0	1	2	3	4
Respiratory (PaO_2/FiO_2)	<400	301–400	201–300	101–200	<101
Renal [serum creatinine (mg/dL)]	<1.4	1.4–1.8	1.9–3.6	3.6–4.9	>4.9
Cardiovascular (systolic blood pressure mm Hg)	>90	<90, fluid responsive	<90, not fluid responsive	<90, pH <7.3	<90, pH <7.2

***Note*: A score of ≥ 2 qualifies as organ failure.**

resuscitation is therefore an important component of management. The optimal fluid volume is still a matter of debate. In general, intravenous crystalloid fluid at a dose of 1.5–3 mL/kg/h is recommended in the first 24–48 hours. In addition, a fluid bolus of 20 mL/kg is given in patients who are overtly fluid deficient or in hypotension. Ringers lactate (RL) is preferred over normal saline (NS) since RL has anti-inflammatory effect and large volume NS infusion entails a risk of hyperchloremic acidosis. Over aggressive fluid resuscitation is marred with the risk of volume overload and consequent increased organ failure particularly in those with severe pancreatitis. Hence, a goal-directed fluid therapy should be used such as a decrease in heart rate <100 bpm, mean arterial pressure between 65 and 85 mm Hg, and urinary output > 0.5–1.0 mL/min as recommended by major society guidelines. There should be frequent check points for periodic assessment for overhydration.

In addition to clinical assessment, pulmonary ultrasonography to look for interstitial edema and inferior vena cava diameter can be used to guide fluid therapy and prevent volume overload.

ANALGESIA

Since the chief presenting complain of patients with AP is severe abdominal pain, adequate analgesia forms a very important part of management. Opioid analgesics such as pentazocine and tramadol are generally preferred over nonsteroidal anti-inflammatory drugs. Rescue analgesia using fentanyl can be provided preferably using a patient-controlled analgesia (PCA) pump. Respiratory depression and ileus may occur due to opioid analgesics and should be kept in mind prior to their use.

NUTRITION

Traditionally, a concept of bowel rest by keeping patients nil by mouth prevailed for quite some time in the hope of giving rest to pancreas. However, this has been found to decrease gut barrier function and lead to increased intestinal permeability with transmigration of bacteria. Hence, the current concept is bowel rousing rather than resting and early enteral nutrition is preferred. Patients with mild AP should be given oral diet as tolerated as soon as pain subsides. The timing of initiation of enteral feeding in patients with severe pancreatitis depends on patients' tolerability. Two randomized controlled trials (RCTs) have shown that early aggressive tube feeding is not superior to gradual oral feeding after 72 hours of onset. Hence, in patients with predicted severe AP, tube feeding should be initiated if there is inadequate oral intake after 3–5 days of onset of AP. Patients who do not tolerate oral or nasogastric feeding require placement of a nasojejunal tube for feeding. Standard polymeric diet is generally recommended and there is no benefit of elemental diet. Parenteral nutrition should be resorted to only in patients with abdominal compartment syndrome (ACS) and persistent ileus in whom enteral nutrition cannot be resumed early.

ANTIBIOTICS AND PROBIOTICS

Multiple RCTs and meta-analyses have shown that use of prophylactic antibiotics is futile. Antibiotics should only be instituted on suspicion of infection particularly infected necrosis. IPN is suspected in patients with no improvement/deterioration in clinical condition in the 2nd to 3rd week of illness, fever, leukocytosis, and imaging evidence of air foci in a fluid collection. It can be confirmed by either Gram stain or culture. Probiotics have been shown to increase the risk of bowel ischemia and mortality in patients with AP and hence should not be used.

EARLY ENDOSCOPIC RETROGRADE CHOLANGIOPANCREATOGRAPHY (ERCP)

Since the likely mechanism of gallstone pancreatitis is obstruction due to a bile duct stone, early ERCP has been suggested to improve outcomes. Although early RCTs showed some mortality benefit, most RCTs have shown that early ERCP is indicated only if the pancreatitis is associated with cholangitis or if there is persistent cholestasis. This is because most of the gallstones which cause biliary pancreatitis are small and pass down the ampulla spontaneously. Improvement in liver function tests over 24–48 hours is a very good clinical guide to suggest that the stone has passed out and there is no need for ERCP.

ABDOMINAL COMPARTMENT SYNDROME

Excessive loss of fluid into the peritoneum, edematous pancreas, peripancreatic fluid collections (PFCs), bowel ileus, and overzealous fluid administration often lead to an elevation in intra-abdominal pressure of >12 mm Hg which is found in up to three-fourths of patients with severe AP and is labeled as intra-abdominal hypertension (IAH). If it is pronounced, known as ACS, it can lead to development of organ dysfunction due to reduced diaphragmatic mobility and reduced renal blood flow. Hence, it is recommended that in patients with suspected ACS, abdominal pressure should be lowered by decompressing the stomach and bowels using a nasogastric tube and drainage of ascites and fluid collections. Laparostomy, a more extreme measure, may occasionally be required.

SUPPORTIVE INTENSIVE CARE

Patients with predicted severe AP should be referred to a higher centre with facilities for intensive care. Patients with organ failure due to severe AP need to be admitted in an ICU for close monitoring and intensive supportive care. Early use of noninvasive ventilation (NIV) may be initiated in patients with respiratory failure. However, invasive mechanical ventilation should be provided in case of worsening hypoxemia, respiratory muscle fatigue, IAH, or altered sensorium. In patients with acute renal failure, the indications for hemodialysis remain the same as in any other patient with acute kidney injury. Cardiovascular failure should be managed with fluid resuscitation and inotropes as appropriate.

MANAGEMENT IN LATE PHASE: LOCAL COMPLICATIONS

The majority of patients with mild AP are discharged from the hospital early within first 2 weeks. Patients with moderate or severe pancreatitis often have a prolonged disease course requiring management of local complications. Most common local complication is development of PFCs.

Peripancreatic fluid collections have been divided into four types depending on the timing and presence or absence of necrotic debris.

1. *Acute peripancreatic fluid collection (APFC)* may develop in patients with interstitial edematous pancreatitis within 4 weeks of illness. The imaging

characteristics on an abdominal contrast-enhanced computed tomography (CECT) scan are homogeneous collection with fluid density without an identifiable wall.

2. The term *pseudocyst* applies to these collections after formation of a well-encapsulated wall which takes usually >4 weeks. These collections develop either due to inflammatory exudate or leak from the pancreatic duct in the absence of significant pancreatic necrosis.
3. *Acute necrotic collections (ANCs)* develop in patients with acute necrotizing pancreatitis. The collection contains variable amounts of fluid and necrotic tissue.
4. A well-defined inflammatory wall is formed around ANCs usually after 4 weeks resulting in a mature encapsulated collection called *walled-off necrosis (WON)*. On a CECT scan, the collection appears heterogeneous with liquid and nonliquid densities with varying degree of loculations.

STERILE FLUID COLLECTIONS

Most patients with sterile acute fluid collections do not require any intervention or drainage procedure since intervening without any definite indication is not without risk of introducing infection into the collection. Hence, the decision to intervene in sterile collections is only undertaken if the collection is symptomatic and causing pain, IAH, and pressure symptoms such as extrahepatic biliary obstruction or gastric outlet obstruction. In patients with non-necrotizing AP, most acute fluid collections resolve and only a minority persists and evolve into a pseudocyst. Most ANCs, on the other hand, persists and evolve into WON. Therefore, drainage is done later in the course of disease after 4–6 weeks when the wall around collections is well-formed. In sterile pseudocysts/WON, internal drainage modality such as endoscopic or surgical cystogastrostomy is preferred as compared to external drainage to avoid risk of external pancreatic fistula.

INFECTED NECROSIS

Treatment of infected necrosis should be initiated on strong suspicion such as persistent fever, leukocytosis, and deteriorating clinical condition. Fine-needle aspiration of contents of necrotic collection to prove infection is no longer recommended.

Traditionally, infected necrosis had been a surgeon's domain with open necrosectomy as the standard of care. However, the paradigm has evolved over the last two decades and majority of the infected collections can be managed by a multidisciplinary team using a step-up approach. On the first suspicion of IPN, intravenous antibiotics preferably carbapenem, quinolone, or third-generation cephalosporin should be started empirically as guided by local sensitivity patterns. In patients with infected ANCs, intervention should be delayed to week 4, but may be required even earlier if there is no response to antibiotics and the patient is deteriorating. Percutaneous drainage of the infected collections should be done in such situations when there is no response to antibiotics. If there is inadequate response, minimally invasive (endoscopic or percutaneous) necrosectomy should be undertaken. The superiority of the step-up approach of percutaneous drainage followed by minimally invasive surgery, e.g., video-assisted retroperitoneal dissection (VARD) over direct open surgery was first shown in the landmark PANTER trial. Around one-third of patients could be effectively treated with drainage alone, hence avoiding the need for necrosectomy and decreasing the rate of consequent complications such as hernia and pancreatic insufficiency.

Although long established in drainage of pseudocysts, feasibility and efficacy of endoscopic drainage and step-up direct endoscopic necrosectomy (DEN) has been demonstrated even in patients with infected necrotic collections. Endoscopic drainage is performed preferably under endoscopic ultrasound (EUS) guidance with placement of two double pigtail plastic stents (7–10 Fr) in cases of pseudocysts and WON with <30% necrosis. Lumen-apposing metallic stents (LAMSs) are preferred over plastic stents in WON with significant solid debris (>30%) which provide better drainage and easy access for necrosectomy, if needed. The plastic stents are removed after 6 months while the LAMS is removed after 2–3 weeks due to concerns of stent migration and other stent-related complications such as bleeding.

Endoscopic versus percutaneous step-up approach: Of late, the endoscopic step-up approach, comprising of endoscopic cystogastrostomy followed by DEN has been compared to percutaneous step-up approach [percutaneous catheter drainage followed by minimally invasive surgery—VARD or percutaneous endoscopic necrosectomy (PEN)]. In the landmark TENSION trial by the Dutch group, both modalities have been shown to be equally effective but with a higher fistula rate in the percutaneous arm. In another landmark trial (MISER), endoscopic approach was shown to be better than percutaneous approach in terms of decreased risk of external fistula as a major complication.

It is important to understand that endoscopic and percutaneous drainage are not mutually exclusive and the choice of treatment depends on many factors such as location, size, and morphology of the collection, expertise available, duration of the disease, and condition of the patient. In fact, in many patients, large collections extend from the lesser sac to paracolic gutters and pelvis and dual modality drainage may be required. Moreover, some patients may be too sick for endoscopic drainage under general anesthesia in whom a percutaneous drainage may be preferred. Hence, the final approach needs to be tailored according to the anatomy of the collections and the patient's condition.

Endoscopic versus laparoscopic cystogastrostomy: Although laparoscopic cystogastrostomy offers a wider drainage and chance for simultaneous cholecystectomy in patients with biliary pancreatitis, endoscopic cystogastrostomy is associated with a shorter hospital stay and a lower cost. A recent RCT comparing both approaches in sterile pseudocyst/WON showed similar efficacy but with a higher need for reintervention in the endoscopic group.

Upfront open surgery may still be needed in patients with major complications such as perforation of viscus with accompanying peritonitis and hemorrhage not amenable to control with interventional radiologic measures.

LONG-TERM CARE AND PREVENTION OF RECURRENCE

There is a risk of developing *impaired glucose tolerance* or diabetes in up to 40% and pancreatic *exocrine insufficiency* in 25% of the patients following AP, particularly in those with a severe course and having undergone necrosectomy. Patients with necrosis of pancreatic parenchyma in the body with a viable distal part may present with *disconnected pancreatic duct syndrome* (DPDS) which may cause persistent external fistula or recurrence of collection. Although long-term placement of plastic stents across cystogastrostomy site or distal pancreatectomy may be required for DPDS, the majority of patients with DPDS are asymptomatic in our experience.

Patients with biliary pancreatitis have 10–20% risk of *recurrent AP* which can be reduced by same admission cholecystectomy in patients with mild AP and interval cholecystectomy after 6–8 weeks in patients with moderate-to-severe AP. Patients with alcoholic pancreatitis should be counseled for abstinence from alcohol. A search for the cause of AP should continue even after the subsidence of acute illness in order to prevent recurrence.

CONCLUSION

The course of AP in the majority of patients is self-limiting. Management in the early phase of the disease should focus on adequate analgesia, optimal goal directed fluid therapy, intensive care for those with persistent SIRS/organ dysfunction, and enteral nutrition. Later in the course of disease, local complications should be managed judiciously. Asymptomatic sterile collections are best left untouched while drainage is required for symptomatic collections. Infected necrosis should be treated aggressively with antibiotics and endoscopic or percutaneous step-up approach tailored to the individual patient. Recurrence should be prevented by adequately addressing the etiology (cholecystectomy/alcohol abstinence) of AP. The early mortality is mainly due to primary organ failure while late mortality is largely governed by infected necrosis. Newer directed treatments for systemic inflammation in AP to prevent/treat organ failure are in development and much awaited.

RECOMMENDED READINGS

1. Boxhoorn L, Voermans RP, Bouwense SA, Bruno MJ, Verdonk RC, Boermeester MA, et al. Acute pancreatitis. Lancet. 2020;396(10252):726-34.
2. Banks PA, Bollen TL, Dervenis C, Gooszen HG, Johnson CD, Sarr MG, et al. Classification of acute pancreatitis—2012: revision of the Atlanta classification and definitions by international consensus. Gut. 2013;62(1):102-11.
3. Garg PK, Madan K, Pande GK, Khanna S, Sathyanarayan G, Bohidar NP, et al. Association of extent and infection of pancreatic necrosis with organ failure and death in acute necrotizing pancreatitis. Clin Gastroenterol Hepatol. 2005;3(2):159-66.
4. Mouli VP, Sreenivas V, Garg PK. Efficacy of conservative treatment, without necrosectomy, for infected pancreatic necrosis: a systematic review and meta-analysis. Gastroenterology. 2013;144(2):333-40.e2.
5. van Brunschot S, van Grinsven J, van Santvoort HC, Bakker OJ, Besselink MG, Boermeester MA, et al. Endoscopic or surgical step-up approach for infected necrotising pancreatitis: a multicentre randomised trial. Lancet. 2018;391(10115):51-8.
6. Jain S, Padhan R, Bopanna S, Jain SK, Dhingra R, Dash NR, et al. Percutaneous endoscopic step-up therapy is an effective minimally invasive approach for infected necrotizing pancreatitis. Dig Dis Sci. 2020;65(2):615-22.
7. Mahapatra SJ, Jain S, Bopanna S, Gupta S, Singh P, Trikha A, et al. Pentazocine, a kappa-opioid agonist, is better than diclofenac for analgesia in acute pancreatitis: a randomized controlled trial. Am J Gastroenterol. 2019;114(5):813-21.
8. Garg PK, Singh VP. Organ failure due to systemic injury in acute pancreatitis. Gastroenterology. 2019;156(7):2008-23.
9. Garg PK, Zyromski NJ, Freeman ML. Infected necrotizing pancreatitis: evolving interventional strategies from minimally invasive surgery to endoscopic therapy-evidence mounts, but one size does not fit all. Gastroenterology. 2019;156(4):867-71.
10. Singh N, Sharma B, Sharma M, Sachdev V, Bhardwaj P, Mani K, et al. Evaluation of early enteral feeding through nasogastric and nasojejunal tube in severe acute pancreatitis: a noninferiority randomized controlled trial. Pancreas. 2012;41(1):153-9.
11. Jain S, Mahapatra SJ, Gupta S, Shalimar, Garg PK. Infected Pancreatic Necrosis due to Multidrug-Resistant Organisms and Persistent Organ failure Predict Mortality in Acute Pancreatitis. Clin Transl Gastroenterol. 2018;9(10):190.
12. Garg PK, Sharma M, Madan K, Sahni P, Banerjee D, Goyal R. Primary conservative treatment results in mortality comparable to surgery in patients with infected pancreatic necrosis. Clin Gastroenterol Hepatol. 2010;8(12):1089-94.e2.

CHAPTER

139 Chronic Pancreatitis

Rupjyoti Talukdar, D Nageshwar Reddy

ABSTRACT

Chronic pancreatitis (CP) is a complex multifactorial disorder characterized clinically by recurrent abdominal pain with exocrine and endocrine insufficiency. The pathological hallmark of the disease is activation of the pancreatic stellate cells that results in progressive pancreatic inflammation and fibrosis. Diagnosis of CP can be confirmed with modalities such as transabdominal ultrasonography (USG) or contrast-enhanced computed tomography (CECT) of abdomen or magnetic resonance cholangiopancreatography (MRCP), and endoscopic ultrasonography (EUS). Even though identification of advanced CP can be done even with plain X-ray of the abdomen or transabdominal USG, diagnosis of early CP is still challenging because of the low sensitivity/specificity of the available modalities and limited availability of the modalities with better sensitivity/specificity.

Methionine-containing antioxidants and neurotropic drugs such as pregabalin are key elements in the long-term management of pain in CP. Pancreatic exocrine insufficiency (PEI) should be treated with enteric-coated (mini) microsphere pancreatic enzyme preparation while treatment of diabetes should be initiated with metformin. Painful ductal calculi and/or stricture should be treated with endoscopic modalities as the first line, failure of which should mandate surgical approaches. However, surgery should be used as a first line if there are stones or multiple strictures all along the pancreatic duct. Appropriate counseling and optimal nutritional management is essential.

"The first step towards change is awareness. The second step is acceptance"

—Nathaniel Branden

INTRODUCTION

Chronic pancreatitis (CP) is a multifactorial and systemic illness that is characterized by progressive inflammation and fibrosis of the pancreas that results in intractable pain, malnutrition and associated metabolic abnormalities, and endocrine insufficiency/diabetes. Comfort and colleagues were the first to describe CP and observe the precipitating factors in 1946. Several risk factors and mechanisms shape the disease progression in a temporal manner over a long period of time. CP contributes to substantial clinical and economic burden and treatment is predominantly directed toward palliation of complications.

EPIDEMIOLOGY

- Even though CP is a global disease, its prevalence is particularly high in India.
- The disease phenotype of CP was first described as "**Tropical Chronic Pancreatitis (TCP)**" by Professor Geevarghese based on his observations in over 1,500 such patients from the state of Kerala in 1962. Based on these observations, a subsequent population-based study from the Quilon district of Kerala estimated a prevalence of 126 CP patients per 100,000 population. Subsequently, CP with a similar phenotype had been reported from other regions of India and nontropics.
- Based on a nationwide Indian study on CP published in 2008 that used well-defined criteria had reported that only 3.8–5.8% of patients with CP satisfied the criteria of TCP.
- Furthermore, in a later study from Kerala, when a cohort of patients with CP from 1994 (n = 220) was compared to another cohort from 2004 (n = 244) in the same geographic area, the mean age of onset of symptoms was found to be nearly 10 years older in the latter cohort, proportion of diabetic patients was nearly 17% lower in the latter cohort, diabetes was easily manageable with diet and oral hypoglycemic agents, and alcohol as a risk factors was higher in the 2004 cohort. Therefore, TCP is now by and large considered to be a variant or an advanced form of idiopathic CP that possibly results from gene–environment interactions.
- *Chronic pancreatitis in India* has a few unique features compared to that from the west. The mean age of onset of CP in India ranges from approximately 15–39 years compared to above 40 years in the Europe and the USA, and approximately 70% of cases in India have an idiopathic etiology compared to a similar proportion of alcoholic etiology in the west.

NATURAL HISTORY

- Chronic pancreatitis is believed to develop after a series of subclinical or clinical episodes of acute pancreatic injury. In a meta-analysis of 14 studies (n = 8,492; 1966–2014), it was shown that 21% of patients with acute pancreatitis (AP) develop recurrent acute pancreatitis

(RAP), out of which 36% progress to CP. 10% patients with AP progressed to CP without any intervening clinical episodes of RAP. A very similar figure has also been observed in an ongoing study that the authors' institute wherein 9.3% patients with AP and 32.3% with RAP progressed to CP (unpublished data).

- The clinical course of CP can be arbitrarily divided into three overlapping and variable phases: (1) early, (2) intermediate, and (3) late, as described in **Table 1**.

RISK FACTORS

- The risk factors of CP can be classified according to the **TIGAR-O** risk classification system (**Box 1**).
- Heavy alcohol consumption is a known risk factor of CP. Meta-analyses have shown that consumption of 60 g/day alcohol increases the risk of CP by over 6-fold.
- Ever cigarette smoking of even less than one pack per day increases the risk of CP, which further increases with an increase in the number of cigarettes. However, abstinence reduces the risk.
- Other factors such as hypercalcemia and hypertriglyceridemia could also result in the progression of AP or RAP to CP if not adequately managed.
- In India, 70% of CP are idiopathic, and several genetic polymorphisms have been implicated. Structural anomaly of the pancreatic duct, namely pancreas divisum have also been associated with RAP and CP. However, recent studies have implicated that PD could be associated with a higher frequency of RAP only in the presence of certain genetic polymorphisms.

TABLE 1 Natural history of progression of chronic pancreatitis.

Stage	Duration (from onset)	Features
Early stage	0–5 years	Recurrent acute pain (with/without clinical acute pancreatitis)
Intermediate stage	5–10 years	• Development of morphologic changes, e.g., pancreatic ductal calculi, calcifications, ductal strictures, and pseudocysts • Onset of pancreatic exocrine insufficiency (PEI)
Late stage	>10 years	Establishment PEI and diabetes

There can be substantial overlap between the three stages among patients and the duration from onset could be variable in Indian patients.

BOX 1 TIGAR-O classification of risk factors for chronic pancreatitis.

- **T** : Toxic-metabolic
- **I** : Idiopathic
- **G** : Genetic/Hereditary
- **A** : Autoimmune
- **R** : Recurrent acute pancreatitis
- **O** : Obstructive-mechanical

PATHOGENIC MECHANISMS

OXIDATIVE STRESS

Figure 1 depicts the role of oxidative stress in generating inflammation in the context of CP.

GENETICS

- The discovery of the association of cationic trypsinogen (*PRSS1*) mutations with hereditary pancreatitis by Whitcomb et al. in 1996 had unveiled an entirely new area in the pathogenesis of pancreatitis.
- Subsequently, several other genes including the pancreatic secretory trypsin inhibitor (*SPINK1*), cystic fibrosis transmembrane conductance regulator (*CFTR*), chymotrypsinogen C (*CTRC*), cathepsin B (*CTSB*), calcium-sensing receptor (*CaSR*), and carboxypeptidase A1 (*CPA1*) were also found to be associated with CP.
- More recently, a strong association of the polymorphisms in the *claudin 2* was described with alcoholic and idiopathic recurrent AP and CP.
- In the Indian context, the *SPINK1* N34S gene is the one most commonly associated with CP.
- Interestingly, the specific polymorphism in the *PRSS1* gene, namely R122H, that has a causal association with hereditary pancreatitis and increased risk of pancreatic cancer in the west, is rare in India.
- On the contrary, the *CTSB* gene polymorphism L26V which is common in India is seldom observed in the west.
- Other recently reported polymorphisms associated with CP in India have been mapped to the *claudin 2*, *PRSS1-PRSS2*, and *CPA* genes.
- The mechanisms by which genetic polymorphisms could result in CP are varied and involve intra-acinar and intraductal mechanisms related to autoactivation of trypsin, failure to inhibit autoactivated trypsin, endoplasmic reticulum stress, and possible missorting of intra-acinar vesicular traffic.

FIBROSIS

- Progressive fibrosis is the pathological hallmark of CP and is mediated by the pancreatic stellate cells (PSCs).
- When PSCs are exposed to prolonged oxidative stress (that results from RAP, exposure to cigarette smoke and alcohol metabolites, hyperglycemia, and pressure) they transform into an activated phenotype and start laying down excess amounts of collagen I in the extracellular matrix. This is mediated in autocrine and paracrine manner via the action of cytokines.

PAIN

- Pain is the most debilitating clinical manifestation of CP which results from several simultaneously occurring discrete mechanisms.
- One of the most important mechanisms that has therapeutic implications is speculated to be persistent oxidative stress.

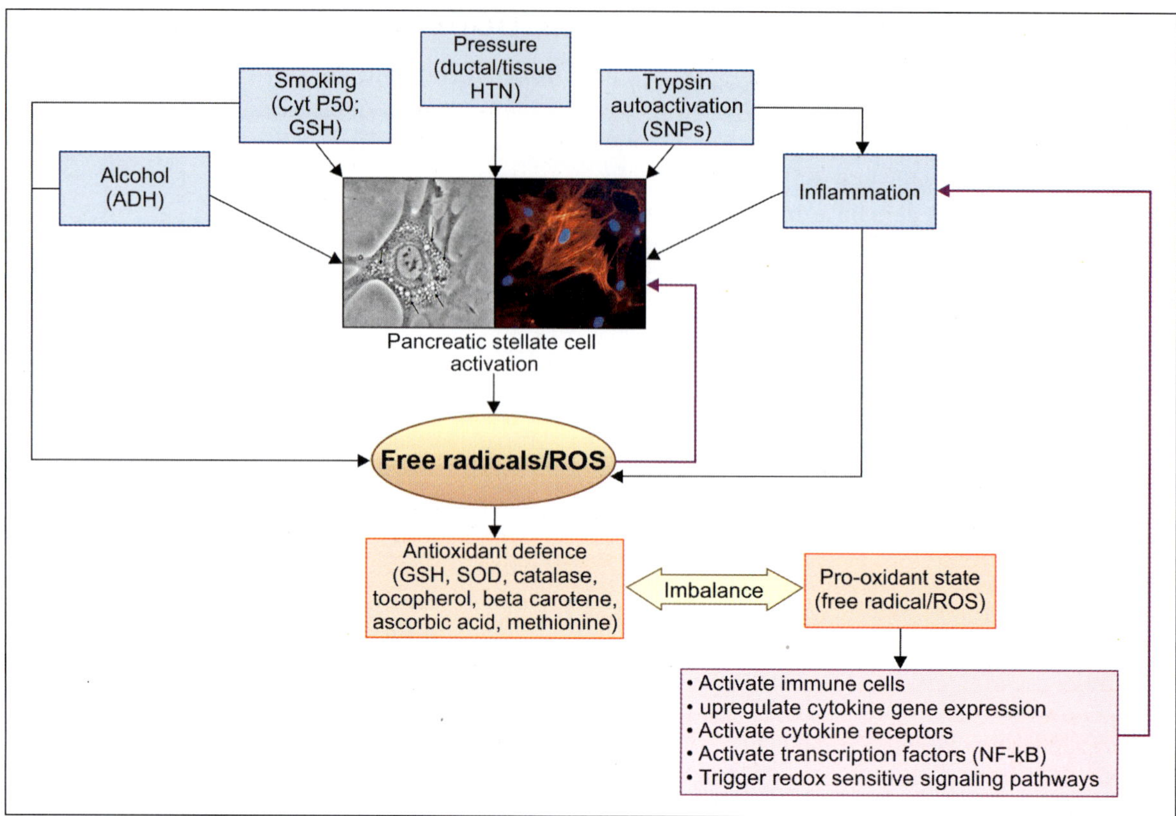

(ADH: alcohol dehydrogenase; Cyt: cytochorome; NF: nuclear factor; GSH: glutathione; ROS: reactive oxygen species; SNPs: single-nucleotide polymorphisms; SOD: superoxide dismutases)

FIGURE 1: Role of oxidative stress in generating inflammation.

- Other mechanisms include activation of pain receptors (nociceptors) by inflammatory mediators, and neuroimmune alterations (neuroplasticity).
- Evidence of neural inflammation in CP has been indicated by histological demonstration of infiltration of inflammatory cells (especially mast cells and eosinophils); neural edema and perineural disruption; Schwann cell (glial cell in peripheral nerves) proliferation; and neural hypertrophy and sprouting. Development of neuroplasticity is marked by the expression of nestin and growth-associated protein (GAP43).
- The persistent inflammation and neuroplastic changes in the pancreatic nerves result in continuous depolarization culminating in a state of spinal hypersensitivity that emanates into phenomenon such as inflammatory hyperalgesia and temporal summation. Spinal hypersensitivity further culminates in central neuroplasticity, in which there is an alteration in the entire pain modulation architecture in the frontoparietal lobe of the brain. There is also alteration of the descending cortical inhibition. **Table 2** summarizes the neuropathic pain mechanisms in CP.

DIABETES

- Diabetes associated with CP is now called type 3c diabetes mellitus (DM) and had been earlier ascribed to be pancreatic parenchymal fibrosis and islet destruction. Diabetes that was previously seen in patients with TCP was called fibrocalculous pancreatic diabetes (FCPD), but this terminology is seldom used currently.
- Recent studies have demonstrated that beta cell becomes dysfunctional while still remaining viable. This lack of response appears to be mediated by the inflammatory milieu contributed by PSCs and infiltrating T-helper subsets into the islets that secrete interferon gamma.
- Furthermore, type 3c diabetes mellitus has also been recently ascribed to alteration in the gut microbiota and gut mucosal barrier that results in translocation of endotoxins. It is known that endotoxins could result in beta cell dysfunction via nuclear factor (NF)-κB and toll-like receptor-4 (TLR4)-mediated pathways.

TABLE 2 Mechanisms of pain in chronic pancreatitis.

Pancreatic neuropathy/neuroplasticity	Central neuropathy/neuroplasticity
• Neural inflammation	• Temporal summation
• Glial activation	• Global sensitization
• Neural regeneration	• Mechanical allodynia
• Neural remodeling	• Inflammatory hyperalgesia
• Autonomic nervous system changes	• Lower latency of central pain processing

CLINICAL FEATURES

- *Abdominal pain* is the dominant clinical manifestation; however, approximately 10% patients may not have pain. Pain in CP can be divided into types A and B. Type A pain is characterized by short episodes of relapsing pain while type B implies constant or prolonged pain. Earlier studies had suggested the types of pancreatic pain could be different depending on the etiology, presence of complications, and time of disease onset. However, a recent nationwide study from the Netherlands has shown that pain patterns in CP do not result from distinctly different pathophysiological entities.

  The pattern of pain could change over time from one type to the other with intermittent acute exacerbations or progression from nociceptive to neuropathic mechanisms. However, currently there are no definitive objective methods to identify pancreatic neuropathic pain. Quantitative sensory testing is a potentially useful tool that is still in the research phase. PainDetect, another tool that is available online, can also be used to assess the pattern of pain, whether nociceptive or neuropathic. Interestingly, 30–40% of patients continue to require analgesics even after total pancreatectomy. This is due to central neuropathic pain mechanisms.
- The pancreas has a significant exocrine secretory reserve. Overt *clinical manifestations of PEI* become evident only after the postprandial output into the duodenum falls to below 10% of normal. This can occur either after development of gross pancreatic atrophy or obstructing ductal calculi predominantly in the head region. However, patients often have subclinical PEI if the output of pancreatic juice is not as low as 10% of normal.
- Even though *steatorrhea* is the hallmark symptom of exocrine insufficiency, it is not common in Indian patients with CP.
- Other manifestation of exocrine insufficiency includes features of fat-soluble vitamin deficiencies and features of malnutrition.
- Even though type 3c diabetes mellitus is pancreatogenic, it may not present with the typical features of polyuria, polydipsia, and polyphagia. Therefore, a high level of suspicion is important. Patients with long-standing CP and those with rapid weight loss are indicators which should trigger evaluation for diabetes.
- *Weight loss* is a frequent manifestation of PEI which results from malnutrition. However, it may also occur even in the absence of PEI, due to poor oral intake as a result of pain and anorexia, uncontrolled diabetes, intestinal dysmotility, small intestinal bacterial overgrowth, gastric outlet obstruction, and underlying pancreatic cancer.
- *Diarrhea* in a patient with CP may occur as a result of fat malabsorption, diabetic autonomic neuropathy, small intestinal bacterial overgrowth, and CP-associated intestinal dysmotility.

DIAGNOSIS

Diagnosis of CP includes evaluation of the morphologic and functional (exocrine and endocrine) alterations.

MORPHOLOGIC CHANGES

Table 3 represents the different modalities to detect morphologic changes of CP. Currently, endoscopic retrograde cholangiopancreatography (ERCP) is not usually used as a diagnostic modality for CP, but has a key role in the treatment. **Figures 2 A** to **D** show representative images of morphologic changes in CP.

EXOCRINE FUNCTION

There are several indirect or direct pancreatic function tests to evaluate PEI. However, most of these are not available widely or lack sensitivity and specificity for detecting early disease. **Table 4** presents the currently available tests for exocrine function of the pancreas.

ENDOCRINE FUNCTION

- Current guidelines recommend evaluation of type 3c diabetes mellitus with fasting blood glucose and HbA1c estimation. If these are abnormal, oral glucose tolerance testing should be performed.
- Presence of glutamic acid decarboxylase (GAD) antibodies and hyperinsulinemia can distinguish type 3c diabetes mellitus respectively from type 1 diabetes mellitus and type 2 diabetes mellitus (T2DM).
- Pancreatic polypeptide response during a mixed-nutrient meal is another test, though not routinely employed in clinical practice, that could differentiate type 3c diabetes mellitus from the other types.
- Estimation of plasma C-peptide levels during an oral glucose tolerance or mixed-nutrient meal testing can ascertain functional beta cell reserve.

COMPLICATIONS

Complications of CP include pancreatic pseudocyst, biliary obstruction due to strictures or pancreatic head pathology (calculi/calcification, inflammation, and head mass), gastric outlet obstruction, and the most ominous pancreatic cancer.

In Indian patients with CP, an idiopathic etiology is a high-risk factor for pancreatic cancer compared to alcohol etiology. Smoking could also increase the risk of pancreatic cancer in these patients. Unfortunately, there are currently no proven ways to do cancer surveillance in these patients, nor there are any specific early diagnostic modalities. However, a few red flags that could point toward a possible pancreatic cancer on the background of CP are: New onset diabetes in a patients after the age of 50 years, sudden deterioration of glycemic control in a patient with type 3c diabetes mellitus in spite of continuing treatment, relapse of abdominal pain or change in the character of pain especially after long-standing disease or higher age, and

TABLE 3 Currently available modalities to evaluate structural abnormalities of the pancreas in chronic pancreatitis.

	Advantages	Disadvantages
Plain X-ray abdomen	• Can detect calcification (high specificity)	• Cannot assess parenchymal volume and ductal changes
Transabdominal ultrasonography	• Most commonly used • Can assess parenchymal atrophy, duct size, duct stone, and parenchymal calcification	• Operator dependent • Poor reliability for early changes of CP • Unreliable for mass lesions on the background of CP • Cannot evaluate MPD strictures
CECT scan	• Can provide reliable evidence of the pancreatic parenchymal volume, localization of pancreatic stones and calcifications, complications such as pseudocyst, bleeding and pseudoaneurysms (better with CT angiography), and presence of a mass lesion	• Risk of radiation of exposure • Not ideal for detecting early changes
MRCP	• Radiation exposure can be avoided • Can identify parenchymal volume changes • Can identify communication between the pancreatic duct and the pseudocysts (not in all patients though); presence of structural ductal anomaly, e.g., pancreas divisum; and early ductal changes in the form of side branch prominence or dilatation • Can detect complications such as pseudocyst, bleeding, and presence of a mass lesion	• Cannot detect presence of calculi and calcifications reliably
EUS	• Can detect changes of early CP • Can detect morphologic changes such as calcification, calculi, ductal changes, and pseudocysts • Can reliably detect pancreatic mass and offers possibility of FNA or Trucut biopsy	• Operator dependent • Tend to over diagnose early CP • Age-related changes reduce the specificity for early CP • EUS during the resolving phase of AP may show false positive diagnosis of early CP

(EUS: endoscopic ultrasonography; FNA: fine needle aspiration; MPD: main pancreatic duct; MRCP: magnetic resonance cholangiopancreatography)

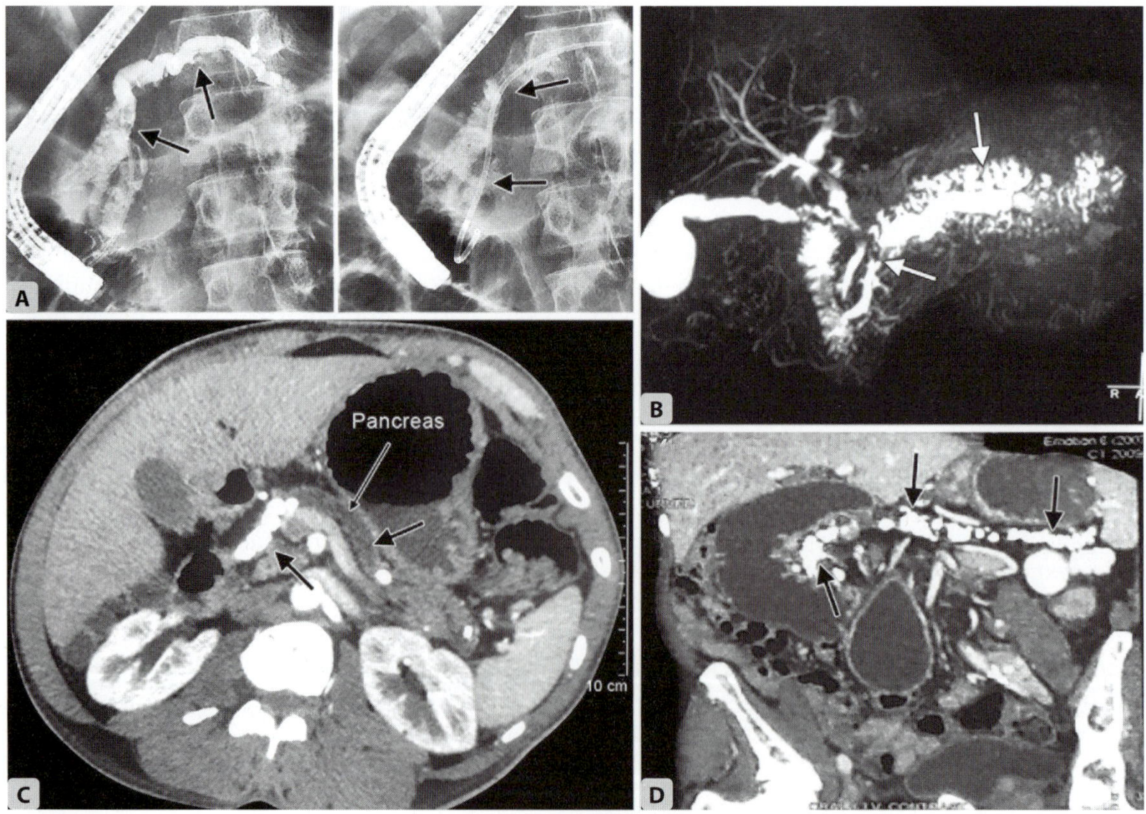

FIGURES 2 A to D: Morphologic changes in chronic pancreatitis.

TABLE 4 **Currently available modalities to evaluate functional abnormalities of the pancreas in chronic pancreatitis.**

Types of test	Test	Characteristics
Indirect tests	72-hours fecal fat estimation	• Gold standard for steatorrhea, but not specific for exocrine insufficiency • Requires adherence to specific diet and needs to be off pancreatic enzyme supplementation for ~7 days • Requires refrigeration of stools collected for over 72 h • Not used in routine practice any longer • Use restricted to research setting
	Fecal elastase test	• Stable enzyme that survives intestinal transit • Levels in stool correlate with levels in pancreatic secretion • No effect of supplemented enzymes on test results • Fair to good sensitivity and specificity for severe disease, but not for mild disease • Presence of diarrhea may result in false positivity • Available in limited centers in India
	13C-Mixed triglyceride test	• Requires mass spectroscopy or infrared-based estimation • >90% sensitivity and specificity • Could also be used to assess response to PERT • Limited availability • Currently not available in India
Direct tests	Secretin/CCK/Combined stimulation test	• Gold standard for exocrine insufficiency • Good sensitivity and specificity for advanced CP, but fair for early disease • Technically challenging [requires prolonged intubation with special tubes (e.g., Dreiling's tube)] • Time consuming • Expensive • Limited availability globally • Dilution by bile may skew results • Potential for CCK-induced adverse events such as nausea/vomiting
	Intraductal secretin stimulation test	• In addition to above, there is a risk of post ERCP pancreatitis • Short time for sample collection
	Endoscopic pancreatic function test	• In addition to above, requires prolonged sedation/anesthesia
	Secretin MRCP test	• Can detect both structural (ductal) and functional changes simultaneously • Less time consuming than other direct tests • Expensive

(CCK: cholecystokinin; PERT: pancreatic enzyme replacement therapy)

sudden weight loss. Patients with these red flags should be investigated further for pancreatic cancer with a pancreas protocol CT scan. If there is still ambiguity in the diagnosis, then a MRCP or EUS could provide additional evidence.

TREATMENT

Treatment of CP requires a multipronged approach and a single modality is unlikely to result in a durable improvement in pain and other structural and functional abnormalities.

MEDICAL TREATMENT

Medical treatment in CP is primarily targeted toward pain management, improving exocrine function and glycemic control.

- The World Health Organization pain ladder, starting with a nonsteroidal anti-inflammatory drug (NSAID), may be used for acute pain relief. Low potency selective μ-opiate receptor agonist such as tramadol hydrochloride has been shown to be as effective as higher potency narcotics but with a significantly better safety profile. High potency narcotics such as morphine and analogues should be avoided.
- Antioxidant combination containing organic selenium, ascorbic acid, β-carotene, α-tocopherol, and methionine has been shown to result in long-term pain relief. The potential mechanism involves restoration of the trans-sulfuration pathway (by donating methyl and thiol groups) in the acinar cells, thereby resulting in zymogen exocytosis and preventing intra-acinar trypsin activation along with the subsequent inflammation.
- About 150–300 mg pregabalin in daily divided doses have been shown to benefit patients with pain in CP. Pregabalin acts by altering the descending cortical inhibition of pain, thereby reducing neuropathic pain. Patients with long-standing disease are more likely to

be benefitted since neuropathic pain develops over time along with the dynamic progression of inflammation.

- Results from a recent Indian double blind, randomized controlled trial have shown efficacy of a combination of antioxidant and pregabalin for pain that recurs after ductal clearance with endotherapy or surgery.
- Based on results of systematic review and meta-analyses, pancreatic enzyme supplementation does not appear to have a role in pain management in CP. Only nonenteric-coated enzyme preparation may have a role in ameliorating pain in a subgroup of patients. However, nonenteric-coated enzyme preparations are not available in India.
- Pancreatic enzyme replacement therapy (PERT) is the mainstay of treatment for exocrine insufficiency. Of the supplemented enzymes, lipase is the most important since it is vulnerable to proteolytic digestion. For the treatment of PEI, pancreatic enzymes preparations should be in enteric-coated (mini) microsphere form, with a daily dose of at least 20,000 units to be taken along with major meals, and 10,000 units with each major snack. The dose can be titrated on the basis of approximate fat content of the meal. The response to PERT can be measured by the c13 mixed triglyceride breath test, but this test is currently not available in India. Fecal fat estimation could also measure the response to PERT, but this test is also not performed routinely by laboratories due to logistical issues. The fecal elastase test, which is available in India, however, cannot assess the response to PERT. Therefore, currently in the Indian context, response to PERT has to be evaluated based on clinical and nutritional parameters.
- In a recent study on Indian patients with CP, nearly a third of patients continued to have malnutrition even after treatment with PERT. The reason for this emerged to be poor oral intake of the calories and the proximate principles. It is important that patients with CP on PERT should take a balanced diet as adequate amount of dietary substrates, especially fat, is mandatory for the supplemented enzymes to work. Therefore, fat restriction is not recommended for a patient who is on PERT. Dietary supplements should include antioxidants-containing food, multivitamins including fat-soluble vitamins, and diets with high complex carbohydrates. Deep frying of food should be avoided since it depletes the naturally occurring antioxidants. Prescription of medium chain triglycerides is not mandatory.
- Treatment of type 3c diabetes mellitus should begin with oral hypoglycemic agents, preferably metformin, in the same manner as treatment for T2DM. In a recently published Indian study, long-term follow-up of patients with CP demonstrated that early ductal clearance interventions (endoscopic or surgical clearance of pancreatic duct of stones) could delay the development of diabetes.
- Patients who consume alcohol, cigarettes, and smokeless tobacco should be encouraged and counseled to abstain from substance use. Young patients with idiopathic CP should be counseled not to resort to consuming alcohol and smoking later in life.
- Patient education regarding their disease is important as this could help them to cope with their disease in a better way.

ENDOSCOPIC TREATMENT

The single most common indication for endotherapy for CP is intractable pain in the presence of pancreatic ductal calculi and/or pancreatic and biliary strictures. Other indications of endotherapy include symptomatic pseudocysts and celiac plexus block.

- Currently endotherapy is the first-line therapy for pancreatic ductal calculi. Small pancreatic ductal stones can be treated by ERCP alone, while larger stones (>5 mm diameter and especially those located in the head and body region) require extracorporeal shock wave lithotripsy (ESWL) with or without pancreatic duct stenting. Best results from ESWL can be obtained by using a third generation lithotriptor with dual focusing system (fluoroscopy with ultrasonography). The third generation system is available only in select centers in India. Patients with calculi located throughout the pancreatic duct or specifically in the tail region are not ideal candidates for ESWL. ESWL is a safe procedure with a small risk of postprocedure AP, and rare incidence of splenic injury (if performed for stones in the tail region) or bleeding.
- Strictures of the pancreatic and bile duct that are associated with symptoms and altered liver function can be treated with stents, and a subgroup of patients will require prior stricture dilation. Even though single plastic stent with repeated exchanges is most commonly used, few centers advocate multiple plastic or metallic stents if stricture resolution is not achieved with single plastic stents. The plastic stents need to be exchanged every 3–6 months as required. Stent migration and stent blockage are common complications of stenting.
- Pancreatic pseudocysts are treated in the presence of symptoms related to pseudocyst infection (pain and fever), intracystic bleeding, biliary obstruction (jaundice), and gastrointestinal compression (pain and vomiting). Endoscopic drainage can be performed through papilla (transpapillary) or gut wall (transmural). Under the guidance of linear echoendoscope, drainage is now possible even for pseudocysts that do not produce a bulge on the stomach or duodenum.
- Management of intractable pain in CP not responding other modalities can be attempted with celiac plexus block. This can be performed under EUS or CT guidance and a local anesthetic (bupivacaine) with or without a combination of steroid (triamcinolone). Even though it is a favorable method of pain relief for patients with unresectable pancreatic cancer, benefit in patients with CP is not as good, with a benefit in only 10% at 24 weeks. Therefore, the threshold for the use of this modality should be kept high and be attempted only if other modalities fail.

SURGICAL TREATMENT

- Procedures for ductal drainage for pain management include lateral pancreaticojejunostomy and Frey's procedure, while pancreatic resection procedures for concomitant mass lesions or refractory strictures include classical (Kausch) Whipple or pylorus-preserving (Traverso-Longmire) pancreaticoduodenectomy and distal pancreatectomy.
- Select centers in the USA and Europe advocate total pancreatectomy with autoislet transplantation (TPIAT) for intractable pain in CP. In India, islet autologous transplantation is currently performed at the Asian Institute of Gastroenterology after distal pancreatectomy in select patients who has painful distal pancreatic ductal strictures that are not amenable to endoscopic therapy.

RECOMMENDED READINGS

1. Dumonceau JM, Delhaye M, Tringali A, Dominguez-Munoz JE, Poley JW, Arvanitaki M, et al. Endoscopic treatment of chronic pancreatitis: European society of gastrointestinal endoscopy (ESGE) Clinical Guideline. Endoscopy. 2012;44:784-800.
2. Talukdar R, Reddy DN. Pain in chronic pancreatitis: managing beyond the pancreatic duct. World J Gastroenterol. 2013;19(38):6319-28.
3. Talukdar R, Sasikala M, Pavan Kumar P, Rao GV, Pradeep R, Reddy DN. T-helper cell mediated islet inflammation contributes to β-cell dysfunction in chronic pancreatitis. Pancreas. 2016;45(3):434-42.
4. Tandon RK, Garg PK. Oxidative stress in chronic pancreatitis: Pathophysiological relevance and management. Antioxid Redox Signal. 2011;15(10):2757-66.
5. Talukdar R, Reddy DN. Endoscopic therapy for chronic pancreatitis. Curr Opin Gastroenterol. 2014;30(5):484-9.
6. Aslam M, Jagtap N, Karyampudi A, Talukdar R, Reddy DN. Risk factors for development of endocrine insufficiency in chronic pancreatitis. Pancreatology. 2021;21(1):15-20.
7. Talukdar R, Reddy DN, Tandan M, Gupta R, Lakhtakia S, Ramchandani M, et al. Impact of ductal interventions on diabetes in patients with chronic pancreatitis. J Gastroenterol Hepatol. 2021;36(5):1226-34.
8. Arutla M, Sarkar S, Unnisa M, Sarkar P, Raj MA, Mrudula MR, et al. Malnutrition after pancreatic enzyme replacement therapy in chronic pancreatitis: Risk factors in real world practice. Pancreatology. 2021;21(1):34-41.
9. Hegyi P, Párniczky A, Lerch MM, Sheel ARG, Rebours V, Forsmark CE, et al. International consensus guidelines for risk factors in chronic pancreatitis. Recommendations from the working group for the international consensus guidelines for chronic pancreatitis in collaboration with the International Association of Pancreatology, the American Pancreatic Association, the Japan Pancreas Society, and European Pancreatic Club. Pancreatology. 2020;20(4):579-85.
10. Phillips AE, Faghih M, Kuhlmann L, Larsen IM, Drewes AM, Singh VK, et al. A clinically feasible method for the assessment and characterization of pain in patients with chronic pancreatitis. Pancreatology. 2020;20(1):25-34.
11. Kempeneers MA, Issa Y, Verdonk RC, Bruno M, Fockens P, van Goor H, et al. Pain patterns in chronic pancreatitis: a nationwide longitudinal cohort study. Gut. 2020;gutjnl-2020-322117.

CHAPTER 140

Gallbladder

Srikant Mohta, Anoop Saraya

ABSTRACT

The gallbladder is an integral part of the digestive system forming the storage unit of the hepatobiliary system. Although predominantly a storage organ, it serves other functions as well. Bile is composed of many components including bile acids and phospholipids. The gallbladder concentrates the bile acids and regulates secretion of bile into the bowel based on the meal stage. Due to anatomical considerations such as proximity to the liver and sphincter of Oddi and physiological alterations in bile composition as well as flow, the gallbladder lies at the center of multiple pathologies in the hepatobiliary system. Gallstones are one of the most common disorders of the gastrointestinal (GI) tract and their management still remains debated in an asymptomatic stage. Gallbladder carcinoma is very common in northern India and is an aggressive disease. In this chapter, we will try to discuss the common pathologies affecting the gallbladder and their management.

"Let food be thy medicine and medicine be thy food"

—Hippocrates

INTRODUCTION

The gallbladder is an integral part of the biliary tract which is located at the fossa on the inferior surface of the liver. It serves as a storage reservoir for bile which is produced in the liver. As a reservoir, it serves the purpose of storage as well as concentration of bile acids in the bile. This allows for it to be gradually released into the duodenum based on the bolus of chime passed into the duodenum and regulated by cholecystokinin (CCK) and other hormones.

ANATOMY

The gallbladder measures about 3 cm by 7 cm and has a capacity of up to 50 mL. The gallbladder has a fundus, body, infundibulum, and a neck. A small outpouching near the infundibulum is a Hartmann's pouch which may be a site of stone impaction leading to cholecystitis.

The gallbladder has a mucosa, lamina propria, tunica muscularis, and a serosa. There are distinct microscopic structures in the gallbladder lining including Rokitansky-Aschoff sinuses which are invaginations of the surface epithelium and ducts of Luschka which are on the hepatic surface and open directly into the intrahepatic bile ducts.

The gallbladder can be malpositioned or duplicated which may lead to diagnostic confusion; however, it has few clinical consequences.

PHYSIOLOGY

Bile is composed of a complex solution composed of bile acids (60–70%), phospholipids (mainly, phosphatidylcholine; 20–25%), and other minor components including cholesterol, bile pigments, and protein. A total of 500–600 mL of bile is secreted per day and the concentration of bile acids gets multiplied in the gallbladder.

In the fasting state, the sphincter of Oddi offers a high-pressure zone preventing bile flow into the duodenum, thus allowing it to concentrate in the gallbladder. This tonic contraction also serves in preventing duodenal content reflux into the pancreatic and bile duct. The sphincter of Oddi is controlled by neurohormonal mechanisms. The gallbladder pours its contents into the duodenum both postprandially and between meals. The secretion is primarily under control of influence of CCK.

GALLSTONE DISEASE

Gallstones are the most common disorders of the biliary system and one of the most common diseases of the digestive system (**Table 1**). It occurs in one of every eight individuals in the world. Indian studies show a lower prevalence. A study of 1,104 patients from India revealed a prevalence of 4.3% with a two to three-fold higher prevalence in North India. The incidence of gallstones is difficult to ascertain due to asymptomatic nature; however, it is likely to be increasing with the rise in obesity and other noncommunicable diseases.

TABLE 1 Diseases of the gallbladder.

Benign	Malignant
• Gallstone • Choledocholithiasis • Cholecystitis • Gallbladder dyskinesia • Gallbladder polyps—majority	• Gallbladder polyps—few • Carcinoma gallbladder

Gallstones are of three main types: (1) cholesterol, (2) pigment, and (3) rare stones. Cholesterol stones are composed of cholesterol monohydrate crystals and occur most frequently accounting for 75% of stones. Pigment stones can be black (~20%) or brown stones (~5%), which are formed in hemolytic anemia. Much higher proportions of cholesterol stones have also been reported in the Indian series.

RISK FACTORS

Risk factors for gallstones include increasing age, female gender (twice as common as males), diet rich in fats and refined sugars, and high-calorie diet. Pregnancy is an independent risk factor due to poor gallbladder motility by progesterone. Rapid weight loss post bariatric surgery is an increasingly recognized factor in the current era. Some implicated drugs in the pathogenesis of gallstones are hormones such as estrogen, ceftriaxone, fibrates, and somatostatin analogs.

FORMATION OF GALLSTONES

Bile is primarily composed of cholesterol and phospholipids. Although phospholipids are soluble in water, cholesterol is usually not. Its solubility in physiological state is dependent on the formation of micelles and vesicles which create an aqueous medium and lead to stable soluble structures in bile. As compared to micelles, vesicles are smaller in size, contain less of bile salts, and are produced in higher number during fasting state. In some situations, the cholesterol:phospholipid ratio in vesicles rises, the vesicle becomes unstable and combines to form liquid crystals, which are unstable and lead to solid plate such as cholesterol monohydrate crystal formation. This process is known as **cholesterol nucleation**. Some molecules such as mucin have been well established to be a pronucleating factor and others such as apolipoproteins have been shown to be inhibitors of nucleation. Imbalance from physiological levels may tilt the scale toward gallstone formation (**Flowchart 1**).

In some cases, the bile becomes *supersaturated*. The solubilization capacity of cholesterol is maximized in the micelles in such cases and the remaining insoluble cholesterol can form liquid crystals or cholesterol monohydrate crystals which are primers for gallstone formation. This phenomenon of supersaturation occurs

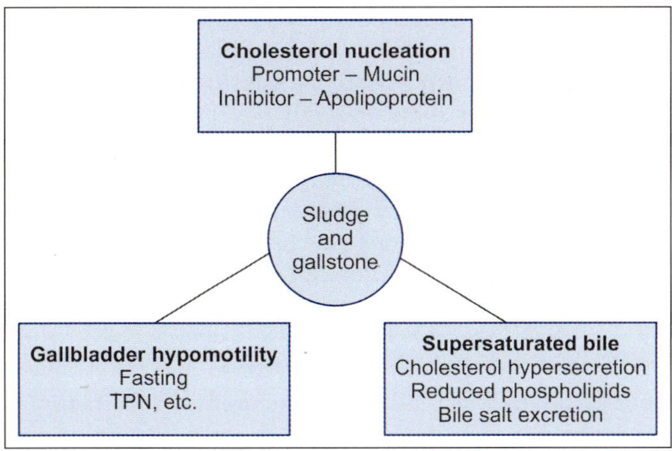

(TPN: total parenteral nutrition)

FLOWCHART 1: Gallstone formation.

due to either hypersecretion of cholesterol by the liver or relative undersecretion of lipids as compared to cholesterol. Increased cholesterol availability may also be present due to increased cholesterol absorption as a result of poor intestinal motility.

Apart from composition of bile, physical factors also play a role. A raised fasting gallbladder volume with incomplete emptying interprandially can lead to residual bile and has been shown to be associated with increased gallstone formation. This is termed as *gallbladder hypomotility*. A similar phenomenon is seen when the patient is on parenteral nutrition when the contraction of the gallbladder is incomplete and formation of gallstones is increased.

Finally, the role of *genetics* is being understood in all diseases. Gallstones occur three times more frequently amongst family members as compared to general population. Few of the genetic abnormalities associated with gallstone formation are the *LITH* genes including mutations in *CYP7A1*, *ABCB4* gene, genes responsible for CCK receptor, and many others.

Pigment stones: The mechanism for pigment stone formation is not as well elucidated as in cholesterol stones. The key abnormality is in the metabolism of bilirubin. There is increased unconjugated bilirubin and the stones are composed of bile pigment along with matrix of mucin glycoproteins. Black stones are composed of polymeric calcium bilirubinate while brown stones contain monomeric calcium bilirubinate. Chronic hemolytic anemias are responsible for most black stones which anatomical anomalies with bile stasis and biliary tract infection are responsible for brown stones.

CLINICAL FEATURES

The most common presenting manifestation of gall stone is biliary colic. The term itself is a misnomer as the pain is not intermittent but rather a continuous sort of pain when it occurs. The pain intensifies gradually over 15 minutes, plateaus over an hour, and then fades away. The pain usually lasts for a maximum of 6 hours and if it lasts longer, cholecystitis must be suspected. The location of the pain is predominantly -in the right upper quadrant or epigastric region. The pain is ill localized due to its visceral nature. There are also associated symptoms such as nausea and vomiting. Jaundice does not occur unless the stone is in the common bile duct (CBD).

There is a significant variation between the natural history of asymptomatic and symptomatic gall stones. A study following up asymptomatic gallstones has shown that over a long-term follow-up, 10, 15, and 18% patients became symptomatic at the end of 5, 10, and 15 years of follow-up. So a rate of 2% chance of symptoms per year is expected. This rate is slightly higher in diabetic patients. Another study had shown that over a follow-up after 24 years, only 28% of patients with asymptomatic gall stones persisted to have gall stones. This study demonstrated the high rate of spontaneous resolution of gallstones. There is no data from India on natural history of asymptomatic gallstones.

In symptomatic gall stones, the rate of recurrent pain is at almost 25–35% patients per year. The long-term rate of other major complications include biliary pancreatitis (5%), cholangitis (5%), and obstruction of the common hepatic duct by stone stuck in the cystic duct (Mirizzis syndrome, 0.1%). Large stones may erode and through into the bowel lumen and cause duodenal obstruction (Bouveret's syndrome) or small bowel obstruction due to distal ileal impaction (gallstone ileus). The most dreaded complication is development of cancer which can occur at 0.1% patients over time.

DIAGNOSIS

Ultrasound: Diagnosis of gallstones is primarily made by imaging modalities. The mainstay of diagnosis is transabdominal ultrasound. Gallstones appear as echogenic foci in the lumen of gallbladder and cast a posterior acoustic shadow. Ultrasound is observer dependent; however, if the gallbladder is properly visualized, there is a high degree of agreement between observers for gallstones. The sensitivity and specificity are both upward of 90% for stones >2 mm. The only limitation is nonvisualization of the gallbladder due to contraction or scarring; in which case another imaging modality is required.

Endoscopic ultrasound: The most accurate modality for evaluation of gallstones in the current era is endoscopic ultrasound (EUS). It can detect small calculi as well as accurately be used to evaluate the bile duct for calculi. Appearance of gallstone on EUS is similar to abdominal USG.

Other modalities to assess gallstones include magnetic resonance cholangiopancreatography (MRCP) which is also very accurate and almost comparable to EUS as well as more widely available.

Abdominal X-ray is not a recommended modality as only about 10–30% of gallstones are radiopaque. CT is also not a good modality for gallstone detection; however, it is useful when complications such as perforation or cholecystitis are suspected.

MANAGEMENT

Treatment options for gallstones include both medical and surgical. The progress in medical therapies has lagged behind endoscopic and surgical modalities. For gallstones alone, surgery remains the most important therapeutic option.

Indications for treatment: As observed from natural history studies, the rates of complications in asymptomatic gallstones are very low over long term. Hence, the standard recommendation is to not treat asymptomatic gallstones. This is based on calculations that compared the advantage of complication prevention by cholecystectomy with the complication rate associated with surgery. They found both to be almost equal; however, these analyses are based on prior data with open surgery.

Sometimes asymptomatic gallstones should also be treated if expected rate of complication is higher or severity of complication if occurs would be high. These scenarios include ethnic groups having high risk of gallbladder carcinoma and heart and lung transplant recipients. Although formerly advocated, diabetes with gallstone is no longer an indication for cholecystectomy. There are also soft pointers which when combined could favor cholecystectomy even in asymptomatic gallstones. These include young age (higher lifetime risk of carcinoma), very large (>3 cm) or very small (<3 mm) stones, calcified or nonfunctioning gallbladder, female gender (due to higher prevalence of malignancy).

Although the standard recommendation is for expectant management of asymptomatic simple gallstones, a case can be made for prophylactic cholecystectomy in ethnic populations having high risk of gallbladder cancer. This is followed in South American countries such as Chile and the policy has shown a reducing trend in incidence of carcinoma. The same is not advocated yet in India; however, the Gangetic belt in India is a high-risk zone.

The most common indication for treatment in symptomatic gallstones is recurrent biliary colic (**Flowchart 2**). Once symptomatic, the rate of complications rises significantly, so treatment must be considered unless there are contraindications. Other indications include complications of gallstone disease such as acute cholecystitis, gallstone pancreatitis, and history of cholangitis.

Medical management: The most established nonsurgical modality of treatment of gallstones includes oral dissolution therapy with ursodeoxycholic acid (UDCA). UDCA works by reducing the cholesterol secretion and thereby prevents the key step of bile supersaturation. Addition of other agents such as chenodeoxycholic acid or prokinetics has not been shown to be beneficial. UDCA is given at a dose of 10–15 mg/kg/day and best given at night time. The prerequisites for oral dissolution therapy alone are uncomplicated small gallstones (<10 mm in size) and a normally functioning gallbladder (by physiological tests). Failure of complete resolution of stones after a trial of 6 months is an indication to consider alternate treatment modality.

Extracorporeal shock wave lithotripsy (ESWL) is another nonsurgical therapy which is used as an adjunct to oral dissolution therapy. It works by breaking down stones and increasing the surface area of stones. Prerequisites

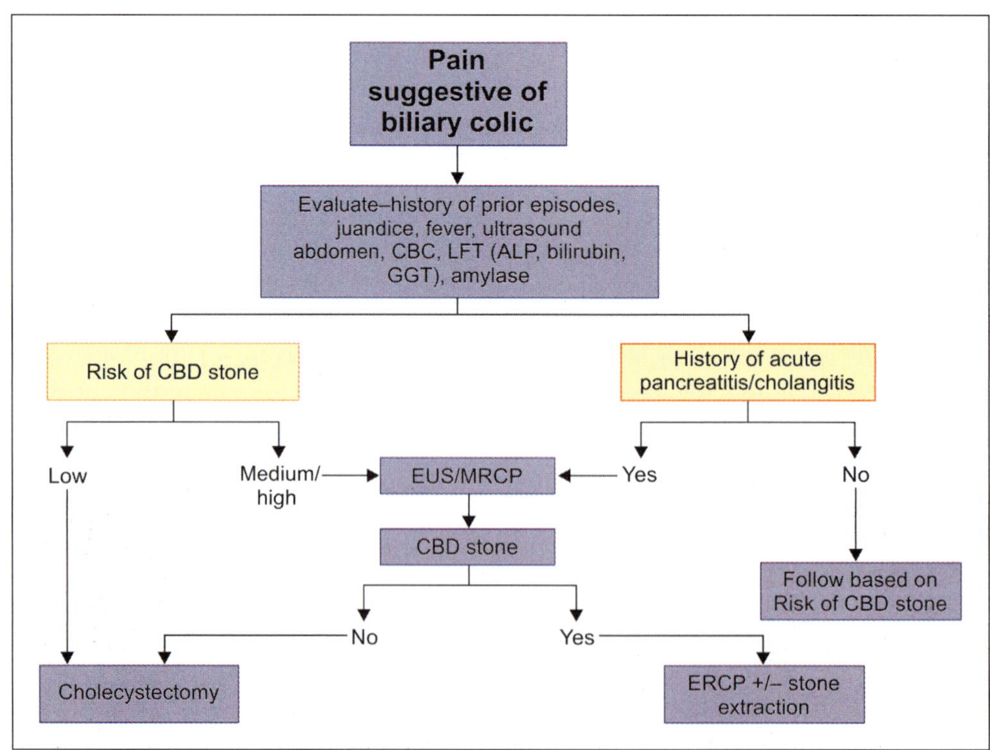

FLOWCHART 2: Approach to a patient with biliary colic.

for ESWL include noncalcified cholesterol stones of size <20 mm and a normally functioning gallbladder. UDCA is to be continued with ESWL; however, the clinical efficacy is only 40–70% at 6 months, in spite of multiple sessions.

Surgery: The limited efficacy of medical management makes surgery the cornerstone of therapy. Surgical techniques have improved significantly over time and complications associated with them have reduced. The laparoscopic approach has gained tremendous popularity and is performed six to seven times more frequently than open cholecystectomy. This approach is encouraged because of lower rate of morbidity and mortality and early recovery. It was limited previously by technical expertise and availability of instruments.

Open cholecystectomy has not lost its importance and conversion rate from laparoscopy to open is 5–10%. Most important reasons include difficult anatomy, injury, and need for exploration of bile duct. The rate of clinical success in amelioration of biliary pain is >90% with surgery and the overall mortality for cholecystectomy for elective surgery is <0.5%.

BILIARY SLUDGE

Biliary sludge is the term used to define the admixing of particulate matter with bile that results due to precipitation of solutes in bile. It consists of cholesterol crystals, calcium salts, protein-lipid complexes, and undefined substances. It is a crucial intermediate stage in the formation of both cholesterol and pigment gallstones. The crystals may also serve as a precursor lesion for stone formation, and sometimes may just remain as sludge. In case of associated stones, the composition is similar to stone, but in their absence the sludge is a representation of bile composition abnormality such as excess cholesterol or mucin. It is a diagnosis made on ultrasonography. Sludge appears as hypoechoic areas in the gallbladder without posterior acoustic shadowing. The sensitivity for sludge is lower than stones and it also cannot define the composition of precipitates. CT scan may also show a layering appearance which appears hyperdense as compared to normal bile due to calcium content. Microscopic examination of the bile by aspiration from duodenum is the method for proper identification of crystals, however, not used frequently. EUS has now become the most sensitive and specific method to detect sludge as for gallstones.

Sludge is seen with gallstones most commonly. Other risk factors include pregnancy, prolonged fasting, total parenteral nutrition (TPN), and use of medications such as ceftriaxone (combined with calcium).

Sludge should be suspected as a cause for typical biliary pain in the absence of documented gallstones on ultrasound. Previously, in such cases, duodenal aspirate of bile after CCK stimulation would be recommended; however, with the advent of EUS and its increasing availability, it is the investigation of choice in acalculous biliary pain.

Treatment of biliary sludge is largely similar to that of gallstones with minor differences. Surgical therapy is best for those with symptomatic sludge. Medical management with UDCA can be tried. In those who have a definite precipitant for sludge formation, removal of the factor may help. So, TPN should be replaced by enteral feed and early postoperative feeding is recommended to prevent biliary stasis. In very high-risk surgical candidates, who have had CBD obstruction or pancreatitis due to sludge, an endoscopic sphincterotomy may be done alone to prevent the dreaded complication of cholangitis and pancreatitis.

CHOLEDOCHOLITHIASIS

Choledocholithiasis is defined as occurrence of stones in the CBD. They are seen in 10–15% patients with gallstones while 95% of patients with CBD stone have gallstones. Although most cases of choledeocholithiasis involve gallstones passing into the CBD, de novo CBD stones are also well documented and may be seen in patients up to years post cholecystectomy. CBD stones may remain asymptomatic; however, stones may get occlude the CBD and lead to obstructive jaundice presenting with pain and jaundice with cholestatic features (in chronic cases). If the bile gets infected, cholangitis occurs which is a life-threatening illness. Due to this possibility of cholangitis and its associated mortality, even asymptomatic CBD stones warrant therapy.

Treatment is in the form of ERCP and stone removal followed by cholecystectomy. In some cases, precholecystectomy, liver function test (LFT) may provide a clue to diagnosis of presence of CBD stone. Raised alkaline phosphatase is a marker and should prompt evaluation with an MRCP or EUS prior to cholecystectomy as ultrasound is only ~50% sensitive for diagnosis of gallstones. In case, large CBD stones are found or in cases of nonavailability of ERCP, intraoperative cholangiogram/ultrasound may be used to decide regarding CBD exploration.

ACUTE CHOLECYSTITIS

Acute cholecystitis belongs to the spectrum of complicated gallstone disease. It occurs as a result of stone getting stuck in the cystic duct leading to chronic obstruction. The bile gets accumulated in the gallbladder and damages the mucosa leading to cell lysis and enzymatic degradation. Consequently, inflammatory pathways are activated leading to acute inflammation, necrosis, and edema.

Patients present with pain in the right upper quadrant that lasts for >6 hours (helps differentiate from biliary colic) with or without fever, nausea, and mild jaundice. The diagnosis is made initially on clinical grounds and supported by examination finding of Murphy's sign. However, sonographic Murphy's sign which is elicited during USG is more specific in the appropriate clinical setting. There is a wide range of differential diagnosis for cholecystitis including peptic ulcer disease, renal calculus, hepatitis etc., and they should be ruled out.

Management includes supportive care with intravenous fluids, balancing electrolytes, and organ support in case of severe disease. Patient is generally kept nil by mouth and diversion of gastric contents by nasogastric (NG) tube may help in abdominal distension. Antibiotics covering gram-negative rods and anaerobes are usually added, and definite therapy is cholecystectomy.

GALLBLADDER POLYP

Polyp is a mucosal projection and can be seen in multiple organs. Polyps in the gallbladder are of various types ranging from completely benign to those having a malignant potential. Most of the times, they are incidentally detected during routine ultrasonography of the abdomen. They increase with age and prevalence ranges from 1 to 5% of the population.

TYPES

Nonneoplastic:

Cholesterol polyp: They are the most commonly found polyps in the gallbladder. They are formed by the deposition of triglycerides and cholesterol esters in the gallbladder mucosa. Fat-laden macrophages are seen in the elongated villi. They are usually small, multiple, and pedunculated. They may break off and behave similarly to small stones.

Adenomyoma: It is the localized form of adenomyomatosis. It is characterized by overgrowth of the mucosa, thickening of the muscle wall, and intramural diverticula. On imaging, a sessile echogenic mass with multiple microcysts (dilated Rokitansky–Aschoff sinuses) or a comet-tail artifact is seen. It is usually solitary and slightly larger than cholesterol polyp.

Inflammatory polyp: They are composed of granulation tissue and inflammatory cells such as plasma cells and lymphocytes. They are less common and can be pedunculated or sessile.

Neoplastic:

Adenomas: They are rare benign epithelial tumors. Usually they are solitary, pedunculated and appear as homogenous isoechoic to liver on ultrasound. Based on pathology, they may be either papillary (branching tree like cytoskeleton of connective tissue) or nonpapillary (glandular proliferation encased by fibrous stroma). The progression to malignancy is based on size of polyp.

DIAGNOSIS

Usually they are asymptomatic and detected incidentally. Symptomatic polyps may cause right upper quadrant pain mimicking biliary pain and rarely a calculous cholecystitis. Clinical factors predicting malignant potential are symptomatic polyps and age >60 years.

Transabdominal ultrasound can detect up to 80% of polyps, however, it is more accurate in the absence of gallstones and even then cannot reliably differentiate between the types of polyps. EUS is a better method for detection as well as characterization. An EUS score including flow on Doppler can predict malignant potential of polyp with reasonable accuracy. Sometimes, when there are large polyps, FDG-PET (fluorodeoxyglucose-positron emission tomography) scan can be used to detect malignant tissue in the gallbladder. Imaging characters associated with high risk of malignant potential are size >10 mm, solitary polyp and concurrent gallstones.

MANAGEMENT

There is lack of good-quality data on natural history of gallbladder polyps. However, the available data suggests that most polyps are benign and premalignant polyps can be reliably identified with high-risk features. A study showed that over 5 years, polyps <10 mm showed no growth in 88% individuals. Another study concluded that size of the polyp is the highest predictor of malignant potential and most malignant polyps were >15 mm.

Symptomatic polyps should be managed with cholecystectomy, if the clinician feels the pain is of a biliary character. Cholecystectomy should also be considered if the polyps are >10 mm in size. The decision to go for surveillance with regular ultrasound can also be taken on an individual basis, depending on patient preference and surgical fitness. Polyps >18 mm should be taken up for surgery without delay and open surgery may be the better choice as these patients often have malignant cells. Frozen section during surgery should be obtained, wherever feasible. Asymptomatic polyps between 3–6 mm and 6–9 mm are management dilemmas. The decision between regular surveillance and elective cholecystectomy is a difficult one and no clear recommendation is available for this size.

CARCINOMA GALLBLADDER

Gallbladder carcinoma is a common malignancy of the GI tract and more so in the Indian subcontinent. The northern and eastern parts of India report a high incidence of carcinoma in gallbladder. The main risk factors for development are gallstone disease, typhoid carriers, low socioeconomic status, aflatoxins, and pancreaticobiliary malunion. Most commonly carcinoma is detected incidentally postoperatively in histopathology or during surgery. Symptomatic patients usually present at a late stage with pain abdomen, lump, or biliary obstruction. More than 50% of symptomatic patients are unresectable at the time of presentation.

Diagnosis is suspected by ultrasonography; however, CT is the most commonly used test which allows assessment of resectability in the form of locoregional anatomy as well as metastasis. In operable cases, preoperative histopathology is not a must but must be obtained before palliative or neoadjuvant therapy. Treatment is primarily surgical whenever possible. Palliative care includes pain relief; managing obstructive jaundice, cholestatic features, and gastric outlet obstruction; and gemcitabine-based chemotherapy if the patient's performance status allows.

RECOMMENDED READINGS

1. Jones MW, Hannoodee S, Young M. Anatomy, abdomen and pelvis, gallbladder. Treasure Island (FL): StatPearls Publishing; 2021.
2. Boyer JL. Bile formation and secretion. Compr Physiol. 2013;3(3):1035-78.
3. Tandon RK. Prevalence and type of biliary stones in India. World J Gastroenterol. 2000;6(Suppl 3):4-5.
4. Sarin SK, Kapur BM, Tandon RK. Cholesterol and pigment gallstones in northern India. A prospective analysis. Dig Dis Sci. 1986;31(10):1041-5.
5. Malet PF, Takabayashi A, Trotman BW, Soloway RD, Weston NE. Black and brown pigment gallstones differ in microstructure and microcomposition. Hepatology. 1984;4(2):227-34.
6. Gracie WA, Ransohoff DF. The natural history of silent gallstones: the innocent gallstone is not a myth. N Engl J Med. 1982;307(13):798-800.
7. Schmidt M, Hausken T, Glambek I, Schleer C, Eide GE, Søndenaa K. A 24-year controlled follow-up of patients with silent gallstones showed no long-term risk of symptoms or adverse events leading to cholecystectomy. Scand J Gastroenterol. 2011;46(7-8):949-54.
8. Ahmed A, Cheung RC, Keeffe EB. Management of gallstones and their complications. Am Fam Physician. 2000;61(6):1673-80.
9. Sanders G, Kingsnorth AN. Gallstones. BMJ. 2007;335 (7614):295-9.
10. Gupta D, Sakorafas GH, McGregor CG, Harmsen WS, Farnell MB. Management of biliary tract disease in heart and lung transplant patients. Surgery. 2000;128(4):641-9.
11. Gupta SK, Shukla VK. Silent gallstones: a therapeutic dilemma. Trop Gastroenterol. 2004;25(2):65-8.
12. Mathur AV. Need for prophylactic cholecystectomy in silent gall stones in North India. Indian J Surg Oncol. 2015;6(3):251-5.
13. Sakpal SV, Bindra SS, Chamberlain RS. Laparoscopic cholecystectomy conversion rates two decades later. JSLS. 2010;14(4):476-83.
14. Scollay JM, Mullen R, McPhillips G, Thompson AM. Mortality associated with the treatment of gallstone disease: a 10-year contemporary national experience. World J Surg. 2011;35(3):643-7.
15. Myers RP, Shaffer EA, Beck PL. Gallbladder polyps: epidemiology, natural history and management. Can J Gastroenterol. 2002;16(3):187-94.
16. Moriguchi H, Tazawa J, Hayashi Y, Takenawa H, Nakayama E, Marumo F, et al. Natural history of polypoid lesions in the gall bladder. Gut. 1996;39(6): 860-2.
17. Xu A, Zhang Y, Hu H, Zhao G, Cai J, Huang A. Gallbladder polypoid-lesions: What are they and how should they be treated? A single-center experience based on 1446 cholecystectomy patients. J Gastrointest Surg. 2017;21(11):1804-12.
18. Mainprize KS, Gould SW, Gilbert JM. Surgical management of polypoid lesions of the gallbladder. Br J Surg. 2000;87(4):414-7.
19. Kubota K, Bandai Y, Otomo Y, Ito A, Watanabe M, Toyoda H, et al. Role of laparoscopic cholecystectomy in treating gallbladder polyps. Surg Endosc. 1994;8(1):42-6.
20. Kubota K, Bandai Y, Noie T, Ishizaki Y, Teruya M, Makuuchi M. How should polypoid lesions of the gallbladder be treated in the era of laparoscopic cholecystectomy? Surgery. 1995;117(5):481-7.

CHAPTER 141

Approach to Management of Jaundice: Obstructive Jaundice/Hepatitis

Subrat K Acharya, Pankaj Puri, Shivanand Gamanogatti

ABSTRACT

Jaundice due to hepatitis and biliary tract obstruction have multiple causes. These etiologies include intrahepatic as well as extrahepatic pathologies. Identification of these broad categories at the initial evaluation of a jaundiced patient provides a possible differential diagnosis of specific etiology causing jaundice. At the initial evaluation, a thorough clinical history, physical examination along with liver function tests (LFTs) and abdominal ultrasonography differentiate the obstructive and hepatitis type of jaundice in most. However, to identify specific etiology causing hepatitis, further tests for serological and molecular diagnostic markers for various hepatitis virus(es) and autoimmune hepatitis (AIH) are needed. Such tests may also be necessary to diagnose reactivation of underlying pre-existing chronic hepatitis. Specific tests for diseases like Wilson's diseases, hemochromatosis may be necessary when clinical suspicion for such etiology exists. Therapy in such cases is directed at the specific etiology as enumerated in the text.

Ultrasonography and LFT indicating possibility of obstructive jaundice need further evaluation with more sophisticated imaging techniques such as magnetic resonance imaging (MRI) with magnetic resonance cholangiopancreatography (MRCP), contrast-enhanced computed tomography (CT) scan and endoscopic ultrasonography. Liver biopsy with evaluation of histology may be necessary, particularly in conditions where etiological diagnosis may be unclear and may be specific for certain diseases such as, chronic viral hepatitis with reactivation, alcoholic hepatitis, intrahepatic nonobstructive cholestatic hepatitis, drug-induced hepatitis, and AIH with or without overlap syndrome. Acute viral hepatitis (AVH) needs only supportive therapy whereas, reactivation of chronic hepatitis due to hepatitis B virus (HBV) should be treated with specific antiviral drugs against HBV. Therapy for AIH and alcoholic hepatitis includes corticosteroids with supportive treatment schedules. Treatment for Wilson's disease and hemochromatosis constitutes specific chelating agents. Liver transplantation may be necessary in some severe hepatitis ailments particularly when associated with features of liver failure, not responding to adequate medical treatment resulting in possibility of high mortality.

Treatment of obstructive jaundice is directed to treat the etiology. Surgical intervention is often necessary in such patients such as in patients with choledocholithiasis with cholelithiasis and cancers causing biliary obstructions. Adjuvant chemo and radiotherapy in later cases as and when necessary is instituted to improve progression free survival or recurrence of the mitotic disease. Often, biliary decompression using various endoscopic or percutaneous radiologic catheter-guided techniques may be needed as an essential component of such therapy. Irrespective of the cause of jaundice appropriate nutritional intervention is needed to improve the quality of life as well as to accelerate recovery in such patients.

"Progress is slow and gradual. Continue putting effort with patience, enthusiasm and faith"

—Anonymous

INTRODUCTION

Jaundice is a clinical manifestation characterized by yellow discoloration of the skin, sclerae, and mucous membranes due to deposition of bilirubin and is usually seen when the serum bilirubin levels are elevated above 3.0 mg% (hyperbilirubinemia). It occurs when liver is unable to metabolize or excrete bilirubin [a breakdown product of hemoglobin (Hb)] and indicates an underlying diseased status the liver or biliary tracts. It can also occur due to various inherited disorder of bilirubin metabolism and hemolytic conditions. Jaundice due to liver or biliary tract disorder needs systematic approach for appropriate management which includes diagnosis and appropriate treatment. Jaundice can occur due to multiple causes and best understood with understanding of bilirubin metabolism.

BILIRUBIN METABOLISM

Bilirubin metabolism primarily occurs in the hepatocytes (**Fig. 1**). Human red blood cells (RBCs) have a half-life of about 120 days and are degraded in the reticuloendothelial (RE) cells residing in spleen. Hb released from broken RBCs are further degraded to heme and globin and the RE enzyme heme oxidase further accts on heme (a cyclic tetrapyrrole ring) at α position of the tetrapyrrole ring to decarbonylate it with resultant biliverdin IX α which is converted to bilirubin IX α (unconjugated bilirubin—it is lipophilic)) by a cytosolic enzyme biliverdin reductase. Approximately 80% of this, bilirubin is derived from the breakdown of Hb of senescent erythrocytes with the remainder coming from various other hemoproteins such as myoglobin and cytochrome as well infrequently from intravascular hemolysis. In hemolytic diseases, this lipophilic unconjugated bilirubin gets elevated. Normally the unconjugated bilirubin comes to plasma where albumin binds it reversibly to transport it to the liver where through a carrier protein on hepatocyte membrane [organic anion transporting polypeptide (OATP)] translocate the free unconjugated bilirubin to hepatocyte cytosol, where glutathione-S transferase transports it to the smooth endoplasmic reticulum to conjugate it to hydrophilic bilirubin (conjugated bilirubin). Uridine diphosphate-glucuronosyltransferase is the enzyme which converts unconjugated bilirubin to conjugated uridine diphosphate monoglucuronide and then bilirubin diglucuronide (conjugated bilirubin). This conjugated bilirubin is transported across the hepatocyte apical plasma membrane to the biliary canaliculi via adenosine triphosphate (ATP)-dependent multidrug resistant-associated protein 2 (MRP2). Then through the bile ductules and bile ducts it is excreted to the duodenum through ampullary opening, subsequently it enters into the duodenum, small intestines, and to colon. In the colon, bacteria hydrolyze and reduce conjugated bilirubin to yield tetrapyrroles known as urobilinogen, approximately 90% of that is excreted in feces. Remaining urobilinogen is reabsorbed and eventually enter the portal circulation in which they are re-excreted by the liver, although a small portion reaches the kidneys and are excreted in the urine. About 4 mg/kg of bilirubin a day is produced in this way. Therefore, in diseases effecting the liver parenchyma or bile ductules or larger bile ducts, conjugated bilirubin gets elevated.

JAUNDICE: A CLINICAL SYNDROME

Jaundice is a clinical condition of yellow discoloration of mucus membrane, skin, and exposed elastic tissues like sclera, and occurs due to multiple systemic disorders in which serum bilirubin is elevated >3 mg/dL (usual normal level (1 mg/dL). Hyperbilirubinemia can occur due to excessive hemolysis (hemolytic jaundice) or hepatic parenchymal disorders (hepatic jaundice) and bilirubin

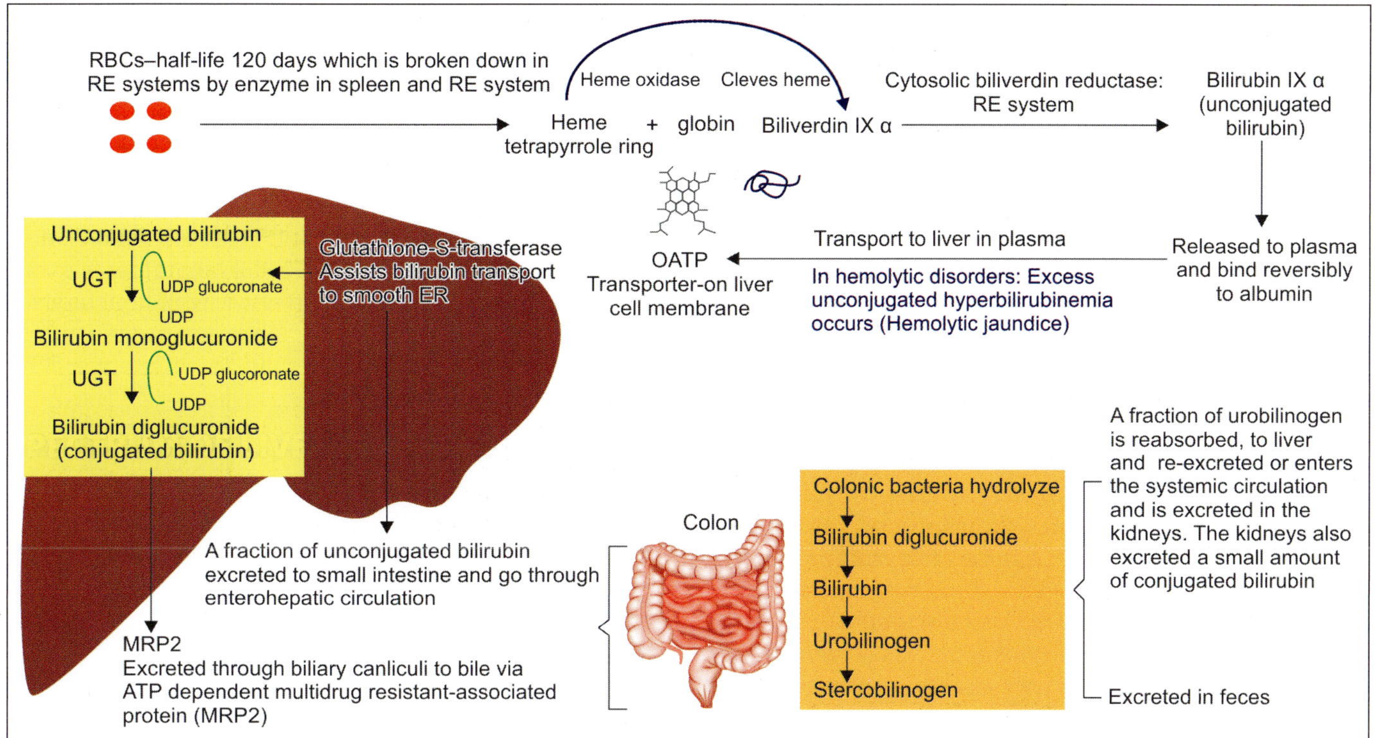

(ATP: adenosine triphosphate; OATP: organic anion transporter protein; RE: reticuloendothelial; UDP: uridine diphospho-glucuronosyltransferase; UGT: urldlne glucuronosyltransferase)

FIGURE 1: Bilirubin metabolism.

excretion disorder (obstructive jaundice). Each of these broad categories of jaundice results due to numerous etiologies causing specific categories of syndromic presentation of jaundice. Such etiologies are accompanied with etiology-specific symptoms and signs resulting in a syndromic disorder.

Therefore, history and physical examination are important components in differentiating these three basic categories of jaundice which in turn assist in achieving specific differential diagnosis under each categories and subsequent laboratory, imaging, and histopathology tests usually confirm specific etiological diagnosis of particular ailment manifesting as jaundice. Present chapter confines to the approach to hepatic and obstructive jaundice. These two broad categories can have overlapping clinical manifestation and yet may have overt or subtle distinct clinical features. Therefore, understanding the different causes and site of the pathogenic condition is important for differential diagnosis of a patient with jaundice.

DIFFERENTIAL DIAGNOSIS AND CAUSES

Jaundice is hyperbilirubinemia. Hyperbilirubinemia may be isolated hyperbilirubinemia and may be associated with other liver function abnormalities such as rise in transaminases, alkaline phosphatase abnormal prothrombin time, or lower serum albumin. Therefore, LFTs along with history and physical examination constitutes the initial approach in evaluation of a jaundiced patients which essentially can segregate intrahepatic as well extrahepatic causes of jaundice in about 60–70% of the cases with an overlap in about 30–40% of patients. Some authors try to approach a patient of jaundice as unconjugated or conjugated hyperbilirubinemia. However, we prefer to approach such patient with an effort to segregate them into broad categories of intrahepatic and extrahepatic causes of jaundice, because each of these categories has distinct etiology, clinical feature, imaging findings, and histology.

INTRAHEPATIC CAUSES OF JAUNDICE

The intrahepatic causes of jaundice can be broadly categorized to four distinct groups:

1. Liver parenchymal injury (primary hepatocyte damage)
2. Liver parenchymal damage with features of cholestasis
3. Intrahepatic biliary tract obstructive pathologies
4. Isolated hyperbilirubinemia without hepatocyte injury

Liver parenchymal injury (primary hepatocyte damage): There are many agents which can cause direct hepatocyte injury leading to bilirubin excretion compromise, such as *hepatitis virus(es)* which when infect human liver due to their hepatotropism initiate host immune-mediated parenchymal injury for clearance of such viral infections. Viral hepatitis is most frequent cause of both acute and chronic liver parenchymal injury.

Hepatitis virus(es) A through E, some nonA-nonE viruses are the usual hepatotropic or hepatitis viruses accounting to 85–90% of AVH presenting typically with hyperbilirubinemia, raised transaminases with or without prolonged International Normalized Ratio (INR), with or without compromise of synthetic functions of liver such as serum albumin levels. Not infrequently cytomegalovirus (CMV) and parvovirus in an immunosuppressed patient, Epstein–Barr virus and herpes simplex viruses (in pregnant females) can induce primary liver parenchymal injury.

Many hemorrhagic fever viruses such as Ebola, Lassa fever, and yellow fever have also been described to cause parenchymal liver injury with jaundice. In such patients, the transaminases are moderate-to-severely raised (up to 5,000 IU/L) along with varying degree of conjugated hyperbilirubinemia depending upon the degree of hepatocyte loss, presence of intrahepatic cholestasis and the duration of liver injury and associate hepatic regenerative capacity.

Other causes of parenchymal liver injury include *drugs* such as paracetamol overdose (>4 g/24 h), cloxacillin, amoxicillin, anticonvulsant (Na-valproate), antithyroid (carbamazepine), major tranquilizers like chlorpromazine, cancer chemotherapeutic agents, dapsones, halothane etc. Drug-induced liver injury (DILI) is a discussion by itself.

Excessive continuous *alcohol abuse* has been identified as an important cause of acute hepatitis, acute on chronic hepatitis with or without liver failure as well cirrhosis with sepsis and jaundice.

Various complementary alternative medicines containing heavy metals and alkaloids have been implicated in acute liver injury and not infrequently with acute liver failure (ALF).

Rarely, *ischemic liver injury* due to hypotension, acute Budd–Chiari syndrome, sinusoidal obstruction syndromes, and severe sepsis may cause liver injury with jaundice. Many etiologies of chronic liver disease such as AIH, Wilson's disease, and chronic hepatitis due to HBV may undergo a phenomenon identified as reactivation causing accelerated hepatocyte injury resulting in rise in conjugated bilirubin with rise in transaminases.

A primary hepatic parenchymal injury due to above-mentioned etiologies classically presents with icterus, tender hepatomegaly, anorexia, nausea, and fatigue and is associated with conjugated hyperbilirubinemia with marked rise in hepatic transaminases [alanine transaminase (ALT) > aspartate transaminase (AST)] with or without prolonged INR, but usually with normal albumin level and an ultrasonography not revealing features suggestive of biliary tract obstruction in the form of dilated intrahepatic biliary channels. A prolonged INR > 1.5 is termed as severe acute liver injury (sALI).

Specific etiology of the injury (acute hepatitis or reactivation of underlying chronic liver disease) is reached through specific diagnostic serological and molecular diagnostic tests. Not infrequently, a liver biopsy is needed to identify the severity of liver injury as well as specific etiology through immunohistochemistry for specific infective peptides present in the liver. The various etiologies and their diagnostic approach have been provided in **Table 1**.

In tropical countries like India, various endemic systemic infective agents such as dengue, malaria, leptospirosis, and scrub typhus may also present with febrile illness with acute hepatitis (icteric or anicteric), in whom fever with constitutional symptoms persists throughout the illness period and specific diagnostic tests determine the etiology in such cases (**Table 2**). In such cases, the febrile illness is dominant and altered liver function in the form of raised AST/ALT (less than five times of upper limit of normal), AST > ALT, lactate dehydrogenase (LDH): AST ratio of more than one with normal INR is the usual laboratory features. Icterus is usually infrequent. Awareness with high index of suspicion combined with specific laboratory tests (**Table 2**) achieves definitive diagnosis in them, facilitating specific management.

Liver parenchymal damage with feature of jaundice and cholestasis: There are many specific etiologies causing parenchymal liver injury with features of cholestasis without any imaging evidence of biliary obstruction. Such patients do have itching and clay colored stool, but usually the features of cholangitis in the form of fever with chills and rigor. Such cholestasis occurs either due to canalicular cholestasis due to ballooning degeneration of hepatocytes typically seen in AVH particularly after first week of the icteric illness or due to injury to cholangioles as in DILI and AIH. Some of the congenital genetic aberrations such as benign recurrent intrahepatic cholestasis (BRIC), cholestasis of pregnancy (COP), and progressive familial intrahepatic cholestasis (PFiC) may also present with cholestatic features, but in them the evidence of parenchymal liver injury in the form of raised hepatic transaminases (AST and ALT) or in histology is infrequent. However, gamma-glutamyl transpeptidase (GGTP) may be raised in them. Their diagnosis is based on typical clinical history, familial predisposition, and histology with exclusion other causes as depicted in **Table 1**.

Intrahepatic biliary tract obstructive pathologies: Intrahepatic biliary tract pathologies such as intrahepatic primary sclerosing cholangitis (PSC), particularly with small duct involvement; vanishing bile duct diseases due to primary biliary cirrhosis (PBC); autoimmune cholangiopathies, sarcoidosis, certain types of lymphoma, post-liver transplant chronic rejection, may clinically present with features of jaundice with features of cholestasis, but without any imaging evidence of biliary obstruction in the form of dilated intrahepatic biliary channels. Usually in such patients, the histology is necessary to provide definitive diagnosis as each of these conditions has characteristic histological features. The LFT typically reveals raised alkaline phosphatase with raised GGTP with or without prolonged INR which improves with injectable vitamin K.

Isolated hyperbilirubinemia without parenchymal liver Injury: Isolated hyperbilirubinemia is typically found in the inherited intrahepatic disorders. The most frequent and well-studied disorders include inherited disorder with isolated unconjugated and isolated conjugated hyperbilirubinemia without raised transaminases or

TABLE 1 Etiologies of liver parenchymal injury (hepatitis) presenting with jaundice and their diagnosis methods.

Broad categories	Specific etiology	Diagnosis
Acute hepatitis virus(es)	HAV, HEV, HBV, nonA nonE, HDV, acute-HCV (rarely cause jaundice)	Specific viral serology by ELISA (IgM HAV; IgM HEV; IgM anti-HBc, HBsAg; HDV-Ag, IgM anti-HDV; anti-HCV/HCV-RNA (PCR); nonA nonE—presentation like acute hepatitis without any above serology positivity
Reactivation of underlying chronic liver disease	Chronic hepatitis-HBV, autoimmune hepatitis, Wilson's disease, hemochromatosis, and cirrhosis with sepsis	HBsAg with raised HBV DNA and anti-HBe positivity; auto antibodies like ANA, ASMA, anti-LKM1, anti-SLA, raised serum IgG; Low serum ceruloplasmin with raised urinary copper/KF ring positivity/*ATPB7* gene mutation; serum ferritin/*HFE* gene mutation. Often liver histology needed
Systemic viral infections	CMV, EB, Ebola, and Lassa fever	IgM CMV, CMV DNA (PCR); EB virus serology (ELISA); Ebola virus antibody by ELISA, RT-PCR for Ebola RNA; IgM antibody to Lassa fever virus, RT-PCR for Lass RNA, Lassa antigen
Drug-induced liver disease	Anti-TB drugs, paracetamol overdose, cloxacillin, Na-valproate, carbamazepine, chlorpromazine, and rat poison containing yellow phosphorus	History of specific drugs with exclusion of other causes
Hepatic ischemia	Hypotension, acute Budd–Chiari syndrome, and sinusoidal obstruction syndrome	History, imaging, and histology
Alcohol abuse	Alcoholic hepatitis, ACLF, and cirrhosis	History and exclusion of other causes
CAMs	Ayurvedic drug and indigenous drugs	History and exclusion of other causes
Rare causes	Tubercular liver, sarcoidosis of liver, amyloidosis, hepatic lymphoma, sepsis, and cystic fibrosis	Histology and imaging
Tropical infections	Dengue, malaria, scrub typhus, and leptospirosis	Specific blood tests in **Table 2**

(ACLF: acute-on-chronic liver failure; ASMA: anti-smooth muscle antibody; CAMs: complementary and alternative medicines; HBc: hepatitis B core; SLA: soluble liver antigen; TB: tuberculosis)

alkaline phosphatase and GGTP. There are three types of inherited, primarily unconjugated hyperbilirubinemias: Gilbert syndrome, Crigler–Najjar syndrome type 1, and Crigler–Najjar syndrome type 2. They are caused by the direct result of mutations in the UGT (**Fig. 1**) gene that code for a defective protein unable to perform the process of conjugation of unconjugated bilirubin to conjugated bilirubin (**Fig. 1**). In contrast, the most common causes of primarily conjugated hyperbilirubinemia (or mixed) include the Dubin–Johnson syndrome (DJS) and Rotor's syndrome. DJS results from impaired bilirubin transport by MRP2 (**Fig. 1**). These patients usually have a characteristic black liver due to a deposition of a melanin like pigment. Rotor's syndrome is a mild, predominately conjugated hyperbilirubinemia thought to stem from functional deficiencies of the organic anion transporter, *OATP* genes. Both of these transporter disorders are benign.

There are a number of miscellaneous disorders such as cystic fibrosis, infiltrative liver diseases like non-Hodgkin's lymphoma, various paraneoplastic syndromes, and severe sepsis can present with jaundice.

EXTRAHEPATIC CAUSES OF JAUNDICE

Biliary tract obstruction due to both benign as well as malignant pathologies, causes excretion defect of bilirubin and results in conjugated hyperbilirubinemia with raised alkaline phosphatase and GGTP. Some of the systemic illness such as PSC associated with inflammatory bowel diseases (IBDs) like ulcerative colitis and Crohn's disease and immunoglobulin G4 (IgG4) systemic illness causing inflammatory changes in the biliary channel (pseudosclerosing cholangitis) may present with features of obstructive jaundice. The obstruction to biliary tract can be intrahepatic as well extrahepatic. These patients typically present with features of cholestasis, right hypochondriac pain with often features of cholangitis as fever with rigor and chills. These causes have been depicted in **Table 3**.

The ultrasound will show dilated intrahepatic biliary channels with CBD dilatation in obstructive jaundice (**Figs. 2 A** and **B**). In patients with CBD stone this is better visible on Magnetic resonance cholangiopancreatography (MRCP) and endoscopic retrograde cholangiopancreatography (ERCP) (**Figs. 3 A to D**). In malignant block of CBD the mass lesion may also be visible (**Figs. 4 A** and **B**).

TABLE 2 Tropical infections causing febrile illness with jaundice.

Disease	Clinical and laboratory distinctiveness	Diagnostic test
Severe falciparum malaria	• Fever and chills and hepatosplenomegaly • Altered sensorium ± seizure • Anemia due to hemolysis • Hemoglobinuria and renal failure • Shock can be present • Unconjugated hyperbilirubinemia, mild increase in AST/ALT with normal INR	• Peripheral blood smear for malaria parasite • Quantitative buffy coat test • Rapid diagnostic kit (ICT) • Combination of tests can detect with a sensitivity and specificity of >95%
Dengue fever	• High-grade persistent fever, headache, and retro-orbital pain • Myalgia, arthralgia, and rash (dengue fever) or • Skin/mucosal bleeds, rise in hematocrit (dengue hemorrhagic fever) or • Hypotension • Wide pulse pressure <20 mm Hg, or • Complications such as encephalitis, myocarditis, hepatitis, renal failure, ARDS (dengue shock syndrome) • Mild rise in bilirubin, AST/ALT raised 5–20 times, AST > ALT • Thrombocytopenia and hematocrit rise • Evidence of muscle injury raised CPK	• NS1 antigen detection • IgM and IgG dengue serology
Leptospirosis	• Fever, headache, myalgia, abdominal pain, conjunctival suffusion, transient skin rash • Severe form, i.e., Weil's disease, with jaundice, proteinuria, hematuria, AKI, pulmonary hemorrhages, ARDS, myocarditis, and hepatomegaly	• Raised creatinine phosphokinase levels • Serologic test, MAT • IgM ELISA
Scrub typhus	• Prolonged fever, headache and myalgia, breathing difficulty, delirium, cough, and jaundice • Hepatomegaly common • Characteristic rash: Eschar early in disease • Jaundice–hepatocellular, AST/ALT raised less than five times • Normal INR	• Indirect fluorescent antibody: "Gold standard" • ELISA IgG and IgM antibodies: Sensitivity and specificity > 90%

(ALT: alanine aminotransferase; AST: aspartate aminotransferase; INR: international normalized ratio; MAT: microscopic agglutination test)

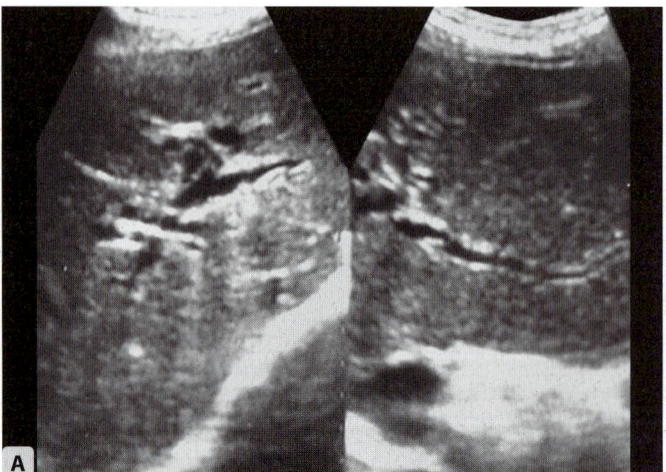

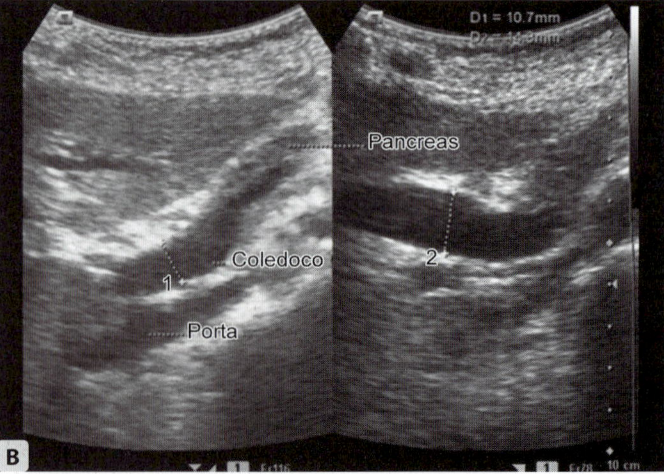

FIGURES 2 A & B: (A) Ultrasound image showing dilated intrahepatic biliary channels suggestive of obstructive jaundice; **(B)** Obstruction at lower end of common bile duct (CBD) causing CBD dilatation.

TABLE 3 **Extrahepatic causes of jaundice and their specific features and diagnostic approach.**

Causes	Specific clinical and laboratory features	Diagnosis
Benign		
Acquired pathologies: • Intrahepatic ductal stones • Choledocholithiasis	Abdominal pain, fever, jaundice, and hepatomegaly	• LFT: Raised conjugated bilirubin/ALP/AST • US–IHBRD + stones • Dilated CBD + stone
Primary sclerosing cholangitis	• Recurrent fever with jaundice • Usually in males	• LFT: Raised ALP, raised bilirubin • MRCP: Typical cholangiography
Benign biliary strictures (postcholecystectomy, anastomotic strictures, tubercular stricture, lower common bile duct strictures due to chronic pancreatitis, pancreatic tuberculosis of head of pancreas or postinflammatory subsequent to passage of gallstones)	Relevant history and cholestatic clinical feature in isolation or combination	Cholestatic LFT, typical cholangiography features in MRCP or ERCP
• Parasitic infections such as Roundworm in Biliary Tract and ruptured hydatid cysts to biliary channel • Pseudocyst of pancreas • Benign tumors such as lipoma, neurofibroma, leiomyoma in extrahepatic bile ducts	Relevant history	Cholestatic LFT, ultrasound and typical cholangiography on MRCP and ERCP
Congenital pathologies: • Choledochal cysts		
Systemic diseases		
• Inflammatory bowel disease causing PSC • IgG4 disease causing pseudosclerosing cholangiopathy		
Malignant		
Proximal or hepatic hilar pathologies: • Carcinoma gallbladder • Cholangiocarcinoma of bile ducts • Metastatic infiltration of carcinoma of antrum of stomach • Lymph nodes in hepatic hilum compressing the common hepatic duct	Constitutional symptoms of mitotic diseases such as anorexia, weight loss with pain abdomen, cholestatic jaundice, and abdominal lumps	Cholestatic LFT, CECT abdomen, contrast-enhanced MRI with MRCP, and histology
Distal biliary tract/lower end common bile duct pathologies: • Periampullary cancer • Pancreatic cancer • Lower bile duct cholangiocarcinoma	Cholestatic jaundice, typical pancreatic pain referred to back, and palpable gallbladder	Cholestatic LFT, cholangiographic picture in MRCP, and ultrasonography

(ALP: alkaline phosphatase; AST: aspartate aminotransferase; IHBRD: intrahepatic biliary radical dilatation; IgG4: immunoglobulin G4; MRCP: magnetic resonance cholangiopancreatography; PSC: primary sclerosing cholangitis)

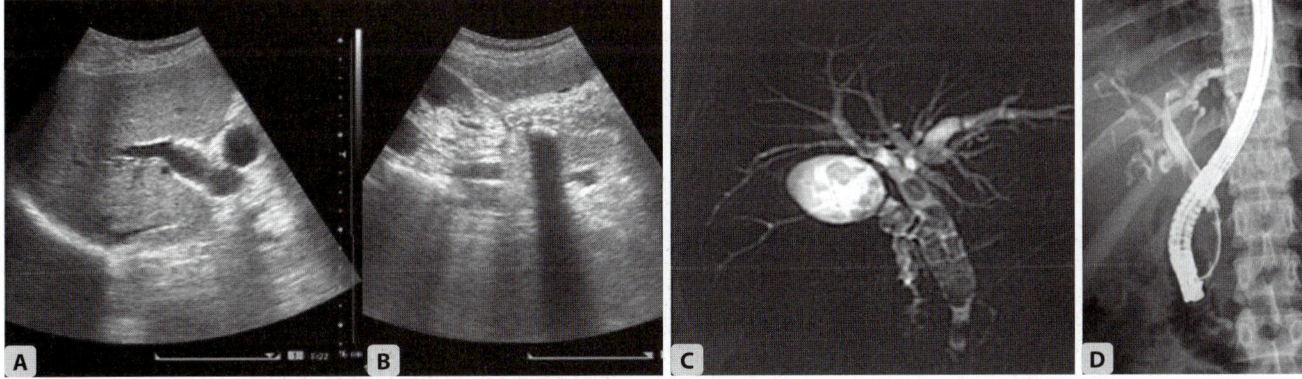

FIGURES 3 A to D: **(A)** Ultrasound image of dilated common bile duct (CBD) till lower end; **(B)** Ultrasound image showing CBD calculus blocking the lower end of CBD; **(C)** Magnetic resonance cholangiopancreatography (MRCP) image showing gallbladder calculi with choledocholithiasis; **(D)** Endoscopic retrograde cholangiopancreatography (ERCP) image showing CBD stone in gallbladder with choledocholithiasis.

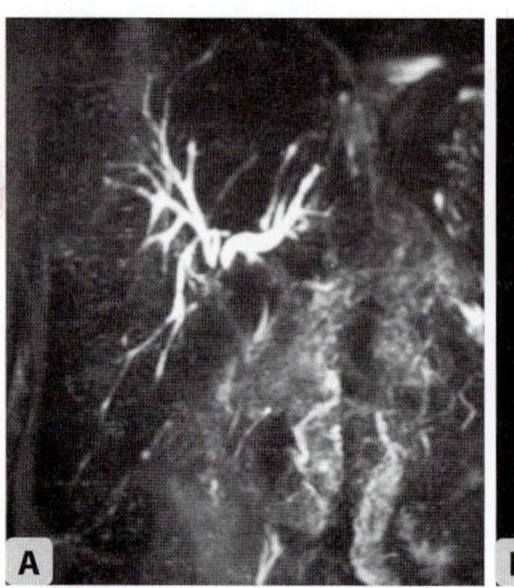

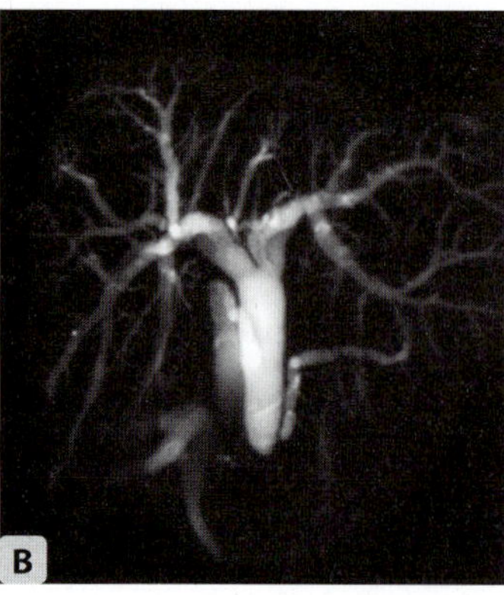

FIGURES 4 A & B: Magnetic resonance cholangiopancreatography (MRCP) image showing **(A)** hilar block due to cholangiocarcinoma and **(B)** lower end common bile duct (CBD) block due to pancreatic head cancer.

CLINICAL APPROACH

Management of any type of jaundice is based on identification of specific broad categories of jaundice and the specific etiology. The management is distinct as per the etiology of jaundice. At the initial clinical management approach, identification of the broad category of jaundice as depicted in earlier paragraphs helps in limiting the differential diagnosis of etiology to certain specific causes and thereby assists in choosing specific diagnostic tests which in turn decides the specific treatment strategy. Such approach in diagnosis includes clinical history and physical examination and investigations or laboratory tests, to establish the broad categories of jaundice followed by specific further tests using various imaging modalities [ultrasonography, contrast enhanced CT scan/MRI with cholangiopancreatography (contrast-enhanced MRI with MRCP)] and when necessary a liver histological study to clinch the etiological diagnosis (**Tables 1** to **4**).

HISTORY AND PHYSICAL EXAMINATION

Detailed history and physical examination can provide vital clues towards the etiology of the jaundice. **Table 4** depicts the various important aspects of clinical features in a jaundiced patient. History elicitation should specifically include a history of prodrome, history of cholangitis/cholestasis, and color of urine and stools. History of travel, ethanol intake, drugs, blood transfusion, needle stick exposure or tattooing, and sexual history are also important. In above paragraphs, a brief but distinct clinical characteristic of each broad categories of jaundice has been provided.

SUGGESTIVE OF HEPATOCELLULAR JAUNDICE

- A history of prodrome of anorexia, nausea, and vomiting suggests AVH.
- History of AVH in other members of the family also suggests a possibility of acute hepatitis.
- History of significant alcohol intake, blood transfusion, needle stick exposure, and history of intravenous (IV) drug use or tattooing may help as additional clinical clue to the hepatitic type of illness (parenchymal injury). The later history of transfusion and other parenteral exposure is relevant for parenterally transmitted hepatitis virus infection such as hepatitis B

TABLE 4 Clinical features in jaundice.

History and symptoms	Physical examination	Interpretation
• Prodrome (anorexia, nausea, fever, myalgia, and fatigue of duration of 7–15 days) • *Risk factors*: Household/neighbor contact, travel to endemic area of hepatitis virus(es), transfusion during previous 6 months, drug abuse, men having sex with men, and pregnancy in endemic area Immunosuppressed patients	Smooth tender hepatomegaly usually <5 cm	• Acute viral hepatitis (AVH) • Drug-induced hepatitis • Reactivation of CH-B • Tropical infections such as dengue, malaria, leptospirosis, and scrub typhus
• Pain abdomen (right hypochondrium/epigastrium) • Fever with chills/rigor • Subsequent itching/pale stool	Hepatomegaly, may be >5 cm with without palpable smooth or irregular gallbladder lump	Obstructive jaundice, benign or malignant
Jaundice with altered sensorium with features of prodrome	Overt encephalopathy	Acute liver failure
Jaundice with ascites (with previous history of diagnosed chronic liver disease, history of variceal bleed, pedal edema, weight loss, fatigue, loss of muscle mass, darkening of skin, and alcohol abuse of >5 years	Ascites, pedal edema, palpable left lobe, splenomegaly, prominent epigastric or flank or back veins	• Acute-on-chronic liver failure (ACLF) • Cirrhosis with acute decompensation

- Certain physical findings may suggest particular liver diseases, such as hyperpigmentation in hemochromatosis, xanthomas in primary biliary cirrhosis, and Kayser–Fleischer rings in Wilson's disease.
- *Jaundice with febrile illness*: Usually in AVH the fever subsides after onset of icterus, but if fever persists even after icterus the tropical infections/biliary obstruction may be suspected and specific tests for them need to be carried out.

and hepatitis C virus infection and excessive alcohol consumption in absence of the hepatitis viral infection (established subsequently with appropriate tests) may suggest alcohol-associated liver diseases.

- Presence of associated autoimmune diseases such as hypothyroidism, rheumatoid arthritis, SLE, or other forms of vasculitis, psoriasis, and celiac disease particularly in female sex points to autoimmune pathology.
- Young adolescent presenting with movement disorders raises suspicion of Wilson's disease and presence of diabetes, darkening of skin/hyperpigmentation, and testicular atrophy may lead to suspicion of hemochromatosis.
- Presence of certain stigmata of chronic liver disease such as ascites and history of hematemesis/melena/encephalopathy, presence of testicular atrophy, loss of secondary sexual characteristics, clubbing, spider naevi, palmar erythema, parotid swelling, sarcopenia, presence of caput medusae (periumbilical dilated vein with flow away from the umbilicus)/distended veins in epigastric region, palpable spleen, and left lobe of liver may suggest presence of underlying cirrhosis of liver.
- Certain physical findings may suggest particular liver diseases, such as hyperpigmentation in hemochromatosis, xanthomas in PBC, and Kayser–Fleischer rings in Wilson's disease.
- Presence of dilated flank and back veins with flow upwards with marked hepatomegaly may suggest hepatic outflow tract obstruction.

SUGGESTIVE OF OBSTRUCTIVE JAUNDICE

- Pruritus and clay-colored stools are the hallmark of cholestatic liver disease.
- Previous biliary surgery with subsequent jaundice suggests strictures, residual stones, or transfusion/surgery-related hepatitis.
- High fever and right upper abdominal tenderness suggest cholangitis due to choledocholithiasis, stricture in common bile duct or chronic rejection resulting in vanishing bile duct syndrome (VBDS).
- History of recent liver transplant may suggest anastomotic stricture in common bile duct, or chronic rejection resulting in VBDS.
- Association of IBD presenting with features of cholestasis may suggest PSC.
- A patient with history of acute pancreatitis in recent past and presenting with features of cholestatic jaundice with or without cholangitis may suggest bile duct obstruction due to pseudocyst of pancreas compressing the bile duct or presence of choledocholithiasis which might have caused pancreatitis.
- A palpable abdominal mass suggests a malignant obstructive jaundice.
- A right upper abdominal scar or palpable gallbladder is a clue to suggest obstructive jaundice.
- Usually, the liver enlargement in obstructive jaundice is marked.

INVESTIGATIONS

In any patients presenting with jaundice, the clinical features need to be corroborated with laboratory investigations and initial ultrasonographic examination to achieve the categorization of such patients to the above-mentioned broad categories of jaundice and then specific imaging or histology may be performed to achieve specific diagnosis. However, other tests including hematological tests, renal function parameters, glycemic status, the lipid profile, and serum electrolytes are necessary as supportive tests for monitoring and assessment of the general well-being and presence of comorbidity in such patient for a holistic management approach. In the form of **Flowchart 1**, a simple approach has been provided to assist the diagnostic algorithm for jaundice due to hepatitis and **Flowchart 2**, in providing the practical brief investigation that can be systematically or simultaneously carried out to achieve the specific diagnosis in obstructive jaundice.

TREATMENT

Once the broad category and specific cause of the jaundice is established, the therapy in individual cases optimally can be structured as follows:

- Treatment of specific causes of the jaundice with treatment for cholestasis and cholangitis when present and palliative treatment for those in whom curative options are limited (particularly malignant obstructive jaundice)
- Nutritional and other supportive therapy

TREATMENT OF SPECIFIC CAUSES OF JAUNDICE

Viral hepatitis: Usually acute viral hepatitis A through E have been implicated in causing acute hepatitis and jaundice due to parenchymatous liver injury indicated by hepatitis type of abnormal LFT—conjugated hyperbilirubinemia with transaminase about 10 times or more than the upper limit of normal. Most AVH (particularly due to HAV, HEV, and HBV) are self-limiting with spontaneous improvement in about 98–99% and 1–2% may develop ALF in whom management and specific therapy are distinct and needs a separate chapter for detailed discussion. AVH-HAV (IgM anti-HAV +ve) and AVH-HEV (IgM anti-HEV +ve) usually need symptomatic treatment and no specific drugs have been recommended in them to reduce the duration of the illness or prevent ALF, despite the fact some agents in cell culture have been shown moderate efficacy in inhibiting viral replication.

About 95% of the acute HBV infections in adults in contrast to 5% infections in pediatric population (at birth or before 5 years) clear the HBV spontaneously. Acute HBV infection indicated by abnormal hepatitis type of LFT, and positive serology IgM anti-hepatitis B core (HBc) antibody positivity with or without hepatitis B surface antigen (HBsAg) positivity, with hepatitis B envelope antigen (HBeAg) negative with or without anti-HBe positivity and HBV-deoxyribonucleic acid (DNA) positive in the early phase (during incubation or first week of rise in transaminases)

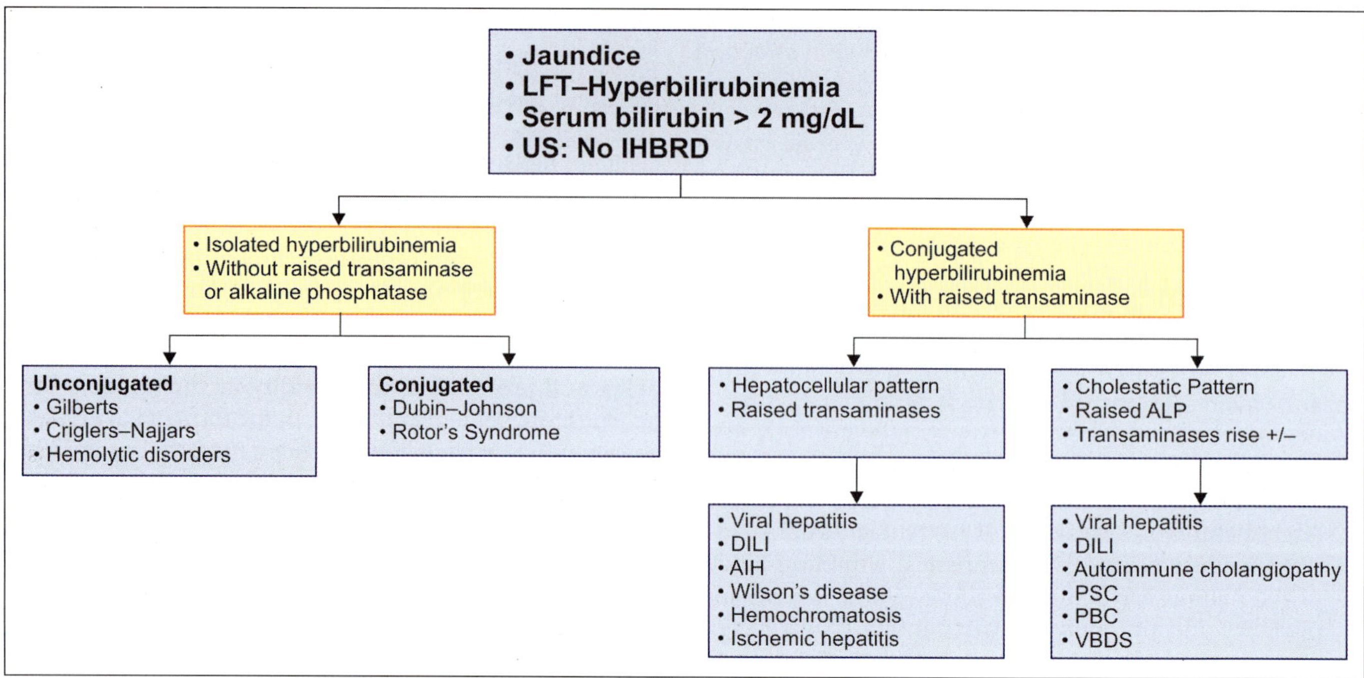

Note: Magnetic resonance cholangiopancreatography (MRCP)/liver biopsy may be necessary in specific cases.

(AIH: autoimmune hepatitis; DILI: drug-induced liver injury; IHBRD: intrahepatic biliary tract dilatation; PBC: primary biliary cirrhosis; PSC: primary sclerosing cholangitis; VBDS: vanishing bile duct syndrome)

FLOWCHART 1: Diagnostic algorithm for hepatitis with jaundice.

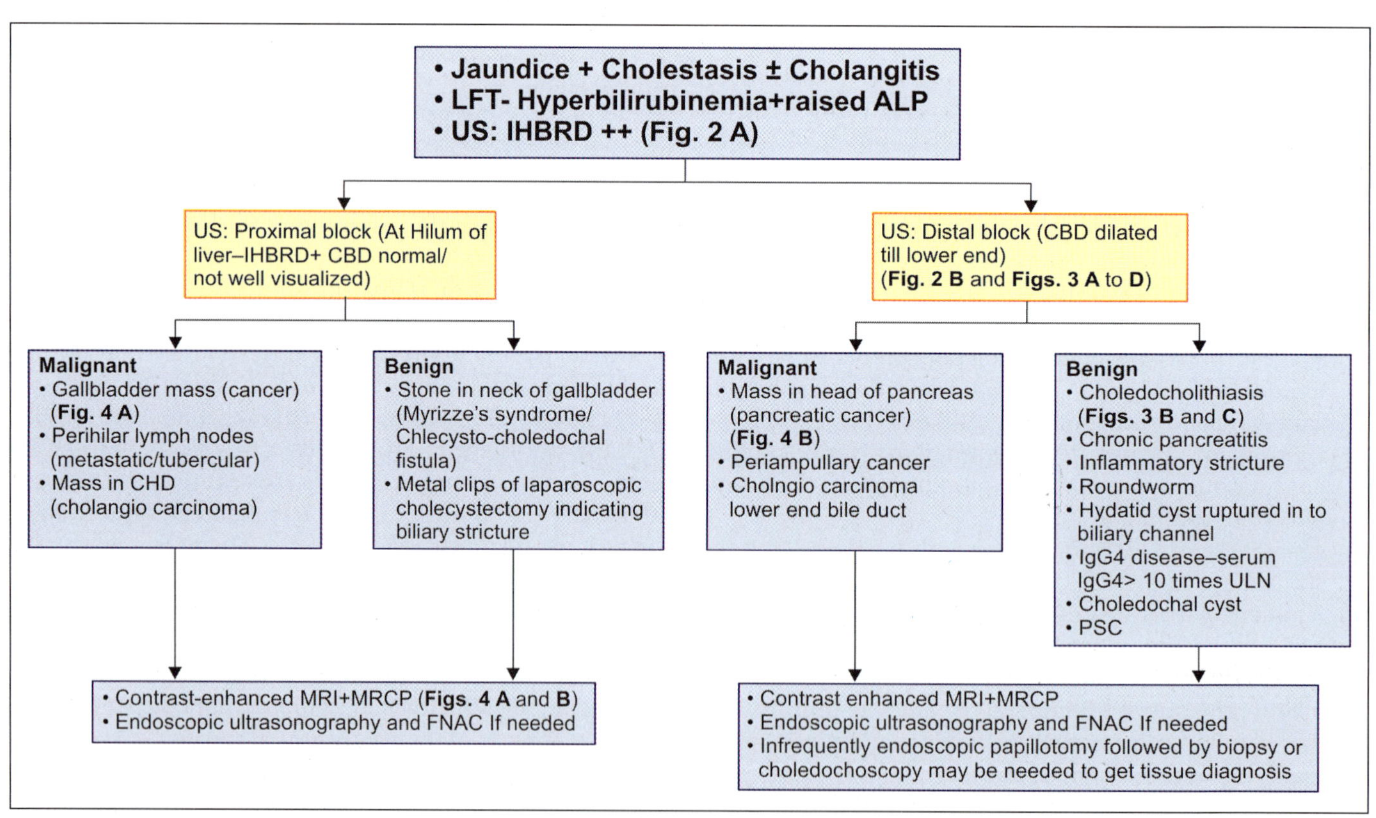

(CHD: common hepatic duct; IgG4: immunoglobulin G4; IHBRD: intrahepatic biliary tract dilatation; PSC: primary sclerosing cholangitis; ULN: upper limit of normal)

FLOWCHART 2: Diagnostic algorithm for obstructive jaundice.

and negative in the later phases and they clear HBsAg with anti-HBs antibody seroconversion during ensuing 6 months of follow-up with complete clinical, biochemical, and virological recovery without specific antiviral therapy.

Acute hepatitis C virus infection is anicteric in about 75% of the patients and presence of jaundice following acute hepatitis C which is infrequent (5–25%), indicates a better outcome. However in such patients, spontaneous clearance during ensuing 6 months is infrequent and about 50–75% of them have been reported to have long-term persistence of HCV with late sequels such as chronic hepatitis, cirrhosis, and even hepatocellular cancer. Therefore, they have been recommended to be treated with pan genotypic direct-acting antiviral (DAAs) like sofosbuvir (400 mg/day) with velpatasvir (100 mg daily) for about 12 weeks.

There are now many effective pan genotypic DAAs for treating HCV infections resistant to above therapy. They include combination treatment with above two drugs with voxilaprevir (100 mg/day) for 12–24 weeks with or without ribavirin (dose as per weight- 1,000 mg/day for <75 kg and 1,200 mg/day >75 kg). Combination of glecaprevir (300 mg/day) with pibrentasvir (120 mg/day) for 12 weeks with or without weight-based ribavirin is also effective. Interferon with ribavirin also has been shown to be effective in such patients, but presently infrequently used because of associated side effects of these two later drugs. Treatment of acute HCV infection with above treatment has been reported to clear the virus in 98–100% of such patients.

Reactivation of other chronic liver disease with hepatitis type of jaundice: Reactivation of other underlying chronic liver disease like Wilson's diseases who presents with icterus infrequently responds to copper chelating agents like D-penicillamine, trientine, or zinc and need frequently liver transplantation to salvage them. In contrast hemochromatosis patients with icterus may more often respond to iron chelating therapy like IV desferrioxamine (40–50 mg/kg/day 5 days/week or oral deferiprone) 25 mg/kg thrice daily or deferasirox (20–30 mg/kg/day) with an aim to keep serum ferritin level around 1,000–1,500 mg/L. But a distinct benefit of such therapy is unclear and often they may need liver transplant because appearance of jaundice in them would indicate advanced liver damage. Phlebotomy in such patients may be an option. However, since jaundice is extremely uncommon in such patient; cirrhosis with portal hypertension, with or without cardiac, pancreas and testicular involvement is more frequent.

Autoimmune liver diseases presenting with jaundice: Three specific autoimmune diseases such as AIH with or without overlap syndrome, PSC, and PBC need specific therapy and because of variable degree of severity or degree of liver involvement or nonresponse/side effects associated with initial first-line treatment often needs individualized approach.

Autoimmune hepatitis: The drug of choice for induction of remission is corticosteroids and drug of choice for maintenance of remission is azathioprine.

Patient intolerant to azathioprine can be treated with 6-MP along with mycophenolate mofetil (MMF) and such combination have been reported to maintain remission in about 80% of the azathioprine intolerant patients (**Flowchart 3**).

Primary sclerosing cholangitis: Treatment in icteric PSC is frequently unsatisfactory. When both intrahepatic and large duct involvement is extensive, drugs or endoscopic decompression through biliary stenting or balloon dilatation is unsatisfactory and often they need liver transplant. Despite lack of survival advantage of UDCA in large randomized controlled trial, controversy exists about its use in PSC. However, some studies documented worsening of liver biochemistry with withdrawal of UDCA. Most clinician despite lack of clear evidence of substantial benefit recommends use of UDCA (17–23 mg/kg/day) in such patients. If an isolated dominant stricture (infrequent) is associated with icterus, biliary stenting helps to ameliorate icterus and cholangitis. Many patients with PSC who were asymptomatic or had abnormal liver biochemistry in past when presents with icterus raises the suspicion of occurrence of cholangiocarcinoma and therefore, such patient need to be investigated to rule out presence of malignancy of the biliary tract by contrast-enhanced MR scan, MRCP, contrast-enhanced CT scan, endoscopic ultrasonography, biliary brush cytology, choledochoscopic examination and biopsy. Use of experimental therapy may be tried as liver transplant is not accessible to most of the patients.

Primary biliary cirrhosis: Primary biliary cirrhosis is infrequently seen in India. Once jaundice occurs in PBC, usually response to medical therapy is suboptimal and most of them needs liver transplant.

Ursodeoxycholic acid (13–15 mg/kg daily) is the first-line treatment, and a 4-year therapy has been reported to lower probability of death or liver transplant. Usually, UDCA is continued for life. It should be started at the earliest and delay in such treatment is associated with inferior response. Recently OCA in a dose of 5–10 mg/day have been cleared in USA and Europe as the second-line drug to be used in patients without having desired biochemical response with UDCA and have been documented in about 40–45% of the patients with improvement in hepatic transaminases as well. However, in PBC a bilirubin of 5 mg or more or having cirrhosis with child's B or C status require liver transplant.

Drug-induced liver disease and cholestasis: Patients with DILI are treated with withdrawal of the offending drug and supportive as well symptomatic treatment. N acetyl cysteine has been used in paracetamol poisoning. DILI patients may often present with cholestasis and symptomatic treatment of cholestasis using microsomal proliferators like rifampicin (300–600 mg/day), bile chelating agents like cholestyramine (4–19 g/day to be given 4 hours apart from other medications), replacing hydrophobic bile acid with hydrophilic UDCA (10–15 mg/kg/day), opioid antagonist naltrexone (50 mg/day; starting dose 12.5 mg/day), serotonin-uptake inhibitors like sertraline (50–100 mg/day)

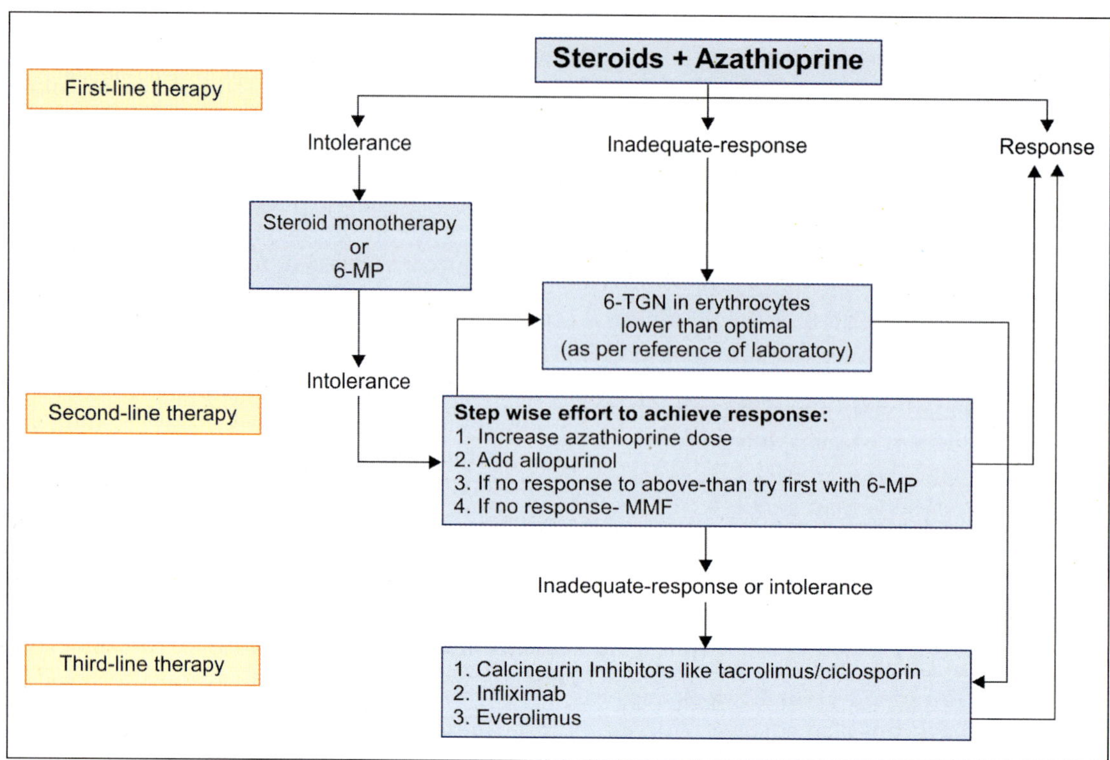

(AIH: autoimmune hepatitis; MMF: mycophenolate mofetil; 6-MP: 6-mercaptopurine; 6-TGN: 6-thioguanine nucleotide)

FLOWCHART 3: Therapeutic approach in AIH.

have been used. In some patients, recent evidence suggests that high volume plasmapheresis may be beneficial.

Alcoholic hepatitis: Alcoholic hepatitis and alcoholic ACLF in recent time have been reported to be a frequent cause of jaundice and frequent cause of liver transplantation globally. Most experts suggest that to achieve definitive diagnosis of alcoholic hepatitis, a liver biopsy [often transjugular liver biopsy (TJLB) because of presence of ascites and coagulopathy] should be performed and histology in them is characteristic (ballooning, neutrophilic infiltration, giant mitochondria, and bilirubinostasis with chicken wire fibrosis).

The present therapeutic strategy in most centers is depicted in **Flowchart 4**.

Obstructive jaundice: The specific diagnosis of obstructive jaundice and its causes have been enumerated earlier in this chapter and have been depicted in **Flowchart 2** and **Table 3**.

The treatment in such cases can be structured into (1) symptomatic relief of cholestasis and cholangitis; (2) assessment of comorbidities such as diabetes, hypertension, cardiac status, and renal dysfunction; (3) definitive curative therapy.

Biliary decompression to alleviate cholestasis and cholangitis using endoscopic methods such as endoscopic retrograde cholangiopancreatography (ERCP)—endoscopic papillotomy and stenting or endoscopic ultrasound-guided techniques (most frequently used at present) or percutaneous transhepatic biliary drainage (PTBD) when the former is technically not feasible are the usual procedure. Use of appropriate antibiotic to treat cholangitis and anticholestatic agents such as UDCA is usual practice in vogue. Simultaneous assessment of comorbidity particularly renal dysfunction not infrequently associated with cholangitis needs particular support with help of nephrologist. Other comorbidities also need special attention and should be controlled when present.

The specific treatment for choledocholithiasis is endoscopic clearance of biliary channel and if associated with gallstone—a subsequent laparoscopic cholecystectomy. Similarly, other benign diseases like parasitic infestation like hydatid cysts or round worm in the bile ducts needs endoscopic clearance of the bile ducts whereas the benign biliary stricture will need biliary dilatation using various biliary dilators and when not amenable with such techniques, a surgical approach as appropriate is usually followed. Drainage of pancreatic pseudocysts (by endoscopic or percutaneous drainage techniques) when it causes obstructive jaundice usually alleviates the jaundice. Other benign diseases as enumerated in **Table 3** needs appropriate combination of specific medical treatment combined with temporarily biliary decompression depending upon the specific etiology.

Malignant etiologies causing obstructive jaundice are assessed for curative resectability which predominantly depends upon absence of distant spread and local vascular involvements. When resectable, postoperative staging of cancer and recommended chemo/radiotherapy when necessary to prevent recurrence are considered. In unresectable cases, the palliation of obstructive

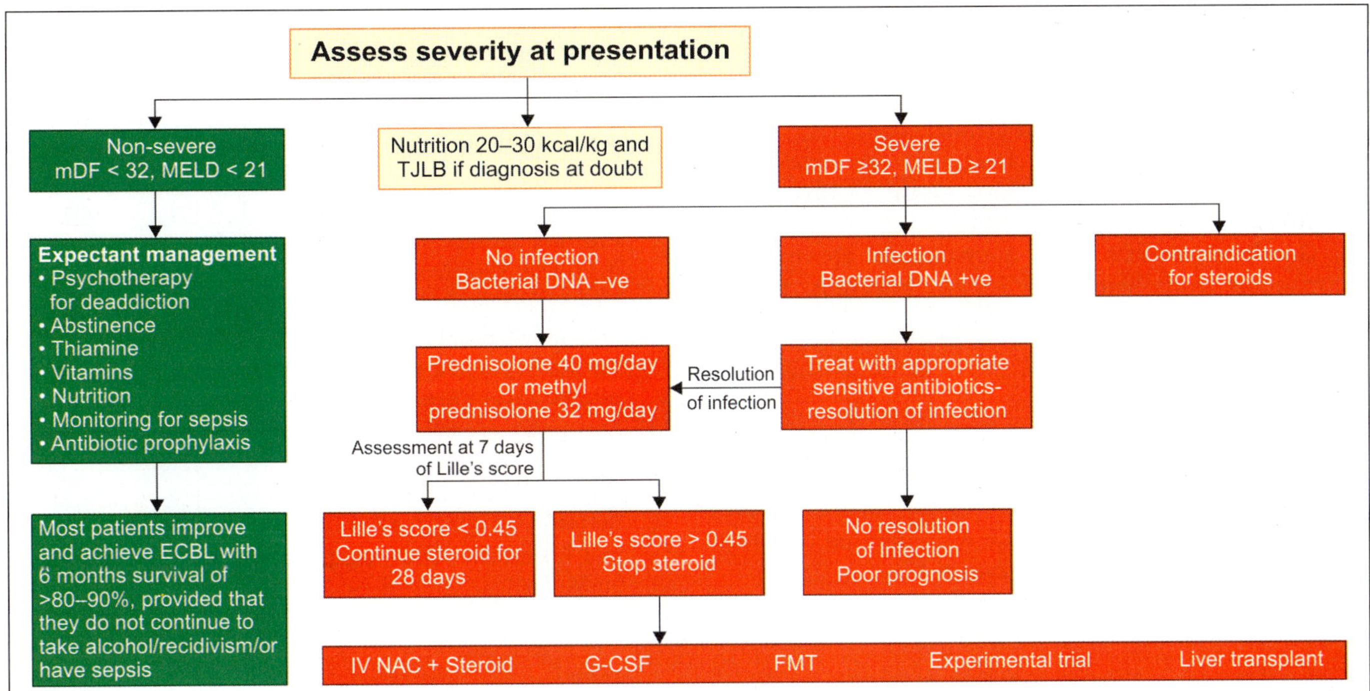

(ECBL: early change in bilirubin level; FMT: fecal microbiota transplantation; G-CSF: granulocyte colony-stimulating factor; IV: intravenous; mDF: Maddrey's discriminant score; MELD: model for end-stage liver disease; NAC: N-acetylcysteine; TJLB: transjugular liver biopsy)

FLOWCHART 4: Therapeutic approach in alcoholic hepatitis.

jaundice is usually attempted through endoscopic biliary decompression particularly using stents like self-expanding metal stents (SEMS) whose durability and patency is markedly longer than the plastic stents which needs frequent changes to avoid their blockage.

NUTRITIONAL AND SUPPORTIVE THERAPY

As mentioned earlier, nutritional therapy during the treatment of specific causes of jaundice is essential to prevent: (1) Immunocompromised state associated with presence of long-standing jaundice irrespective of cause. Liver is an important immune organ and prevent gut derived endotoxemia and is the source of opsonic proteins such as fibronectin and vitronectin (necessary for phagocytosis of neutrophils and macrophages) innate immune system, as well as complements; (2) Sarcopenia is associated with long-standing jaundice irrespective of cause. Loss of muscle protein due to anorexia and intolerance to food is associated with most cases of jaundice; (3) Cholangitis and infection-induced hypercatabolism, and cachexia associated with malignant condition needs adequate nutrition; (4) Alcoholic hepatitis associated with malnutrition and increased risk of infection need adequate nutritional supplement.

Further, prolonged cholestasis may be associated with deficiency of fat-soluble vitamins like vitamin A, D, E, and K and may need parenteral replacement. Additionally, steatorrhea associated with bile acid deficiency and pancreatic diseases, maldigestion, small intestinal bacterial overgrowth and protein loosing enteropathies may need specific treatment approach and specific nutritional supplements. Such nutritional therapy preferably is introduced using enteral route which is physiological and helps in maintaining gut barrier functions to prevent transmigration of gut bacteria; however, when oral therapy is not feasible due to oral intolerance or due to bowel obstructions such as in pancreatic carcinoma or metastatic peritoneal or omental deposits parenteral nutrition may be preferred.

Usually nutritional supplement of 25–30 kcal/kg with adequate protein supplement of 1–1.5 g/kg with supplement of necessary electrolytes, vitamins constitute the essential nutritional therapy. Specific involvement of a nutritionist and monitoring of nutritional parameters, assessment of sarcopenia should be undertaken as an integral management strategy in all patients with jaundice.

CONCLUSION

The etiology of jaundice due to both hepatitic and obstructive jaundice is multiple. Management of such cases includes understanding of bilirubin metabolism, specific diagnostic algorithms of broad categories as well as specific causes of jaundice. The treatment constitutes specific therapy for etiology, cholestasis as well as cholangitis associated with such etiology. Evaluation of nutritional deficiency with nutritional therapy and improvement of nutritional status enhance the recovery of such patients. Team approach including gastroenterologists, surgeons, nutritionists, and radiologists is necessary for an optimal therapy and improvement as well as cure of such patients.

RECOMMENDED READINGS

1. Colmenero J, Forner A, Londona MC, Bruix J, Forns X, Gracia-Pagan JC, et al. Therapy in Liver Disease. New Delhi: Ichinen Medical Publishing; 2019.
2. Sullivan JI, Rockey DC. Diagnosis and evaluation of hyperbilirubinemia. Curr Opin Gastroenterol. 2017;33:164-70.
3. Gondal B, Aronsohn A. A systematic approach to patients with jaundice. Semin Intervent Radiol. 2016;33(4):253-8.
4. Kathpalia P, Ahn J. Assessment of jaundice in the hospitalized patient. Clin Liv Dis. 2015;19:155-70.
5. Gossard AA, Talwalkar JA. Cholestatic liver disease. Med Clin North Am. 2014;98(1):73-85.
6. Mieli-Vergani G, Vergani D, Czaza AJ, Manns MP, Krawitt EL, Vierling JM, et al. Autoimmune hepatitis. Nat Rev Dis Primers. 2018;12;4:18017.
7. European Association for the Study of Liver. EASL Clinical Practice Guidelines: Autoimmune Hepatitis. J Hepatol. 2015;63:971-1004.
8. Karlesen TH, Folseraas T, Thorburn D, Vesterhus M. Primary Sclerosing Cholangitis—A Comprehensive Review. J Hepatol. 2017;67:1298-323.
9. Lindor KD, Bowlus CL, Boyer J, Levy C, Mayo M. Primary Biliary Cholangitis:2018 Practice Guidance from the American Association for the Study of Liver Diseases. Hepatology. 2019;69;394-419.
10. European Association for the Study of Liver. EASL Clinical Practice Guideline: Management of alcohol-related Liver Disease. J Hepatol. 2018;69:154-81.
11. European Association for the Study of Liver. EASL Practice Guideline: Management of Cholestatic Liver Diseases. J Hepatol. 2009;51:237-67.
12. Beuers U, Kremer AE, Bolier R, Elferink RP. Pruritus in Cholestasis. Facts and Fiction. Hepatology. 2014; 60:399-407.

CHAPTER 142

Acute Liver Failure

Shalimar, Subrat K Acharya

ABSTRACT

Acute liver failure (ALF) is a rare, potentially fatal complication of severe hepatic illness resulting from various causes. Significant geographical and regional differences exist in the definitions, etiologies, and prognostic models across the globe. The clinical presentation of severe hepatic injury includes jaundice, encephalopathy, and coagulopathy. The main clinical event in ALF is hepatic encephalopathy (HE) and cerebral edema. The pathogenesis of encephalopathy and cerebral edema in ALF is unique and multifactorial. Ammonia plays a central role in the pathogenesis. The role of newer ammonia-lowering agents is still evolving. Liver transplant (LT) is the only effective therapy that has been identified to be of promise in those with poor prognostic factors. Apart from LT, aggressive intensive medical management can salvage a substantial proportion of patients. Due to the shortage of donor liver organs, only a small fraction of patients receive LT, and the remaining are managed with medical therapy. Multiple prognostic models are available to help identify ALF patients at risk of poor outcomes. This review discusses the global differences in ALF etiologies, prognostic scores, and the management options.

"Every cause produces more than one effect"

—Herbert Spencer

INTRODUCTION AND DEFINITIONS

Acute liver failure is a fatal complication of acute hepatic injury and occurs unpredictably. It is a rare clinical entity marked by the sudden loss of hepatic function and a severe life-threatening course in a person with no prior history of liver disease. ALF represents a syndrome rather than a specific disease, having multiple causes that vary in course and outcome. Significant geographical and regional differences exist in the definitions, etiologies, and prognostic models across the globe. A recent systematic review that evaluated 1,233 published articles on ALF reported 41 different definitions with varying diagnostic characteristics to define ALF.

In 1969, Trey and Davidson defined ALF as the occurrence of encephalopathy with or without coagulopathy within 8 weeks of the onset of symptoms of acute hepatitis in an individual without any history of preexisting liver disease. Patients who develop ALF within 7 days of the onset of icterus have significantly better survival than those who develop encephalopathy later. O'Grady classified ALF as hyperacute if encephalopathy develops within 7 days of the onset of the icterus; acute, if it occurs between 7 days and 4 weeks of the onset of jaundice and subacute if jaundice to encephalopathy interval is between 4 and 12 weeks. However, in India, ALF is defined as the occurrence of encephalopathy within 4 weeks of the onset of jaundice in an individual without any history of preexisting liver disease. The American Association for the Study of Liver Diseases (AASLD) practice guidance document defines ALF as "liver diseases characterized by the development of HE and coagulation abnormality, usually characterized by an International Normalized Ratio (INR) of ≥1.5 in patients without preexisting cirrhosis, and an illness of <26 weeks duration" (**Box 1**).

The occurrence of progressive ascites with or without encephalopathy after 4 weeks but within 6 months of acute hepatic illness is termed as subacute hepatic failure (SHF). The International Association for the Study of the Liver Subcommittee provided nomenclature and defining criteria for ALF and SHF which are shown in **Box 2**. The term SHF is uncommonly used these days, possible reason may be that a subset of such patients are now diagnosed as acute-on-chronic liver failure. (ACLF)

ETIOLOGIES

Differences in the etiologies of ALF between different parts of the world are striking (**Box 3**). Published reports from the Indian subcontinent have identified hepatitis viruses as the etiological agent in >90% of ALF patients. Non-A, Non-E hepatitis accounts for 38% (although this is not further defined) and HEV is responsible for 31% of cases. There are relatively few drug-induced cases and antituberculosis drugs cause the majority of these. Other causes such as paracetamol overdose, drug-induced liver failure, Wilson disease, and acute fatty liver of pregnancy are infrequent.

In contrast, the etiology of ALF among Western countries is somewhat heterogeneous as shown in **Table 1**. In the UK, paracetamol overdose was the etiology in 57% of ALF patients, whereas in the USA, France, Germany, and Australia, paracetamol was the reported etiology of ALF in 46%, 7%, 9%, and 36% cases, respectively. The common etiologies of ALF in different parts of the world are highlighted in **Table 1**.

Amanita poisoning (*Amanita phalloides*) causing ALF is uncommon and is observed when amateur mushroom hunters fail to recognize the poisonous variety. Cases have been reported from Africa, Australia, Central and South America, and west Asia. However, only rare cases have been reported from the Indian subcontinent.

BOX 1 ALF: Definition.

- Despite differences in the definition of ALF—rapid development of jaundice, coagulopathy, and encephalopathy in the absence of underlying chronic liver disease are the key components of the syndrome
- Time duration to the onset of encephalopathy after the onset of symptoms varies across different definition:
  - *UK*: Up to 8 weeks
  - *USA*: Up to 26 weeks
  - *India*: Up to 4 weeks
  - *France*: Up to 12 weeks
  - *Japan*: Up to 8 weeks

BOX 2 IASLS definition and classification of acute hepatic failure (AHF) and subacute hepatic failure (SHF).

Key points: Nomenclature

AHF: Synonyms such as fulminant hepatitis, fulminant hepatic failure, and acute yellow atrophy should not be used

SHF: Synonyms such as subfulminant hepatitis, SHF and late-onset hepatic failure should not be used

Diagnostic criteria of liver failure:

AHF: Encephalopathy

SHF: Encephalopathy and/or progressive ascites

Maximum interval between onset of icterus and features of liver failure:

AHF < 4 weeks

SHF > 4–24 weeks

Subclassification:

- Etiological to indicate specific cause of AHF
- Temporal to indicate the rapidity of encephalopathy
  - Hyperacute: Encephalopathy within 10 days of icterus
  - Fulminant: Encephalopathy between 10 and 30 days of the onset of jaundice
- Not otherwise specified

Example (AHF, hyperacute-A)

(IASLS: International Association for the Study of the Liver Subcommittee)

BOX 3 Acute liver failure: Etiology.

- **East:**
  - India, Pakistan, Somalia: Hepatitis A and E
  - Japan, Korea and China: Hepatitis B and herbal remedies
- **West:**
  - US and Europe: Drugs (paracetamol/acetaminophen and prescription drugs, principally antibiotics)
- **Rarer causes:** Autoimmune hepatitis, Wilson's, Budd–Chiari syndrome, *Amanita* poisoning

TABLE 1	Different etiologies of ALF across the world.									
Country	(N)	Drugs		Viral					Indeterminate	Others
	Number of cases	Paracetamol	Other drugs	HAV	HBV	HEV	Other viral	Non A, Non E		
India	1,223		6% (ATT)	1%	16%	31%	6%	38%		2% (data not available)
USA	1,696	46%	12% (antimicrobial agents: ATT, antibiotics, antifungals, antiepileptics, NSAIDs and antimetabolites)	2%	7%				13%	• Autoimmune 6.5% • Ischemic 5% • Wilson's 1% • Budd–Chiari 1% • Pregnancy 1% • Other causes 5%
Japan	856		10% (ATT, acetaminophen), anticancer agents, allopurinol and acarbose	6%	42%	1%	2%		3%	• Autoimmune 7% • Unknown 30%
UK	422	57%	11%	2%	5%	1%			17%	7%
France	363	7%	21%	5%	28%				18%	21%
Germany (total % >100: Overlap in some cases)	109	9%	32% phenprocoumon, valproate, NSAIDs, sertraline, clindamycin	4%	10%	4%	3%		24%	• Autoimmune 3% • Wilson's 3% • Budd–Chiari 2% • Malignancy 3% • Pregnancy 3% • *Amanita* 2% • Others 4%
Australia	80	36%	6% (nitrofurantoin, sodium valproate, isoflurane and ketorolac)	4%	10%			34% (Non A Non B)		• Wilson's 7% • Budd–Chiari 3%

Alcoholic liver disease has never been included as the cause of ALF since most acute alcoholic hepatitis occurs in the setting of cirrhosis.

PATHOGENETIC DRIVERS

The underlying pathogenesis of encephalopathy, consequent cerebral edema, and raised intracranial hypertension (ICH) in ALF is complex and has been extensively studied. Ammonia has been implicated as the major neurotoxin in ALF. In addition, systemic inflammatory response syndrome (SIRS) and loss of autoregulation of cerebral blood flow (CBF) have been implicated as other important pathogenetic events in accentuating encephalopathy and cerebral edema in ALF.

ROLE OF AMMONIA

In animal models as well as in patients with ALF, marked swelling of astrocytes has been documented. In animal models of ALF, the expression of various astrocytic proteins has been reported. Astrocytes are specialized neuroglial cells, initially considered passive supporters of the neuronal framework, which are now recognized to play crucial roles in brain metabolism, maintaining the blood–brain barrier (BBB), and modulating synaptic transmission in neural inflammation. Changes in astrocytes are documented to be due to hyperammonemia in ALF. Astrocyte swelling due to increased brain water and alteration in the astrocytes' functional property causes encephalopathy and cerebral edema resulting in ICH, which often results in brain herniation, which is the most important mechanism of death in ALF. In ALF, the liver's ability to metabolize ammonia is grossly compromised, resulting in hyperammonemic state, which exerts deleterious effects contributing to HE. The arterial ammonia level measured within 24 hours of patient presentation has also been demonstrated to correlate with patient outcomes in ALF. An arterial ammonia level of >124 mmol/L was found to predict mortality with 78.6% sensitivity and 76.3% specificity. Patients with higher ammonia levels also develop more complications, including deeper encephalopathy, cerebral edema, need for ventilation, seizures and mortality (**Box 4**).

INFECTIONS AND SIRS

Liver is an important component of the immune system. In ALF, rapid immune paralysis is well known, which predisposes to sepsis. A strong association between the occurrence of infection and the course of encephalopathy has been clearly documented. In addition, the risk of progression of encephalopathy also increases with the number of systemic inflammatory response syndrome (SIRS) components.

LOSS OF CEREBRAL AUTOREGULATION

Usually, CBF is independent of change in systemic blood pressure, and blood flow to the various regions of the brain varies depending upon the metabolic need of neurons (glucose and oxygen). This delicate balance of regional CBF and the metabolic requirement is lost in ALF. This may cause an increase in CBF and cerebral congestion, which aggravates cerebral edema. CBF correlates very closely with the brain water and intracranial pressure (ICP) in experimental ammonia-induced brain edema. Normally, the brain autoregulation can maintain a normal CBF at arterial pressures from 65 to 140 mm Hg. This loss of CBF autoregulation in ALF signifies that even mildly elevated cerebral perfusion pressure (CPP) will increase CBF and hydrostatic pressure across the BBB, while episodes of arterial hypotension may stop capillary blood flow, leading to cerebral hypoxia. This phenomenon has been called "dissociated cerebral vasoparalysis." CBF is reduced in most patients with grade 3 or 4 encephalopathy, even with maintained mean arterial pressure. However, increased CBF precedes high ICP and cerebral herniation. This loss of CBF autoregulation is rare in patients with cirrhosis or sepsis. Even though the exact mechanism of loss of CBF autoregulation is poorly understood, it is a definite event in ALF perpetuating the process of cerebral edema. This loss of autoregulation is restored within 1 day of LT and within 4 days of spontaneous recovery.

BOX 4	ALF: Neurotoxic effects of ammonia.
• Alteration in cell (astrocyte) volume regulation	
• Alteration in cerebral energy homeostasis	
• Alteration in astrocytic and neuronal protein expression affecting its structure and functions	
• Oxidative and nitrosative stress	

MANAGEMENT

All patients with ALF should be managed in the intensive care unit. The essential steps of management of the ALF can be categorized as: (1) General supportive measures; (2) Specific therapy directed to control encephalopathy and cerebral edema; (3) Other forms of therapy directed to control and prevent complications such as sepsis, hemodynamic instability, renal failure, coagulopathy, hypoglycemia, and respiratory failure; and (4) LT.

GENERAL SUPPORTIVE MEASURES

The general supportive measures to be followed in management in ALF are shown in **Box 5.** Blood sugar should be monitored at 2-hour intervals. Whenever the blood glucose level is lower than 60 mg/dL, an intravenous bolus of 50–100 mL of 50% dextrose should be administered. The amount of water administered as a solvent for dextrose should be minimized by providing solutions concentrated to 25–50%. Interventions that have not been useful in the management of ALF are shown in the **Box 6.** The algorithmic approach to a patient with ALF is shown in **Flowchart 1.**

BOX 5	ALF: General supportive measures.
• Correct fluid status and avoid hypo- or hypervolemia	
• Strict aseptic precautions should be practiced while handling catheters and tubes	
• Administer supplemental oxygen in case of hypoxemia and avoid hypercapnia	
• Avoid hypertension/hypotension	
• Manage fever with surface cooling	
• Neck should be kept in the neutral position	
• Minimize external stimuli	
• Monitor blood glucose 2 hourly and maintain between 140 and 180 mg%	
• Monitor serum electrolytes and maintain corrected levels	
• Nutrition—nasogastric feeding should be started early. Protein 1–1.5 g/kg. No need to restrict protein	

BOX 6	ALF: Interventions not useful.
• Corticosteroids	
• L-ornithine	
• Branched-chain amino acids	
• Fresh frozen plasma transfusion in the absence of bleeding	
• Enteral decontamination	
• Prophylactic phenytoin	
• Hypothermia	
• Prophylactic hyperventilation for raised intracranial hypertension	

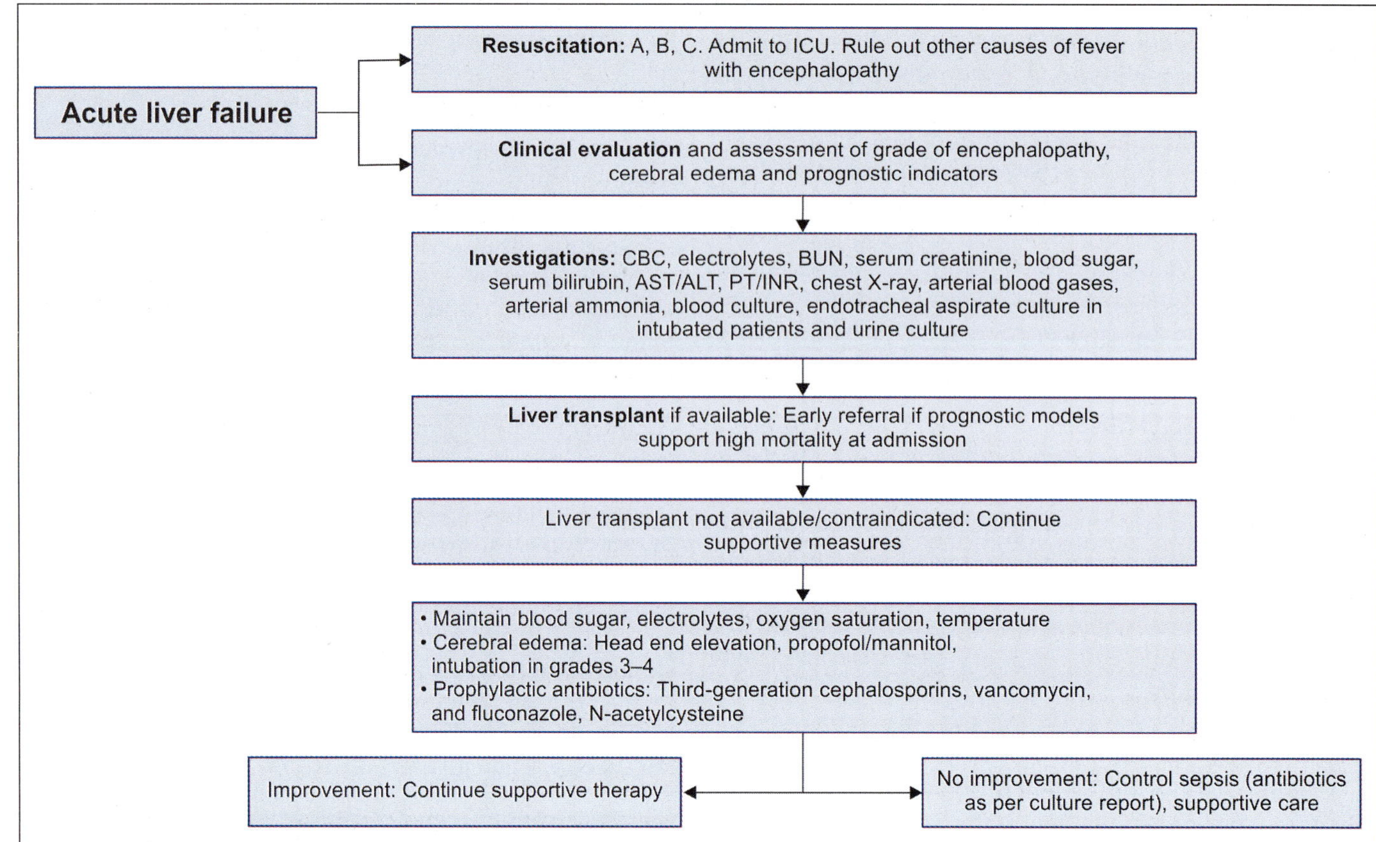

(ALT: alanine aminotransferase; AST: aspartate aminotransferase)

FLOWCHART 1: Algorithmic approach to a patient with acute liver failure.

THERAPY TO CONTROL ENCEPHALOPATHY AND CEREBRAL EDEMA

Neurologic support: All patients should be nursed in a 20–30° head-up tilt to improve venous drainage. Patient turning and other tactile stimulation should be minimized. Respiratory suctioning should be limited to <15 seconds duration at a time. About 1–2 mL of lidocaine instilled in the endotracheal tube and ventilation with 100% oxygen prior to suctioning may help prevent surges of raised ICP. Control of agitation is essential, as Valsalva maneuver from psychomotor agitation may elevate the ICP. A diligent search for treatable causes of agitation such as distended bladder and bedsores should be made.

Intracranial pressure monitoring: Traditional signs (bradycardia, hypertension, and widened pulse pressure) of elevated ICP are unreliable in ALF. Computed tomography of the head is not a reliable way to estimate ICP in ALF. The direct measurement of ICP is associated with risk. Subdural bolts and parenchymal monitors carry complication rates (mainly bleeding) of 20% and 22%, respectively. Colonization of ICP devices increases significantly after about 5 days of insertion, and the risk of superficial wound infection and meningitis rises. Therefore, most experts avoid invasive monitoring as a routine.

Noninvasive tools for assessing raised ICP include optic nerve sheath diameter, and middle carotid artery Doppler. However, these techniques need further validation.

Reverse jugular venous monitoring: Jugular bulb venous saturation is frequently used in neurosurgical intensive care and involves the insertion of a fine catheter in a retrograde fashion until its tip lies in the jugular bulb. Blood returning from the cerebral circulation can then be sampled. A jugular venous saturation of <55% represents an ischemic brain, while saturation of >85% represents a hyperemic brain. Measures to improve oxygen supply are indicated in the former situation, and measures to reduce CBF in the latter situation.

Osmotherapy: Mannitol lowers the ICP by reducing the brain water and changing the rheological characteristics of blood. When the ICP rises to over 20–25 mm Hg for >5 minutes, an intravenous bolus of mannitol should be given (0.5–1 g/kg, 20% solution, over 5 min). Repeated boluses may be administered as long as the serum osmolality is <320 mOsm/L. The response to a mannitol bolus may be expected 15–60 minutes post injection. In about 20% of patients, a paradoxical increase in ICP occurs after mannitol infusion. High doses can result in acute renal failure and damage to the BBB. Mannitol works best in mild-to-moderate ICH and is less effective when the ICP is >60 mm Hg. In oliguric/anuric patients, mannitol should only be given in combination with continuous venovenous or arteriovenous hemodiafiltration.

Hypothermia: Moderate hypothermia (32–35°C) using cooling blankets reduces CBF, cerebral metabolism, ammonia uptake by the brain, and glutamine synthesis and reduces ICP in patients with ALF. However, hypothermia as therapy has not shown any improvement in survival among ALF patients but has been used as a therapeutic bridge to transplantation. Prolonged hypothermia is well known to cause cardiac arrhythmia and coagulopathy.

Prophylactic phenytoin: Prophylactic use of phenytoin has not been shown to prevent cerebral edema and seizures or improve survival.

Hyperventilation: Patients with ALF often hyperventilate spontaneously and attempts to control this are of no use. Hyperventilation reduces CBF and may be useful in the subgroup of patients with cerebral hyperemia as reflected by jugular bulb venous saturation of >75%. Prophylactic hyperventilation does not reduce the frequency of ICH in ALF, but a moderate reduction in pCO_2 to 25–30 mm Hg helps decrease the ICP once cerebral edema has begun to develop. Excessive hyperventilation may lead to cerebral vasoconstriction.

OTHER MEASURES

Lactulose: Lactulose has a definite role in the management of HE in patients with chronic liver disease. The role of lactulose in the management of ALF is unclear. The side effect of bloating may interfere with the LT procedure.

L-ornithine L-aspartate: L-ornithine L-aspartate (LOLA) is a stable salt of the amino acids ornithine and aspartic acid. These two amino acids get converted to glutamate in the muscles and hepatocytes. Glutamate is the substrate on which the enzyme glutamine synthase (present in the muscle as well as liver) acts and combines it with ammonia to make glutamine and thereby reduces blood ammonia levels. In liver failure, the enzyme glutamine synthase in the muscle is upregulated and therefore it is hypothesized that in liver failure, LOLA by the mechanism as mentioned above may reduce arterial ammonia levels. It has been shown that LOLA reduces arterial ammonia levels accompanied by improvement in mental status in patients with HE associated with chronic liver disease. In the animal model of ALF, LOLA has been shown to prevent brain edema and HE. However, in a randomized placebo-controlled double-blind trial of LOLA in patients with ALF, LOLA therapy was not associated with a decrease in ammonia levels or improvement in encephalopathy or survival.

L-ornithine phenyl acetate: Phenyl acetate combines with glutamine to form phenylacetylglutamine which is water soluble and is excreted in the urine. One molecule of phenyl acetate removes two molecules of glutamine. In a pig model of ALF, L-ornithine phenyl acetate (LOPA) has been shown to prevent the rise of plasma and brain ammonia concentration and rise in ICP. LOPA has been shown to be safe when used in ALF patients. The therapeutic efficacy of LOPA in ALF in humans needs evaluation.

Rifaximin: Rifaximin is an oral antibiotic with a broad spectrum of activity against enteric bacteria. It is minimally absorbed from the gut (<0.4%). Current data suggests that rifaximin is as effective as established therapies such as lactulose or neomycin in the treatment of HE and has a better safety profile and tolerability in patients with chronic liver disease. Its possible benefit in lowering ammonia in patients with ALF has yet not been explored appropriately.

N-acetylcysteine: In a recently published trial by the USALF study group, 21 days of transplant-free survival among grade I and II coma nonparacetamol ALF patients were significantly better in the N-acetylcysteine (NAC) treated than the placebo-treated patients. However, there was no difference in the survival in those with grade III and IV coma grades.

Maintenance of serum sodium levels between 145 and 155 mmol/L has been shown to decrease ICP.

High-volume plasma exchange: A recent, multicenter, randomized control trial reported that high-volume plasma exchange improves survival in patients with ALF. The likely mechanisms are removal of plasma cytokines and adhesion molecules, replacement of plasma factors and immune modulation. However, further studies are needed.

MANAGEMENT OF COMPLICATIONS

Renal failure: Renal failure has been described in 40–80% of patients from the Western series depending upon the etiology and is associated with a poor prognosis. Renal failure occurs more frequently in patients with acetaminophen-induced ALF (70%) and in 30% of patients with other causes in Western series, suggesting that there is a direct toxic effect of acetaminophen on the renal tubules. Renal failure is less frequent (10%) in ALF patients in India. The indications of renal replacement therapy (RRT) include metabolic acidosis, fluid overload, hyperkalemia, and oliguria. Continuous RRT is preferred over intermittent RRT. The additional benefit of continuous RRT is the reduction of ammonia levels and may benefit in improving outcomes.

Sepsis: Infection is a common complication (50–90% of patients) in ALF that has been documented across the globe. A recent study reported the most common site of infection is the respiratory tract and the most common organisms are gram-negative bacilli. The profile and site of organism may vary from center to center. All ALF patients should undergo regular surveillance cultures, and antibiotics need to be modified as per the culture reports. Intravenous catheters should be changed every 72 hours and removed catheter tips cultured. Majority of bacterial infections occur within 72 hours of admission. Hence prophylactic broad-spectrum parenteral antibiotics should be started at admission. Any unexplained decrease in blood pressure, drop in urinary output, worsening encephalopathy, and development of severe acidosis or disseminated intravascular coagulation should be considered as signs of sepsis. Fungal infection should be strongly considered in the setting of unresponsive fever, leukocytosis, and deterioration of neurologic status after initial improvement and presence of renal failure.

Hemodynamic support: Acute liver failure patients have a high cardiac output, low systemic vascular resistance, and relative arterial hypotension. An adequate cardiovascular filling pressure [pulmonary capillary wedge pressure (PCWP): 8–14 mm Hg] must be assured. The goal is to maintain the mean arterial pressure (MAP) above 60 mm Hg. Vasopressor agents are indicated if the MAP is <60 mm Hg, despite the adequate intravascular volume. Arterial hypotension, despite an adequate intravascular volume, should be considered a sign of bacterial or fungal sepsis and treated accordingly.

Coagulopathy: Prophylactic transfusion of fresh frozen plasma is not recommended for correction of internal normalized ratio. Infusion of FFP is indicated only for active bleeding or before invasive procedures.

Mechanical ventilation of patients with liver failure: The lungs are relatively spared in ALF and standard modes of mechanical ventilation can be used, when indicated. Traumatic intubation may induce a sudden rise in the ICP and provoke herniation. Hence tracheal intubation must be gentle. Standard ventilation modes, most commonly synchronized intermittent mandatory ventilation (SIMV), are used. Avoid high positive end-expiratory pressure (PEEP) levels (>10–15 mm Hg), as it leads to worsening or facilitating the development of cerebral edema and a decrease in hepatic arterial blood flow. Propofol is the preferred agent prior to intubation and sedation as it has an additional benefit in reducing ICP and has anticonvulsant properties.

Treatment of underlying etiology: Both HEV and HAV-ALF have better outcomes as compared to other etiologies. Antituberculosis therapy (ATT)-induced ALF is associated with a high mortality of 70%. Paracetamol-induced ALF has a better outcome than most other etiologies, even after development of hepatic failure. In some specific etiologies, drugs have been shown to be effective. In patients with hepatitis B virus (HBV)-ALF, antivirals have been recommended. The choice of antivirals is between tenofovir and entecavir, the former being preferred in patients with renal failure due to its safety profile. The doses of antivirals need to be modified as per the creatinine clearance. In patients with antituberculosis drug-induced or any other suspected drug-induced ALF, the suspected drug should be immediately stopped. In HEV-ALF, presently, there is no data on the use of ribavirin, though this has been shown to be effective in managing chronic HEV in solid organ transplant patients and selected patients with HEV-related ACLF. In patients with paracetamol toxicity, activated charcoal has been shown to be effective in gastric decontamination. High doses of NAC are recommended in such patients and should be started within 48 hours of ingestion.

Pregnancy and acute liver failure: The ALF frequency is higher (10–22%) among pregnant women with HEV infection than among men and nonpregnant women (1–2%). Hence, the mortality rate is significantly higher among pregnant women who develop hepatitis during epidemics (10–39%) than in the general population affected with hepatitis (0.06–12%). The attack rate among pregnant women during epidemics is 1–4%. In the sporadic setting, evidence of HEV infection has been detected in 30–45% of patients with ALF.

There is an increased risk of maternal and fetal complications in pregnant patients with ALF. The management of abortions, preterm labor, premature rupture of membranes, and stillbirth remains unchanged. Termination of pregnancy is not indicated. There is an increased risk of bleeding due to associated coagulopathy. Management of pregnant patients with ALF is similar to other ALF patients. Complications need to be managed on a case-to-case basis.

Liver transplantation: Overall, the 1-year and 5-year survival after liver transplantation has been reported as 79% and 72%, respectively. Survival is substantially reduced among patients with sepsis and multi-organ failure before orthotopic liver transplantation (OLT). Assessment for candidates for LT should be dynamic—clinical evaluation and parameters should be monitored continuously. LT should not be performed in case of improving clinical status, in presence of three or more organ failures, especially those with respiratory and circulatory failure or those on extracorporeal membrane oxygenation (ECMO). In addition, ongoing sepsis and invasive fungal infections are relative contraindications.

Bioartificial liver support systems: Liver support systems work on the principle of removing toxins and albumin-bound substances. Till date, none of the bioartificial and other extracorporeal liver assist devices, including Molecular Adsorbent Recirculating System (MARS) have shown to improve survival among patients with ALF.

PROGNOSTIC MODELS

The ability to predict which patients with ALF will recover with medical management alone and succumb without liver transplantation is paramount. Static variables that correlate with survival are age and etiology. Patients with hepatitis A virus (HAV), hepatitis E virus (HEV), and acetaminophen toxicity and acute fatty liver of pregnancy have better survival rates; those with drug-induced, autoimmune, hepatitis B, and cryptogenic ALF have spontaneous survival of <30%.

Acute liver failure is a dynamic process where variables determining prognosis at admission change over time, and thus the clinical course varies accordingly. The ALF early dynamic (ALFED) model is based on whether the predictive variables' levels remain persistently high or increase over 3 days above the discriminatory cutoff values. The model has four variables: (1) arterial ammonia ≥123 μmol/L, (2) serum bilirubin ≥15 mg/dL, (3) INR ≥5, and (4) HE > Grade

TABLE 2 Prognostic models in ALF.	
Non-paracetamol-induced	**Paracetamol-induced**
Prothrombin time (PT) >100 s or	Plasma pH < 7.30 or
Any three of the following:	Arterial lactate level > 3.5 mmol/L at 4 h or
• Age < 10 or > 40 years	Arterial lactate level >3.0 mmol/L at 12 h
• Etiology—non-A, non-B hepatitis	Or
• Drug-induced hepatitis • Icterus–encephalopathy interval > 7 days • PT > 50 s (INR > 3.5) • Serum bilirubin > 17.5 mg/dL	PT > 100 s (INR > 6.5) and serum creatinine > 3.4 mg/dL in patients with grade 3–4 encephalopathy
Clichy criteria (France):	
• Factor V levels < 20% of normal in patients < 30 years of age	
• Factor V levels < 30% of normal in patients > 30 years of age	
ALF early dynamic (ALFED) model-variables assessed over 3 days:	
• Arterial ammonia, persistent or increased to ≥123 μmol/L	ALFED score ≥ 4–88.5% mortality
• INR, persistent or increased to ≥5	
• Serum bilirubin, persistent or increased to ≥15 mg/dL	
• Hepatic encephalopathy, persistent or increased to grade > 2	

II. These values if present on day 3 of presentation are independent predictors of mortality. The scores have been depicted in **Table 2**; total scores vary from 0 to 6.

The ALFED model's performance was superior to the King's College Hospital criteria and the Model for End-stage Liver Disease score, even when their 3-day serial values were taken into consideration. An ALFED score of ≥4 had a high positive predictive value (85%) and negative predictive value (87%) in the validation cohort. The most widely used prognostic model is the King's college criteria (**Table 2**). However, in the Indian scenario, its relevance is questionable. In India, paracetamol poisoning-associated ALF is practically nonexistent, the prognostic criteria for paracetamol poisoning are not practiced. The King's prognostic criteria for non-paracetamol poisoning include five parameters (**Table 2**), of which three parameters are not prevalent in Indian cases. Most Indian patients with ALF are 20–30 years old at presentation; almost all patients have an I-E interval of <7 days, and Non-A, Non-B virus (its exact nature is not known) and drug idiosyncrasy as etiology of ALF are absent among the Indian patients. Therefore, the ALFED model may be more applicable in countries such as India and probably in other developing countries in Asia and Africa, where two-thirds of the world's population lives.

CONCLUSION

Acute liver failure is uncommon and associated with high mortality. Cerebral edema and infection are the major causes of death in this disease. A specific strategy for neurological support, prevention of infection and its treatment, ammonia-lowering therapies, maintenance of acid–base balance, close monitoring in an ICU setup with adequate support for failing organs remain the mainstay of medical management of encephalopathy in ALF. Patients with ominous prognostic criteria benefit from a LT. However, liver support devices till date have not been very beneficial in ALF.

RECOMMENDED READINGS

1. Anand AC, Nandi B, Acharya SK, Arora A, Babu S, Batra Y, et al. Indian National Association for the Study of the Liver Consensus Statement on Acute Liver Failure (Part 1): Epidemiology, Pathogenesis, Presentation and Prognosis. J Clin Exp Hepatol. 2020;10(4):339-76.
2. Anand AC, Nandi B, Acharya SK, Arora A, Babu S, Batra Y, et al. Indian National Association for the Study of Liver Consensus Statement on Acute Liver Failure (Part-2): Management of Acute Liver Failure. J Clin Exp Hepatol. 2020;10(5):477-517.
3. Wlodzimirow KA, Eslami S, Abu-Hanna A, Nieuwoudt M, Chamuleau RA. Systematic review: acute liver failure - one disease, more than 40 definitions. Aliment Pharmacol Ther. 2012;35(11):1245-56.
4. Aggarwal R. Hepatitis E: Historical, contemporary and future perspectives. J Gastroenterol Hepatol. 2011;26 Suppl 1:72-82.
5. Kumar R, Shalimar, Bhatia V, Khanal S, Sreenivas V, Gupta SD, et al. Antituberculosis therapy-induced acute liver failure: magnitude, profile, prognosis, and predictors of outcome. Hepatology. 2010;51(5):1665-74.
6. Kumar R, Shalimar, Sharma H, Goyal R, Kumar A, Khanal S. et al. Prospective derivation and validation of early dynamic model for predicting outcome in patients with acute liver failure. Gut. 2012;61(7):1068-75.

CHAPTER

143 Approach to Management of Chronic Hepatitis

Akash Roy, Sunil Taneja

ABSTRACT

Chronic hepatitis refers to a state of chronic inflammation in the liver as evidenced by abnormalities in liver function tests and/or histology and continuing without improvement for at least 6 months. Multiple causes lead to the development of chronic hepatitis, the most common of which include chronic viral hepatitis, nonalcoholic fatty liver disease (NAFLD), autoimmune hepatitis (AIH), and drug-induced liver injury. The challenge in the diagnosis of chronic hepatitis remains in the establishment of etiology and to assess the degree of fibrosis secondary to the chronicity. Liver biopsy, although a gold standard is less commonly indicated in the present day and remains the go-to-test in cases of diagnostic uncertainty. Once the diagnosis is established, specific therapy can be instituted depending upon the degree of liver damage.

"When you confront a problem you begin to solve it"

—Rudy Giullani

INTRODUCTION

DEFINITION

Traditionally, the term chronic hepatitis has been used to define a state of chronic inflammation in the liver as evidenced by abnormalities in liver function tests and/or histology and continuing without improvement for at least 6 months. This classical definition primarily serves to differentiate between an providing a cutoff time acute and a chronic pathologic process, limit. However, in practice, there remain gray zones as acute processes may have a smoldering course, and contrarily, chronic processes may have an acute presentation. Various subclassifications have been used for chronic hepatitis in the past including terms such as "chronic persistent hepatitis," "chronic active hepatitis," and "chronic lobular hepatitis," which are currently not used in practice.

ETIOLOGY

A spectrum of chronic liver diseases may have an inflammatory aspect but the specific term *chronic hepatitis* is often used in the following conditions:

- Viral hepatitis:
  - Chronic hepatitis B (CHB)
  - Chronic hepatitis C (CHC)
  - Hepatitis B virus (HBV) + hepatitis D virus coinfection
  - Atypical viruses: Epstein–Barr virus, cytomegalovirus
- Chronic AIH
- Wilsons Disease
- Alpha-1 antitrypsin deficiency
- Chronic drug-induced liver injury
- Idiopathic chronic hepatitis

APPROACH TO CHRONIC HEPATITIS

STEP 1: CONFIRMATION

The first step in the approach to a case of chronic hepatitis presenting with elevated aminotransferase levels is to reconfirm the presence of liver test abnormality with a sequential test and to confirm that the abnormalities truly reflect a hepatic abnormality. A common scenario for this is to document a simultaneous increase in ALT (alanine transaminase) levels in cases with an elevated AST (aspartate transaminase). Multiple nonhepatic causes of AST elevations exist, such as hemolysis, muscle disease, myocardial infarction, and hypothyroidism, which should be excluded prior to initiating a workup for underlying liver disease.

STEP 2: ANALYSIS OF HISTORY

Once a suspicion of underlying liver disease is made, the next step involves the analysis of the patient's history in detail.

- **History** of anorexia, generalized weakness, low-grade fever, arthralgia, rashes, and associated autoimmune conditions
- History of cholestasis (clay-colored stools, pruritus)
- History of alcohol use, intravenous drug usage, illicit substance usage, sexual promiscuity, tattooing, needle pricks, unsterilized shaving instrument sharing, and ear piercings
- Detailed drug history with particular attention to complementary and alternative medicine intake
- History of chronic medical comorbidities (type 2 diabetes mellitus, hypertension, obesity, hyperuricemia, and dyslipidemia)

- Family history of chronic hepatitis, history of liver failure in siblings, liver disease in the family and or known death due to liver disease in the family
- Family history of hepatic or nonhepatic cancers

STEP 3: DETAILED PHYSICAL EXAMINATION

General examination:

- Anthropometry [height, weight, body mass index (BMI) assessment, and recording of maximum premorbid body weight]
- Tattoo marks, evidence for intravenous drug usage, nail changes, and Kayser–Fleischer rings
- Stigmata of chronic liver disease (palmar erythema, gynecomastia, Duputryen's contracture, parotid enlargement, paper money skin, testicular atrophy etc.)
- Signs for liver cell failure (icterus, ascites, and hepatic encephalopathy)

Ancillary systems examination: Ancillary systems examination should include a thorough evaluation of the cardiorespiratory and neurological system for additional clues to aid in the diagnosis.

STEP 4: INTERPRETATION OF ENZYME ELEVATION

The transaminases mediate the transfer of amino groups of amino acids (aspartate and alanine) to ketoglutaric acid. AST is an enzyme that is nonspecific to the liver. In contrast, ALT serves as an index of liver cell injury. An AST increase in the absence of an ALT increase reflects cardiac, muscle disease, or hemolysis as described earlier. A rare cause of isolated AST elevation is the presence of macroAST in which there is a development of complexes of AST with immunoglobulins, which leads to its reduced clearance from the blood. The ratio of AST to ALT is useful in certain situations.

Alcoholic hepatitis: Since the alcohol-mediated damage leads to significant mitochondrial dysfunction, the rise in AST (present both in mitochondria and cytosol) is higher than that of the ALT (confined to cytosol). Furthermore, alcoholics have pyridoxine deficiency. ALT is more sensitive to pyridoxine deficiency; hence ALT is comparatively lower. Consequently, in patients with alcoholic hepatitis, the AST:ALT ratio is usually >1.5 and the AST increase is not >400 U/L.

Chronic viral hepatitis-related cirrhosis: The AST:ALT ratio is comparatively less sensitive in cases with chronic viral hepatitis as the presence of cirrhosis per se can alter and increase the AST:ALT ratio to >1.0.

Drug-induced liver disease: Multiple drugs causes a hepatocellular pattern of injury. The R-value gives the indicator of the pattern of injury.

$$R\ value = ALT/ULN \div AP/ULN$$

(AP: alkaline phosphatase; ULN: upper limit of normal)

- Hepatocellular injury ($R \geq 5$ and ALT > 2× ULN)
- Cholestatic injury ($R \leq 2$ and AP > 2× ULN)
- Mixed injury ($5 > R > 2$ and ALT, AP both >2× ULN)

TABLE 1 Tests for assessment of liver fibrosis.

Serum-based tests	Elastography	Invasive tests
• Platelet count • APRI (AST/platelet ratio index) • FIB-4 • European liver fibrosis Panel (ELF) test • Fibro test	• Transient elastography • ARFI (acoustic radiation force impulse) • MR elastography	• Liver biopsy: ◦ Percutaneous ◦ Trans jugular ◦ Laparoscopic

(AST: aspartate transaminase; FIB-4: fibrosis 4; MR: magnetic resonance)

STEP 5: ASSESSMENT OF DEGREE OF FIBROSIS

The severity of fibrosis forms a critical assessment once a diagnosis of chronic hepatitis has been made. In certain specific situations (nondiagnostic noninvasive tests, suspicion of dual pathology, AIH/Overlap syndromes)], invasive modalities are advised. Multiple noninvasive tests are available, of which the common ones in clinical practice are given in **Table 1**.

APRI: Aspartate aminotransferase/platelet ratio index (APRI) is the index calculated based upon the AST and platelet count. An APRI ≥ 1.5 has an AUROC (area under the receiver operating curve) of 0.8 and 0.89 for advanced fibrosis (F3–F4) and cirrhosis, respectively

Formula for APRI: (AST value of patient ÷ upper limit of the normal range)/platelet count

Fibrosis 4: The fibrosis 4 (FIB-4) is a score that uses the parameters of age, AST, ALT, and platelet count. The score has an AUC of 0.85 and 0.81 for predicting severe fibrosis in HCV and HBV infection, respectively.

STEP 6: LIVER BIOPSY

The role of liver biopsy is manifold in the setting of chronic hepatitis when extensive workup has been inconclusive. It helps in:

- Establishment of the diagnosis
- Evaluation of the types of necrosis
- Assessment of histological activity and (grading) evaluation of structural changes (staging): The two commonly used staging systems are the METAVIR and the ISHAK staging systems.

Additionally, liver biopsies may also yield additional clues regarding possible superinfection and provide an immunohistochemical assessment of viral antigens in the liver tissue core.

ETIOLOGIES OF CHRONIC HEPATITIS

CHRONIC HEPATITIS B

Any patient with HBsAg (hepatitis B virus surface antigen) present for at least 6 months are designated as CHB. The chronicity of HBV is dependent upon the age of acquisition of the virus, with higher rates of chronicity when acquired during the neonatal period (90%) in comparison to those that acquire HBV during adulthood (5%). The clinical manifestations in cases of chronic HBV range from asymptomatic, to nonspecific complaints (fatigue, right upper quadrant pain), to complications of cirrhosis. Certain extrahepatic manifestations (arthralgias, polyarteritis nodosa, glomerulonephritis, and cryoglobulinemia) can be seen associated with chronic HBV infection.

Classically, the stages of HBV had been divided into four distinct phases which include:

1. Immune-tolerant phase
2. Immune-active phase
3. Immune-control phase
4. Immune reactivation phase

However, recently this nomenclature has been modified (**Table 2**).

Treatment of CHB: There is considerable heterogeneity in various society guidelines regarding the initiation of treatment in CHB. As per the current American Association of study of Liver Disease (AASLD) guidelines, treatment of HBV should be offered in the following circumstances:

- *HBeAg-positive CHB*: HBV DNA > 20,000 IU/mL, ALT > 2 × ULN
- *HBeAg-negative CHB*: HBV DNA > 2,000 IU/mL, ALT > 2 × ULN
- *Compensated cirrhosis and decompensated cirrhosis*: All patients with CHB, if there is a presence of cirrhosis, should be treated.
- Furthermore, in certain selected cases such as adults >40 years of age, normal ALT with HBV
- DNA ≥ 1,000,000 IU/mL and with significant necroinflammation or fibrosis treatment is recommended.
- Additionally, patients with a family history of cirrhosis or HCC as well as those with extrahepatic manifestations, should be treated as per the recent AASLD guidelines.

The preferred treatment options for patients for naïve CHB according to the European Association for the Study of the Liver (EASL) are entecavir (ETV), tenofovir disoproxil fumarate (TDF), and tenofovir alafenamide (TAF).

CHRONIC HEPATITIS C

The development of chronic hepatitis with HCV is high. Of those who develop acute HCV infection, 55–89% develop chronic HCV infection. Up to 2–24% of patients with CHC develop cirrhosis over 20 years. Around 3% of patients with HCV cirrhosis develop decompensating events each year. The predominant mode of transmission is blood borne, with other less common routes being sexual and perinatal.

Most patients with CHC are asymptomatic. The most common symptom is fatigue, with other symptoms being abdominal discomfort, anorexia, musculoskeletal pain, pruritus, sicca syndrome, depression, impaired concentration, and reduced quality of life.

A majority of the patients with CHC have persistent or intermittent elevations of aminotransferases, although they may be normal in up to one third of the cases. Once cirrhosis develops, complications of portal hypertension form the predominant presentations. The most common extrahepatic manifestation of HCV is cryoglobulinemia, which must be excluded.

Evaluation and management of chronic hepatitis C:

- *Diagnose HCV infection*: Anti-HCV and quantitative HCV RNA
- *Evaluation for comorbidities/coinfections*: Renal function, HBsAg/HIV coinfection, and pregnancy assessment
- *Virological assessment*: HCV RNA with HCV genotype in selected cases
- *Assessment of fibrosis*:
  - Transient elastography (TE) [TE LSM (liver stiffness measure) >12.5 KPa suggests cirrhosis]
  - Serum tests: APRI, FIB-4
- *Any evidence of decompensation*:
  - USG/CT scan to rule out HCC
  - Simplified Indian National Guidelines for management of HCV
- *Confirmed HCV infection (HCV RNA+)*:
  - No cirrhosis: Treat with Sofosbuvir (400 mg) + Daclatasvir (60 mg) × 12 weeks
  - Check HCV RNA 12 weeks after treatment completion.
  - HCV RNA not detected: Treatment completed and sustained virological response (SVR) achieved
- *Cirrhosis (compensated Child-Pugh A)*:
  - Treat with Sofosbuvir (400 mg) + Velpatasvir (100 mg) × 12 weeks
  - Check HCV RNA 12 weeks after treatment completion
  - HCV RNA not detected: Treatment completed
  - If HCV RNA detectable: Refer to a higher center for expert opinion and management.
- *Decompensated cirrhosis (Child-Pugh B/C)*:
  - Sofosbuvir (400 mg) + Velpatasvir (100 mg) + Ribavirin (600–1200 mg) for 12 weeks
  - If Ribavirin intolerant: Sofosbuvir (400 mg) + Velpatasvir (100 mg) for 24 weeks

TABLE 2 Newer recommendations for phases of HBV infection.

Phase	ALT	HBV DNA	HBeAg	Liver biopsy
HBeAg-positive chronic infection	Usually normal	$>10^7$	Positive	Minimal inflammation
HBeAg-positive chronic hepatitis	Elevated	10^4–10^7	Positive	Moderate inflammation
HBeAg -negative chronic infection	Normal	<2,000	Negative	None
HBeAg-negative chronic hepatitis	Elevated	>2,000	Negative	Moderate-to-severe inflammation/fibrosis

(ALT: alanine aminotransferase; HBV: hepatitis B virus; HBeAg: hepatitis B e-antigen)

NONALCOHOLIC FATTY LIVER DISEASE

The diagnosis of NAFLD depends on two essential characteristics, which include:

1. Evidence of hepatic steatosis, either by imaging or histology, and
2. Lack of secondary causes such as significant alcohol consumption, long-term use of a steatogenic medication, or monogenic hereditary disorders

NAFLD exists in two predominant forms: (1) NAFL (nonalcoholic fatty liver) and (2) NASH (nonalcoholic steatohepatitis). NAFL is defined as the presence of >5% hepatic steatosis without evidence of hepatocellular injury. NASH is defined as the presence of >5% hepatic steatosis and inflammation with hepatocyte injury with or without any fibrosis.

The initial suspicion for attributing chronic hepatitis due to NASH should be suspected in patients having traditional risk factors for NASH (**Table 3**).

Clinical presentation and assessment of fibrosis: Patients with NAFL or NASH are usually asymptomatic. Up to one third of the patients may describe a vague right upper quadrant pain possible due to stretching of the liver capsule. Physical examination of patients with NAFLD is often unremarkable except for hepatomegaly, which again can be masked due to obesity. Peripheral signs of insulin resistance such as acanthosis nigricans, although rare in adults, should be looked for while evaluating such patients.

Liver biopsy is the gold standard for hepatic steatosis assessment but is rarely needed in clinical practice. Ultrasound is the initial imaging test for patients with suspected steatosis.

Transient elastography (with M probe and XL probe, especially in obese patients) has become a widely available tool for measuring liver stiffness. Other newer modalities in the assessment of fat in the liver and fibrosis include magnetic resonance elastography (MRE) and magnetic resonance imaging proton density fat fraction (MRIPDFF).

The key steps in the management of patients suspected to have NASH include:

- *Lifestyle modifications*:
  - To achieve a gradual weight loss of 7–10%
  - Caloric restriction: 1,200–1,600 calories-restricted diet with preferable consumption of a Mediterranean diet
  - Exercise: 150–200 min/week of aerobic and resistance training
- *Pharmacotherapeutics*: Vitamin E, pioglitazone, obeticholic acid, and saroglitazar
- *Surgical interventions for obesity*: Roux-en-Y gastric bypass (RYGB), adjustable gastric banding (AGB)
- *Endoscopic weight loss methods*: Intragastric balloons

TABLE 3 Risk factors for NAFLD.

Established risk factors	Evolving risk factors
• Metabolic syndrome	• Obstructive sleep apnea
• Obesity#	• Endocrinopathies
• Type 2 diabetes mellitus/ insulin resistance	• Polycystic ovarian disease not related to obesity
• Dyslipidemia	• Psoriasis
• Hypertension	• Osteoporosis
• Age	• Colorectal cancer
• Controversial: Sex, ethnicity	

It is important to note that that the BMI limits for obesity/overweight are lower than that of conventional cutoffs for Asians-Indians. Normal: 18–22.9 kg/m^2, overweight: 23–24.9 kg/m^2, and obesity: >25 kg/m^2.

(NAFLD: nonalcoholic fatty liver disease)

AUTOIMMUNE HEPATITIS

The classic setting for a case of AIH is a young female with a history of intermittent jaundice, significantly elevated transaminases, and a positive autoimmune serology with the possibility of concomitant associated autoimmune conditions (e.g., autoimmune hypothyroidism, vitiligo, pernicious anemia). AIH may present in various forms, which include severe acute presentation, asymptomatic cases, chronic hepatitis, and cirrhosis.

A simplified scoring system makes the bedside clinical diagnosis for chronic AIH (**Table 4**).

Characteristics of AIH patients with chronic hepatitis:

- Seen in one third of the patients
- Most commonly present with fatigue, malaise, arthralgias, or amenorrhea
- Most common presentation is easy fatigability.
- Jaundice may be present in certain cases.

Histological hallmarks in classical autoimmune hepatitis:

- Interface hepatitis is accompanied by lobular (panacinar) hepatitis (50%) and plasma cell infiltration (two-thirds).
- Emperipolesis (65%)
- Hepatocyte rosettes (33%)

TABLE 4 Simplified International Scoring System for the diagnosis of autoimmune hepatitis.

Criteria	Interpretation	Score
• ANA or SMA	• >1:40	+1
	• >1:80	+2
• Anti-LKM	• >1:40	+2
• Anti-SLA	• Positive	+2
Immunoglobulin G Levels	>ULN	+1
	>1.1 ULN	+2
Histology: • Interface hepatitis with no incompatible findings	• Compatible with AIH	+1
• Interface hepatitis with lymphoplasmacytic infiltration	• Typical of AIH	+2
Viral markers (HBV, HCV, HAV)	Negative	+2
Aggregate score: • Definite diagnosis: ≥7 • Probable diagnosis: 6		

(anti-LKM: anti-liver-kidney microsomal antibody; anti-SLA: anti-soluble liver antigen; SMA: smooth muscle antibodies; ULN: upper limit of normal)

Treatment of autoimmune hepatitis: All patients with AIH are candidates for therapy, except individuals with inactive disease by clinical, laboratory, and histological assessment. The first-line recommended treatment is prednisolone/prednisone alone or in combination with azathioprine.

- Prednisone: When used alone 40–60 mg daily in adults or a lower dose of prednisone, 20–40 mg daily, in combination with azathioprine
- Azathioprine: 50–150 mg daily or 1–2 mg/kg daily

Alternative agents include budesonide, mycophenolate mofetil, and tacrolimus in cases which are intolerant/failure to first-line therapy.

CONCLUSION

Chronic hepatitis is a diagnostic challenge and needs a detailed clinical evaluation. The etiological workup should initially be focused on common causes, and in specific cases, additional investigations for rarer causes need to be ascertained in detail. Besides, etiological workup assessment of the severity of liver disease is essential to prognosticate and plan therapeutic decisions. Early establishment of etiology as well as adequate risk stratification pave the way of initiating appropriate therapy.

RECOMMENDED READINGS

1. Sherlock S. Chronic hepatitis. Gut. 1974;15(7):581-97.
2. Kamath PS. Clinical approach to the patient with abnormal liver test results. Mayo Clin Proc. 1996;71(11):1089-94.
3. Andriulli A, Festa V, Leandro G, Rizzetto M. Usefulness of a liver biopsy in the evaluation of patients with elevated ALT values and serological markers of hepatitis viral infection. Digestive diseases and sciences. 2001;46(7):1409-15.
4. Terrault NA, Lok AS, McMahon BJ, Chang KM, Hwang JP, Jonas MM, et al. Update on prevention, diagnosis, and treatment of chronic hepatitis B: AASLD 2018 hepatitis B guidance. Hepatology. 2018;67(4):1560-99.
5. Ghany MG, Marks KM, Morgan TR, Wyles DL, Aronsohn AI, Bhattacharya D, et al. Hepatitis C guidance 2019 update: AASLD-IDSA recommendations for testing, managing, and treating hepatitis C virus infection. Hepatology. 2019;71(2):686-721.
6. Dhiman RK, Grover G, Premkumar M, Rathi S, Chopra M, Kaur R, et al. Decentralized care is effective in the management of patients with hepatitis C in a public health care setting: The Punjab model. J Hepatology. 2018;68:S50.
7. Mack CL, Adams D, Assis DN, Kerkar N, Manns MP, Mayo MJ, et al. Diagnosis and management of autoimmune hepatitis in adults and children: 2019 practice guidance and guidelines from the American Association for the study of liver diseases. Hepatology. 2020;72(2):671-722.
8. Chalasani N, Younossi Z, Lavine JE, Diehl AM, Brunt EM, Cusi K, et al. The diagnosis and management of non-alcoholic fatty liver disease: Practice Guideline by the American Association for the Study of Liver Diseases, American College of Gastroenterology, and the American Gastroenterological Association. Hepatology. 2012;55(6):2005-23.

CHAPTER 144 Treatment of Hepatitis (B, C, and Autoimmune)

Pankaj Puri, Bimal Kumar Sahu

ABSTRACT

Hepatitis B virus (HBV), hepatitis C virus (HCV), and autoimmune hepatitis (AIH) are the common causes of chronic hepatitis. Treatment of HBV is indicated in patients with active viral replication and evidence of liver dysfunction. The typical indication for treatment requires HBV DNA > 2,000 IU/mL, elevated ALT, and/or at least moderate histological lesions though all cirrhotic patients with detectable HBV DNA should be treated. The long-term administration of a potent nucleos(t)ide analog with high barrier to resistance, i.e., entecavir, tenofovir, disoproxil, or tenofovir alafenamide, represents the treatment of choice. All individuals who are infected with HCV and show viral replication should be treated. Treatment with combination therapy of direct-acting antiviral agents (DAA) has superseded pegylated interferon-based therapy in the management of hepatitis C. AIH is managed with immunosuppressive therapy with oral steroids and/or azathioprine (AZA). The combination regimen is preferred. Treatment should be instituted with prednisolone (starting with 30 mg daily and tapering down to 10 mg daily within 4 weeks) in combination with AZA (50 mg daily or 1–2 mg/kg body weight) or a higher dose of prednisolone alone (starting with 40–60 mg daily and tapering down to 20 mg daily within 4 weeks) in adults with AIH. Treated patients should be monitored for therapy response and adherence. All patients should be monitored for risk of disease progression and development of hepatocellular carcinoma (HCC).

"Twenty two million cases of hepatitis B spread every year because of the reuse of syringes. The WHO says one in two injections given is unsafe"

—Marc Koska

INTRODUCTION

While chronic hepatitis can arise from a diverse number of etiologies, HBV, HCV, and AIH are the most common causes of chronic hepatitis. Untreated patients can develop progressive liver disease resulting in cirrhosis, HCC, and can have a high mortality. The current chapter gives an approach to management of HBV, HCV, and AIH.

TREATMENT OF HEPATITIS B

Globally, approximately 240 people have been infected with HBV. India has a HBV carrier rate of approximately 3.0% with a high prevalence rate in the tribal population. HBV accounts for a large number of deaths due to liver cirrhosis and/or HCC. The goal of therapy is to prevent disease progression and HCC development, and improve survival. Besides this, the therapy helps to prevent mother-to-child transmission, hepatitis B reactivation, and helps in prevention and treatment of HBV-associated extrahepatic manifestations.

Treatment of HBV is indicated in patients with active viral replication evaluated by hepatitis B e antigen (HBeAg) and HBV DNA and features of liver dysfunction as evidenced by derangement of alanine aminotransferase (ALT), increased liver fibrosis on liver biopsy, or noninvasive tests such as transient elastography or clinical/ultrasonological evidence of cirrhosis. The recent guidelines for Prevention, Diagnosis, and Management of Hepatitis B Virus Infection include those issued by the European Association for the Study of the Liver (EASL) in 2017 practice guidelines, the American Association for the Study of Liver Diseases (AASLD) in 2018, and the Indian National Association for Study of the Liver (INASL) in 2018.

INDICATIONS

Treatment of chronic hepatitis B (CHB) is indicated in patients with elevation of ALT > 2 times the upper limit of normal (ULN) or evidence of significant histologic disease plus elevated HBV DNA > 2,000 IU/mL (in HBeAg negative) or > 20,000 IU/mL (in HBeAg positive). Noninvasive tests such as transient elastography can be used to assess liver fibrosis. Using transient elastography, patients with CHB can be considered to have severe fibrosis if the liver stiffness is >9 kPa with normal ALT, and >12 kPa elevated ALT but below 5 × ULN.

- HBV treatment is indicated in HBeAg-positive chronic hepatitis, if:
  - ALT > 80 U/L, or
  - If ALT 40–80 U/L and moderate necroinflammation, or fibrosis on noninvasive test for liver fibrosis, or liver biopsy
- HBV treatment is indicated in HBeAg-negative chronic hepatitis, if:
  - HBV DNA > 20,000 IU/mL, or
  - HBV DNA > 2,000 IU/mL and ALT > 80 U/L, or
  - HBV DNA > 2,000 IU/mL and moderate necroinflammation, or fibrosis on noninvasive test for liver fibrosis, or liver biopsy.
- Besides these, the following group of adult patients can be treated even if typical treatment indications are not fulfilled:
  - Patients with compensated or decompensated cirrhosis with any detectable HBV DNA, regardless of ALT levels, HBeAg status, or HBV DNA levels
  - Patients with liver failure (acute liver failure or acute-on-chronic liver failure), regardless of ALT levels, HBeAg status, or HBV DNA levels,
  - Patients with extrahepatic manifestation of HBV, regardless of ALT levels, HBeAg status, or HBV DNA levels,
  - Patients with family history of cirrhosis or HCC, with HBV DNA > 2,000 IU/mL, regardless of ALT levels or HBeAg status.
- HBeAg-positive patients with normal ALT and high HBV DNA levels > 20,000 IU/mL, may be treated if they are older than 30 years.

Patients not started on antiviral therapy should be closely monitored for the need of the therapy. Patients with HBeAg-positive CHB infection who are <30 years should be followed at least every 3–6 months. Patients with HBeAg-negative CHB infection with HBV DNA < 2,000 IU/mL should be followed every 6–12 months. Patients with HBeAg-negative CHB infection and serum HBV DNA ≥ 2,000 IU/mL should be followed every 3 months for the 1st year and every 6 months thereafter.

OPTIONS

Currently, there are two main treatment options for CHB patients: Nucleos(t)ide analogs (NAs) or pegylated interferon alpha (PegIFNα). The main concepts and features of current treatment strategies of CHB are depicted in **Table 1**.

The NAs that have been approved for HBV treatment are lamivudine (LAM), adefovir dipivoxil (ADV), entecavir (ETV), telbivudine (TBV), tenofovir disoproxil fumarate

TABLE 1 Main concepts and features of current treatment strategies of chronic hepatitis B.

Features	PegIFNα	ETV, TDF, TAF
Strategy	Induction of a long-term immune control	Inhibiting viral replication
Route of administration	Subcutaneous injections	Oral
Treatment duration	Finite therapy: 48 weeks	Long-term therapy: Until HBsAg loss (stopping NA can be considered in selected cases after a few years)
Tolerability	Low	High
Long-term safety concerns	Rare persistence of on-treatment adverse events (thyroid, psychiatric, neurological)	Renal safety and bone disease concerns with tenofovir
Contraindications	Decompensated liver disease, cytopenias, comorbidities etc.	None but dose may need to be adjusted according to eGFR
Level of viral suppression	Moderate (variable response pattern)	Universally high
Effect on HBeAg loss	Moderate, depending on baseline characteristics	Low in the 1st year, increases to moderate during long-term treatment
Risk of relapse after treatment cessation	Low for those with sustained response 6–12 months after therapy	• Moderate if consolidation treatment provided after HBeAg seroconversion • High for HBeAg-negative disease
Early stopping rules	Yes	No
Risk of viral resistance development	No	Minimal to none

(ETV: entecavir; HBeAg: hepatitis B e antigen; NA: nucleos(t)ide analog; PegIFNα: pegylated interferon alpha; TAF: tenofovir alafenamide; TDF: tenofovir disoproxil fumarate)

(TDF) and tenofovir alafenamide (TAF). However, LAM, ADV, and TBV frequently develop drug resistance. The potent NAs with high barrier to resistance include ETV, TDF, and TAF and have high antiviral efficacy leading to undetectable HBV DNA levels as well as its favorable safety profile. These drugs are the only treatment option for patient with decompensated liver disease, liver transplant (LT), extrahepatic manifestations, and acute hepatitis B or severe chronic HBV exacerbation, and for prevention of HBV reactivation in patients under immunosuppression.

Pegylated interferon alpha therapy for treatment of CHB patients: Pegylated interferon alpha can be considered as an initial treatment option for patients with mild-to-moderate HBeAg-positive/negative CHB. The standard dose of PegIFNα2a is 180 µg once weekly and that for PegIFNα2b is 1.5 µg/kg once weekly and the standard duration of PegIFNα therapy is 48 weeks. PegIFNα is more effective in HBeAg-positive patients with high pretreatment ALT, lower HBV DNA levels and genotype A (vs. genotype D). The rationale for a PegIFNα-based approach is to induce long-term immunological control with a finite duration treatment. The main advantage of PegIFNα therapy is that it is a finite therapy with absence of resistance and achievement of higher rates of HBeAg and HBsAg loss. The main disadvantages of PegIFNα treatment are its high cost, low efficacy (HBeAg seroconversion rates of 20–31% and sustained off-treatment HBV-DNA suppression of <2,000 IU/mL in 65% of persons who achieve HBeAg to anti-HBe seroconversion), need for administration by injection, frequent adverse effects, and numerous contraindications. Contraindications to PegIFNα include decompensated cirrhosis, hypersplenism, thyroid disease, autoimmune diseases, severe coronary artery disease, transplant recipients, pregnancy, seizure disorder, psychiatric illness, and cytopenias. Patients treated with PegIFNα require periodic monitoring of blood counts and thyroid functions for adverse effects. CHB patients with virological response after PegIFNα therapy should remain under long-term follow-up because of the risk of relapse.

Since there is a low efficacy of PegIFNα, there are predictors for stopping rules rather than continuing the drug for 1 year.

In HBeAg-positive patients, PegIFNα should be stopped if:

- At 12 weeks: HBsAg levels at 12 weeks of therapy are >20,000 IU/mL in genotype B and C or, no decline in HBsAg levels for genotype A and D.
- At 24 weeks: HBsAg levels > 20,000 IU/mL at 24 weeks in genotype A-D.

  In HBeAg-negative patients with genotype D, PegIFNα should be stopped, if:
- There is a combination of no decline in HBsAg levels and <2 log IU/mL decline in HBV DNA levels at 12 weeks.

Nucleos(T)ide analogs for treatment-naïve CHB patients: The long-term administration of a potent NA with high barrier to resistance is the treatment of choice, regardless of the severity of liver disease. The preferred regimens are ETV, TDF, and TAF as monotherapies at doses of 0.5, 300, and 25 mg, respectively. ETV is preferred over TDF in patients > 60 years, patients with bone disease, and patients with renal dysfunction. TAF is preferred over ETV in patients with previous exposure to NA.

Nucleos(t)ide analogs should be continued until there is confirmed HBsAg loss, with or without anti-HBs seroconversion. However, in selected noncirrhotic cases, NA discontinuation may be considered even without HBsAg less. However, these would require close monitoring after stoppage of NAs.

- In noncirrhotic HBeAg-positive CHB patients who achieve undetectable HBV DNA and stable HBeAg seroconversion, NAs can be discontinued after they complete at least 12 months of consolidation therapy.
- In selected noncirrhotic HBeAg-negative patients who have achieved long term (≥3 years) virological suppression under NA(s), discontinuation of may be considered, only if close post NA monitoring is possible.

Management of patients with nucleos(t)ide analog failure: Compliance to NA therapy should be checked in all cases of treatment failure. Treatment of NA resistance depends on previous drug exposure and is summarized in **Table 2**.

TREATMENT OF HEPTATIS B IN SPECIAL SITUATION

Prevention of HBV recurrence after liver transplantation: All patients on the transplant waiting list with HBV-related liver disease should be treated with NAs to reduce the HBV DNA load and risk of reactivation. They should continue lifelong NA therapy after transplant. While most cases are managed with NA therapy, combination of hepatitis B immunoglobulin (HBIg) and a potent NA is recommended in high-risk patients with detectable HBV DNA at liver transplantation, drug-resistant HBV, and human immunodeficiency virus or hepatitis delta virus (HIV or HDV) coinfection. HBsAg-negative patients receiving livers from donors with evidence of past HBV infection (anti-HBc positive) should receive antiviral prophylaxis with a NA without HBIg.

HIV coinfected patients: Antiretroviral therapy (ART) should be started, irrespective of CD4-cell count. All patients with HBV and HIV coinfection should receive HIV ART that includes two drugs with activity against HBV [(TAF or TDF) + (emtricitabine or LAM) + third agent active against HIV recommended]. We should not use TDF, LAM, or ETV as single agents. ETV should only be used in combination with a fully suppressive HIV regimen.

TABLE 2 Management of chronic hepatitis B patients who develop nucleos(t)ide analog resistance.

Resistance pattern	Recommended rescue strategies
LAM, TDV, or TBV resistance	• Switch to TDF or TAF
ADV resistance	• If LAM-naïve: Switch to ETV or TDF or TAF • If LAM-resistance: Switch to TDF or TAF • If HBV DNA plateaus: Add ETV or switch to ETV
TDF or TAF resistance	• If LAM-naïve: Switch to ETV • If LAM-resistance: Add ETV
Multidrug resistance	• Switch to ETV plus TDF or TAF combination

(ADV: adefovir; ETV: entecavir; LAM: lamivudine; TAF: tenofovir alafenamide; TBV: telbivudine; TDF: tenofovir disoproxil fumarate)

HDV coinfected patients: In patients with HBV and HDV coinfection, PegIFNα for at least 48 weeks is the current treatment of choice in compensated liver disease. Treatment success defined as undetectable HDV RNA 24 weeks after completing the treatment. In patients with elevated HBV DNA, concurrent treatment with ETV, TAF, or TDF is recommended.

HCV coinfected patients: Treatment of HCV infection in patients with HBV can result in a flare of the HBV. Patients fulfilling the standard criteria for HBV treatment should receive NA treatment. Patients with HBV and HCV coinfection with mild-to-moderate liver disease not meeting the treatment threshold for HBV should undergo close monitoring of the HBV load during DAA treatment for an early diagnosis of HBV reactivation. Cirrhotic patients should be treated with NA started before or together with DAA, regardless of the HBV load because HBV reactivation may be serious or life-threatening.

Acute hepatitis B: Only patients with severe acute hepatitis B, characterized by coagulopathy or protracted course, should be treated with NA.

Pregnancy: Besides treatment for maternal liver disease, treatment is also indicated to decrease transmission of HBV to the child. In pregnant women already on NA therapy, TDF should be continued while ETV or other NA should be switched to TDF. In pregnant women with high HBV DNA levels (>200,000 IU/mL), antiviral prophylaxis with TDF should start at week 24–28 of gestation and continue for up to 12 weeks after delivery. Breastfeeding is not contraindicated in HBsAg-positive untreated women or those receiving TDF therapy.

Patients undergoing immunosuppressive therapy or chemotherapy: All HBsAg-positive patients should receive prophylactic therapy with ETV or TDF or TAF. HBsAg-negative, anti-HBc-positive subjects should either receive prophylactic NA therapy or close monitoring of ALT, HBV DNA, and HBsAg. If monitoring is chosen, measure HBV DNA every 1–3 months and treat with NA upon first sign of reactivation (i.e., HBV DNA elevation, HBsAg seroconversion). All patients receiving anti-CD20 therapy (e.g., rituximab) or undergoing stem cell transplantation should receive anti-HBV prophylaxis, regardless of HBsAg status. Prophylactic therapy should be continued for 6–12 months after stoppage of immunosuppressive therapy.

Dialysis and renal transplant patients: HBsAg-positive dialysis patients who require treatment should receive ETV or TAF. The dose of ETV needs to be adjusted based on the estimated glomerular filtration rate (eGFR). TAF does not need any dose modification if eGFR is >15 mL/min. All HBsAg-positive renal transplant recipients should receive prophylactic ETV or TAF. HBsAg-negative, anti-HBc-positive subjects should be monitored for HBV infection after renal transplantation.

Extrahepatic manifestations: Patients with extrahepatic manifestations and raised HBV DNA should receive antiviral treatment with NA. PegIFNα should be avoided in patients with immune-related extrahepatic manifestations.

TREATMENT OF HEPATITIS C

The estimated prevalence of HCV infection in India is 0.5–1.5%, which translates to approximately 12–18 million HCV-infected individuals in the country. All individuals who are infected with HCV and show viral replication should be treated, except in patients with a life expectancy of ≤1 year.

TREATMENT OPTIONS

Direct-acting antiviral agents have replaced PegIFNα in the management of chronic hepatitis C (CHC). DAA target the NS3/4A serine protease, the NS5A replicase/assembly moiety, and the NS5B RNA-dependent polymerase of the HCV. The DAA are used in drug combinations which ensures efficacy and prevents the development of resistant variants. The choice of the DAA regimen is dependent upon genotype, resistance-associated variants, availability, and cost. Pangenotypic and genotype-specific DAA combinations are highlighted in **Tables 3** and **4**.

The AASLD recommendations for management of HCV as per genotype in patients with or without compensated cirrhosis are abridged in **Table 5**. The AASLD also recommends simplified therapy in adults with CHC (any genotype) who do not have cirrhosis and have not previously received hepatitis C treatment. The recommended regimen for simplified therapy for HCV are:

- Glecaprevir (GLE) (300 mg)/pibrentasvir (PIB) (120 mg) to be taken with food for a duration of 8 weeks
- Sofosbuvir (SOF) (400 mg)/velpatasvir (VEL) (100 mg) for a duration of 12 weeks

MANAGEMENT OF TREATMENT-NAÏVE CHC

Many of the drugs recommended by the AASLD and the EASL guidelines are not available in India.

TABLE 4 Genotype-specific DAA combinations.

Drugs	Formulation	Dosage
Sofosbuvir and ledipasvir for genotypes 1,4, 5 and 6	*Coformulated tablet*: Sofosbuvir 400 mg + Ledipasvir 90 mg	One tablet per day
Elbasvir and grazoprevir for genotype 1,4, and 6	*Coformulated tablet*: Elbasvir 50 mg + Grazoprevir 100 mg	One tablet per day

(DAA: direct-acting antiviral agents)

TABLE 5 AASLD recommendations for management of chronic hepatitis C in patients without cirrhosis or with compensated cirrhosis.

Genotype	Recommended regimen
Genotype 1 or 4	• Elbasvir (50 mg) + Grazoprevir (100 mg) × 12 weeks • Glecaprevir (400 mg) + Pibrentasvir (120 mg) × 8 weeks • Sofosbuvir (400 mg) + Ledipasvir (90 mg) × 12 weeks* • Sofosbuvir (400 mg) + Velpatasvir (100 mg) × 12 weeks
Genotype 2 or 3	• Glecaprevir (400 mg) + Pibrentasvir (120 mg) × 8 weeks • Sofosbuvir (400 mg) + Velpatasvir (100 mg) × 12 weeks#
Genotype 5 and 6	• Glecaprevir (400 mg) + Pibrentasvir (120 mg) × 8 weeks • Sofosbuvir (400 mg) + Ledipasvir (90 mg) × 12 weeks* • Sofosbuvir (400 mg) + Velpatasvir (100 mg) × 12 weeks

*In genotype 1a or genotype 4 patients without cirrhosis or HIV coinfection and HCV RNA levels < 6 million IU/mL, Ledipasvir-Sofosbuvir therapy can be decreased to 8 weeks.

#Patients with genotype 3 who have compensated cirrhosis should undergo resistance testing. Patients with NS5A RAS Y93H for velpatasvir should have weight-based ribavirin added to the regimen or be treated with fixed-dose combination of sofosbuvir (400 mg)/velpatasvir (100 mg)/voxilaprevir (100 mg) for 12 weeks.

TABLE 3 Pangenotypic DAA combinations.

Drugs	Formulation	Dosage
Sofosbuvir (NS5B polymerase inhibitor) and daclatasvir (NS5A inhibitor)	• Sofosbuvir 400 mg • Daclatasvir 60 mg	One tablet each per day
Sofosbuvir (NS5B polymerase inhibitor) and velpatasvir (NS5A inhibitor)	*Coformulated tablet*: Sofosbuvir 400 mg + Velpatasvir 100 mg	One tablet per day
Sofosbuvir (NS5B polymerase inhibitor), velpatasvir (NS5A inhibitor) and voxilaprevir (NS3/4A protease inhibitor)	*Coformulated tablet*: Sofosbuvir 400 mg + Velpatasvir 100 mg + Voxilaprevir 100 mg	One tablet per day
Glecaprevir (NS3/4A protease inhibitor) and pibrentasvir (NS5A inhibitor)	*Coformulated tablet*: Glecaprevir 100 mg + Pibrentasvir 40 mg	Three tablets (i.e., 300 mg/120 mg total dose) per day

(DAA: direct-acting antiviral agents)

Genotype-wise recommendations for management of treatment-naïve CHC with or without compensated cirrhosis in India are given in **Table 6**.

MANAGEMENT OF HCV IN SPECIAL SITUATIONS

Management of treatment failures:

PegIFNα-RBV-experienced, DAA-naïve HCV-infected patients with or without compensated cirrhosis: These patients can be managed with standard treatment as per genotype.

Prior treatment failures to regimen-containing DAA without NS5A inhibitors with or without compensated cirrhosis: These patients can be treated with SOF (400 mg) with VEL (100 mg) for 12 weeks. In genotype 3-infected patients with cirrhosis or Y93H substitution, weight-based ribavirin (RBV) should be added.

Prior treatment failures to DAA regimen-containing NS5A inhibitors with or without compensated cirrhosis: Ideally treatment could be modified according to resistance testing. Therapy should preferably be deferred till newer DAA are available in India. However, patients with advanced fibrosis can be treated with SOF (400 mg) and VEL (100 mg) along with weight-based RBV for 24 weeks.

IN DECOMPENSATED CIRRHOSIS

Patients with decompensated HCV-related cirrhosis should be treated with SOF with one of the NS5A inhibitors and RBV for 12 weeks. However, if the patient is ineligible/intolerant to RBV, the treatment should be for 24 weeks. While VEL-based regimen can be used across all genotypes, alternative regimen which can be used are DCV based in genotypes 2–3 and LDV-based regimen in genotypes 1, 4–6. The initial dose of RBV should be 600 mg and should be increased as tolerated.

AFTER LIVER TRANSPLANT

Successful therapy of HCV infection after LT has been shown to improve both graft and patient survival. The optimal timing to initiate therapy is usually after 3 months of LT by which time the patient's postoperative issues have been addressed and the immunosuppression is stable. Addition of low initial dose RBV should be considered in patients with cirrhosis.

IN HIV COINFECTION

Antibody test for HCV can be false negative in HIV patients with low CD4 counts and the presence of HCV infection may need to be confirmed by HCV RNA. HIV-coinfected patients should be treated with the same principles as those without HIV. However, drug interactions between ART and DAA are important.

Sofosbuvir/velpatasvir should not be used with efavirenz, atazanavir, nevirapine, or ritonavir. SOF should not be used with tipranavir. Ribavirin should not be used with didanosine, stavudine, or zidovudine. Tenofovir levels may increase with SOF/LDV or SOF/VEL and renal functions should be closely monitored.

PATIENTS WITH RENAL IMPAIRMENT

Glecaprevir-pibrentasvir and elbasvir/grazoprevir (EBR-GZR) have been recommended in patients with renal impairment and these do not require any renal modification. However, these are not available in India. SOF predominantly has renal excretion. Patients with mild or moderate renal dysfunction (eGFR ≥ 30 mL/min/1.73 m^2) do not require any modification of dosages. Several studies have demonstrated the safety of SOF-based regimen in patients with renal impairment. SVR12 (sustained virologic response at 12 weeks after treatment) of 95% has been reported with 12 weeks of therapy with SOF/VEL.

MANAGEMENT OF ACUTE HCV

Acute HCV is defined as HCV infection which presents within 6 months of exposure. Following HCV exposure, HCV RNA can be negative during the first 6 weeks. Before starting therapy, HCV RNA should be monitored for at least 6 months so as to look for spontaneous clearance. If there is no spontaneous viral clearance, the patients can be treated as per genotype.

IN PREGNANCY

Pregnancy should be avoided for 6 months after completion of therapy if ribavirin is included in the therapy. DAA should be avoided due to lack of safety data.

TABLE 6 Management of for treatment-naïve CHC with or without compensated cirrhosis in India.

	Patients without cirrhosis	Patients with compensated cirrhosis
GT 1, 4–6	• SOF (400 mg) + VEL (100 mg) × 12 weeks • SOF (400 mg) + LDV (90 mg) × 12 weeks* • SOF (400 mg) + DCV (60 mg) × 12 weeks	• SOF (400 mg) + VEL (100 mg) × 12 weeks Alternative regimen: • SOF (400 mg) + LDV (90 mg) × 12 weeks • SOF (400 mg) + DCV (60 mg) × 12 weeks
GT 2,3	• SOF (400 mg) + VEL (100 mg) × 12 weeks • SOF (400 mg) + DCV (60 mg) × 12 weeks	• SOF (400 mg) + VEL (100 mg) + weight-based RBV# × 12 weeks • SOF (400 mg) + DCV + weight-based RBV# × 24 weeks

*8 weeks if HCV RNA < 6 million IU/mL and no advanced fibrosis.

#*For genotype 3*: In patients with cirrhosis, weight-based RBV (1,000 mg if weight < 75 kg and 1,200 mg if >75 kg, as tolerated) to be added to SOF and VEL or DCV regimen.

(CHC: chronic hepatitis C; DCV: daclatasvir; GT: genotype; LDV: ledipasvir; RBV: ribavirin; SOF: sofosbuvir; VEL: velpatasvir)

Breastfeeding is not contraindicated unless the nipples are cracked and bleeding or the mother is HIV positive. As anti-HCV may be positive due to maternal antibodies till 18 months, the child should undergo anti-HCV testing after 18 months of age. If the child has anti-HCV antibodies, HCV RNA should be deferred till 3 years of age due to lack of approved drugs for children.

HCV RNA of the mother should be tested at 9–12 months after delivery to assess for spontaneous clearance (10–25%) prior to therapy of HCV.

IN CHILDREN

Adolescents between age 12 and 17 years and weighing >35 kg can be treated with same regimen as for genotype-specific CHC. Data support 12 weeks of SOF/LDV for adolescents infected with genotypes 1, 4, 5, and 6, and SOF/RBV for adolescents infected with genotype 2 (for 12 weeks) or genotype 3 (for 24 weeks). The US Food and Drug Administration has approved GLE/PIB for the treatment of genotype 1–6-infected adolescents with or without compensated cirrhosis and SOF/LDV for children aged 3 years and older who have genotype 1, 4, 5, and 6 HCV infections.

TREATMENT OF AUTOIMMUNE HEPATITIS

Autoimmune hepatitis is an unresolving inflammation of the liver of unknown cause. It is a relatively rare condition with prevalence of 15–25 cases per 100,000 population. The aim of treatment is to achieve complete clinical, biochemical and histological remission. Biochemical remission is defined as normalization of IgG and transaminases level. Histological remission is characterized by normal histology or minimal hepatitis with histological activity index (HAI) < 4.

Autoimmune hepatitis patients who need therapy are those with symptoms (fatigue, arthralgia, and jaundice), significant rise in transaminase levels, raised immunoglobulin levels, and liver biopsy showing active disease (interface hepatitis, bridging necrosis, or multiacinar necrosis). Currently the main stay of therapy for AIH is oral steroid monotherapy or a combination of steroids with AZA. Studies have shown to have similar survival with prednisone monotherapy as compared to prednisone/AZA combination therapy. However, combination regimen is associated with fewer side effects and is therefore preferred.

DOSING OF IMMUNOSUPPRESSION THERAPY

- Prednisone alone (60 mg daily) or a lower dose of prednisone (30 mg daily) in conjunction with AZA (50 mg or 1–2 mg/kg body weight) daily is used. Prednisolone can be used in place of prednisone in equivalent doses.
- Prednisone may be tapered down weekly to a level sufficient to maintain a remission from 20 mg daily onward. In steroid monotherapy, prednisone is tapered down to ≤20 mg/day while in combination therapy it is tapered down to 10 mg/day. The maintenance regimen is then continued until resolution of the disease, treatment failure, or drug intolerance.
- The initial dose of AZA should be 50 mg/day and should be increased depending on toxicity and response until a maintenance dose of 1–2 mg/kg. AZA is often started 2 weeks after starting steroids to confirm steroid responsiveness, evaluate thiopurine methyltransferase (TPMT) status, and exclude rare possibility of AZA-associated hepatitis.
- Once biochemical remission is achieved, immunosuppression should be continued for atleast 24 months before attempting withdrawal prior to which liver biopsy should be considered.

The dosing of immunosuppression in AIH has been summarized in **Table 7**.

TABLE 7 Immunosuppressive treatment regimens for autoimmune hepatitis.

	Monotherapy	Combination therapy		
	Prednisone only*	Prednisone*	Azathioprine	
	(mg/day)	(mg/day)	USA (mg/day)	EU (mg/kg/day)
Week 1	60	30	50	1–2
Week 2	40	20	50	1–2
Week 3	30	15	50	1–2
Week 4	30	15	50	1–2
Maintenance until endpoint	20 and below	10	50	1–2
Reasons for preference	• Cytopenia • Thiopurine methyltransferase deficiency • Pregnancy • Malignancy • Short course (≤6 months)	• Postmenopausal state • Osteoporosis • Brittle diabetes • Obesity • Acne • Emotional lability • Hypertension		

*Prednisolone can be used in place of prednisone in equivalent doses.

ALTERNATIVE REGIMEN

Budesonide (3 mg thrice daily, reduced to twice daily following remission) combined with weight-based AZA (1–2 mg/kg daily) can be used and has the potential of preserving bone mineral density. Mycophenolate mofetil (MMF) has been used in place of AZA. There is also limited data on the use of calcineurin inhibitors, cyclosporine, and tacrolimus. Anti-TNF and anti-CD20 have been tried as alternative therapies after failure of standard regimens have failed, but they require more to support their use.

ROLE OF LIVER TRANSPLANTATION

Liver transplantation should be considered if immunosuppression is unlikely to improve the patient and improve mortality. The indications of liver transplantation in AIH are:

- Acute liver failure
- Decompensated cirrhosis with a MELD score ≥ 15
- HCC meeting transplant criteria

CONCLUSION

HBV, HCV, and AIH are common causes of chronic hepatitis and liver-related morbidity. NA are the mainstay of management of HBV. Combination therapy with DAA have replaced PegIFNα as the mainstay of therapy for hepatitis C. However, in patients with AIH, the preferred regimen is combination therapy of steroid and AZA.

RECOMMENDED READINGS

1. European Association for the Study of the Liver. EASL 2017 clinical practice guidelines on the management of hepatitis B virus infection. J Hepatol. 2017;67(2): 370-98.
2. Terrault NA, Lok ASF, McMahon BJ, Chang K-M, Hwang JP, Jonas MM, et al. Update on Prevention, Diagnosis, and Treatment of Chronic Hepatitis B: AASLD 2018 hepatitis B guidance. Hepatology. 2018;67(4):1560-99.
3. Arora A, Singh SP, Kumar A, Saraswat VA, Aggarwal R, Bangar M, et al. c. J Clin Exp Hepatol. 2018;8(1):58-80.
4. Puri P, Anand AC, Saraswat VA, Acharya SK, Dhiman RK, Aggarwal R, et al. Consensus statement of HCV task force of the Indian National Association for Study of the Liver (INASL). Part I: Status report of HCV infection in India. J Clin Exp Hepatol 2014;4(2):106-16.
5. Ghany MG, Morgan TR, AASLD-IDSA Hepatitis C Guidance Panel. Hepatitis C guidance 2019 update: American Association for the Study of Liver Diseases–Infectious Diseases Society of America recommendations for testing, managing, and treating hepatitis C virus infection. Hepatology. 2020;71(2): 686-721.
6. European Association for the Study of the Liver. EASL recommendations on treatment of hepatitis C: Final update of the series. J Hepatol. 2020;73(5):1170-218.
7. European Association for the Study of the Liver. EASL Clinical Practice Guidelines: Autoimmune hepatitis. J Hepatol. 2015;63(4):971-1004.
8. Mack CL, Adam D, Assis DN, Kerkar N, Manns MP, Mayo MJ, et al. Diagnosis and management of autoimmune hepatitis in adults and children: 2019 Practice Guidance and Guidelines From the American Association for the Study of Liver Diseases. Hepatology. 2020;72(6):671-722.

CHAPTER 145

Spectrum of Alcoholic Liver Disease and Management of Alcoholic Hepatitis

Shekhar Singh Jaduan, Kaushal Madan

ABSTRACT

Alcoholic liver disease (ALD) is one of the main causes of chronic liver disease worldwide. ALD constitutes a spectrum of disease that includes fatty liver, alcoholic hepatitis (AH), alcoholic cirrhosis, and complications of cirrhosis and portal hypertension (HTN) including hepatocellular carcinoma (HCC). Clinical diagnosis of AH is made in a patient with rapid development or worsening of jaundice and liver-related complications with serum total bilirubin > 3 mg/dL alanine aminotransferase (ALT) and aspartate aminotransferase (AST) elevated > 1.5 times the upper limit but <400 U/L with AST/ALT ratio >1.5, documentation of heavy alcohol use until 8 weeks before onset of symptoms and exclusion of other liver diseases. Transjugular biopsy is not done routinely and considered if diagnosis is in doubt.

Severe AH is identified by Maddrey's discriminant function (mDF) score ≥32 or GAHS (Glasgow Alcoholic Hepatitis Score) ≥9 or MELD (Model for End-stage Liver Disease) score >20. Sever AH is associated with high mortality and patient should be admitted in hospital for management. Patient should be given adequate nutritional supplementation including high-protein diet. Infections are common, have high mortality in these patients, and should be actively treated. If no contraindications, then patients with severe AH should be treated with oral steroids for 4 weeks followed by gradual tapering. Lille score should be calculated at day 4–7 and steroids should be discontinued if Lille score is ≥0.45. Alternative therapies such as pentoxifylline, N-acetyl cysteine (NAC), and fecal microbiota transplant (FMT) can be considered in steroid-nonresponsive patients. Carefully selected severe AH patients not responding to steroids or ineligible for steroid therapy can be considered for early liver transplantation. Patients nonresponsive to corticosteroids, ineligible for early liver transplant, and with multiple organ failures have very poor prognosis and may be considered for palliative therapy.

"First you take a drink, then the drink takes a drink, then the drink takes you"

—FS Fitzgerald

INTRODUCTION

Alcohol consumption has been prevalent all over the world since ancient times and at present is ubiquitous, but patterns of alcohol use and its socioeconomic and health consequences have markedly changed in last few decades. About 2.3 billion people in the world drink alcohol and >50% people in Europe, North America, South America, and western Pacific regions drink actively.

According to the World Health Organization (WHO) global status report, harmful use of alcohol caused approximately 3 million deaths in 2016, and about 5.3% of overall deaths in the world that year. Alcohol is supposed to be the fourth leading cause of preventable death in developed nations after smoking, HTN, and obesity. Harmful alcohol intake results in more deaths as compared to diabetes mellitus (DM), HIV/AIDS, HTN, and tuberculosis.

Alcohol-related liver disease is a significant cause of morbidity and mortality and economic burden around the world. Alcohol is the most common cause of cirrhosis in developed countries and also has become leading cause of cirrhosis in countries such as India. About half of all cirrhosis-related deaths globally are due to alcohol. About 45.8 males and 14.7 females per 100,000 population die in India yearly because of cirrhosis, while alcohol contributed to 60 and 33.3% of them, respectively. Alcohol-related liver diseases result in about 140,632 deaths in India yearly.

ALCOHOL CONSUMPTION

Daily intake of 40–80 g alcohol in males and 20–40 g in females for at least 10 years can lead to significant liver damage. Accurate assessment of alcohol consumption is difficult in clinical practice. Quantification of alcohol intake in grams per day is a precise method but it is cumbersome and difficult in practice as most patients do not remember the different types of drinks and exact amount they were consuming. Alcohol intake can also be measured in terms of drinks per day. However, what defines a "drink" is quite variable. A standard drink is considered about 10–14 g of alcohol. Some internet-based tools can be helpful for measurement of alcohol intake. Amount of alcohol in common alcohol beverages is given in **Table 1**.

TABLE 1 Amount of alcohol in common alcohol beverages.

Beverage type	Beer	Wine	Hard liquor (whisky, rum)
Alcohol content (%)	5 %	12%	40%
One standard drink size (12–14 g alcohol)	350 mL	150 mL	30–40 mL

Harmful drinking is considered when alcohol use is causing damage to health that may be either physical or mental. *Heavy episodic drinking* has been defined as consumption of >60 g of pure alcohol on one occasion. *Binge drinking* is the consumption within about 2 hours of four or more drinks for women and five or more drinks for men.

RISK OF LIVER INJURY

Although consumption of 100 g alcohol per week has been associated with increased all-cause mortality, various studies have shown that regular drinking of 40–80 g alcohol per day in males and 20–40 g per day in females leads to significantly increased risk of chronic liver diseases. Dose–effect relationship between amount of alcohol intake and risk of liver disease is present but there is a marked variability. The effect of drinking pattern like binge drinking and type of beverage on risk of liver disease is controversial. Binge drinking is thought to increase the risk of alcohol-related liver disease including AH but has been unproven by recent studies.

GENETICS AND ENVIRONMENT

Among the patients with chronic heavy alcohol abuse, only 10–20 % will develop advanced liver disease. This indicates that along with dose and duration of alcohol intake, various other factors such as genetic, environmental, and behavioral play an important role in development of alcohol-related liver disease. Females have lower threshold of development of ALD. This is supposed to be due to their higher body fat content and lower activity of alcohol dehydrogenase enzyme in stomach.

Important factors that increase the risk for progressive fibrosis and cirrhosis in chronic drinkers are obesity, chronic hepatitis B, chronic hepatitis C, and smoking. On the other hand, coffee drinking has shown to be protective against cirrhosis in heavy drinkers.

Genetic factors that affect the susceptibility for advanced liver diseases include modifiers of genes involved in neurotransmission such as gamma-aminobutyric acid (GABA) and alcohol metabolism such as alcohol dehydrogenase and acetaldehyde dehydrogenase enzymes. Polymorphism and wide allelic variations of these genes may affect the individual susceptibility for alcohol-related liver damage. Polymorphisms in genes encoding inflammatory mediators, endotoxin response, and oxidative stress have also been shown to have a role in ALD progression. Patatin-like phospholipase domain-containing protein 3 (PNPLA-3) is involved in lipid metabolism. Alterations in this protein have been shown to play an important role in nonalcoholic fatty liver disease, HCC, and ALD.

SPECTRUM OF LIVER DISEASE

Recently, terminology of alcohol-associated liver disease has been changed in the EASL (European Association for the Study of the Liver) guidelines due to the stigma associated with term alcoholic. New and old terminologies with abbreviations have been mentioned in **Table 2**.

The term alcohol-related liver disease includes a broad spectrum of diseases that range from fatty liver to decompensated liver disease. Early asymptomatic ALD includes fatty liver or alcohol-related steatosis. This is the earliest and most common liver abnormality seen in >90% chronic alcohol abusers. With continued alcohol abuse, alcohol-related steatosis can progress to alcohol-related steatohepatitis (ASH) and advanced ALD. Advanced ALD includes AH and compensated and decompensated cirrhosis. Patients with cirrhosis can also develop complications such as HCC, variceal bleed, ascites, and hepatic encephalopathy (HE).

Natural history and clinical course of ALD is strongly determined by the alcohol abstinence or relapse. Fatty liver is a benign condition and resolves with abstinence of alcohol. While with continuous heavy drinking, steatosis can progress to cirrhosis in 10% cases over the course of 5 years. Alcohol-related steatohepatitis can be developed in 10–35% of chronic alcohol abusers (**Fig. 1**). It is characterized by presence of necroinflammation and fibrosis and has much higher mortality compared to steatosis alone. About 8–20% of chronic drinkers will develop micronodular cirrhosis with time that progresses to macronodular cirrhosis. Macronodular cirrhosis can be complicated by HCC and decompensation events such as ascites, variceal bleeding, and HE.

TABLE 2 New terminology for alcohol-related disorders.

Previous term	Current term	Abbreviation
Alcoholic	Alcohol use disorder	AUD
Alcoholic liver disease	Alcohol-related/associated liver disease	ALD
Alcoholic cirrhosis	Cirrhosis due to alcohol-related liver disease	ALD cirrhosis
Alcoholic steatohepatitis	Steatohepatitis due to ALD	ASH
Alcoholic fibrosis	Fibrosis due to ALD	ALD fibrosis
Alcoholic hepatitis	Alcoholic hepatitis	AH

Source: Adapted from EASL Clinical Practice Guidelines: Management of alcohol-related liver disease 2018.

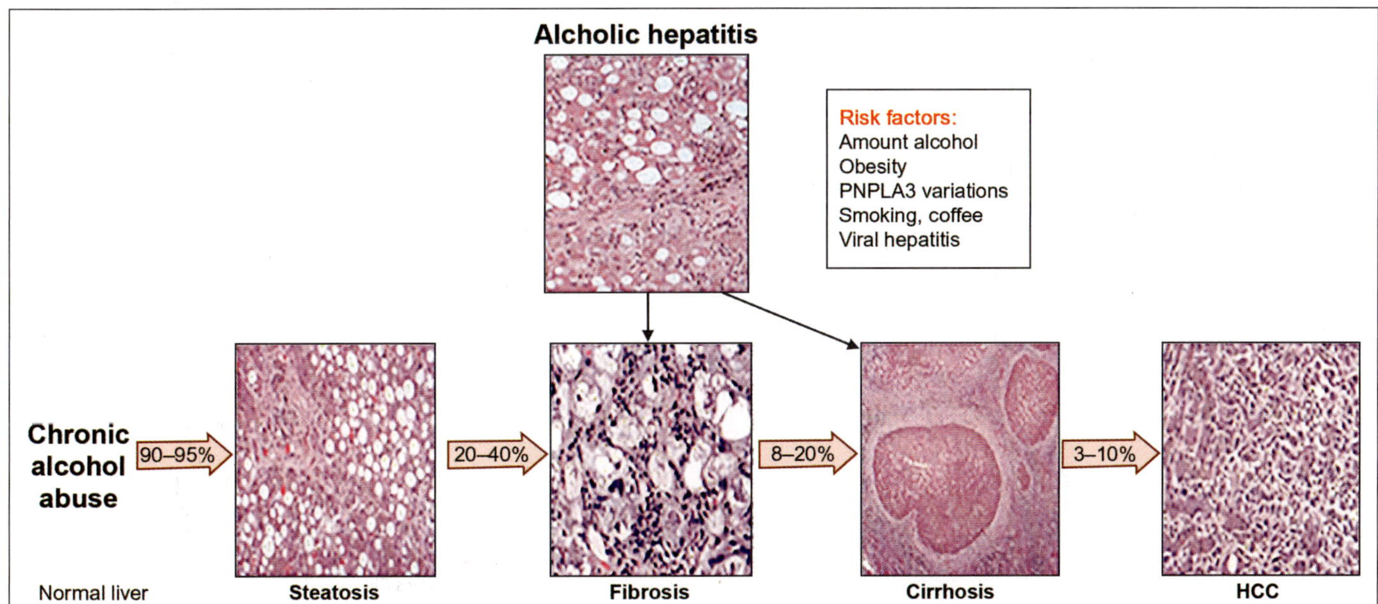

FIGURE 1: Spectrum of alcohol-associated liver disease.

Source: Adapted from ACG Clinical Guideline: Alcoholic Liver Disease 2018.

ALCOHOLIC HEPATITIS

Alcoholic hepatitis is a serious event in spectrum of liver disease associated with very high mortality in its severe form. It is a clinical syndrome with new onset of jaundice and raised International Normalized Ratio (INR) with or without HE and ascites. AH is preceded by ongoing alcohol abuse. Its presence is often ignored in patients where is it superimposed on decompensated ALD-related cirrhosis, so prevalence is difficult to predict. AH can be present at any stage of ALD and severe AH can have underlying cirrhosis in >80 % cases. AH is associated with histologically defined steatohepatitis characterized by inflammatory infiltrates, steatosis, and hepatocyte ballooning.

PATHOGENESIS

Liver is the principal site of ethanol metabolism while other organs such as stomach and skeletal muscle contribute to lesser degree only. Ethanol is metabolized by three-enzyme systems: (1) the cytosolic alcohol dehydrogenase (ADH) system, (2) microsomal ethanol-oxidizing system (MEOS) also called as cytochrome P450 2E1, and (3) peroxisomal catalase system. By all three-enzyme systems, ethanol is converted to acetaldehyde, which is then further metabolized to acetate by acetaldehyde dehydrogenase (ALDH). Acetaldehyde is a reactive metabolite and a principal mediator of liver injury via multiple pathways. Acetaldehyde-modified proteins and lipids on the cell surface may behave as neoantigens and trigger immunologic injury. Acetaldehyde also deplete glutathione reserve of liver, thus impairing its antioxidant defense. Free radicals, superoxides, and hydroperoxides are generated as byproducts of ethanol metabolism that can lead to liver injury. Chronic alcoholics are often depleted in nutritional source of antioxidants such as selenium, zinc, and vitamin E leading to increased risk of oxidative injury.

DIAGNOSIS

It is important to identify patients who have pure AH rather than AH superimposed on advanced cirrhosis because pure AH patients stand a chance to be treated with steroids. On the other hand, patients who have AH superimposed on decompensated cirrhosis will have poor response and will be predisposed to infectious complications if treated with steroids. Such patients should be referred for liver transplantation early.

History and physical examination: The most important feature is progressive jaundice which can be associated with nonspecific symptoms such as fever, malaise, and dull aching right hypochondrial pain. Alcohol withdrawal symptoms (tachycardia, tremors, and restlessness) can be seen at presentation or during admission. On clinical examination, tender hepatomegaly can be seen along with features of chronic liver failure and portal HTN such as jaundice, ascites, and splenomegaly. Sign and symptoms of malnutrition and sarcopenia can also be present. Commonly present laboratory abnormalities are increased leukocyte count even in absence of infection, marked hyperbilirubinemia, and raised aspartate AST and ALT levels. AST and ALT levels although elevated but usually remains <400 IU/mL. AST/ALT ratio is usually in between 1.5 and 3. Severe AH can also have raised prothrombin time and low serum albumin level.

Histology: Diagnosis of AH usually made clinically based on history, physical examination, and laboratory values. Histology provides the definitive diagnosis but not necessary and avoided due to associated cost and bleeding risk. Liver biopsy, preferably by transjugular route, is needed when diagnosis is uncertain or for prognostication. Histological features of AH are macrovesicular steatosis, Mallory-Denk bodies, hepatocyte ballooning, lobular infiltration of neutrophils, cholestasis, and liver fibrosis. Liver fibrosis is mainly pericellular and sinusoidal known as chicken-wire appearance.

Radiology: A large swollen liver usually suggests pure AH, whereas presence of a nodular liver with florid features of portal HTN suggests a long-standing underlying cirrhosis with superadded AH.

ASSESSMENT OF SEVERITY AND PROGNOSIS

Various model scores are available to identify the patients with severe AH that has high risk of death (**Table 3**). These scores also help to select patients who are less likely to respond to conservative means and therefore have to be prepared for aggressive therapies (e.g., liver transplantation) early on in their course. mDF is one of the earliest and most

TABLE 3 Most common prognostic scores (and their components) used in alcoholic hepatitis.

Prognostic scores	Creatinine	Bilirubin	PT/INR	Albumin	Total leukocyte counts	Age
Maddrey's DF	–	+	+	–	–	–
GAHS	+	+	+	–	+	+
ABIC	+	+	+	+	–	+
MELD	+	+	+	–	–	–
Lille	+	+	+	+	–	+

(ABIC: age, serum bilirubin, INR, and serum creatinine score; GAHS: Glasgow alcoholic hepatitis score; Maddrey's DF: Maddrey's discriminant function; MELD: model for end-stage liver disease)

Source: Adapted from EASL Clinical Practice Guidelines: Management of alcohol-related liver disease 2018.

commonly used model scores in AH patients. Score of ≥32 is used to define severe AH. Patients with score ≥32 have 1-month mortality of 35–50% while mortality is only <10% in the patients with score of <32.

Other commonly used scores that have been found to be helpful in prediction of severity in AH are ABIC (age, serum bilirubin, INR, and serum creatinine), MELD, and GAHS. MELD score of >20 is suggestive of severe AH with 1-month mortality of 20%. Lille model is used to identify the severe AH patients who are responsive to steroid therapy. Reduction in serum bilirubin by day 7 has been shown to predictive of steroid response. Lille score of ≥0.45 at day 7 suggests nonresponse to steroids and therapy should be stopped and patients should be considered for liver transplantation or experimental therapies. Recently, it has been suggested that Lille score can be used to assess the steroid nonresponse as early as day 4 and waiting till day 7 may not be required. In recent studies, combination of Lille and MELD score has also been shown as a good indicator of survival.

MANAGEMENT

General measures and supportive treatment: Regardless of severity of AH, all patients should receive supportive treatment including nutritional supplementation, treatment of infections, and management of complications of cirrhosis and portal HTN. In all patients of ALD including AH, alcohol abstinence remains the single most important step. A short-term survival in severe AH is determined by degree of liver injury (as indicated by various prognostic scores) while long-term prognosis is strongly influenced by the alcohol abstinence.

Patients with HE should be treated with rifaximin and lactulose. Ascites is managed with diuretics, albumin, and paracentesis. ALD patients commonly have B-complex vitamin deficiencies, especially thiamine and should receive supplementation. Sepsis is common and important cause of mortality in AH patients and should be treated aggressively.

Nutritional therapy: Malnutrition and sarcopenia are common problems in patients with ALD. Almost every patient with ALD-related cirrhosis and AH will have some degree of malnutrition. Malnutrition not only affects the ICU stay and length of hospitalization but also patient survival. Adequate nutritional support has been shown to improve the survival in AH patients.

Accurate assessment of malnutrition is difficult in CLD patients due to low serum proteins, presence of edema, and ascites. Subjective global assessment tool, hand grip strength, and mid arm circumference are relatively reliable tests for assessment of malnutrition and sarcopenia in patients with liver disease.

Daily energy intake of 35–40 kcal/kg of body weight (BW) and a daily protein intake of 1.2–1.5 g/kg of BW in patients with AH has been recommended by the European Society for Clinical Nutrition and Metabolism (ESPEN) and the Indian National Association for Study of Liver (INASL). These patients often failed to reach target intake of daily protein and caloric requirements due to loss of appetite, various dietary restrictions (e.g., salt, water), and prolonged fasting needed for various procedures. Nasogastric tube feeding should be strongly considered if patients fail to achieve daily targeted requirement due to poor oral intake. Nighttime snack (9 PM) and morning breakfast prevent starvation and proteolysis leading to improved muscle mass. Protein restriction should not be done even in the presence of encephalopathy. Branched-chain amino acids (BCAA) supplementation can be beneficial for the patients with HE and also improves muscle mass. Along with thiamine and other B-complex vitamins, these patients commonly have fat-soluble vitamin and mineral deficiencies (Mg, Se, and Zn) which should be supplemented. Parenteral nutrition is associated with sepsis and other complications and is not preferable.

Specific pharmacological therapies:

Steroids: Glucocorticoid therapy has a beneficial role in severe AH, although some studies have shown conflicting results. Newer evidences suggest only modest survival benefit at 1 month. Steroids provide only short-term survival benefit at 1 month, while no benefit was seen at 3 months or beyond that. Use of steroids in AH patients may be associated with increased risk of sepsis and GI bleed. So, selection of appropriate candidate for steroids therapy should be carefully done. Therapy should be stopped early if patient is unlikely to respond. Steroid treatment is contraindicated in patients with sepsis, acute kidney injury, and gastrointestinal Bleed. Steroids are only given in patients who fulfil the criteria for severe AH. In appropriately selected patients, prednisolone 40 mg/day or methylprednisolone 32 mg/day is given for 4 weeks followed by tapering over next 2–3 weeks. Lille score is use to identify the patients not responding to steroids at day 7. If Lille score is ≥0.45 at day 7, steroids can be stopped. Some recent studies have described the use of Lille score at day 4 to identify steroid-nonresponder patients.

Pentoxifylline: Pentoxifylline is a phosphodiesterase inhibitor that inhibits the activity of tumor necrosis factor alpha (TNF-α). TNF-α is supposed to play a role in AH pathogenesis. Although an initial study showed benefit, most randomized controlled trials (RCTs) have not shown survival benefit in severe AH. A network meta-analysis reported low-quality evidence of short-term mortality reduction at 28 days with pentoxifylline. Use of pentoxifylline in steroid nonresponders or in combination with steroid has not proven beneficial. In few studies, pentoxifylline reduced the incidence of acute kidney injury, hepatorenal syndrome, and death due to hepatorenal syndrome. Use of pentoxifylline may be considered in a subgroup of severe AH with kidney injury, although more prospective studies are required. The largest trial [STOPAH (Steroids or pentoxifylline for alcoholic hepatitis) trial] which compared corticosteroids, with pentoxifylline either alone or in combination against placebo, in AH patients has not shown any survival advantage over short- or long-term with either of the agent.

N-acetyl cysteine and other antioxidants: Oxidative stress plays a major role in alcohol-induced liver injury and use of antioxidants may have a theoretical advantage. NAC restores glutathione levels in liver and so combats oxidative stress. Most of the studies of NAC use in AH failed to provide evidence of significant advantage over standard medical therapy. In a multicentric trial, combination of NAC and prednisolone in AH patients had lower incidence of hepatorenal syndrome, infection, and better survival at 4 weeks compared to prednisolone alone.

Other antioxidants such as silymarin, S-adenosyl methionine, and vitamin E have been evaluated in various studies. Despite having a good safety profile, evidences of potential benefit and survival advantage are very limited or absent.

Newer therapies: Only a proportion of patients with severe AH are eligible for steroids and there is a strong unmet need for newer therapies to improve survival and outcome in AH patients.

- *Granulocyte colony stimulating factor (GM-CSF):* Use of GM-CSF have shown positive results in few studies in patients with AH and acute-on-chronic liver failure. GM-CSF stimulates the bone marrow and mobilizes CD34-positive stem cells into blood circulation. CD34-positive stem cells then home into the liver and contribute to liver regeneration leading to improved survival.
- *Fecal microbiota transplant:* Gut–liver axis and gut dysbiosis play an important role in liver diseases including ALD. Use of FMT has shown promising and encouraging results in patients with severe AH. In a small pilot study, use of FMT resulted in significantly better survival at 1 year as compared to control group. Although data is still very limited, more evidence is needed before FMT can be recommended as an established therapy for AH. Various pharmacological therapies used in AH has been described in **Table 4**.

Liver transplantation: Alcohol-related cirrhosis is a well-established and one of the most common indication of liver transplant worldwide. Early liver transplant in patients with severe AH not responding to medical therapy used to be considered contraindicated in past. This was because of the requirement of a 6-month alcohol abstinence period before being considered for liver transplant. An initial small pilot study in 26 patients showed excellent survival in severe AH patients with early liver transplant. In a large recent multicenter study from US, early liver transplantation (mean abstinence duration of 55 days) resulted in good survival rates (94% and 84% at 1 and 3 years, respectively). Relapse of alcohol drinking remains a challenge and patients selection should be done carefully. Clinical tools and markers are needed to identify the patients who are likely to have relapse of drinking behavior.

TABLE 4 Pharmacological therapies for management of alcoholic hepatitis.

Therapies with proven efficacy	Therapies with potential benefits	Therapies with no proven benefits
• Steroids • Nutrition supplementation	• Pentoxifylline • N-acetyl cysteine • Granulocyte colony stimulating factor • Fecal microbiota transplant	• TNF-α inhibitors • Antioxidants, vitamin E • Insulin, glucagon, anabolic steroids • Propylthiouracil

(TNF-α: tumor necrosis factor alpha)

CONCLUSION

Alcohol use disorder, in addition to being a social and public health problem, is a major cause of morbidity and mortality due to alcohol-related liver diseases. The spectrum of ALD ranges from simple steatohepatitis to fatal severe AH, from compensated cirrhosis to acute-on-chronic liver failure with complications of decompensated cirrhosis and liver cancer. The treatment of cirrhosis and its complications is similar to other cause of cirrhosis. AH is a unique condition driven by inflammatory response and having a high short-term mortality in severe cases. The treatment of AH is both frustrating and less than optimal. All patients should be treated with nutritional therapy. Corticosteroids benefit only a subset of patients who should be selected carefully. Patients with severe AH who are ineligible for steroid therapy or are intolerant to steroids should be considered for early liver transplantation. Significant research in this area has paved way for promising therapy with newer anti-inflammatory molecules which may improve survival in these patient and hold promise in the future.

RECOMMENDED READINGS

1. Qayed E, Srinivasan S, Shahnavaz N. Alcohol associated liver disease. Sleisenger and Fordtran's Gastrointestinal and liver disease, 10th edition. China: Saunders; 2015.
2. European Association for the Study of the Liver. EASL Clinical Practice Guidelines: Management of alcohol-related liver disease. J Hepatol. 2018;69(1):154-81.
3. Singal AK, Bataller R, Ahn J, Kamath PS, Shah V. ACG Clinical Guideline: Alcoholic liver disease. Am J Gastroenterol. 2018;113(2):175-94.
4. Lucey MR, Mathurin P, Morgan TR. Alcoholic hepatitis. N Engl J Med. 2009;360(26):2758-69.
5. Louvet A, Labreuche J, Artru F, Boursier J, Kim DJ, O'Grady J, et al. Combining data from liver disease scoring systems better predicts outcomes of patients with alcoholic hepatitis. Gastroenterology. 2015;149(2):398-406.e8.
6. Singal AK, Charlton MR. Nutrition in alcoholic liver disease. Clin Liver Dis. 2012;16(4):805-26.
7. Plauth M, Cabré E, Riggio O, Assis-Camilo M, Pirlich M, Kondrup J, et al. ESPEN guidelines on enteral nutrition: Liver disease. Clin Nutr Edinb Scotl. 2006;25(2):285-94.

8. Cheung K, Lee SS, Raman M. Prevalence and mechanisms of malnutrition in patients with advanced liver disease, and nutrition management strategies. Clin Gastroenterol Hepatol. 2012;10(2):117-25.
9. Singh S, Murad MH, Chandar AK, Bongiorno CM, Singal AK, Atkinson SR, et al. Comparative effectiveness of pharmacological interventions for severe alcoholic hepatitis: A systematic review and network meta-analysis. Gastroenterology. 2015;149(4):958-70.e12.
10. Sarin SK, Sharma S. Predictors of steroid non-response and new approaches in severe alcoholic hepatitis. Clin Mol Hepatol. 2020;26(4):639-51.
11. Thursz MR, Richardson P, Allison M, Austin A, Bowers M, Day CP, et al. Prednisolone or pentoxifylline for alcoholic hepatitis. N Engl J Med. 2015;372(17):1619-28.
12. Sarin SK, Pande A, Schnabl B. Microbiome as a therapeutic target in alcohol-related liver disease. J Hepatol. 2019;70(2):260-72.

CHAPTER

146 Cirrhosis of Liver and Its Complications

Manav Wadhawan

ABSTRACT

The natural history of end-stage liver disease (cirrhosis) is characterized by progressive decompensation over a period of time. Various complications such as variceal bleeding, ascites, renal dysfunction, and hepatic encephalopathy (HE) occur as the liver dysfunction progresses. Timely identification and appropriate management of these complications improve prognosis and increase survival of these patients. The current management protocols for each of these complications are detailed in this chapter. The role of liver transplantation in each of these complications is also discussed.

"Is life worth living? It all depends on the liver"

—William James

INTRODUCTION

Cirrhosis is end-stage liver disease that happens due to various causes. Alcohol-induced liver disease is the most common cause of cirrhosis in India, closely followed by nonalcoholic steatohepatitis (NASH) and viral hepatitis. Various complications of cirrhosis include variceal bleeding, ascites, spontaneous bacterial peritonitis (SBP), hepatorenal syndrome (HRS), and HE. In this chapter, we will discuss each of these complications along with the respective management protocols.

VARICEAL BLEEDING

The lifetime prevalence of varices in a patient with cirrhosis varies from 40 to 70%. Patients with compensated cirrhosis have a prevalence of 40%, which goes up to 70% in decompensated. New development of varices in cirrhosis range from 5–8 % per year. Varices develop once hepatic venous pressure gradient (HVPG) crosses a threshold HVPG value of 10 mm Hg. The usual threshold where variceal bleeds happen is ≥12 mm Hg. Varices may rupture and bleed at rate of 5–15% per year, with a higher risk in patients with large esophageal varices and red signs.

Variceal bleeding in a patient with cirrhosis is a critical emergency in medicine, with a mortality rate of 10–20%. Variceal bleeding may stop spontaneously in 40–50% of patients and treatment achieves control of bleeding within 24 hours from admission in nearly 90 %. Nearly 5% of patients may die from uncontrolled bleeding. If untreated, rebleeding and death occur in approximately 60 and 30% of patients, respectively.

The clinical diagnosis of variceal bleeding is usually straightforward. The patient (previously known or unknown cirrhosis) presents with either hematemesis or melena, or both.

Following features may help achieve a diagnosis of variceal bleed in emergency itself:

- Signs of underlying liver disease (jaundice, ascites, encephalopathy etc.)
- *Physical examination*: Following findings indicate variceal bleed—
  - Firm liver
  - Left-lobe hypertrophy
  - Splenomegaly
  - Stigmata of alcohol abuse (spider nevi)

Every patient presenting with upper gastrointestinal (UGI) bleed requires an UGI endoscopy (that is the primary modality to diagnose and treat variceal bleeding).

MANAGEMENT

- Patients with acute variceal bleed should preferably be managed in an intensive care unit (ICU) or high dependency unit (HDU).
- Immediate volume restitution should be initiated to restore and maintain hemodynamic stability (preferably with crystalloids).
- Blood transfusions should be given to maintain a hemoglobin between 7 and 9 g/dL
- Correction of prothrombin time/international normalized ratio (INR) or platelet counts by the use of fresh frozen plasma and platelets is not required in every patient and needs to be individualized.
- Antibiotic prophylaxis should be given in patients with cirrhosis presenting with acute variceal bleed.
- Intravenous (IV) ceftriaxone (1–2 g/24 h) for a maximum of 7 days is preferred. However, initial antibiotic choice should be dictated by local antibiogram.
- Proton-pump inhibitors (PPIs) are not routinely recommended in treatment of variceal bleeds. However, PPIs can be justified if there is a doubt about diagnosis of varices as a cause of bleed. In contrast, PPIs are the drug of choice in case of erosive gastric/ulcer bleeding.
- *Use of vasoactive agents*: Vasoactive agents such as somatostatin, octreotide, and terlipressin have been shown to significantly lower mortality and improve hemostasis in patients with cirrhotic UGI bleed. Hence these medications should be started as early as possible in a patient presenting with acute variceal bleed. The efficacy of all three available vasoactive drugs (somatostatin, terlipressin, and octreotide) in controlling variceal bleed is similar. Choice of agent should, therefore depend of availability and cost of these medicines. However, patients who present with variceal bleed and acute kidney injury (AKI) may benefit from use of terlipressin (over somatostatin or octreotide). Terlipressin is better avoided in patients with significant cardiac disease. The optimum duration of therapy with vasoactive agents is 2–5 days. In view of significant cardiac side effects of these medicines, baseline ECG and continuous hemodynamic monitoring are recommended. Contraindications to usage of these agents are peripheral vascular disease, arrhythmias, ischemic heart, or cerebral disease.
- *Use of beta-blockers*: Beta-blockers should not be started in the acute setting; introduction of beta-blocker should be after stopping vasoactive drugs (2–5 days after acute bleed). In patients on beta-blockers presenting with bleed, beta-blockers should be stopped at presentation.
- *Endoscopy*: Upper gastrointestinal endoscopy should be done within 24 hours of admission and earlier if there is excessive bleeding. A good attempt at resuscitation and pharmacological treatment before the endoscopy improves the outcomes after endoscopy. Although endoscopic band ligation (EBL) and sclerotherapy are both effective in controlling variceal bleeding, EBL is the preferred endoscopic method. *Sclerotherapy* has higher complications compared with EBL and should no longer be offered in acute variceal hemorrhage.
- *Balloon tamponade*: This age-old method is highly effective and controls acute bleeding in up to 90% of patients although >50% rebleed when the balloon is deflated. It may be a life-saving treatment in massive uncontrolled variceal hemorrhage where immediate UGI is not possible. Also it allows for resuscitation and safe transportation to a center where endoscopic facilities are available. Sengstaken–Blakemore tube can be kept inflated for a maximum of 24 hours.
- *Transjugular intrahepatic portosystemic stent-shunt (TIPSS)*: TIPSS is an effective salvage measure for failure of endoscopic treatment in acute variceal bleeding. In various studies, control of bleeding was achieved in 90–100%, with rebleeding in 6–16%. However, the expertise for TIPSS is only available at a few centers in the country.

ASCITES

Ascites is defined as accumulation of fluid in the abdomen. A majority of ascites (>80%) is due to cirrhosis, malignant ascites being the other common cause. Ascites is one of the most common complications of cirrhosis. It is often the first complication predating other serious problems such as SBP, HRS, and HE.

All patients with clinically apparent ascites should undergo a diagnostic paracentesis, analysis of peritoneal fluid is mandatory for the evaluation of the cause of ascites. The aspirated fluid should be tested for a total and differential leukocyte count (TLC and DLC), a total protein level, albumin level, and a serum-ascites albumin gradient (SAAG). Other tests such as adenosine deaminase (ADA) and malignant cytology should also be done to rule out other etiologies such as tuberculosis (TB) and malignancy. The TLC and DLC of ascitic fluid is important in diagnosing SBP (to be discussed subsequently).

SAAG of ascitic fluid indicates the portal pressure; it is calculated by subtracting the ascitic albumin level from the serum albumin level obtained on the same day not more than a few hours apart. A SAAG value equal to or greater than 1.1 g/dL indicates a high likelihood of portal hypertension. A value <1.1 g/dL virtually rules out portal hypertension and other causes of ascites should be considered. The classical description of ascitic fluid as transudative (protein <2.5 g/dL) and exudative (protein ≥2.5 g/dL) is considered outdated these days, especially in context of portal hypertension. For example, in patients with hepatic venous outflow obstruction or cardiac failure leading to portal hypertension and ascites, protein content is high.

MANAGEMENT

The first-line treatment for cirrhotic ascites is salt restriction (<3 g/day), along with a combination of spironolactone (potassium sparing diuretic) and loop diuretic (furosemide or torsemide). Nowadays, fluid restriction is not recommended unless serum sodium is <125 mmol/L. Patients not responding to salt restriction and diuretics (either maximum dose or developing complications on diuretics) are labeled as refractory ascites.

The treatment options for refractory ascites are very limited. Repeated large-volume paracentesis (LVP) along with albumin infusions can be considered. It is important to replace albumin @ 5–8 g/L of fluid removed during LVP. Appropriate replacement can prevent development of post paracentesis circulatory dysfunction (PPCD), which can be fatal in worse cases. TIPSS can be considered in selected patients with refractory ascites [those with preserved liver functions and Model for End-Stage Liver Disease (MELD) score ≤12]. The best treatment option for these patients is often a liver transplantation (best survival rates for refractory ascites are with liver transplant compared to all other therapies). Nowadays, oral vasoconstrictive agent, midodrine, with weekly albumin infusions has been found to be effective in some patients with refractory ascites (with preserved liver functions).

SPONTANEOUS BACTERIAL PERITONITIS

Spontaneous bacterial peritonitis is defined as ascitic fluid cell count >500 cells/mm^3 with >50% neutrophils or an absolute neutrophil count ≥250 cells/mm^3 without any intra-abdominal surgical treatable source of infection (**Table 1**). Empirical antibiotic therapy with either cefotaxime or ceftriaxone is recommended in these patients without waiting for the culture reports. Also patients with SBP should be given daily albumin infusions to prevent development of HRS. The duration of IV antibiotic as well albumin should be 5–7 days.

Recurrence of SBP after the first episode is seen in majority of these patients (up to 70%). Risk factors for recurrent SBP include ascitic total protein < 1 g/dL, impaired renal functions (creatinine ≥1.2 or serum sodium ≤130). It is recommended that a fluoroquinolone (norfloxacin 400 mg once daily) should be used in prevention of recurrent SBP.

TABLE 1 Testing of ascitic fluid and definition of SBP.

Tests to be done for ascitic fluid	Definition of SBP
• Total and differential count of ascitic fluid cells • Serum-ascites albumin gradient (SAAG) • Biochemistry (total protein, albumin, glucose) • Adenosine deaminase • Malignant cytology	• Total ascitic cell count >500 cells/mm^3 with >50% PMNs or • Absolute PMN count in ascitic fluid >250 cells/mm^3

(SBP: spontaneous bacterial peritonitis; PMN: polymorphonuclear neutrophil)

HEPATORENAL SYNDROME

Hepatorenal syndrome is classically seen in cirrhotic patients with ascites (especially refractory ascites). It is defined as functional renal dysfunction in cirrhosis with normal kidneys. The pathophysiologic mechanism is intense renal vasoconstriction leading to decreased GFR and low urine output and rising creatinine. Occurrence of HRS signifies high short-term mortality in patients with cirrhosis. Traditionally, HRS was defined as rise in serum creatinine (sCr) above 1.5 mg/dL. But recently the criteria for AKI in cirrhosis have been changed to following (**Table 2**):

- Rise in creatinine ≥50% from baseline
- Rise by ≥0.3 mg/dL in <48 hours

Acute kidney injury has further been divided in three stages:

- *Stage 1*: Rise in creatinine ≥ 50% from baseline or rise by ≥0.3 mg/dL in <48 hours
- *Stage 2*: Increase in sCr rising to 2–3 times the baseline (within 7 days)
- *Stage 3*: Increase of sCr >3-fold from baseline or sCr ≥4.0 mg/dL with an acute increase ≥0.3 mg/dL or initiation of renal replacement therapy

Accordingly, HRS is now defined as in a patient with cirrhosis and ascites (**Box 1**):

- Diagnosis of AKI according to the International Club of Ascites-Acute Kidney Injury (ICA-AKI) criteria

TABLE 2 Definition of AKI in cirrhosis.

Stage of AKI	Definition
1	Rise in creatinine ≥50% from baseline or rise by ≥0.3 mg/dL in <48 h
2	Increase in serum creatinine (sCr) rising to 2–3 times the baseline (within 7 days)
3	Increase of sCr >3-fold from baseline or sCr ≥4.0 mg/dL with an acute increase ≥0.3 mg/dL or initiation of renal replacement therapy

BOX 1 Definition of HRS (all the following criteria should be fulfilled).

- Patient has cirrhosis and ascites
- Diagnosis of AKI according to the ICA-AKI criteria
- No response after two consecutive days of diuretic withdrawal and plasma volume expansion with albumin 1 g/kg of body weight
- Absence of shock
- No current or recent use of nephrotoxic drugs (NSAIDs, aminoglycosides, iodinated contrast media etc.)
- No macroscopic signs of structural kidney injury, defined as:
  - Absence of proteinuria (>500 mg/day)
  - Absence of microhematuria (>50 RBCs per HPF)
  - Normal findings on renal ultrasonography

(HRS: hepatorenal syndrome; ICA: International Club of Ascites)

- No response after two consecutive days of diuretic withdrawal and plasma volume expansion with albumin 1 g/kg of body weight
- Absence of shock
- No current or recent use of nephrotoxic drugs [nonsteroidal anti-inflammatory drugs (NSAIDs), aminoglycosides, iodinated contrast media etc.]
- No macroscopic signs of structural kidney injury, defined as:
  - Absence of proteinuria (>500 mg/day)
  - Absence of microhematuria (>50 RBCs per hpf)
  - Normal findings on renal ultrasonography

Hepatorenal syndrome types 1 and 2: The cutoff of creatinine ≥ 2.5 mg/dL has been removed to diagnose HRS type 1. Stages 2 and 3 of AKI-HRS has been categorized as HRS type 1. Stage 1 of HRS-AKI would correspond to type 2 HRS.

MANAGEMENT

Hepatorenal syndrome is a life-threatening complication of cirrhosis associated with a very high short-term mortality. Hence all efforts should be made to prevent HRS. Use of albumin infusions along with antibiotics during treatment of SBP has been shown to help prevent HRS and improve prognosis in SBP. Also replacement of 5–8 g of albumin for each liter of ascitic fluid tapped during LVP has been shown to prevent PPCD/HRS (discussed earlier in the ascites section).

Vasoconstrictive agents: The most effective treatment for HRS is use of vasoconstrictive agents such as terlipressin along with albumin infusions. Various studies have shown that terlipressin improves renal function in 40–50% of patients of type 1 HRS with improved short-term survival. The starting dose of terlipressin is usually 1 mg/4–6 h which can be subsequently increased to a maximum of 2 mg/4–6 h. Recently, it has been proposed that terlipressin is used as a continuous infusion and is better tolerated with lower dosages and less side effects. Most of the centers including ours have shifted to using terlipressin infusion than boluses. Treatment is continues till sCr below 1.5 mg/dL is achieved.

Other vasoconstrictors such as noradrenaline and midodrine plus octreotide, both in combination with albumin have also been used in treatment of HRS. Although these have shown to improve renal function in some patients, the trials reported are in small number of patients.

Transjugular intrahepatic portosystemic stent-shunts has shown to improve renal function in HRS type 1 patients.The number of patients who can safely undergo TIPSS in the setting of HRS is very low (considering extremely sick status and poor liver reserve).

Early liver transplantation: The best treatment option for HRS is early liver transplantation. It reverses the pathophysiology of HRS and simultaneously cures the liver disease. High survival rates of 65–87% have been reported in type 1 HRS. The kidneys in these patients usually recover after liver transplant. Hence, combined liver–kidney transplant is not advised in patients with HRS, except in patients are on renal support for >12 weeks before liver transplant.

HEPATIC ENCEPHALOPATHY

Hepatic encephalopathy in cirrhosis refers to decrease in sensorium (often reversible) precipitated by factors such as GI bleed, metabolic abnormalities such as hyponatremia, infections, sedative medicine intake, fluid losses, constipation, and diuretic overdose. HE can be further classified into minimal or overt. Overt HE is seen in 30–40% of all patients with cirrhosis whereas prevalence of minimal hepatic encephalopathy (MHE) has been reported to be 60–80%. MHE can only be diagnosed by specialized tests as patients have no overt symptoms. The importance of MHE is in predicting future occurrence of overt HE and preventing motor accidents. We will discuss only overt HE in this chapter, those interested in reading about MHE can refer to the consensus published by the Indian National Association for Study of the Liver (INASL).

MANAGEMENT

Serum ammonia levels have an important implication in the diagnosis of HE. If ammonia value is normal, it virtually rules out hepatic cause of altered sensorium. But elevated ammonia levels do not confirm HE as ammonia may be raised in cirrhosis patients even without encephalopathy.

However, despite all the fallacies of ammonia, all treatment options of HE are directed toward lowering ammonia in these patients. All patients with HE should be investigated for potential precipitating factors (discussed above) and treated accordingly.

Lactulose is the first-line therapy; dose should be titrated for patient to pass 2–4 soft stools in a day. If patients are not able to tolerate oral lactulose, enemas can be given. Lactulose is helpful in treating ongoing HE as well as preventing future episodes (secondary prophylaxis of HE).

Rifaximin (oral nonabsorbable antibiotic) is often added to lactulose at a dose of 550 mg twice a day. It is not required for treating grade 1–2 encephalopathy but may be useful in higher grades of HE. However, in secondary prophylaxis (preventing future episodes in recovered patient), a combination of lactulose and rifaximin is better than lactulose alone.

Other therapies that can be used in refractory cases include oral branched-chain amino acids (BCAA), probiotics and intravenous L-ornithine L-aspartate. Intravenous BCAA have not been found to be effective in overt HE and hence are not recommended.

RECOMMENDED READINGS

1. D'Amico G, Garcia-Tsao G, Pagliaro L. Natural history and prognostic indicators of survival in cirrhosis: a systematic review of 118 studies. J Hepatol. 2006;44(1): 217-31.
2. Groszmann R, Garcia-Tsao G, Bosch J, Grace ND, Burroughs AK, Planas R, et al. Beta-blockers to prevent

gastroesophageal varices in patients with cirrhosis. N Engl J Med. 2005;353(21):2254-61.
3. D'Amico G, Pasta L, Madonia S, Tarantino G, Mancuso A, Malizia G, et al. The incidence of esophageal varices in cirrhosis. Gastroenterology. 2001;120(5):A2.
4. Merli M, Nicolini G, Angeloni S, Rinaldi V, De Santis A, Merkel C, et al. Incidence and natural history of small esophageal varices in cirrhotic patients. J Hepatol. 2003;38(3):266-72.
5. Chavez-Tapia NC, Barrientos-Gutierrez T, Tellez-Avila F, Soares-Weiser K, Mendez-Sanchez N, Gluud C, et al. Meta-analysis: antibiotic prophylaxis for cirrhotic patients with upper gastrointestinal bleeding—an updated Cochrane review. Aliment Pharmacol Ther. 2011;34(5):509-18.
6. Wells M, Chande N, Adams P, Beaton M, Levstik M, Boyce E, et al. Meta-analysis: vasoactive medications for the management of acute variceal bleeds. Aliment Pharmacol Ther. 2012;35(11):1267-78.
7. Ginés P, Quintero E, Arroyo V, Terés J, Bruguera M, Rimola A, et al. Compensated cirrhosis: natural history and prognostic factors. Hepatology. 1987;7(1):122-8.
8. Singh V, Dhungana SP, Singh B, Vijayverghia R, Nain CK, Sharma N, et al. Midodrine in patients with cirrhosis and refractory or recurrent ascites: a randomized pilot study. J Hepatol. 2012;56(2):348-54.
9. Hoefs JC, Canawati HN, Sapico FL, Hopkins RR, Weiner J, Montgomerie JZ. Spontaneous bacterial peritonitis. Hepatology. 1982;2(4):399-407.
10. Sort P, Navasa M, Arroyo V, Aldeguer X, Planas R, Ruiz-del-Arbol L, et al. Effect of intravenous albumin on renal impairment and mortality in patients with cirrhosis and spontaneous bacterial peritonitis. N Engl J Med. 1999;341(6):403-9.
11. Titó L, Rimola A, Ginès P, Llach J, Arroyo V, Rodés J. Recurrence of spontaneous bacterial peritonitis in cirrhosis: frequency and predictive factors. Hepatology. 1988;8(1): 27-31.
12. Runyon BA; AASLD. Introduction to the revised American Association for the Study of Liver Diseases Practice Guideline management of adult patients with ascites due to cirrhosis 2012. Hepatology. 2013;57(4): 1651-3.
13. Goyal O, Sidhu SS, Sehgal N, Puri S. Noradrenaline is as effective as terlipressin in hepatorenal syndrome type 1: A prospective, randomized trial. J Assoc Physicians India. 2016;64(9):30-5.
14. Mattos AZ, Schacher FC, Mattos AA. Vasoconstrictors in hepatorenal syndrome - A critical review. Ann Hepatology. 2019;18(2):287-90.
15. Brensing KA, Textor J, Perz J, Schiedermaier P, Raab P, Strunk H, et al. Long-term outcome after transjugular intrahepatic portosystemic stent shunt in non-transplant cirrhotics with hepatorena syndrome: a phase II study. Gut. 2000;47(2):288-95.
16. Dhiman RK, Saraswat VA, Sharma BK, Sarin SK, Chawla YK, Butterworth R, et al. Indian National Association for Study of the Liver. Minimal hepatic encephalopathy: consensus statement of a working party of the Indian National Association for Study of the Liver. J Gastroenterol Hepatol. 2010;25(6):1029-41.
17. Vilstrup H, Amodio P, Bajaj J, Cordoba J, Ferenci P, Mullen KD, et al. Hepatic encephalopathy in chronic liver disease: 2014 practice guideline by the European Association for the Study of the Liver and the American Association for the Study of Liver Diseases. J Hepatol. 2014;60(2):715-35.
18. Agrawal A, Sharma BC, Sharma P, Sarin SK. Secondary prophylaxis of hepatic encephalopathy in cirrhosis: an open-label, randomized controlled trial of lactulose, probiotics, and no therapy. Am J Gastroenterol. 2012;107(7):1043-50.

CHAPTER 147

Nonalcoholic Fatty Liver Disease

Arka De, Ajay Duseja

ABSTRACT

Nonalcoholic fatty liver disease (NAFLD) refers to the presence of hepatic steatosis in the absence of significant alcohol consumption and other etiologies. It is a metabolic liver disease that has snowballed into a significant public health problem in the background of increased urbanization, sedentary lifestyles, and easy access to calorie-dense foods. Most patients are detected incidentally on ultrasound or while workup for elevated transaminases, although they may also present with cirrhosis and its complications. There is an intrinsic relation between NAFLD and metabolic comorbidities, and as such NAFLD may be considered to be the hepatic component of metabolic syndrome. NAFLD is an umbrella term and the histologic spectrum includes nonalcoholic fatty liver (NAFL), nonalcoholic steatohepatitis (NASH), cirrhosis, and hepatocellular carcinoma (HCC).

NASH is generally considered to be the progressive form and its differentiation from NAFL requires liver biopsy. The degree of underlying fibrosis is the main determinant of clinical outcomes and can be reliably estimated using noninvasive techniques. Management of NAFLD centers around the management of metabolic risk factors and lifestyle measures for weight loss. Pharmacotherapeutic options are currently limited and include vitamin E, pioglitazone, and saroglitazar. Several new drugs are in different phases of clinical trials. The indications and outcome of liver transplantation for NASH-related cirrhosis and HCC are same as for other etiologies.

"Your diet is a bank account. Good food choices are good investments"

—B Frankel

INTRODUCTION

Nonalcoholic fatty liver disease refers to the accumulation of "fat" in >5% hepatocytes in the absence of significant alcohol intake or other alternate etiologies of steatosis (**Box 1**). NAFLD is an overarching term that includes a histologic spectrum ranging from NAFL to NASH, cirrhosis, and HCC. As discussed later, the differentiation between NAFL and NASH is based on histologic findings in liver biopsy. In simplified terms, NASH denotes the presence of active inflammation with ongoing hepatic injury and is usually considered to portend a higher risk of progressive fibrosis, cirrhosis, and HCC, as compared to NAFL. Nonetheless, it is important to emphasize that it is the severity of underlying fibrosis that is the ultimate determinant of clinically relevant outcomes (**Flowchart 1**).

NAFLD has been described as the hepatic component of the metabolic syndrome. Indeed, there is an intrinsic and bidirectional relationship between NAFLD and metabolic risk factors such as obesity, type 2 diabetes mellitus (T2DM), hypertension, and dyslipidemia. The more the number of metabolic risk factors, higher is the risk of having not just NAFLD but also NASH. Moreover, patients with NAFLD also have a higher propensity of emergent or worsening of metabolic comorbidities.

Recently, an international team of experts have suggested the new nomenclature of metabolic dysfunction-associated fatty liver disease (MAFLD). There is much debate in the Hepatology community about the pros and cons of this change in nomenclature. A detailed discussion about this is beyond the scope of this chapter. As such, the term MAFLD is not yet widely accepted and may well be premature and confusing to the hepatologists and other medical subspecialties. Hence, we will be using the term NAFLD in the remainder of the chapter.

BOX 1	Alternate etiologies of fatty liver.
• Alcoholic liver disease	
• Drug-induced fatty liver (e.g., amiodarone, corticosteroids)	
• Chronic hepatitis C (particularly genotype 3)	
• Autoimmune hepatitis	
• Wilson's disease	
• Celiac disease	
• Hemochromatosis	
• Starvation	
• Parenteral nutrition	
• Abetalipoproteinemia, Wolman's disease or cholesteryl ester storage disease (CESD)	

EPIDEMIOLOGY

Worldwide, roughly a quarter of the general population suffers from NAFLD. The prevalence is highest in the Middle Eastern and South American countries (~30%) and low in Africa (~10%). Data on the prevalence of NASH is limited but it is estimated to be around 5–6% in the general population. NAFLD prevalence in India ranges from 9 to 53%. Estimates suggest that in excess of 25 million Indians have NAFLD. Given the close association of lifestyle factors with NAFLD, it is not surprising that the prevalence is higher in urban areas compared to rural areas.

The concomitant epidemics of obesity and T2DM together with increasing urbanization, calorie-dense diets, and sedentary lifestyles have catapulted NAFLD into a substantial public health problem not just in the Western world but also in developing countries such as India. Earlier data from India had suggested a mild disease at presentation in patients with NAFLD. The recent data, however suggests that a significant number of patients with NAFLD in India present with NASH and significant fibrosis and NASH are an important cause of cirrhosis and HCC.

ETIOPATHOGENESIS

Originally, a two-hit hypothesis was proposed for the pathogenesis of NAFLD. The first hit is hepatic steatosis occurring as a consequence of insulin resistance. Inflammatory and oxidative injury to the steatotic liver constitutes the second hit which leads to progressive damage to hepatocytes. Presently, a multi-hit hypothesis is implicated in the pathogenesis. There appears to be a complex parallel interplay of genetic predilection [e.g., patatin-like phospholipase domain-containing 3 (*PNPLA3 I148M*) and transmembrane 6 superfamily 2 (*TM6SF2 E167K*) gene variants], imbalance of calorie intake and expenditure, insulin resistance, dysfunctional and expanded visceral adipose tissue with altered adipokine levels (decreased adiponectin and increased leptin), lipotoxicity of intrahepatic lipids, changes in gut microbiome, oxidative stress, and activation of innate immunity. All these contribute to inflammation, hepatocyte apoptosis, and progressive fibrosis.

Insulin resistance is central to the pathogenesis of NAFLD. Usually, insulin suppresses peripheral lipolysis.

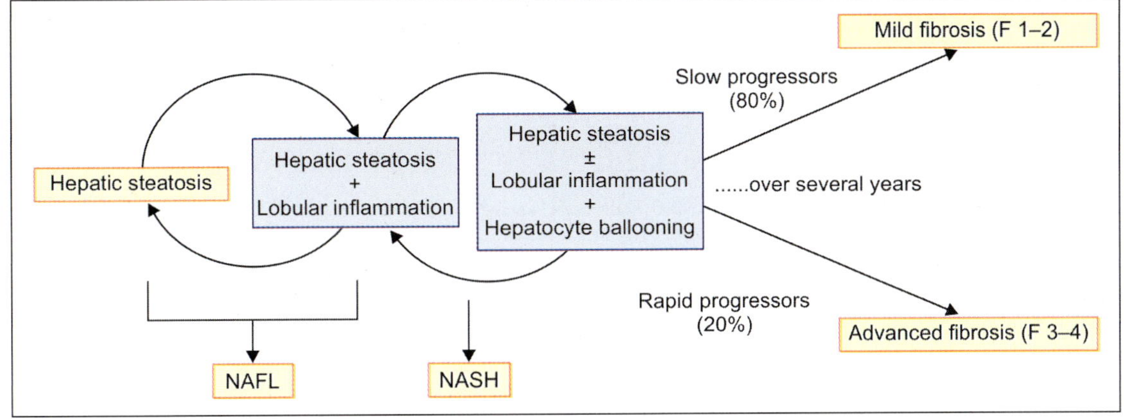

FLOWCHART 1: Spectrum and progression of NAFLD.

Source: Adapted from De A, Duseja A. Natural history of simple steatosis or nonalcoholic fatty liver. J Clin Exp Hepatol. 2020;10(3):255-62.

In insulin resistance, there is increased lipolysis from the adipose tissue with release of free fatty acids. Additionally, insulin resistance also increases expression of hepatic fatty acid translocase which promotes the uptake of free fatty acids by the liver.

De novo lipogenesis in the liver also increases insulin resistance. This is mediated via sterol regulatory element-binding protein (SREBP-1c) and carbohydrate responsive element binding protein (ChREBP). Thus, there is a net increase in intrahepatic fatty acids which are then esterified to triglycerides. Very low-density lipoprotein (VLDL) is the main route for extrusion of triglycerides from the liver. Although, the secretion of triglycerides in VLDL is increased in NAFLD, this cannot keep pace with the increased triglyceride formation. The excess triglycerides accumulate in the hepatocytes as histologically demonstrable steatosis.

However, lipotoxicity of triglycerides per se is limited. Rather certain intermediates such as ceramides, diacylglycerol, and lipophosphatidylcholine, which are produced during hepatic fatty acid metabolism, are the major contributors toward lipotoxicity. These intermediates promote insulin resistance by activating protein kinase C, mammalian target of rapamycin (mTOR), and nuclear factor kinase B (NFκB), and inhibiting Akt 25. Thus, insulin resistance promotes NAFLD and in turn NAFLD promotes insulin resistance, thereby setting up a vicious cycle. Chronic inflammation and injury ultimately lead to activation of stellate cells and progressive fibrosis.

NATURAL HISTORY

As mentioned previously, NAFL is usually considered to be relatively innocuous and NASH is associated with a higher risk of progression of fibrosis to cirrhosis and HCC. However, NAFL is not completely benign and may evolve into NASH overtime. Indeed, the current evidence suggests that there may be a dynamic cycling between NAFL and NASH in the initial stages of the disease (**Flowchart 1**). Those with age > 45 years and male patients with metabolic comorbidities/metabolic syndrome are at a higher risk of having NASH.

The onset of fibrosis is another landmark event in the natural history of NAFLD. Majority of the patients (80%) have slow progression of fibrosis. However, around 20% patients have rapid progression of fibrosis and may develop advanced fibrosis in 5–10 years (**Flowchart 1**). Presence or the new development of metabolic comorbidities, particularly T2DM and obesity, may serve as clinical clues to identify patients who are more likely to have rapid progression of fibrosis. As such, the degree of underlying fibrosis is the most important determinant of clinical outcomes and liver-related mortality increases substantially with advancing fibrosis stage.

Nonalcoholic steatohepatitis appears to be the most important cause of cryptogenic cirrhosis and cryptogenic (non-HBV and non-HCV) HCC. Roughly half of the cases of cryptogenic cirrhosis may be attributed to NASH. Most NAFLD patients with HCC have a background cirrhotic liver. Much less commonly, HCC can also develop in NASH patients without cirrhosis or even advanced fibrosis.

Overall, the most common cause of mortality in patients with NAFLD is cardiovascular disease followed by liver disease and malignancies.

CLINICAL FEATURES

Most patients with noncirrhotic NAFLD are asymptomatic at presentation and are detected to have "fatty liver" on ultrasound during workup for dyspepsia, other abdominal complaints, or for raised transaminases. About 30% of patients may have malaise or fatigue, patients may also complain of vague right upper quadrant discomfort (due to stretching of the capsule of the enlarged steatotic liver). Patients can also present with cirrhosis and its complications or HCC.

Although obesity is one of the most common risk factors for NAFLD, 10–15% patients of NAFLD have normal BMI. This phenotype is termed lean NAFLD. Insulin resistance is more prevalent in these patients as compared to healthy individuals. Current evidence suggests that lean NAFLD may have less severe disease on histology as compared to NAFLD patients with obesity.

It is important to note that apart from the classical components of metabolic syndrome (T2DM, obesity, hypertension, and dyslipidemia) NAFLD is also associated with a multitude of other extrahepatic conditions. These include coronary atherosclerosis and cardiovascular disease, chronic kidney disease, polycystic ovarian syndrome, obstructive sleep apnea, hypothyroidism, osteoporosis, and extrahepatic malignancies and thus require workup for these conditions in the clinical context.

History and clinical examination: Exclusion of alternate causes of steatosis should be attempted in the history. Importance of adequate history of alcohol intake and drug history cannot be overemphasized. Enquiry should be made about the duration and amount of alcohol intake. The American Association for the Study of Liver Disease (AASLD) guidelines define significant alcohol intake as more than 21 and 14 standard drinks in a week in males and females, respectively. However, the position paper jointly published by the Indian National Association for the Study of the Liver, Endocrine Society of India, Indian College of Cardiology and Indian Society of Gastroenterology recommends a cutoff of <20 g/day of alcohol in both males and females. Dietary and exercise habits should be gleaned from the history.

Waist circumference and body mass index (BMI) should be measured routinely. In India, obesity is defined as BMI ≥ 25 kg/m^2 while BMI ≥ 23 kg/m^2 is considered as overweight. Central obesity in Indians is defined by waist circumference ≥ 90 cm in males and ≥ 80 cm in females. Hepatomegaly is present in approximately 50% of the patients. Xanthomas and xanthelasmas may be present in patients with dyslipidemia. Peripheral stigmata of insulin resistance such as acanthosis nigricans should be searched for. Stigmata of cirrhosis and portal hypertension such as spider nevi, gynecomastia, splenomegaly, and ascites, should also be looked for as per the clinical setting.

DIAGNOSTIC APPROACH

Nonalcoholic fatty liver disease is a diagnosis of exclusion. Hence, together with the demonstration of steatosis (usually on imaging), other etiologies of fatty liver should be ruled out on history or investigations (**Box 1**).

Noninvasive assessment of hepatic steatosis: Ultrasound (USG) abdomen is the most commonly used and preferred initial imaging for hepatic steatosis. It is cheap, widely available, and does not entail any radiation hazard. Another advantage is that the degree of steatosis can be qualitatively graded on USG (**Table 1**). Presence of a nodular liver with irregular outline, splenomegaly, ascites, or collaterals suggest the presence of underlying cirrhosis. However, USG has limited diagnostic accuracy for steatosis of <20–30%. Further, it may not provide information about the stage of fibrosis in noncirrhotic patients.

TABLE 1 Grades of fatty liver on USG.

Grade of fatty liver	USG findings
Grade 1	Liver is more echogenic than spleen and kidneys
Grade 2	Intravascular structures are blurred
Grade 3	Deep attenuation of ultrasound signal; diaphragm cannot be readily discerned from posterior surface of liver

Normally, liver and spleen have similar attenuation on noncontrast CT abdomen. However, in presence of steatosis, the liver appears hypoattenuated as compared to the spleen. Liver attenuation index (LAI) (defined as difference in attenuation between liver and spleen on noncontrast CT) has been used as a surrogate measure of hepatic steatosis. LAI < −10 HU is highly specific for moderate-to-severe macrovesicular steatosis while a LAI > +5 HU suggests the absence of significant steatosis. Like USG, CT also provides us additional evidence such as the presence of cirrhosis and is better in delineating the nature of solid liver space-occupying lesions (particularly triple-phase CT). However, with respect to the diagnostic accuracy for hepatic steatosis per se, CT is comparable to that of USG. As such, it is not usually preferred as an initial investigation in noncirrhotic patients due to higher costs and radiation exposure.

MRI-based techniques include magnetic resonance spectroscopy (MRS) and magnetic resonance proton density fat fraction (MR-PDFF). Though highly accurate, MRS is not widely available and requires considerable expertise. MR-PDFF measures the fraction of fat-bound protons to total protons (bound to fat and water) and this technology can be incorporated into routine MRI machines. Further, MRI-based techniques can be incorporated with elastography [magnetic resonance elastography (MRE)] for simultaneous assessment of fibrosis. As such, MRI-based techniques are the most accurate techniques that are currently available for detecting and quantifying steatosis and possibly fibrosis. However, the use of these techniques remains largely confined to research settings.

Controlled attenuation parameter (CAP) obtained using FibroScan is another commonly used noninvasive indicator of hepatic steatosis. Its accuracy is higher than that of USG abdomen. Grading of the degree of hepatic steatosis is also possible using CAP values (**Table 2**).

Various non-imaging-based indices such as hepatic steatosis index (HSI) and fatty liver index (FLI) based on anthropometry and biochemical parameters for prediction of hepatic steatosis are rarely used in clinical practice but may still have utility for screening large communities for hepatic steatosis in the absence of USG.

Exclude alternate causes of fatty liver and deranged liver functions: Presence of raised serum transaminases have a poor correlation with histological activity in NAFLD and should not be used to diagnose NASH which truly is a histological diagnosis. However, AST/ALT ratio > 1 usually suggests the presence of advanced fibrosis or cirrhosis. In fact, a detailed etiologic workup should be done to exclude other causes of raised transaminases (if present) in NAFLD. Depending on the clinical scenario, this usually include but is not limited to HBsAg, anti-HCV, workup for autoimmune hepatitis, serum ceruloplasmin, IgA tTg, and iron profile. Autoimmune antibodies such as antinuclear antibody (ANA) and anti-smooth muscle antibody (ASMA) may be present in around 25% of patients with NAFLD. This is an epiphenomenon and should be interpreted after giving due to consideration to the clinical background. While it may be prudent to go ahead with further investigations including serum IgG (total) and liver biopsy in a young female with significantly elevated transaminases and with evidence of another autoimmune disease; this would be completely unnecessary in a septuagenarian diabetic with transaminases < 2 × upper limit of normal (ULN).

Noninvasive assessment of fibrosis: Noninvasive assessment of hepatic fibrosis include many free "online" nonproprietary tests and proprietary panels. Some of the commonly used nonproprietary tests are NAFLD fibrosis score (NFS), AST-platelet ratio index (APRI), and Fibrosis-4 (FIB-4). The components of these scores and the suggested cutoffs are depicted in **Table 3**. Important proprietary tests include FibroTest and enhanced liver fibrosis (ELF) test. The components of these tests are shown in **Table 4**. More than the biomarkers, elastographic techniques are now frequently being used in clinical practice for the assessment of hepatic fibrosis. The basic principle of these techniques is based on the velocity of the propagated shear wave through a solid medium which is proportional to the stiffness of that solid medium which is also known as the elasticity modulus. In case of liver elastography, this implies that higher the velocity of the shear wave while passing through the liver, higher is the liver stiffness.

Liver stiffness (measured in kilopascal or kPa) is a surrogate for the degree of underlying fibrosis. However, liver stiffness measurement (LSM) values may be elevated in a number of other conditions such as hepatic congestion due to heart failure, chronic renal failure, cholestasis, and in patients with significantly elevated transaminases or bilirubin. In such patients, LSM should be interpreted with caution. Transient elastography (FibroScan) has been widely validated for predicting fibrosis in NAFLD. Cutoffs for FibroScan are shown in **Table 5**.

The availability of a special XL probe permits the performance of FibroScan even in obese patients. However, the performance of FibroScan becomes unreliable in the presence of ascites. Other USG-based elastographic techniques include point shear wave elastography and 2D-shear wave elastography. Unlike FibroScan, these techniques allow localization of the region of interest as they are mounted on conventional ultrasound machines. They can also be performed in the presence of ascites or obesity. MRE is the most accurate method for detecting and staging fibrosis; however, cost and infrastructure requirement limit its routine use.

It is worthwhile to remember that the specificity and positive predictive values of these noninvasive tests is only 60–80% while their specificity and negative predictive values are impressive (90%). Thus, they are better at ruling out advanced fibrosis rather than ruling it in. By combining two noninvasive tests, we can improve the specificity, predictive value, and diagnostic accuracy. As such these tests are best

TABLE 4 Proprietary clinical panels for fibrosis assessment.

Name of test	Variables for calculating score
ELF test	Hyaluronic acid, aminoterminal propeptide of Type III procollagen, tissue inhibitor of metalloproteinase 1
FibroTest	Bilirubin, GGT, α2-macroglobulin, apolipoprotein A1 and haptoglobin

(ELF: enhanced liver fibrosis)

TABLE 2 Grading of hepatic steatosis using controlled attenuation parameter (CAP).

Steatosis severity	CAP value
S0 (no steatosis)	<248 dB/m
S1 (mild steatosis)	248 to <268 dB/m
S2 (moderate steatosis)	268 to <280 dB/m
S3 (severe steatosis)	>280 dB/m

TABLE 5 Staging of fibrosis using LSM values obtained by FibroScan.

Stage of fibrosis	LSM value
F0–F1	<7 kPa
≥F2	7 to <8.7 kPa
≥F3	8.7 to <10.3 kPa
F4	≥10.3 kPa

(LSM: liver stiffness measurement)

TABLE 3 Nonproprietary, noninvasive scores for detection of advanced fibrosis (F3–F4).

Name of score	Variables for calculating score	Rule-in cutoff	Rule-out cutoff
APRI	AST, platelet count	>1.5	<0.5
FIB-4	AST, ALT, age, platelet	>2.67	<1.3
NFS	Age, BMI, AST, ALT, albumin, platelet count, diabetes or impaired fasting glucose	>0.676	<–1.455

(APRI: AST to platelet ratio index; FIB-4: Fibrosis-4; NFS: NAFLD fibrosis score)

utilized for risk stratification. Patients deemed to be of low risk can be followed up at a primary care level while those at high risk of advanced fibrosis should be ideally confirmed by liver biopsy.

Noninvasive diagnosis of NASH: Differentiating NASH from NAFL noninvasively is a much-required unmet need in the field of NAFLD. Cytokeratin-18 (CK-18) is a marker of apoptosis and has been used for the diagnosis of NASH but is limited by its availability and validation. The recently envisaged FibroScan-AST (FAST) score amalgamates serum AST (surrogate of inflammation) with CAP (surrogate of steatosis) and LSM (surrogate of fibrosis) parameters obtained on FibroScan. It was shown to have high accuracy in discriminating those with fibrotic NASH among patients with biopsy proven NAFLD. Although promising, the FAST score needs further validation, particularly in Indian patients, before its routine use can be advocated and as of now liver biopsy remains the gold standard for the diagnosis of NASH.

LIVER BIOPSY

Histologic features of NAFLD in general include presence of steatosis in >5% hepatocytes, which are usually macrovesicular (lipid droplet pushes the nuclei and cellular organelles to the periphery) or mixed. Microvesicular steatosis alone goes against the diagnosis of NAFLD. In NAFL, steatosis is not accompanied by features of hepatocyte damage such as ballooning and there is minimal or no inflammation and fibrosis. In NASH, in addition to hepatic steatosis, there is evidence of hepatocyte ballooning, lobular inflammation with or without significant fibrosis (**Flowchart 1**). Ballooned hepatocytes are enlarged hepatocytes with a diameter of >30 μm with pale staining cytoplasm and indicates damage to microtubules with loss of intermediate filaments. Other findings that can sometimes be present in NASH include Mallory hyaline bodies, apoptotic hepatocytes, megamitochondria and glycogenated nuclei.

It is interesting to note that many of these features may also be present in alcoholic liver disease. This highlights the need for a thorough history about alcohol intake as discussed previously. Unlike chronic viral hepatitis, fibrosis in NAFLD often involves the perivenular areas (zone 3) initially. This fibrosis is often pericellular/perisinusoidal and is described as "chicken-wire" pattern. Portal and periportal fibrosis may also be present. Ultimately this progresses to bridging fibrosis and micronodular cirrhosis.

Many histologic scoring systems have been suggested for standardizing the interpretation and reporting of liver biopsy in NAFLD. The NASH Clinical Research Network (CRN) system and the Steatosis-Activity-Fibrosis (SAF) score are two semiquantitative, validated scoring systems that are commonly used (**Tables 6** and **7**).

Indications for liver biopsy: Liver biopsy is an invasive procedure with a small but definite risk of complications such as pain and bleeding. Thus, its use should be restricted to patients who are deemed to be at high risk of having

TABLE 6 NAFLD Activity Score (NAS) as per the NASH-CRN system.

Histologic feature	Score	Definition
Steatosis	0	<5%
	1	5–33%
	2	34–66%
	3	>66%
	+	
Hepatocyte ballooning	0	None
	1	Few
	2	Many
	+	
Lobular inflammation	0	None
	1	1–2 foci per 20 × field
	2	2–4 foci per 20 × field
	3	>4 foci per 20 × field
= NAFLD Activity Score (NAS); range 0–8		
Fibrosis stage	0	No fibrosis
	1a	Zone 3 mild perisinusoidal fibrosis
	1b	Zone 3 moderate perisinusoidal fibrosis
	1c	Portal or portal fibrosis only
	2	Zone 3 + portal/periportal fibrosis
	3	Bridging fibrosis
	4	Cirrhosis

(CRN: Clinical Research Network)

NASH or advanced fibrosis (suggestive on noninvasive test results, age > 45 years and presence of multiple metabolic comorbidities), inconclusive or indeterminate results on noninvasive assessment of fibrosis, diagnostic dilemma or suspicion of coexistent etiologies and as a part of clinical trials.

MANAGEMENT

GENERAL MEASURES

It is worthwhile to remember that the most common cause of mortality in patients with NAFLD is cardiovascular disease. Thus, a holistic approach to management needs to be emphasized. Central to the management of NAFLD is detection and adequate management of metabolic comorbidities such as T2DM, obesity, hypertension, and dyslipidemia. Statins, if indicated, can be used safely even in the presence of elevated transaminases. Alcohol consumption should be discouraged. Recent studies suggest that even modest alcohol consumption can worsen histology and noninvasive parameters in NAFLD.

TABLE 7 Steatosis-Activity-Fibrosis (SAF) score for NAFLD.

Histologic feature	Score	Definition
Steatosis	0	<5%
	1	5–33%
	2	34–66%
	3	>66%
= Steatosis score (S 0–3)		
Hepatocyte ballooning	0	None
	1	Clusters of round hepatocytes with pale cytoplasm
	2	Same as above with enlarge hepatocytes (>2 times than normal)
	+	
Lobular inflammation	0	None
	1	<2 foci per 20 × field
	2	>2 foci per 20 × field
= Activity score (A 0–4)		
Fibrosis	0	No fibrosis
	1a	Zone 3 mild perisinusoidal fibrosis
	1b	Zone 3 moderate perisinusoidal fibrosis
	1c	Portal or portal fibrosis only
	2	Zone 3 + portal/periportal fibrosis
	3	Bridging fibrosis
	4	Cirrhosis
= Fibrosis score (F 0–4)		

DIET, EXERCISE, AND WEIGHT LOSS

The amount of weight loss predicts improvement in liver histology; weight loss of 3–5% improves hepatic steatosis while higher degrees of weight loss are required for improvement in features of NASH (≥7%) and fibrosis (≥10%). Aerobic exercises such as brisk walking, jogging, running, swimming, and cycling, for at least 45–60 minutes, at least 5 days per week, to achieve a target heart rate of 60–70% of their maximal heart rate are usually advised. It has been shown that exercise alone can improve insulin sensitivity and possibly steatosis even if it does not lead to a loss in body weight. Resistance exercise may be used to supplement aerobic exercise. Dietary restriction in calories by 30% or 500–1,000 kcal/day should go hand-in-hand with exercise. Many specific diets have been advocated and there is some evidence that the Mediterranean diet may be beneficial. However, these diets have not been extensively evaluated for improvement in NAFLD per se. Overall, the attainment of a calorie restriction to obtain a negative energy balance appears to be more important than the specific type of diet. Hypocaloric diets and rapid weight loss are not advisable because of the possibility of worsening of liver functions.

Additional strategies for weight loss in NAFLD: Only around 10% patients are able to attain a weight loss of >10% with lifestyle interventions alone. Sustaining this weight loss is even more difficult and only 5% patients are able to sustain it over a period of 12 months. Currently, the drugs approved for weight loss by the FDA include orlistat, liraglutide, phentermine-topiramate, and naltrexone-bupropion. As such pharmacologic therapies for decreasing body weight are not recommended in NAFLD.

Bariatric surgery has been shown to improve liver histology, survival, and cardiovascular outcomes. Although not recommended for the management of NAFLD per se, it can be considered in otherwise eligible obese patients with NAFLD (BMI > 35 kg/m^2). However, caution should be exercised to avoid surgery in patients with underlying cirrhosis. There is much recent interest in endoscopic techniques for weight loss and glycemic control including endoscopically placed gastric balloons and duodenal mucosal resurfacing. The field of metabolic endoscopy is rapidly evolving and is likely to be a part of the future armamentarium for managing NAFLD. As of now, however, the data is limited and these techniques are not yet recommended for managing NAFLD.

PHARMACOTHERAPY FOR NASH

A number of drugs such as UDCA (ursodeoxycholic acid), metformin, and omega-3-fatty acids have been evaluated for the treatment of NAFLD/NASH. Although there are reports of improvement in liver enzymes with these drugs, there is no improvement in liver histology and are therefore not recommended for management of NAFLD/NASH.

Pioglitazone: The PIVENS (Pioglitazone versus Vitamin E versus Placebo for the Treatment of Non-diabetic Patients with Nonalcoholic Steatohepatitis) trial was a landmark study in NAFLD. In this study, 247 biopsy-proven NASH patients without diabetes mellitus (DM) were randomized to either pioglitazone (30 mg/day), vitamin E (800 IU/day), or placebo for 96 weeks. Both vitamin E and pioglitazone improved steatosis, lobular inflammation, and NASH resolution as compared to placebo. Pioglitazone has also been shown to improve NASH resolution in diabetic and prediabetic patients.

Vitamin E: The current guidelines recommend vitamin E or pioglitazone only in biopsy-proven noncirrhotic NASH patients. While pioglitazone is recommended in both diabetics and nondiabetics, vitamin E is recommended only in those without DM. There is a possibility of increased risk of prostate cancer with long-term use of vitamin E although concerns with increased all-cause mortality have been disproved in a recent meta-analysis. The biggest concern with the use of pioglitazone is weight gain which may offset its beneficial effects. There is also a concern about osteoporosis, particularly in females, and a possible increased risk of carcinoma of the urinary bladder.

Saroglitazar: Unlike pioglitazone, which is a peroxisome proliferator-activated receptor-gamma (PPAR-γ) agonist, saroglitazar, is a dual PPAR-α/γ agonist with predominant PPAR-α effect and moderate PPAR-γ effect. Because of a different pyrrole ring and absence of thiazolidine ring, saroglitazar is not associated with the side effects seen with other glitazars and glitazones. The drug has been in use in India for many years for patients with diabetic dyslipidemia and based on the noninvasive and histological efficacy data, saroglitazar in a dose of 4 mg/day has recently been approved by the Drug Controller General of India (DCGI) for the treatment of patients with NASH with F1–F3 fibrosis.

FUTURE DRUGS FOR NASH

Obeticholic acid (OCA): A number of other drugs for NASH are currently being evaluated in phase II and phase III clinical trials. A lot of interest is centered around OCA, a farnesoid X receptor (FXR) agonist. An interim analysis of the phase III REGENERATE (Randomized Global Phase 3 Study to Evaluate the Impact on NASH With Fibrosis of Obeticholic Acid Treatment) study in NASH patients with stage 2 or 3 fibrosis showed that the primary outcome of ≥1 stage improvement in fibrosis without worsening of NASH was significantly more common in patients treated with 25 mg (23.1%, $p = 0.0002$) of OCA compared to placebo (11.9%). However, pruritus was seen in nearly half of the patients on 25 mg of OCA with treatment discontinuation in 13%. Dyslipidemia requiring the use of statins is another common side effect of OCA and the drug has still not been approved for the treatment of patients with NASH.

Cenicriviroc: Other drugs in phase III clinical trials for the treatment of NASH include cenicriviroc (chemokine 2 and 5 inhibitor), resmetirom (thyroid hormone receptor beta-agonist) and aramchol (synthetic fatty acid/bile-acid conjugate).

Liraglutide: It is a glucagon-like-peptide-1 (GLP-1) receptor agonist, was shown to improve resolution of NASH and decrease progression of fibrosis in the phase II LEAN trial. Additionally, liraglutide was also associated with significantly more weight loss as compared to placebo. Similar observations with respect to improvement in histologic resolution of NASH and weight loss have also been made with semaglutide, another GLP-1 receptor agonist. Future may lie with the combination of drugs targeting different pathways involved in the pathogenesis of NASH.

MANAGEMENT OF NASH-RELATED CIRRHOSIS AND HCC

Histologic evidence of NAFLD in patients with cirrhosis may be difficult to demonstrate due to the decrease in hepatic steatosis with advancing hepatic fibrosis. Presence of two or more components of metabolic syndrome in the absence of other etiologies of liver disease supports the diagnosis of NASH in these patients with cryptogenic cirrhosis or HCC.

As weight loss is common in cirrhosis, past history of being overweight or obese should also be considered as a risk factor while evaluating these patients. Cirrhosis is also associated with perturbations in other metabolic parameters. For instance, the development of cirrhosis may worsen insulin resistance leading to the development of new-onset DM. Further, cirrhotics often have low blood pressures and serum lipid levels. Thus, a meticulous history regarding the presence of long-standing T2DM, hypertension, and dyslipidemia may be more helpful in establishing the diagnosis of NAFLD than screening for metabolic risk factors in those presenting with cryptogenic cirrhosis or HCC.

NASH-specific therapies such as pioglitazone, vitamin E or saroglitazar are not recommended in patients with underlying cirrhosis. Some retrospective evidence suggests that vitamin E and metformin reduces the risk of decompensation and improves transplant-free survival in patients with NASH-related advanced fibrosis or compensated cirrhosis. However, pending further evidence, this is not yet recommended in routine clinical practice. As such, management of cirrhosis and HCC in NAFLD should be along the same lines as for other etiologies. Decompensated cirrhotics should be evaluated for liver transplantation. Patients with NASH cirrhosis/HCC while being evaluated for liver transplantation require special attention due to commonly associated comorbidities of obesity and diabetes mellitus. Even though the recurrence of hepatic steatosis is very common in NASH-related cirrhosis, post-transplant graft and patient survival outcomes at 1, 3, and 5 years are comparable to liver transplants for other etiologies.

RECOMMENDED READINGS

1. Chalasani N, Younossi Z, Lavine JE, Charlton M, Cusi K, Rinella M, et al. The diagnosis and management of nonalcoholic fatty liver disease: Practice guidance from the American Association for the Study of Liver Diseases. Hepatology. 2018;67(1):328-57.
2. Marchesini G, Day CP, Dufour JF, Canbay A, Nobili V, Ratziu V, et al. EASL-EASD-EASO Clinical Practice Guidelines for the management of non-alcoholic fatty liver disease. J Hepatol. 2016;64(6):1388-402.
3. Duseja A, Singh SP, Saraswat VA, Acharya SK, Chawla YK, Chowdhury S, et al. Non-alcoholic fatty liver disease and metabolic syndrome-position paper of the Indian National Association for the study of the liver, Endocrine Society of India, Indian College of Cardiology and Indian Society of Gastroenterology. J Clin Exp Hepatol. 2015;5(1):51-68.
4. Eslam M, Newsome PN, Sarin SK, Anstee QM, Targher G, Romero-Gomez M, et al. A new definition for metabolic associated fatty liver disease: an international expert consensus statement. J Hepatol. 2020;73(1):202-9.
5. Duseja A, Taneja S. Changing nomenclature from nonalcoholic fatty liver disease to metabolic dysfunction-associated fatty liver disease – Not only premature but also confusing. J Clin Exp Hepatol. 2021;11(2):278-9.

6. De A, Duseja A. Natural history of simple steatosis or nonalcoholic fatty liver. J Clin Exp Hepatol. 2020;10(3):255-62.
7. Younossi ZM, Koenig AB, Abdelatif D, Fazel Y, Henry L, Wymer M. Global epidemiology of nonalcoholic fatty liver disease—Meta-analytic assessment of prevalence, incidence, and outcomes. Hepatology. 2016;64(1):73-84.
8. Castera L, Chan HLY, Arrese M, Afdhal N, Bedossa P, Mireen Friedrich-Rust, et al. EASL-ALEH Clinical Practice Guidelines: Non-invasive tests for evaluation of liver disease severity and prognosis. J Hepatol. 2015;63(1):237-64
9. Wong VWS, Adams LA, de Lédinghen V, Wong GLH, Sookoian S. Noninvasive biomarkers in NAFLD and NASH — current progress and future promise. Nat Rev Gastroenterol Hepatol. 2018;15(8):461-78.
10. Sanyal AJ, Chalasani N, Kowdley KV, McCullough A, Diehl AM, Bass NM, et al. Pioglitazone, Vitamin E, or Placebo for Nonalcoholic Steatohepatitis. N Eng J Med. 2010;362(18):1675-85.
11. Younossi Z, Loomba R, Rinella M, Bugianesi E, Marchesini B. Current and future therapeutic regimens for non-alcoholic fatty liver disease (NAFLD) and non-alcoholic steatohepatitis (NASH). Hepatology. 2017;777(5):1-36.

CHAPTER 148

Toxic and Drug-induced Liver Injury

Mallikarjun Patil, Harshad Devarbhavi

ABSTRACT

Drug-induced liver injury (DILI) is an uncommon, and under recognized cause of liver injury that carries significant morbidity and mortality. It is a leading cause of drug withdrawal during drug development and following marketing. DILI can occur from a large number of prescribed medicines, and complementary and alternative medicines (CAM). The clinical spectrum of DILI varies from asymptomatic liver biochemical test abnormalities, to acute and chronic hepatitis, cholestatic liver disease and acute on chronic liver failure leading to death or necessitating liver transplantation. Antitubercular therapy (ATT) drugs are the most common cause of DILI and drug-induced acute liver failure (ALF) in India whereas antibiotics and paracetamol are the leading causes of DILI and ALF in the Western world.

There are no diagnostic markers for the diagnosis of DILI and hence DILI is predominantly a diagnosis of exclusion of viral and autoimmune hepatitis and biliary obstruction. Causality assessment scales such as the Roussel Uclaf Causality Assessment Method (RUCAM) aid in the diagnosis. Prompt identification of the implicated drug is key minimize injury and aid recovery. The presence of jaundice, ascites, encephalopathy, and coagulopathy indicates severe disease with associated high mortality. Treatment is largely supportive and only few antidotes are available for DILI such as N-acetylcysteine for paracetamol poisoning, cholestyramine for leflunomide DILI, and L-carnitine for valproate DILI. This review provides an overview of the epidemiology, clinical presentation, pathogenesis, diagnosis, and treatment of toxic and DILI.

Liver is the major organ which regulates the metabolism of internal compounds and administered medications. Liver is a tolerogenic organ and adverse drug reaction leading to liver injury is rare. The spectrum DILI varies from asymptomatic liver biochemical test abnormalities to acute hepatitis, chronic hepatitis, and ALF sometimes leading to death or liver transplantation. DILI is often under-reported and unrecognized due to the lack of diagnostic tests. Hence it is a diagnosis of exclusion. DILI is a major cause for the withdrawal of drugs from the market.

"One way of testing the toxicity of the drug is how you feel the next day?"

—Terence McKenna

EPIDEMIOLOGY

The exact incidence and prevalence of DILI is lacking; estimates range from 1:10,000 to 1: 100,000. In prospective, population-based studies, the incidence varied from 13 to 19 per 100,000 population but could be more common in India. DILI is the most common cause of ALF in Western countries largely due to paracetamol toxicity. However, paracetamol toxicity is very rare in India. In a single center study from St. John's Medical College, Bangalore, DILI contributed to 1.4% of all admissions in gastroenterology and 2.5% of admissions due to hepatobiliary diseases.

The common drugs responsible for DILI vary geographically. In the United States, antimicrobial drugs are the most common cause of idiosyncratic DILI, followed by herbal and dietary supplements (HDS), cardiovascular drugs, and central nervous system agents. Amoxicillin-clavulanate was the most common drug causing DILI.

According to the Indian DILI network, ATTs were the most common cause of DILI responsible for 46.4% cases followed by CAM in 13.9%, antiepileptic drugs in 8.1%, antimicrobial drugs (other than ATT) in 6.5%, and others.

DEFINITION

An international expert working group proposed the following thresholds for a diagnosis of DILI:

- Elevation of alanine aminotransferase (ALT) and/or aspartate aminotransferase (AST) > 5 times the upper limit of normal (ULN) without symptoms
- Rise in AST or ALT ≥ 3 with symptoms such as nausea, vomiting, abdominal pain, anorexia, and fatigue
- Rise in alkaline phosphatase (ALP) value ≥ 2 × ULN or
- Rise in AST or ALT value ≥ 3 × ULN and total bilirubin (TB) ≥ 2 × ULN.

Further, DILI is classified as hepatocellular, mixed, or cholestatic pattern by determining the R ratio which is the ratio of ALT to ALP relative to their respective upper limits of normal (ALT/ULN)/(ALP/ULN). An R ≥ 5 identifies the hepatocellular pattern of injury; R ≤ 2 cholestatic pattern, while an R between 2 and 5 defines mixed pattern. Hepatocellular injury is associated with increased risk of death especially in younger individuals while cholestasis is more common in the elderly.

PATHOGENESIS

Liver is the major site of metabolism/detoxification of administered drugs; hence it is an important target of drug toxicity. The drugs after absorption from the gut are taken up by the hepatocytes. During the phase I reaction, the parent drug is converted into water-soluble metabolite by oxidation/reduction or by hydrolysis using the cytochrome P450 group of enzymes. In phase II reaction, the drug metabolite is converted into more water-soluble compound by conjugation/acetylation or sulfation. The resultant water-soluble drug metabolites are either excreted into the bile through the export proteins located on the biliary canaliculi or effluxed into systemic circulation for subsequent renal excretion.

Drug-induced liver injury is classified into three types: (1) intrinsic/direct, (2) idiosyncratic, and (3) indirect types based on the pathogenesis.

Intrinsic DILI is caused by the agents, which are intrinsically toxic to the liver and is predictable, dose-dependent and occurs after short latency period of few days. This is exemplified by paracetamol toxicity. Direct toxicity to hepatocytes may lead to hepatocyte necrosis and ALF while direct toxicity to sinusoidal endothelial cells may cause sinusoidal obstruction syndrome (e.g., busulfan and other myeloablative agents) which presents with abdominal pain, hepatomegaly, and jaundice that can progress to liver failure. Chronic direct injury to the hepatic microvasculature may result in nodular regenerative hyperplasia (NRH). Usual implicated drugs in causing NRH are azathioprine and oxaliplatin.

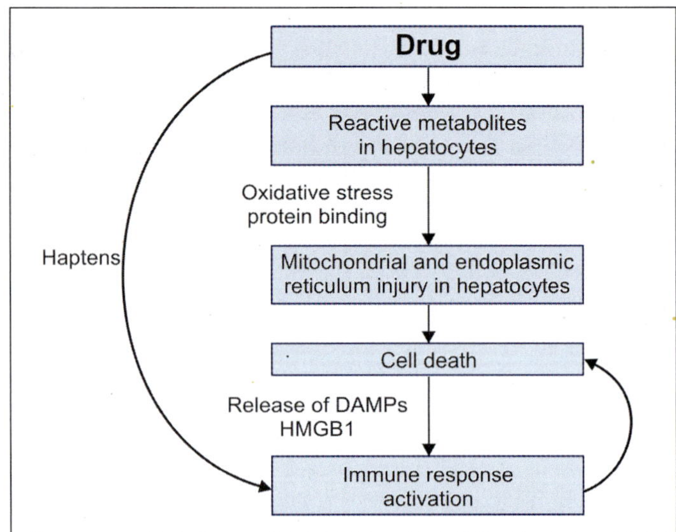

(DAMP: damage-associated molecular pattern; HMGB1: high mobility group box 1 protein)

FLOWCHART 1: Pathogenesis of idiosyncratic DILI.

Idiosyncratic DILI is caused by the agents, which have little or no intrinsic toxicity to the liver and is not dose-dependent and hence is unpredictable. The reactive metabolites formed during the phase I and II reaction during the drug metabolism in the liver may covalently bind to the cellular proteins in the endoplasmic reticulum and mitochondria and may lead to the hepatocyte injury/death. The injured hepatocyte may also release damage-associated molecular patterns (DAMPs) such as high mobility group box 1 protein (HMGB1) which in turn activates toll-like receptors causing cytokine secretion and proinflammatory response (**Flowchart 1**). For example, diclofenac causes DILI due to the formation of toxic quinine and acyl glucuronides metabolites during phase I reaction. The drug metabolites may lead the formation of haptanes which are immunogenic that can cause immune stimulation and cellular injury (**Flowchart 1**). Some drug metabolites can cause the inhibition of bile salt export pumps on the biliary canaliculi, leading to stasis of toxic bile salts, and bile acids resulting in damage to mitochondria. The drugs like cyclosporine A and bosentan are examples of drugs causing cholestasis.

Indirect hepatotoxicity causing DILI is not due to the inherent toxic effect of the drug but due to its action. For example, chemotherapeutic agents due to its immuno-suppressive effect may cause reactivation of hepatitis B/ hepatitis C infection. Glucocorticoid therapy is another example of drug-induced fatty liver due to insulin resistance.

RISK FACTORS

Susceptibility to DILI depends on interplay between host, drug, and environmental factors as mentioned below.

- **Age:** The risk of developing DILI increases with advancing age, particularly cholestatic pattern of DILI. The risk of developing DILI was five times higher in patients aged 70 years as compared to those between 15 and 29 years age group in large population base study conducted in Iceland. Impaired renal functions in elderly might increase the drug/drug metabolite concentration in the blood which may the cause of increased susceptibility to develop DILI in aged people.
- **Sex:** Women are at a higher risk of developing DILI as compared to men, but not in all studies. The risk of developing DILI to certain medications is different between men and women. Autoimmune—DILIs (caused by minocycline, nitrofurantoin etc.) are commonly seen in women, whereas men have increased risk of developing azathioprine related DILI. Females are at high risk of developing severe DILI and fulminant liver failure.
- **Daily dose:** Although idiosyncratic DILI is not dose dependent, relationship to dose has been observed for example with certain medications such as diclofenac, flucloxacillin, and amoxicillin/clavulanate. Drugs given in daily dose of > 50 mg/day accounts for 70–80% of DILI. Drugs such as paracetamol cause direct hepatotoxicity when taken in higher dose (>6 g/day).
- **Alcohol:** Chronic alcohol consumption predisposes to DILI for certain medications like isoniazid (INH), methotrexate, and halothane and paracetamol. Chronic alcohol consumption induces CYP450 enzymes and causes depletion of glutathione thereby predisposing to DILI.
- **Chronic liver disease:** Although the liver is a major site of metabolism of drugs, chronic liver disease predisposes to DILI only to certain medications such as ATTs, methotrexate, and others. However, consequences from DILI in chronic liver disease may result in severe DILI and a higher mortality.
- **Genetic factors:** Single nucleotide polymorphism of genes involved in the metabolism of drugs predisposes to DILI. For example, HLA-B*5701 genotype is associated with flucloxacillin DILI and HLA-DRB1*15:01 and DQB1*0602 are associated with amoxicillin-clavulanate DILI.

CLINICAL FEATURES

The clinical manifestations are usually nonspecific and appear after latency period of days to months. The clinical features are often indistinguishable from other liver disease. Hence a high index of suspicion should be entertained in all cases of liver disease. Patients may present with asymptomatic liver test abnormalities. Others may present with nausea, vomiting, decreased appetite, fatigue, and jaundice. Some patients may present with features of cholestasis like jaundice, pruritus, and light-colored stools after exposure to drugs such as amoxicillin-clavulanate. A few patients may develop allergic manifestations like fever, skin rashes, lymphadenopathy, and eosinophilia accompanied with DILI. Drugs such as dapsone, phenytoin, carbamazepine, and sulfonamides are prime examples for development of drug rash, eosinophilia, and systemic symptoms (DRESS). The same drugs may cause Stevens–Johnson syndrome/toxic epidermal necrolysis (SJS/TEN) in other individuals. Liver injury is less commonly seen in patients with SJS/TEN than and DRESS.

TABLE 1 Patterns of drug-induced liver injury.

Acute hepatitis	Isoniazid, rifampicin, pyrazinimide, phenytoin
Cholestatic	Amoxicillin-clavulanate, flucloxacillin, carbamazepine
Autoimmune	Minocycline, nitrofurantoin
Bland cholestasis	Anabolic steroids, danazol
Granulomatous hepatitis	Dapsone, sulfonamides
Nodular regenerative hyperplasia	Didanosine, stavudine
Vanishing bile duct syndrome	Carbamazepine
Peliosis hepatitis	Anabolic steroids, azathioprine

Many drugs produce the typical pattern of DILI called "drug signature" which may help in the identifying the implicated drug and aid in early diagnosis (**Table 1**).

DIAGNOSIS

There are no specific clinical features or test for the diagnosis of DILI; diagnosis needs exclusion of other causes by appropriate investigations. Thorough history particularly about exposure to prescribed and nonprescribed drugs including complimentary and traditional medicines in the past 1–3 months should be obtained. Some drugs may cause DILI after longer latency period (e.g., minocycline, nitrofurantoin, and alpha-methyldopa). The diagnostic approach in suspected DILI is as shown in the **Flowchart 2**.

Causality assessment tools help in the diagnosis of DILI. The RUCAM is the most common liver specific tool used in clinical practice. The other tools are Maria and Victorino method and DILIN expert opinion. In RUCAM, points are assigned to certain variables, which are totaled to get a final score, leading to the likelihood or certainty scales of DILI (**Table 2**).

TREATMENT

Once DILI is suspected, the suspected drug needs to be discontinued immediately. In majority of the patient spontaneous and gradual fall leading to recovery of liver biochemical abnormalities occurs. Treatment is largely supportive. Specific treatment as antidotes is available only to a few drugs causing injury. These are the following:

- **N-acetylcysteine (NAC):** In patients with paracetamol-induced ALF/severe acute liver injury, NAC therapy improves the transplant free survival. Paracetamol in higher doses generates the hepatotoxic reactive metabolite—N-acetyl-p-benzoquinoneimine (NAPQI)

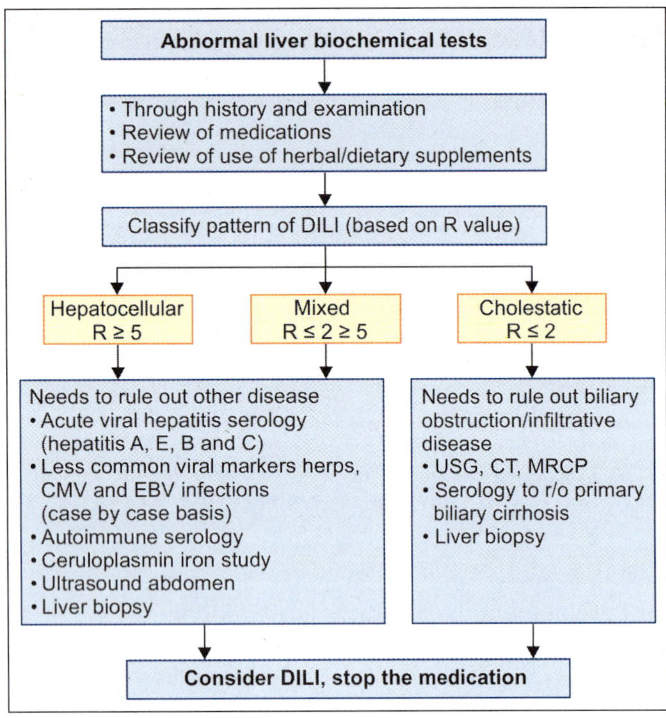

FLOWCHART 2: Approach to a patient with suspected DILI.

which binds with cellular proteins called adducts which in turn cause hepatocyte necrosis. Normally, NAPQI is conjugated with glutathione and excreted in the urine. In toxic dose, paracetamol generates excessive amounts of NAPQI and body's glutathione stores are exhausted. NAC is precursor of the glutathione, increases the concentration of the available glutathione for conjugation with NAPQI. The recommended dose of NAC in acute paracetamol-induced liver failure is:

- Loading dose of 150 mg/kg body weight given over 15–60 minutes (IV)
- About 12.5 mg/kg body weight given over 4 hours (IV)
- About 6.25/ kg body weight given over 16 hours (IV)

N-acetylcysteine therapy has also been shown to be helpful in other causes of ALF including drug-induced ALF but only in early stages of disease.

- **Cholestyramine therapy:** Certain drugs undergo extensive enterohepatic circulation thereby increasing the circulating drug levels even after stopping the drug. Examples include leflunomide, teriflunomide, and terbinafine. Cholestyramine is a bile acid binding resin and interrupts the enterohepatic circulation by binding with bile acids thereby reduces the circulating drug levels. Cholestyramine in the dose of 4 g every 8 hours for <2 weeks is indicated in leflunomide-induced DILI.
- **Carnitine:** L-carnitine therapy improves survival in severe DILI due to sodium valproate. Carnitine regulates the mitochondrial acetyl-CoA and leads to increased fatty acid uptake and β-oxidation. Intravenous carnitine 100 mg/kg over 30 minutes followed by 15 mg/kg body weight every 4 hours is indicated in valproate induced DILI until clinical recovery.

TABLE 2 Roussel Uclaf Causality Assessment Method (RUCAM).

Variables	Score
Latency	0 to +2
Course after de-challenge	– 2 to +3
Risk factors	0 to +2
Comedications	– 3 to 0
Exclusion of other etiologies	– 3 to +2
Data on drug hepatotoxicity	0 to +2
Re-challenge	– 2 to +3

Total score:

1. Highly likely ≥8 **3. Possible 3–5**

2. Probable 6–7 **4. Unlikely ≤2**

Source: Danan G, Benichou C. Causality assessment of adverse reactions to drugs--I. A novel method based on the conclusions of international consensus meetings: application to drug-induced liver injuries. J Clin Epidemiol. 1993;46:1323-30.

- **Corticosteroids:** Corticosteroid therapy is indicated in drug-induced autoimmune hepatitis, drugs associated with hypersensitivity reaction or DRESS syndrome, and DILI secondary to immune check point inhibitors.

ATT-INDUCED DILI

Tuberculosis (TB) is a major health issue in India with estimated prevalence of 256/100,000 population. The first-line drugs used in the treatment of TB namely INH, rifampicin (RIF), pyrazinamide (PZA), and ethambutol (EMB) are generally well tolerated in majority of the patients. Up to 20% patients exposed to anti-TB drugs may develop mild increase in AST and ALT without symptoms which improves with continuation of medications. This asymptomatic elevation of aminotransferases is called adaptation; treatment with anti-TB drugs may be continued especially if there are no symptoms. Awareness about adaptation is important in order to avoid inadvertent stoppage of anti-TB drugs. ATT drugs needs to be stopped only when AST/ALT is increased > 5 × ULN or AST/ALT is increased > 3 ULN with symptoms.

RISK FACTORS

The various host, environmental, and genetic factors that contribute to the development of anti-TB DILI include:

- *Age*: ATT DILI is four times more common in patients older than 35 years of age.
- *Gender*: Females are at high risk of developing severe DILI and death as compared to men.
- *Malnutrition*: Malnutrition predisposes to ATT DILI; patients with hypoalbuminemia (<3.5 g/dL) are at 3-fold higher risk of developing ATT DILI.
- *Alcohol*: Alcohol predisposes to ATT DILI due to associated malnutrition and reduced glutathione store.
- *Hepatitis B and C infection*: Both hepatitis B and C infection predispose to ATT DILI, risk of which increases with increase in hepatitis B and C viral load.

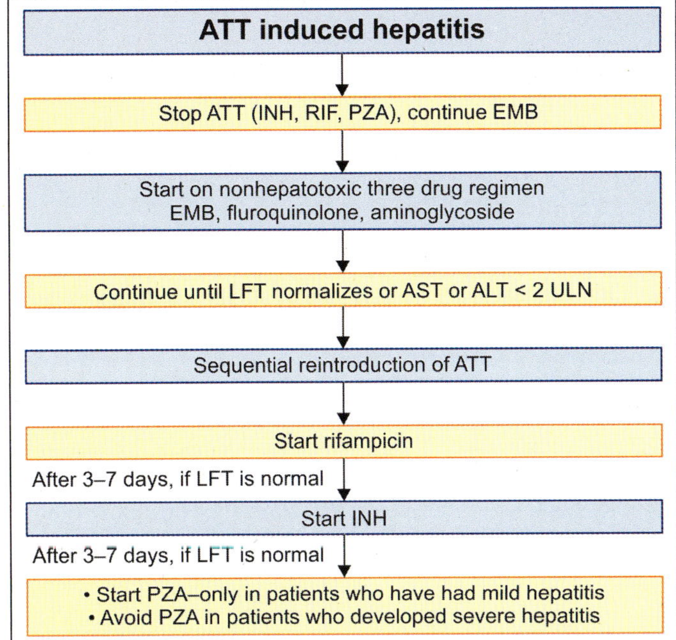

(INH: isoniazid; PZA: pyrazinamide; RIF: rifampicin; ULN: upper limit of normal; EMB: ethambutol)

FLOWCHART 3: Management of antituberculosis therapy (ATT) induced DILI.

- *Genetic polymorphism*: The enzyme polymorphism predisposes to ATT DILI by altering the drug metabolism. The enzymes involved in the metabolism of INH are extensively studied which include N-acetyltransferases 2 (NAT2), CYP2E1, and glutathione S-transferases.

Slow and ultraslow acetylator genotype (NAT2) involved in the metabolism of INH is implicated in causing DILI in some studies but not others.

DIAGNOSIS AND MANAGEMENT

Drug-induced liver injury needs to be considered in patients receiving ATT when patients develop symptoms of nausea, anorexia, vomiting, fatigue, and jaundice associated with elevation of AST/ALT > 3 times and bilirubin > 2 times or any asymptomatic elevations of AST/ALT > 5 times normal. ATT needs to be stopped immediately after suspicion and all other competing causes such as viral and autoimmune and biliary obstruction needs to be ruled out by appropriate investigations. While the first-line drugs are discontinued, patients need to be placed on three nonhepatotoxic drugs such as EMB, fluoroquinolones, aminoglycoside or cycloserine until liver functions normalizes or ALT is < 2 times normal. As INH and RIF are the crucial medications required in the treatment of TB, these drugs can be reintroduced sequentially with staggered doses in majority of the people while monitoring liver biochemical tests and clinical symptoms (**Flowchart 3**). During reintroducing, if DILI develops, the last added drug needs to be stopped.

RECOMMENDED READINGS

1. Aithal GP, Watkins PB, Andrade RJ, Larrey D, Molokhia M, Takikawa H, et al. Case definition and phenotype standardization in drug-induced liver injury. Clin Pharmacol Ther. 2011;89:806-15.
2. Fontana RJ, Seef LB, Andrade RJ, Björnsson E, Day CP, Serrano J, et al. Standardization of nomenclature and causality in drug-induced liver injury: summary of a clinical research workshop. Hepatology. 2010;52:730-42.
3. Chalasani N, Fontana RJ, Bonkovsky HL, Watkins PB, Davern T, Serrano J, et al. Causes, clinical features, and outcomes from a prospective study of drug-induced liver injury in the United States. Gastroenterology. 2008;135:1924-34.
4. Devarbhavi H, Dierkhising R, Kremers WK, Sandeep MS, Karanth D, Adarsh CK. Single-center experience with drug-induced liver injury from India: causes, outcome, prognosis, and predictors of mortality. Am J Gastroenterol. 2010;105:2396-404.
5. Devarbhavi H. An update on drug-induced liver injury. J Clin Exp Hepatol. 2012;2(3):247-59.
6. Kumar R, Shalimar, Bhatia V, Khanal S, Sreenivas V, Gupta SD, et al. Antituberculosis therapy induced acute liver failure: magnitude, profile, prognosis, and predictors of outcome. Hepatology. 2010;51:1665-74.
7. Devarbhavi H. Antituberculous drug-induced liver injury: current perspective. Trop Gastroenterol. 2011;32(3):167-74.
8. Saukkonen JJ, Cohn DL, Jasmer RM, Schenker S, Jereb JA, Nolan CM, et al. An official ATS statement: hepatotoxicity of antituberculosis therapy. Am J Respir Crit Care Med. 2006;174:935-52.
9. European Association for the Study of the Liver. EASL Clinical Practice Guidelines: Drug-induced liver injury. J Hepatol. 2019;70(6):1222-61.
10. Chalasani NP, Hayashi PH, Bonkovsky HL, Navarro VJ, Lee WM, Fontana RJ, et al. ACG Clinical Guideline: The Diagnosis and Management of Idiosyncratic Drug-Induced Liver Injury. Am J Gastroenterol. 2014;109:950-66.
11. Danan G, Benichou C. Causality assessment of adverse reactions to drugs--I. A novel method based on the conclusions of international consensus meetings: application to drug-induced liver injuries. J Clin Epidemiol. 1993;46:1323-30.

CHAPTER

149 Hepatocellular Carcinoma

Dharmesh Kapoor, Anil Kumar Mannava

ABSTRACT

Hepatocellular carcinoma (HCC) is the most common primary liver malignancy and is the fourth most common cause of cancer-related death worldwide. Cirrhosis remains the most important risk factor for the development of HCC, regardless of etiology. Hepatitis B and C are independent risk factors for the development of cirrhosis. Alcohol consumption remains an important additional risk factor. HCC is an aggressive cancer that occurs in the setting of cirrhosis and commonly presents in advanced stages, but screening protocol adopted based on ultrasound and serological markers such as alpha-fetoprotein (AFP) at 6-monthly interval are leading to early detection and better management of HCC. Diagnosis of HCC is confirmed with dynamic computerized tomography (CT) or magnetic resonance imaging (MRI).

Multiple treatment modalities exist but surgical resection or liver transplantation (LT) are curative. LT is available for patients who meet the Milan criteria. Additional treatment modalities include transarterial chemoembolization, radiofrequency ablation, microwave ablation, percutaneous ethanol injection, cryoablation, radiation therapy, systemic chemotherapy, and molecularly targeted therapies. Selection of a treatment modality is based on tumor size, location, extrahepatic spread, and underlying liver function, age, and performance status. Rational deployment of preventive measures, programs for viral hepatitis eradication, and new advances in the treatment of viral hepatitis along with improvement in HCC surveillance and continued improvement in both surgical and nonsurgical approaches have demonstrated significant benefits in overall survival.

"Cancer is a word, not a sentence"

— John Diamond

EPIDEMIOLOGY

Hepatocellular carcinoma, also known as Hepatoma, is the most common liver malignancy arising from the hepatocytes and accounts for >80% of primary liver cancers.

Worldwide, liver cancer is the fourth most common cause of cancer-related death and sixth in terms of incident cases. The data on epidemiology of HCC in India is sparse and available data shows crude incidence rate of 2.8 cases per 100,000 population per year (males: 3.9, females: 1.6), and the crude mortality rate of 2.7 per 100,000 population per year.

RISK FACTORS

Hepatocellular carcinoma is rare among patients without liver disease and is twice as common in men as in women. Cirrhosis of any cause increases the risk of HCC, with an annual incidence between 2 and 4%, depending on the etiology of cirrhosis (**Box 1**).

Worldwide, hepatitis B virus (HBV) infection is the main cause of HCC. The same holds true for India too. Other risk factors include excessive alcohol consumption, hepatitis C virus (HCV) infection, nonalcoholic steatohepatitis (NASH), exposure and ingestion of aflatoxin, diabetes mellitus, tobacco, and sporadic genetic diseases such as alpha-1 antitrypsin deficiency, hemochromatosis, tyrosinemia, porphyria, and Wilson's disease.

BOX 1 Risk factors for hepatocellular carcinoma.

- Chronic hepatitis C infection with advanced fibrosis or cirrhosis
- Chronic hepatitis B infection with/without cirrhosis
- Alcoholic liver disease with cirrhosis
- Hereditary hemochromatosis with cirrhosis
- Alpha-1 antitrypsin deficiency with cirrhosis
- Autoimmune hepatitis with cirrhosis
- Porphyrias
- Wilson's disease
- Nonalcoholic fatty liver disease
- Nonalcoholic steatohepatitis with cirrhosis
- Primary biliary cholangitis
- Type 1 hereditary tyrosinemia
- Type 1 and 2 glycogen storage disease
- Hereditary ataxia-telangiectasia
- Hypercitrullinemia
- Aflatoxin exposure
- Other carcinogens
    - Thorotrast
    - Polyvinyl chloride
    - Carbon chloride

Patients who have cirrhosis due to hepatitis C or hepatitis B have the highest risk of developing HCC as compared to chronic hepatitis or cirrhosis due to other etiologies.

In patients with chronic HBV infection, hepatitis e antigen (HBeAg) positivity carries higher risk of developing HCC compared to HBeAg negativity. In addition, late HBeAg seroconversion (to anti-HBe positivity) also increases the risk of HCC.

In addition, the HCC occurrence in Indian patients with chronic hepatitis B is more often associated with:

- HBV genotype D infection/mixed genotype infections
- High HBV DNA levels (>2,000 IU/mL)
- Persistently elevated serum ALT (alanine transaminase) levels
- High level of hepatitis B surface antigen

In patients with chronic HCV infection:

- HCC is most often associated with advanced fibrosis; however, in up to 10% of cases, it may occur even with mild degrees of fibrosis. In Indian patients with chronic hepatitis C, HCC is more often associated with:
  - HCV genotype 3 infection
  - High serum HCV RNA levels

Hepatitis B and C coinfection have a cumulative effect in contributing to the formation of HCC.

With the obesity epidemic and increasing prevalence of diabetes, NASH appears to be a major factor which predisposes to the development of HCC. Just as with chronic hepatitis B, patients may develop HCC in the absence of cirrhosis.

PATHOGENESIS

In patients with chronic liver disease, there is persistent hepatic inflammation which leads to liver fibrosis and aberrant hepatocyte regeneration. Over time, these abnormalities lead to cirrhosis and series of genetic and epigenetic changes that culminate in the formation of dysplastic nodules, which are pre-neoplastic lesions. Additional molecular alterations provide the dysplastic cells with proliferative, invasive, and survival advantages and leads to full-blown HCC. HCC can also arise in patients who have chronic liver disease but do not have established cirrhosis or marked inflammation (e.g., patients with HBV infection).

Patients with HCC at the same clinical stage can have different molecular subtypes. These subtypes correlate with clinical features. The molecular subtypes can be grouped in two main classes: The proliferative class and the non-proliferative class (**Fig. 1**).

The proliferative class which is more commonly seen in patients with HBV infection, is characterized by molecular and histologic features that result in aggressive clinical behavior, including high serum levels of AFP, poor cell differentiation, chromosomal instability, *TP53* mutations, and activation of oncogenic pathways. Tumors of the non-proliferative class have more *CTNNB1* (beta-catenin) mutations, and their gene-expression pattern resembles that of normal hepatocytes. Understanding the interaction between cancer cells and their micro-environment is crucial for developing new therapies and identifying biomarkers, as also targeting the tumor with the best possible therapy—appropriately christened "Precision Oncology."

CLINICAL FEATURES

The presentation of HCC varies according to the size of the lesion(s). With use of ultrasound surveillance, small lesions are increasingly discovered incidentally. In most of the cases, the clinical manifestations are of underlying cirrhosis or chronic hepatitis. Large tumors may cause pressure effects and may present with ill-defined upper abdominal pain, malaise, weight loss, fatigue, and sometimes an awareness of an abdominal mass or fullness. Jaundice may result due to the compression of the common bile duct, or occasionally tumor embolization, and ascites may occur and suggest advanced disease or co-existing cirrhosis. Other presentations include the paraneoplastic syndrome, (hypercalcemia and hyperglycemia), gastrointestinal or esophageal variceal bleeding and tumor necrosis-induced fever. Sudden decompensation in the form of ascites or variceal bleeding in a stable cirrhotic suggests the development of HCC or portal vein thrombosis and should be looked for.

SURVEILLANCE

Screening interval for HCC is based on the average tumor doubling time of 3–5 months. Any patient with cirrhosis should be screened for HCC.

Exception to this rule may be patients with advanced/decompensated cirrhosis who are not transplant candidates. Their life expectancy is too short to offer any survival benefit from surveillance. The goal of surveillance for patients on the transplant waiting list is to ensure that a tumor does not develop that would preclude transplantation according to the established criteria. Surveillance is also recommended in patients with chronic hepatitis due to HBV and HCV infection who are non-cirrhotics as the risk of HCC in these patients is high even without the development of liver cirrhosis. Abdominal ultrasonography every 6 months is the recommended method for surveillance, with or without measurement of serum levels of AFP. The results are operator dependent, with a sensitivity of 47–84% and a specificity >90%. CT or MRI is not recommended as a surveillance tool for cirrhosis.

DIAGNOSIS

A focal liver lesion identified in a patient (especially cirrhotic) on ultrasound needs further evaluation in order to differentiate between benign and malignant tumors.

Vascular shift occurs during malignant transformation of hepatocytes, in which benign lesions (e.g., regenerative and dysplastic nodules) are supplied by branches of the portal system, whereas malignant nodules are supplied blood from the hepatic artery. This shift results in a distinctive pattern of hyper-enhancement in the

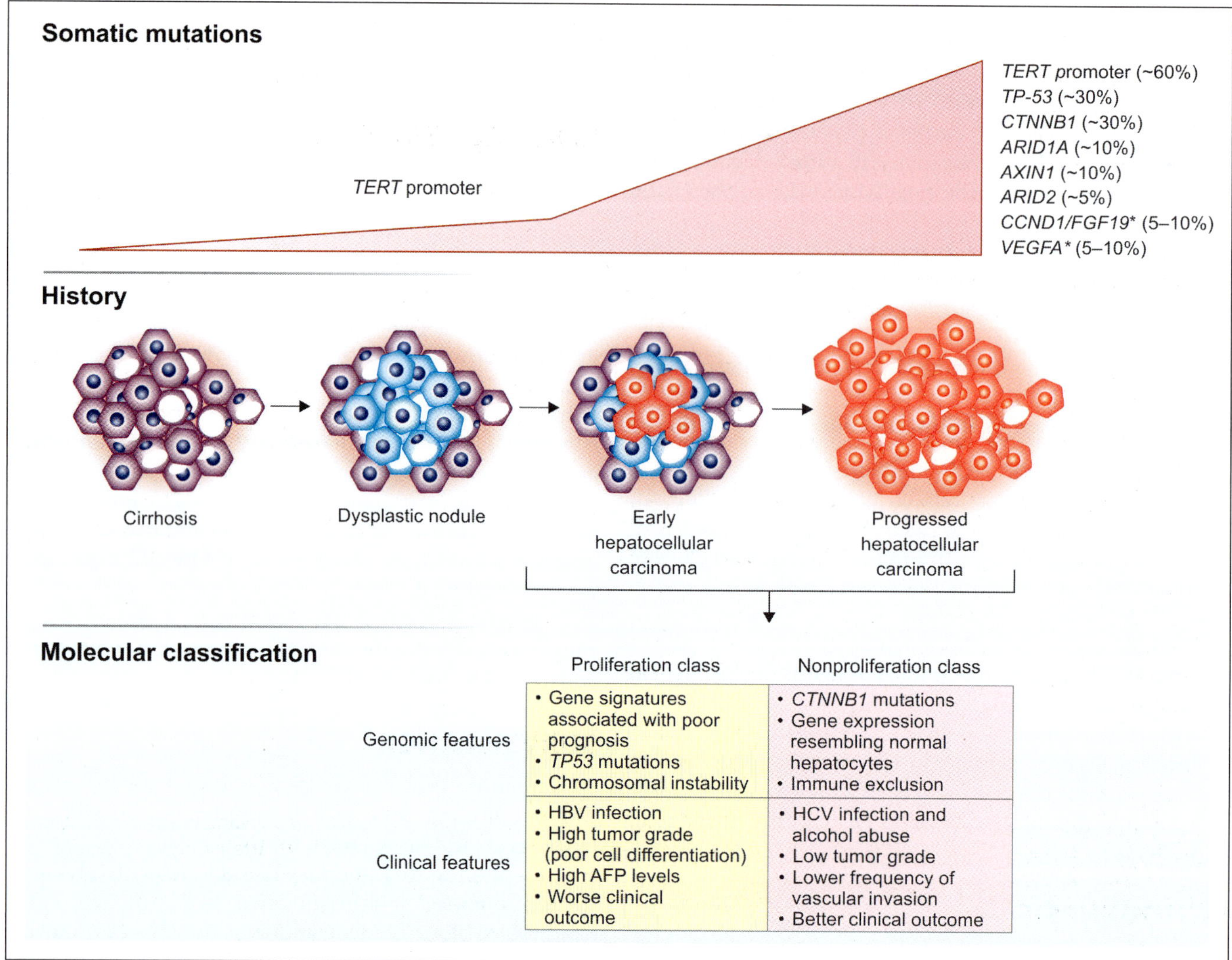

FIGURE 1: Genetic alterations and molecular classification of hepatocellular carcinoma.

Source: Adapted from Villanueva A. Hepatocellular carcinoma. N Engl J Med. 2019;380(15):1450-62.

arterial phase and washout in venous or delayed phases on contrast-enhanced CT or MRI (**Fig. 2**). This pattern has a sensitivity between 66 and 82% and a specificity >90% for the diagnosis of HCC in patients with cirrhosis and nodules >1 cm in diameter. The AASLD (American Association for the Study of Liver Diseases) and the EASL (European Association for the Study of the Liver) guidelines endorse the diagnosis of HCC radiologically (in a cirrhotic patient), if this pattern of imaging is seen on dynamic CT or MRI.

If an imaging study does not reveal this typical vascular pattern, then another imaging study with enhancement using a different modality should be performed, or tissue diagnosis must be pursued.

If a nodule of size <1 cm is detected in the liver:

- A 3-monthly follow-up is recommended for 1 year using ultrasound for any enlargement in size. If there is any change in pattern or growth, dynamic CT/dynamic MRI should be done.
- Nodules <1 cm may also be evaluated for HCC with gadolinium-ethoxybenzyl, diethylenetriamine penta-acetic acid (Gd-EOBDTPA)-/Gd-BOPTA-enhanced MRI scan (**Fig. 3**)

LIVER IMAGING REPORTING AND DATA SYSTEM

The Liver Imaging Reporting and Data System (LI-RADS) was introduced to standardize the reporting and data collection of CT and MRI for HCC. LI-RADS classifies new hepatic lesions into five classes based on their size, extent of interval growth, and patterns of enhancement (**Fig. 4**). Of note, lesions with a low LI-RADS class 1–2 should also be followed carefully as the system has low specificity for the prediction of benign lesions.

Tissue diagnosis of HCC is not required in majority of cases. The indications of tissue diagnosis include:

- When imaging and other findings are equivocal or not typical
- May be indicated in larger lesions in non-cirrhotic livers

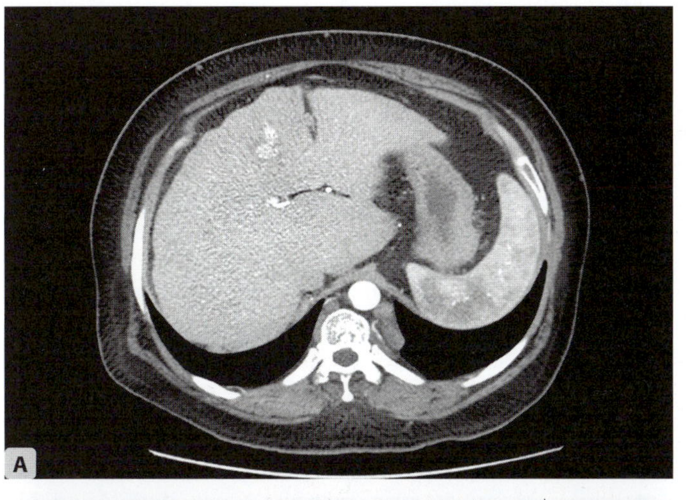

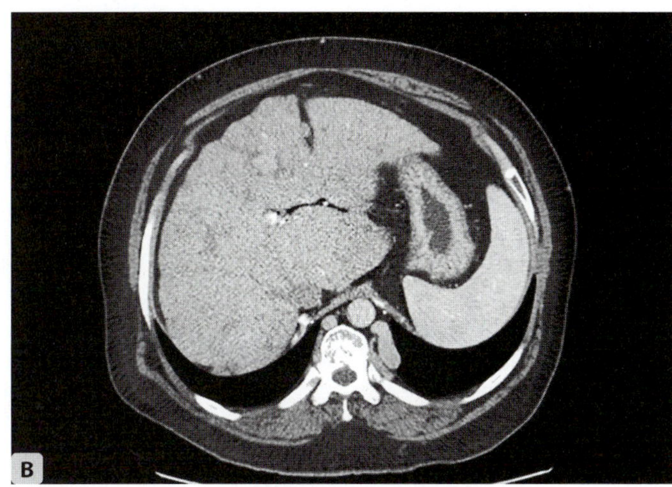

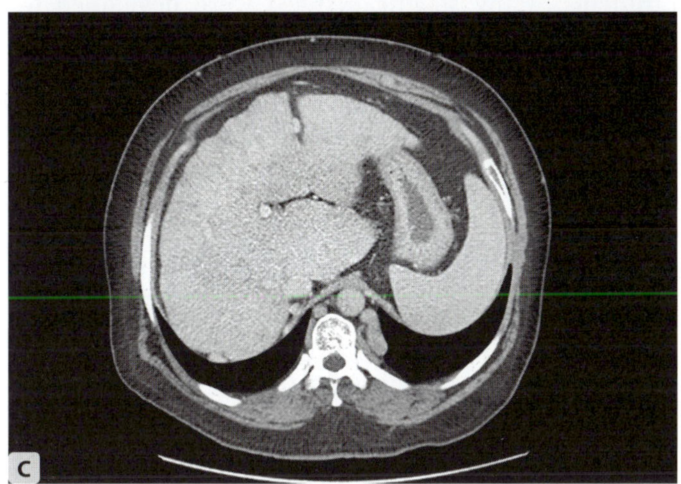

(CT: computerized tomography; HCC: hepatocellular carcinoma)

FIGURES 2 A to C: Dynamic CT showing classical enhancement pattern in a patient with HCC. **(A)** Arterial phase showing hyper enhancement; **(B)** portal venous phase; **(C)** delayed venous phase showing contrast washout.

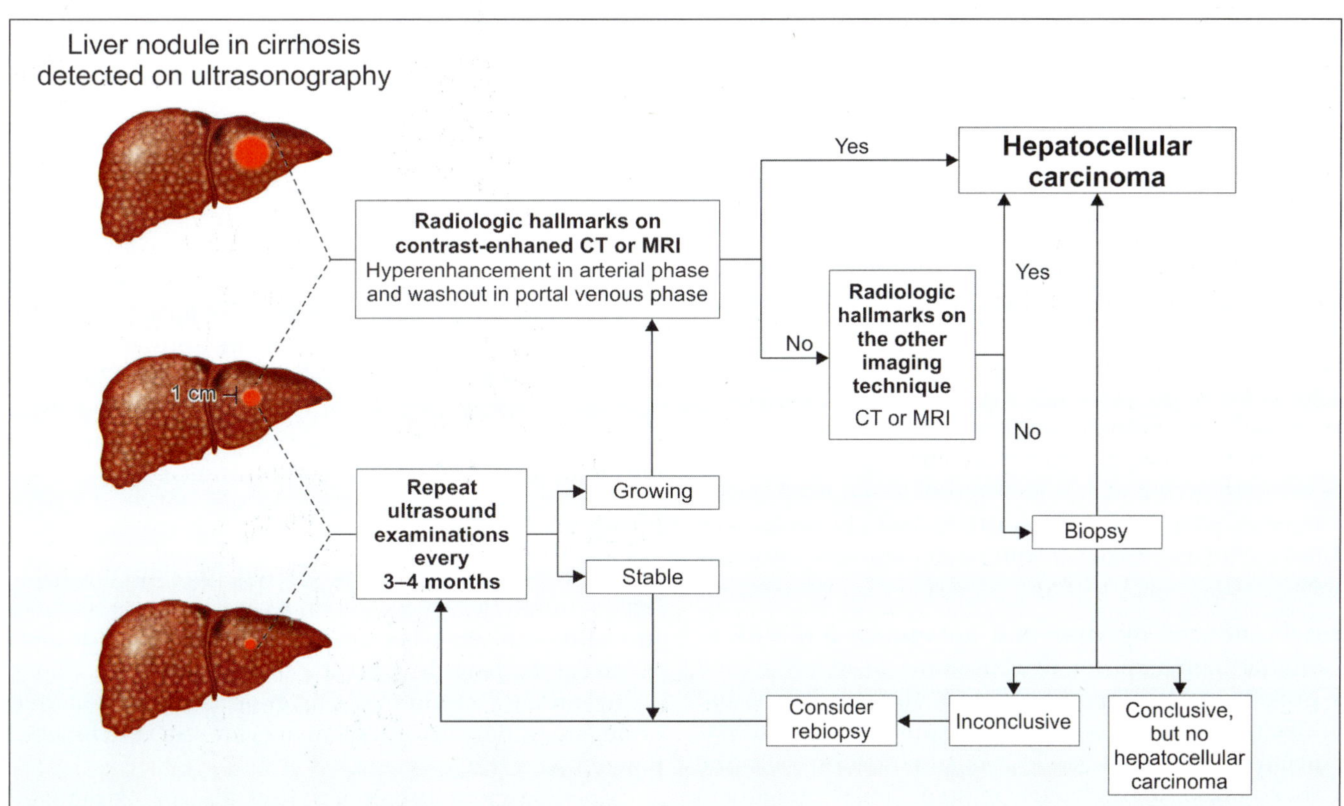

FIGURE 3: Diagnostic algorithm for a liver nodule in a patient with cirrhosis.

Source: Adapted from the guidelines of the European Association for the Study of the Liver.

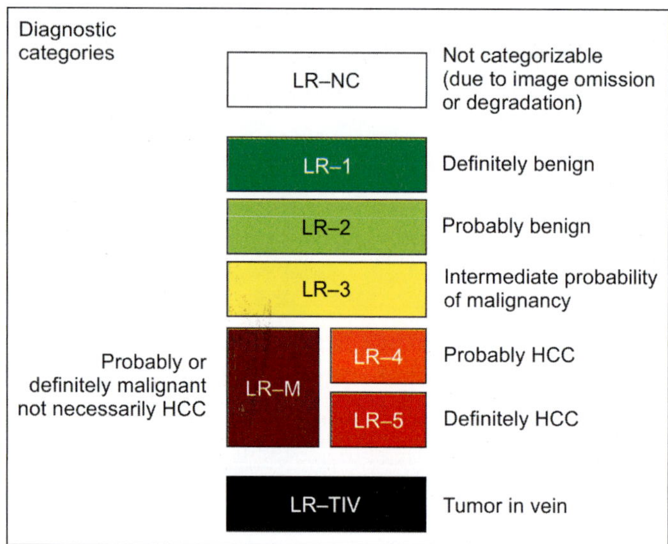

FIGURE 4: Liver Imaging Reporting and Data System (LI-RADS).
Source: Adapted from CT/MRI LI-RADS® v2018 CORE.

Immunohistochemistry is necessary for confirming the diagnosis and prognostic sub-classification in most cases.

There is no significant role of fluorodeoxyglucose-positron emission tomography (FDG PET)/CT in diagnosis of HCC, except for detection of distant metastases. FDG PET/CT may play an important role in prognostication of HCC. Higher the standardized uptake value (SUV), poorer is the prognosis.

DIAGNOSTIC AND PROGNOSTIC BIOMARKERS

Alpha-fetoprotein is the only tumor marker that has undergone extensive evaluation. AFP alone is not recommended either in surveillance or diagnosis of HCC. Serum AFP, when used with the conventional cut-off point of 500 ng/mL, has a sensitivity of about 50% and a specificity of >90% in detecting the presence of HCC in a patient with co-existing liver disease. Serum AFP estimation is useful in monitoring response to therapy. There is preliminary evidence that changes in serum AFP may be a more accurate and sensitive way of determining the degree of response to treatment than conventional imaging procedures that rely on physical determination of tumor size. Hence baseline AFP should be done along with the imaging for estimating the response to therapy. High levels of tumor markers are associated with worse prognosis in HCC patients. AFP >1,000 ng/mL is associated with poorer outcomes from LT for HCC.

Protein induced by vitamin K antagonist-II (PIVKA-II) is another biomarker for HCC used for diagnosis as well as prognosis. Combined with AFP, the sensitivity and specificity of HCC diagnosis can be improved to 94 and 98%, respectively. PIVKA-II alone or in combination with AFP has been shown to be effective in predicting the treatment response.

Neutrophil-to-lymphocyte ratio (NLR) *and platelet-to-lymphocyte ratio (PLR)* have been evaluated as tumor markers and both the NLR and PLR were identified as independent risk factors for predicting overall survival and recurrence-free survival in HCC patients.

Long noncoding RNAs (lncRNAs) have also been evaluated as tumor markers in HCC. Data showed that *lncRNAs* were of high diagnostic value for HCC and their expression could potentially be used as an auxilliary biomarker in confirming HCC.

STAGING

Staging of HCC is necessary for guiding the management decision, prognostication, and uniformity of research protocols. Many staging systems were developed for prognostication and for management of patients with HCC. The Barcelona Clinic Liver Cancer (BCLC) classification is currently the most commonly used standard staging system for HCC. This provides an algorithmic approach for the management of HCC and is the only staging system that has been prospectively validated.

The Indian guidelines (INASL) modified the BCLC staging and one of the most important modifications of the BCLC system proposed was with regard to end-stage cirrhosis. Patients with end-stage liver cirrhosis with heavily impaired liver functions (Child–Pugh class C) but with tumor size within Milan criteria and PS ≤ 2 should be considered for LT.

TREATMENT

The treatment of HCC depends on the tumor extent, patient co-morbidities, and the severity of liver dysfunction (**Fig. 5**). HCC management requires a multidisciplinary team approach to achieve the best outcome.

SURGICAL RESECTION

The ideal candidates for resection are patients with a solitary tumor at an early stage (BCLC stage 0 or A), regardless of tumor size with good performance status, well-preserved liver function and with no clinically significant portal hypertension. With resection in a properly selected patient, the survival is >60% at 5 years, with low post-operative mortality (<3%); around 70% of these patients have tumor recurrence at 5 years. Adjuvant therapies have not been shown to reduce tumor recurrence.

LIVER TRANSPLANT

Liver transplant can be offered for patients with a limited tumor burden who are not candidates for resection. In addition to removing the tumor, LT has the advantage of curing the liver disease. The Milan criteria for LT (i.e., a single nodule ≤5 cm in diameter or up to three nodules, none larger than 3 cm in diameter) are the benchmark in patients with HCC.

Macrovascular tumor invasion and/or extrahepatic spread are a contraindication for transplantation because

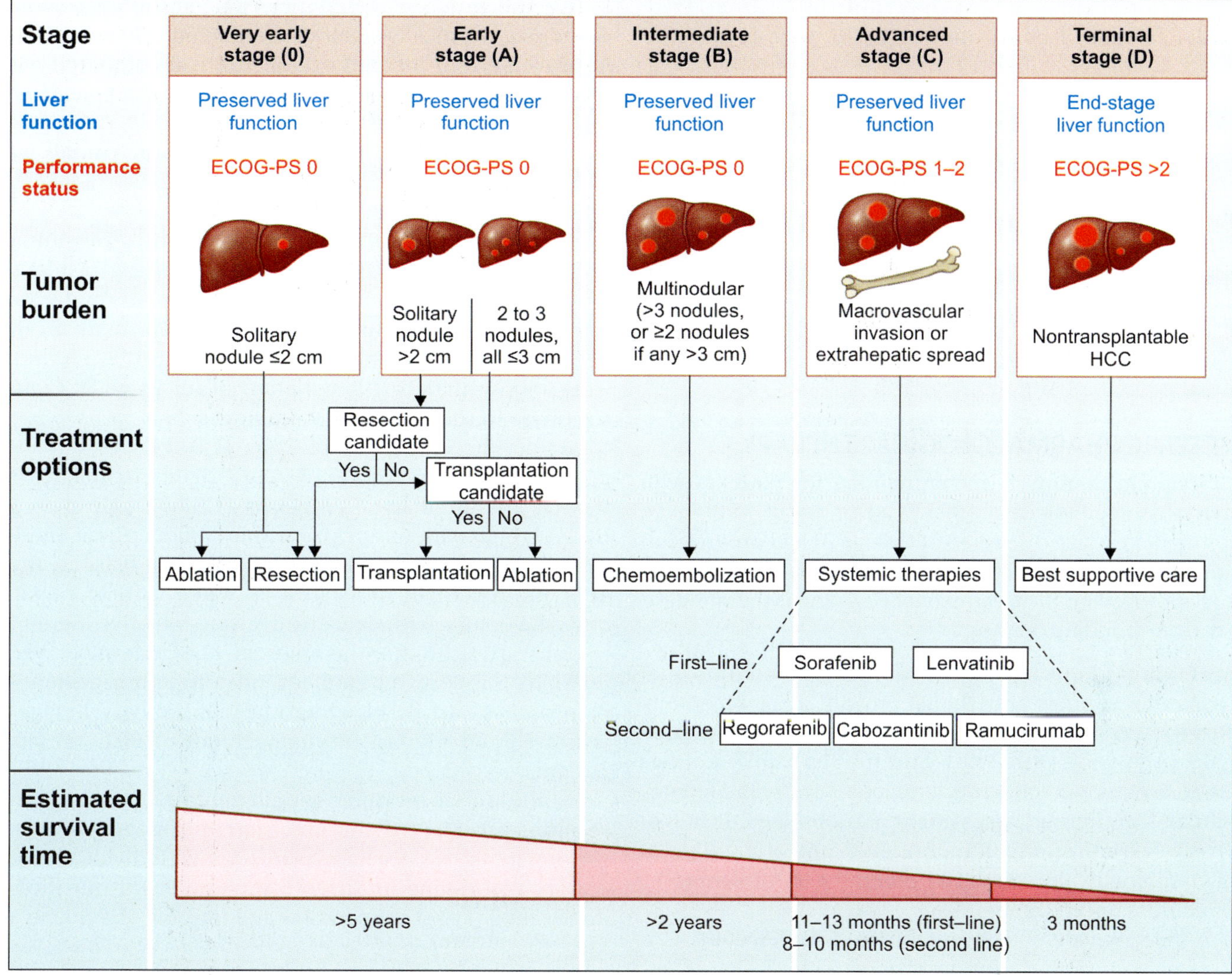

FIGURE 5: Management of hepatocellular carcinoma based on Barcelona clinic liver cancer algorithm.

Source: Adapted from Villanueva A. Hepatocellular carcinoma. N Engl J Med. 2019;380(15):1450-62.

of the high risk of tumor recurrence. Transplantation in patients with tumors that meet the Milan criteria is associated with survival of 60–80% at 5 years and 50% at 10 years, with post-transplantation tumor recurrence lower than 15%.

Transplantation in patients with tumors that do not meet the Milan criteria has worse outcomes.

Neo-adjuvant therapies such as ablation or transarterial therapies are administered while patients are on the wait list for LT to reduce the number of dropouts due to tumor progression when the expected waiting time is longer than 6 months. The use of these therapies to downstage some tumors exceeding the Milan criteria (i.e., reducing the tumor burden to meet the criteria) is a way of making ineligible patients eligible for transplantation.

TUMOR ABLATION

Ablation is recommended in patients with BCLC stage 0 or A tumors who are not candidates for surgery. The main method is image-guided percutaneous radiofrequency ablation, which results in tumor necrosis by inducing a high intratumoral temperature. The extent of tumor necrosis is negatively correlated with tumor size and efficacy reduces significantly in tumors larger than 3 cm in diameter. As compared with resection, ablation has fewer complications but provides worse local control for larger tumors. Other ablative options include microwave ablation, cryoablation, and ethanol injection.

TRANSARTERIAL THERAPY

In patients with intermediate stage tumors (BCLC stage B), transarterial therapy can be considered. The main treatment method is transarterial chemoembolization (TACE), in which intra-arterial cytotoxic agent is infused followed by embolization of the vessels that feed the tumor. Studies showed survival benefits with TACE as compared with the best supportive care. The mortality associated with TACE is below 1%, with most deaths due to liver failure. TACE should not be considered in patients with decompensated cirrhosis. TACE performed with drug-eluting beads has antitumoral activity similar to that of conventional TACE, with fewer side effects.

Selective internal radiation therapy (SIRT) or trans-arterial radioembolization (TARE) is another locoregional treatment approach for BCLC stage B tumors in which radioisotope Yttrium-90 microspheres are infused intra-arterially. The radiation emitted by Yttrium-90 is responsible for its antitumoral activity. SIRT is a safe procedure with an objective response similar to that seen with TACE. In contrast to TACE, this has minimal embolic effects in the hepatic artery distribution and can, therefore, be used in patients with portal vein thrombosis or tumor invasion.

SYSTEMIC PHARMACOLOGICAL THERAPY

Systemic therapy is recommended for patients who have advanced disease (BCLC stage C) or who have intermediate-stage disease (BCLC stage B) and progression with transarterial therapies. Sorafenib was the first systemic drug approved for the treatment of HCC and is the standard of care for frontline therapy.

Sorafenib is a small molecule multikinase inhibitor that targets the vascular endothelial growth factor receptors, VEGFR1, VEGFR2 and VEGFR3; platelet-derived growth factor receptor-β (PDGFRβ); and the Raf family kinases (predominantly C-Raf). In the pivotal Sorafenib Hepatocellular Carcinoma Assessment Randomized Protocol (SHARP) trial, survival increased from a median of 7.9 months with placebo to 10.7 months with sorafenib.

Sorafenib is not recommended:

- As neoadjuvant or adjuvant therapy with resection
- As neoadjuvant or adjuvant therapy with LT
- As bridging therapy for patients on transplant wait list
- As a downstaging therapy either alone or in combination with locoregional therapy.

The usual dose of sorafenib is 400 mg twice daily with optimal management of adverse effects to improve survival. However, Sorafenib should be initiated at reduced dose to minimize the adverse events and increase tolerability.

Adverse effects of sorafenib*:* Although sorafenib has demonstrated many benefits, the most common treatment-related toxicities seen with its usage are diarrhea, fatigue, cutaneous lesions especially hand-foot skin reaction, and hypertension. Most of these toxicities are considered mild-to-moderate and manageable to varying degrees.

Lenvatinib is noninferior to sorafenib and is an alternative first-line therapy for:

- Advanced HCC (BCLC C)
- Intermediate-stage HCC (BCLC-B) with preserved liver function (Child A; selected Child B), not suitable for or progressing despite loco regional therapy.

Regorafenib*,* an inhibitor of multiple kinases, increases survival, as compared with placebo, from 7.8 to 10.6 months and is recommended as second-line treatment for patients tolerating but progressing on sorafenib with well-preserved liver function (Child–Pugh A class) and good performance status.

Another multikinase inhibitor, **cabozantinib**, was shown to induce statistically significant and clinically meaningful improvement in median overall survival compared with placebo in patients with advanced HCC who had previously received sorafenib.

Antiangiogenic VEGFR2 antagonist, **ramucirumab**, was shown to improve overall survival in patients with advanced HCC and serum AFP levels ≥400 ng/mL.

Immune checkpoint inhibitors (such as nivolumab and pembrolizumab) have shown promising results in phase I and II trials, and phase III studies are underway. Recently, atezolizumab [programmed cell death ligand (PD-L1) antagonist] and bevacizumab (VEGFR inhibitor) were approved for first-line therapy of advanced HCC after the phase III trials showed favorable results.

As per the INASL modification of BCLC-based management, patients with end-stage liver cirrhosis with heavily impaired liver functions (Child–Pugh class C, BCLC-D) but with tumor size within Milan criteria and PS ≤2 should be considered for LT. If LT is not feasible, then after improvement of ascites, jaundice, and/or hepatic encephalopathy with conservative care, ablative therapies or trans-arterial tumor therapies may be performed, when possible. Supportive treatment including management of pain, ascites, variceal bleeding, nutrition, and psychological issues should be part of management of BCLC-D HCC patients.

Routine oral nutrition supplementation (ONS) is not recommended for patients in the terminal-stage HCC when the oral intake is satisfactory. However, in individual cases, dietary counseling and ONS can slow down nutritional deprivation, avoid dehydration and improve the quality of life.

Management of psychosocial and "futility of care" issues should be a part of the care of terminal HCC patients.

CONCLUSION

Hepatocellular carcinoma is a major contributor to the cancer-related morbidity and mortality. Hence, prevention and treatment of viral hepatitis and minimizing risk factor exposure are crucial elements in decreasing the global burden of HCC. HCC surveillance leads to early detection of cancer and improves overall survival. Thus, implementation of programs for viral hepatitis screening, HCC surveillance in high-risk patients, and effective treatment of HCC are important to improve the current dismal outcomes of patients with this disease. The marked improvement in community awareness, health advocacy, public health and civil society's efforts in the past few years has given hope for the prospect of substantially decreasing the global burden of illness and death from HCC within the next few decades.

RECOMMENDED READINGS

1. Villanueva A. Hepatocellular Carcinoma. N Engl J Med. 2019;380(15):1450-62.
2. Yang JD, Hainaut P, Gores GJ, Amadou A, Plymoth A, Roberts LR. A global view of hepatocellular carcinoma:

trends, risk, prevention, and management. Nat Rev Gastroenterol Hepatol. 2019;16(10):589-604.
3. Waller LP, Deshpande V, Pyrsopoulos N. Hepatocellular carcinoma: A comprehensive review. World J Hepatol. 2015;7(26):2648-63.
4. Sleisenger MH, Feldman M, Friedman LS, Brandt LJ. Sleisenger and Fordtran's Gastrointestinal and Liver Disease: Pathophysiology, Diagnosis, Management, 9th edition. Philadelphia, PA: Saunders/Elsevier; 2010.
5. El-Serag, HB, Rudolph, KL. Hepatocellular carcinoma: epidemiology and molecular carcinogenesis. Gastroenterology. 2007;132:2557-76.
6. Jemal A, Bray F, Center MM, Ferlay J, Ward E, Forman D. Global cancer statistics. CA Cancer J Clin. 2011;61:69-90.
7. Kumar A, Acharya SK, Singh SP, Arora A, Dhiman RK, Aggarwal R, et. al. 2019 Update of Indian National Association for Study of the Liver Consensus on Prevention, Diagnosis, and Management of Hepatocellular Carcinoma in India: The Puri II Recommendations. JCEH. 2020;10(1):43-80
8. Heimbach JK, Kulik LM, Finn RS, Sirlin CB, Abecassis MM, Roberts LR, et al. AASLD guidelines for the treatment of hepatocellular carcinoma. Hepatology. 2018;67(1):358-80.
9. European Association for the Study of the Liver. EASL Clinical Practice Guidelines: Management of hepatocellular carcinoma. J Hepatol. 2018;69(1):182-236.

CHAPTER

150

Liver Transplantation

Abhideep Chaudhary, Gaurav Sood, Ajay Kumar

ABSTRACT

The field of liver transplantation (LT) has undergone remarkable advances in the last three decades. From an essentially experimental procedure in the early 1980s, LT has progressed to become the treatment of choice for patients with liver failure and liver cancer. The 1-year patient survival rates have increased from 30% in the early 1980s to >90% at present. The major reasons for this dramatic increase include refined surgical techniques, better immunosuppressive regimens, more effective treatment of infections, and improved care during the critical perioperative period. Yet LT remains a major undertaking, with the continuing potential for complications affecting every major organ system. This chapter will provide basic information on indications and timing of liver transplant, pretransplant assessment, technical issues regarding the recipient operation, posttransplant care, surgical and medical complications, and long-term care of transplant patients.

"We cannot live only for ourselves. A thousand fibers connect us with our fellow men"

—Herman Melville

INTRODUCTION

Liver transplantation is a time-honored treatment for patients with end-stage liver disease. The results have markedly improved since 1963, when Professor Thomas Starzl performed the first liver transplant. The technical advancement gained over the years, improvement in the intensive care, as well as the development of newer immunosuppressant drugs have made it a successful surgical procedure, with 1-year survival of >90%.

In India, the first LT was performed in 1998 and after an initial slow start, both deceased donor and living donor programs have picked up all over the country. Still the disease burden is huge, and it is estimated that 25,000 transplants are needed per year whereas only 1,400–1,800 transplants are being done per year.

INDICATIONS

CHRONIC LIVER DISEASE

Cirrhosis with end-stage liver disease is the most common indication for LT. **Box 1** lists the common etiological factors of chronic liver disease (CLD) and diseases amenable to treatment by LT. The diagnosis of cirrhosis per se does not mean that transplantation is indicated. LT is justifiable only if projected survival is <90% at 1 year. Model for end-stage liver disease (MELD) score uses serum bilirubin, international normalized ratio (INR), and creatinine for calculation and is a useful tool to predict 3 months mortality. This score is used to list patients for LT. A score of >15 is an indication for LT. However, the family counseling and transplant evaluation should typically start

BOX 1 Diseases amenable to treatment by liver transplantation (LT).

Chronic liver disease

Noncholestatic
- Hepatitis B and C
- Alcohol-induced cirrhosis
- Autoimmune hepatitis

Cholestatic
- Primary biliary cirrhosis
- Secondary biliary cirrhosis
- Primary sclerosing cholangitis

Metabolic
- Wilson's disease
- Hemochromatosis
- Alpha-1 antitrypsin deficiency
- Amyloidosis
- Tyrosinemia
- Cystic fibrosis

Vascular
- Budd-Chiari syndrome

Others
- Primary oxalosis
- Glycogen storage diseases

Acut liver failure
- Hepatitis A/E
- Hepatitis B
- Acetaminophen toxicity
- Wilson disease
- Autoimmune hepatitis
- Budd-Chiari syndrome

Malignant disease
- Hepatocellular carcinoma (HCC, within Milan criteria)
- Hepatoblastoma
- Epithelioid hemangioendothelioma
- Neuroendocrine liver metastases

Cryptogenic

BOX 2 MELD score–3 months mortality.

- 40 or more 71.3% observed mortality
- 30–39 52.6% observed mortality
- 20–29 19.6% observed mortality
- 10–19 6.0% observed mortality
- <9 1.9% observed mortality

BOX 3 Indications for a liver transplant in patients with chronic liver disease.

Clinical indications:
- Refractory ascites
- Spontaneous bacterial peritonitis
- Recurrent or severe hepatic encephalopathy
- Hepatorenal syndrome
- Significant weakness, fatigue, or progressive malnutrition
- Recurrent cholangitis or severe pruritus
- Progressive bone disease

Biochemical indications:
- Serum albumin < 3.0 g/dL
- Serum INR > 1.7
- Serum bilirubin > 2 mg/dL (>4 mg/dL for cholestatic disorders)

TABLE 1 Child–Pugh score.

Parameter	Score		
Ascites	None	Slight	Moderate to severe
Encephalopathy	None	Slight to moderate	Moderate to severe
Bilirubin (mg/dL)	<2	2–3	>3
Albumin (g/dL)	>3.5	2.8–3.5	<2.8
Prothrombin time (Prolonged in seconds)	1–3 s	4–6 s	>6
Class A score 5–6; Class B score 7–9; Class C score 10–15			

once patient has a MELD score >10. **Box 2** shows 3 months mortality associated with the MELD score.

Child-Turcotte-Pugh (CTP) score is also a valuable tool in assessing severity of disease (**Table 1**). A cumulative score of 7 meets the minimal listing requirement for a transplant.

Patients with cirrhosis should be referred to a transplant center when they experience their first major complication or develop synthetic dysfunction (**Box 3**). Waiting to refer patients until they develop terminal illness frequently results in death before a transplant can even occur. Any significant decompensation, such as variceal bleed, hepatic encephalopathy, ascites, spontaneous bacterial peritonitis, and hepatorenal syndrome (HRS), dramatically decreases the 1-year survival and are indications for LT.

In some diseases such as primary sclerosing cholangitis (PSC) and primary biliary cirrhosis (PBC), poor quality of life due to fatigue, weakness, and intractable itching are also indications of transplant.

ACUTE LIVER FAILURE

Acute liver failure (ALF) is defined as development of severe acute liver injury leading to encephalopathy and impaired synthetic function with no preexisting CLD. It can progress within 2–8 weeks to encephalopathy or even hepatic coma. These patients have limited treatment options such as steroids for autoimmune hepatitis and N-acetyl cysteine for paracetamol overdose. Timely LT is lifesaving in this setting. The challenge for clinicians in this setting is to

TABLE 2 King's College criteria.	
Paracetamol overdose	**Nonparacetamol overdose**
• pH < 7.30 Or all of the following: • PT > 100 seconds • Creatinine > 300 µmol/L • Grade III/IV encephalopathy	• PT > 100 seconds Or three of the following: • Time from jaundice to encephalopathy >2 days • Non-A, non-B hepatitis, halothane or drug induced liver failure • Age < 10 or > 40 years • PT > 50 seconds • Bilirubin > 300 µmol/L

(PT: prothrombin time)

TABLE 3 Dynamic ALFED risk score.	
Predictors of mortality at admission	**Points assigned**
HE > grade II	1
INR > 5	1
Arterial ammonia > 123 µmol/L	1
Bilirubin > 15 mg/dL	1
Variable over 3 days	
HE persistent or progressive over 3 days	2
INR persistent or increased to >5	1
Arterial ammonia persistent >123 µmol/L	2
Bilirubin increased to or persistent >15 mg/dL	1
Alfed score	**Risk group**
0–1	Low
2–3	Moderate
4–6	High

(HE: hepatic encephalopathy; INR: international normalized ratio)

perform LT at the right time before the onset of irreversible complications such as raised intracranial pressure (ICP), brain stem herniation, and at the same time avoiding LT in patients with potentially reversible liver failure. Prognostic assessment should begin at the site of first presentation and decisions in relation to patient transfer to a specialist center must be made at the earliest opportunity.

King's criteria (**Table 2**) is most commonly followed worldwide to decide the timing of liver transplant, however it is limited by low sensitivity. A more dynamic criterion (**Table 3**) which includes assessment at the time of admission and after 48 hours is a useful predictor of outcome in patients with ALF that helps in clinical decision making regarding the timing of transplant.

HEPATOCELLULAR CARCINOMA

Hepatocellular carcinoma (HCC) is associated with cirrhosis in 90% of the cases and liver cirrhosis predisposes to HCC. In this setting, LT potentially cures the disease and removes the underlying precancerous cirrhotic liver. The best results of LT in HCC are seen in patients within the Milan or University of California San Francisco (UCSF) criteria (**Box 4**). With this stringent criterion, a relapse rate of <20% and a 5-year survival equivalent to those in which transplant is done for other benign indications of LT can be achieved. With increased experience the criteria for transplantation for patients suffering from HCC is constantly being expanded, with different criteria using biochemical (e.g., alpha-fetoprotein) as well as biological behavior of the tumor.

BOX 4 HCC listing criteria.

- **Milan:** Single HCC nodule ≤5 cm
  Criteria: ≤3 lesions each ≤3 cm
- **UCSF:** Solitary HCC lesion ≤6.5 cm
  Criteria: ≤3 nodules each ≤4.5 cm with total diameter of ≤8 cm

BOX 5 Contraindications to liver transplantation.

Absolute
- Severe cardiac and/or pulmonary diseases and severe pulmonary hypertension (mPAP > 45 mm Hg)
- Hepatocellular carcinoma with extra hepatic metastases
- Extrahepatic malignancies
- Sepsis

Relative
- Untreated alcohol abuse and other drug-related addiction
- Cholangiocarcinoma
- Hepatic metastatic neuroendocrine tumors (NET), metastatic hemangioendothelioma
- Morbid obesity

(mPAP: mean pulmonary artery pressure)

METABOLIC LIVER DISEASES

Several metabolic diseases such as glycogen storage diseases, tyrosinemia, galactosemia, and Gaucher's disease present with inborn errors of metabolism and chronic liver failure. LT corrects both the cirrhosis and metabolic deficiency present in the native liver.

CONTRAINDICATIONS

With improving result and experience, contraindications to LT are shrinking and diseases which were previously considered absolute contraindications are now undergoing successful transplant.

Box 5 summarizes the various contraindications of LT.

TYPES OF LIVER TRANSPLANTATION

DECEASED DONOR LIVER TRANSPLANTATION

Deceased donor form most of the organ pool in the west compared to the east, where cultural and regional differences have led to living donations as the primary source of organs.

Deceased donation can be both after "brain death" or "cardiac death". Brain death is defined as cessation of

BOX 6	Criteria for brain death diagnosis.
• **Prerequisite:**	
◦ Known irreversible cause of coma	
◦ Exclude potentially reversible condition (drug intoxication, poisoning, electrolyte, and acid-base imbalance)	
◦ Core body temperature > 35°	
◦ Systolic BP > 90 mm Hg	
• **No spontaneous movements**	
• **No response to deep painful stimulus**	
• **Absent brainstem reflexes:**	
◦ Pupillary reflex	
◦ Oculovestibular reflex	
◦ Corneal reflex	
◦ Pharyngeal reflex	
◦ Tracheal reflex	

activities of the brain stem. The diagnosis of brain death is made clinically, supplemented by brain stem tests conducted by dedicated doctors in the hospital. The criteria of establishing the diagnosis of brain death are summarized in **Box 6**. Donation after cardiac death (DCD) is now gaining acceptance due to the gap in the organ donation and patient waitlist. These patients have severe neurologic injury, such as anoxia and intracranial hemorrhage, but do not meet brain death criteria.

LIVING DONOR LIVER TRANSPLANT

In living-related liver donation, a part of the normal liver from a related family member is removed and implanted in the recipient. This remaining liver and the transplanted liver both regenerate and take over the normal functions. Living-related LT is appealing because it allows elective transplantation after optimizing the health of the recipient, reduces cold ischemia time, and potentially shortens the waiting time for a patient. The disadvantage includes morbidity and rare mortality in the donor.

The liver transplant in India mainly started with living donor liver transplant (LDLT) and deceased donation was sporadic and limited to a few regions. With improving public awareness and government support, in the last 20 years, cadaveric programs have picked up. From 2013 to 2018, 9,383 liver transplants were reported in India, which included 6,416 living-donors and 2,967 deceased-donor organ recipients. India is now a regional transplant center for South East Asia and a major hub for medical tourism. About 25–30% of the total transplants per year are performed on patients from other countries. In 1994, Transplantation of Human Organs Act was passed which was aimed at regulation of removal, storage, and transplantation of human organs for therapeutic purposes and for prevention of commercial dealings in

BOX 7	Evaluation for liver transplant recipient.
• **History and examination:**	
– Any decompensation in the form of ascites, jaundice, variceal bleeding, encephalopathy, SBP, and hepatorenal syndrome	
– Significant previous medical or surgical history	
– Vaccinations for hepatitis A and B	
– Assessment by psychiatrist	
• **Blood tests:**	
– *ABO and typing, CBC, INR, aPTT, and electrolytes,*	
• **Other tests:**	
– Microbiology/Virology	
– Hepatitis serology (hepatitis A/B/C/D), CMV IgG/IgM, VZV, IgG/IgM, HIV, and tuberculosis	
– Maxillofacial/Dental examination	
– ENT examination	
– Gynecology/Urology examination, and esophagogastroduodenoscopy	
• **Preparation for surgery:**	
– Pulmonary function test and blood gas analysis	
– ECG and echocardiography	
– Cardiac catheterization in patients at risk or >65 years	
– Assessment by transplant anesthetist	
• **Radiologic assessment:**	
– X-ray of paranasal sinuses	
– Thoracic and abdominal triple-phase CT angiography	
– Mammography in female patients at risk or >40 years	
– Duplex-sonography of the liver (if CT not possible)	
• **Final assessment:**	
– Interdisciplinary review by transplant board (hepatologist, transplant surgeon, transplant anesthetist, and psychiatrist)	

(Ig: immunoglobulin; VZV: varicella zoster virus)

human organs. It was later modified in 2011 and finally to transplantation of Human Organs and Tissue Act in 2014. The amendments allowed for swapping of organs and widened the donor pool by including grandparents and grandchildren in the list.

EVALUATION AND WORKUP

Transplant recipient: All patients should be thoroughly evaluated as early as possible after the onset of cirrhosis. This allows for complete etiological workup, assessment of candidacy for LT, detection of HCC, and management of decompensation. **Box 7** summarizes the basic evaluation for a patient suffering from liver disease before being listed for LT.

Living donor evaluation: The potential donor is evaluated by multidisciplinary team in three phases to make sure that there is no risk to the donor (**Box 8**). Also, the potential donor is counseled to ensure donor commitment, motivation, and understanding of the risks involved.

BOX 8	Donor evaluation.
• **Phase 1:**	
◦ Comprehensive history and physical examination	
◦ Laboratory profile, viral serology, and blood type	
◦ Initial counseling to ensure donor commitment, motivation, and understanding of the risks involved	
• **Phase 2:**	
◦ Triphasic CT of the abdomen with liver volumetry	
◦ MRI for biliary duct anatomy and evaluation of fat fraction	
• **Phase 3:**	
◦ Evaluation by multidisciplinary team	

TECHNIQUE

A detailed description of the operative procedure is beyond the scope of this chapter. A basic understanding of the intraoperative course is necessary, however, to aid in postoperative care and in monitoring for possible complications. In this chapter, the technique of right lobe LDLT would be described, which forms the most common type of living-related liver donation in India.

Donor surgery: The left or right lobe of the liver can be used for transplantation depending upon anatomic considerations, the volume of the donor liver, and the size of the recipient.

Back table preparation—preparing the liver for implantation:

- *Organ preservation*: Graft is perfused with cold perfusion fluids such as histidine-tryptophan-ketoglutarate (HTK) or University of Wisconsin (UW) solution.
- Hepatic vein outflow reconstruction

Recipient hepatectomy: The first part of the recipient operation is removing the diseased liver which can often be the most challenging part of the transplant due to portal hypertension and adhesions from previous surgeries or episodes of spontaneous bacterial peritonitis.

Implantation: The process of implantation involves three vascular anastomosis followed by biliary reconstruction (**Box 9**).

BOX 9	Steps of graft implantation.
• RHV with MHV (ePTFE) to IVC—venous outflow	
• Graft portal vein to recipient main portal vein—portal inflow	
• Graft artery to right or left hepatic artery—arterial inflow	
• Graft duct to recipient bile duct or hepaticojejunostomy—biliary reconstruction	

(ePTFE: expanded polytetrafluoroethylene; MHV: middle hepatic vein; RHV: right hepatic veins)

EARLY POSTTRANSPLANT CARE

The care of all such patients involves (1) stabilization of the major organ systems (e.g., cardiovascular, pulmonary, and renal); (2) evaluation of graft function and achievement of adequate immunosuppression; and (3) monitoring and treatment of complications directly and indirectly related to the transplant.

IMMEDIATE POSTOPERATIVE CARE

The initial care is performed in an intensive care unit (ICU) setting. Recipients generally require mechanical ventilatory support for the first 12–36 hours. The goal is to maintain adequate oxygen saturation, acid-base equilibrium, and stable hemodynamics. Continuous hemodynamic monitoring should be maintained by an arterial line. Fluid management, electrolyte status, and renal function require frequent evaluation after surgery. Most liver recipients have an increased extravascular volume but a reduced intravascular volume. Magnesium levels should be kept above 2 mg/dL to prevent seizures; phosphate levels between 2 mg/dL and 5 mg/dL for proper support of the respiratory and alimentary tracts.

Serum transaminase levels will usually rise during the first 48–72 hours secondary to preservation injury, and then should fall rapidly over the next 24–48 hours. Regular Doppler ultrasound monitoring of vascular anastomosis is done in the initial few days to detect early thrombosis.

IMMUNOSUPPRESSION

The risk of acute rejection is highest in the initial few days following transplantation due to the added insult of surgical trauma and reperfusion injury. Aim of immunosuppression is to adequately decrease the T cell activity and at the same time maintain the body defenses to not inappropriately increase the risk of infections. Most patients are started on a three-drug protocol: a calcineurin inhibitor (tacrolimus), a mycophenolate mofetil (MMF), and corticosteroids. Most commonly, the dose of the calcineurin inhibitor is decreased, the MMF is withdrawn at 6–12 months posttransplant, and the prednisone is withdrawn at 3–6 months posttransplant.

COMPLICATIONS

Complications resulting from LT can be early or late (**Table 4**). Early complications are mainly related to technical issues and early nonfunction or delayed function of the graft whereas late complications may be due to rejection, infection, and adverse effects of immunosuppressants.

EARLY COMPLICATIONS

Hemorrhage: Bleeding is common during and after recipient hepatectomy because of the need to remove the hard cirrhotic liver in a coagulopathic, rundown patient with portal hypertension. Meticulous hemostasis and timely correction of coagulopathy are essential to minimize the risk of intraoperative and postoperative hemorrhage and the need for re-exploration.

TABLE 4 Timeline of major complications after liver transplant.

Common complications	Timeline
Primary graft nonfunction	1st week
Biliary complications	
Acute kidney injury	
Infections—surgical, chest	1–4 weeks
Acute liver allograft rejection	
Hepatic artery thrombosis	
CMV	1–3 months
Fungal infection	
Acute liver allograft rejection	
Biliary complications	
Hepatic artery thrombosis	
Acute liver allograft rejection	3–6 months
Biliary complications	
EBV hepatitis	
Chronic rejection	Over 6 months
EBV hepatitis	
Portal vein thrombosis	
Disease recurrence	
Late hepatic artery thrombosis	
Posttransplant lymphoproliferative disease	

(CMV: cytomegalovirus; EBV: Epstein–Barr virus)

Hepatic artery thrombosis: Liver has dual blood supply; the hepatic artery provides oxygenated blood to the liver and exclusively supplies the bile duct. Hepatic artery thrombosis (HAT) is associated with the increased incidence of graft loss, long-term biliary complications, and patient death. The incidence of HAT is in the range of 5–10%. It may present as a rise in serum transaminase levels, unexplained fever, or bile leak. Timely and early detection of thrombosis and thrombolysis (within 24 hours) may salvage the graft. If thrombolysis fails, surgical thrombectomy or early retransplantation is advocated as a lifesaving measure.

Portal vein thrombosis: Fortunately, this is a rare phenomenon and occurs in around 1% cases. Patients present with features of portal hypertension, ascites being the most common. Complete portal vein thrombosis (PVT) can lead to parenchymal injury, graft loss, and death. In early cases thrombolysis by intervention radiologist or surgical thrombectomy may be done.

Biliary complications: The spectrum of biliary complications includes bile leak and isolated or diffuse biliary strictures. Incidence is variable in different series and ranges from 10% to 30%. The reason for biliary complications can be technical as well as be related to donor factors including the number and size of ducts, DCD, and HAT.

Strictures can often be managed with endoscopic or percutaneous interventional radiology techniques, but occasionally surgical revision with hepaticojejunostomy is required.

LATE COMPLICATIONS

Acute rejections: Acute rejection mostly within the first 90 days but can be seen any time after LT. In an analysis from two large transplant databases, about 15% of transplant recipients had at least one episode of acute rejection. It initially presents as an asymptomatic rise in liver enzymes and biopsy is diagnostic. Diagnosis is difficult as hepatitis, viral diseases, drugs, and autoimmune recurrence can all have similar clinical and histopathological features. Treatment is intravenous methylprednisolone followed by a corticosteroid taper, as well as augmentation of maintenance immunosuppression.

Chronic rejection: Chronic rejection is relatively rare in the setting of LT. The histologic characteristic of chronic rejection is progressive bile duct injury leading to ductopenia. This is also known as "vanishing bile duct syndrome" as there is paucity of bile ducts on histopathological examination. Retransplant is the only effective treatment option in patients with chronic rejection.

Infections: Transplant recipients are more prone to infections because of malnutrition, chronic illness, and the use of immunosuppressants to prevent rejection.

Infections have been found to be responsible for 15–25% of deaths of all liver transplants. It is directly responsible for over half of deaths in the first year, remaining the most common cause of death during the first 3 years following transplant.

Bacterial infection: Gram negative bacilli are the most common infectious organisms in the early postoperative period. Common sources of bacteremia are pneumonia, bile leak, other abdominal infections, and wound sepsis. Source control forms the nucleus of treatment along with starting sensitive antibiotics. The emergence of multidrug resistant strains can make the management of these patients difficult.

Viral infection: Cytomegalovirus (CMV) infection can occur following liver transplant as either new primary infection or reactivation of latent infection. Almost two-thirds of CMV episodes occur between 2 months and 6 months. Recipients who are CMV seronegative (i.e., those who have not been infected previously with CMV) and receive an organ from a CMV-seropositive donor, are most at-risk to develop CMV infection. CMV infection can manifest as fever, leukopenia, and weakness. Organ systems most infected are lungs, liver, colon, and rarely brain and eyes. High-risk patients need prophylaxis with antivirals like valganciclovir.

Herpes simplex virus and herpes zoster infections can recur due to latent virus activation. Management of herpes simplex is with topical acyclovir and systemic therapy. Herpes zoster is rare and difficult to treat.

Fungal infections: Although less common but fungal infections are the most lethal and difficult to treat in an LT recipient. *Pneumocystis jiroveci* is a common fungal pathogen after LT and presents with respiratory symptoms. Chemoprophylaxis after transplant is given for 3–6 months.

Other invasive fungal infections such as *Candida* spp. and *Aspergillus* can be lethal and difficult to treat. Early aggressive debridement and sensitive antifungal drugs offer the only chance of survival.

Metabolic complications: It includes either or combination of hypertension, diabetes, dyslipidemia, and obesity. It may be present in the preoperative period or exacerbated by immunosuppressants following transplant. **Table 5** describes various metabolic complications and associated treatment strategies.

Noninfectious medical complications: After LT, almost every major organ system may be affected. Awareness about the potential complications and their management is essential for best results.

Neurologic complications: Neurologic complications posttransplant are common, affecting >20% of liver recipients. Complications generally manifest as a decreased level of consciousness, seizures, or focal neurologic deficits.

Cardiovascular complications: Several cardiovascular complications (including arrhythmia, ischemia, changes in blood pressure, and cardiac arrest) can be seen intra- and postoperatively. Systemic arterial hypertension necessitating treatment is the most common vascular complication posttransplant. The incidence of postoperative myocardial ischemia is 5–13%.

Pulmonary complications: The pulmonary system is one of the most common sites of complications posttransplant. Infectious complications predominate after the first posttransplant week, but noninfectious complications [such as pulmonary edema, pleural effusion, atelectasis, and adult respiratory distress syndrome (ARDS)] predominate during the first week.

Renal complications: Some degree of renal dysfunction is common posttransplant, affecting almost all liver recipients. About 10% have renal failure severe enough to require dialysis. Postoperative renal problems that may have been present pretransplant are most commonly due to HRS or acute tubular necrosis (ATN).

Posttransplant malignancy: Immunosuppressive state associated with transplant leads to an increased risk of development of malignancies. Squamous cell carcinoma is the most common malignant disease in transplant recipients. Other skin tumors, posttransplant lymphoproliferative diseases, and Kaposi sarcoma are known to occur and require delayed and regular follow-up.

TABLE 5 List of metabolic complications and management strategy.

Symptoms	Follow-up	Management in step wise manner
Hypertension (70%)	Every week for 6 months	• Limited salt intake • Dose modification of immuno-suppression • Calcium channel blocker • Beta blocker
Diabetes mellitus (5–20%)	1 year	• Diet and weight loss • Insulin initially, tapering of immunosuppression • Switch to oral hypoglycemics
Obesity (30%)	1 year	• Calorie restriction • Exercise • Decrease steroids
Dyslipidemia (16–43%)	1 year	• Calorie restriction • Exercise • Decrease steroids
Metabolic bone diseases	6 months	• Reduction in steroids • Bisphosphontes

OUTCOMES

Surgical techniques and perioperative management for transplant patients have improved and undergone

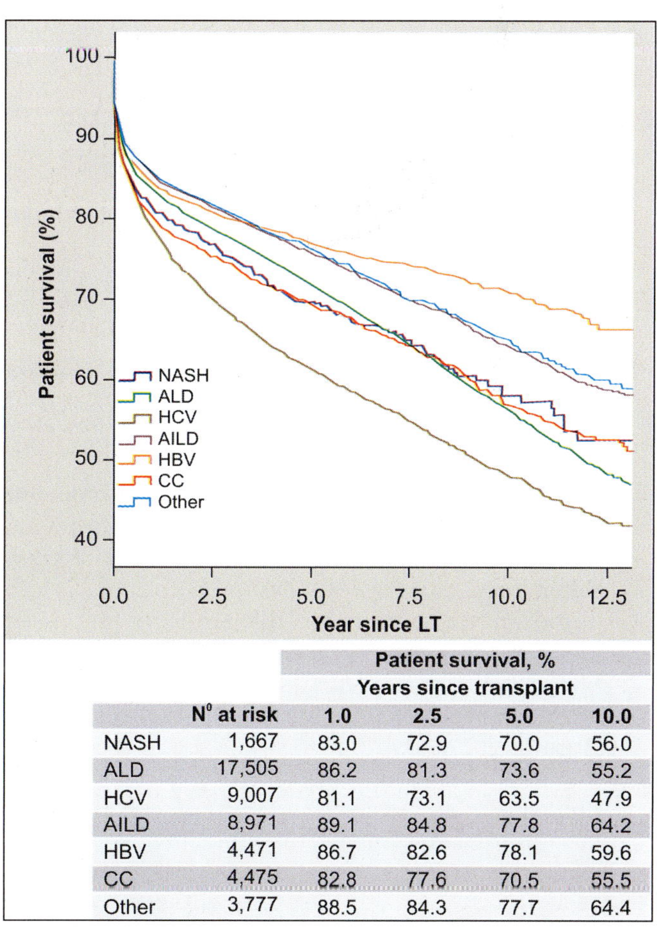

		Patient survival, %			
		Years since transplant			
	N° at risk	1.0	2.5	5.0	10.0
NASH	1,667	83.0	72.9	70.0	56.0
ALD	17,505	86.2	81.3	73.6	55.2
HCV	9,007	81.1	73.1	63.5	47.9
AILD	8,971	89.1	84.8	77.8	64.2
HBV	4,471	86.7	82.6	78.1	59.6
CC	4,475	82.8	77.6	70.5	55.5
Other	3,777	88.5	84.3	77.7	64.4

(ALD: alcohol-related liver disease; AiLD: autoimmune liver diseases; CC: cryptogenic cirrhosis; LT: liver transplantation; NASH: nonalcoholic steatohepatitis)

FIGURE 1: Overall allograft survival analysis for patients undergoing primary liver transplantation for different indications.

Source: Haldar D, Kern B, Hodson J, Armstrong MJ, Adam R, Berlakovich G, et al. Outcomes of liver transplantation for non-alcoholic steatohepatitis: A European liver transplant registry study. J Hepatol. 2019;71(2):313-22.

standardization over time. Many centers worldwide report a 1- and 10-year survival of 90% and 70%, respectively and this is consistent for both deceased donor liver transplantation (DDLT) and LDLT. As per the Scientific Registry of Transplant Recipients (SRTR) data, the 1-year and 3-year patient survival is 91.8% and 82.9%, respectively with graft survival of 91.2% and 84%, respectively. Similar results are shown in the European liver transplant registry data base. **Figure 1** shows the overall allograft survival for different indications over a 12-year period.

CONCLUSION

Liver transplantation is an important treatment option for patients with end-stage liver disease. Most of the complications after transplant like rejection, disease recurrence etc., (from hepatitis B and C) are easier to manage now, than ever before. With appropriate patient selection, meticulous detail to perioperative management and prolonged follow-up, excellent results can be achieved.

RECOMMENDED READINGS

1. Berg CL, Steffick DE, Edwards EB, Heimbach JK, Magee JC, Washburn WK, et al. Liver and intestine transplantation in the United States 1998-2007. Am J Transplant. 2009;9(4):907-31.
2. Poonacha P, Sibal A, Soin AS, Rajashekar MR, Rajakumari DV. India's first successful pediatric liver transplant. Indian Pediatr. 2001;38(3):287-91.
3. Soin AS, Thiagarajan S. Liver transplant scene in India. MAMC J Med Sci. 2016;2(1):6-11.
4. Keeffe EB. Patient selection and listing policies for liver transplantation. J Gastroenterol Hepatol. 1999;14(Suppl):S42-7.
5. D'Amico G, Garcia-Tsao G, Pagliaro L. Natural history and prognostic indicators of survival in cirrhosis: a systematic review of 118 studies. J.Hepatol. 2006;44(1):217-31.
6. Kamath PS, Wiesner RH, Malinchoc M, Kremers W, Therneau TM, Kosberg CL, et al. A model to predict survival in patients with end-stage liver disease. Hepatology. 2001;33(2):464-70.
7. European Association for the Study of the Liver; Wendon J, Cordoba J, Dhawan A, Larsen FS, Manns M, Samuel D, et al. EASL Clinical Practical Guidelines on the management of acute (fulminant) liver failure. J Hepatol. 2017;66(5):1047-81.
8. Kumar R, Shalimar, Sharma H, Goyal R, Kumar A, Khanal S, et al. Prospective derivation and validation of early dynamic model for predicting outcome in patients with acute liver failure. Gut. 2012;61(7):1068-75.
9. Mazzaferro V, Regalia E, Doci R, Andreola S, Pulvirenti A, Bozzetti F, et al. Liver transplantation for the treatment of small hepatocellular carcinomas in patients with cirrhosis. N Engl J Med. 1996;334(11):693-9.
10. Yao FY, Ferrell L, Bass NM, Watson JJ, Bacchetti P, Venook A, et al. Liver transplantation for hepatocellular carcinoma: expansion of the tumor size limits does not adversely impact survival. Hepatology. 2001;33(6):1394-403.
11. Kute V, Ramesh V, Shroff S, Guleria S, Prakash J. Deceased-donor organ transplantation in india: Current Status, Challenges, and Solutions. Exp Clin Transplant. 2020;18(Suppl 2):31-42.
12. Miyagi S, Kawagishi N, Kashiwadate T, Fujio A, Tokodai K, Hara Y, et al. Relationship between bile duct reconstruction and complications in living donor liver transplantation. Transplant Proc. 2016;48(4):1166-9.
13. Shamsaeefar A, Nikeghbalian S, Kazemi K, Motazedian N, Geramizadeh B, Malekhosseini SA. Thirteen-year evaluation of the management of biliary tract complication after deceased donor liver transplantation. Prog Transplant. 2017;27(2):192-5.
14. Levitsky J, Goldberg D, Smith AR, Mansfield SA, Gillespie BW, Merion RM, et al. Acute rejection increases risk of graft failure and death in recent liver transplant recipients. Clin Gastroenterol Hepatol. 2017;15(4):584-93.e2.
15. Vera A, Contreras F, Guevara F. Incidence and risk factors for infections after liver transplant: single-center experience at the University Hospital Fundación Santa Fe de Bogotá, Colombia. Transpl Infect Dis. 2011;13(6):608-15.
16. Kim SI, Kim YJ, Choi JY, Yoon SK, Choi HJ, Na GH, et al. Strategies to reduce infectious complication using epidemiologic data analysis in liver transplant recipients. Transplant Proc. 2013;45(8):3061-4.
17. Yi NJ, Suh KS, Suh SW, Chang YR, Hong G, Yoo T, et al. Excellent outcome in 238 consecutive living donor liver transplantations using the right liver graft in a large volume single center. World J Surg. 2013;37(6):1419-29.
18. Kwak BJ, Kim DG, Han JH, Choi HJ, Bae SH, You YK, et al. Clinical outcome of 1,000 consecutive cases of liver transplantation: A single center experience. Ann Surg Treat Res. 2018;95(5):267-77.
19. Kwong A, Kim WR, Lake JR, Smith JM, Schladt DP, Skeans MA, et al. OPTN/SRTR 2018 annual data report: Liver. Am J Transplant. 2020;20:193-299.
20. Haldar D, Kern B, Hodson J, Armstrong MJ, Adam R, Berlakovich G, et al. Outcomes of liver transplantation for non-alcoholic steatohepatitis: A European liver transplant registry study. J Hepatol. 2019;71(2):313-22.

CHAPTER

151 Gastrointestinal Manifestations of COVID-19

Neha Berry, Amrish Sahney, Ajay Kumar

ABSTRACT

The latest novel coronavirus [severe acute respiratory syndrome-coronavirus-2 (SARS-CoV-2)] was first recognized in Hubei, China outbreak in December 2019, where it was identified to cause a pneumonic disease, now termed as COVID-19, which has since then become a worldwide pandemic. Though fever and cough are its typical symptoms, a considerable number of patients present with gastrointestinal (GI) symptoms, including diarrhea, vomiting, and nausea. This virus has shown to affect the GI tract via the angiotensin-converting enzyme 2 (ACE2) receptors found abundantly on the enterocytes, and has been detected in the stool samples of those infected with the virus, with stool specimens remaining positive even after negative respiratory samples. Hence GI involvement by COVID-19 has important implications in patients with underlying diseases, particularly inflammatory bowel disease (IBD) and chronic liver disease (CLD). Elective endoscopic procedures should be delayed, but the urgent procedures should be performed. The aim of this review is to focus on the GI and hepatic manifestations of COVID-19 and to understand their pathophysiological background, as well as the effect of this infection on patients with underlying chronic GI diseases.

"It might be stormy now but the rain doesn't last forever"

—Anonymous

INTRODUCTION

The SARS-CoV-2, a novel coronavirus, was isolated in an outbreak in the city of Wuhan, Hubei Province of China and named by the International Committee on Taxonomy of Viruses in January, 2020. The pneumonia disease caused by this virus was named coronavirus disease-2019 (COVID-19) by the World Health Organization and has evolved into a pandemic affecting almost every country with massive global health crisis. Although the usual symptoms include fever, cough, difficulty in breathing, and myalgia or fatigue, a large proportion of patients demonstrated GI manifestations such as nausea, vomiting, abdominal pain and diarrhea as well as abnormal liver enzymes, with few reporting only GI symptoms.

Studies have shown the presence of viral ribonucleic acid (RNA) in anorectal swabs as well as stool samples despite the virus having disappeared from the upper respiratory tract samples. ACE2, believed to be the target entry receptor for SARS-CoV-2, is abundantly expressed in GI epithelia, thereby implicating ACE2 as a vehicle for possible fecal-oral transmission. It can also be expressed in hepatocytes and cholangiocytes, potentially allowing direct infection of hepatic cells. In fact, it is hypothesized by some that enteric infection by SARS-CoV-2 might modulate the severity of pulmonary and systemic illness through alterations in the microbiome, dysregulated intestinal immunity, and/or increased gut permeability.

The aim of this review is to focus on the GI and hepatic manifestations of COVID-19 and to understand their pathophysiological background, as well as the effect of this infection on patients with underlying chronic GI diseases, so that physicians consider SARS-CoV-2 even when the "gastroenteritis" type symptoms predominate.

GASTROINTESTINAL SYMPTOMS

Gastrointestinal symptoms are common in COVID-19 and can be seen in up to 26% of patients.

- The most common GI symptom in patients with COVID-19 is diarrhea (3.8–34%), followed by nausea and/or vomiting (3.9–10.1%) and abdominal pain (1.1–2.2%).
- Other GI symptoms reported by patients with COVID-19 include anorexia, anosmia, and dysgeusia.
- While earlier studies from China and few meta-analyses showed a lower prevalence of GI symptoms in up to 10% patients, recent studies have shown a much higher proportion ranging from 30% to 60%, with abnormal liver function tests (LFTs) in 15–50% patients.
- Diarrhea is usually mild and nondehydrating, usually up to three times per day. Up to 5–8% patients have diarrhea at initial presentation to the hospital, with a median duration of symptoms about 4 days (range 1–9 days). However, unusual presentations, such as hemorrhagic colitis and voluminous diarrhea with electrolyte disturbances, sometimes preceding respiratory symptoms, have also been reported, highlighting the variable GI manifestations of COVID-19. Vomiting is more common in the pediatric population.

- Up to 16% patients may present with GI symptoms only in the absence of respiratory symptoms, with loss of appetite and nausea being the most common symptoms. However, majority of these patients (96%) had lung infiltrates on chest computed tomography (CT) scan. It has also been seen that patients with GI symptoms take a longer time from COVID-19 onset to admission compared to those without GI symptoms (9.0 vs. 7.3 days). Thus, GI symptoms alone demand a high level of awareness among clinicians, because patients get admitted in non-COVID-19 wards for GI symptoms and hence could represent a potential infection hazard.
- Though, a large meta-analysis has suggested GI symptoms to be more common in patients with severe COVID-19 disease, the results were not replicated in other descriptive data, probably due to low patient number.
- Gastrointestinal manifestations are usually mild in the majority of cases and not found to be independently associated with the need for mechanical ventilation or death. However, recently a pooled analysis of studies has shown that abdominal pain was significantly associated with COVID-19 severity. This could be related to the degree of viral replication in the gut, with increased severity of illness related to a high viral load and subsequent viremia.

MECHANISMS OF GI INFECTION

- SARS-CoV-2 enters and replicates into cells by binding of the S protein component of the virus to the ACE2 receptor.
- Bioinformatics analysis based on single-cell transcriptome showed that ACE2 is highly expressed in the stomach and absorptive enterocytes from the ileum and colon, besides the lungs. Staining of viral nucleocapsid protein has been visualized in the cytoplasm of gastric, duodenal, and rectum glandular epithelial cell.
- Studies on human small intestinal organoids have shown that enterocytes can be infected by SARS-CoV-2 which then replicates in ACE2+ mature enterocytes.
- Furthermore, TMPRSS2 and TMPRSS4, two transmembrane protease serines, can promote SARS-CoV-2 infection of human small intestinal enterocytes. A high coexpression of ACE2 and TMPRSS2 has been detected in enterocytes, esophagus, and lungs.
- On histology, the epithelium of the digestive tract shows plasmacytic and lymphocytic infiltration with interstitial edema, mainly in the stomach, duodenum, and rectum and more patchy lymphocytic infiltration in the esophagus.
- Elevated fecal calprotectin in patients with COVID-19 suggests that SARS-CoV-2 causes an inflammatory response in the intestine.
- Currently, the exact mechanism of SARS-CoV-2 interaction with the GI tract is still not fully understood. Absorptive enterocytes may be infected and destroyed by SARS-CoV-2, potentially leading to malabsorption, unbalanced intestinal secretion, and an activated enteric nervous system resulting in symptoms like diarrhea. GI symptoms could also be related to infection-induced respiratory complications causing tissue hypoxia and cell injury, or drug-related side effects.

FECAL–ORAL TRANSMISSION

- A recently published systematic review found a pooled prevalence of stool samples positive for viral RNA to be 48.1% [95% confidence interval (CI) 38.3–59.7%] in 12 studies, with stool RNA positive in 70.3% of patients after respiratory specimens became negative for the virus.
- The duration of stool positivity usually ranges between 1 and 28 days, with average duration of fecal positivity about 11 days higher than in respiratory samples, with highest rate of fecal shedding in the first week of infection. The median viral load in the feces of patients with diarrhea has been found to be higher than in patients without diarrhea.
- In most studies, the authors were unable to isolate infectious virus, despite a high stool viral RNA load, thus concluding that stool is not a primary source for spread of infection. However, one study using electron microscopy on stool samples with high viral copies did detect live virus in a very small number of cases, thus leaving the question of feco-oral transmission unsettled.
- This also expands the possibility of utilizing the stool viral RNA testing for diagnosing COVID infection, particularly late in the diseases course, and where obtaining oropharyngeal swabs may be a challenge, like in children.
- Presence of virus in GI tract raises concern in patients with preexisting digestive diseases as well as those who are potential fecal microbiota transplant (FMT) donors, in whom additional screening strategies may now be incorporated in the usual protocol.
- In addition, the GI endoscopy departments face significant risk of viral transmission during endoscopy, particularly to healthcare workers, not only by respiratory droplets, but also by aerosols generated during endoscopy and contact with contaminated body fluids and fecal material. Hence, various organizations, particularly the American and European societies of GI endoscopy, have provided recommendations for performing endoscopies during the COVID pandemic.
- Therefore, strict disinfection in the treatment of feces and other sewage from patients with COVID-19 should be followed.

IMPACT ON GUT MICROBIOME

Primary inflammatory stimuli trigger the release of microbial products and cytokines, which cause microbial dysbiosis that can further induce an inflammatory environment thereby releasing intestinal cytokines into the circulatory system and increasing the systemic inflammation of COVID-19. A small study from Hong Kong used shot-gun metagenomics to identify the changes in gut microbiome in COVID-19. The abundance of *Coprobacillus, Clostridium ramosum*, and *Clostridium hathewayi* correlated with COVID-19 severity, and an inverse correlation was observed between the abundance of *Faecalibacterium prausnitzii* (an anti-inflammatory bacterium). Reduced microbiome diversity, as observed in elderly, could also be responsible for a more significant inflammatory state and a higher number of fatalities seen in this age group. The use of prebiotics and probiotics to regulate the balance of the intestinal microbiota could be an effective treatment to reduce the severity of COVID-19 infection by reducing the inflammatory response, and it would be worthwhile to investigate the effect of high-fiber diets and/or probiotics on the outcome of SARS-CoV-2 infection. However, currently there is no evidence that can associate the efficacy of probiotics in reducing symptoms or time of hospitalization, and exploring modulation of gut microbiome through diet, prebiotics, probiotics, or fecal transplants warrants further investigation.

IMPACT ON UNDERLYING GI DISORDERS

There is concern that the course, outcome, and treatment of certain preexisting GI disorders, e.g., IBD, may be modified by COVID-19. Also, the operation of several GI procedures and treatments has been affected in large unforeseen manner due to COVID pandemic. Studies have documented an increased expression of ACE2 in histological specimens of IBD with an upregulation of trypsinases, which may aid in the solubilization of viral S protein to aid assimilation of the virus in the human host intestinal cells. The use of ACE-blocking agents used for control of hypertension, may upregulate the expression of ACE2 receptors and might predispose patients with COVID-19 to more severe manifestations with poor outcomes. Investigators from different parts of the world have joined hands to initiate a collaborative voluntary online registry, known as the Surveillance Epidemiology of Coronavirus Under Research Exclusion-IBD (SECURE-IBD) database to understand the effect of COVID-19 on underlying IBD, and to drive treatment recommendations for IBD during the pandemic (**Flowchart 1**). SECURE has also invited data regarding celiac disease, eosinophilic gastroenteritis, and other GI diseases; however, data regarding these is scanty, with maximum data available for IBD.

COVID AND INFLAMMATORY BOWEL DISEASE

- Despite the fact that patients with IBD may be at an increased risk for COVID-19, due to use of immunosuppressants and immune-modifying therapy to control chronic inflammation, and increased exposure by hospital visits or endoscopic procedures, available data and expert opinion suggest that patients with IBD are not at a baseline increased risk of infection with SARS-CoV-2 or development of COVID-19. However, patients with severe IBD and COVID-19 are more likely to be hospitalized due to their IBD or COVID or both.
- Patients should continue their treatment regimens with the goal to stay in remission and avoid unnecessary relapse due to nonadherence to therapy. This also includes continued visits to infusion centers using all screening protocols.
- In a situation where the patient is known to be infected with the virus but does not have the disease, they should be actively moved to lower doses of prednisone (<20 mg/day) or shifted to budesonide when feasible, and thiopurines, methotrexate, and tofacitinib should be held temporarily. The doses of biologicals (infliximab, adalimumab, and vedolizumab) should be postponed for at least 2 weeks while monitoring for development of COVID-19.
- Patients with IBD who develop COVID-19 should hold thiopurines, methotrexate, tofacitinib, and biological therapies during the illness, which can be restarted after complete symptom resolution or when follow-up viral testing is negative. Careful risk benefit assessment is required keeping in mind the severity of COVID and IBD.
- Only urgent and emergent endoscopic procedures should be performed with full precaution, such as in following scenarios to diagnose new severe IBD, to exclude cytomegalovirus infection if noninvasive tests are equivocal, or in patients with severe activity or suspected malignancy where mucosal inspection might direct surgical intervention.

COVID vaccine in inflammatory bowel disease: The IBD Section of the British Society of Gastroenterology and the IBD Clinical Research Group strongly support SARS-CoV-2 vaccination for patients with IBD. The risks of SARS-CoV-2 vaccination in IBD patients are anticipated to be very low, and should accept whichever approved SARS-CoV-2 vaccination is offered to them. No serious GI side-effects to SARS-CoV-2 vaccinations have yet been reported. In those taking immunosuppressive drugs, including biologics and small molecule inhibitors, the key concerns are related to the theoretical risk of suboptimal vaccine response rather than vaccine side effects. Though currently there is no data, but SARS-CoV-2 vaccine responses in IBD patients receiving infliximab or vedolizumab will be assessed in the CLARITY IBD study.

COVID AND PANCREAS

Angiotensin-converting enzyme 2 expression is noted both in the exocrine pancreatic glands and in the islets. Pathogenesis of pancreatic injury in COVID is multifactorial: (A) direct virus-mediated injury via ACE2 receptors; (B) systemic inflammation and pancreatic injury in severe COVID; (C) virus-mediated injury to the islet cells; (D) damage by proinflammatory cytokines (IL-1b, MCP-1) and immune dysregulation; (E) virus-induced lipotoxicity from unsaturated fatty acids causing hyperlipasemia; (F) drug-induced pancreatic injury [from nonsteroidal anti-inflammatory drugs (NSAIDs) and corticosteroids].

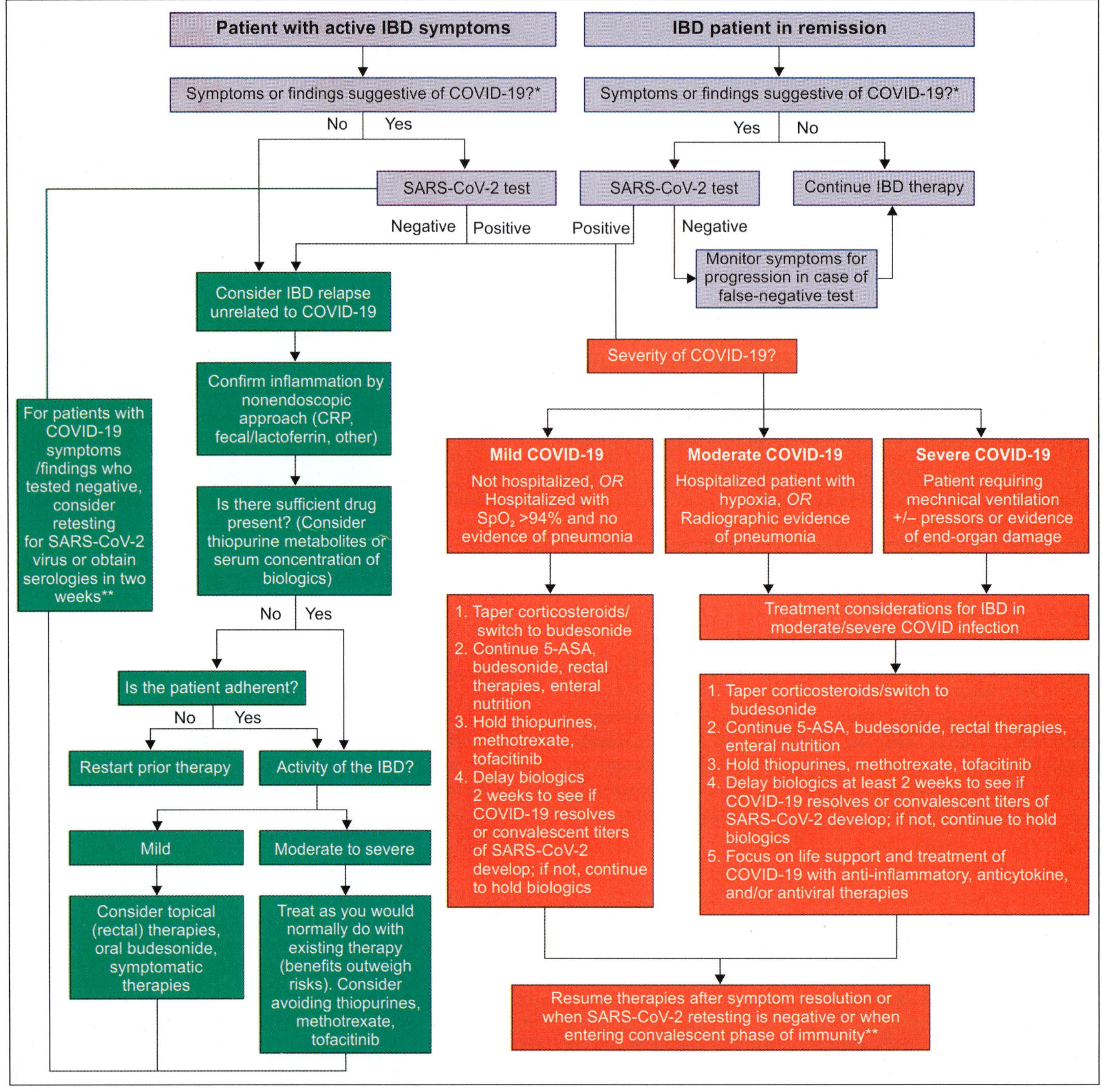

* New onset or increased frequency of diarrhea, fever, nausea and vomiting, or respiratory symptoms. ** Covid IgG antibodies.

(5-ASA: 5-aminosalicylic acid)

FLOWCHART 1: Management of IBD during COVID-19 pandemic.

- Pancreatic injury was found to be higher in severe diseases compared to milder one.
- Raised serum amylase and lipase, suggestive of pancreatic injury, have been seen in 8.5–17.3% of cases; however, elevation of more than three times to suggest acute pancreatitis was seen in only about 2.8% cases. Elevated pancreatic enzymes could also be due to cytokine storm and multiorgan dysfunction, as well as due to hypoxic pancreatic injury.
- COVID-19 infection can worsen the glycemic control in patients by damage to the pancreatic beta cells either directly by SARS-CoV-2 or via cytokine-mediated damage.
- Whenever deciding for any surgical or endoscopic intervention in these patients, important parameters that need to be reviewed include threat to patient's life, risk of disease progression, or risk of metastasis. Hence, procedures to be done on a priority basis include

endoscopic retrograde cholangiopancreatography (ERCP) for obstructive jaundice or cholangitis, endoscopic ultrasonography (EUS)-guided drainage for infected pancreatic fluid collections, or for fine needle aspiration/biopsy for pancreatic lesion/cyst without metastatic lesions. Endotherapy for chronic pancreatitis, celiac plexus block, evaluation for idiopathic/recurrent pancreatitis etc. may be deferred.

COVID AND LIVER

- Liver involvement in COVID-19 disease presents a special challenge to the clinician.
- First, there is often uncertainty whether liver function derangement is due to COVID-19 or due other cause and if there is preexisting undiagnosed liver disease. Second, medications used to treat moderate and severe disease may lead to liver toxicity. Finally, in the subset of severe critically ill COVID-19 patients, multiple factors may influence the level of liver injury.

Epidemiology and pattern of liver injury:

- COVID-19-associated liver injury is defined as any liver damage occurring during disease course with or without preexisting liver disease (**Fig. 1**).
- Liver biochemistries do not appear to be associated with GI manifestations in COVID-19. Liver injury is seen in 14–53% of COVID-19 positive hospitalized patients. Mild elevation of bilirubin (<5 mg%) is in up to 10% of patients only.
- Though ACE2 receptors are predominantly located at cholangiocytes, the pattern of liver injury in COVID-19 disease is hepatocellular (raised transaminases) mainly rather than cholestasis. This indicates that liver involvement in COVID-19 disease is due to "bystander hepatitis" and is transient.
- Aspartate aminotransferase (AST) is usually elevated more than alanine aminotransferase (ALT). On the basis of ALT/AST levels, liver injury is classified as (1) Mild—ALT/AST more than upper limit normal (ULN) but <2 times ULN, (2) Moderate—AST/ALT is between 2 and 5 times the ULN, and (3) Severe—AST/ALT >5 times ULN.
- A large cohort study of COVID-19 patient reported mild, moderate, and severe liver injury in 45%, 21%, and 6.4% of patients, respectively.
- Aspartate aminotransferase >5 times ULN is associated with severe COVID-19, ICU stay, and mortality, which may reflect nonhepatic injury. Predictors of peak abnormal liver tests >5 times ULN include age, male gender, body mass index, diabetes mellitus, medications (e.g., lopinavir/ritonavir, hydroxychloroquine, remdesivir, and tocilizumab), and inflammatory markers [interleukin-6 (IL-6), ferritin].
- This pattern of liver injury is unlike that commonly observed in other forms of viral hepatitis, such as hepatitis A, E, B, and C. In prior SARS outbreak during influenza A/H1N1 influenza infection of 2003, a similar pattern of liver injury was observed.
- The pattern of abnormal liver biochemistries characterized by AST level greater than ALT, but with accompanying GGT elevation, is also commonly encountered in both alcoholic liver disease and ischemic or congestive liver injury. Approach to liver function abnormality is presented in **Flowchart 2**.
- The prevalence of abnormal LFTs among asymptomatic patients with SARS-COV-2 infection is unknown.

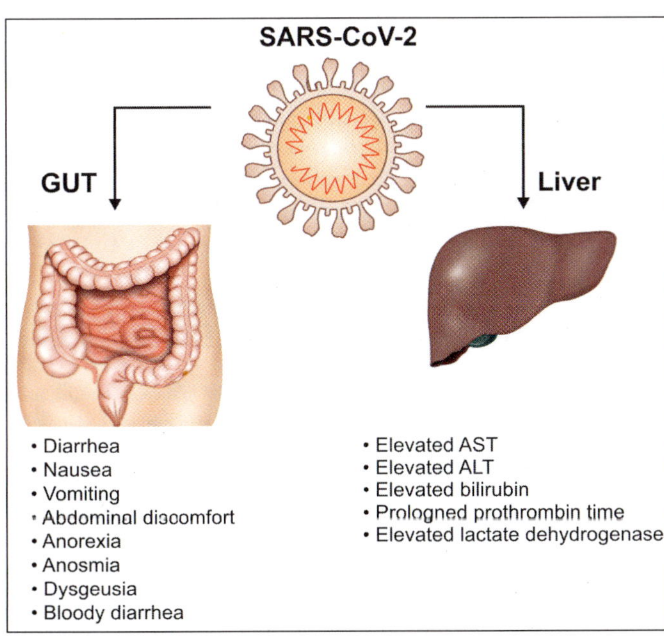

(ALT: alanine aminotransferase; AST: aspartate aminotransferase)

FIGURE 1: Pattern of GI and liver injury.

Mechanisms of liver injury in COVID-19:

Direct cytotoxicity: Published data suggest that liver injury in COVID-19 is most likely mediated by systemic inflammation rather than direct cytopathic effect of viral infection of liver cells. The low prevalence of clinically significant liver injury in patients without CLD suggests that direct infection of hepatocytes or cholangiocytes is unlikely a major mechanism of liver injury.

Immune-mediated liver injury: Severe COVID-19 disease is associated with severe liver injury. The human antiviral response is mediated by the innate and the acquired immune system which recognize specific viral antigens, release inflammatory molecules such as cytokines and chemokines and activate macrophages and T-cells to clear the virus and kill virus-infected cells. In all patients with COVID-19, higher levels of several inflammatory cytokines have been observed. Patients with severe COVID-19 have higher levels of proinflammatory type 1 cytokines, type 2 cytokines mediating anti-helminthic effects, and type 3 cytokines activating mononuclear macrophages, recruiting neutrophils and inducing epithelial antimicrobial responses. In summary, severe COVID-19 leads to systemic inflammation, early massive cytokine release, which does not regress over the disease course and trigger multiorgan failure.

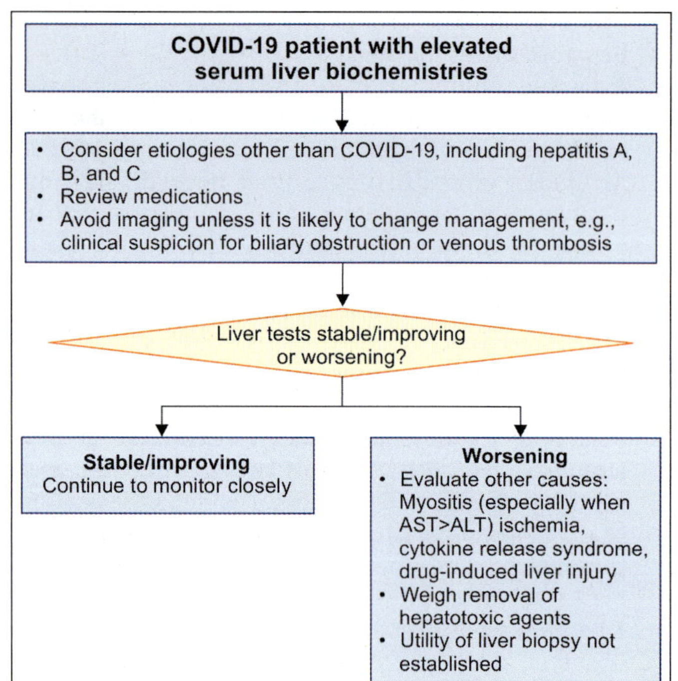

(AASLD: American Association for the Study of Liver Diseases; ALT: alanine aminotransferase; AST: aspartate aminotransferase)

FLOWCHART 2: AASLD approach to the patient with COVID-19 and elevated liver enzymes.

Liver injury related to COVID-19 clinical care:

- *Hypoxic liver injury/hepatic congestion*: Patients with severe forms of COVID-19 are frequently admitted to the ICU and require mechanical ventilation and/or vasopressor support which alters liver hemodynamic and adversely affects hepatic function by decreasing cardiac output, increasing hepatic vascular resistance, and portal vein pressure reducing portal and arterial blood flow.
- *Drug-induced liver disease (DILI)*: It is likely an important cause of liver injury in hospitalized COVID-19 patients. A recent meta-analysis reported a pooled incidence of DILI of 25.4% in COVID-19 patients. DILI was reported in 15.2% of patients treated with remdesivir and in 37.2% of patients treated with lopinavir/ritonavir. Furthermore, immunosuppressive drugs, such as tocilizumab and tofacitinib, used for the treatment of severe COVID-19, can potentially induce liver injury via hepatitis B virus (HBV) reactivation in patients with occult infections. It is recommended that remdesivir should not be started if AST/ALT >5 ULN.

LIVER CIRRHOSIS

- COVID-19 infection in patients with cirrhosis is associated with worsening Model for End-Stage Liver Disease (MELD) score, acute-on-chronic liver failure (ACLF), and death. A multinational (APOCOLIS) study comparing liver-related outcomes between 185 noncirrhotic patients with CLD (i.e., F1-F3) and 43 cirrhotic patients of mostly metabolic and viral etiology, reported a significantly higher rate of severe liver injury and death with more advanced stage of liver disease following COVID-19 infection, especially in patients with Child–Pugh score of ≥9. One-fifth of patients with cirrhosis developed either ACLF or acute decompensation. Moreover, mortality was significantly higher among cirrhotic patients with COVID-19 compared to a control group of cirrhotics admitted for bacterial infections.
- Data from two combined international reporting registries (COVID-Hep and Secure-Cirrhosis) reported a high mortality rate of 39.8% in patients of cirrhosis with COVID-19 infection. Cause of death in patients with cirrhosis was liver related in 12.2%, compared to 78.7% pulmonary, and 4.3% cardiac. Mortality strongly correlated with Child–Turcotte–Pugh (CTP) class: About 23.9% CTP class A, 43.4% CTP class B, and 63.0% CTP class C died.
- Hepatic decompensation during COVID-19 was strongly associated with subsequent risk of death (63.2% with new decompensation died vs. 26.2% without decompensation). Importantly 24.3% with new hepatic decompensation had no respiratory symptoms of COVID-19 at the time of diagnosis.

HEPATITIS B AND C

- The published evidence suggests that chronic HBV and hepatitis C virus (HCV) infection patients are neither at increased risk of COVID-19 disease nor there is any increase in worse outcomes compared to those without HBV/HCV infection.
- There is theoretical risk that COVID-19 infection induces lymphopenia which may trigger HBV reactivation in patients coinfected with SARS-CoV-2/HBV. Also tocilizumab and corticosteroids can trigger HBV reactivation. American Association for the Study of Liver Diseases (AASLD) recommends that patients with SARS-CoV-2/HBV coinfection should be treated with antiviral therapy for HBV if there is suspicion of HBV flare, patient is already having significant fibrosis/cirrhosis, or patient is started on immunosuppressive therapy for COVID-19 disease (corticosteroids/tocilizumab).
- For HCV/SARS-CoV-2 coinfection, initiating treatment for HCV can be deferred till recovery from COVID-19 disease.
- If chronic HCV/HBV-infected patient already on antiviral treatment acquires COVID-19 disease, antiviral treatment should be continued.

NONALCOHOLIC FATTY LIVER DISEASE

- Nonalcoholic fatty liver disease (NAFLD) is associated with 4-fold increased risk of severe COVID-19 disease. A published study from the US showed an increased risk of ICU admissions and need for mechanical ventilation among patients with CLD primarily due to NAFLD.
- It is difficult to separate NAFLD from known metabolic risk factors for severe COVID-19 (obesity, diabetes, and hypertension); however, the available data suggests that NAFLD is an independent risk factor for severe

COVID-19. The risk of severe COVID-19 increases with the number of metabolic risk factors present, such as obesity or diabetes.

- Most studies have not distinguished between NAFLD and nonalcoholic steatohepatitis (NASH). Thus, whether the more severe outcomes are predominantly in patients with NASH remains to be determined.

AUTOIMMUNE HEPATITIS

- Published data suggests neither autoimmune hepatitis (AIH) nor corticosteroids use in AIH increase the risk of COVID-19 disease. Hence in AIH patients on corticosteroids and/or antimetabolites [azathioprine and mycophenolate mofetil (MMF)], no dose reduction is recommended to prevent COVID-19 disease.
- In AIH patients with COVID-19 disease no change in corticosteroids or antimetabolites dosage is recommended unless a patient has lymphopenia, fungal or bacterial infection.
- If patient with COVID-19 disease develops AIH flare, it is prudent to consider using budesonide for treatment of flare, to limit total glucocorticoids exposure in circumstance where dexamethasone is given for respiratory treatment for COVID-19 disease.

COVID-19 AND LIVER TRANSPLANT

- Earlier published data shows that post-transplant immunosuppression was not a risk factor for mortality associated with SARS (2002–2003) or MERS (2012)
- A recently published multicentric study reported that in a cohort of 151 liver transplant recipients with COVID-19 disease, 124 (82%) were hospitalized, 47 (31%) required intensive care, and 28 (19%) died. In propensity score-matched analysis comparing liver transplant recipients to nontransplant recipients liver transplant status did not significantly increase the risk of death in patients with COVID-19 disease. Further, the immune response is the main driver for pulmonary injury attributable to COVID-19 and that immunosuppression may be protective. There is mortality benefit with the use of corticosteroids for the treatment of critically ill patients with COVID-19.
- In view of these findings AASLD recommends no reduction in dosage of immunosuppression in liver transplant recipients without COVID-19. In liver transplant recipients with COVID-19 disease lowering dosage of antimetabolites (MMF/azathioprine) should be considered.
- Patients with acute liver failure, decompensated CLD, and ACLF should be worked up for liver transplantation as and when indicated.

VACCINATION IN CHRONIC LIVER DISEASE

- Prior experience with influenza, pneumococcal, and HBV vaccines shows that vaccines are less effective in patients with CLD and those with postliver transplant. But, there is no data specifically with the COVID-19 vaccines. Also vaccine trials have not looked specifically at safety in patients with liver disease; there is no data to suggest harm for people with CLD.
- Although it is likely that the vaccine will offer some level of protection, at present it is not known whether the vaccines will be equally effective in transplant patients or those who are immunosuppressed.
- Hence it is important that everyone who has the COVID-19 vaccine, does not change their behaviors and continues to take precautions against COVID-19.
- We will only get information about the safety and efficacy of COVID-19 vaccines in CLD and postliver transplant patients once the same are being used in clinical practice.

IMPACT ON ENDOSCOPY UNITS

As endoscopy is an aerosol-generating procedure, with potential to spread infection, it places both healthcare professionals and patients at risk. This led most national societies to produce guidelines on how to improve safety in endoscopy during the pandemic with one of the key recommendations being to drastically reduce procedure numbers, restricting to urgent and life-saving procedures. Thus, elective endoscopy ceased on a global scale, thus delaying diagnosis of various benign and malignant disorders. However, as we recover from the pandemic and with availability of vaccine, endoscopy services need to be restarted in a safe setting.

CONCLUSION

While SARS-CoV-2 is an established respiratory tract pathogen, it can also be responsible for the GI manifestations that accompany COVID-19, with patients developing symptoms such as diarrhea, nausea, vomiting, and abdominal pain (**Table 1**). Additionally, laboratory abnormalities, hepatic injury, and pancreatic injury have been noted in a subset of patients, ranging on a spectrum with the severity of disease. As the viral receptor ACE2 has been confirmed in the GI tract, it may play a pivotal role in the virus's ability to dysregulate the digestive system, hepatobiliary function, and pancreatic function, thereby resulting in GI symptoms. As SARS-CoV-2 RNA can remain in stool longer than respiratory specimens, it may serve as evidence for GI viral replication and subsequent shedding, having important implications in development of stool test for COVID, and screening of donors for FMT. Currently, though fecal-oral transmission has not been definitively proven, there is evidence to support its possibility, warranting the need for additional precautions. Therefore, a high index of suspicion is needed to diagnose COVID-19 in patients presenting with predominantly, and sometimes only GI symptoms.

TABLE 1 Gastrointestinal (GI) manifestations in patients with COVID-19.

Study reference	No. of patients	Anorexia/Loss of appetite (%)	Diarrhea (%)	Nausea (%)	Vomiting (%)	Abdominal pain (%)	GI bleed (%)
Wang et al.	138	39.9	10.1	10.1	3.6	2.2	NA
Guan et al.	1,099	NA	3.8	5	5	NA	NA
Pan et al.	103	78.64	33.98	NA	3.88	1.94	NA
Zhang et al.	140	12.2	12.9	17.3	5	5.8	NA
Fang et al.	305	50.2	49.5	29.4	15.9	6	NA
Lin et al.	95	17.9	24.2	17.9	4.2	2.1	2.1
Xiao et al.	73	NA	35.6	NA	NA	NA	13.7

RECOMMENDED READINGS

1. Zhang C, Shi L, Wang FS. Liver injury in COVID-19: management and challenges. Lancet Gastroenterol Hepatol. 2020;5(5):428-30.
2. Fix OK, Hameed B, Fontana RJ, Kwok RM, McGuire BM, Mulligan DC, et al. Clinical Best Practice Advice for Hepatology and Liver Transplant Providers During the COVID-19 Pandemic: AASLD Expert Panel Consensus Statement. Hepatology. 2020;72(1):287-304.
3. Boettler T, Marjot T, Newsome PN, Mondelli MU, Maticic M, Cordero E, et al. Impact of COVID-19 on the care of patients with liver disease: EASL-ESCMID position paper after 6 months of the pandemic. JHEP Rep. 2020;2(5):100169.
4. Sultan S, Altayar O, Siddique S, Davitkov P, Feuerstein JD, Lim JK, et al. AGA Institute Rapid Review of the Gastrointestinal and Liver Manifestations of COVID-19, Meta-Analysis of International Data, and Recommendations for the Consultative Management of Patients with COVID-19. Gastroenterology. 2020;159(1):320-34.e27.
5. Rubin DT, Feuerstein JD, Wang AY, Cohen RD, et al. AGA Clinical Practice Update on Management of Inflammatory Bowel Disease During the COVID-19 Pandemic: Expert Commentary. Gastroenterology. 2020;159(1):350-7
6. Cha MH, Regueiro M, Sandhu DS. Gastrointestinal and hepatic manifestations of COVID-19: A comprehensive review. World J Gastroenterol. 2020;26(19):2323-32

MULTIPLE CHOICE QUESTIONS

To access the multiple choice questions of this Section online, kindly scan the QR code.

CHAPTER

152 Disorders of RBCs: How to Approach?

Afaq Ahmad Khan, Prashant Sharma, Reena Das

ABSTRACT

Disorders of red blood cells (RBCs) are extremely common in clinical practice and include inherited as well as acquired diseases with etiologies ranging from reduced or dysfunctional production, peripheral destruction, and excess losses as well as a separate group of disorders characterized by RBC overproduction (erythrocytosis). Clinical presentations range from asymptomatic or mild to life-threatening, and often are linked to coexisting pathologies or morbidities in the patient. A detailed history (including family, dietary, and drug histories) and the physical examination can provide many clues to the underlying etiology.

Patients in whom the cause is not immediately apparent require hematological laboratory workup, which must always be guided by the clinical findings. The initial and often the most rewarding test is a complete blood count (CBC) including red cell indices and peripheral smear examination. An add-on reticulocyte count indicates the status of marrow erythropoiesis and in cases of unexplained anemia with low reticulocyte count, or those in whom hematological malignancies or marrow infiltrations are suspected/need to be excluded, a bone marrow examination is helpful.

In polycythemic patients, once spurious, residence-related and smoking-related erythrocytosis are excluded, investigation for underlying hypoxic states (pulmonary disease, cyanotic heat disease, sleep apnea etc.), neoplasms, and inherited mutations need to be considered. This chapter sequentially discusses the myriad disorders characterized by anemia and erythrocytosis, their definition, clinical approach and classification, history and examination findings, and the use of laboratory tests for their accurate diagnosis and therapy.

"Blood alone moves the wheels of history"

—Martin Luther

INTRODUCTION

Disorders of RBCs can be broadly divided into those presenting with anemia, and those that result from an increase in hemoglobin, RBC count, or hematocrit (conventionally called erythrocytosis). These are discussed separately in the following text.

CLINICAL APPROACH TO ANEMIA

INTRODUCTION

Anemia is a sign of a disease and not a disease in itself. It is one of the most common hematological abnormalities seen worldwide in virtually all practice settings. It is imperative to correctly identify the precise cause of anemia, as it may be a clue to or an initial presentation of another systemic disorder. Anemia from different causes has vastly diverse treatment options including oral and parenteral iron and vitamin B-complex supplementation, immunosuppression (e.g., corticosteroids, cyclosporine), erythropoietin, immunomodulation (e.g., lenalidomide), eculizumab, epigenetic modification (e.g., 5-azacytidine, decitabine), RBC transfusions, and stem cell transplantation. Many of them are expensive, inconvenient and/or carry significant toxicities, underlining the importance of a correct diagnosis.

Anemia is defined quantitatively based on reduction of hemoglobin levels at least two standard deviations below the mean normal hemoglobin for that age, sex, and altitude of residence. The World Health Organization (WHO) cutoffs for anemia are 13 g/dL for adult males, 12 g/dL for nonpregnant females, 11 g/dL for pregnant females and children <5 years and 11.5 g/dL for children between 5 and 12 years of age.

SYMPTOMS AND SIGNS

Mild or even moderate anemia can go undetected, especially if gradual in onset, and in the absence of access to healthcare. Typical symptoms include fatigue, effort intolerance, breathlessness, palpitations, giddiness, pounding in the ears, and headache. Signs include pallor and signs of congestive cardiac failure.

CLASSIFICATION

Anemia is classified in two ways:

1. Kinetic approach, based on the mechanism(s) responsible for the decline in hemoglobin
2. Morphologic approach, categorizing anemias based on alterations in RBC size [i.e., mean corpuscular volume (MCV)], variation in cell size [i.e., red cell distribution width (RDW)], and the reticulocyte response

Mechanism of fall in Hb: Based on the *mechanism of fall in Hb*, anemia is classified into anemia of blood loss, hypoproliferative anemia, and hyperproliferative anemia. Hypoproliferative anemia is due to the marrow's inability to produce adequate number of RBCs in response to an appropriate stimulus. Examples are nutritional anemias, anemia of chronic disease or inflammation, anemia of renal disease, hematologic malignancies, myelophthisis, and bone marrow hypoplasia. Hyperproliferative anemias are characterized by a brisk bone marrow erythropoietic response to peripheral destruction of RBCs. This response is recognizable as reticulocytosis in peripheral blood. Examples include thalassemias, sickle cell disease, unstable hemoglobinopathy, enzymopathies, autoimmune hemolytic anemia, hereditary spherocytosis, paroxysmal nocturnal hemoglobinuria (PNH), and microangiopathic anemia.

Morphological classification is based on red cell size (MCV) and variation in red cell size, i.e., red cell distribution width (RDW) on autoanalyzers, or anisocytosis on a peripheral blood film (PBF). These two RBC indices have etiological relevance and help narrow down the possibilities so that the specific diagnosis is reached with minimal testing. The reticulocyte percentage and more specifically, the corrected reticulocyte production index (RPI) is an important parameter to differentiate hyperproliferative anemias from hypoproliferative anemias (calculation shown in **Fig. 1**). An increased RPI (RPI > 3) is seen in hemolytic anemias, following hemorrhage, and as a marrow response to therapy. RPI < 2 is a feature of hypoproliferative disorders such as aplastic anemia, pure red cell aplasia, and inherited and acquired dyserythropoietic anemias. The usefulness of MCV and RDW to classify anemias into six categories helps a physician categorize patients and facilitates further evaluation (**Table 1**). Additional information may also be obtained by analysis of red cell histograms obtained from automated hematology analyzers (**Table 2**).

Types of approaches to anemia: In evaluating an anemic patient, the aim is to render an appropriate diagnosis, including the type of anemia and its primary cause, in the shortest possible time with the fewest possible number of laboratory tests at the lowest cost and causing the least discomfort to the patient.

There are two basic approaches:

1. Where the CBC is not available and the approach is more general
2. Where the CBC is available and approach is more specific

The steps in reaching to proper diagnosis include history, examination, and specific laboratory testing.

HISTORY

Detailed medical history with main emphasis on following points:

Age: Inherited anemias are commoner in childhood. Examples include β-thalassemia major, sickle cell disease, congenital sideroblastic anemia, congenital dysery-

Corrected reticulocyte count

$$= \% \text{ reticulocyte count} \times \frac{\text{Hematocrit of the patient}}{\text{Expected hematocrit for patient's age and sex}}$$

Reticulocyte production index (RPI)

= Corrected reticulocyte count ÷ Maturation factor (MF)

MF: 1.0 (Hct > 36%), 1.5 (Hct 26–35%), 2.0 (Hct 16–25%), 2.5 (Hct < 15%)

RPI: <2 in hypoproliferative anemia; >3 in hyperproliferative anemia

Note: The absolute reticulocyte count does not require correction for anemia. (Hct: hematocrit)

FIGURE 1: Formulae for the calculation of the corrected reticulocyte count and the reticulocyte production index.

TABLE 1 MCV and RDW based classification of causes of anemia.

	Microcytic, i.e., low MCV (<80 fL)	Normocytic, i.e., normal MCV (80–99 fL)	Macrocytic, i.e., high MCV (>100 fL)
High RDW	• Iron deficiency • β-thalassemia major • Sideroblastic anemia • Lead poisoning • Sickle cell-β-thalassemia • Hemoglobin E-beta (HbE-β)-thalassemia	• Early iron, folate, or vitamin B12 deficiency • Dimorphic anemia • Myelodysplasia • Sickle cell disease • Chronic liver disease	• Folate or vitamin B12 deficiency • Myelodysplasia • Immune hemolytic anemia • Chemotherapy • RBC agglutination (artifact)
Normal RDW	• Anemia of chronic disease • α- or β-thalassemia trait • HbE-trait	• Anemia of chronic disease • Anemia of renal disease • Acute blood loss	• Aplastic anemia • Chronic liver disease • Chemotherapy/antivirals/alcohol

(MCV: mean corpuscular volume; RDW: red cell distribution width)

TABLE 2 Automated hematology analyzer derived RBC histogram abnormalities in anemia.

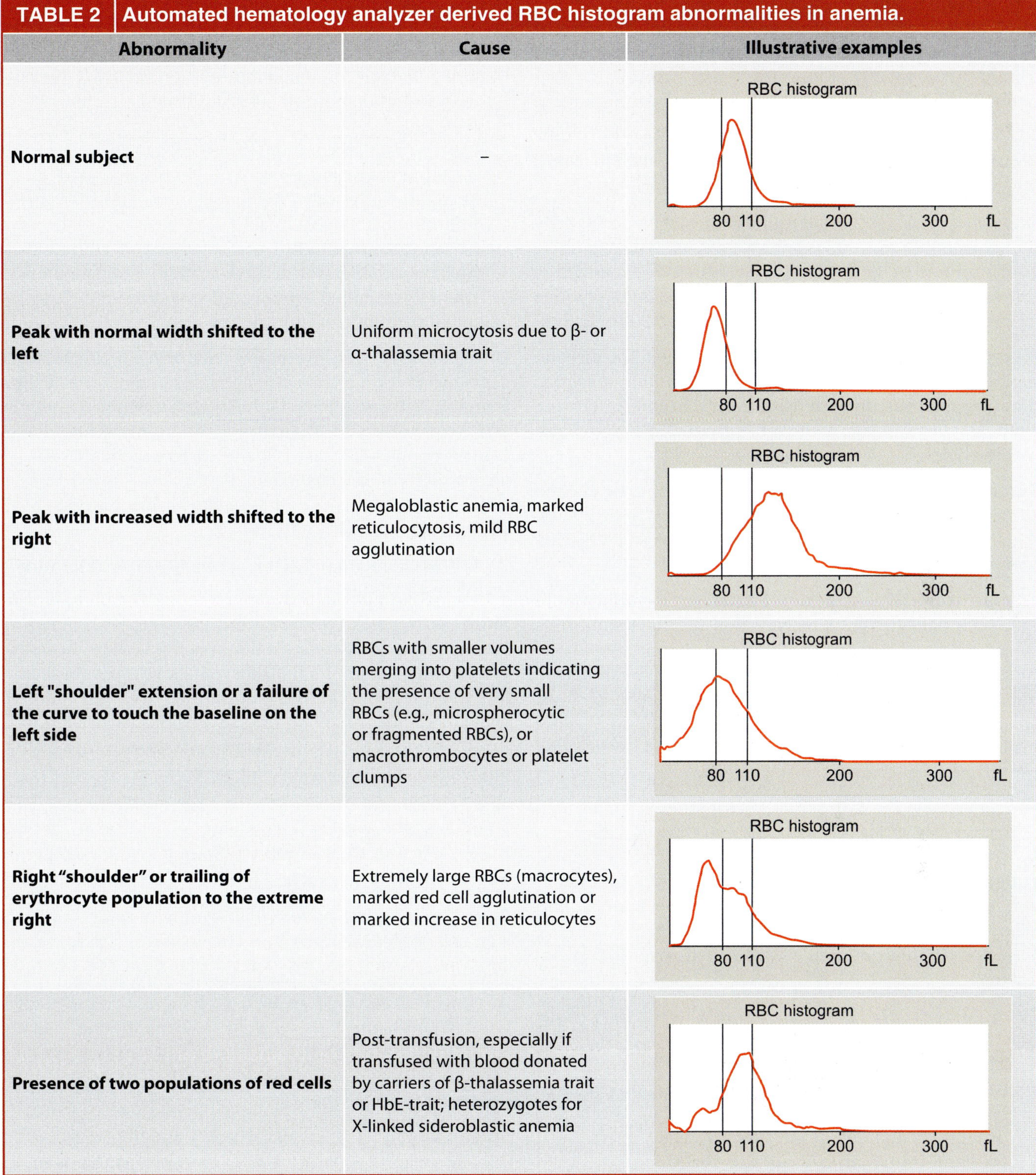

Abnormality	Cause	Illustrative examples
Normal subject	–	
Peak with normal width shifted to the left	Uniform microcytosis due to β- or α-thalassemia trait	
Peak with increased width shifted to the right	Megaloblastic anemia, marked reticulocytosis, mild RBC agglutination	
Left "shoulder" extension or a failure of the curve to touch the baseline on the left side	RBCs with smaller volumes merging into platelets indicating the presence of very small RBCs (e.g., microspherocytic or fragmented RBCs), or macrothrombocytes or platelet clumps	
Right "shoulder" or trailing of erythrocyte population to the extreme right	Extremely large RBCs (macrocytes), marked red cell agglutination or marked increase in reticulocytes	
Presence of two populations of red cells	Post-transfusion, especially if transfused with blood donated by carriers of β-thalassemia trait or HbE-trait; heterozygotes for X-linked sideroblastic anemia	

(HbE: hemoglobin E; RBC: red blood cell)

thropoietic anemia (CDA), hereditary and spherocytosis. Autoimmune hemolytic anemia, anemia of chronic disease, myelodysplastic syndrome, malignancies, PNH etc. are more common in adults. Iron deficiency and megaloblastic anemia are common across all ages, but more frequent at ages of increased demand.

Sex: Glucose-6-phosphate dehydrogenase (G6PD) deficiency and congenital sideroblastic anemia being X-linked are seen mostly in boys. Women, due to menstrual blood losses and potentially, poorer dietary intake, are more likely to have iron deficiency. Other anemias may be seen in either sex.

Ethnicity: Beta-thalassemia is more prevalent among Punjabis and Sindhis, sickle cell hemoglobin in eastern Maharashtra, Odisha, and Chhattisgarh (especially among tribals), CDA type II among the Vaish community, and hemoglobin E-beta (HbE-β) in the north-eastern parts of India.

Blood loss: History of blood loss, especially hematemesis, melena, or menorrhagia, is important.

Diet: Dietary history should probe details of the usual daily diet consumed, especially pure vegetarianism, veganism, consumption of green leafy vegetables, red meat etc. Chronic alcohol drinking may lead to anemia due to various mechanisms. Excessive tea intake impairs iron absorption.

Medical history: Many medical conditions are directly linked to anemia, e.g., cardiac; renal and liver diseases; diabetes mellitus; hypertension; and chronic infections such as tuberculosis, collagen vascular diseases, and malignancies.

Surgical history: History of gastrectomy should be elicited as it can lead to vitamin B12, iron, and folic acid deficiencies. A history of cholecystectomy or splenectomy can give a clue about hemolytic anemia.

Travel history: While a history of travel may reveal exposure to specific parasites potentially responsible for anemia, this is less informative in India. Hemolytic anemia in malaria, iron deficiency in hookworm infestation, megaloblastic anemia in *Diphyllobothrium latum* infection and hemolysis, splenomegaly and gastrointestinal blood loss in visceral leishmaniasis are some of the examples of locale- and travel-related infections causing anemia.

Family history: This is important in inherited anemias such as thalassemia, sickle cell anemia, CDA, Diamond–Blackfan syndrome (autosomal recessive); G6PD deficiency, congenital sideroblastic anemia (X-linked), hereditary spherocytosis (autosomal dominant inheritance), and Pearson syndrome (mitochondrial DNA mutations). Congenital malformations with anemia suggest Fanconi anemia.

Drug history: Drugs cause anemia through various mechanisms, e.g.,
- Bleeding and iron deficiency: NSAIDs
- Immune hemolytic anemia: Diclofenac, piperacillin, levofloxacin, ceftriaxone, other beta-lactam antibiotics, oxaliplatin, fludarabine, levodopa, lorazepam etc.
- Oxidant injury and/or methemoglobinemia: Amyl nitrite, chlorpropamide, dabrafenib, dapsone, fluoroquinolones, methylene blue, nalidixic acid, nitrofurantoin, nitrofurazone, primaquine, tafenoquine, rasburicase, sulfonylureas, benzocaine, lidocaine etc.
- Aplastic anemia: Chloramphenicol, anticonvulsants, sulfonamides, cytotoxic drugs etc.
- Megaloblastic anemia: Metformin, phenytoin, hydroxyurea, isoniazid (also sideroblastic) etc.
- Thrombotic microangiopathy: Cyclosporine, tacrolimus etc.

Review of systems:
- Central nervous system (CNS): Vitamin B12 deficiency megaloblastic anemia causes peripheral neuropathy and subacute combined degeneration of cord. Patients may experience numbness and tingling in hands and feet.
- Cardiovascular system (CVS): Breathlessness and orthopnea may suggest congestive cardiac failure.
- Skeletal: Bony pains may suggest myeloma, marrow infiltration, and leukemia.
- Gastrointestinal: Anorexia, dysphagia, weight loss, melena, and blood with stools may suggest malignancy-related anemia. History of steatorrhea suggests malabsorption-related anemia.

Occupational and personal history: Inquiry about exposure to toxic chemicals, metal dust, paint, or radiation is appropriate in individuals with pancytopenia, hemolysis, and lead poisoning. Cigarette smoking increases risk of cancer, peptic ulcer disease, and cardiovascular disease—all of which can cause anemia.

PHYSICAL EXAMINATION

Complete physical examination with special emphasis on following points:

Skin: Skin color, texture, and presence of bleeding (petechiae or ecchymoses) should be looked for. In severe megaloblastic anemia, the skin may have a lemon-yellow tint. In myxedema, the skin is coarse and dry. Petechiae and ecchymotic spots may be seen in anemias associated with thrombocytopenia or disturbance in coagulation or renal failure-related platelet function disorder.

Nails: Brittleness, flattening, longitudinal ridging, and koilonychia suggest iron deficiency anemia. Chronic liver disease stigmata such as spider angiomas, palmar erythema, and loss of body hair suggest liver disease-related anemia.

Eyes: Conjunctival pallor suggests anemia. Jaundice is a sign of hemolytic anemia and chronic liver disease.

Mouth: Atrophy of the papillae of the tongue can occur in chronic iron, vitamin B12, or folic acid deficiencies. Gum hypertrophy is seen in AML, especially acute myelomonocytic leukemia. Mouth ulcerations may be seen in infectious mononucleosis, agranulocytosis, and hematological malignancies.

Splenomegaly: It is unclear whether anemia *per se* causes enlargement of spleen or not. However, splenomegaly and its degree of enlargement may suggest the etiology of anemia. Examples include:
- Mild splenomegaly: Megaloblastic anemia, rheumatoid arthritis, and systemic lupus erythematosus
- Moderate splenomegaly: Lymphoma, acute leukemia, chronic myeloid leukemia, chronic lymphocytic leukemia, chronic liver disease with portal hypertension, and hemolytic anemia
- Massive splenomegaly: Myelofibrosis, hairy cell leukemia, thalassemia major, and amyloidosis.

Hepatomegaly: The liver is firm and has a sharp border in cirrhosis. It is nodular in secondary carcinoma. The liver is smooth and mildly tender in anemia-related cardiac failure.

Abdominal masses: Epigastric mass may suggest carcinoma stomach as a cause of anemia. A right iliac fossa mass is indicative of carcinoma cecum.

Superficial lymph nodes: Lymphadenopathy is seen in leukemias, lymphomas, and secondary cancers as well as in chronic infections.

Bony tenderness: It is observed in acute leukemia and metastatic bone disease and less commonly in myeloma and chronic myeloid leukemia.

Rectal examination: It is important to exclude hemorrhoids and any rectal growths.

CVS examination: Signs of congestive cardiac failure may be seen in severe anemia. Cardiac traumatic hemolysis may result from damaged or prosthetic heart valves. Restrictive cardiomyopathies may result from hemochromatosis, amyloidosis, connective tissue disorders, and chemo-radiation exposure.

CNS examination: Loss of position and vibration sense may be an early indicator of vitamin B12 deficiency. Rare neurodegenerative disorders with acanthocytosis and hemolysis like the autosomal recessive chorea-acanthocytosis and X-linked McLeod syndrome present with chorea, dystonia and peripheral myoneuropathies with seizures.

LABORATORY TESTING

A battery of tests are available to elucidate the cause of anemia, including CBC, PBF, reticulocyte count, erythrocyte sedimentation rate (ESR), detailed biochemistry, iron profile, endoscopies, CT scan abdomen/chest, bone marrow aspiration/biopsy, flow cytometry, USG abdomen, Hb HPLC (high-performance liquid chromatography), direct Coombs test (DCT) and indirect Coombs test (ICT), RBC enzyme levels, osmotic fragility test, sickling tests, cytogenetics, vitamin B12 levels, folic acid levels, genetic mutation testing, screen for chronic diseases etc. Test selection should never be broad and blind, rather specific for the type of anemia. The CBC, PBF, and reticulocyte count are almost always useful. Further investigations in microcytic group include iron profile, endoscopies, USG abdomen, Hb HPLC etc. Normocytic anemias need detailed chemistry, chronic disease screen, iron profile, vitamin B12 levels, folic acid levels, sickle test, screening for malignancies and PNH, bone marrow evaluation etc. In macrocytic anemia, relevant testing includes vitamin B12 levels, folic acid levels, bone marrow, thyroid and liver function, hemolytic workup and genetic testing. Bone marrow examination is important for the diagnosis of acute leukemias, myelodysplastic syndromes, myelofibrosis, aplastic anemia, marrow infiltration, myeloma etc.

DIFFERENTIAL DIAGNOSIS

Differential diagnostic clues in common anemia scenarios are given below:

Iron deficiency anemia:
- Microcytic hypochromic anemia with high RDW
- Low serum iron, high total iron-binding capacity (TIBC), low transferrin saturation, and low ferritin (**Table 3**)
- Assess for blood loss, especially menorrhagia, other genitourinary and gastrointestinal bleeds
- Treat with oral iron or intravenous (IV) iron

Megaloblastic anemia:
- Macrocytic anemia with high RDW, macroovalocytes, and hypersegmented neutrophils
- Low vitamin B12 or folic levels
- CNS manifestations
- Bone marrow shows megaloblastic anemia picture
- Responds to parental hydroxocobalamin or cyano-cobalamin and folic acid

Dual deficiency anemia:
- Microcytes and macrocytes seen in PBF
- Usually nutritional
- Responds to iron, folic acid, and vitamin B12 supplements

Anemia of chronic disease:
- Underlying chronic disease is usually obvious.
- Produces mild anemia with low normal MCV and normal RDW
- Iron profile shows low iron, low TIBC, normal or low transferrin saturation, and normal or high ferritin (**Table 3**)

TABLE 3 Interpretation of the iron profile in anemia and iron overload.

Test	Iron deficiency	Anemia of inflammation	Iron overload	Iron-refractory iron deficiency anemia
Serum iron	Low	Low	Low	Low
Total iron binding capacity	High	Normal or low	Normal	High
% transferrin saturation	Low	Low	High	Low
Serum ferritin	Low	Normal or high	High	Variable
Serum transferrin receptor/ log(ferritin) ratio	>2	<1	Low	Variable
Hepcidin	Low	High	Low	High

- Treatment focuses on treating the underlying cause. It may also require erythropoietin, IV iron for associated iron deficiency

Congenital sideroblastic anemia:
- Usually X-linked, seen in boys
- Microcytic hypochromic anemia
- Early age, i.e., childhood
- May present with transfusion-dependent anemia, hepatosplenomegaly
- Pappenheimer bodies in PBF
- Ring sideroblasts are seen in bone marrow.
- Treatment includes pyridoxine trial and stem cell transplant.

Beta-thalassemia major:
- Child symptomatic from 6 months of age, predominantly with transfusion-dependent anemia, hepatosplenomegaly, failure to thrive, and hemolytic facies
- Microcytic hypochromic anemia with high RDW with anisopoikilocytosis, nucleated RBCs, target cells, polychromasia
- Hb HPLC or capillary electrophoresis provide the diagnosis (70–98% HbF, nearly absent adult Hb); parental studies can help if the diagnosis is unclear, or child already transfused.
- Genetic mutation analysis is confirmatory.
- Definitive treatment is allogenic stem cell transplant, otherwise lifelong blood transfusion with iron chelation.

Beta-thalassemia trait:
- This comes in the differential diagnosis of iron deficiency anemia in adults.
- Microcytic hypochromic anemia of mild intensity with normal RDW, high RBC count and disproportionately low MCV
- Hb HPLC or capillary zone electrophoresis are diagnostic (elevated HbA2%).
- Family counseling required (testing of spouse), may need folic acid, if anemic

Sickle cell disease:
- Predominantly normocytic anemia with high RDW
- Vaso-occlusive crisis, organ damage, and leg ulcers
- Sickling test and Hb HPLC provide the diagnosis.
- Treatment includes hydroxyurea, blood transfusions, exchange transfusion, allogenic stem cell transplant and newer therapies (L-glutamine, crizanlizumab, voxelotor)

Alpha-thalassemia:
- May involve deletions of one or more α-*globin* genes
- Asymptomatic types of α-thalassemia include silent carriers and α-thalassemia trait.
- HbH disease (thalassemia intermedia phenotype) and Hb Bart's hydrops fetalis (in utero death) show microcytic hypochromic anemia and high RDW.
- Molecular genetic tests needed for diagnosis (exception: HbH disease can be picked up on HPLC).

Pure red cell aplasia:
- May be primary (idiopathic) or secondary to autoimmune disorders, drugs, neoplasms (thymoma, natural killer-cell leukemias, others), infections [Parvovirus B19, Epstein–Barr virus (EBV), cytomegalovirus (CMV), others] etc.
- Anemia with normal MCV and normal RDW
- Reticulocytopenia
- Bone marrow: Absent erythroid precursors
- Treatment: Steroids, blood transfusion, immunosuppressants, and addressing underlying cause

Congenital dyserythropoietic anemia:
- Predominantly macrocytic anemia with high RDW
- Bone marrow shows pathognomonic internuclear bridging, binucleate, or multinucleate erythroid cells
- Genetic mutation testing is useful.
- May require blood transfusions, interferon, and splenectomy

Myelodysplastic syndromes:
- Anemia with normal-to-high MCV with normal-to-high RDW
- Other cytopenias
- Elderly age group
- PBF shows pseudo-Pelger–Huët neutrophils and in poor-risk cases, it shows circulating blasts.
- Bone marrow examination with cytogenetic analysis is diagnostic.
- Treatment options include supportive care, erythropoietin, hypomethylating agents, and stem cell transplant.

Aplastic anemia:
- Pancytopenia with high MCV and normal RDW
- Reticulocytopenia
- Bone marrow biopsy hypocellular
- Allogenic stem cell transplant and immunosuppressive therapy alleviate the problem.

Immune hemolytic anemia:
- May be primary or secondary to autoimmune diseases, chronic lymphocytic leukemia, non-Hodgkin lymphoma, infections (EBV, CMV, *Mycoplasma pneumoniae* etc.)
- Anemia, jaundice, and splenomegaly
- Unconjugated jaundice, reticulocytosis, high LDH, and low haptoglobin
- High MCV and high RDW
- PBF: Nucleated RBCs (nRBCs), polychromasia, and spherocytes. IgM type shows RBC agglutinates.
- DCT positive
- Treatment options: Steroids, rituximab, and immunosuppressive agents

G6PD deficiency:
- X-linked recessive inheritance (mostly men are affected)

- Predominantly intermittent episodes of intravascular hemolysis following some drug intake or infection
- Normal-to-high MCV with raised RDW with PBF showing bite and blister cells
- Treatment is supportive with folic acid and blood transfusion.

Hereditary spherocytosis:

- Autosomal dominant history
- Normocytic anemia with high mean corpuscular hemoglobin concentration (MCHC), high RDW, and raised reticulocyte count
- Clinically anemia, jaundice, and splenomegaly
- PBF shows nRBCs, spherocytes, and polychromasia
- DCT negative; flow cytometric eosin-5'-maleimide (EMA) test shows reduced fluorescence.
- Folic acid, blood transfusion, and splenectomy may be needed

Myeloma:

- Elderly
- Usually normocytic anemia, lytic bone lesions with bone pains, hypercalcemia, and renal failure
- High ESR and Rouleaux formation in PBF
- M-band positive
- Bone marrow show plasmacytosis >10%.
- Chemotherapy newer agents and autologous transplant are the treatment options.

Myelofibrosis:

- Elderly
- Anemia, pancytopenia, and massive splenomegaly
- PBF shows leucoerythroblastic picture and teardrop cells.
- Bone marrow aspirate dry tap
- Bone marrow biopsy shows fibrosis with megakaryocyte abnormalities.
- Myeloproliferative mutation panel may show JAK2, cMPL, or CAL-R mutations.
- Allogenic stem cell transplant, JAK2 inhibitors, and symptomatic treatment

Microangiopathic hemolytic anemia:

- Classical examples are thrombotic thrombocytopenic purpura (TTP) and hemolytic uremic syndrome (HUS), which may be drug induced or due to cardiac valve-related RBC trauma.
- PBF: Schistocytes (pathognomonic), thrombocytopenia, nRBC, and polychromasia, anemia
- DCT and ICT negative
- High LDH and low haptoglobin
- Coagulogram normal
- In TTP: Low ADAMTS13 or anti-ADAMTS13 antibodies
- Treatment includes plasma exchange, steroids, rituximab, and caplacizumab (for TTP)

Paroxysmal nocturnal hemoglobinuria:

- Acquired bone marrow failure syndrome, usually young adults
- Cause: Deficiency of GPI-anchored cell surface proteins
- Episodic intravascular hemolysis, large vessel thrombosis, and marrow hypoplasia
- Diagnosis: Demonstrating absence of GPI-anchored proteins (CD55, CD59, CD157, CD24, CD14 etc.) or FLAER (fluorescein-labeled proaerolysin) by flow cytometry, hemosiderinuria, Ham's test, low neutrophil alkaline phosphatase (NAP) score
- Treatment: Eculizumab and ravulizumab (complement factor C5 inhibitors), supportive care (transfusions, iron, folate, and anticoagulation), immunosuppression, or stem cell transplant if progression to aplastic anemia.

POLYCYTHEMIA/ERYTHROCYTOSIS

INTRODUCTION

An increase in hematocrit, hemoglobin, or red cell mass is most accurately and unambiguously termed "erythrocytosis", since the term "polycythemia" can be incorrectly inferred as referring to elevated numbers ("poly-") of all blood components ("= cythemia"). Hematocrit > 0.49 and Hb > 16.5 g/dL in adult males and hematocrit > 0.48 and Hb > 16 g/dL in adult females are considered elevated. This condition is rare in children.

CLASSIFICATION AND CAUSES

Polycythemia is classified into two groups:

Relative polycythemia: It is because of contraction of plasma volume. The causes include decreased plasma volume (e.g., in vomiting, diarrhea), overfilling of blood in collection vacuum tubes, and Gaisbock syndrome (seen in obese, hypertensive, and middle-aged male smokers).

True or absolute polycythemia: The causes of true or absolute polycythemia include:

- *Primary familial and congenital polycythemia*:
  - Autosomal dominant
  - Isolated erythrocytosis
  - *JAK2* mutation negative
  - Low erythropoietin
  - Normal oxygen hemoglobin dissociation curve
  - May present with headaches and thrombotic tendencies
  - Erythropoietin receptor (*EPOR*) mutation is seen.
  - Phlebotomy is the treatment.
- *Polycythemia vera (also referred to as primary acquired polycythemia)*:
  - Elderly
  - Erythrocytosis, sometimes with leuko- and/or thrombocytosis
  - Often have splenomegaly
  - *JAK2* mutation positive (V617F or exon 12), low or normal erythropoietin
  - Bone marrow panmyelosis (hyperplasia of all three lineages)
  - Thrombotic tendency
  - Aspirin, phlebotomy with goal ≤45% hematocrit, and cytoreduction are treatment options

- *Secondary polycythemia*:
  - *Secondary acquired polycythemia*:
    - Causes include hypoxic pulmonary disease, congenital cyanotic heat disease, sleep apnea, Pickwickian syndrome, and high altitude and smoker's polycythemia.
    - Usually have low pO2 or oxygen saturation
    - Predominantly have high erythropoietin levels
    - *JAK2* mutation negative
    - Treat the underlying disease and phlebotomy when symptomatic or too high hematocrit.

      Another set of patients have aberrant erythropoietin production, e.g., renal cell carcinoma, Wilms' tumor, hepatocellular carcinoma, uterine leiomyomata, cerebellar hemangioblastomas, solitary renal cysts, polycystic kidney disease, and renal artery stenosis. This group of patients display:
    - High erythropoietin levels
    - Normal blood oxygen levels
    - Negative *JAK2* mutation
    - Imaging studies (CT, MRI) reveal the above lesions.

    Other rare causes in acquired group include post-renal transplant erythrocytosis, Cushing syndrome, primary hyperaldosteronism, and androgen use.
  - *Secondary congenital polycythemia:* The congenital etiology includes high oxygen-affinity hemoglobin variants, 2,3-DPG deficiency, Chuvash polycythemia (von Hippel Lindau mutations), and congenital methemoglobinemia. Usually, these present with high or normal erythropoietin levels.

High-affinity hemoglobin variants are autosomal dominant and present with p50 values below 17 mm Hg. 2,3-DPG deficiency and Chuvash polycythemia are autosomal recessive.

- *Idiopathic/unexplained erythrocytosis:*
  - Usually young persons, no identifiable cause
  - *JAK2* mutation negative
  - Erythropoietin not very helpful (may be low, normal or high).
  - Needs introspection into dietary history, environmental exposure, and expanded genetic testing
  - Aspirin and phlebotomy in selected cases

CONCLUSION

Red cell disorders are extremely common, multifarious in their etiologies, and may be simple or challenging to diagnose. Anemias are rarely a primary hematologic disorder but more commonly represent the manifestation of a systemic process. Erythrocytosis, on the other hand, are due to a direct driver effect on erythropoiesis. A systematic approach to the clinical evaluation, including careful history and examination, followed by the CBC with PBF and reticulocyte count facilitates an efficient diagnosis and minimizes unnecessary testing.

RECOMMENDED READINGS

1. Adamson JW, Longo DL. Anemia and polycythemia. In: Jameson JL, Fauci AS, Kasper DL, Hauser SL, Longo DL, Loscalzo J (eds.). Harrison's Principles of Internal Medicine, 20th edition. USA: McGraw Hill; 2018.
2. Bunn HF. Approach to the anemias. In: Goldman L, SchaferA (eds.). Cecil Medicine, 24th edition. Netherlands: Elsevier; 2011.
3. Lin JC. Approach to anemia in the adult and child. In: Hoffman R, Benz EJ, Silberstein LE, Heslop HE, Weitz JI, Anastasi J, Salama ME, Abutalib SA (eds.). Hematology, 7th edition. USA: Elsevier; 2018. pp. 458-67.
4. Kremyanskaya M, Najfeld V, Mascarenhas J, Hoffman R. The polycythemias. In: Hoffman R, Benz EJ, Silberstein LE, Heslop HE, Weitz JI, Anastasi J, Salama ME, Abutalib SA (eds.). Hematology 7th edition. USA: Elsevier; 2018. pp. 1071-105.
5. Russo R, Marra R, Rosato BE, Iolascon A, Andolfo I. Genetics and genomics approaches for diagnosis and research into hereditary anemias. Front Physiol. 2020;11:613559.
6. Anand S, Burkenroad A, Glaspy J. Workup of anemia in cancer. Clin Adv Hematol Oncol. 2020;18(10):640-6.
7. Powell DJ, Achebe MO. Anemia for the primary care physician. Prim Care. 2016;43(4):527-42.
8. Williams MD, Wheby MS. Anemia in pregnancy. Med Clin North Am. 1992;76(3):631-47.
9. Koury MJ, Rhodes M. How to approach chronic anemia. Hematology Am Soc Hematol Educ Program. 2012;2012(1):183-90.
10. Cascio MJ, DeLoughery TG. Anemia: Evaluation and diagnostic tests. Med Clin North Am. 2017;101(2): 263-84.

CHAPTER
153 Approach to Disorders of Leukocytes

Tushar Sehgal

ABSTRACT

Blood abnormalities can be broadly classified into disorders of leukocytes, erythrocytes, and platelets. One of the most common among these abnormalities is disorders of leukocytes. These can be further divided into leukocytosis and leukopenia. Leukocytosis simply refers to an increase in the white blood cell (WBC) count. Leukopenia is defined as reduction in WBC count. The increase or decrease in the WBC count is based on reference intervals based on patient's age and hospital population. Leukocytosis and leukopenia consist of a wide spectrum of disorders encompassing both benign and malignant entities. So the approach in diagnosis should be very systematic starting from meticulous peripheral smear examination and then proceeding with further special tests for clinching the diagnosis. Here in this chapter we discuss the approach to various types of disorders of leukocytes.

A leukocyte is further classified into five major types: (1) neutrophils, (2) lymphocytes, (3) monocytes, (4) eosinophils, and (5) basophils. An increase in a particular leukocyte is suffixed by "philia" as in neutrophilia, eosinophilia, and basophilia or by "cytosis" as in lymphocytosis and monocytosis. Likewise a decrease in number is suffixed by "penia" for example neutropenia, lymphopenia, monocytopenia, eosinopenia, and basopenia. **Table 1** shows a classification of disorder of leukocytes with the examples of disease conditions in which they occur.

"Stay committed to your decisions, and stay flexible in your approach"

—Tony Robbins

DISORDERS OF NEUTROPHILS

NEUTROPENIA

Neutropenia is further divided depending on absolute neutrophil count (ANC) into mild (ANC <1.5 but >1.0 × 10^9/L), moderate (ANC <1.0 but >0.5 × 10^9/L), and severe (ANC <0.5 × 10^9/L).

Approach to disorders of neutropenia:

Step 1: Complete blood count (CBC): CBC shows pancytopenia with neutropenia or isolated neutropenia. These are frequently seen in:

- Aplastic anemia:
  - Inherited bone marrow failure syndromes, e.g., Fanconi anemia, dyskeratosis congenita, Shwachman-Diamond syndrome, and Diamond-Blackfan anemia
  - Acquired—drugs, paroxysmal nocturnal hemoglobinuria (PNH), autoimmune disorders, viral infections, chemicals, radiation, and myelodysplastic syndrome (MDS)
- Nutritional—vitamin B12, folic acid, and copper deficiency
- Ethnic neutropenia—African-Americans, Jews
- Hypersplenism
- Congenital:
  - Severe congenital neutropenia (Kostmann syndrome)
  - Cyclic neutropenia
  - Glycogen storage disorder Ib
  - WHIM syndrome (warts, hypogammaglobulinemia, immunodeficiency and myelokathexis)
  - Shwachman-Diamond syndrome
  - Chédiak-Higashi syndrome
  - Griscelli syndrome II
  - Hermansky-Pudlak syndrome
  - Cartilage-hair hypoplasia

Step 2: Peripheral blood film (PBF):

- Scenario 1: Neutropenia with relative lymphocytosis—perform bone marrow examination (BME).
  - If BME shows dry tap, hypocellularity with absence of blasts—likely aplastic anemia.
  - Workup for cause of aplastic anemia:
    - Drugs (penicillin, β-lactams, valproate, carbamazepine, propylthiouracil), chemicals, and radiation
    - Connective tissue disorders
    - Viral markers—human immunodeficiency virus (HIV), hepatitis C virus (HCV), hepatitis B virus (HBV)
    - Chromosome breakage studies for Fanconi anemia
    - Lymphocytic telomere length using FISH (fluorescence in situ hybridization) for dyskeratosis congenita

TABLE 1 Classification of disorders of leukocytes.

Disorders of neutrophils	Disorders of lymphocytes	Disorders of monocytes	Disorders of eosinophils	Disorders of basophils
Neutropenia: *Benign*: • Aplastic anemia (inherited and acquired) • Benign ethnic neutropenia • Nutritional deficiency • Congenital neutropenia • Hypersplenism • Pseudoneutropenia (antipsychotic drugs, cold agglutinins) • Neonatal alloimmune neutropenia	**Lymphopenia:** *Benign*: • Congenial immunodeficiency • Infection • Rheumatoid arthritis • Sarcoidosis • Lupus • Irradiation • Hypercortisolism	**Monocytopenia:** *Benign*: • Drugs, e.g., corticosteroids and cytotoxic drugs • Stress • Infections • Severe thermal injuries • Autoimmune disorders	**Eosinopenia:** *Benign*: • Acute infection • Acute stress • Drugs • Autoimmune disorders • Endocrine disorders	**Basopenia:** • Hyperthyroidism • Hypersensitivity reactions • Corticosteroids • Autoimmune disorders
Malignant: • Acute leukemia • MDS • Large granular lymphocytic leukemia	*Malignant*: • Solid tumors and lymphomas • Acute leukemias	*Malignant*: • Hairy cell leukemia		
Neutrophilia: *Benign*: • Neonates • Infection • Myocardial infarction • Drugs • Burns • Splenectomy • Chronic idiopathic neutrophilia (smoking and obesity) • Familial neutrophilia-mutation in G-CSF receptor • TAM associated with Down syndrome	**Lymphocytosis:** *Benign*: • Infections—bacterial and viral • Young female smokers	**Monocytosis:** *Benign*: • Infections (bacterial, viral, protozoal, and rickettesial) • Inflammatory bowel diseases • Granulomatous inflammations—sarcoidosis • Vasculitides • Iatrogenic • Myocardial infarction • Hemoglobinopathies and hemolytic anemia	**Eosinophilia:** *Benign*: • Allergic disorders • Dermatological disorders (nonallergic) • Parasitic and fungal • Drugs • Gastrointestinal disorders • Vaculitides • Rhematological diseases • Respiratory disorders • Miscellaneous (GVHD, atheroembolic disease, Gleich syndrome)	**Basophilia:** *Benign*: • Hypothyroidism • IBD, RA • Allergy • Infections (chicken pox and TB)
Malignant: • Chronic myeloid leukemia • Chronic neutrophilic leukemia	*Malignant*: • Chronic lymphoproliferative disorders • Monoclonal B-cell lymphocytosis • Acute lymphoblastic leukemia • Lymphoma with leukemic phase	*Malignant*: • MPN • MDS/MPN neoplasms • AML • Carcinoma-associated monocytosis	*Malignant*: • AML • ALL • Chronic eosinophilic leukemia • Neoplasms with PDGFRA/B • Neoplasms with FGFR1 • Hypereosinophilic syndrome • Solid tumors • Systemic mastocytosis • MDS/MPN	*Malignant*: • MPN • MDS/MPN • AML (t;6,9) • Acute basophilic leukemia • Mast cell leukemia

(FGFR: fibroblast growth factor receptor; G-CSF: granulocyte colony-stimulating factor; LAD: leukocyte adhesion deficiency; MDS: myelodysplastic syndrome; MPO: myeloperoxidase; MPN: myeloproliferative neoplasms; PDGF: platelet-derived growth factor receptor; TAM: transient abnormal myelopoiesis)

- Scenario 2: Blasts on PBF with or without dysplasia, perform BME
  - Likely diagnosis acute leukemia or MDS—perform flow cytometry and genetic testing
- Scenario 3: Hypersegmented neutrophils, macrocytes, ovalocytes, and Howell–Jolly bodies
  - Perform serum vitamin B12/folic acid assay, methyl malonic acid (urine and blood)
- Scenario 4: Anemia (microcytic, macrocytic, or macrocytic) and neutropenia
  - Perform copper levels in blood
- Scenario 5: Numerous large granular lymphocytes (LGLs) on blood film
  - Evaluate for reactive conditions—viral fever or do flow cytometry to rule out LGL leukemia
- Scenario 6: Infective causes—examples include malarial parasite/Leishman–Donovan bodies/toxic granules/ reactive lymphocytes
- Scenario 7: Giant granules in neutrophils, eosinophils, and monocytes—suspect Chédiak–Higashi syndrome
- Scenario 8: Oculocutaneous albinism with neutropenia—suspect Griscelli syndrome II or Hermansky–Pudlak syndrome
- Scenario 9: Neutropenia with metabolic crisis with hepatomegaly—suspect glycogen storage disease
- Scenario 10: Short limbs—dwarf, fine hair with neutropenia suspect cartilage hair hypoplasia
- Scenario 11: Healthy newborn with neutropenia and no other cause identifiable—do genotyping of granulocytes from patient and mother and serum assays for granulocyte-specific antibody for neonatal alloimmune neutropenia

Step 3: Bone marrow examination:
Specific findings for various disorders:
- MDS—blasts <20% with dysplasia in megakaryocytes or erythroids or granulocytes
- Acute leukemia—blasts >20% with or without dysplasia
- Vitamin B12/folic acid deficiency—hypercellular bone marrow with megaloblasts (sieve-like chromatin)
- Kostmann syndrome—arrest at promyelocyte/ myelocyte stage with absence of mature neutrophils

Step 4: Flow cytometry (includes specific CD markers):
- PNH panel—CD55, CD59, fluorescent aerolysin (FLAER)
- Acute leukemia panel:
  - B-cell markers—CD10, CD19, CD79a, CD22, and CD20
  - Myeloid markers—CD13, CD33, CD117, MPO (myeloperoxidase), CD14, CD64, CD41, CD61, and CD235
  - T-cell markers—CD3, CD7, CD2, and CD1a
  - Immaturity markers—CD34, HLA DR, and TdT
  - LGL panel—CD3, CD4, CD7, CD8, CD16, CD56, CD57, TCR $\alpha\beta$, and TCR $\gamma\delta$

Step 5: Genetic testing:
- Neutrophil elastase gene (*ELA2*), HS-1-associated protein X (*HAX1*) gene, *WASP* gene, and *GF11* genes for severe congenital neutropenia
- *RPS*, *GATA1* gene testing for Diamond–Blackfan anemia
- *FANC* genes or *BRCA* gene testing for Fanconi anemia
- *SBDS* gene for Shwachman–Diamond syndrome
- *RAB27A* gene for Griscelli syndrome II
- *AP3B1* gene for Hermansky–Pudlak syndrome
- *LYST* gene for Chédiak–Higashi syndrome
- *RMRP* gene for cartilage-hair hypoplasia
- Cytogenetic and molecular tests for MDS and acute leukemia
- Clonality testing for T-cell receptor gene for LGL
- Polymerase chain reaction with sequence-specific primers (PCR-SSP) for granulocyte typing

NEUTROPHILIA

Neutrophilia refers to an increase in the absolute number of neutrophils in the PBF (ANC > 14,000 at birth, ANC > 6,000 at 6 months of age, ANC > 7,000 at 1 year of age, and ANC > 8,000/µL at 2 years and above).

Step 1: CBC:
Leukocytosis with neutrophilia:
- Infection—bacterial, viral, and parasitic
- Myocardial infarction
- Granulocyte colony-stimulating factor (G-CSF) therapy
- Trauma, surgery, and burns
- Drug, e.g., steroids
- Stress (postoperative), exercise
- Heat stroke
- Splenectomy
- Chronic idiopathic neutrophilia (smoking and obesity)
- Familial neutrophilia—mutation in G-CSF receptor
- Transient abnormal myelopoiesis (TAM) associated with Down syndrome

Step 2: PBF:
- Neutrophils with increase in immature cells (myelocyte, metamyelocyte, and promyelocytes) having toxic granulation, cytoplasmic vacuolation, and Döhle bodies—perform workup for infection/inflammation or check for G-CSF therapy.
- Leukocytosis (particularly when $\geq 50.0 \times 10^9$/L) with neutrophilia and increase in immature cells (promyelocytes, metamyelocyte, myelocyte) with blasts and basophilia—suspect chronic myeloid leukemia (CML)
- Leukocytosis (particularly when $\geq 25.0 \times 10^9$/L) with neutrophilia ($\geq$80%) with <10% immature cells (promyelocytes, metamyelocyte, and myelocyte), no blast, no monocytosis, and no dysplasia—suspect chronic neutrophilic leukemia (CNL)
- Neutrophilia with spherocytes, red cell fragmentation, irregular contracted cells, and pseudothrombocytosis (due to marked RBC fragmentation)—check for burns
- Neutrophilia with thrombocytosis, acanthocytes, pappenheimer bodies, target cells, Howell–Jolly bodies, lymphocytosis, and giant platelets—check for splenectomy
- Neonate with Down syndrome with leukocytosis, neutrophilia, and variable blasts—suspect TAM

Step 3: Bone marrow examination:

- Hypercellular bone marrow, megakaryocytes increased with dwarf forms, granulocytic proliferation, variable blasts (depending on the phase of disease), and increased basophils—likely CML
- Hypercellular bone marrow, increased neutrophils with normal maturation, no dysgranulopoiesis, and no increase in blasts—likely CNL

Step 4: Genetic testing:

- *CSF3R* T6181 or another activating *CSF3R* mutation for CNL
- BCR-ABL1 mutation for CML
- GATA1 mutation for TAM
- G-CSF receptor mutation for familial neutrophilia

DISORDERS OF NEUTROPHILIC FUNCTION

- Myeloperoxidase deficiency—inherited and acquired:
  - Inherited: Mostly asymptomatic and a small percentage suffer from *Candida* infections.
  - Acquired: Pregnancy, lead intoxication, Hodgkin lymphoma, AML, myeloproliferative neoplasms, and MDS
- Leukocyte adhesion deficiency (LAD): Neutrophilia, recurrent bacterial infections, and delayed wound healing
  Deficiency of CD11/CD18 integrins on neutrophils
- Chronic granulomatous disease: Recurrent infections, neutrophilia, flow cytometry-based dihydrorhodamine (DHR) test
- Job syndrome (hyperimmunoglobulinemia E syndrome): Infections, high IgE levels, blood eosinophilia, dysmorphic facial features, and mutation of *STAT3*

DISORDERS OF LYMPHOCYTES

LYMPHOPENIA

Lymphopenia is defined as absolute lymphocyte count (ALC < 3,000/μL at birth, ALC < 4,000/μL at 6 months of age, ALC < 3,500/μL at 1 year of age, and ALC < 1,000/μL in adults).

Table 2 enlists the disorders associated with lymphopenia and tests to diagnose them.

TABLE 2 Disorders associated with lymphopenia.

Disorders	Examples	Tests
Congenital immunodeficiency	Severe combined immunodeficiency	Measure concentration of T-cell receptor excision circles using real-time qPCR
	DiGeorge syndrome	Detection of del22q by FISH/qPCR
Infection	Influenza, measles, HIV	Serology for HIV, CD4:CD8 count by flow cytometry
Autoimmune disorders	Lupus, sarcoidosis, and rheumatoid arthritis	ANA, ACE, anti-CCP
Illness/Infection	Hypercortisolism	Serum cortisol
Irradiation (X-rays/ gamma rays)		
Malignancies	• Solid tumors and lymphomas • Acute leukemia	

(CCP: cyclic citrullinated peptide; FISH: fluorescence in situ hybridization; qPCR: quantitative polymerase chain reaction)

LYMPHOCYTOSIS

Lymphocytosis is an increase in the ALC above that expected in a healthy subject of the same age. Since the lymphocyte counts of infants and children are considerably higher than those of adults, it is particularly important to use age-adjusted reference ranges. (ALC > 8,000/μL at birth, ALC > 12,000/μL at 6 months of age, ALC > 1,100/μL at 1 year of age, and ALC > 5,000/μL in adults).

Step 1: CBC and PBF:

- Lymphocytosis with atypical/abnormal lymphocytes:
  - Epstein–Barr virus (EBV) infectious mononucleosis
  - Cytomegalovirus (CMV)
  - Hanta virus
  - Hepatitis
  - HIV
  - Lymphoma with leukemic phase (human T-lymphotropic virus-1, hepatosplenic T-cell lymphoma)
- Neutrophilia, thrombocytopenia, increased hematocrit, and circulating lymphoblast—suspect hantavirus
- Small lymphocytosis in children—suspect infections like pertussis or lymphoid leukemia
- Small mature lymphocytosis (<5 $\times 10^9$/L) in a young to middle-aged asymptomatic women—ask for history of smoking
- Small mature lymphocytes (>5 $\times 10^9$/L) in >50 years patient—suspect chronic lymphocytic leukemia (CLL)
- Small mature lymphocytes (<5 $\times 10^9$/L) in >50 years patient—suspect monoclonal B-cell lymphocytosis

Step 2: Serological studies for viral infections

Step 3: Bone marrow studies for lymphoid leukemia, lymphomas

Step 4: Flow cytometry:

- To differentiate between reactive lymphocytes from leukemic blasts
- To differentiate polytypic B-cells in young female smoker from lymphoma
- To differentiate CLL (characteristically shows coexpression of CD5 and CD23, weak CD20, weak surface immunoglobulin, and positive CD200) from other lymphomas

Step 5: Genetic tests:

- FISH studies for CLL and other lymphomas
- Cytogenetics and molecular studies for lymphoblastic leukemia.

DISORDERS OF MONOCYTES

MONOCYTOPENIA

Monocytopenia is the reduction of the monocyte count below that expected in a healthy subject of the same age (ALC < 500/μL at birth, ALC < 200/μL at 3 months of age and in adults).

Table 3 shows list of disorders associated with monocytopenia with tests needed to diagnose them.

MONOCYTOSIS

Monocytosis is an increase of the monocyte count above that expected in a healthy subject of the same age. The absolute monocyte count is higher in neonates than at other stages of life. Monocytosis is defined as absolute monocyte count $>2 \times 10^9$/L at birth, $>1.2 \times 10^9$/L at 6 months, and $>1 \times 10^9$/L at 1 year of age.

Table 4 shows list of disorders associated with monocytosis with tests needed to diagnose them.

DISORDERS OF EOSINOPHILS

EOSINOPENIA

It is defined as absolute eosinophil count <100 cells/μL.

Table 5 enlists the disorders associated with eosinopenia and tests to diagnose them.

EOSINOPHILIA

It is defined as absolute eosinophil count >500 cells/μL.

Flowchart 1 shows investigations to evaluate the cause of eosinophilia.

DISORDERS OF BASOPHILS

BASOPENIA

It can be defined as absolute basophil count <10 cells/μL.

Table 6 enlists the disorders associated with basopenia and tests to diagnose them.

BASOPHILIA

It is defined as absolute basophil count $>200 \times 10^9$/L.

TABLE 3 Disorders associated with monocytopenia.

Disorders	Examples	Test
Drugs	Corticosteroids, cytotoxic drugs	
Infections	HIV	ELISA, and Western blot
Autoimmune disorders	Systemic lupus erythematosus and rheumatoid arthritis	ANA, anti-CCP, and dsDNA
Severe thermal injuries		
Stress		
Neoplasms	Hairy cell leukemia	Bone marrow examination, flow cytometry, and molecular test for BRAFV600E mutation

(CCP: cyclic citrullinated peptide; dsDNA: double-stranded deoxyribonucleic acid;)

TABLE 4 Disorders associated with monocytosis.

Causes	Disorders	Tests
Infections	Bacterial, viral, protozoal, and rickettesial	• Tuberculosis—culture, NAAT • Brucella—RT-PCR • Syphilis—VDRL, FTA-ABS • Malaria—microscopy
Inflammatory bowel disease	Ulcerative colitis and Crohn's disease	Upper gastrointestinal endoscopy, small bowel endoscopy, and/or colonoscopy/sigmoidoscopy
Myocardial infarction		ECG, biochemical markers like myoglobin, cardiac troponin T, cardiac troponin I, CK-MB, LDH
Vasculitidies	Temporal arteritis and polyarteritis nodosa	• Antineutrophil cytoplasmic antibodies (ANCA) • Viral markers (HIV, hepatitis B, C) • Biopsy • Imaging
Granulomatous disorders	Sarcoidosis	Serum calcium, ACE levels, and biopsy
Iatrogenic	Corticosteroids, cytokine therapy, radiation therapy, and chemotherapy	
Solid tumors	Renal, colorectal, and lung	Biopsy and imaging
Hematological neoplasms	MPN, MDS/MPN neoplasms, AML with monocytic differentiation	See **Table 7**

(CK-MB: creatinekinase-muscle brain; FTA-ABS: fluorescent treponemal antibody absorption; MDS: myelodysplastic syndrome; MPN: myeloproliferative neoplasm; NAAT: nucleic acid amplification tests; VDRL: venereal disease research laboratory)

TABLE 5 Disorders associated with eosinopenia.

Conditions	Cause/Examples	Tests
Acute stress	Mediated by adrenal glucocorticoids and epinephrine	
Endocrine disorders	• Cushing syndrome	Cortisol levels in blood and urine, imaging studies
	• Acromegaly	Growth hormone and insulin-like growth factor-1 measurement. Growth hormone suppression test
Autoimmune disorders	Systemic lupus erythematosus	ANA, antibodies to dsDNA
Drugs	Corticosteroids, epinephrine, and histamine	
Acute infections	Bacterial, viral	

(ANA: antinuclear antibody; dsDNA: double-stranded deoxyribonucleic acid)

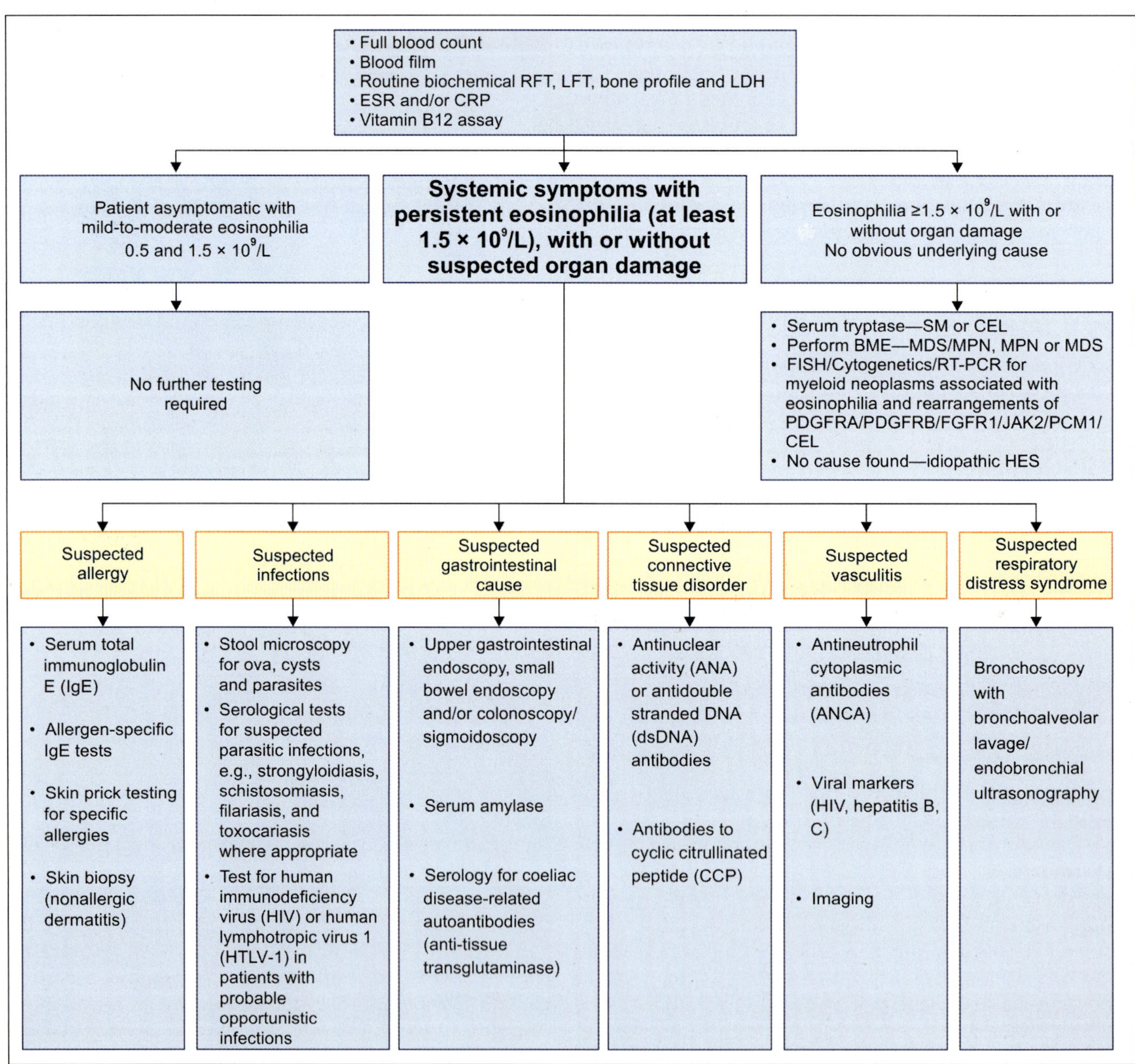

(BME: bone marrow examination; MDS: myelodysplastic syndrome; MPN: myeloproliferative neoplasm; SM: systemic mastocytosis; CEL: chronic eosinophilic leukemia)

FLOWCHART 1: Investigations to evaluate the cause of eosinophilia.

TABLE 6	Disorders associated with basopenia.	
Disorders	**Examples**	**Test**
Autoimmune disorders	SLE	ANA, antibodies to dsDNA
Thyroid disorders	Hyperthyroidism	T3, T4, TSH
Drugs	Steroid	
Hypersensitivity reactions	Urticaria, anaphylaxis	

(ANA: antinuclear antibody; dsDNA: double-stranded deoxyribonucleic acid)

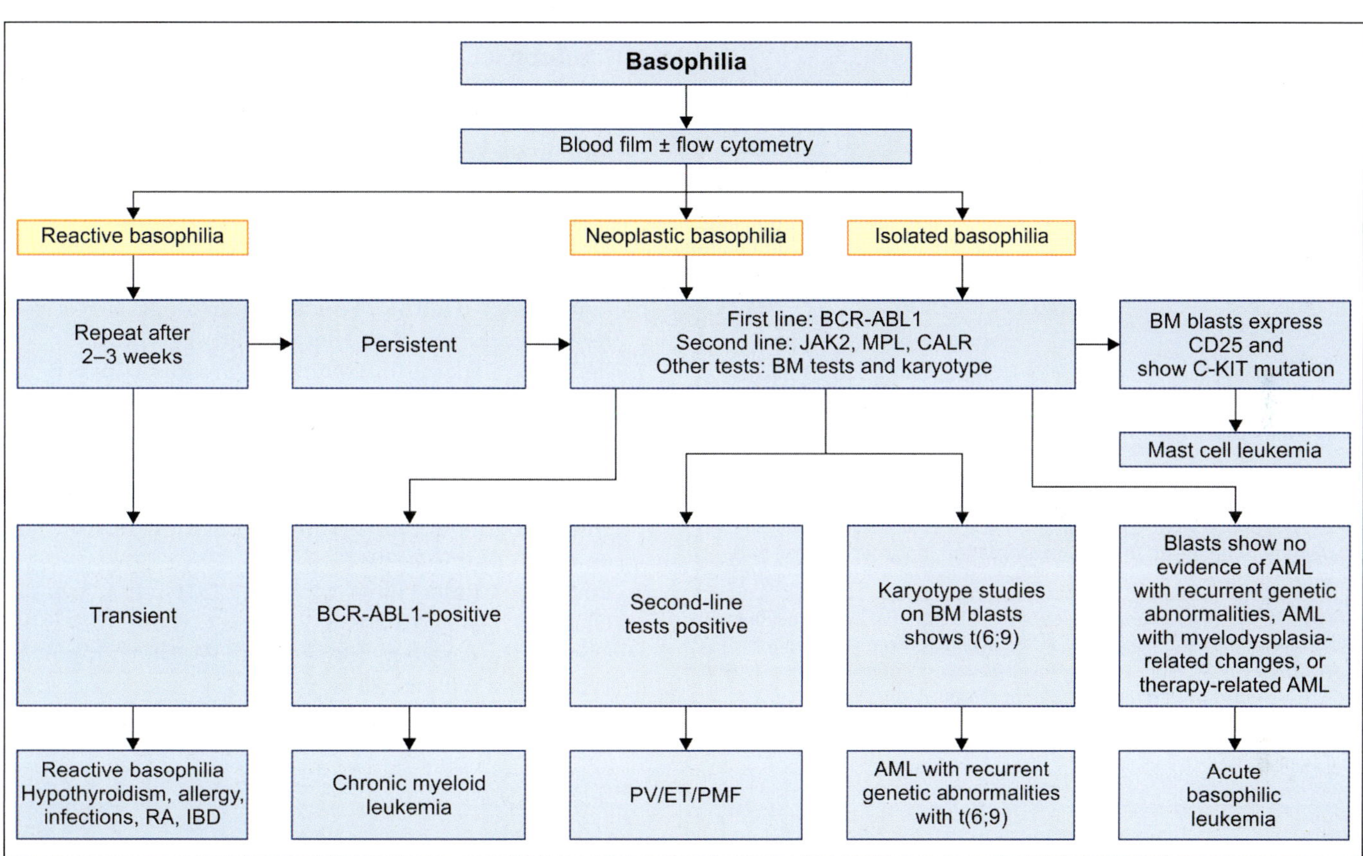

(ET: essential thrombocythemia; PV: polycythemia vera; PMF: primary myelofibrosis)

FLOWCHART 2: Disorders associated with basophilia.

Flowchart 2 depicts the disorders associated with basophilia and tests to diagnose them.

If monocytosis is sustained, unexplained, and/or features concerning for a hematologic neoplasm are present (**Table 7**), then further clinicopathologic workup should be considered including bone marrow examination with cytogenetic analysis and other testing as necessary: Flow cytometry, immunohistochemistry, cytochemical stains, special stains, and molecular genetic studies.

To conclude, disorders of leukocyte are one of the most common blood disorders. They relate to various conditions ranging from benign infectious or inflammatory to malignant proliferative disorders. It is important that disorders of leukocyte be approached in a methodical manner. The first step is usually the examination of CBC and blood film to confirm the automated differential and identification of the abnormality. The abnormality identified or suspected is confirmed by further appropriate special tests including genetic investigations. Identification and confirmation of disorders is imperative in managing and treating patients appropriately.

TABLE 7 Determining the need for further hematologic workup for monocytosis.

Blood/Clinical findings	Finding	Finding
Peripheral blood monocytosis ≥1 × 10^9/L	Yes	Yes
Monocytes at least 10% of total leukocytes	Yes	+/–
Presence of granulocytic dysplasia	Yes	No
Cytopenias	Yes	No
Promonocytes	+/–	No
Blasts	Yes	+/–
Eosinophilia	+/–	+/–
Left-shifted neutrophilia	+/–	+/–
Thrombocytosis	No	+/–
Basophilia	No	+/–
Polycythemia	No	+/–
Splenomegaly	Yes	Yes
All other reactive causes excluded	Yes	Yes
Possible diagnosis	**MDS/MPN (CMML); AML with monocytic differentiation; myeloid neoplasm with PDGFRB**	**MPN (CML, ET, PV, PMF) and SM**
Recommended: Bone marrow examination, flow cytometry, and genetic testing		

(CMML: chronic myelomonocytic leukemia; ET: essential thrombocythemia; MDS: myelodysplastic syndrome; MPN: myeloproliferative neoplasm; PV: polycythemia vera; PMF: primary myelofibrosis; PDGFRB: platelet-derived growth factor receptor beta; SM: systemic mastocytosis)

RECOMMENDED READINGS

1. Bain BJ. Qualitative changes in blood cells In: Bain BJ (Ed). Blood Cells: A Practical Guide, 5th edition. UK: John Wiley & Sons, Ltd.; 2015.
2. Arber D, McCurley T, Greer J. Diagnostic approach to malignant and nonmalignant disorders of the phagocytic and immune systems. In: Greer J, Arber D, Glader B, List A, Means R, Rodgers G (Eds). Wintrobes Clinical Hematology, 13th edition. PA, USA: Lippincott Williams & Wilkins; 2014. p. 1259-77.
3. Bates I. Reference Ranges and Normal Values. In: Bain BJ, Bates I, Laffan M (Ed). Dacie and Lewis Practical Hematology, 12th edition. Elsevier; 2012. p. 17-26.
4. Jacobson C, Berliner N. Neutropenia. In: Greer J, Arber D, Glader B, List A, Means R, Rodgers G (Eds). Wintrobes Clinical Hematology, 13th edition. PA, USA: Lippincott Williams & Wilkins; 2014. p. 1279-87.
5. Butt NM, Lambert J, Ali S, Beer PA, Cross NCP, Duncombe A, et al. Guideline for the investigation and management of eosinophilia. Br J Haematol. 2017;176(4):553-72.
6. Lynch DT, Hall J, Foucar K. How I investigate monocytosis. Int J Lab Hematol. 2018;40:107-14.
7. Feriel JJ, Depasse F, Genevieve F. How I investigate basophilia in daily practice. Int J Lab Hem. 2020;42(3):237-9.
8. Swerdlow SH, Campo E, Harris NL, Jaffe ES, Pileri SA, Stein H, et al. WHO Classification of Tumours of Haematopoietic and Lymphoid Tissues, Revised 4th edition, Volume 2. 2017.
9. Porwitt A. Clinical Flow cytometry. In: Greer J, Arber D, Glader B, List A, Means R, Rodgers G (Eds). Wintrobes Clinical Hematology, 13th edition. PA, USA: Lippincott Williams & Wilkins; 2014. p. 19-44.

CHAPTER

154 Bleeding Disorders

Pooja Prasad, Nabhajit Mallik

ABSTRACT

Normal hemostasis is a complex interplay of several components including platelets, vessel wall, coagulation factors, and fibrinolytic system. Bleeding manifestations are one of the most common reasons for a hematology referral and managing these patients is a challenge. A complete history, physical examination, and stepwise laboratory workup are essential for evaluation. Bleeding disorders can be classified on the basis of mechanism of defect and can have varied causes, both inherited and acquired.

Disorders of primary hemostasis present with platelet-type bleeding showing mucocutaneous manifestations. Inherited platelet function disorders include Bernard–Soulier syndrome, Glanzmann thrombasthenia, and storage pool defects among others. Platelet dysfunction can also be acquired, most commonly due to drugs. These disorders are managed by the use of desmopressin, antifibrinolytics, platelet transfusions, and recombinant factor VIIa for severe cases. Thrombocytopenia can be inherited or acquired and can be caused by decreased production, increased destruction or sequestration.

Among disorders of secondary hemostasis, hemophilia A and B and von Willebrand disease (vWD) are the inherited causes. vWD is the most common inherited bleeding disorder and has features of both primary and secondary hemostatic disorders. Hemophilia requires a multidisciplinary approach to treatment. Clotting factor concentrates, both plasma-derived and recombinant, are available for prophylaxis and on-demand treatment. Extended half-life factor concentrates are increasingly being used to decrease treatment burden. Management of hemophilic patients who develop inhibitors is one of the most difficult aspects in hematology practice.

"As to diseases, make a habit of two things — to help, or at least, to do no harm"

—Hippocrates

OVERVIEW OF HEMOSTASIS

The chief functions of the hemostatic system are: (1) To ensure that blood stays in the fluid state while circulating in vasculature and (2) to stop bleeding at the site of injury to the blood vessels. The various components which help in achieving these goals are:

- Blood vessels
- Platelets
- Coagulation factors and their inhibitors
- Fibrinolytic system

These components work in collaboration with each other to create a fine balance of normal hemostasis, and a tilt of balance toward one or the other side leads to either bleeding or thrombosis.

PRIMARY HEMOSTASIS

Damage to vessel wall leads to exposure of structures of the subendothelium, including basement membrane and collagen. von Willebrand factor (vWF), a multimeric high molecular weight glycoprotein (produced by endothelial cells, megakaryocytes, and platelets), binds to exposed collagen at the endothelial injury site, and interacts with platelet glycoproteins (GpIba and GpIIb-IIIa) to initially form a platelet monolayer (adhesion). This is followed by platelet–platelet interaction (aggregation) with help of fibrinogen and fibronectin, leading to formation of platelet plug, the first line of defense against bleeding.

SECONDARY HEMOSTASIS

In addition to formation of platelet plug, vessel wall damage also leads to exposure of blood to cells which express tissue factor. Tissue factor activates coagulation factor VII and a series of reactions involving various coagulation factors ensue, leading to formation of thrombin, which converts soluble fibrinogen to insoluble fibrin, and eventual hemostatic plug (clot) formation.

TERTIARY HEMOSTASIS

After the hemostatic plug stops bleeding at site of vessel wall injury and healing is complete, the clot needs to be eventually removed so that there is resumption of normal blood flow. This function is carried out by the fibrinolytic system, wherein plasminogen activators (t-PA and u-PA) convert plasminogen to plasmin, which finally breaks down fibrin into soluble fragments.

APPROACH TO BLEEDING DISORDERS

Diagnosing and managing a patient with a suspected bleeding disorder is a challenge and a step-by-step approach is the key to evaluation.

CLINICAL HISTORY

- A complete bleeding history, outcome of bleeding challenges (such as surgery, dental extractions, and trauma), menstrual history, pregnancy history, family history, medication use, and past history of any underlying disease are the essential first step in narrowing down the type of disorder (primary vs. secondary hemostasis) (**Table 1**).
- *Bleeding score or bleeding assessment tool (BAT)*: It is a standardized score used to quantify bleeding by site and severity as a means for predicting the likelihood of a bleeding disorder and/or to compare bleeding in clinical studies.

PHYSICAL EXAMINATION

Examine for bleeding manifestations including petechiae (**Fig. 1**), purpura, bruise/ecchymosis, telangiectasias, hematoma, epistaxis, gum bleeding, and menorrhagia. Look for skin and hair changes, joint laxity, and splenomegaly.

LABORATORY EVALUATION

Laboratory confirmation is required for a precise diagnosis and treatment. No single test is adequate. A typical evaluation begins with a complete blood count (CBC) with peripheral smear examination followed by a screening coagulogram comprising prothrombin time (PT), activated partial thromboplastin time (APTT), thrombin time (TT), and fibrinogen levels. Detailed diagnostic testing will be discussed with the individual disorder.

CLASSIFICATION

Bleeding disorders can be classified on the basis of mechanism of defect and further subtyped as inherited or acquired (**Table 2**).

TABLE 1 Comparison of features of disorders of primary and secondary hemostasis.

Findings	Primary hemostatic disorder	Secondary hemostatic disorder
Prototype disorders	Thrombocytopenia, platelet function disorders	Hemophilia
Gender predilection	Relatively more common in females	80–90% of inherited forms occur in males
Inheritance	Autosomal dominant	Autosomal or X-linked recessive
Positive family history	Rare (except in vWD and HHT)	Common
Timing of bleeding	Immediate	Delayed
Petechiae	Yes	No
Epistaxis	Common	Uncommon
Superficial ecchymoses	Characteristic; usually small and multiple	Common; usually large and solitary
Bleeding from superficial cuts and scratches	Persistent, often profuse	Minimal
Intramuscular hematomas	Uncommon	Common
Hemarthroses	Rare	Characteristic
Menorrhagia	Common	Uncommon

(HHT: hereditary hemorrhagic telangiectasia; vWD: von Willebrand disease)

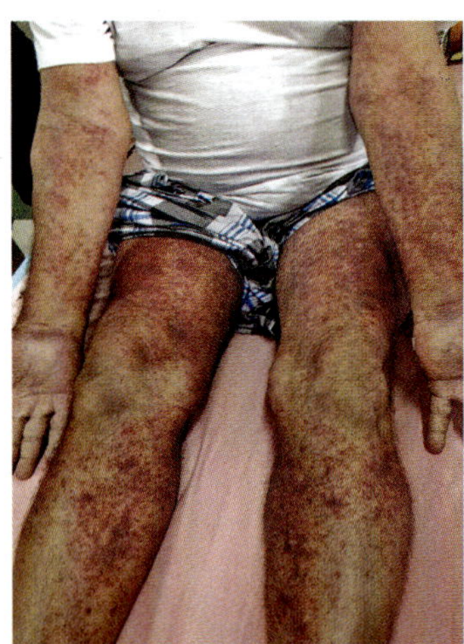

FIGURE 1: Diffuse petechiae and purpuric spots over extremities in a case of immune thrombocytopenia.

PLATELET DISORDERS

These are characterized by variable mucocutaneous bleeding manifestations (ranging from minor, e.g., limited bruising, epistaxis, heavy menstrual bleeding to severe, e.g., petechiae, purpura, gastrointestinal bleeding, intracranial bleeding causing significant anemia) and hemorrhage following surgery (including dental procedures) and trauma.

DISORDERS OF PLATELET FUNCTION

Defects in platelet function may be inherited or acquired, with the latter being more common.

INHERITED

These are due to defects at any of the steps of platelet function (adhesion, aggregation, activation, and secretion). They can be classified as shown in **Table 3**.

Bernard–Soulier syndrome: It is an autosomal recessive platelet function disorder resulting from an abnormality in the platelets GpIb-IX complex (mediates binding of vWF to platelets).

Diagnosis:
- Prolonged bleeding time, giant platelets, and thrombocytopenia are seen on peripheral smear.
- Platelet function test (light transmission aggregometry)—normal aggregation to adenosine diphosphate (ADP), epinephrine, thrombin, and collagen. Decreased or absent response to ristocetin
- Flow cytometry: Decreased platelet GpIb (loss of CD42b expression).

Glanzmann thrombasthenia: It is an autosomal recessive platelet function disorder resulting from a quantitative or qualitative defect in the GpIIb-IIIa complex (required for platelet aggregation).

Diagnosis:
- Prolonged bleeding time, normal platelet count.
- Platelet function test (light transmission aggregometry) - absent or markedly decreased aggregation to all agonists (ADP, epinephrine, thrombin and collagen) except ristocetin.
- Flow cytometry: Decreased platelet GpIIb-IIIa (absent CD41 and CD61 expression)

Storage pool disorders: Refers to deficiency in platelet content of dense granules (δ-SPD), alpha granules (α-SPD), or both types of granules.
- δ-SPD has been reported in association with other inherited disorders, such as Hermansky–Pudlak syndrome (HPS) (oculocutaneous albinism and increased reticuloendothelial ceroid), Chédiak–Higashi syndrome, Wiskott–Aldrich syndrome (WAS), thrombocytopenia with absent radius (TAR) syndrome, and Griscelli syndrome.

TABLE 2 Classification of bleeding disorders.

Disorders of primary hemostasis (platelet disorders)	Disorders of secondary hemostasis (coagulation disorders)	Disorders of tertiary hemostasis
Quantitative defects	**Inherited**	**Inherited**
• Inherited: WAS, CAMT, MYH9-related, BSS • Acquired: ITP, drug induced, HIT, DIC, TTP/HUS, SLE	• Hemophilia A and B • vWD* • Rare bleeding disorders	• Deficiencies of PAI-1 • Deficiency of a2 antiplasmin
Platelet function defects	**Acquired**	**Acquired**
• Inherited: BSS, GT, SPD • Acquired: drugs, MPNs, CKD, CLD	• DIC • Vitamin K-related • Acquired inhibitors • Coagulopathy of blood loss and trauma • AV malformation (HHT)	• Liver disease • Snake bites • Metastases • Artificial surfaces (cardiopulmonary bypass, cardiac assist devices)

* vWD may be considered as disorder of both primary and secondary hemostasis.

(AV: arteriovenous; BSS: Bernard–Soulier syndrome; CAMT: congenital amegakaryocytic thrombocytopenia; GT: Glanzmann thrombasthenia; HIT: heparin-induced thrombocytopenia; HHT: hereditary hemorrhagic telangiectasia; HUS: hemolytic uremic syndrome; MPNs: myeloproliferative neoplasms; SPD: storage pool defect; TTP: thrombotic thrombocytopenic purpura; WAS: Wiskott–Aldrich syndrome; vWD: von Willebrand disease)

TABLE 3 Causes of inherited disorders of platelet function.

Defects in platelet vessel wall interaction (disorders of adhesion)	• von Willebrand disease • Bernard–Soulier syndrome • GP VI deficiency
Defects in platelet–platelet interaction (disorders of aggregation)	• Congenital afibrinogenemia • Glanzmann thrombasthenia
Disorders of platelet secretion and granule abnormalities	• Storage pool deficiencies (delta, alpha granules) • Quebec platelet disorder
Disorders of platelet secretion and signal transduction (including receptor defects)	• ADP, thromboxane A2, collagen, epinephrine • Phospholipase and cyclooxygenase deficiency
Disorders of platelet coagulant–protein interaction	• Scott syndrome
Defects related to cyto-skeletal/structural proteins	• Wiskott–Aldrich syndrome • Tubular deficiency
Abnormalities of transcription factors	• RUNX1, GATA1, FLI1 mutations

(ADP: adenosine diphosphate; GP: glycoprotein)

- Isolated deficiency of α granules manifests as gray platelet syndrome (platelets have a gray appearance with paucity of granules on peripheral smear).
- Mild-to-moderate bleeding diathesis are associated with a prolonged bleeding time
- Platelet aggregation studies are highly variable.

WAS: X-linked recessive disorder caused by mutations in the *WAS* gene. It is characterized by immunodeficiency (susceptibility to infections associated with adaptive and innate immune deficiency), severe platelet dysfunction, thrombocytopenia with small platelets (4-5fL), and eczema.

- Bleeding manifestations: Thrombocytopenia at birth in majority patients with the classical phenotype and can lead to petechiae and/or prolonged umbilical stump bleeding or after circumcision.

BOX 1 Causes of acquired disorders of platelet function.

- Liver disease
- End-stage renal disease
- Myeloproliferative neoplasms (MPNs)
- Acute leukemia and MDS
- Dysproteinemia (MM and WM)
- Extracorporeal perfusion
- Acquired von Willebrand disease
- Cardiopulmonary bypass
- Diabetes mellitus and hyperlipidemias
- Trauma
- Drugs, food, and additives

(MDS: myelodysplastic syndromes; MM: multiple myeloma; WM: Waldenstrom macroglobulinemia)

ACQUIRED

They are among the most common hematologic abnormalities and reflect the sensitivity of platelets to external and internal perturbations. Alterations in platelet function can occur in many acquired disorders of diverse etiology (**Box 1**), of which drugs are the most common cause.

Management: Therapeutic decisions need to be individualized and should not be based solely on laboratory testing.

- Discontinuation of implicated drug
- Iron supplementation to prevent iron deficiency anemia
- Platelet transfusions are indicated in the management of significant bleeding and in preparation for surgical procedures
- Desmopressin (DDAVP) is effective in preventing bleeding after dental extraction and minor surgery.
- Antifibrinolytic agents can be used in minor mucosal bleeding.
- Hormonal contraceptives and/or antifibrinolytics for menorrhagia
- Recombinant factor VIIa

THROMBOCYTOPENIA

These result from one or more of the three mechanisms:

1. Decreased bone marrow production
2. Increased peripheral destruction
3. Sequestration in spleen

DECREASED PLATELET PRODUCTION

Hereditary thrombocytopenia: These are rare disorders and require a high index of suspicion for diagnosis. These should be considered in any patient with anatomic defects (skeletal, cardiac, hearing loss, early-onset cataracts, interstitial nephritis) or family history of thrombocytopenia, or in patients with long-standing disease not responding to standard therapy for immune thrombocytopenia (ITP). Peripheral blood film (PBF) examination helps to identify platelet morphology and gives a clue about potential hereditary thrombocytopenia. Genetic testing may be used to confirm the diagnosis. **Table 4** enumerates the hereditary causes of thrombocytopenia based on platelet size.

Autosomal dominant MYH9-related disorders are the most frequent of the inherited macrothrombocytopenias. They consist of:

- May–Hegglin syndrome
- Fechtner syndrome
- Sebastian syndrome
- Epstein syndromes

These are caused by mutations in the *MYH9* gene, which codes for nonmuscle myosin heavy chain and are characterized by sensorineural hearing loss, cataracts and nephritis, and leukocyte inclusions (Döhle bodies). Bleeding symptoms are mild to moderate.

Acquired thrombocytopenia: Platelet production may be impaired due to infections causing bone marrow suppression such as EBV, CMV, HIV, varicella, dengue, bacterial sepsis etc., or bone marrow failure and infiltrative disorders such as aplastic anemia, leukemia, MDS (myelodysplastic syndrome), lymphomas and nutritional deficiencies such as iron, B12, and folate.

INCREASED PLATELET DESTRUCTION (BOX 2)

Immune thrombocytopenia: Immune thrombocytopenia is a common acquired bleeding disorder caused by autoantibodies against platelet antigens leading to thrombocytopenia (platelet count < 100,000/mL). Annual ITP incidence is 1–6 per 100,000 adults. In children, it is usually an acute disease, most commonly following an infection, and with a self-limited course. In adults, it usually runs a more chronic course.

Major diagnostic concern is to distinguish ITP from other causes and to determine whether it is primary or secondary to an underlying condition. ITP is a diagnosis of exclusion, characterized by isolated thrombocytopenia.

According to the time elapsed since diagnosis, ITP can be referred to as:

- Newly diagnosed: Up to 3 months since diagnosis
- Persistent: 3–12 months since diagnosis
- Chronic ITP: >12 months since diagnosis

Pathogenesis: Reduced platelet lifespan due to antibody-mediated destruction is the predominant mechanism. However, autoreactive T-cells, as well as humoral and cellular autoimmunity directed at megakaryocytes has also been postulated.

BOX 2	Causes of thrombocytopenia due to increased platelet destruction.
• Immune thrombocytopenia	
• Disseminated intravascular coagulation	
• Heparin-induced thrombocytopenia	
• Other drug-induced thrombocytopenia	
• Systemic lupus erythematosus	
• Thrombotic microangiopathies (thrombotic thrombocytopenic purpura/hemolytic-uremic syndrome)	

TABLE 4 Causes of inherited thrombocytopenia due to decreased platelet production.

Normal-sized platelets	Large-sized platelets	Small-sized platelets
• Congenital amegakaryocytic thrombocytopenia (CAMT) • Thrombocytopenia with absent radii (TAR) • Radioulnar synostosis with amegakaryocytic thrombocytopenia (RUSAT) • Familial platelet disorder with predisposition to acute myeloid leukemia (FPD/AML) • Paris–Trousseau/Jacobsen syndrome • ETV6-related thrombocytopenia	• Bernard–Soulier syndrome • Platelet-type von Willebrand disease • MYH9-related disease • Gray platelet syndrome • DiGeorge syndrome (velocardiofacial syndrome) • *GATA-1* mutation of X-linked thrombocytopenia and thalassemia	• Wiskott–Aldrich syndrome

Clinical presentation: It can be incidentally detected in routine CBC, two-thirds patients present with bleeding, and few patients experience fatigue and impaired quality of life.

Bleeding manifestations: It seen in skin and mucous membranes (platelet-type bleeding), ranging from mild bleeds such as petechiae, purpura, ecchymoses, and epistaxis to severe hemorrhage. Life-threatening bleeds such as intracranial hemorrhage (1.4%), gastrointestinal, and hematuria are uncommon. Spontaneous bleeding is uncommon at platelet counts > 30,000/mL.

Diagnosis: A good clinical history, physical examination, CBC, and PBF examination and exclusion of other causes of thrombocytopenia are needed for diagnosis of ITP (**Table 5**).

Whom to treat?

- Treatment should be individualized to the patient and phase of disease, should prevent severe bleeding, should have minimal toxicity, and should optimize health-related quality of life.
- Asymptomatic patients with mild or moderate thrombocytopenia (≥30 × 10^9/L) and no bleeding—observation only
- In adults with newly diagnosed ITP and a platelet count of <30 × 109/L who are asymptomatic or have minor mucocutaneous bleed—short course (<6 weeks) of corticosteroids (prednisone 0.5–2 mg/kg/day or dexamethasone 40 mg/day for 4 days given over one to six cycles every 2 weeks)
- Use of intravenous immunoglobulin (IVIg) (1 g/kg on 1 or 2 consecutive days or 0.4 g/kg/day for 5 days), or IV anti-D (50–75 mg/kg once) where available, may be appropriate in patients with bleeding, at high risk for bleeding, who require a surgical procedure and rapid rise in platelet count or those having relative contraindications to corticosteroids.
- For life-threatening bleeds (e.g., intracranial bleeding), a combination of initial treatments including IV corticosteroids (dexamethasone or methylprednisolone) and IVIg should be used along with platelet transfusions.
- Second-line therapy (for persistent or chronic ITP): For adults who are corticosteroid dependent or do not have response with corticosteroids, any of the following may be used—thrombopoietin-receptor agonist (TPO-RA) (eltrombopag or romiplostim or avatrombopag), fostamatinib, rituximab, or splenectomy. Each of these second-line agents may be effective and choice of therapy should be individualized and based on duration of ITP, frequency of bleeding episodes, comorbidities, age, medication adherence, financial constraints, patient preference, cost, and availability.
- Other medical therapies having less robust evidence such as immunosuppressive agents (cyclosporine A, mycophenolate mofetil, azathioprine), danazol, dapsone and vinca alkaloids may also be tried in some patients.

Drug-induced immune thrombocytopenia: These are caused by drug-dependent antibody-mediated platelet destruction and diagnosed by temporal association between drug exposure and thrombocytopenia (<2 weeks), exclusion of other causes of thrombocytopenia and reoccurrence after drug rechallenge. Patients usually present with severe thrombocytopenia with nadir platelet count < 20,000/mL and major bleeding episodes occurring in 9% and fatal bleeding is seen in 0.8% cases. Discontinuation of the offending drug will lead to platelet recovery after four to five half-lives of the culprit drug. Severe cases may be treated with IVIg or corticosteroids.

Heparin-induced thrombocytopenia: It is another cause of thrombocytopenia; however, it mainly presents with thrombotic manifestations than bleeding. It is a drug reaction caused by antibodies against multimolecular complexes of platelet factor 4 (PF4) and heparin.

Thrombotic microangiopathies: These include micro-angiopathies with hereditary and acquired causes associated with diffuse microvascular coagulation and/or thrombosis. Examples include thrombotic thrombo-cytopenic purpura (TTP), hemolytic uremic syndrome (HUS), and disseminated intravascular coagulation (DIC). Bleeding manifestations include petechiae and purpura occurring due to thrombocytopenia (seen in nearly 50% cases). However, overt bleeding is rare.

TABLE 5 Recommendations for the diagnostic work-up of ITP in adults (Adapted from ASH 2019 guidelines).

Basic evaluation in all patients	Tests of potential utility
• Patient history	• Antiphospholipid antibodies (anti-cardiolipin and lupus anticoagulant)
• Family history	• Anti-thyroid antibodies and thyroid profile
• Physical examination	• Antinuclear antibodies
• CBC, reticulocyte count, and peripheral smear	• Direct Coombs test
• Viral serology (HBV, HCV, HIV)	• *Helicobacter pylori*
• Blood group (Rh)	• Bone marrow examination (in selected patients)*
• Nutritional profile (B12, folate, iron profile)	• Glycoprotein-specific antibody (not a primary diagnostic test)

* Bone marrow examination: Indicated in elderly >60 years, in patients with systemic symptoms, abnormal signs or suspicion of different diagnosis, before considering splenectomy and refractory cases.

(ASH: American Society of Hematology; Rh: Rhesus)

DUE TO SPLENIC SEQUESTRATION

Splenic enlargement, most commonly from cirrhosis and portal hypertension, results in sequestration of platelets in the splenic vascular network, results in mild-to-moderate thrombocytopenia. Typically, platelet counts range from 60,000 to 100,000/μL. Severe thrombocytopenia or bleeding in the setting of splenomegaly should prompt workup for these causes.

COAGULATION DISORDERS

HEMOPHILIA A

It is the second most common inherited bleeding disorder (after vWD), with an estimated prevalence of approximately 1 in 10,000 males. The World Federation of Hemophilia report on the annual global survey 2019 reveals that there are 195,263 hemophilia patients in the world, of which 80% suffer from hemophilia A and 20% from hemophilia B. The report states that India harbors the highest number of hemophilia patients—23,666— a number which is probably an underestimate.

ETIOLOGY

Hemophilia A is caused by a deficiency/functional abnormality of coagulation Factor VIII. *F8* gene (which produces factor VIII) is located on the long arm of the X chromosome (Xq28), and the disease is inherited as X-linked recessive. Males with affected X chromosome (hemizygous) present with clinical features of bleeding. The sons of affected males are normal (as they receive the X chromosome from their mother), while the daughters are obligate carriers (heterozygous, as they get one affected X chromosome from their father). The sons of the carrier females have a 50% chance of getting the disease. Thus, the disease is carried from a male to his grandsons through his daughters (**Fig. 2**).

Although more than 2,000 mutations have been identified in the *F8* gene, only two appear to be common in severe hemophilia A. Inversion of intron 22 is noted in 45% of these patients, while inversion of intron 1 is noted in 5%.

CLINICAL FEATURES

Depending on the level of Factor VIII deficiency and severity of symptoms, hemophilia A is categorized as:

- Severe: Factor VIII levels <1 IU/dL. Spontaneous bleeding present
- Moderate: Factor VIII levels 1–5 IU/dL. Minimal trauma causes bleeding, and spontaneous bleeding, occasional
- Mild: Factor VIII levels 5–40 IU/dL. Major trauma causes bleeding and spontaneous bleeding, rare

In severe hemophilia A, bleeding manifestations may begin in the neonatal period or infancy, while some kids may not have any symptoms till they start walking. Mild hemophilia A patients, on the other hand, may be asymptomatic till they face trauma or surgery.

Hemarthrosis or joint bleeding (Fig. 3): Hemarthrosis is the most common and characteristic manifestation of hemophilia A. Hinge joints such as knees, ankles, and elbows are more commonly involved compared to multiaxial joints such as shoulder and hip. Bleeding may be spontaneous in severe cases but is rarely so in mild and moderate ones. In acute phase, there is bleeding into the synovial space and patients may experience extreme pain. Some "target joints" may experience multiple episodes of bleeding and remain painful and swollen for months. Eventually, ankylosis and joint destruction leads to permanent deformity and termed chronic hemophilic arthropathy. MRI is the best tool for assessment of hemophilic arthropathy.

Muscle and soft-tissue bleeding: Spontaneous or trauma-induced bleedings into muscle or soft tissue are a common finding. Some bleeds (e.g., in the neck) may compress vital organs and become life threatening. Calf, thigh, and buttock muscles are commonly involved, and may cause

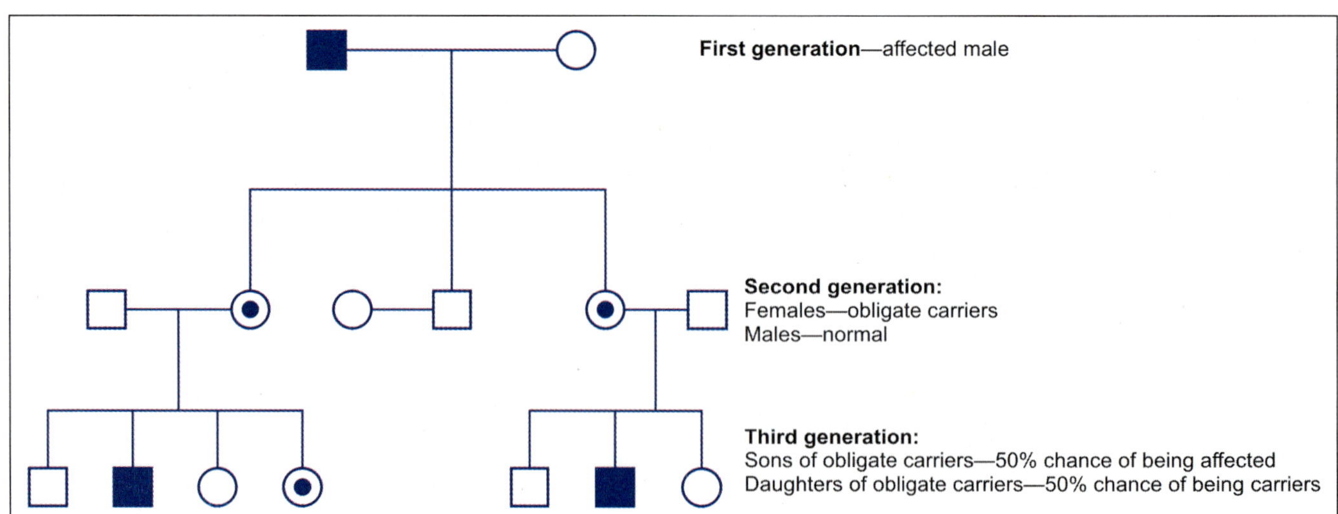

FIGURE 2: Pedigree chart showing X-linked recessive inheritance in hemophila A.

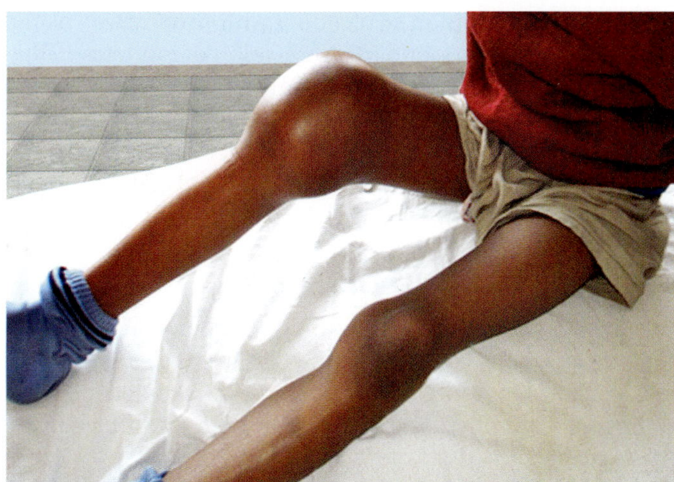

FIGURE 3: Joint swelling due to hemarthrosis of right knee in a 7-year-old boy with severe hemophilia A.

Courtesy: Dr Richa Jain.

"compartment syndrome." Iliopsoas bleeds are particularly problematic.

Genitourinary and gastrointestinal bleeding: Hematuria is relatively common and is mostly spontaneous. Gastrointestinal bleeds may occur commonly in patients taking nonsteroidal anti-inflammatory drugs (NSAIDs) for arthropathy.

Central nervous system bleeding: Although occurring in <5% cases, intracranial hemorrhage is the most dangerous and life-threatening manifestation of hemophilia A. It is predominantly trauma-related, and is the major cause of death in neonates and children.

LABORATORY DIAGNOSIS

Screening tests:

- Complete blood count is essentially normal. However, anemia, neutrophilia, and thrombocytosis may be present if there is acute bleeding/hemorrhage.
- Screening coagulogram: Isolated prolongation of APTT
- Mixing study: APTT is normalized if the test is performed after mixing patient's plasma with normal pooled plasma (1:1 ratio). If the APTT stays prolonged, it points toward an inhibitor (antibody against factor VIII)

Confirmatory tests: Clotting factor assay for factor VIII (FVIII:C) reveals the activity of Factor VIII. Low levels (<40 IU/dL) confirm the diagnosis of hemophilia A, and also classifies the patients as mild, moderate, or severe.

HEMOPHILIA B

Hemophilia B is caused by deficiency of factor IX and is approximately five times less common compared to hemophilia A. It has X-linked recessive inheritance with clinical features similar to hemophilia A. Screening coagulogram shows prolonged APTT which corrects with normal plasma (1:1) and factor IX levels are reduced. No frequent single mutation is noted, and missense mutations are common.

TREATMENT OF HEMOPHILIA A AND B

Management of hemophilia requires treatment and comprehensive care provided by a multidisciplinary team. The key components are:

- Prevention of bleeding and joint damage
- Prompt management of bleeding episodes: RICE measures (rest, ice pack application, compression, and elevation), analgesics, and factor replacement
- Physical therapy and rehabilitation after joint bleeds and other musculoskeletal complications
- Pain management
- Prevention and management of inhibitors
- Dental care
- Psychosocial support
- Genetic counseling

The main goal of treatment is for the patients to not experience any bleeds.

Treatment approach can be divided into two main categories: (1) *On-demand*—replacement with plasma-derived or recombinant clotting factor concentrates, and (2) *prophylaxis*—regular infusion of factor replacement therapy to prevent bleeding events. A wide variety of factor concentrates (plasma-derived or recombinant, standard half-life or extended half-life) are commercially available.

Episodic or on-demand treatment (standard half-life clotting factor concentrates):

- Factor VIII: Each IU of the concentrate/kg bodyweight infused intravenously will raise the plasma factor VIII level by 2 IU/dL.
  Half-life: 12 hours
- For factor VIII: Dose calculation—multiply patient's weight (in kilograms) by desired factor VIII level*, then multiply by 0.5.
- Factor IX: Each IU of the concentrate/kg bodyweight infused intravenously will raise the plasma factor IX level by 1 IU/dL.
  Half-life: 18–24 hours.
- For factor IX: Dose calculation—multiply patient's weight (in kilograms) by desired factor IX level*, then multiply by 1.0.*

Extended half-life products: Developed to address the need to reduce treatment burden of prophylaxis (by reducing frequency of infusions) and to maintain higher factor trough levels to improve bleeding prevention.

Mechanisms: Fusion technologies and PEGylation have increased the half-life to 1.4–1.6-fold for factor VIII and three to 5-fold for factor IX products.

Other plasma products (when clotting factor concentrates are not available):

- Fresh frozen plasma: Contains all coagulation factors and can be used for treatment of both hemophilia A and B.

---

* The desired peak factor levels of clotting factor concentrate replacement differs according to anatomical site of hemorrhage and also depends on available resources.

- Cryoprecipitate: Contains significant quantities of factor VIII, vWF, fibrinogen, and factor XIII and can be used for treatment of hemophilia A.

Other pharmacological agents:
- Desmopressin: Useful treatment option for patients of mild or moderate hemophilia A and for prevention of bleeding in carriers of hemophilia A.
- Antifibrinolytics: Tranexamic acid and epsilon aminocaproic acid (EACA)
- Emicizumab is the first and only licensed substitution agent, a chimeric bispecific antibody directed against the enzyme factor IXa and the zymogen factor X that mimics the cofactor function of factor VIII in patients with hemophilia A, with or without inhibitors.

Inhibitors in hemophilia: Development of neutralizing antibodies (inhibitors) that bind factor VIII or IX after exposure to replacement therapy is a significant complication and poses a challenge for management as they render standard treatment ineffective and are associated with increased risk of morbidity and mortality.

Prevalence: 10% in factor VIII deficiency and 3–5% in factor IX deficiency.

Many a times, they are clinically silent and are discovered when factor infusions become ineffective in treating or preventing bleeding or raising the factor level.

They are divided into two categories using the Bethesda assay (with Nijmegen modification) as:
1. Low titer or low responding: <5 Bethesda units
2. High-titer or high responding: >5 Bethesda units

Treatment:
- Patients with low titres are managed with higher doses or increased frequency of factor replacement therapy to achieve a hemostatic factor level.
- For high responding titers, a multipronged approach is needed comprising (1) management of bleeding episodes with bypassing agents [activated prothrombin complex concentrates (aPCC) and recombinant factor VIIa], (2) prevention of bleeding with prophylaxis using by passing agents, and (3) eradication of inhibitor using immune tolerance induction (ITI).
- A variety of ITI protocols are available starting from use of a higher dose of factor VIII to addition of an immunosuppressive agent such as rituximab and/or mycophenolate mofetil.

VON WILLEBRAND DISEASE

Von Willebrand disease is the most common inherited bleeding disorder, with an estimated prevalence of 0.1–1%. It is caused by a quantitative and/or functional defect of vWF, and predominantly has autosomal dominant inheritance. The two chief functions of vWF are:
1. Platelet adhesion—by binding platelets to the subendothelial collagen.
2. Stabilizing factor VIII and acting as its carrier protein.

Thus, vWF plays a role in both primary and secondary hemostasis.

CLASSIFICATION

Von Willebrand disease is classified into various subtypes, depending on whether the defect in vWF is quantitative or qualitative, as shown in **Table 6**.
- *vWD type 1*: These patients have partial quantitative deficiency of vWF. It is the most common subtype comprising 70–80% vWD cases. Most patients have mild symptoms. A subgroup (type 1c) is caused by an increased and rapid clearance of vWF from circulation.
- *vWD type 2*: This is characterized by functional defects of vWF and has four subtypes as shown in **Table 6**.
- *vWD type 3*: These patients show a total deficiency of vWF antigen and markedly reduced factor VIII levels.

CLINICAL FEATURES

Patients with vWD typically present with mucocutaneous bleeding—epistaxis, gum bleeds, easy bruising, and menorrhagia are some of the most common symptoms.

TABLE 6 Classification and salient features of von Willebrand disease (vWD).

vWD Type	Inheritance	Description	Lab features
Type 1	Autosomal dominant	Partial quantitative defect of VWF	Low vWF:Ag, with concordant reduction in vWF:GPIbR (vWF:GPIbr/vWF:Ag ratio >0.6)
Type 2A	Autosomal dominant	Reduced vWF-dependent platelet adhesion due to selective loss of HMW multimers	Low/normal vWF:Ag, with discordant reduction in functional assays (GPIbR/Ag and CB/Ag ratios <0.6). Loss of HMW multimers
Type 2B	Autosomal dominant	Increased vWF-platelet GpIb interaction, leading to increased clearing from circulation	Low/normal vWF:Ag, with discordant reduction in vWF:GPIbR (vWF:GPIbr/vWF:Ag ratio < 0.6). RIPA positive
Type 2M	Autosomal dominant	Reduced vWF-dependent platelet adhesion without selective loss of HMW multimers	Low/normal vWF:Ag, with discordant reduction in vWF:GPIbR (GPIbR/Ag ratio <0.6). CB:Ag ratio usually normal. No selective loss of HMW multimers
Type 2N	Autosomal recessive	Reduced Factor 8 binding affinity	Reduced vWF:FVIIIB. Low FVIIIB/Ag ratio
Type 3	Autosomal recessive	Near-total quantitative defect of vWF	Markedly reduced vWF:Ag, moderately reduced FVIIIC

[Ag: antigen; (CB:Ag): collagen binding to antigen; GP: glycoprotein; HMW: high molecular weight]

Young girls are often diagnosed during their menarche. Dental procedures, oral surgeries such as tonsillectomy and childbirth might cause the first episode of bleeding in some patients. However, in type 3 and type 2N vWD where the factor VIII levels are very low, symptoms similar to those seen in hemophilia are noted, e.g., hemarthrosis and intramuscular hematomas. Some vWD patients remain virtually asymptomatic.

LABORATORY DIAGNOSIS

Screening tests:

- Complete blood count: Usually normal. Thrombocytopenia may be noted in some subtypes (e.g., vWD type 2B). Prolonged bleeding episodes may cause anemia.
- Screening coagulogram: APTT may be prolonged or normal. PT, TT, and fibrinogen levels are normal.

First-level tests: These tests are performed when the clinical history and screening coagulogram suggest a possibility of vWD and include:

- vWF antigen level (vWF:Ag): Normal values lie between 50 and 200 IU/dL. Various physiological factors such as blood group may influence the levels of vWF:Ag, with blood group O individuals having almost 25% lower vWF levels compared to those with blood group A.
- vWF functional assay (vWF:GPIbR): The functional assessment of vWF glycoprotein is usually done by measuring its ability to bind to platelet GPIba. Traditionally, ristocetin cofactor assay was performed; now most laboratories perform the ristocetin triggered GPIba binding assay (vWF:GPIbR).
- vWF:GPIbR/vWF:Ag ratio: In type 1 vWD, the vWF:Ag and vWF:GPIbR are reduced proportionately. However, in type 2 vWD, there is a disproportionate reduction in the vWF:RCo compared to the vWF:Ag. The ratio of vWF:RCo to vWF:Ag may be used to differentiate between type 1 (ratio > 0.6) and type 2 vWD (ratio < 0.6).
- Factor VIII assay (FVIII:C): FVIII:C may be mildly reduced in vWD type 1 and most cases of type 2. However, in type 3 and type 2N vWD, the levels may be as low as that seen in moderate-to-severe Hemophilia A.

Second-level tests: These tests are performed to further define and subclassify the disease after the first level tests reveal a diagnosis of vWD.

- Ristocetin-induced platelet aggregation (RIPA): Used to distinguish type 2B vWD from other types
- Collagen binding activity (vWF:CB) is used to differentiate type 2M from 2A vWD.
- vWF multimer analysis: There is selective loss of high molecular weight multimers in types 2A and 2B vWD. Types 1 and 3 have mild and severe loss, respectively, in all the multimers, irrespective of molecular weight.

Genetic testing: The gene encoding vWF is very large and hence mutation analysis is quite cumbersome and usually performed only in specialized laboratories. However, in certain cases, they may assist in the diagnosis and subclassification.

TREATMENT

The cornerstone of management in vWD is to increase or replace vWF to achieve hemostasis, and it depends on the type of vWD, severity and location of bleeding and the need for invasive procedures.

Major options are:

- Desmopressin causes secretion of stored vWF from Weibel–Palade bodies in endothelial cells into the plasma. Intranasal or intravenous preparation may be used for management of mild-to-moderate bleeding episodes.
- vWF concentrates—plasma derived
- Recombinant vWF
- Antifibrinolytic agents
- Hormonal contraceptives

ACQUIRED VON WILLEBRAND SYNDROME

Any patient who has a noninherited qualitative, structural, or functional defect of vWF which leads to an increased risk of bleeding is said to be suffering from acquired von Willebrand syndrome (AVWS). Late onset of bleeding symptoms and a negative family history are two crucial features of this syndrome. Patients with AVWS usually have an associated underlying disorder—commonly lymphoproliferative, myeloproliferative, cardiovascular, other neoplastic, and autoimmune disorders.

RARE BLEEDING DISORDERS

These include deficiencies of:

- Fibrinogen
- Prothrombin
- Factor V
- Combined factor V and factor VIII
- Factor VII
- Factor X
- Factor XI
- Factor XIII
- Vitamin k-dependent factors

These disorders are usually autosomal recessive. Factor VII is the most common among these, with a prevalence of 1 in 500,000. Bleeding manifestations are varied and do not always correlate with the degree of factor deficiency; however, life-threatening bleeds (e.g., CNS bleeds) are rarer compared to hemophilia. These patients should be treated with purified blood product which contains the missing factor—solvent/detergent-treated plasma is commonly recommended.

DISORDERS OF FIBRINOLYTIC SYSTEM

Congenital deficiencies of α2-antiplasmin and plasminogen activator inhibitor-1 (PAI-1) can cause bleeding manifestations. These are rare causes of bleeding; hence their exact prevalence is unknown. Bleeding due to acquired defects in fibrinolysis may be seen in liver disorders, acute promyelocytic leukemia, snake bite etc.

RECOMMENDED READINGS

1. Gomez K, Tuddenham EDG, McVey JH. Normal hemostasis. In: Hoffbrand AV, Tuddenham EDG, Catovsky D, Green AR (eds). Postgraduate Hematology, 6th edition. Chichester, Endland: Wiley-Blackwell; 2011. pp. 746-71.
2. Weitz JI. Overview of hemostasis and thrombosis. In: Hoffman R, Benz E, Silberstein LE, Heslop H, Weitz J, Anastasi J. Hematology basic principles and practice, 6th edition. Philadelphia: Elsevier; 2012. pp. 1774-83.
3. Ma A. Approach to the adult with a suspected bleeding disorder. [online] Available from https://www.uptodate.com/contents/approach-to-the-adult-with-a-suspected-bleeding-disorder.
4. Lambert M, Cuker A, Greinacher A. Disorders of platelet number and function. In: Cuker A, Altman JK, Gerds AT, Wun T (eds). USA: American Society of Hematology Self-Assessment Program, 7th edition. pp. 291-320.
5. Neunert C, Terrell DR, Arnold DM, Buchanan G, Cines DB, Cooper N, et al. American Society of Hematology 2019 guidelines for immune thrombocytopenia. Blood Adv. 2019;3(23):3829-66.
6. Powell JS, Rodgers GM. Inherited coagulation disorders. In: Greer JP, Arber DA, Glader B,. List AF, Means Jr. RT, Paraskevas F, Rodgers GM. Wintrobe's Clinical Hematology. Philadelphia, PA: Wolters Kluwer, 13th edition. pp. 1143-85.
7. Srivastava A, Santagostino, E, Dougall, A, Kitchen S, Sutherland M, Pipe SW, et al. WFH Guidelines for the Management of Hemophilia, 3rd edition. Haemophilia. 2020;26(Suppl.6):1-158.
8. Sachdeva A, Gunasekaran V, Ramya HN, Dass J, Kotwal J, Seth T, et al. Consensus in Diagnosis and Management of Hemophilia' Committee, Indian Academy of Pediatrics. Consensus Statement of the Indian Academy of Pediatrics in Diagnosis and Management of Hemophilia. Indian Pediatr. 2018;55(7):582-90.
9. Kumar R, Kempton LC. Bleeding disorders. Cuker A, Altman JK, Gerds AT, Wun T. American Society of Hematology Self-Assessment Program, 7th edition. USA: American Society of Hematology; 2019. pp. 260-90.
10. Sharma R, Flood VH. Advances in the diagnosis and treatment of Von Willebrand disease. Blood. 2017;130(22):2386-91.

CHAPTER 155

Thrombotic Disorders

Preethi Jeyaraman, Pulkit Rastogi

ABSTRACT

Thrombotic disorders encompasses a varied spectrum of clinical manifestations characterized by a common pathogenetic process of occlusion of vessel lumen by clot. Broadly, it can be divided into venous or arterial subtype. A variety of inherited and acquired risk factors predispoes an individual to the development of thrombosis. These risk factors either augment the prothrombotic mechanisms or weaken the antithrombotic ones and hence lead to the imbalance in normal hemostatic process. The most common manifestations of venous thrombosis are deep vein thrombosis (DVT) of leg vein and pulmonary thromboembolism. For arterial thrombosis, acute myocardial infarction and stroke are the most common events. A careful evaluation by appropriate clinical scores, imaging methods, and laboratory assays helps in guiding the management of these patients so as to prevent recurrence and complications.

"Cure sometimes, treat often and comfort always"

—Hippocrates

INTRODUCTION

Thrombosis is defined as the development of a blood clot within the lumen of blood vessel (venous or arterial), leading to the obstruction of blood flow, which may lead to tissue hypoxia and damage. Physiologically, there is an intricate balance between the various components of hemostasis which prevent uncontrolled hemorrhage following an injury, and also excessive clotting in certain challenging situations. A variety of inherited or acquired risk factors, called thrombophilic states, predispose an individual to the development of thrombosis which can be either arterial or venous or both.

Thrombotic disorders are one of the significant causes of morbidity and mortality worldwide. To enumerate, the major thrombotic disorders are DVT and pulmonary embolism (PE), collectively termed as venous thromboembolism (VTE). Besides, thrombosis in arteries may lead to acute vascular events such as myocardial infarction (MI) and stroke.

EPIDEMIOLOGY

The factors influencing the epidemiology of thrombosis are:

- Anatomic location: Venous *versus* arterial
- Underlying predisposing factor: Provoked *versus* unprovoked
- Frequency: First episode *versus* subsequent episode

The average age- and sex-adjusted annual VTE incidence in the West is 117/100,000 (for DVT; 48/100,000 and for PE; 69/100,000). Males are affected slightly more than females (M : F = 1.2:1); however, both of them are equally affected by the first episode of VTE. Age is a significant risk factor for DVT, and it is predominantly considered as a disease of the elderly. Racial differences have been noticed for VTE. The highest risk groups are African Americans, followed by Caucasians. Recurrent episodes of VTE are also less common in Caucasians than for African-American and Hispanic people. The exact incidence of DVT in India as reported from the South is 1.79/1,000 population.

The average age- and sex-adjusted annual incidence of acute MI in the West is 139.3/100,000. Males have consistently been affected more than females (M : F = 1.5:1). Stroke comprises two types, *viz.*, ischemic and hemorrhagic. Ischemic stroke is a thrombotic condition and accounts for about 67% of all strokes and 50% of stroke-related mortality. The average age- and sex-adjusted annual incidence of ischemic stroke in the West is 114.3/100,000 and for India is 154/100,000. Peculiar aspects of the Indian population are early age of onset, accelerated buildup, and high case fatality rate.

ETIOPATHOGENESIS

The classical three conditions which lead to thrombosis has been described by *Virchow's triad*—the endothelial injury, stasis, and blood hypercoagulability. A variety of inherited or acquired risk factors predispose an individual to one of these conditions and can lead to the development of either venous or arterial thrombosis, or both. When thrombosis occurs in the setting of any of these risk factors, it is called provoked. A brief overview of the normal coagulation cascade is essential to understand the pathogenesis of thrombosis.

COAGULATION CASCADE

The key mechanism for regulating hemostasis is the coordinated sequence of coagulation cascade events where the inactive substrates called as zymogens/coagulation proteins are converted into the active serine proteases. These enzymatic reactions are governed by the principle of amplification at each step. The end result is the formation of sufficient quantities of fibrin which can stop hemorrhage at the site of vascular injury.

The prime steps leading to a clot formation can be recapitulated as under:

1. Exposure of tissue factor (TF) due to injury or from blood cell-derived microparticles
2. Binding of inactivated factor VII to TF leading to its activated form (FVIIa)
3. TF/FVIIa complex activates factor X (FXa) and IX (FIXa)
4. FXa on TF-bearing cell interacts with activated Factor V (FVa) released from activated platelets at the site of injury to form FXa/FVa complex (prothrombinase), leading to the generation of thrombin (FIIa)
5. Thrombin converts fibrinogen to fibrin in the presence of factor XIII, leading to a stable hemostatic plug.

Regulation of coagulation cascade: It is managed by several antithrombotic factors (**Fig. 1**) such as:

- Antithrombin (AT): Broad-spectrum inhibitor (blocks thrombin, FXa, FIXa, FXIa, FXIIa, plasma Kallikrein, TF/FVIIa)
- Tissue factor pathway inhibitor (TFPI): Inhibits TF/FVIIa complex
- Heparin cofactor II: Inactivates thrombin
- Protein C/protein S: Activated protein C in the presence of protein S leads to inhibition of FVa and FVIIIa

These factors get activated once a sufficient quantity of clot is formed and prevent its perpetuation into the adjacent normal endothelium.

VENOUS THROMBOSIS

The risk factors for venous thrombosis relate to either hypercoagulability or stasis. These can be inherited or acquired.

Acquired:

- Advancing age
- Major trauma
- Surgery, mainly orthopedic, abdominal, and neurologic
- Immobilization
- Obesity
- Pregnancy and postpartum state
- Oral contraceptives
- Hormone replacement therapy
- Chemotherapeutic agents such as tamoxifen, thalidomide, lenalidomide, and asparaginase
- Heavy smoking
- Malignancy
- Central venous catheterization
- Long air travel
- Antiphospholipid syndrome (APS)
- Heparin-induced thrombocytopenia and thrombosis (HITT)
- Myeloproliferative neoplasm
- Rheumatologic states
- Paroxysmal nocturnal hemoglobinuria (PNH)
- Nephrotic syndrome
- Inflammatory bowel disease

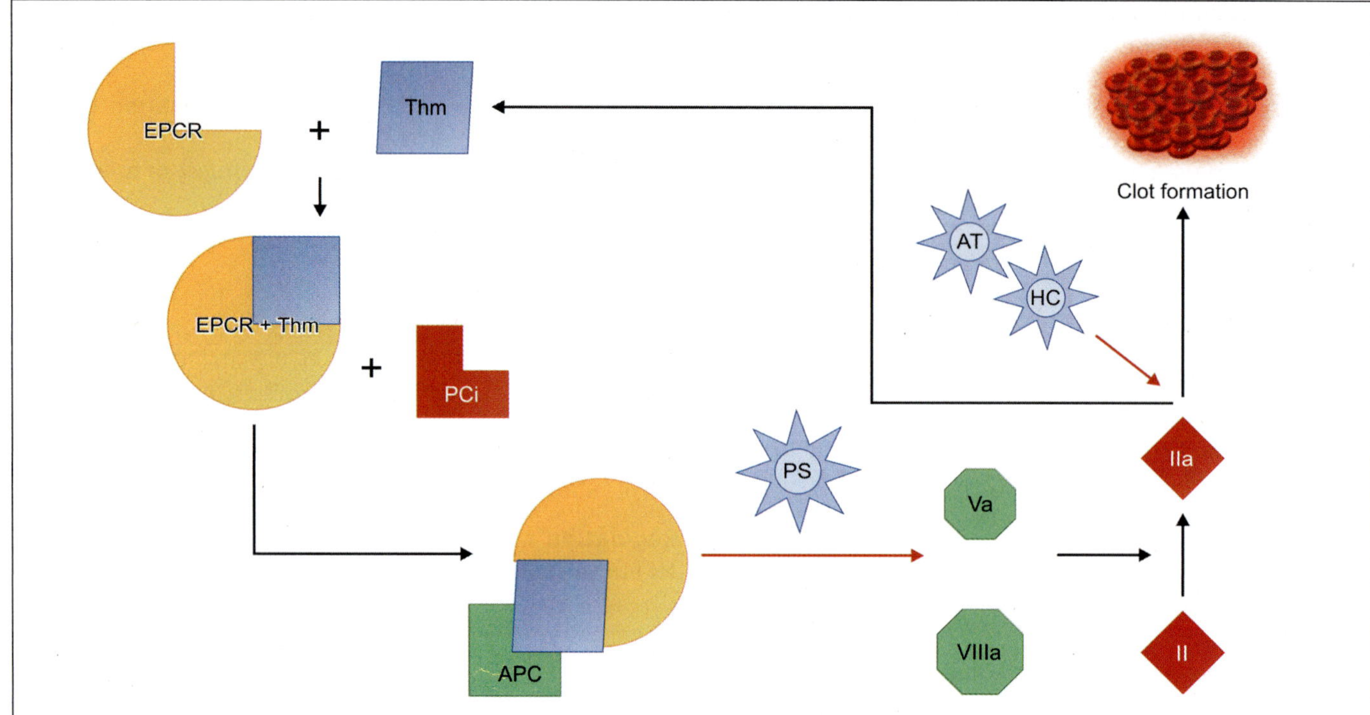

FIGURE 1: Sequence of event depicting regulation of coagulation by protein C pathway. Thrombin (IIa) formation as a result of coagulation cascade gets bound to thrombomodulin (Thm) at the advancing front of clot. Thm combines with endothelial-cell protein C receptor (EPCR) to activate protein C (APC). The APC then inactivates activated factor V and factor VIII in the presence of protein S (PS). This ultimately results in reduced generation of IIa. The thrombin is also neutralized by antithrombin (AT) bound to heparin cofactor II (HC).

Inherited:

- Strong factors:
  - AT deficiency
  - Abnormalities in protein C and S system (protein C deficiency, protein S deficiency)
- Moderately strong factors:
  - Resistance to activated protein C (*Factor V Leiden* mutation)
  - Hyperprothrombinemia (*PT G20210A* mutation)
  - Non-O blood group
  - *Fibrinogen 10034T* mutation
- Weak factors:
  - Fibrinogen, factor XIII, and factor XI variants
  - Hyperhomocysteinemia

ARTERIAL THROMBOSIS

The risk factors for developing arterial thrombosis relate more to endothelial injury and an atherosclerotic process often acts as a nidus.

Acquired:

- Hypertension
- Smoking
- High levels of low-density lipoprotein cholesterol
- Diabetes mellitus
- Pregnancy
- Advancing age
- Severe infections
- Hormone replacement therapy
- Rheumatologic states such as systemic lupus erythematosus (SLE) and rheumatoid arthritis
- APS
- HITT
- PNH

Inherited:

- Platelet receptor mutations (GPIb, β3 and α2 integrins)
- Hyperhomocysteinemia

To note, HITT, APS, myeloproliferative neoplasms, and PNH can predispose both to arterial and venous thrombosis.

Any of the above risk factors in an individual can perturb the homeostasis of coagulation system and leads to thrombus formation. More than one risk factor may be present in the same patient and further augments the risk.

CLINICAL FEATURES

Patients with thrombosis manifest with a variety of signs and symptoms depending on the site and acuity.

DVT:

- Involved extremity becomes painful (usually calf or thigh), swollen, warm, and red.
- Pain worsens with walking and is described as crampy.

PE:

- Common: Dyspnea on exertion, pleuritic chest pain, tachypnea, and cough

- Less common: Fever, hemoptysis, cyanosis, hypotension, shock, palpitations, anxiety, and light-headedness
- Massive PE: Dyspnea at rest, hypotension, syncope, central and peripheral cyanosis, gallop rhythm due to heart failure; distended jugular veins due to right-sided heart failure; widely split second heart sound and a loud pulmonic component; right ventricle heave.

Thrombosis of superficial lower extremity veins:
- Pain, tenderness, induration, and erythema along the course of superficial vein
- Palpable cord-like vein; low-grade fever
- Can be complicated by suppuration or DVT/PE

Venous thrombosis of the upper extremities: It is usually associated with central venous catheters, acquired/inherited risk factors, or thoracic-outlet syndrome.
- Acute presentation:
  - Sudden, severe pain and swelling in upper extremity following vigorous activity in a young athletic male
  - Edema and cyanosis of the affected extremity
  - Low-grade fever +/–
  - Palpable venous cord of superficial veins +/–
  - Dilated subcutaneous collaterals over upper chest and proximal upper extremity +/–
  - Brachial plexus compression signs in the form of paresthesias +/-
  - Signs of PE +/-
- Intermittent symptoms:
  - Minimal pain/edema
  - Prominent collaterals over the chest

Mesenteric vein thrombosis:
- Acute: Periumbilical colicky pain, nausea, vomiting, abdominal distension, and occult blood in the stool
- Subacute: Nonspecific abdominal pain for days to weeks
- Chronic: Usually asymptomatic; incidentally diagnosed by imaging studies; can present with symptoms of portal hypertension.

Cerebral vein and dural sinus thrombosis:
- Headache: Usually gradual, severe type and worsens with Valsalva maneuver
- Isolated intracranial hypertension syndrome: Presents in patient with chronic state, headache associated with papilledema.
- Focal/generalized seizures, encephalopathy, mono-/hemiparesis

Arterial thrombosis of lower extremity:
- Caused by acute thrombosis of an atherosclerotic artery, or a stent or graft, or from direct trauma or can be an embolus from a proximal source
- The classic signs of acute arterial occlusion (embolus) are 6 Ps (pain, pallor, pulselessness, paresthesia, paralysis, and poikilothermia)
- Collaterals development causes minimal symptom if thrombus forms in an atherosclerotic artery.

Mesenteric ischemia:
- Postprandial abdominal pain in case of thrombotic mesenteric arterial occlusion
- Sudden, severe, periumbilical pain with nausea/vomiting in case of embolic phenomenon

Retinal artery and vein occlusion:
- Arterial occlusion: Painless sudden loss of vision in an acute event
- Vein occlusion: Blurring of vision in the area of occlusion

Stroke and MI: (Refer to Chapters 107, 108, 186 & 187).

Antiphospholipid syndrome (APS): It refers to a clinical state characterized by the presence of anti-phospholipid antibodies, which predominantly results in a hypercoagulable state. The three most common antiphospholipid antibodies are: (1) lupus anticoagulant (LA), (2) anticardiolipin antibody (ACA), and (3) anti-β2-glycoprotein I antibodies (B2GPI). These antibodies are found in 1–5% of the general population, and their prevalence increases as age advances. SLE patients have a high prevalence of antiphospholipid antibodies, with 12–30% having ACA and 15–34% having LA antibodies. Of these SLE patients, about 50–70% may develop the APS.

"Sydney Investigational Criteria for the Diagnosis of the Antiphospholipid Syndrome" defines the various required criteria for a definitive diagnosis of APS. A patient of APS must satisfy at least one of the clinical criteria and one of the laboratory criteria.

The criteria are outlined below:
- Clinical criteria:
  - Vascular thrombosis:
    - "One or more clinical episodes of arterial, venous, or small-vessel thrombosis, occurring within any tissue or organ"
  - Complications of Pregnancy:
    - "Three or more otherwise unexplained recurrent spontaneous miscarriages before 10 weeks of gestation, or
    - One or more fetal losses after the 10th week of gestation, or
    - Stillbirth, or
    - Episodes of preeclampsia, preterm labor, placental abruption, intrauterine growth restriction, or oligohydramnios those are otherwise unexplained."
- Laboratory criteria:
  - "Medium- or high-titer ACA or B2GPI IgG or IgM antibody present on two or more occasions, at least 12 weeks apart, measured by standard enzyme-linked immunosorbent assays, or
  - LA in plasma on two or more occasions at least 12 weeks apart detected according to the guidelines of the International Society on Thrombosis and Hemostasis—Scientific and Standardization Committee on LA and phospholipid-dependent antibodies."

The most common clinical manifestation of the APS is DVT of the legs. Arterial thrombosis is less common than venous thrombosis, and these can manifest in any form as described earlier. Other common manifestations are livedo reticularis, thrombocytopenia, transient ischemic

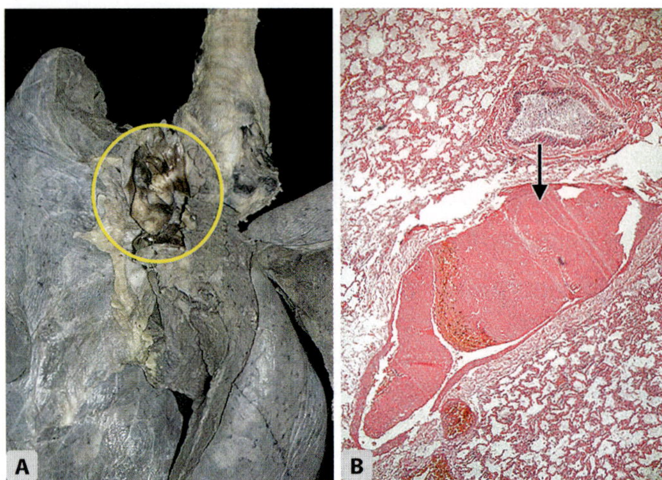

FIGURES 2 A & B: (A) Gross pathology of pulmonary embolism at autopsy showing a large-saddle thrombus (yellow circle) in the lumen of right main pulmonary artery; **(B)** Microscopy of the lung showing presence of fibrin-rich thrombus (black arrow) in lumen of pulmonary artery.

attacks, valvular heart disease, and acute or chronic renal failure. In rare cases, multiorgan failure due to small-vessel thrombosis can occur, and this condition is termed as "catastrophic APS."

Miscellaneous manifestations:

- Neonatal purpura fulminans, warfarin-induced skin necrosis in homozygous protein C/S deficiency

PATHOLOGY OF THROMBOSIS

The pathology of thrombosis is usually seen at autopsy as most of the times diagnosis is made on imaging studies. The gross pathology of venous or arterial thrombosis is a cord-like red structure within the lumen of vessel and focally attached to the endothelial layer. On cross-section, they typically show laminated appearance called as lines of Zahn. On microscopy, a thrombus is composed of layer of fibrin with entrapped red blood cells, platelets, and few leukocytes (**Figs. 2 A** and **B**). Arterial thrombosis in addition usually shows evidence of atherosclerosis.

EVALUATION

DIAGNOSIS OF DEEP VEIN THROMBOSIS

Pretest probability of deep vein thrombosis: In case of clinical suspicion of DVT, pretest probability of DVT can be assessed by Wells score (**Table 1**). Wells score in addition to D-dimer, helps in deciding the need for further evaluation with compression ultrasound for DVT. If the D-dimer test is negative and Wells score < 3, no other investigations are needed. If the D-dimer test is positive or score 3 or higher, compression ultrasonography is indicated.

There is activation of the fibrinolytic system in presence of thrombosis which results in elevation of D-dimer levels in plasma. However, elevated D-dimer can be present in other conditions such as severe infection/inflammation, cancer, trauma, surgery, or pregnancy. Therefore, a normal D-dimer test (<500 µg/L) result has a good negative predictive value to rule out DVT, whereas an elevated D-dimer can be nonspecific.

TABLE 1 Wells score for clinical probability of DVT.

Clinical condition	Points
Active cancer (treatment ongoing, within 6 months or palliative)	1
Paralysis, paresis, or recent plaster immobilization of a lower limb	1
Recently bedridden for longer than 3 days or major surgery within 4 weeks	1
Localized tenderness along the distribution of the deep venous system	1
Entire leg swollen	1
Calf swelling > 3 cm compared with the asymptomatic leg (measured 10 cm below the tibial tuberosity)	1
Pitting edema (greater in the symptomatic leg)	1
Collateral superficial veins (nonvaricose)	1
Alternative diagnosis as likely or greater than that of DVT	– 2
Probability	
3 points or more	High probability, about 75% risk of DVT
1–2 points	Moderate probability, about 17% risk of DVT
0 points	Low probability, about 3% risk of DVT

Source: Adapted from Wells PS, Anderson DR, Rodger M, Forgie M, Kearon C, Dreyer J, et al. Evaluation of D-dimer in the diagnosis of suspected deep-vein thrombosis. N Engl J Med. 2003;349(13):1227-35.

Ultrasonography: Duplex ultrasound of the extremities has a 95% sensitivity and specificity for DVT (less for distal DVT). Features of thrombosis include (**Fig. 3**):

- Noncompressibility of the venous segment
- Loss of phasic flow with Valsalva maneuver
- Lack of flow augmentation with calf squeeze
- Absent color flow if completely occlusive

DIAGNOSIS OF PULMONARY EMBOLISM

In patients with suspected acute PE, clinical likelihood is calculated by the Wells rule, which consists of 7 variables (**Table 2**).

Patients are classified based on Wells score as:

- PE unlikely: ≤4 points; 2.3–9.4% PE risk (in these patients, a normal D-dimer test can be applied to rule out PE)
- PE likely: >4 points, 28–52% PE risk

The negative predictive value for this assessment is 99.7%.

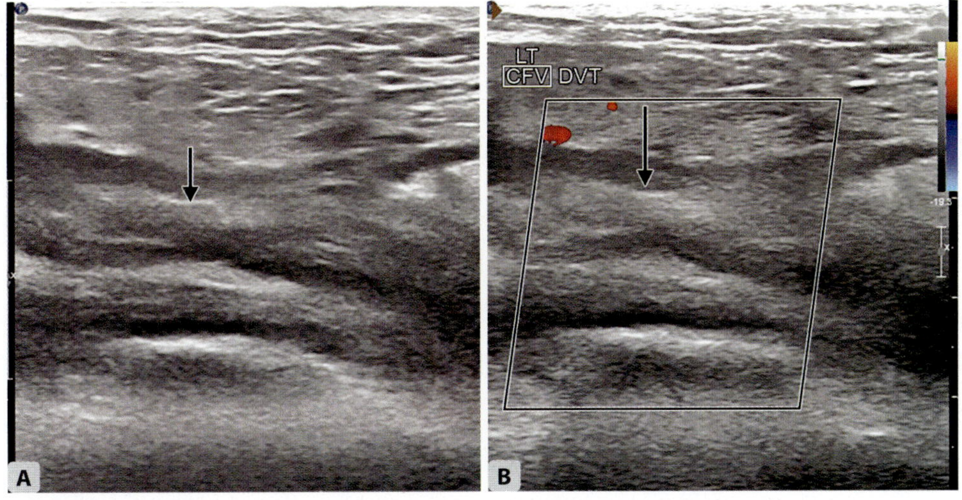

FIGURES 3 A & B: Gray scale image **(A)** shows echogenic contents in the left common femoral vein (arrow); **(B)** There is no color flow (arrow) on Doppler evaluation.

Courtesy: Dr Pankaj Gupta, Department of Radiodiagnosis and Imaging, PGIMER, Chandigarh.

TABLE 2 Wells score for clinical probability of PE.

Clinical condition	Points
Previous PE or DVT	1.5
Heart rate > 100/min	1.5
Surgery or immobilization < 4 weeks	1.5
Hemoptysis	1
Active malignancy	1
Clinical signs of DVT	3
Alternative diagnosis less likely than PE	3
Probability	
PE unlikely	≤4
PE likely	>4

Source: Adapted from van Belle A, Buller HR, Huisman MV, Huisman PM, Kaasjager K, Kamphuisen PW, et al. Effectiveness of managing suspected pulmonary embolism using an algorithm combining clinical probability, D-dimer testing, and computed tomography. JAMA. 2006;295(2):172-9.

Imaging modalities for diagnosis of Pulmonary Embolism

- Gold standard imaging modality for assessing patients with clinically suspected acute PE is invasive pulmonary angiography by *Computed tomography pulmonary angiography (CTPA)*. Sensitivity ranges from 20 to 30% for small, distal, and subsegmental emboli using single-row CTPA to >95% for segmental, lobar, and centrally located pulmonary emboli using multirow-detector (MD) CTPA (**Fig. 4**).
- *Ventilation-perfusion scan (V-Q scan):* A normal V-Q scintigram (one with no perfusion defects) virtually rules out PE. A V-Q scintigram showing at least one segmental perfusion defect combined with a normal ventilation scan, the so-called high-probability lung scan, has an 85–90% predictive value for PE.
- *Magnetic resonance pulmonary angiography*: It has a sensitivity of 85% and specificity of 96% for central, lobar, and segmental emboli; MRI is inadequate for the diagnosis of subsegmental emboli.
- *Echocardiography:* Right ventricular enlargement and/or hypokinesis of the free wall, leftward septal shift, and evidence of pulmonary hypertension can be identified. If right ventricular dysfunction is seen on cardiac ultrasonography, the diagnosis of acute submassive or massive PE is supported. Transesophageal echocardiography may identify central PE, and the sensitivity for central PE is reported to be 82%. Overall sensitivity and specificity for central and peripheral PE are 59% and 77%, respectively.

Electrocardiography: The most common ECG abnormalities in the setting of pulmonary embolism are tachycardia and nonspecific ST-T wave abnormalities. The finding of S1 Q3 T3 is nonspecific and insensitive in the absence of clinical suspicion for PE.

DIAGNOSIS OF CORTICAL VENOUS THROMBOSIS

Noncontrast CT of the brain can show generalized or localized hyperdensity areas, indicative of hemorrhagic infarctions in 40%. Three signs of cortical venous thrombosis (CVT) in CT include string sign (elongated hyperdense image relating to the brain parenchyma), dense triangle sign (spontaneous superior sagittal sinus opacification from fresh coagulated blood), and empty delta sign (intraluminal filling defect surrounded by contrast in posterior portion of the superior sagittal sinus). CT venography is a reliable method to confirm CVT with 95% sensitivity. MR venography can be used in place of CT venography with similar sensitivity.

DIAGNOSIS OF ARTERIAL THROMBOSIS

Imaging study required will depend on site of thrombus. Contrast CT angiography has a sensitivity of 71–96% and specificity of 89–94% for diagnosis of acute mesenteric ischemia. MR angiography has similar sensitivity and specificity for mesenteric ischemia.

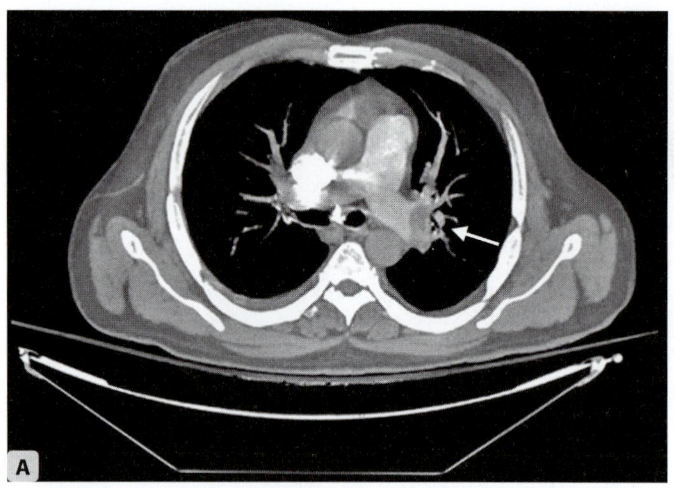

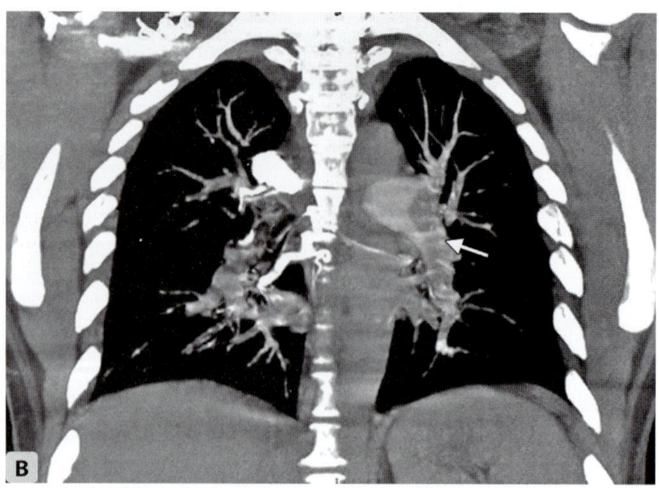

FIGURES 4 A & B: Axial **(A)** and coronal **(B)** CT pulmonary angiography images showing filling defect in the left branch of the pulmonary artery extending into inferior lobar branch.

Courtesy: Dr Pankaj Gupta, Department of Radiodiagnosis and Imaging, PGIMER, Chandigarh.

LABORATORY EVALUATION OF HYPERCOAGULABLE STATE

Timing: Before treatment is started and at least 6 weeks after an acute episode of thrombosis or 1 month after discontinuation of anticoagulant therapy (a few tests such as protein C, free protein S, AT and lupus anticoagulant are clot-based assays and to be done 6 weeks after an acute episode of thrombosis, if the patient is not on anticoagulation or 4 weeks after completion of anticoagulant therapy).

Indications of evaluation:

- Age < 50 years
- Family history of VTE
- VTE in unusual sites (Abdomen, CNS)
- Extensive VTE
- Idiopathic VTE
- Recurrent VTE
- Warfarin-induced skin necrosis
- Autoimmune disorders

Testing for venous thromboembolism: The following tests are routinely advised for the conditions as mentioned above when associated with VTE:

- Protein C assay
- Free protein S antigen assay
- AT assay
- For antiphospholipid syndrome:
  - Lupus anticoagulant: by silica clotting time or diluted Russell's viper venom test (dRVVT)
  - Anticardiolipin (ACA) IgG/IgM antibody assay
  - Anti-beta-2-glycoprotein 1 (B2GPI) IgG/IgM antibody
- Factor V Leiden mutation
- Prothrombin gene mutation (rare in Indian population)
- Assays for dysfibrinogenemia (screening by thrombin time, reptilase time, and confirmation by fibrinogen activity-antigen ratio)

Testing for arterial thromboembolism: Antiphospholipid syndrome, dysfibrinogenemia

TREATMENT

Treatment of venous and arterial thrombosis differs significantly. This section deals with the treatment aspects of VTE. For arterial thrombosis, (Refer to Chapters 107, 108 & 187). Not all patients of VTE need inpatient therapy. Home management can be considered in uncomplicated DVT without additional comorbidities or risk factors with adequate social support.

CHOICE OF ANTICOAGULANT THERAPY

Low molecular weight heparin:

- *Dalteparin* by subcutaneous injection 100 units/kg twice daily or 200 units/kg once daily
- *Enoxaparin* by subcutaneous injection 1 mg/kg twice daily or 1.5 mg/kg once daily.
- *Tinzaparin* by subcutaneous injection 175 IU/kg once a day—the effect of tinzaparin can be reversed with protamine more completely than when using the other drugs mentioned above.

Low molecular weight heparin (LMWH) is the preferred anticoagulation in pregnancy. Fondaparinux is an alternative for LMWH. It is suitable for patients with heparin allergy and for the treatment of HITT.

Vitamin K antagonists: Warfarin is started concomitantly at the dose of 5 mg/day. In elderly patients and patients with heart or liver failure, the recommended initial dose is 3 mg/day. International normalized ratio (INR) readings guide further dosage. Heparin/LMWH is continued until INR has been within the target range (2.0–3.0) for at least 1 day (24 hours) in any case for at least 5 days (taking the risk of bleeding and the INR readings into account).

Direct oral anticoagulants: *Direct factor Xa inhibitors (rivaroxaban, apixaban, and edoxaban) and direct thrombin inhibitor (Dabigatran)*: These do not require laboratory monitoring to adjustment dosage and may be used as alternatives to warfarin. These agents are not recommended in patients with renal insufficiency (creatinine clearance

<30 mL/min), moderate-to-severe liver disease, or APS. Rivaroxaban and apixaban treatments are initiated directly without heparin treatment. For dabigatran and edoxaban, a preceded treatment by LMWH (for a minimum of 5 days) is recommended.

OTHER TREATMENT

These are required only in special circumstances.

Fibrinolytic therapy: Catheter-directed thrombolysis may be attempted in DVT in the following scenarios:

- Recent (symptoms for <2 weeks) DVT
- Limb-threatening DVT (phlegmasia cerulea dolens) involving the iliac and common femoral veins
- Extension of thrombosis proximally in upper limb thrombosis

Systemic thrombolysis can be considered in PE if there is a hemodynamic compromise (in case of massive PE)

Inferior vena cava filters:

Indications:

- Contraindication to anticoagulation
- Complication of anticoagulation necessitating cessation
- Failure of anticoagulation
- Propagation/progression of DVT during therapeutic anticoagulation

Surgical treatment: Surgical intervention can be considered if the limb's viability is threatened, particularly if both thrombolytic and anticoagulant therapy are contraindicated.

Duration of therapy: Anticoagulation is typically given for a 3–6 months for primary therapy for VTE (**Table 3**). The decision to continue anticoagulation beyond 3–6 months will differ from patient to patient. Factors to be considered include the extent of the thrombosis, bleeding risk factors, and compliance. All patients on secondary prevention should be re-evaluated regularly to review the benefits and risks of continued anticoagulant therapy.

Management of breakthrough and recurrent DVT/PE: For patients with breakthrough DVT and/or PE during therapeutic vitamin K antagonist (VKA) treatment, LMWH can be used. These patients require an indefinite duration of anticoagulation.

COMPLICATIONS

- Post-thrombotic syndrome: Seen in 20–50% cases of DVT within 1–2 years of initial presentation; patient complains of chronic pain, cramps, heaviness, and increased swelling after exercise, which get relieved on rest.
- Pulmonary hypertension: Seen in 0.1–9% of cases of PE
- Spontaneous hemorrhage: Maybe within or outside cranium; as a result of anticoagulation
- Arterial thrombosis: Morbidity due to cardiac or cerebrovascular diseases

TABLE 3 Duration of anticoagulant therapy: DVT and PE (ASH Guidelines 2020).

Indications	Duration
• First episode of thrombosis with a transient risk factor present (e.g., surgery, trauma, immobility, hormonal contraception or replacement therapy, pregnancy)	3–6 months
• First episode of unprovoked thrombosis	At least 3–6 months
• First episode of thrombosis in a patient with:	
◦ Active cancer	Permanent
◦ Antiphospholipid antibodies in repeated tests (with a 3-month interval)	Permanent
◦ Factor V or prothrombin (factor II) homozygous gene mutation	Permanent
◦ Established antithrombin or protein C deficiency	Permanent
◦ Established protein S deficiency and venous thrombosis in close relatives	Permanent
◦ Combination of two or more thrombophilias	Permanent
◦ Based on individual assessment, if there are some other risk factors of permanent nature	Permanent
• Recurrent unprovoked thrombosis	Permanent
• First life-threatening thrombosis without a predisposing factor	Permanent
• First thrombosis without a predisposing factor at an atypical location (e.g., veins of the abdominal area or venous sinus thrombosis)	Permanent

(ASH: American Society of Hematology Guidelines)

RECOMMENDED READINGS

1. Silverstein MD, Heit JA, Mohr DN, Petterson TM, O'Fallon WM, Melton LJ 3rd. Trends in the incidence of deep vein thrombosis and pulmonary embolism: a 25-year population-based study. Arch Intern Med. 1998;158(6):585-93.
2. Lee AD, Stephen E, Agarwal S, Premkumar P. Venous thrombo-embolism in India. Eur J Vasc Endovasc Surg. 2009;37(4):482-5.
3. Nguyen D, Coull BM. Thrombosis. Primer on Cerebrovascular Diseases, 2nd edition. USA: Elsevier; 2017. pp. 108-13.
4. Freed J, Bauer KA. Thrombophilia. Consultative Hemostasis and Thrombosis, 4th edition. USA: Elsevier; 2019. pp. 242-65.

5. Rosendaal FR. Risk factors for venous thrombosis: prevalence, risk, and interaction. Semin Hematol. 1997;34(3):171-87.
6. Miyakis S, Lockshin MD, Atsumi T, Branch DW, Brey RL, Cervera R, et al. International consensus statement on an update of the classification criteria for definite antiphospholipid syndrome (APS). J Thromb Haemost. 2006;4(2):295-306.
7. Wells PS, Anderson DR, Rodger M, Forgie M, Kearon C, Dreyer J, et al. Evaluation of D-dimer in the diagnosis of suspected deep-vein thrombosis. N Engl J Med. 2003;349(13):1227-35.
8. van Belle A, Büller HR, Huisman MV, Huisman PM, Kaasjager K, Kamphuisen PW, et al. Effectiveness of managing suspected pulmonary embolism using an algorithm combining clinical probability, D-dimer testing, and computed tomography. JAMA. 2006;295(2):172-9.
9. Ortel TL, Neumann I, Ageno W, Beyth R, Clark NP, Cuker A, et al. American society of hematology 2020 guidelines for management of venous thromboembolism: Treatment of deep vein thrombosis and pulmonary embolism. Blood Adv. 2020;4(19):4693-738.

CHAPTER 156 Transfusion Medicine: Principles and Application

Suchet Sachdev, Hari Krishan Dhawan, Ratti Ram Sharma

ABSTRACT

Postgraduate residents need to obtain, an overall concept of the functioning of blood centre, since a dialogue between the clinical and the transfusion residents is most important for the proper management of the blood components need of patients. The basics of selection of a safe blood donor, the blood components, the proper storage of blood components and the safety of the blood component which includes blood grouping, transfusion transmissible infections testing and pretransfusion compatibility testing, the best and next compatible options of blood components that could be transfused to the patients. The need of a written consent and order for blood transfusion for the right indication in right dose, the steps involved in right identification of the patient, right identification of the blood component, the right method of starting blood transfusion along with the right monitoring of transfusion, the right identification of adverse transfusion reactions and the right action to be taken in the event of a transfusion reaction. The knowledge of patient blood management, hemovigilance and that therapeutic interventions which could be conducted by the transfusion specialists.

"An ounce of blood is worth more than a pound of friendship"

—Proverb

INTRODUCTION

Blood Transfusion Services (BTS) play a vital role in healthcare delivery system of a country. In India, blood has been categorized as a "Drug," in section 3 (b) of the Drugs and Cosmetics Act (1940) and the Rules (1945) therein as amended from time to time. Over a period of time blood banking has evolved into a specialty called transfusion medicine, having multiple facets starting from donor to recipient and includes stem cell and other regenerative therapies.

Blood and its components require a written informed consent to be obtained prior to administration, and transfusion without consent has been considered akin to "assault" as per the judgment of the National Consumer Commission, India. The branch has deep roots within the society, primarily because the blood (source material) can only be obtained from a human volunteer. The branch has evolved from a predominantly laboratory-based functioning (blood bank) to more clinical interface with acquisition of the apheresis technology [therapeutic plasma exchange (TPE)]. It has transitioned from evidence-based transfusion (transfusion triggers, guidelines, and consensus statements) to individual patient-centric approach (PBM), most importantly from managing the delicate balance between the sufficiency with safety, to total quality management with incorporation of surveillance in the entire chain from the donors' vein to the recipients' vein (hemovigilance) and third-party assurance (proficiency assessment). It works akin to pharmaceutical industry with intricate critical control at each step in its functioning and follows the principles of good manufacturing practices (GMP) and is unique in that each blood component of it is a batch in itself because the source is from a unique biological entity.

In order to collect the input, the blood donation activities are carried out simultaneously from the blood donation center to the outdoor blood donation drives using mobile blood collection facilities. Subsequently, the blood is transported under controlled temperature conditions to the laboratory where blood components are prepared [packed red blood cells (PRBCs), platelet concentrate (PC), fresh frozen plasma (FFP), and cryoprecipitate] and are tested for blood grouping and TTIs. After all testing reports on donated blood are compiled, the blood components are marked, labeled, and shifted to the stocks in the blood components inventory.

There is a separate section that has special cell separator machines (apheresis) that separate platelets [single donor apheresis platelets (SDAP), plateletpheresis], granulocytes (granulocyte collection), or stem cells (peripheral blood stem cell collections) from donors connected online and can also be used to perform therapeutic procedures (TPE, leukapheresis, plasmapheresis, and erythrocytapheresis).

Finally, the blood components are issued to patients after a positive identification of their samples with the blood requisitions after pretransfusion testing (compatibility testing). The maintenance of all records of the blood center (formerly blood bank) is a mandatory requirement under lens of drug control organization. An overall idea about the functioning of the blood center will open scope for a dialogue between the clinical and the blood bank services.

CENTRAL DOGMA OF TRANSFUSION MEDICINE

The branch revolves on a unique blend of the fundamentals of immunology, hematology, biochemistry, and microbiology with genetics as the elite controller. The genetic material inherited from parents encodes messenger RNA that translates the proteins that are responsible for the characterization of unique antigens that stimulate antibody response consequent upon allogenic blood transfusion.

The ability of recognition of one own as "self" and things that are not one's own as "nonself" is the holy grail of transfusion medicine. At the first instance of the transfusion of allogenic blood, which is recognized as nonself, a set of immunological defense is instigated resulting in the production of antibodies and memory cells as harbingers of future defense upregulation.

All this is based on the subtle recognition of differences in structure of certain proteins on cell and in plasma constituents. The human leukocyte antigens (HLAs) have a very important role to play in this recognition as self, nonself. The entire journey of the red blood cell (or other cells and plasma constituents) from donors' vein to recipients' vein forms a chain that undergoes characterization and processing for maximum safety (**Fig. 1**). However, the unique biological nature makes it impossible to make it free of the inherent immunological or infectious risk, contrary the expectation of patients and public at large.

For a safe blood component, the selection of a safe blood donor and testing for infections markers in quality assured manner is equally important as is the pretransfusion compatibility testing for immunological harmony. Nevertheless, despite the best of aforementioned, neither is it possible to avert the transmission of known and unknown infections, nor is it possible to blunt the immunological response. This is where the transfusion experts try to dwell to excel, despite the known and unknown limitations. Therefore, blood transfusion has been on a lighter note compared to "marriage" in literature, and it is advised not to transfuse without a risk-benefit assessment. It is recommended to try avoid single unit transfusions as far as possible, and the best transfusion has described as no transfusion on a lighter note.

BLOOD COLLECTION AND PROCESSING

Safe blood donor: A safe blood component can only begin with a safe blood donor. The blood donor must pass through extensive questioning, and a mini examination that includes a hemoglobin check (>12.5 g/dL) and pulse and blood pressure measurement. The questioning is structured and includes many items that ascertain the safety of donor, and many items that ascertain the safety of blood component, as far as possible. These range from simple questions like presence of cough, cold, sore throat, fever, history of infections like influenza, dengue, jaundice to risk factors for infections like human immunodeficiency virus (HIV)/acquired immunodeficiency syndrome (AIDS), hepatitis, and usage of medications that may either point

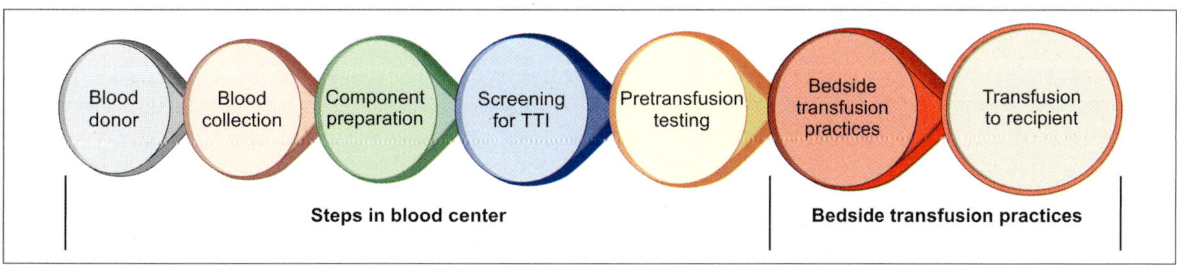

(TTI: transfusion transmissible infection)

FIGURE 1: Blood transfusion chain from vein to vein. The chain demarcates blood centers interface with the clinical transfusion, to highlight that errors can occur at each step from donors' vein to recipients' vein. The strength of chain is as strong as its weakest link.

to underlying disease or infections. Apart from these, presence of asthma, epilepsy, coronary artery disease etc. is considered prior to certification of fitness to donate.

Whole human blood (WB) is collected in blood bags made of polyvinyl chloride (PVC) with CPDA-1 (citrate-phosphate-dextrose adenine) as anticoagulant preservative solution and Di-(2-ethylhexyl) phthalate (DEHP), as plasticizer. The pilot evacuated tubes collected with the blood are tested for blood group, TTIs, and processed into blood components, PRBCs, random donor platelets (RDPs or PCs), FFP, and cryoprecipitate (Cryo) (**Fig. 2**).

WB is processed to components based on the principle of differential centrifugation, where cells settle in the blood bag as layers depending on their specific gravity. WB is centrifuged at relative centrifugal force (RCF) of 1,000 g (soft spin) to get two layers, of red blood cells and platelet-rich plasma or at 5,000 g (hard spin) to get three layers as red cells, buffy coat layer (WBC and platelets) and plasma. Programing based on these two centrifugation programs is used for the preparation of blood components. Cryoprecipitates are prepared by thawing FFP at 4°C where proteins like fibrinogen, factor VIII, and von Willebrand factor (vWF) precipitate and are separated by hard spin. The component processing optimizes the usage of scare human resource.

TRANSFUSION TRANSMISSIBLE INFECTIONS TESTING

The mandatory screening for TTIs in our country includes, testing for HIV/AIDS, hepatitis B, hepatitis C, syphilis, and malaria. This screening has improved from testing for the antibodies for HIV and hepatitis C virus (HCV) and hepatitis B surface antigen (HBsAg) for HBV initially using the rapid diagnostic tests (RDTs), to testing for simultaneous presence for antigen and antibody for HIV and HCV, to higher sensitive HBsAg assays for HBV using enzyme-linked immunosorbent assay (ELISA) and the more sensitive technology of chemiluminescence immunoassay (CLIA).

However, despite the best testing there is still a possibility for residual risk of infections, which depends on the window period for infection, described better as time from the acquisition of infection to time required for screening test to pick up the antigen or antibody. The molecular testing [nucleic acid testing (NAT)] has shortened this window period since it directly detects the presence of DNA or RNA. The window period and residual risk as per current estimates are depicted in **Table 1**.

The blood components can be further processed for *reduction in number of leukocytes*, as these are the main culprits behind many immunological reactions like alloimmunization, transfusion-related acute lung injury (TRALI), febrile nonhemolytic transfusion reactions (FNHTRs), and transfusion-related immuno-modulation (TRIM) and infections (cytomegalovirus). The simplest way to do this is to use buffy-coat removal methodology to prepare PRBCs and PCs. This can be better done using leukofilters at the bedside, but is best done using in-line filters in the blood bags for leukoreduction in

TABLE 1 Window period and residual risk of transmission of infections.

Infection	ELISA* (weeks)	NAT** (days)	Residual risk*** (per donations)
HIV	2–3	2–12	1 in 1–2 million
HCV	2–8	2–12	1 in 1–2 million
HBV	3–5	12–24	1 in 2–3 lakh# or 1 in 8 lakh to 1 million##

* Third generation antibody only to fourth generation antigen and antibody together or highly sensitive reagents, may vary as per sensitivity of kits.
** Individual donation (ID) to minipool (MP) testing platforms and the pool size of 6, 16, 24 etc., may vary as per sensitivity of kits.
*** Donations (#HBsAg or anti-HBc, ##NAT, may vary as per the sensitivity of kits).

[ELISA: enzyme-linked immunosorbent assay; HBV: hepatitis B virus (HBsAg); HCV: hepatitis C virus (anti-HCV antibodies); HIV: human immunodeficiency virus, (anti-HIV 1 and 2 antibodies and/or P24 antigen); NAT: nucleic acid testing]

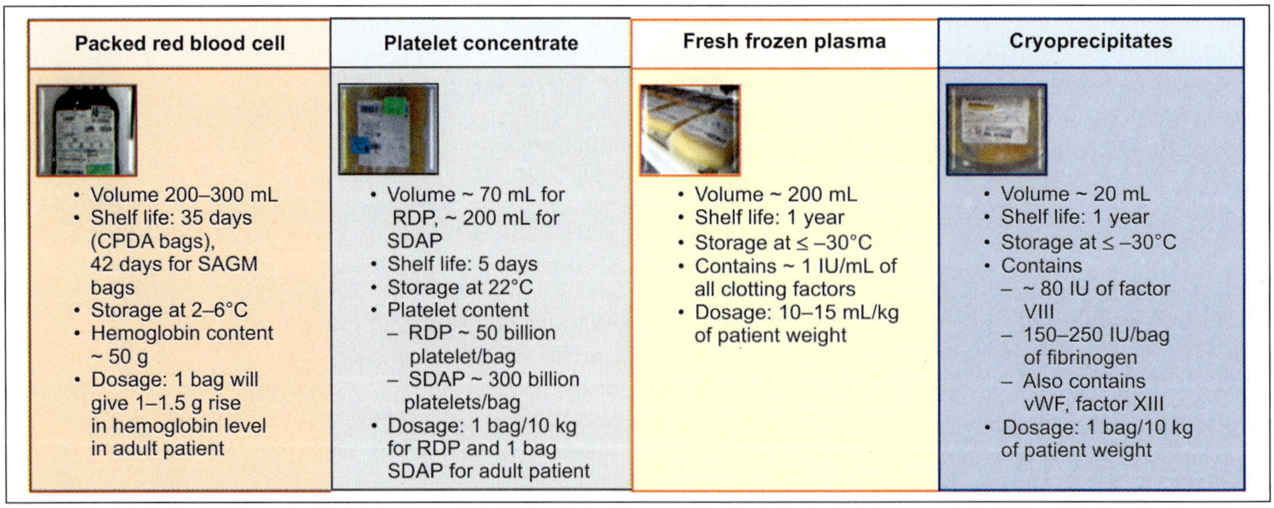

Packed red blood cell	Platelet concentrate	Fresh frozen plasma	Cryoprecipitates
• Volume 200–300 mL • Shelf life: 35 days (CPDA bags), 42 days for SAGM bags • Storage at 2–6°C • Hemoglobin content ~ 50 g • Dosage: 1 bag will give 1–1.5 g rise in hemoglobin level in adult patient	• Volume ~ 70 mL for RDP, ~ 200 mL for SDAP • Shelf life: 5 days • Storage at 22°C • Platelet content – RDP ~ 50 billion platelet/bag – SDAP ~ 300 billion platelets/bag • Dosage: 1 bag/10 kg for RDP and 1 bag SDAP for adult patient	• Volume ~ 200 mL • Shelf life: 1 year • Storage at ≤ –30°C • Contains ~ 1 IU/mL of all clotting factors • Dosage: 10–15 mL/kg of patient weight	• Volume ~ 20 mL • Shelf life: 1 year • Storage at ≤ –30°C • Contains – ~ 80 IU of factor VIII – 150–250 IU/bag of fibrinogen – Also contains vWF, factor XIII • Dosage: 1 bag/10 kg of patient weight

(CPDA: citrate-phosphate-dextrose adenine; RDP: random donor platelet; SAGM: saline adenine glucose mannitol; SDAP: single donor apheresis platelet; vWF: von Willebrand factor)

FIGURE 2: Characteristics of blood components, volume, shelf life, storage temperatures, and contents.

laboratory during processing to avoid release of biological amines from leukocytes till the reduction is carried out.

The blood components can also be manipulated for *reduction of plasma volume* by normal saline washing to reduce repeated allergic reactions and irradiated for reduction of transfusion-associated graft-versus-host disease (TA-GVHD). The final component is then labeled in line with the regional requirements, but mandatory information like blood group, TTI status, and type of component with date of collection and expiry is written before being included in the inventory of ready to issue stock.

SEROLOGIC TESTING OF BLOOD GROUPING

The serologic testing of blood grouping antigens and antibodies using the knowledge of genetics, biochemistry, immunology, and hematology is taken up together on one platform of immunohematology (IH) in transfusion medicine. This deals with detection of antigen-antibody interaction in vitro as the closest aide to understand as to what would happen in vivo, knowing that the in vivo interactions may or may not simulate the results in vitro testing. The fascinating study of IH started with discovery of the ABO blood groups by Karl Landsteiner, 1900–1901 and the Rh blood group by Weiner and Landsteiner, 1937.

The genetic inheritance of major blood groups is Mendelian, codominant, and autosomal (Xg^a being X-borne). The *ABO* gene is on chromosome 9, while the *Rh* gene complex is on chromosome 1. These genes produce glycosyl transferases for enzymatic addition of specific antigenic carbohydrates. Naturally occurring antibodies against red cell antigens are present from birth and are of immunoglobulin M (IgM) specificity, and can cause compliment activation and hemolysis. Other IgM type antibodies, called autoantibodies (antibodies against autologous blood group antigens) or cold agglutinins, are clinically insignificant as they have low affinity at human body temperature; however, some may have large thermal amplitude and may cause clinical manifestation due to intravascular red cell lysis.

Cold agglutinins in lymphoproliferative disorders and cold agglutinin disease usually have "I" specificity, an antigen found on adult red cells, while those that appear postinfections (mycoplasma, infectious mononucleosis) have "i" specificity, an antigen on red cells in the cord blood.

Red blood cell antigens are antigenic and result in production of antibodies upon the exposure of antigens that they lack during allogenic transfusion. These antibodies are of IgG specificity and upon binding with the antigen react best at warmer temperatures (37°C) and cause extravascular lysis that is cleared by the reticuloendothelial system. IgG antibodies can also cross placenta and bind fetal red cells.

ABO blood group system: The system has four major blood groups: A, B, AB, and O—based on the presence of antigen of red cell surface. The ABO groups are due to the *ABO* genes, and each individual has two such genes. Therefore, the genotype of group B can be BB or BO, similarly for A. The A and B molecules have terminal carbohydrate moieties and proteins as integral part of a base unit made up of band 3 molecule.

The H substance is immediate precursor and is formed by addition of fucose to base unit (two galactose residues on either side of N-acetyl glucosamine). The H gene codes for L-fucose transferase that adds a molecule of fucose on terminal galactose of unit. The addition of N-acetyl D-galactosamine by enzyme N-acetylglucosamine (NAG) transferase (A gene) to terminal galactose results in antigen A, whereas addition of D-galactose by enzyme D-galactosyltransferase (B gene) to terminal D-galactose results in antigen B. Therefore, activity of both H and A gene result in production of group A, similarly for B. Activity of H, A, and B genes is required for group AB. Absence of both A and B genes or their enzymatic activity results in group O (H is formed).

The ABO system is unique in that individuals lacking one antigen that produce corresponding antibodies. These are formed by exposure to carbohydrate mimics in nature, and do not produce memory cells (independent of T cell response). They are IgM type, can bind compliment, and initiate red blood cell lysis (intravascular) resulting in acute hemolytic transfusion reaction (AHTR). Therefore, these are of prime concern during blood transfusion (basis for group-specific whole blood transfusion).

The absence of H alleles results in homozygous state (hh) and the resultant blood group is called as Bombay blood group. The serum of this group has antibodies to H substance; this makes it very difficult to find compatible blood. Only Bombay (Oh) blood can be transfused to such people.

Rh blood group system: This is the second most important blood group consideration in day-to-day pretransfusion compatibility testing. The presence of D antigen dictates Rh positive phenotype, and its absence is phenotyped as Rh negative. The system also has two other allelic antigens E, e and C, c. The D antigen is highly immunogenic, and exposure of D antigen in Rh-negative person can immunize production of anti-D alloantibodies in about 90% of the recipients, either through transfusion or pregnancy. These alloantibodies can cause delayed hemolytic transfusion reaction (DHTR) due to extravascular hemolysis of red cells. It is the most common cause of hemolytic disease of fetus and newborn (HDFN) in RhD negative mothers carrying an RhD positive fetus.

Other clinically significant blood group: There are many antigens and blood group systems apart from the ABO and Rh systems. Normally they are not typed for routine blood transfusion. But for patients receiving regular blood transfusion matching for some of the more immunogenic ones may be a better strategy to avoid alloimmunization and the consequent difficulty in blood compatibility due to requirement of the antigen negative blood due to alloimmunization.

Apart from routine ABO and Rh typing, extended Rh typing, and typing for the minor blood group antigens of Kell (K), Kidd (Jk^a and Jk^b), and Duffy (Fy^a and Fy^b), the other

TABLE 2 Blood group, antigens, antibodies, and options available to transfuse.

Blood type	Antigen present on RBC	Antibodies present on plasma	Safe to receive RBC from	Safe to receive plasma and platelet from
O	None*	Anti-A, anti-B	O only	O, A, B, AB
A	A	Anti-B	A and O	A, AB
B	B	Anti-A	B and O	B, AB
AB	Both A and B	None	AB, B, A, O	AB only

* There is only precursor H chain on RBC.

(RBC: red blood cell)

immunogenic blood group systems have been proposed a better matched blood supply in some thalassemia transfusion programs to reduce the development of alloimmunization. Specifically, the antibodies to Kidd antigens may disappear rapidly in alloimmunized patients, presenting a challenge on subsequent transfusion with Kidd antigen positive red cells, when there is anamnestic response and a consequent DHTR.

Blood grouping: This is performed to detect both antigen and antibodies and the results verified to confirm the blood grouping as depicted in **Table 2**. Forward grouping for detection of antigens on red blood cells is done using commercially available antisera (anti-A, anti-B, anti-AB, and anti-D). Reverse grouping for detection of antibodies in serum is done using pooled suspension of red blood cells prepared freshly at the blood center using volunteer samples (O, A, and B pooled cells).

An autocontrol may be incorporated for best practice that uses washed autologous red cells and the serum for ruling out autoantibodies. Traditionally all immune-hematological tests were being done in test tube called tube technique. These days we have sensitive techniques like gel technique and microplate assays which have more objective, rapid, consistent results, and are amenable to automation.

Compatibility testing: Crossmatching is an in vitro test performed in blood bank serology laboratory. It entails testing compatibility between donor's RBCs and recipient's plasma, to primarily check if there is any preformed IgM (immediate spin crossmatching) or IgG [antihuman globulin (AHG) crossmatch] antibodies to an antigen present on RBCs being transfused (**Table 3**).

Antigens on platelets: Platelets express ABO antigens (at much lower density), while they do not carry Rh antigens. However, the chances of red cell contamination in platelets dictate the preference of ABO and Rh compatible platelets transfusion as far as possible. If in exigency across the Rh barrier platelets are to be transfused in women of reproductive age group, then it is advisable to give prophylaxis of anti-D (RhoGAM) to provide passive immunity and prevent sensitization. Platelets also express certain HLA class I molecules. However, platelets have their own antigens called as human platelet antigens (HPA).

TABLE 3 Urgent (immediate spin) versus routine crossmatching.

Immediate spin crossmatching	Antihuman globulin (AHG)/ Coombs crossmatch
• Detects immunoglobulin M (IgM) antibodies and ABO compatibility	• Detects IgG type of antibodies in addition to IgM
• Also detect anti-Le^a , -Le^b, -I, -P_1, -M and N antigen	• AHG testing detects anti-D, -C, -E, -c, -e, -K, -Jk, -Fy, -S, -s, -Le^a and Le^b
• May not detect clinically significant antibodies	• Detects most of the clinically significant antibodies

TRANSFUSION COMPONENTS AND INDICATIONS

Whole blood: In developing countries due to limited availability of blood components, whole blood may be used in an acutely bleeding patient especially of trauma.

Packed red cells: These are indicated in patients with symptomatic anemia. In chronic anemia, avoid volume overload. One unit raises hemoglobin by 1 g/dL or hematocrit by 3%. There is no absolute transfusion trigger, but transfusion is recommended when the hemoglobin is <6–7 g/dL in normovolemic patients with stable cardiac status, and based on the clinical assessment when the hemoglobin is between 6 and 10 g/dL. In older patients and those with cardiac disease a higher threshold of 10 g/dL is recommended. There is evidence that restrictive versus liberal transfusion based on the transfusion triggers does not have any superiority or inferiority. In nutritional anemia (iron, B12, and folate deficiency), it is best to avoid transfusions unless there is symptomatic decompensated anemia.

Platelets: Platelet transfusions may be prophylactic (to prevent bleeds) or therapeutic (during bleed). The transfusion thresholds are as low as 5,000/μL in stable chronic thrombocytopenic patients, e.g., aplastic anemia, 10,000/μL in stable acute leukemic patients, 20,000/μL in patients with fever, 50,000/μL in invasive diagnostics, and 100,000/μL in neurosurgical interventions. The rule of thumb dosage is one RDP/10 kg in adults. One unit of RDP (component derived from WB using centrifugation) and SDAP (prepared on apheresis machine) raises platelet count by 5,000–1,0000/μL and 30,000–60,000/μL in an adult stable patient weighing 70 kg.

Platelets are contraindicated in thrombotic thrombocytopenic purpura (TTP), heparin-induced thrombocytopenia (HIT), whereas may be given in life-threatening bleeds or for splenectomy in idiopathic thrombocytopenic purpura (ITP) patients. A corrected count increment (CCI) of >10,000 at 1 hour or 7,500 at 24 hours is considered as a successful platelet transfusion. In poor response, refractoriness is expected, and HLA-matched or crossmatch compatible platelets are the options, after nonimmune causes like sepsis, fever, disseminated intravascular coagulation (DIC), splenomegaly and medications are ruled out.

Fresh frozen plasma: It is indicated in DIC, congenital bleeding disorders, liver disease, and for reversal of warfarin therapy. The rule of thumb dose is 10–15 mL/kg body weight in adults and is expected to increase coagulation factors by 8–10%. Transfusion is guided by prothrombin time [international normalized ratio (INR)] and partial thromboplastin time testing. Caution is needed in known IgA deficient recipient, plasma from IgA deficient donor is needed to avoid anaphylaxis.

Cryoprecipitate: In developing countries, it is a source of factor VIII in hemophilia A, in nonavailability of factor concentrate as each unit contains 80 IU of factor VIII. It is a good source of fibrinogen and vWF. One unit of cryoprecipitate increases fibrinogen level by 10 mg/dL and is one option in volume-sensitive patients.

TRANSFUSION TRIAGE

The routine practice is to issue ABO Rh (D)-matched crossmatch compatible blood (on Coombs phase) in most cases but this process takes time (1–4 h) keeping in view the throughput of laboratory and modality of testing like batch testing. In case of life-threatening bleed where transfusion is required on urgent basis following strategies are the options.

Blood request in extreme emergency (life-threatening bleed): These strategies must be restricted to life-threatening emergencies and reason must be documented in the medical record.

Blood group specific but uncrossmatched blood: This option is when sample of the patient is available. This is done after performing the blood grouping of patient and the donor blood bag. The ABO Rh (D) matched, however uncrossmatched, blood can be issued as early as in 15 minutes, but may take a little longer based on workload, throughput, and working shift of the blood center. As a standard practice blood center continues with crossmatching and any eventual incompatibility is immediately informed to clinician.

Emergency O Rh (D) negative/O Rh (D) positive, uncrossmatched blood: This option is when there is no time to obtain and test a sample, "O Rh (D) negative PRBC" [if not available "O Rh (D) positive PRBC"] can be issued within minutes after consent from clinician as a life-saving measure (**Flowchart 1**).

Next compatible blood group: Blood components can be transfused across ABO and Rh blood groups, when group-specific [ABO Rh (D) matched] blood component is not available, next compatible available group component can be transfused based on the options detailed in **Table 2**. RDPs can be transfused across ABO group in adult patients but Rh (D) caution is important in case of females of reproductive age to prevent Rh isoimmunization. For FFP transfusion Rh (D) group is advisable, though not necessary. Cryoprecipitate can be safely transfused across ABO and Rh blood group barrier.

THE TRANSFUSION PROCESS (FIG. 3)

Informed consent: As blood transfusion is intervention, separate informed consent must be taken regarding the need for blood transfusion, after explaining the alternatives available, as well as risks involved in transfusion and no transfusion. This is a regulatory requirement in our country and has medicolegal implications in case patient develops a serious adverse event due to blood transfusion.

Physicians order: Physician order is written and signed order for specific blood component transfusion in patient file by the treating physician as is usually done for any other drug. It has been observed that decision to transfuse blood component is usually verbal and is not documented in patient file/treatment chart leading to irrational

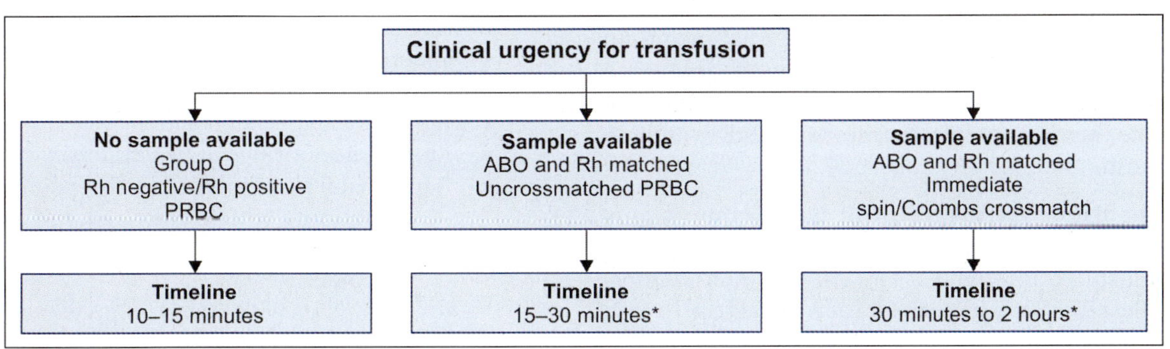

* Time will vary depending on technology used for blood grouping and crossmatching, workload and the level of care medical facility where blood center functions.

(PRBC: packed red blood cell)

FLOWCHART 1: Transfusion triage.

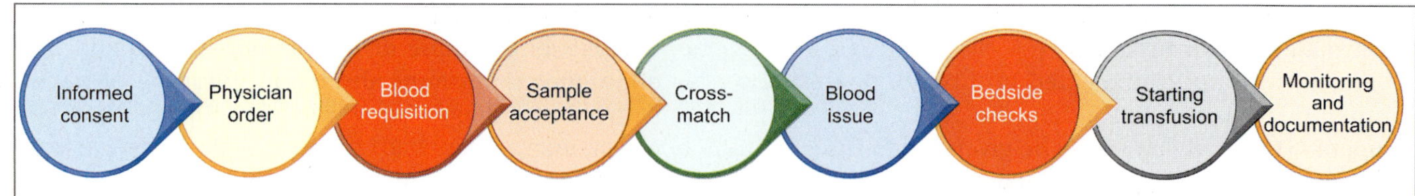

FIGURE 3: **Correct transfusion process flow.**

blood transfusion and exposing the patient to hazards of transfusion.

Blood requisition and bedside checks: These are two most important steps in transfusion chain where positive identification of patient is of paramount importance. Most of the hemolytic transfusion reactions occur due to the errors during these steps. While requisitioning blood, the patient sample labeling must be done in immediate area around the patient called as sample circle. Labeling sample away from patient greatly increases the chance of wrong labeling and consequent problem of wrong blood in the tube (WBIT), which can lead to AHTR. The protocol of bedside checks before initiation of transfusion is the last opportunity to catch any errors in the chain from donor's vein to recipient's vein. It is critical to ensure that the blood component received is intended for the patient and blood group is compatible for transfusion. This check must be done by two bedside staff and documented in patient file. Never omit or deviate from these steps to ensure patient safety.

Need for warming of blood before transfusion: There is no need of warming of blood in elective transfusion where a unit of blood is transfused over 2–4 hours. However, warming of blood is useful when rapid transfusion of components is required, especially in trauma or surgery settings, because the infusion of cold components can cause hypothermia and cardiac complications, increasing morbidity and mortality for the patient.

Warmed blood is most commonly indicated in:

- Large volume rapid transfusions
- Transfusions to neonates
- Exchange transfusion in infants
- Patients with clinically significant cold agglutinins

Never warm blood by placing it in a microwave, on a heat source, or in hot water or by using other devices not specifically approved for blood warming. Inappropriate warming of blood can lead to nonimmune hemolytic transfusion reaction. Blood should only be warmed in a blood warmer having a visible thermometer and an audible warning alarm.

Blood transfusion set (BT set): All blood components (red blood cells, platelets, plasma, and cryoprecipitate) must be transfused through BT set (170–260 micron filter) (**Table 4**). Best is to use a new set for each blood bag. In case of multiple transfusions, change after every 2–4 transfusions and/or 12-hourly depending on temperature and humidity. Do not transfuse platelets through a set used for PRBC transfusion to avoid adherence to fibrin captured in filter.

TABLE 4 **Intravenous (IV) access required for transfusion.**

Blood product	IV access
Red blood cells	16–22 G*
Other blood products	Any size
Pediatrics	22–25 G

*Gauge of cannula needs to be determined by the rate, as transfusion of red cell through smaller cannula rapidly can lead to hemolysis.

Prolonged periods of use may allow bacterial overgrowth in nosocomial environments. It must never be left attached to the patient.

Before starting blood: Identify the patient again, check baseline vitals.

- Temperature
- Blood pressure
- Pulse
- Respiration
- Oxygen saturation if available
- Auscultation for patients at risk for overload (elderly, pediatric, and cardiovascular disease)

Monitoring during blood transfusion:

- *For the first 15 minutes*: Start initially with a slow rate unless transfusion is extremely urgent.
  Monitor your patient closely for any sign and symptom of adverse event. All serious reaction like hemolytic reaction, bacterial contamination, anaphylactic reactions present during this phase.
- *After the first 15 minutes*:
  - Reassess your patient and repeat vital signs
  - Increase flow to prescribed rate if no reaction observed
  - Monitor the patient:
    - At least every hour during transfusion
    - On completion of the transfusion
    - 4 hours after completing the transfusion
    - If there is suspected reaction
    - Repeat monitoring with each subsequent unit
    - Repeat vital signs more often for patients:
      - In patients with greater risk for circulatory overload (elderly, pediatric, and cardiovascular disease)
      - In patients with history of previous reactions
      - In patients who are unstable
  - Instruct your patient to notify you if they experience:
    - Hives or itching
    - Fever, chills, or rigors

- Difficulty breathing
- Back pain or pain at the infusion site
- Any unusual presentation

MANAGEMENT OF TRANSFUSION REACTION

1. Stop the transfusion immediately

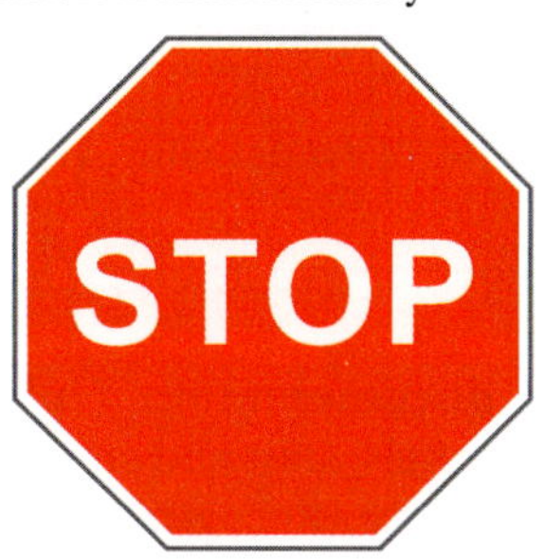

2. Maintain intravenous (IV) access
3. Check vital signs
4. Take necessary resuscitative measures to stabilize the patient
5. Verify that patient ID matches the compatibility label and compatibility report on blood bag
6. Notify blood center
7. Send the BT set with the blood bag and post-transfusion samples to blood center

Investigations to be done as per symptoms:

- Complete hemogram, with peripheral blood film for schistocytes/spherocytes
- Plasma hemoglobin
- Coagulation profile
- Bilirubin (unconjugated/conjugated)
- Urea
- Creatinine
- Electrolytes
- Next voided urine for hemoglobin testing
- Urine output (and for hemolysis)
- Chest X-ray (respiratory symptoms)
- Blood cultures (patient/blood bag)

The diagnosis of transfusion reaction is reached by ruling out reactions one by one. The signs and symptoms of acute transfusion reactions often overlap as depicted in **Table 5**. Delayed reactions include iron overload, delayed hemolytic transfusion reaction, transfusion transmitted infections, TRIM etc.

HEMOVIGILANCE

This is a set of surveillance procedures, to collect and assess information on unexpected or undesirable effects resulting from the therapeutic use of labile blood products and to prevent their occurrence or recurrence.

On lines of pharmacovigilance where all drug reactions should be reported to assess safety of drug, all transfusion reactions should be reported to blood center so as to generate national data regarding safety of blood component.

In India there is a National Hemovigilance Program of India, since 2012. The major aim of the program is to

TABLE 5 Adverse transfusion symptom and the differential diagnosis.

Signs and symptoms	Possible transfusion reaction	Other supportive evidence
Fever, chills, or rigor	Febrile nonhemolytic transfusion reaction (FNHTR)	1°C rise in temperature from baseline within 4 h of transfusion
	Bacterial contamination	Usually within 15 min, associate with rigors and chills
	Transfusion-related acute lung injury (TRALI)	
	Acute hemolytic transfusion reaction (AHTR)	
Dyspnea Or Decrease in SpO_2 below 90% or below	Transfusion-associated circulatory overload (TACO)	Typically associated with hypertension, within several hours of transfusion
	TRALI	Typically associated hypotension, within 6 h of transfusion
	Anaphylaxis	Usually very early in transfusion
	Bacterial contamination	Usually presents within first 15 min
Urticaria and other allergic symptoms	Minor allergic reaction	During or up to 4 h of transfusion, no other symptoms
	Anaphylaxis	Usually presents very early in transfusion and associated with dyspnea and hypotension
Pain	AHTR (at intravenous site and lumber region)	Can be associated with hemoglobinuria
	TACO (chest)	
Hypotension	Bradykinin mediated hypotension	Usually occur in patients on ACE inhibitors
	Bacterial contamination	Usually present very early during transfusion and can be associated with high grade fever
	Other differential diagnoses are AHTR, TRALI, and anaphylaxis	Corelate with other symptoms
Hypertension	TACO	Associated with dyspnea
Hemoglobinuria	AHTR	

track adverse events related to blood transfusion and help to identify trends and recommend best practices and interventions required to improve blood safety in the country.

PATIENT BLOOD MANAGEMENT

It is a patient-focused, multidisciplinary, evidence-based, and systematic approach to optimize the transfusion of blood in individual patient. The primary aim is to improve patient safety and clinical outcomes by appropriately managing the patient's own blood and by minimizing unnecessary exposure to allogenic blood products.

There are four core principles of PBM program:

1. It is patient centric: Involves a dialogue with patient in decision making weighing the potential risk and benefit keeping the alternatives available (pharmacological etc.) as options.
2. Management of red cell mass: Detect etiology of anemia and explore nontransfusion alternative as first option before any clinical decision to transfuse blood is taken.
3. Multidisciplinary blood conservation strategies which may include but are not limited to techniques like autologous transfusion, acute normovolemic hemodilution (ANH), intraoperative red cell salvage, blood sparing surgical techniques, and strategies to limit blood loss as soon as detected.
4. Maintaining homeostasis of coagulation parameters to decrease coagulopathy and uses of point-of-care viscoelastic testing technologies to guide transfusion of blood components.

THERAPEUTIC APHERESIS

Therapeutic apheresis is a novel treatment modality for various clinical conditions which include either harvesting of cellular elements for therapeutic use such as platelets, granulocytes, lymphocytes, and stem cells or removal of toxic substances from the plasma. TPE is an extracorporeal technique designed to remove high molecular weight substances (causing disease) from plasma using apheresis technology. The most commonly removed macromolecules are immunoglobulins/immune complexes and low-density lipoproteins (hyperlipidemia).

TPE is either standard or adjunct therapy in hematological disorders (TTP, hemolytic uremic syndrome, and hyper-viscosity syndromes), autoimmune disorders (Goodpasture syndrome), and neurological disorders (myasthenia gravis and Guillain-Barré syndrome) apart from many other conditions. Red cell exchange is one option in tackling sickling crisis in sickle cell disease, poisonings and cerebral malaria and certain poisonings. Therapeutic cytapheresis reduces white cell/platelets load prior to decrease symptoms due to hyperleukocytosis/thrombocytosis.

TWELVE SALIENT POINTS FOR BEST PRACTICE

1. Ensure avoidance of single transfusion (No transfusion is best transfusion!)
2. Ensure the need of second transfusion (Why give two when one will do!)
3. Ensure right indication for transfusion (PBM!)
4. Ensure right blood product (Clinical indication!)
5. Ensure right patient receives transfusion (Positive identification!)
6. Ensure right dose (Appropriate for patient's condition and weight!)
7. Ensure right time of transfusion (Issue only when to transfuse!)
8. Ensure right mode of transfusion (Dedicated IV access and BT set!)
9. Ensure right documentation (Informed consent, physician order, vitals, start and stop time!)
10. Ensure right response (Recognize and manage adverse reactions!)
11. Ensure right reporting of transfusion reactions (Strengthen hemovigilance!)
12. Ensure right therapy of early plasma exchange in atypical hemolytic uremic syndrome (Utilize the therapeutic interface of blood center!)

RECOMMENDED READINGS

1. Simon TL, McCullough J, Snyder EL, Solheim BG, Stowell CP, Strauss RG. Rossi's Principles of Transfusion Medicine (Eds), 5th edition. Wiley Blackwell Publishing; 2016.
2. Klein HG, Anstee DJ (Eds). Mollisons's Blood Transfusion in Clinical Medicine, 12th edition. Wiley Blackwell Publishing; 2014.
3. Harmening DM (Ed). Modern Blood Banking & Transfusion Practices, 7th edition. F.A. Davis Company; 2018.
4. The Clinical Use of Blood: Handbook. Blood Transfusion Safety. Geneva: World Health Organization; 2009.
5. A Guide to Transfusion Medicine. Bloody easy 4; Blood Transfusions, Blood Alternatives and Transfusion reactions. Ontario Regional Blood Coordinating Network; 2016.
6. Marwaha N, Dolly D. Transfusion Medicine: In: Kamath S (Ed). API Textbook of Medicine, 11th edition. New Delhi: CBS Publishers & Distributors Pvt. Ltd.; 2019.
7. Naidu NK, Bharucha ZS, Sonawane V, Ahmed I. Nucleic acid testing: Is it the only answer for safe Blood in India? Asian J Transfus Sci. 2016;10:79-83.
8. Galel SA, Simon TL, Williamson PC, AuBuchon JP, Waxman DA, Erickson Y, et al. Sensitivity and specificity of a new automated system for detection of hepatitis B virus, hepatitis C virus and human immunodeficiency virus nucleic acid in blood and plasma donations. Transfusion. 2018;58:649-59.
9. Sanford KA. Transfusions. In: Guide to Infection Control in the Healthcare Setting. International Society for Infectious Diseases. [online] Available from https://isid.org/guide/

10. Retter A, Wyncoll D, Pearse R, Carson D, McKechnie S, Stanworth S, et al. BCSH guidelines on the management of anemia and red cell transfusion in critically ill adult patients: Br J Haematol. 2013;160:445-64.
11. Liumbruno G, Bennardello F, Lattanzio A, Piccoli P, Rossetti G, Italian Society of Transfusion Medicine and Immunohaematology (SIMTI) Work Group. Recommendations for the use of plasma and platelets. Working group of Italian Society of Transfusion Medicine and Immunohematology. Blood Transfus. 2009;7:132-50.
12. Stroncek D, Rebulla P. Platelet Transfusions. Lancet. 2007;370:427-38.
13. Padmanabhan A, Connelly-Smith L, Aqui N, Balogun RA, Klingel R, Meyer E, et al. Guidelines on the Use of Therapeutic Apheresis in Clinical Practice - Evidence-Based Approach from the Writing Committee of the American Society for Apheresis: The Eighth Special Issue. J Clin Apher. 2019;34:171-354.
14. Serious Hazards of transfusion. Annual report 2016. Manchester, UK: SHOT office; 2016. [online] Available from https://www.shotuk.org/shot-reports/report-summary-supplement-2016/2016-shot-annual-report-individual-chapters/
15. Haemovigilance Programme of India. [online] Available from http://nib.gov.in/haemovigilance.html

CHAPTER 157

Hematological Malignancies: Classification and Approach

Vijayalakshmi Aravindan Arun, Pankaj Malhotra

ABSTRACT

The hematopoietic neoplasms consist of acute and chronic leukemias, Hodgkin lymphoma (HL) and non-Hodgkin lymphoma (NHL), plasma-cell tumors, and the rare histiocytic and dendritic neoplasms. Each of these disease categories is now recognized to represent various heterogeneous disease groups that include a large number of distinct biologic entities. Although the diagnosis and classification of these tumors were originally based primarily on morphologic features and cytochemical studies, their diagnosis now requires a complex battery of tests including immunophenotyping, and cytogenetic and molecular studies.

Management of hematological malignancies today is based on the pathophysiological pathways driving these disorders in most cases and consists of targeted therapy, immunotherapy, and chemotherapy. The goals of these therapies are personalized and based on performance status, comorbid illnesses, disease stage and risk stratification, and last but not the least the financial and social support. Cure or complete remission (CR) is achievable in two-thirds of hematological malignancies today due to advances in diagnosis and therapeutics. The availability of generics and biosimilars ensures that these results are achieved in resource-constrained setting too, including our country.

"The human body is the most complex system ever created. The more we learn about it, the more appreciation we have about what a rich system it is"

—Bill Gates

CLASSIFICATION

Hematological malignancies encompass a repertoire of >100 entities today. It is therefore, pertinent that we segregate them into relatively homogenous groups to ensure ease of nomenclature and uniformity in scientific reporting. Classification is the language of medicine: Diseases must be described, defined, and named before they can be diagnosed, treated, and studied.

The 2008 World Health Organization (WHO) classification of hematological malignancies was a major attempt to classify these disorders into selected groups based on morphological criteria. However, new information accumulated since then and the need to incorporate clinical relevance for the diagnosis, prognosis, and therapy of patients resulted in the WHO 2016 revision which is currently used globally.

The WHO 2016 revision more accurately reflect the true heterogeneity of hematological malignancies incorporating morphology, immunophenotyping, genomics, and clinical features and helps the clinician in choosing the treatment strategy as well. The "WHO Classification of Tumours of Haematopoietic and Lymphoid Tissues" is one of the "blue book" monographs published by the International Agency for Research on Cancer (IARC; Lyon, France) and is the reference standard for classification of hematological cancers. Briefly, the classification uses all available information—morphology, cytochemistry, immunophenotype, genetics, and clinical features—to define clinically significant disease entities. It is a consensus classification in which a number of experts have agreed on the classification and the diagnostic criteria used for defining the entities that compose it.

In the WHO classification, the term "*myeloid*" includes all cells belonging to the granulocytic (neutrophil, eosinophil, and basophil), monocytic/macrophage, erythroid, megakaryocytic, and mast cell lineages. The term *Leukemia* is applied to neoplasms that typically involve the bone marrow (BM) and the peripheral blood (PB), whereas *lymphoma* is used to describe lymphoid tumors that commonly present as masses within lymph nodes or other soft tissues. Some lymphomas are named based on the resemblance of the tumor cells to a normal counterpart; for example, the malignant B cells of follicular lymphoma (FL) closely resemble the normal cells found within the B-cell follicles of lymph nodes. Other descriptors relate to the natural history of the disease in question. Acute leukemias, if untreated, are lethal within weeks to several months, whereas chronic leukemias may be compatible with survival for many years without treatment.

The WHO criteria for myeloid neoplasms apply to initial diagnostic PB and BM specimens obtained prior to any definitive therapy for a suspected hematologic neoplasm. Morphologic, cytochemical, and/or immunophenotypic features are used for establishing the lineage of the neoplastic cells and for assessment of their maturation. The *blast percentage* remains a practical tool for categorizing myeloid neoplasms and judging their progression. In the WHO scheme, a myeloid neoplasm with 20% or more blasts in the PB or BM is considered to be acute myeloid leukemia (AML). In some cases associated with specific genetic abnormalities, however, the diagnosis of AML may be made regardless of the blast count in the PB or BM. The 20% blast threshold is not a mandate to treat the patient as having AML or blast transformation; therapeutic decisions must always be based on the clinical situation after all information is considered. **Box 1** lists the major subgroups of myeloid neoplasms and acute leukemia in the WHO

BOX 1 Major subgroups of myeloid neoplasms and acute leukemia in the WHO classification.

Myeloproliferative neoplasms (MPN):
- Chronic myeloid leukemia (CML), *BCR-ABL11*
- Chronic neutrophilic leukemia (CNL)
- Polycythemia vera (PV)
- Primary myelofibrosis (PMF)
- Essential thrombocythemia (ET)
- Chronic eosinophilic leukemia, not otherwise specified (NOS)
- MPN, unclassifiable

Mastocytosis

Myeloid/Lymphoid neoplasms with eosinophilia and rearrangement of:
- *PDGFRA, PDGFRB,* or *FGFR1*, or with *PCM1-JAK2*
- Myeloid/lymphoid neoplasms with *PDGFRA* rearrangement
- Myeloid/lymphoid neoplasms with *PDGFRB* rearrangement
- Myeloid/lymphoid neoplasms with *FGFR1* rearrangement
- Provisional entity: Myeloid/lymphoid neoplasms with PCM1-JAK2

Myelodysplastic/Myeloproliferative neoplasms (MDS/MPN):
- Chronic myelomonocytic leukemia (CMML)
- Atypical chronic myeloid leukemia (aCML)
- Juvenile myelomonocytic leukemia (JMML)
- MDS/MPN with ring sideroblasts and thrombocytosis (MDS/MPN-RS-T)

Myelodysplastic syndromes (MDS)
- MDS with single lineage dysplasia
- MDS with ring sideroblasts (MDS-RS)
- MDS-RS and single lineage dysplasia
- MDS-RS and multi-lineage dysplasia
- MDS with multi-lineage dysplasia
- MDS with excess blasts
- MDS with isolated del(5q)

Continued...

Continued...

- MDS, unclassifiable
- Provisional entity: Refractory cytopenia of childhood

Acute myeloid leukemia (AML) and related neoplasms:
- AML with recurrent genetic abnormalities
- AML with t(8;21)(q22;q22.1);RUNX1-RUNX1T1
- AML with inv (16)(p13.1q22) or t(16;16)(p13.1;q22);CBFB-MYH11
- APL with *PML-RARA*
- AML with t(9;11)(p21.3;q23.3);MLLT3-KMT2A
- AML with t(6;9)(p23;q34.1);DEK-NUP214
- AML with inv(3)(q21.3q26.2) or t(3;3)(q21.3;q26.2); GATA2, MECOM
- AML (megakaryoblastic) with t(1;22)(p13.3;q13.3);RBM15-MKL1
- Provisional entity: AML with BCR-ABL1
- AML with mutated NPM1
- AML with biallelic mutations of CEBPA
- *Provisional entity*: AML with mutated RUNX1
- AML with myelodysplasia-related changes
- Therapy-related myeloid neoplasms
- AML, NOS
- AML with minimal differentiation
- AML without maturation
- AML with maturation
- Acute myelomonocytic leukemia
- Acute monoblastic/monocytic leukemia
- Pure erythroid leukemia
- Acute megakaryoblastic leukemia
- Acute basophilic leukemia
- Acute panmyelosis with myelofibrosis
- Myeloid sarcoma
- Myeloid proliferations related to Down syndrome

Blastic plasmacytoid dendritic cell neoplasm:
- Acute leukemias of ambiguous lineage

Continued...

Continued...

Blastic plasmacytoid dendritic cell neoplasm:
- Acute undifferentiated leukemia
- Mixed phenotype acute leukemia (MPAL)

B-lymphoblastic leukemia/lymphoma:
- B-lymphoblastic leukemia/lymphoma, NOS
- B-lymphoblastic leukemia/lymphoma with recurrent genetic abnormalities
- B-lymphoblastic leukemia/lymphoma with t(9;22)(q34.1;q11.2); BCR-ABL1
- B-lymphoblastic leukemia/lymphoma with t(v;11q23.3);KMT2A rearranged
- B-lymphoblastic leukemia/lymphoma with t(12;21)(p13.2;q22.1); ETV6-RUNX1
- B-lymphoblastic leukemia/lymphoma with hyperdiploidy
- B-lymphoblastic leukemia/lymphoma with hypodiploidy
- B-lymphoblastic leukemia/lymphoma with t(5;14)(q31.1;q32.3) IL3-IGH
- B-lymphoblastic leukemia/lymphoma with t(1;19)(q23;p13.3); TCF3-PBX1
- Provisional entity: B-lymphoblastic leukemia/lymphoma, *BCR-ABL1*–like
- Provisional entity: B-lymphoblastic leukemia/lymphoma with iAMP21

T-lymphoblastic leukemia/lymphoma:
- Provisional entity: Early T-cell precursor lymphoblastic leukemia
- Provisional entity: Natural killer (NK) cell lymphoblastic leukemia/lymphoma

classification, and the specific entities of which they are composed. Lymphoid neoplasms are stratified according to their cell lineage and their derivation from precursor or mature lymphoid cells. **Box 2** lists the major subgroups of lymphoid neoplasms.

APPROACH TO TREATMENT

GENERAL PRINCIPLES OF MANAGEMENT

The broad principles of management consist of initial induction therapy (achieving remission), followed by consolidation phase (further cytoreduction) and in some situation maintenance phase (prolonged low-dose therapy). The treatment is further modified based on monitoring of disease parameters by complete blood counts, biomarkers, BM examination, minimal residual disease (MRD) assessment, and imaging at regular interval either alone or in combination.

Induction phase: The goal of induction is to improve marrow function by inducing CR which means an approximate 2-log reduction in tumor burden. CR represents a BM that appears normal morphologically and is functionally able to produce normal numbers of hematopoietic cells. Induction protocols may use conventional chemotherapeutic agents alone like 7 + 3 regimen of daunorubicin + cytarabine in AML or in combination with targeted therapy such as use of tyrosine kinase inhibitor (TKI) dasatinib in Philadelphia

BOX 2 Major subgroups of lymphoid neoplasms.

Mature B-cell neoplasms:
- Chronic lymphocytic leukemia/small lymphocytic lymphoma
- Monoclonal B-cell lymphocytosis
- B-cell prolymphocytic leukemia
- Splenic marginal zone lymphoma
- Hairy cell leukemia
- Splenic B-cell lymphoma/leukemia, unclassifiable
- Splenic diffuse red pulp small B-cell lymphoma
- Lymphoplasmacytic lymphoma
- Waldenstrom macroglobulinemia
- Plasma-cell myeloma
- Solitary plasmacytoma of bone
- Extraosseous plasmacytoma
- Extranodal marginal zone lymphoma of mucosa-associated lymphoid tissue
- Nodal marginal zone lymphoma
- Follicular lymphoma
- Large B-cell lymphoma with *IRF4* rearrangement
- Primary cutaneous follicle center lymphoma
- Mantle cell lymphoma
- Diffuse large B-cell lymphoma (DLBCL), not otherwise specified (NOS)
- T-cell/histiocyte-rich large B-cell lymphoma
- Primary DLBCL of the central nervous system (CNS)
- Primary cutaneous DLBCL, leg type
- Epstein-Barr virus 1(EBV1) DLBCL, NOS
- EBV1 mucocutaneous ulcer
- DLBCL-associated with chronic inflammation
- Lymphomatoid granulomatosis
- Primary mediastinal (thymic) large B-cell lymphoma
- Intravascular large B-cell lymphoma
- Anaplastic lymphoma kinase 1 (ALK1) large B-cell lymphoma
- Plasmablastic lymphoma
- Primary effusion lymphoma
- Human herpesvirus 81 (HHV81) DLBCL, NOS
- Burkitt lymphoma
- High-grade B-cell lymphoma, with *MYC* and *BCL2* and/or *BCL6* rearrangements
- High-grade B-cell lymphoma, NOS

Mature T and NK neoplasms:
- T-cell prolymphocytic leukemia
- T-cell large granular lymphocytic leukemia
- Chronic lymphoproliferative disorder of NK cells
- Aggressive NK-cell leukemia
- Adult T-cell leukemia/lymphoma
- Extranodal NK-/T-cell lymphoma, nasal type
- Enteropathy-associated T-cell lymphoma
- Hepatosplenic T-cell lymphoma
- Subcutaneous panniculitis-like T-cell lymphoma
- Mycosis fungoides

Continued...

Continued...

Mature T and NK neoplasms:
• Sezary syndrome
• Primary cutaneous CD301 T-cell lymphoproliferative disorders
• Lymphomatoid papulosis
• Primary cutaneous anaplastic large-cell lymphoma
• Primary cutaneous T-cell lymphoma
• Primary cutaneous CD81 aggressive epidermotropic cytotoxic T-cell lymphoma
• Peripheral T-cell lymphoma, NOS
• Angioimmunoblastic T-cell lymphoma
• Anaplastic large-cell lymphoma, *ALK1*
• Breast implant-associated anaplastic large-cell lymphoma
Hodgkin lymphoma:
• Nodular lymphocyte predominant Hodgkin lymphoma
• Classical Hodgkin lymphoma
• Nodular sclerosis classical Hodgkin lymphoma
• Lymphocyte-rich classical Hodgkin lymphoma
• Mixed cellularity classical Hodgkin lymphoma
• Lymphocyte-depleted classical Hodgkin lymphoma
Posttransplant lymphoproliferative disorders (PTLD)
Histiocytic and dendritic cell neoplasms
• Histiocytic sarcoma
• Langerhans cell histiocytosis
• Langerhans cell sarcoma
• Indeterminate dendritic cell tumor
• Interdigitating dendritic cell sarcoma
• Follicular dendritic cell sarcoma
• Fibroblastic reticular cell tumor
• Disseminated juvenile xanthogranuloma
• Erdheim–Chester disease

chromosome-positive acute lymphoblastic leukemia (ALL). Achievement of remission is linked with prolonged life expectancy. Infections and BM suppression are the major causes of morbidity and mortality in this phase.

Consolidation phase: After achieving CR, the next priority is to prevent disease relapse through further chemotherapy which is termed as "consolidation." The aim is to achieve further cytoreduction. Two options are usually available: More chemotherapy at induction level of intensity, chemotherapy with autologous or allogeneic hematopoietic cell transplantation (HCT).

Maintenance phase: This phase targets the minimal or microscopic residual disease that remains after the initial two phases and is a quintessential part of ALL therapy for patients who have not undergone an allogeneic HCT as part of their treatment. Maintenance therapy is not the standard of care in AML today, while it is used in patients with ALL, multiple myeloma (MM), and FL.

Hematopoietic cell transplantation: Two major forms of HCT can be distinguished. In autologous HCT, the stem cells are collected from the recipient and are reinfused at a later time. In allogeneic HCT, the cells originate from a different person who can be related or unrelated to the patient. The major benefit of autologous HCT is consolidation, achieved via the effects of the conditioning treatment.

The infusion of autologous hematopoietic cells allows the delivery of high-intensity therapies (conditioning regimen), which would result in irreversible myelosuppression in absence of hematopoietic cell infusion. It permits dose-intense chemotherapy/radiotherapy to be delivered to "debulk" or eradicate the tumor and "rescue" of the resultant marrow aplasia with recipient-derived hematopoietic cells derived from blood or BM. As the stem cells are recipient-derived, no immunosuppression is required. Common indications for this procedure are MM, NHL, and HL.

In allogeneic transplant, the donor immune system significantly contributes to the elimination of disease via the development of the graft versus leukemia or tumor effect. The graft versus leukemia effect can fully eradicate the underlying disease and is significantly exploited in achieving cure or eradicating MRD in ALL or AML.

ACUTE MYELOID LEUKEMIA

Improving outcomes in AML is one of the unmet needs in hematology practice today. Most patients are elderly at presentation with comorbid illnesses and functionally unfit for intense chemotherapy. For the young and fit patients, the *induction therapy* consists of combination of daunorubicin and cytarabine with the aim of achieving CR. About a two thirds of patients achieve CR and proceed to *consolidation therapy* which consists of high-dose cytarabine-based chemotherapy or allogeneic stem cell transplantation depending upon the cytogenetics and molecular risk stratification of patient. *Maintenance therapy* has not been shown clear survival benefit and hence it is rarely used after consolidation in AML. Infections are a major cause of induction mortality which is seen in at least 15–20% of AML patients in our country.

Prohibitive costs of induction regimen, treatment-related complications, and need for allogenic HCT lead to optimal treatment in <10 % of AML patients in our country. Nonetheless, it is promising to note that treatment of AML has changed substantially in the last 5 years. New targeted drugs have emerged, including venetoclax to target B-cell lymphoma 2 (BCL-2), midostaurin and gilteritinib to target FLT3, and ivosidenib and enasidenib to target mutant isocitrate dehydrogenase 1 and 2, respectively. Other additions include gemtuzumab and ozogomycin to target CD33, glasdegib to target the hedgehog pathway, and a liposomal formulation of daunorubicin and cytarabine.

Prognosis: The 3-year overall survival (OS) rates of AML have remained dismal and vary from 40% for good-risk patients to 4% for patients with poor risk stratification. Clinical trials with new agents may transform the outcome of AML patients in future.

Acute promyelocytic leukemia (APL) is a distinct subtype of AML that is cytogenetically characterized by a balanced reciprocal translocation between chromosomes 15 and 17, which results in the fusion of the promyelocytic leukemia and retinoic acid receptor alpha (*RARa*) genes. Because patients with APL are at high risk of bleeding diathesis and infection APL was historically considered to be one of the most fatal forms of acute leukemia till the advent of targeted chemo-free therapy. The cure of APL is achievable today with the use of all-transretinoic acid (ATRA) and arsenic trioxide (ATO)-containing regimens in at least 90% patients today.

ACUTE LYMPHOBLASTIC LEUKEMIA

The aim of initial treatment is to achieve CR similar to AML and complete eradication of ALL cells from the blood, BM, and extramedullary sites. The treatment of ALL has evolved into "complex protocols" that essentially consist of corticosteroid prephase, one to two phases of induction therapy, consolidation with high-dose methotrexate, reinduction or late intensification, and prolonged maintenance therapy. *The regimens* usually consist of the following core agents in addition to steroids: Vincristine, anthracyclines alkylating agents, and L-asparaginase. CR rates following induction therapy are high with over 90% of ALL patients achieving morphological remission. *Consolidation therapy* in ALL is administered following CR with the aim of eliminating residual leukemia cells and to prevent the emergence of drug-resistant disease. This usually consists of several cycles of treatment chemotherapy, including central nervous system (CNS)-directed therapy. *Maintenance therapy* is essential for childhood ALL patient while the clear evidence of its use in adult ALL is lacking though it is given to most patient. 6-mercaptopurine, methotrexate, and pulses of vincristine and steroids usually constitute the maintenance therapy cocktail and is usually given for a period of approximately 2–2.5 years after consolidation. The aim of maintenance is to eliminate MRD and dosing of the chemotherapeutic agents needs to be titrated to trade off moderate myelosuppression with treatment-related toxicity, especially neutropenic sepsis or hemorrhage. Allogeneic stem cell transplant is considered standard for high-risk ALL patients or ALL patients who relapse after initial remission.

Significant scientific advances in recent years have improved the outcome in ALL. Emergence of the concept of measurable residual disease has fine-tuned our prognostic models and guides our treatment decisions today. The use of TKIs targeting *BCR-ABL1*, monoclonal antibodies targeting CD20 (rituximab), antibody–drug conjugates targeting CD22 (inotuzumab ozogamicin), bispecific antibodies (blinatumomab), and CD19 chimeric antigen receptor T-cell therapy (tisagenlecleucel) have revolutionized treatment outcomes in both frontline and relapse setting of ALL. Novel approaches with these agents have indeed reduced reliance on intensive cytotoxic chemotherapy and hematopoietic stem cell transplantation in first remission, especially in resource-rich settings.

Prognosis: Nonetheless unlike pediatric ALL, which is curable in >90% of cases, adult ALL has historically had a dismal prognosis with cure rates <40%.

CHRONIC MYELOID LEUKEMIA

Chronic myeloid leukemia (CML) is a myeloproliferative neoplasm characterized by rearrangement of the long arms of chromosome 9 and 22, resulting in the Philadelphia chromosome, creating the fusion oncogene *BCR-ABL1*. The fusion gene encodes for a constitutively active tyrosine kinase that occurs in a hemopoietic progenitor and confers proliferative and antiapoptotic effects.

CML is among the first malignancies where targeted therapy with TKI was used which increased the survival of chronic phase (CP)-CML patients to at par with normal population. In the pre-TKI era, the annual mortality in CML was 10% in the first 2 years and 15–20% thereafter. The median survival time in CML was 3–7 years. With TKI therapy, the annual mortality in CML has decreased to 2% and 10-year survival rates are ~85%.

More than two-thirds of patients present in CP of the disease but about a third present in advanced phases, namely accelerated phase (AP) and blast crisis (BC). Monotherapy with a first-generation TKI, imatinib, has been the standard of care for CML patients for almost two decades now. Initially considered to be lifelong therapy, a proportion of patients may be able to cease their TKI therapy entirely without losing their remissions status referred to as treatment-free remission (TFR). The availability of generic version of second-generation TKI such as dasatinib and their rapid and deeper responses have resulted in them being preferred agents upfront, especially in high-risk CML patients; patients presenting in AP/BC and those desiring earlier TFR such as in women planning pregnancy.

Prior to the introduction of TKIs, CML was one of the most common indications for allogeneic HCT. Today, HCT is now reserved for patients with advanced phase disease or in case of therapeutic failure of two or more TKIs.

Prognosis: Although the great majority of patients with CP-CML has an excellent prognosis, intolerance to currently available TKI is not uncommon and resistance to TKI therapy due to *BCR-ABL* mutations occurs invariably in most patients.

LYMPHOMAS

Treatment strategy in lymphomas is based on their histological type, staging of the disease, performance status of patient, and various prognostic models. For example, in low-grade lymphomas such as FL even in advanced-stage asymptomatic disease, watch-and-wait strategy is acceptable but in high-grade lymphomas such as diffuse large B-cell lymphomas (DLBCL) treatment is invariably mandated. Depth of response to treatment has also been used to provide prognostic information with the evidence to show that patients achieving CR after treatment have significantly longer duration of response than patients achieving only partial remission (PR). Remission status determined by FDG-PET (fluorodeoxyglucose-positron emission tomography) has also been shown to be more predictive of outcome than by conventional imaging.

There are four main groups of therapeutic modalities for treatment of lymphomas: Conventional chemotherapeutic agents, combination chemoimmunotherapy, radiotherapy, and novel agents. Surgery is rarely used to treat lymphomas.

Chemotherapy regimens used for treatment of HL are: (1) ABVD (adriamycin, bleomycin, vinblastine, and dacarbazine) and (2) the more intense escalated BEACOPP (bleomycin, etoposide, adriamycin, cyclophosphamide, vincristine, procarbazine, and prednisolone) regimen. Combination chemoimmunotherapy like RCHOP (rituximab, cyclophosphamide, doxorubicin, vincristine, prednisolone) is one of the frontline therapeutic options today in treating aggressive lymphomas such as DLBCL. It combines the immune-mediated cytotoxicity of rituximab targeting CD20 with conventional multi-agent chemotherapy.

Radiotherapy is a highly effective modality for the treatment of HL and FL. Indeed, radiotherapy alone was used in 1960s as curative therapy for HL till the advent of effective chemotherapy regimens such as ABVD. Nonetheless, involved field radiotherapy (IFRT) and, more typically, involved node radiotherapy (INRT) are now used, resulting in a dramatically lower volume of normal tissue irradiated compared to the more extensive historical fields. IFRT is also curative in early-stage FL and is now recommended as one of the treatment options.

Novel agents or targeted therapy have also improved treatment outcomes, especially in the relapse of refractory settings of lymphoma treatment. For example, brentuximabvedotin (BV) is an antibody–drug conjugate, which consists of an anti-CD30 antibody conjugated to an antimicrotubule agent monomethyl auristatin E (MMAE) and has revolutionized treatment outcomes in relapse or refractory HL. The specificity of the anti-CD30 antibody is used to guide the cytotoxin (MMAE) to the Reed Sternberg cells in HL, where binding of the anti-CD30 antibody–drug conjugate is followed by receptor-mediated endocytosis and delivery of the cytotoxic agent upon hydrolysis of the linker molecule by lysosomal enzymes. Checkpoint inhibitors such as nivolumab and pembrolizumab are increasingly used either alone or in combination in relapsed refractory HL and primary mediastinal large B-cell lymphoma.

For patient's refractory to first-line therapy as above and for those with disease relapse salvage chemotherapy followed by autologous HCT is recommended.

Prognosis: Median survival rates in lymphomas are highly variable. Hodgkin's lymphoma has one of the best outcomes and 10-year survival figures now exceed 80%, compared with <50% 40 years ago. On the other hand, aggressive NHLs such as DLBCL have modest outcomes with a progression-free survival of 35% and a 10-year OS of 43.5% following RCHOP therapy.

MULTIPLE MYELOMA

The approach to treatment of symptomatic newly diagnosed MM is dictated by eligibility for autologous HCT and risk stratification. Transplant-eligible patients are treated with approximately 3–4 cycles of induction therapy followed by autologous HCT. The *induction therapy* generally consists of combination of three drugs (triplet), e.g., proteasome inhibitor (bortezomib, carfilzomib) with immunomodulatory drug (e.g., thalidomide/lenalidomide) or alkylator (e.g., cyclophosphamide) and steroid (e.g., dexamethasone or prednisolone). In high-risk patients, especially those with double-hit or triple-hit myeloma, quadruplet regimens incorporating novel agents such as daratumumab is added to triplet regimen as described above for 3–4 cycles followed by auto HCT. *Maintenance therapy* is given indefinitely following auto HCT. Transplant ineligible patients are generally treated with 12–18 cycles of triplet therapy followed by low-dose maintenance therapy indefinitely. Lenalidomide is the standard of care for maintenance therapy for standard-risk patients and bortezomib for high-risk myeloma. Almost all patients with MM eventually relapse. The choice of a treatment regimen at relapse is usually decided by considering the timing of the relapse, response to prior therapy, aggressiveness of the relapse, and performance status of patient.

Prognosis: Patients with standard-risk MM have a median OS of >7 years while those with high-risk disease have a median OS of approximately 3 years, despite autologous HCT. The availability of monoclonal antibodies and targeted therapy may improve the outcomes in future.

CHRONIC LYMPHOCYTIC LEUKEMIA

Chronic lymphocytic leukemia (CLL) is generally seen in older adults and may not cause symptoms for years. Many people live for a long period of time without treatment. Further, early treatment in asymptomatic patients has not shown any benefit and thus treatment is advised only in symptomatic patients. *CLL patients with symptomatic or active disease as defined by* at least one of the following criteria needs treatment:

- Evidence of progressive marrow failure as manifested by the development of, or worsening of, anemia and/or thrombocytopenia
- Massive (i.e., ≥6 cm below the left costal margin) or progressive or symptomatic splenomegaly
- Massive nodes (i.e., ≥10 cm in longest diameter) or progressive or symptomatic lymphadenopathy
- Progressive lymphocytosis with an increase of ≥50% over a 2-month period, or lymphocyte doubling time (LDT) of <6 months
- Autoimmune complications including anemia or thrombocytopenia poorly responsive to corticosteroids
- Symptomatic or functional extranodal involvement (e.g., skin, kidney, lung)

- Disease-related symptoms as defined by any of the following:
    - Unintentional weight loss ≥10% within the previous 6 months.
    - Significant fatigue (i.e., ECOG PS ≤ 2)
    - Fever ≥100.5°F for 2 or more weeks without evidence of infection
    - Night sweats for ≥1 month without evidence of infection

The *management of CLL* has undergone dramatic changes over the previous two decades with the introduction of targeted therapy. The following options either alone or in combination exist: Ibrutinib monotherapy, chemoimmunotherapy combination of venetoclax with rituximab or obinutuzumab, bendamustine and rituximab, chlorambucil and prednisolone, mini-RCHOP or CVP (cyclophosphamide, vincristine, and prednisolone). When deciding treatment, patient's age, performance status, presence of comorbidities, and cytogenetics and *IGHV* mutation status are taken into account. For physically fit patients younger than 65, especially those patients with a mutated *IGVH* gene, chemoimmunotherapy with fludarabine, cyclophosphamide, and rituximab remains a standard therapy, since it may have curative potential. Patients with a del (17p) or *TP53* mutation constitute a high-risk category and should be treated with targeted agents such as inhibitors of Bruton tyrosine kinase (ibrutinib/acalabrutinib) or Bcl2-antagonists (venetoclax). Allogeneic HCT may be considered in relapsing patients with *TP53* mutations or del (17p), or patients that are refractory to targeted therapy.

Prognosis: The median survival of patients with CLL has improved over the last decade and is now around 10 years.

RECOMMENDED READINGS

1. Swerdlow SH, Campo E, Harris NL, Jaffe ES, Pileri SA, Stein H, et al. WHO Classification of Tumours of Haematopoietic and Lymphoid Tissues. Lyon, France: IARC; 2008.
2. Hoffbrand AV, Moss PAH. Hoffbrand's Essential Hematology, 7th edition. USA: John Wiley & Sons Ltd; 2015.
3. Rodgers GP, Young NS. The Bethesda Handbook of Clinical Hematology, 4th edition. USA: Wolters Kluwer; 2018.
4. Yanamandra U, Malhotra P. CML in India: Are We There Yet? Indian J Hematol Blood Transfus. 2019;35(1):1-2.
5. Jain A, Jain A, Malhotra P. Re-defining prognosis of hematological malignancies by dynamic response assessment methods: Lessons learnt in chronic myeloid leukemia, Hodgkin lymphoma, diffuse large B cell lymphoma and multiple myeloma. Indian J Hematol Blood Transfus. 2020;36(3):447-57.
6. Yanamandra U, Malhotra P. Myeloma at cross roads in India. Indian J Hematol Blood Transfus. 2018;34(4):593-4.
7. Tejaswi V, Lad DP, Jindal N, Prakash G, Malhotra P, Khadwal A, et al. Chronic lymphocytic leukemia: Real-world data from India. JCO Glob Oncol. 2020;6:866-72.
8. Nair R, Kakroo A, Bapna A, Gogia A, Vora A, Pathak A, et al. Management of lymphomas: Consensus Document 2018 by an Indian Expert Group. Indian J Hematol Blood Transfus. 2018;34(3):398-421.

Oncology

CHAPTER 158 Cancer: Hallmarks and Prevention

Davinder Paul, Subhadeep Bose

ABSTRACT

The hallmarks of cancer provide us with the framework, as to how a normal cell gets transformed into a cancer cell. There are six such classical hallmarks, i.e., sustaining proliferative signaling, evading growth suppressors, resisting cell death, enabling replicative immortality, inducing angiogenesis, and activating invasion and metastasis. The acquisition of these hallmark phenotypical changes is in turn made possible by the ever-increasing genomic instability in the cancer cells, which are propagated from progeny to progeny. Understanding these hallmarks has given us number of targets through which we can hit cancer cells. Of course, over last 20 years, an ever-increasing list of targeted drugs including immunotherapy have ushered an era of great fight and success against cancer, resulting in saving millions of lives.

Further, fight against cancer cannot be fought by just improving cancer therapies: Cancer prevention plays an equal or may be a more important role. Cancer prevention remains an urgent public health priority on a global scale. Till date, the greatest success in dealing with cancer has not been through a particular drug, but through cancer prevention in the form of tobacco control and vaccination against hepatitis B virus and human papillomavirus. Cancer screening against breast, cervical, and colorectal cancer has made considerable impact on cancer incidence and mortality in the developed countries, but their implementation has been poor in the developing and poor countries, which constitutes the major burden of such patients. Bridging this gap of effective implementation is a global challenge of utmost priority.

"You beat cancer by how you live, why you live, and in the manner in which you live"

—Stuart Scott

INTRODUCTION

There are six hallmarks of cancer (**Fig. 1**), which provide the basic framework for deciphering the remarkable diversity and biology of this disease. These six hallmarks are sustaining proliferative signaling, evading growth suppressors, resisting cell death, enabling replicative immortality, inducing angiogenesis, and activating invasion and metastasis. During transformation from normal to malignant cell, there are successive acquisitions of these hallmark capabilities that help them to become malignant.

Now over the last few years, increasing studies and ongoing research have suggested that there are two additional hallmarks of cancer involved in the tumorigenesis (**Fig. 2**). The first one involves the ability to modify and reprogram the cellular metabolism in such a way to most effectively help the proliferation of cancer cells. The second additional hallmark capability allows the cancer cells to escape the destruction mediated by the immunological cells, especially by T and B lymphocytes. As these additional hallmark capabilities and not yet fully validated, so they are labeled as emerging hallmarks.

Further, there are two more characteristics, which have been labeled as cancer enabling characteristics. These are not hallmarks in their own right, but they help the cancer cells in acquisition of both the core as well as the emerging hallmarks. These are genomic instability and tumor promoting inflammation. Genomic instability empowers the cancer cells by producing genetic alterations that propagate tumor progression. Inflammation produced by the immune cells is designed to fight infections in the body. But it can indirectly support the acquisition of various cancer hallmarks. Now we will discuss all these properties individually.

CANCER HALLMARKS

SUSTAINING PROLIFERATIVE SIGNALING

The most primitive and basic trait of cancer cell is immortality, which means the capability of endless proliferation. In normal homeostasis, tissue controls their size by meticulously controlling the production of new cells. This is done by carefully managing the production and release of growth promoting signals that instructs the cell to enter and navigate through the various phases of cell cycle. Cancer cells by causing dysregulation of these growth signals, acquires the property of chronic proliferation. These empowering signals are conveyed by growth factors, which bind to the cell surface receptors. This binding leads to downstream signaling through branched intracellular signaling pathways that regulate the journey through the

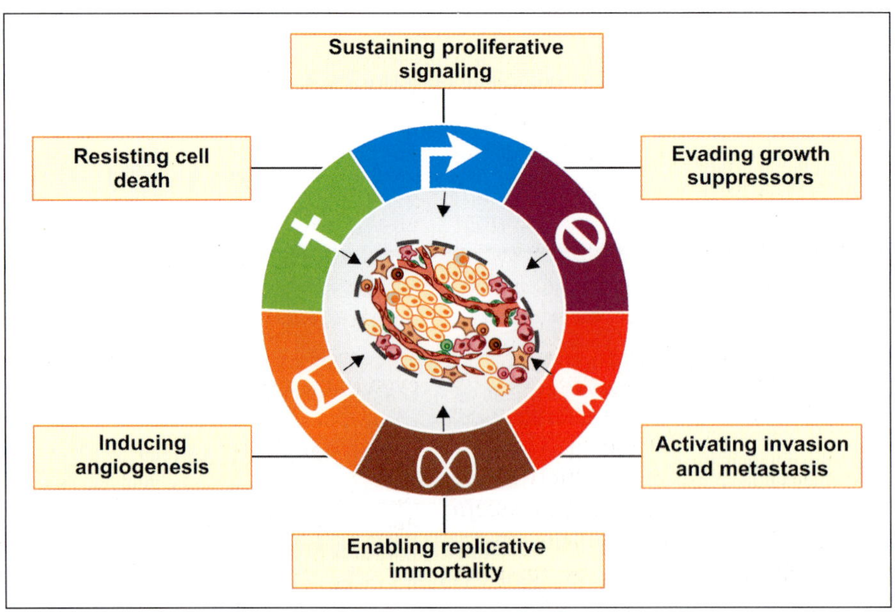

FIGURE 1: The hallmarks of cancer.

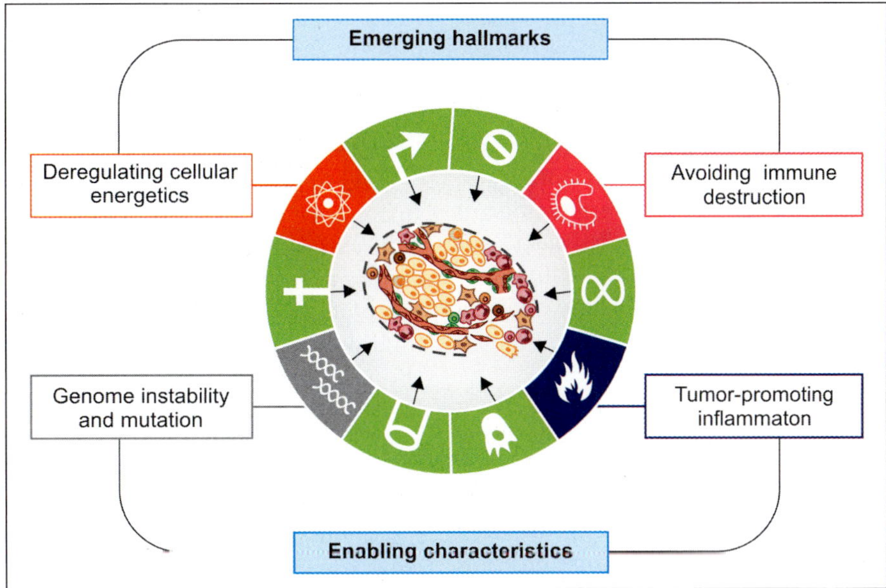

FIGURE 2: The emerging hallmarks and enabling characteristics.

cell cycle. There are some alternate ways also of attaining chronic proliferative capacity.

Cancer cells can produce growth factor themselves, which go and attach to the receptor on the cell surface resulting in autocrine proliferation. Alternatively, cancer cells can send signals to stimulate surrounding normal cells to produce various growth factors and then these growth factors help in cancer cell proliferation. Another important mechanism for sustained proliferation is the growth factor independence, which is attained by constitutive activation of certain components of the signaling pathways operating downstream to these receptors, negating the need to stimulate these pathways by ligand-mediated receptor activation. For example, about 40% of malignant melanoma contains activating mutations targeting the structure of the B-Raf protein, which results in constitutive signaling through the Raf to mitogen-activated protein (MAP)-kinase pathway, without any stimulation from the upstream ligand-mediated receptor activation.

Another important mechanism is the dysregulation of the negative feedback loops, which under normal situation operate to downgrade or stop various types of signaling and thereby ensuring homeostasis. Defects in these feedback mechanisms enhance the capability of proliferation in cancer cells. An example of this type of negative feedback loop involves the Ras oncoprotein. The tumorigenic effect of Ras does not result from an overstimulation of its upstream or downstream signaling pathway. Instead, the oncogenic mutations targeting the *Ras* genes compromise Ras GTPase activity. Now the Ras GTPase operates as an intrinsic negative feedback mechanism, which under normal condition ensures that stimulation of the Ras system remains transitory only. So, when this Ras GTPase activity is compromised, the stimulation of Ras system becomes constitutively active leading to sustained proliferation.

EVADING GROWTH SUPPRESSORS

Under normal homeostasis in the body, there are many tumor suppressor genes, which control powerful programs that negatively regulate cell proliferation and thus limiting cell growth. The two most important *tumor suppressor genes* are those encoding for RB (retinoblastoma-associated) protein and TP53 protein. These two proteins are the central keynote switches in the two key complementary cellular regulatory pathways that govern the decisions for the cells to proliferate or alternatively activate apoptotic programs and die.

The RB protein receives proliferative signals from various extracellular and intracellular sources. It then processes these signals and then decides whether, or not the cell should proceed through the cell growth cycle. Due to this reason, *RB* gene is called the gatekeeper gene of the cell cycle. Many cancer cells have defects in the RB pathway function, which allows persistent cell proliferation as there is no gatekeeper to stop it anymore. *The TP53 protein* plays the role of a sensor judging about the level of damage happening to the cell. It receives inputs from various stress and abnormality sensors within the cell. If TP53 finds that the damage to the cellular genome is excessive, it triggers the apoptotic pathway which ultimately leads to cellular death. Cancer cells with mutation in the *TP53* gene loose this property; thereby sustain continuous proliferation, even in the presence of excessive genomic damage.

RESISTING CELL DEATH

Apoptosis, which is also known as programmed cell death, serves as a barrier for controlling unnecessary cell proliferation and cancer development. The apoptotic pathway is composed of two components: The upstream regulators and the downstream effectors. The upstream regulators are further divided into two major components. First one receiving and processing extracellular death inducing signals, known as extrinsic apoptotic program. Second one receiving and processing intracellular death inducing signals, known as intrinsic apoptotic program. Both of these programs finally culminate in the activation of the downstream effector protease enzymes called caspase-8 and caspase-9. These enzymes normally remain latent and dormant, but once activated, they execute the final phase of apoptosis, in which the cell is progressively disassembled and finally consumed by phagocytic cells.

The interplay between the regulators and effectors is managed by a counterbalancing pro- and antiapoptotic members of the Bcl-2 family of proteins. The antiapoptotic members are Bcl-2, Bcl-xl, Bcl-w, and Mcl-1. They inhibit apoptosis by binding to and then inhibiting two proapoptotic proteins, Bax and Bak, which are present in the outer membrane of mitochondria. When these proapoptotic proteins are relieved of this inhibition by the proapoptotic proteins, they in turn cause disruption of the outer mitochondrial membrane, which leads to release of multiple proapoptotic signaling proteins, most important among them being cytochrome c. Cytochrome c in turn activates series of proteolytic enzymes called caspases, which executes the final cellular changes of the apoptosis.

Cancer cells acquire number of strategies to prevent apoptosis. Most common being the loss of TP53 gatekeeper tumor suppressor gene function, which removes this critical damage sensor protein from the apoptosis-inducing mechanism. Alternatively, cancer cells can circumvent apoptosis by increasing the expression of antiapoptotic proteins or by downregulating the expression of proapoptotic proteins.

ENABLING REPLICATIVE IMMORTALITY

The unlimited replicative potential is prerequisite for the cancer cells to grow and spread. Multiple lines of evidence have now proved that telomeres present at the ends of chromosomes are centrally involved in attaining the capability of unlimited proliferation.

The telomeres consist of multiple tandem hexanucleotide repeats and in normal cells, they keep on progressively shortening in size with each cell cycle. After certain number of cell cycles, the telomeres size reduces to such an extent that they finally lose the ability to protect the ends of chromosomes from end-to-end fusion. Such end-to-end fusion leads to formation of dicentric chromosomes, which are genetically unstable and ultimately leads to activation of apoptosis leading to cell death. So, the length of telomeric deoxyribonucleic acid (DNA) in a cell holds the key as to much replicative potential that particular cell has.

Telomerase are specialized DNA polymerase; whose function is to add telomere repeat segments to the ends of the telomeric DNA. This particular DNA polymerase is almost absent in normal human cell, but in >90% cancer cells it is expressed at a significantly higher level. By adding to the telomeric DNA length, these telomerases are able to prevent the progressive telomere erosion, which in turn provide the replicative immortality to the cancer cells.

INDUCING ANGIOGENESIS

Like in normal human tissues, tumor tissue also requires sustenance in the form of food and oxygen as well as the ability to evacuate metabolic wastes and carbon dioxide. During normal human embryogenesis, the development of vasculature involves the birth of new endothelial cells and their assembly into tubes (vasculogenesis) in addition to sprouting (angiogenesis) of new vessels from existing ones. Once these blood vessels are formed, these properties of vasculogenesis and angiogenesis become largely quiescent. During normal human life, as a response to events such as wound healing and female reproductive cycling, only transient activation of angiogenesis happens. On the contrary, in cancer cells a phenomenon called "*angiogenic switch*" is almost always activated, whereby normally quiescent blood vessels are continuously stimulated to sprout new blood vessels that help sustain expanding cancer tissues. This angiogenic switch is in turn regulated by opposing factors which either induce or oppose angiogenesis. Example of such angiogenesis inducers and inhibitors are *vascular endothelial growth factor-A (VEGF-A) and thrombospondin-1 (TSP-1)*, respectively. Unlike the normal human blood vessels, the blood vessels produced within the cancer tissue are typically aberrant, poorly formed with marked leakiness. This happens because of unbalanced and uncoordinated interplay of various proangiogenic signals.

ACTIVATING INVASION AND METASTASIS

The final journey of most of the cancer involves their invasion into the surrounding structures and ultimately their spread to distant sites in the body. The underlying property which bestows the cancer cells these properties involves alterations in their shape as well as their attachments to other cancer cells and to extracellular matrix (ECM). The most studied alteration involves the downregulation and ultimate *loss of E-cadherin*, a key cell-to-cell adhesion molecule by cancer cells. In normal tissues, role of E-cadherin is to form and maintain adherent junctions between adjacent epithelial cells. Increased expression of E-cadherin by normal cell has been proved to be a natural barrier for invasion and metastases, whereas reduced expression of this molecule by the cancer cells helps them in causing invasion and metastases.

Further there are some more adhesion molecules, which are concerned with cell adhesion and migration normally seen during embryogenesis and inflammation. These molecules are also upregulated in the cancer cells. For example, N-cadherin, a molecule which during normal organogenesis helps in migration of neurons and mesenchymal cells, has been found to be upregulated in many cancer cells.

The multistep process of invasion and metastasis is called the *invasion-metastasis cascade*. It consists of multiple sequences of well-defined steps enumerating the progressive gain of phenotypical changes in the cancer cells. These consists of local invasion, followed by intravasation into surrounding blood and lymphatic vessels leading to hematogenous and lymphatic migration of cancer cells to distant tissues, followed by escaping of cancer cells through the lumina of vessels into distant tissues (extravasation), followed by formation of small colonies of cancer cells in such tissue (micrometastases), and finally the consequent growth of these micrometastatic lesions into macroscopic tumors (colonization).

ENABLING CHARACTERISTICS

GENOME INSTABILITY AND MUTATION

The underlying principle for acquisition of all the hallmarks enumerated till now is the continuous acquisition of alterations in the genomic profile of cancer cells. During the process of converting from normal genotype to mutant genotype, cancer cells pass on these genomic alterations to their progeny and at each subclone level, few more genetic alterations are added. This in turn confer these cancer cells with progressively increasing survival advantage as compared to surrounding normal cells, enabling their profound growth, and eventual dominance in local tissue environment. Thus, in nut shell, the multistep tumor progression can be seen as succession of clonal expansion by progeny after progeny of cancer cells, enabling a mutant genotype.

However, in normal human body, there are number of extraordinary systems whose sole purpose is to detect and resolve such spontaneous genomic alterations, and thus preventing the formation of mutant genotype. These are called genomic surveillance machinery. Cancer cells can circumvent this surveillance machinery in two ways. First, they can increase rate of mutation to such a limit, that *genomic surveillance machinery* is not able to cope up the challenge. Secondly, cancer cells can produce breakdown in one or the several components of this surveillance machinery.

TUMOR-PROMOTING INFLAMMATION

It has long been recognized by the pathologist, that some cancer tissues are profoundly infiltrated by cells involved in both innate and adaptive immunity, mimicking an inflammatory condition in normal tissues. Now lot of research has finally concluded that inflammation can definitely help in acquiring multiple hallmark capabilities by supplying various bioactive ingredients to the tumor microenvironment, such as growth factors, proangiogenic factors, factors limiting cell death, and extracellular matrix-modifying enzymes that help in angiogenesis, invasion, and metastasis.

EMERGING HALLMARKS

REPROGRAMMING ENERGY METABOLISM

The continuous and uncontrolled proliferation in the cancer cells cannot happen without corresponding changes in energy metabolism which can provide fuel for cell growth and division. In normal tissues under aerobic conditions, glucose is first processed to pyruvate via glycolysis in cytoplasm, which goes to mitochondria and gets converted to carbon dioxide.

In normal tissues, the metabolism of glucose through glycolysis leads to generation of energy in the form of adenosine triphosphate (ATP). The end product of this process can be two types. Under normal aerobic conditions, full oxidation of glucose happens via respiration in the mitochondria, leading to generation of CO_2. Under anaerobic conditions, due to unavailability of O_2, fermentation happens leading to generation of lactate. In cancer cells, it has been observed that even in the presence of oxygen and fully functional mitochondria, second process of fermentation is favored. This is known as Warburg effect or aerobic glycolysis. Although by this process, the number of ATP molecules generated are less as compared to full oxidation in mitochondria, but cancer cells compensate this loss in other ways. In cancer cells, rate of glucose uptake increases dramatically and following the Warburg metabolism, an equally increased amount of lactate and other glycolytic intermediates are generated. The cancer cells divert these intermediates into various biosynthetic pathways which are required for assembling new cells, like those generating nucleosides and amino acids. So, cancer cells compensate the low rate of energy generation by increasing the rate of generation of basic molecules required for cell growth and division.

EVADING IMMUNE DESTRUCTION

An enigmatic issue concerned with cancer development is regarding the role played by body's immune system in resisting or eliminating the cancer cells to grow and metastasize. The long-held theory of immune surveillance says that cells and tissues in human body are constantly monitored by an alert immune system, whereby incipient cancer cells are rapidly recognized and eliminated from the body. But still cancer develops in many patients. Cancer cells can do this by two ways. First, by avoiding detection by immune surveillance machinery. Secondly, although they get detected by immune system, but they are able to either limit or totally avoid the extent of immunological killing, thus avoiding total eradication. This hypothesis is given strength by strikingly increased incidence of certain cancers in immunocompromised individuals.

THERAPEUTIC TARGETING

Over the last few decades, decoding the cancer genomic and molecular profile has yielded astounding success stories by providing remarkable progress in cancer therapeutics. Many cancers which were considered totally incurable are nowadays cured by simple targeted medications. Of course, these all are made possible after understanding the basic hallmarks of cancer which have been enumerated above. The rapidly increasing list of targeted anticancer therapies can be enumerated according to the cancer hallmark capabilities against which they are acting upon (**Fig. 3**).

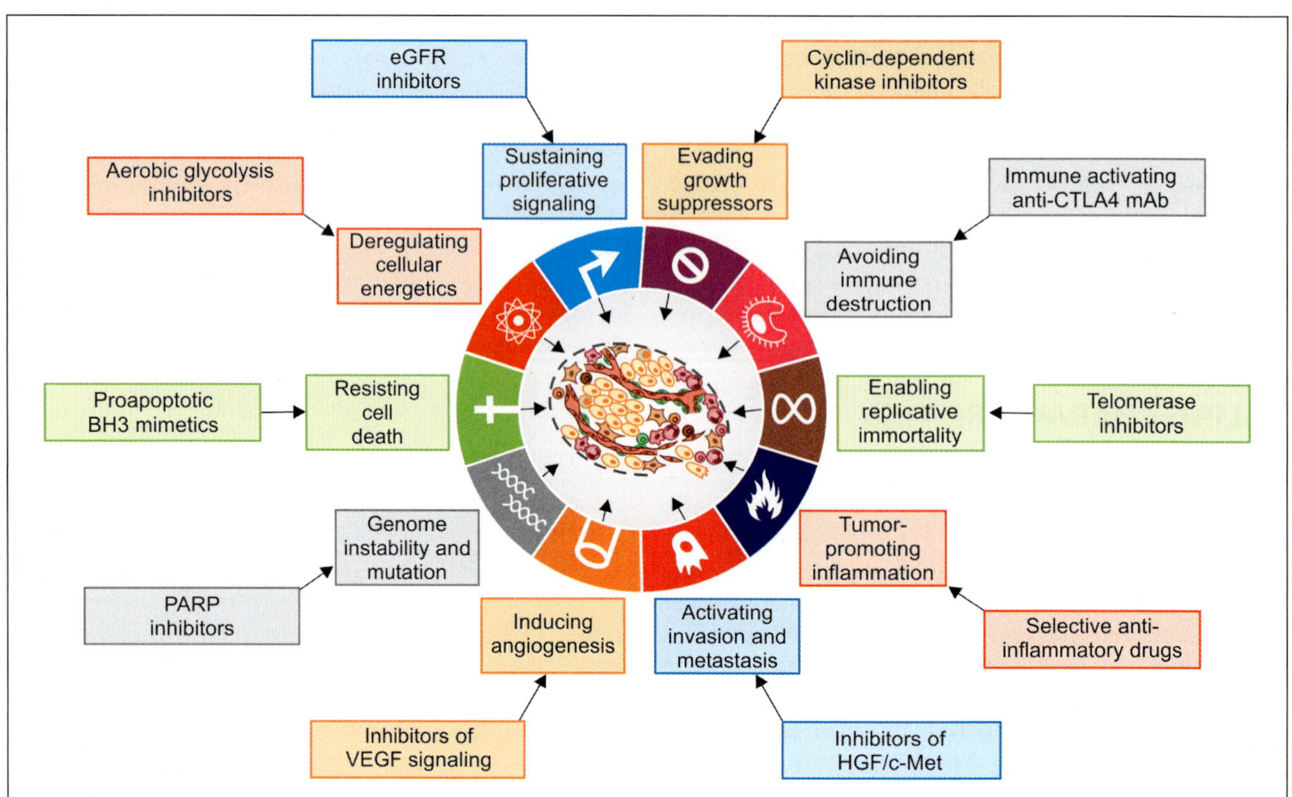

(eGFR: epidermal growth factor receptor; HGF/c-Met: hepatocyte growth factor/c-mesenchymal-epithelial transition; VEGF: vascular endothelial growth factor)

FIGURE 3: Therapeutic targeting of the hallmarks of cancer.

The advantage of such targeted therapies is their specificity, that is they act against only the cancer cells, while having virtually minimal or no effects on the normal cells.

CANCER PREVENTION

INTRODUCTION

Worldwide cancer remains an ever-increasing threat to the mankind, both in terms of increasing number and increasing deaths. The World Health Organization predicts that by 2025, the number of new cases per year will increase from 14 million to 19 million, by 2030 to 21.7 million, and by 2035 up to 24 million. This global problem cannot be dealt with by just improving the cancer treatment, but more importantly requires effective preventive strategies, both at primary and secondary levels. Cancer research from around the world has proved that cancer risk reduction is best achieved by adopting a healthy lifestyle, regular screening, and by avoiding exposure to carcinogens. Primary and secondary prevention is the basic approach to control cancer, and it is estimated that at least one-third of all cancers are preventable.

PRIMARY PREVENTION

Cancer prevention was mainly concerned with early diagnosis of disease, mostly at a precancerous stage. Later it was understood that controlling the causative factors of some cancers are preferred in the general population and also in particular occupational groups. Since primary prevention is directed at large population groups, the cost can be high and program difficult to conduct. Some of the primary preventive measures include:

- *Control of tobacco and alcohol consumption* has remained one of the major primary preventive interventions over last four decades and it has resulted in saving millions of lives.
- *Maintaining good personal hygiene* and avoiding obesity reduces the risk of many cancers such as cervical cancer, head and neck cancer, and gastrointestinal tract cancer.
- *Avoiding exposure to occupational carcinogens* such as asbestos, radon, arsenic, chromium, silica, beryllium, nickel, cadmium,, and diesel exhaust.
- Immunization against the hepatitis B virus helps in preventing primary liver cancer, and immunization against HPV helps in preventing cervical cancer.
- *Early detection and prompt treatment* of precancerous lesions such as cervical tears, intestinal polyposis, warts, chronic gastritis, chronic cervicitis, and adenoma.
- Enforcing stringent *legislation against environmental carcinogens* such as tobacco, alcohol, and air pollution.
- *Cancer education* is an important area of primary prevention. This helps to promote awareness of cancer and helps the individuals to know the early warning

signs or danger signals of cancer. Also, this cancer education motivates people to undergo early diagnosis and early treatment.

SECONDARY PREVENTION

Secondary preventive measures comprise of:

- *Cancer registration*: It is necessary for any kind of cancer control program. This promotes the base for assessing the magnitude of problem and helps in planning the necessary services. Basically, cancer registries are of two types:
  - i. *Hospital-based registries*: This registry includes information of all patients treated by a particular institution. The collected information can be helpful in evaluating the diagnostic and treatment program. As this registry only includes the selected population, it is only helpful for epidemiological purposes.
  - ii. *Population-based registries*: This registry includes information of a complete cancer situation in a given geographic area. It provides incidence rate of cancer and serves as an initiating tool for epidemiological inquiries into causes of cancer, surveillance of time trends, planning, and evaluation of operational activities in all main areas of cancer control.
- *Early detection of cases*:
  - Cancer screening is an important step for early detection of cancer at a preinvasive or premalignant stage.
  - Effective screening programs have been developed for cervical, breast, and oral cancer.
- *Treatment*:
  - Treatment facilities should be available to all cancer patients.
  - Certain forms of cancer are manageable by surgical removal, while some others favorably respond to radiation or chemotherapy or both.

CONCLUSION AND FUTURE VISION

The concepts of cancer hallmarks have provided us with the framework for deciphering and understanding the complexities involved in this enigmatic disease. These hallmarks have started yielding astounding results in the form of new targeted therapies and immunotherapy, which have saved millions of lives. Further refinement in these hallmark capabilities will surely be made in the foreseeable future and thus the coming few decades will provide us with an ever-increasing potent and safe armamentarium of therapies against this disease. Cancer research has now taught us beyond any doubt that we can never defeat cancer by just focusing on the treatment. Prevention of cancer plays an even more important role. Cancer prevention applies to both the primary prevention and the secondary prevention. Improvement in cancer prevention strategies coupled with staggering progress in understanding cancer genomics and ever-increasing list of targeted anticancer therapies including immunotherapy over next few decades will usher the golden period of our fight against this disease.

RECOMMENDED READINGS

1. Hanahan D, Weinberg RA. The hallmarks of cancer. Cell. 2000;100:57-70.
2. Cheng N, Chytil A, Shyr Y, Joly A, Moses HL. Transforming growth factor-beta signaling-deficient fibroblasts enhance hepatocyte growth factor signaling in mammary carcinoma cells to promote scattering and invasion. Mol Cancer Res. 2008;6:1521-33.
3. Burkhart DL, Sage J. Cellular mechanisms of tumour suppression by the retinoblastoma gene. Nat Rev Cancer. 2008;8:671-82.
4. Adams JM, Cory S. The Bcl-2 apoptotic switch in cancer development and therapy. Oncogene. 2007;26: 1324-37.
5. Lowe SW, Cepero E, Evan G. Intrinsic tumour suppression. Nature. 2004;432:307-15.
6. Blasco MA. Telomeres and human disease: ageing, cancer and beyond. Nat Rev Genet. 2005;6:611-22.
7. Folkman J. Role of angiogenesis in tumor growth and metastasis. Semin Oncol. 2002;29(6, Suppl 16):15-8.
8. Jackson SP, Bartek J. The DNA-damage response in human biology and disease. Nature. 2009;461: 1071-8.
9. Warburg O. On respiratory impairment in cancer cells. Science. 1956;124:269-70.
10. Wiszniewska M, Magnuska J, Lipińska-Ojrzanowska A, Pepłońska B, Hanke W, Kalinka J, et al. The prophylactic operational model integrated with occupational healthcare–Prophylactic of some types of cancers among women. Med Pr. 2018;69(4):439-55.
11. Fitzmaurice C, Dicker D, Pain A, Hamavid H, Moradi-Lakeh M, MacIntyre MF, et al. The global burden of cancer 2013. JAMA Oncol. 2015;1(4):505-27.

CHAPTER
159 Cancer Biomarkers: Role and Relevance

Davinder Paul, Subhadeep Bose

ABSTRACT

Cancer biomarkers (CBs) are the unique biomolecules which are either produced by the cancer cells themselves or by the normal cells of the body in response to the cancer. Over the years, the role of cancer biomarkers has evolved from diagnosis to screening and further to determine prognosis and detecting recurrence of cancer. Although many cancer biomarkers have been discovered till date, but only few have made to clinical practice. The aim of this chapter is to provide an updated knowledge and review regarding the cancer biomarkers. Integrating these cancer biomarkers in the clinical utility helps in screening, diagnosis, follow-up, and therapeutic stratification of cancer patients. An ideal cancer biomarker should have high sensitivity and high specificity, so that maximum number of patients can draw benefit from them and at the same time normal subjects are excluded, so that they should not be subjected to further unnecessary investigations. With the advent of cancer genomic era, many new cancer biomarkers are being evaluated in prospective studies and over next few years, they are likely to help in the propagation of precision and personalized cancer care.

"The human spirit is stronger than anything that can happen to it"

—CC Scott

INTRODUCTION

The US Food and Drugs Administration (FDA) definition of biomarkers is "any measurable diagnostic indicator which can be used to assess the risk or presence of a disease". Similarly, CBs are biomolecules which are produced either by the cancer cells or by other normal cells of the body in response to the cancer. CB can be used in multiple manners, as screening tool for early detection, for diagnosis, for determining prognosis or as a predictor for overall survival of a patient. CB can enzymes, hormones, proteins, genes or gene products and they can be found in blood, urine, tissues, or other body fluid.

HISTORICAL BACKGROUND

Bence-Jones protein was the first CB discovered by Sir Bence Jones in 1847, as a protein in the urine of multiple myeloma patient which is detected by heat denaturation. Then in 1867, Sir Michael Foster discovered increased serum amylase levels in patients of carcinoma pancreas. Over next 100 years, numerous CB were discovered such as human chorionic gonadotropin (hCG) in choriocarcinoma, catecholamines in pheochromocytoma and neuroblastoma, acid phosphatase in prostate cancer, and alkaline phosphatase in bone tumors. Unfortunately, despite the discovery of so many CB till date, only few CB have been approved as diagnostic or prognostic cancer markers.

MECHANISMS FOR PRODUCTION

Cancer is a genetic disease. The genetic alteration leads to a cancerous phenotype. These genetic alterations, which include activation of proto-oncogenes, suppression of tumor suppressor genes, abnormality of deoxyribonucleic acid (DNA) repair genes or epigenetic changes in DNA, all these leads to disturbances in cell division and proliferation, which in turn is manifested by release of biomarkers in majority of patients with that particular type of cancer. Genetic, molecular, and metabolic biomarker can be identified by applying the sequence of events occurring in cancer cells from gene mutation following its effects on cellular proliferation and metabolism, as illustrated in **Flowchart 1**.

Serum, biological fluid, and tissue cancer biomarkers: There are three mechanisms which explain for the elevation of CB in various cancers. The first mechanism is amplification or overexpression of a gene product, or enhancement of epigenetic changes such as DNA methylation, which leads to release of CB. Such an example is human epididymal secretory protein 4 (HE4) in ovarian cancer. The second mechanism involves secretion of cellular proteins or shedding of membrane proteins by the cancer cells. An example is alpha-fetoprotein (AFP), which is an oncofetal protein elevated in hepatocellular carcinoma and human epidermal growth factor receptor 2 (HER2)-neu in certain breast cancer. The third mechanism is through cell

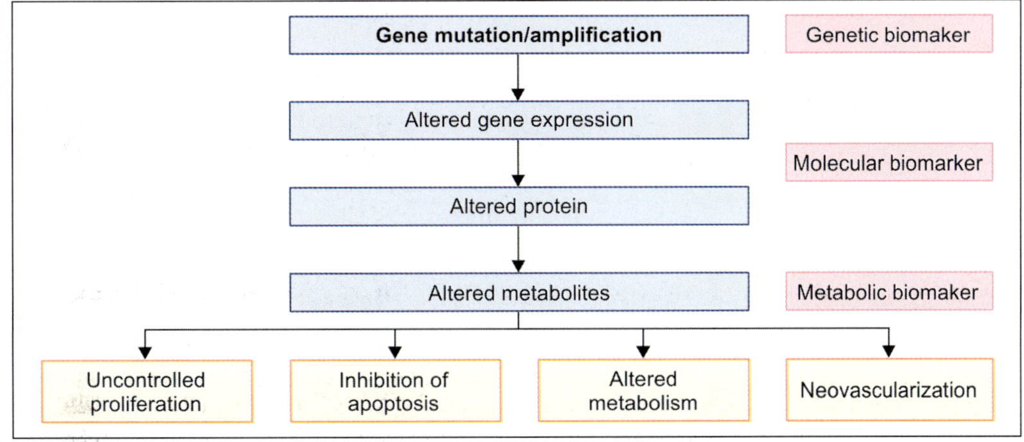

FLOWCHART 1: Identification of biomarkers in the process of carcinogenesis.

invasion and angiogenesis and typical example is prostate-specific antigen (PSA). PSA is normally expressed by prostatic epithelium but elevation of PSA levels occurs due to disruption of basement membrane of prostatic cell. CB can be detected in cancer cells or tissue of origin in solid tumors, bone marrow, and lymph node or as circulating cells. CB can also be detected in biological body fluids such as serum, ascitic fluid, pleural fluid, cerebrospinal fluid, urine, and stool or nipple discharge.

PERFORMANCE INDICATORS

The official definition of tumor markers have been adopted from the fifth International Conference on Human Tumor Markers held in Stockholm, Sweden, in 1988. It states that *"Biochemical tumor markers are substances developed in tumor cells and secreted into body fluids in which they can be quantitated by noninvasive analyses. Because of a correlation between marker concentration and active tumor mass, tumor markers are useful in the management of cancer patients. Markers, which are available for most cancer cases, are additional and valuable tools in patient prognosis, surveillance, and therapy monitoring, whereas they are presently not applicable for screening. Sero-diagnostic measurements of markers should emphasize on relative trends instead of absolute values and cut-off levels."* Despite this, CB have been used for screening general population or certain risk groups. Further, CB have been used to estimate tumor burden.

SENSITIVITY AND SPECIFICITY

Diagnostic value of any test or biomarker is performed in terms of sensitivity and specificity of that test or biomarker. Specificity refers to the ability of the marker to detect nondiseased subjects whereas, sensitivity refers to the ability of that test to identify diseased subjects. At a definitive cutoff value, a test or biomarker may be found above that value (positive), but actually not all positives are diseased subjects.

Therefore, sensitivity is calculated, as the ratio of the all positives who are found by that test, above the cutoff value to the total number of abnormal known to have the disease

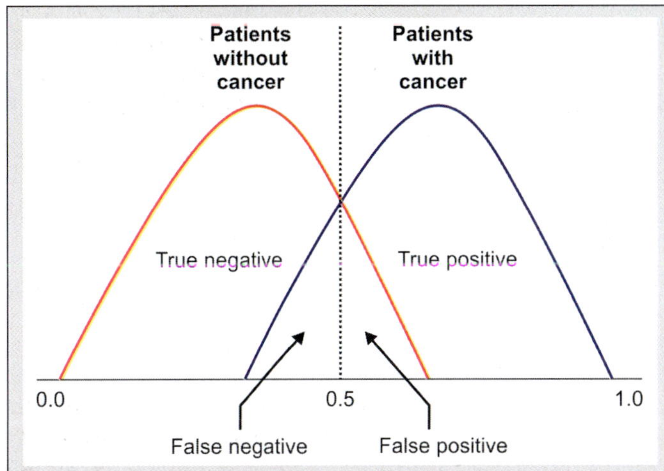

FIGURE 1: Cancer biomarker range of results among cancer and noncancerous patients.

(true positive). In nut shell, sensitivity refers to the true positive rate (TPR). Similarly, by applying the same cutoff value, some people with normal results below cutoff value are actually normal (true negative) but not all of them are not having the disease (false negative). Therefore, the true negative rate or specificity can be calculated as the ratio of the all negatives found by the test below cutoff value to the total number of normal known not to have the disease (true negative).

Thus, a CB with 70% specificity can identify only 70% of the noncancerous as being negative (true negatives), but remaining 30% noncancerous subjects will be falsely identified as positive (false positives). Similarly, a CB with 90% sensitivity means that it can detect 90% of patients with cancer (true positives), but still fail to detect it in 10% of cancer patients (false negatives). So, sensitivity and specificity are inversely related to each other, as depicted in **Figure 1**.

IDEAL BIOMARKER

An ideal tumor marker should fulfill the following general properties:

- *High clinical sensitivity*: Produced by all patients with that specific cancer (100% TPR).

- *High clinical specificity*: Low false negative rate (100% true negative rate).
- Should be specific to that particular organ or tissue.
- The quantitative value of that marker should be proportional to the tumor burden.
- Should have a short half-life, so that early changes in tumor burden are reflected quickly.
- Should be present (if any) at low levels in healthy individuals and those with benign disease.
- Sharply discriminating metastasis.
- Should exist in quantitative, standardized, reproducible, and validated assay.
- Should be inexpensive or low costing method.
- Should be obtained in a noninvasive manner, such as serum, urine, body fluids or in an easily accessible tissue.

Obviously, no tumor marker can fulfill all these requirements, so there is no ideal tumor marker discovered till date.

CLINICAL UTILITY AND LIMITATIONS

Traditionally used CB may directly not be involved in the process of carcinogenesis or development of cancer, rather they can be byproducts of malignant transformation. There are several classifications for CB depending on their different aspects relating to their chemical nature, proposed mechanisms for their release, and applications. For example, CB can be categorized into prediction biomarkers as DNA biomolecules, detection biomarkers as ribonucleic acid (RNA) molecules, diagnostic biomarkers as protein biomarkers, and prognosis biomarkers as glyco-biomarkers. Clinical applications and uses of CB are illustrated in **Figure 2**. CB are used for screening and early detection, for confirmation of diagnosis, prognosis and prediction of therapeutic response, and for monitoring disease and recurrence. Another important use of CB is its role in identifying people who are at a high risk of developing cancer. **Table 1** illustrates most of FDA approved and clinically relevant CB with their uses in various cancer types.

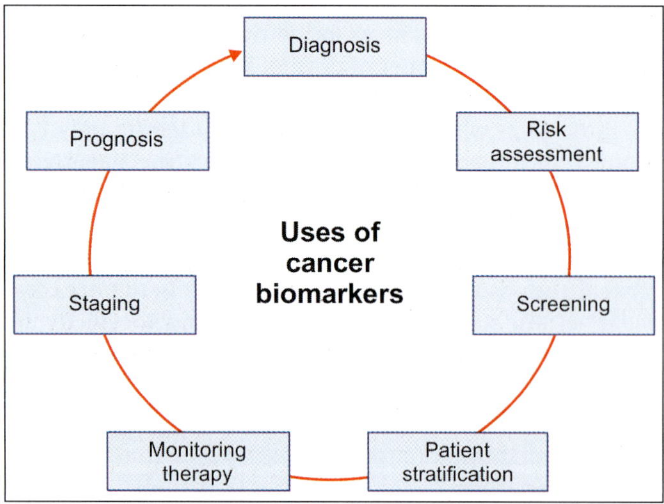

FIGURE 2: Clinical utility and uses of cancer biomarkers.

SCREENING/EARLY DETECTION

Screening is defined as "the systematic application of a test to identify subjects at sufficient risk of a specific disorder to benefit from further investigation or direct preventive action, among persons who have not sought medical attention on account of symptoms of that disorder". The main aim of screening is to detect the disease when a person is asymptomatic, which differ from diagnosis of the symptomatic patients. The ultimate objective of screening remains early detection of cancer leading to better cure rates and prognosis. Screening test must be highly specific, so as to minimize the false positive rate as much as possible. This high specificity is very much important for screening test, because even a small false positive rate will lead to a large number of unnecessary other diagnostic procedures, including invasive procedures that may be unnecessary and just add to the psychological burden and excess costs. Ideal screening test needs to be noninvasive and inexpensive and should definitely lead to reduction in morbidity and mortality and increase in survival rate. Major limiting factors for screening biomarker are the low diagnostic sensitivity and specificity of most of the currently used biomarkers. However, few biomarkers have good specificity and sensitivity, such as AFP in screening for hepatocellular cancer in high-risk subjects, PSA in screening for prostate cancer, and vanillylmandelic acid (VMA) in screening for neuroblastoma in newborns.

DIAGNOSIS

In contrast to screening biomarker which is applicable for asymptomatic subjects, a diagnostic biomarker is applied only for symptomatic patients. However, the characteristics of an ideal diagnostic biomarker are similar to the characteristics for screening biomarker. Many of the well-established biomarkers for screening can be used as diagnostic biomarkers. PSA is the pivotal example of this. PSA along with digital rectal examination, is the most commonly used diagnostic tool for prostate cancer. In contrast to screening biomarker, which needs to be of high specificity, a good diagnostic biomarker should have high sensitivity (TPR). However, some CB helps in confirming the cancer in conjunction with a panel of other markers, like in diagnosis of metastatic disease with unknown primary.

PROGNOSIS

Prognosis refers to probability of cure or likely outcome of any patient. It provides information about the natural history of the disease or the likely outcome. A predictive biomarker on the other hand, predicts the response to different therapeutic modalities. Thus, predictive biomarker is the basic concept for personalized medicine. The amount of elevation in levels of CB usually reflects tumor burden, hence higher elevation of CB mostly relates to bad prognosis and vice versa. By reflecting overall tumor burden, certain CB are used in staging of cancer. For example, in testicular germ cell tumors, very high levels of a CB such as AFP, lactate

TABLE 1 Current cancer biomarkers and uses in clinical practice.

Cancer biomarker	Organ specificity/cancer type	Application/Uses
Prostate specific antigen (PSA)	Prostate	Screening, diagnosis, and monitoring
Carbohydrate antigen 125 (CA125)	Ovary	Diagnosis, prognosis, detecting recurrence, and monitoring treatment
Carcinoembryonic antigen (CEA)	Colorectal/Hepatic	Monitoring therapy, prognosis, detecting recurrence, and screening for hepatic metastases
Carbohydrate antigen 15.3 (CA15.3)	Breast	Monitoring therapy
Estrogen receptor and progesterone receptor (ER and PgRs)	Breast	Prognosis and stratification/selecting patients for endocrine therapy
HER2	Breast	Prognosis and monitoring trastuzumab therapy
Carbohydrate antigen 27.29 (CA27.29)	Breast	Monitoring therapy
Human chorionic gonadotropin-β (HCG-β)	Testicular	Diagnosis, staging, detecting recurrence, and monitoring therapy
Alfa-fetoprotein (AFP)	Hepatocellular carcinoma	Diagnosis, detecting recurrence, and monitoring therapy
Calcitonin	Medullary carcinoma of thyroid	Diagnosis and monitoring therapy
Thyroglobulin	Thyroid	Monitoring therapy
CA19.9	Pancreatic	Monitoring therapy
Nuclear matrix protein-22 (NMP-22)	Urinary bladder	Screening, monitoring therapy, and prognosis
Prostate cancer antigen 3 (PCA3)	Prostate	Prognosis

(HER2: human epidermal growth factor receptor 2)

dehydrogenase (LDH), and HCG-β are indicative of an aggressive cancer with poor prognosis and outcome. These biomarkers are used for staging in tumor-node-metastasis (TNM) system as a site-specific prognostic factor (S is for site-specific prognostic factors). Estrogen receptor (ER) is one of the widely used prognostic and predictive tissue biomarker. As a predictive tissue biomarker, ER is used for selecting the patients likely to respond to hormonal therapy in carcinoma breast. Patients with ER positive breast cancer will mostly respond to selective ER modulators or aromatase inhibitors independent of the stage of breast cancer. ER is also considered a prognostic marker, because once ER is negative, that indicates a poor prognosis and when it is positive, it indicates a better prognosis. Similarly, high serum levels of HER2 in serum of breast cancer patients correlates with a poor prognosis. KRAS is a predictive biomarker for colorectal cancer (CRC), because patients with somatic mutations in KRAS have poor response to chemotherapy and antiepidermal growth factor receptor-targeting therapies.

THERAPEUTIC MONITORING

Therapeutic monitoring may in fact constitute the most common applications of CB in clinical practice. Clinically useful biomarkers usually fluctuate in their value according to the tumor behavior, size, or burden, so that its level increases with progressive disease, decreases with remission, and do not change significantly with stable disease. Further, recurrence of cancer may be detected biochemically via rise in CB levels even before appearance of any clinical or radiological evidence of cancer recurrence. Continued follow-up for cancer patients during and after therapy can mirror their condition if the levels of CB were not elevated or remain at basal level, indicating successful therapy or remission. On the other hand, rising CB levels above the basal level indicates recurrence of the disease. CB can be a warning sign of recurrence, usually it rises 3–12 months before any other diagnostic method can detect the recurrence.

Many CB are used for monitoring therapy or detection of recurrence or metastasis. For example, carcinoembryonic antigen (CEA) in CRC, cancer antigen 125 (CA 125) in ovarian cancers, or PSA in prostatic cancer. Some patients who encounter resistance to a therapeutic modality will experience rising levels of CB, and in that case, reconsideration of alternative therapy is mandatory. Monitoring CB needs to be both diagnostically sensitive and specific to ensure proper assessment of effective therapy and continuation of such beneficial therapies and early discontinuation/replacement of ineffective therapy or resistant cancer to those therapies. For example, carbohydrate antigen (CA19-9) was approved by the FDA in 2002 as a monitoring marker for pancreatic cancer. However, it is not recommended as a screening biomarker.

APPLICATIONS IN COMMON CANCERS

BREAST CANCER

Breast cancer is the most common malignancy among females. Therefore, it is critical to use all available tools for early diagnosis and better treatment of these patients. The role of CB in breast cancer is primarily of helping with prognosis, monitoring of therapy, and for follow-up. Assessment of ER and progesterone receptors (PRs) in tissue for newly diagnosed breast cancers is recommended for predicting response to hormone therapy in early and advanced breast cancer cases.

HER-2 is another such prognostic marker, most useful for selecting patients with either early or metastatic breast cancer for the treatment with Trastuzumab (Herceptin) or predicting resistance to tamoxifen therapy in early stage of breast cancer. Determination of risk groups for the development of breast cancer, who must be included in screening program, involves the detection of genetic mutation of *BRCA1* or *BRCA2* genes, which account for up to 5% of breast cancer cases. Due to their high susceptibility to breast and ovarian cancer, it is strongly recommended that women carrying *BRCA1* or *BRCA2* mutations undergo routine cancer screening.

Certain CB such as CA15.3, CEA, and BR 27-29 are used in postoperative surveillance in breast cancer in conjunction with other radiological and clinical tools. Elevation in serum levels of these markers may indicate recurrence or progression of the disease.

PROSTATE CANCER

Prostate cancer is one of the most common cancer in men and most common causes of male cancer-related deaths. Numerous studies and strong evidence suggest that PSA testing has revolutionized the prostate cancer screening and diagnosis landscape and has helped immensely in reducing mortality from prostate cancer. Later, many studies have demonstrated significant improvement in sensitivity of PSA as a diagnostic marker using a PSA subtractions and isoforms (–2) (proPSA) and its percentage derivative % proPSA (percent value relative to PSA) as these fractions may help for the discrimination between benign and malignant prostatic tumors in patients with PSA values ranging from 4 to 10 µg/L. Other novel and promising biomarkers under investigation include human kallikrein type 2, prostate cancer antigen 3 (PSA 3), and prostate stem cell antigen (PSCA). Elevated levels of metalloproteinase 2 and 9 (MMP-2 and MMP-9) has also been associated with diagnosis of prostate cancer. MMPs have also been studied as biomarker of therapeutic monitoring in prostate cancer.

OVARIAN CANCER

Most of the patients with epithelial ovarian cancer are diagnosed late and as such they have clinically advanced stage III or stage IV at the time of diagnosis. Therefore, we need to have a sensitive and specific biomarker which can help such patients. CA 125 is one of the most widely and conventionally used CB. It is recommended as a screening biomarker for women who have positive family history or are at high-risk for the development of ovarian cancer. Besides this, CA125 has also been used in conjunction with vaginal ultrasound as a well-established, diagnostic biomarker. CA125 is also used as a monitoring biomarker. Fall in the levels after surgery or chemotherapy correlates to favorable response. Similarly, rise in level during the follow-up period after treatment completion usually relates to disease recurrence. So periodic monitoring of carcinoma ovary patients with CA125 is highly recommended during the post-treatment surveillance period to detect recurrence.

COLORECTAL CANCER

Colorectal cancer is ranked third among all cancers all over the world. As per various recommendations, screening program for CRC should be directed to all asymptomatic individuals above 50 years of age. Multiple screening procedures exist for CRC. Fecal occult blood test (FOBT) is the most widely used CB in stool. Testing for blood in the stools involves either detecting globin fraction of blood (hemoglobin) by fecal immunochemical test or the guaiac test which measures pseudoperoxidase activity of heme fraction of hemoglobin. CEA was characterized and introduced into clinical practice in 1965. CEA is not used in screening of CRC due to its low sensitivity and specificity, beside the low prevalence of CRC among asymptomatic population; however, it is very efficient prognostic and therapy monitoring biomarker. CEA estimation is recommended at the beginning of therapy, then every 1–3 months during treatment and also after treatment completion. CA19-9 has also been used as prognostic marker, in surveillance of CRC after surgical resection and as monitoring marker for therapeutic intervention in advanced cases. Other CB under investigations are CA242 and tissue inhibitor of metalloproteinases type 1 (TIMP-1) and both may complement CEA in the surveillance of patients with CRC.

CONCLUSION AND PROSPECTIVE

Cancer biomarkers play an important role as markers for risk assessment, screening, diagnosis (usually along with other diagnostic tools), and most importantly as tools for determining the prognosis and response to a particular treatment modality. It is absolutely essential for the clinicians and researchers to have a comprehensive understanding of the molecular aspects, clinical utility, and reliability of biomarkers in order to determine whether and in what setting a biomarker is clinically useful for the patient care or in what setting, an additional evaluation is required. CB, by facilitating the combination of cancer therapeutics with cancer diagnosis, promise to play an important part in the development of personalized medicine.

RECOMMENDED READINGS

1. Rhea JM, Molinaro RJ. Cancer biomarkers: surviving the journey from bench to bedside. MLO Med Lab Ob. 2011;43(3):10-2.
2. Kulasingam V, Diamandis EP. Strategies for discovering novel cancer biomarkers through utilization of emerging technologies. Nat Clin Pract Oncol. 2008;5(10):588-99.
3. Camp BW. What the clinician really needs to know: questioning the clinical usefulness of sensitivity and specificity in studies of screening tests. J Dev and Behav Pediatr. 2006;27(3):226-30.
4. Mishra A, Verma M. Cancer biomarkers: are we ready for the prime time? Cancers (Basel). 2010;2(1):190-208.
5. Wald NJ. Guidance on terminology. J Med Screen. 2008;15(1):50.
6. Heidenreich A, Bellmunt J, Bolla M, Joniau S, Mason M, Matveev V, et al. EAU guidelines on prostate cancer. Part I: screening, diagnosis, and treatment of clinically localised disease. Actas Urol Esp. 2011;35(9):501-14.
7. Szymendera JJ, Zborzil J, Sikorowa L, Kaminska JA, Gadek A. Value of five tumor markers (AFP, CEA, hCG, hPL and SP1) in diagnosis and staging of testicular germ cell tumors. Oncology. 1981;38(4):222-9.
8. Rosty C, Goggins M. Early detection of pancreatic carcinoma. Hematol Oncol Clin North Am. 2002;16(1):37-52.
9. Mirza AN, Mirza NQ, Vlastos G, Singletary SE. Prognostic factors in node-negative breast cancer: a review of studies with sample size more than 200 and follow-up more than 5 years. Ann Surg. 2002;235(1): 10-26.
10. Benson AB 3rd, Schrag D, Somerfield MR, Cohen AM, Figueredo AT, Flynn PJ, et al. American Society of Clinical Oncology recommendations on adjuvant chemotherapy for stage II colon cancer. J Clin Oncol. 2004;22(16):3408-19.

CHAPTER 160 Solid Tumors: An Overview

Sujith Kumar Mullapally

ABSTRACT

This chapter introduces the approach to oncology, especially solid tumors, in a clinic. A detailed description of individual tumors is out of the scope of the chapter. Hence, the focus is on understanding the basic concepts in management of solid tumors such as multidisciplinary management of cancer, oncologic emergencies, palliative care, and survivorship issues. In India, most common cancers in males are (in descending order) head and neck, lung, stomach, colorectum, esophagus etc., and in females are (in descending order) breast, uterine cervix, ovary, head and neck, colorectum etc.

Solid tumors present with symptoms pertaining to their site of origin and metastatic sites. In most cases, they tend to present in advanced stages and cancer screening is essential especially in cervix, breast and colon cancers. Evaluation involves history, clinical examination, and histopathological studies including molecular tests and imaging for staging. Multidisciplinary team (MDT) approach is the standard of care for all cancers even if in early stages. Early palliative care and survivorship issues are also part of optimal care in oncology.

"Once you choose hope, anything's possible"

—C Reeve

INTRODUCTION

Cancer is diverse but unique for each individual. The molecular basis, genotype, phenotype, clinical presentation, the response to treatment, side effects, and the final outcomes can differ between the same type of cancers which makes them clinically challenging. Solid tumors are those which origin from solid organs such as lung, breast, liver, kidney, brain, and genitourinary system. In this chapter, we will discuss basic concepts in management of solid tumors with focus on common cancers in India.

COMMON CANCERS IN INDIA

The most common cancers are as given in **Table 1**. The data regarding incidences of different cancers are collected from various hospital-based cancer registries (HBCR) and population-based cancer registries (PBCR) worldwide. Cancer registries help in understanding the magnitude of cancer and trends over years in incidence and mortality in each country, and thereby helps to plan cancer prevention and screening and focus on improving the treatment of common cancers. In India, there are currently

36 PBCRs and 236 HBCRs under the National Cancer Registry Programme (NCRP)—National Centre for Disease Informatics and Research (NCDIR) of the Indian Council of Medical Research (ICMR; ICMR-NCDIR-NCRP), Bengaluru.

ETIOLOGY AND GENETIC FACTORS

Cancer is a multifactorial disease and various environmental factors including infectious (E) and genetic or hereditary (H) factors have been implicated in their etiopathogenesis. They result in gradual accumulation of driver gene mutations causing increased cellular proliferation and cancer. Apart from this, random mistakes in DNA replication (R) have been shown to be responsible for two-thirds of mutations in human cancer. This was shown by cancer genome sequencing and epidemiological data on stem cell divisions in 17 cancer types from 69 different countries. Primary prevention works best in cancers due to epidemiological factors whereas secondary prevention is more relevant in cancers caused by random mutation. The main etiological factors (environmental and hereditary/genetic) for common solid tumors are enlisted in **Table 2.** In India, a major concern is use of smokeless oral tobacco in various forms. More patients are getting diagnosed with age < 30 years pointing to early onset of abuse.

TABLE 1 Most common cancers as per the Globocan 2020 data in order of incidence.

Sex	World	India
Females	1. Breast	Breast
	2. Colorectum	Uterine cervix
	3. Lung	Ovary
	4. Cervical	Head and neck
	5. Thyroid	Colorectum
Males	1. Lung	Head and neck
	2. Prostate	Lung
	3. Colorectal	Stomach
	4. Stomach	Colorectum
	5. Liver	Esophagus

CLINICAL PRESENTATION

Symptoms due to solid tumors pertain to the specific organ or system involved in early stages and depend on metastatic sites in advanced stages. Most common symptoms are painless lumps or ulcers (may turn painful if bone or nerve involvement), bleeding, pain, seizures, constipation/diarrhea, prolonged cough, dysphagia, hoarseness etc. There also often are nonspecific constitutional symptoms such as fever, weight loss, anorexia, generalized mild body ache, and fatigue.

Even in the era of advanced imaging, detailed history-taking and meticulous clinical examination are crucial in oncology. History-taking needs to focus on both cross-sectional and longitudinal assessments of symptoms (onset, duration, and progress), and pain assessment is especially important [site, intensity, timing, character, aggravating, relieving factors (SITCAR)]. Most cancers follow a rapid course, except for few, such as skin cancers, prostate cancer, and estrogen-positive breast cancer. The aim is to

TABLE 2 Etiology and genetic/hereditary aspects of common solid tumors.

Common cancers	Risk factors	Genetic/Hereditary/Molecular factors
Breast cancer	• Female gender, high age, early menarche, late menopause, late parity, or nulliparity, prolonged HRT • Benign conditions such as atypical ductal or lobular hyperplasia • High BMI, Family history, smoking, alcohol consumption, prior thoracic irradiation	• Breast cancer (BRCA) 1 and 2 mutation: 56–84% lifetime risk of breast CA • Other familial/hereditary breast cancer: TP53 (Li–Fraumeni), *PALB2, PTEN* (Cowden syndrome), ATM gene (Ataxia Telangiectasia) mutations
Lung cancer	• Cigarette smoking: 85% cases, intensity and duration of smoking (pack years ≥ 30), use of filter cigarettes linked to more peripheral located cancers. Passive smoking increases risk by 20–30% when compared to nonsmokers • Polycyclic aromatic hydrocarbons, radon, metals, asbestos	• Epidermal growth factor receptor (EGFR) mutation: 21% of adenocarcinoma, 43% in never-smokers, exon 19 deletions (45%), exon 21 L858R confers Tyrosine kinase inhibitors (TKI) sensitivity, and acquired T790M mutation-resistance • *Anaplastic lymphoma kinase (ALK)* rearrangements: 2–7%, young males, never and light smoking history, signet-ring adenocarcinoma • Other actionable aberrations: *ROS1* rearrangements, *BRAF, RET* Fusions, *HER2* amp/mutation, *PIK3CA*
Head and neck cancers	• Tobacco: Oral use in combination with betel leaf, slaked lime, areca nut (paan, gutka, mawa): Major cause in India • Alcohol • Human papilloma virus (HPV): HPV-16 (>90%), HPV-18, most commonly oropharyngeal, Younger patients without smoking, alcohol • Nasopharynx: >90% associated Epstein–Barr Virus • Environmental factors: High intake of salt-preserved foods	• Fanconi—most common *Others*: Bloom, Li–Fraumeni, xeroderma pigmentosum • p16: Overexpressed in HPV-associated cancers (E7 protein blocks Rb function, leading to compensatory p16 upregulation) *EGFR*: poorer prognosis • Second cancers: "Field cancerization"—risk cancer of lung and aerodigestive tracts (3% per year)

Continued...

Common cancers	Risk factors	Genetic/Hereditary/Molecular factors
Gynecological cancers	• *Ovarian cancer*: Increased in advancing age, obesity, PCOS, nulliparity • *Endometrial cancer*: Unopposed estrogen—endogenous (obesity, PCOS, nulliparity), exogenous (tamoxifen, hormone replacement therapy) • *Cervical cancer*: Persistent HPV infection—high risk (early age of sexual intercourse, multiple sexual partners, h/o sexually transmitted disease (including genital warts); increased risk in low economic status, immunocompromised (HIV), smokers • *Risk reduction*: By prophylactic bilateral oophorectomy (ovary, endometrium-TAH also), HPV Vaccination (quadrivalent /polyvalent against high-risk subtypes 6,11,16,18)	• About 24% with ovary cancer have a germline mutation: All epithelial ovarian cancer patients should be referred for genetic risk evaluation • *BRCA1 or 2 mutation*: 18% of ovarian cancers. BRCA1: Risk of ovarian cancer 40%, *BRCA2*: Risk of ovarian cancer in 10–20% (also involved in breast, prostate cancers) • *Lynch syndrome*: (ovary, stomach, colorectal, uterine); germline mutation of MMR genes *(MLH1, MSH2, MLH6, PMS2)*. Lifetime risk ovary cancer: 5–15% and uterine cancer: 40–60% • Both are autosomal dominant
Gastrointestinal cancers	• *Colorectal cancer*: Age (above 45 years), history of polyps, inflammatory bowel disease (ulcerative colitis), diabetes, alcohol, tobacco, high red meat intake etc. • *Gastric cancer*: Helicobacter pylori, tobacco (oral/smoking), high B MI/obesity, alcohol, smoked/salted food • *Hepatocellular carcinoma*: Viral hepatitis—HBV and HCV (75% cases); alcoholic cirrhosis, aflatoxin, autoimmune hepatitis, tobacco, nonalcoholic steatohepatitis, hereditary hemochromatosis etc.	• *Colon cancer*: Familial syndrome (Familial adenomatous polyposis (APC gene), Lynch syndrome (mutation in MMR genes, microsatellite instability high), Peutz– Jeghers etc. • *Gastric cancer*: 15% of all gastric CA are familial. Lynch syndrome, diffuse hereditary gastric cancer: Germline e-cadherin (CDH1) mutation, high penetrance • *Pancreatic cancer*: 5–15% genetic predisposition, Hereditary breast cancer syndrome, BRCA2/BRCA1, Lynch syndrome, Germline mutations in PRSS1, SPINK1 and CDK2N1

(BMI: body mass index; h/o: history of; HRT: hormone replacement therapy; PCOS: polycystic ovarian syndrome)

identify whether an underlying malignancy is the cause of symptoms and if so, which is the probable primary site. To rule out metastatic disease, questions regarding bone pains and chronic cough are also asked.

HISTORY-TAKING

- Assessment of patient's physical fitness is based on patient's ability to do daily activities or take care of himself/herself. These are defined by "Performance status" (PS) and **Table 3** gives details on the same. PS of a patient influences the treatment decision and also is an important prognostic factor for many cancers. In special cases such as hematopoietic stem cell transplant and geriatric oncology, more specific scales are in use.
- Exposure to risk factors: Emphasis on smoking history (pack years/type of smoking/ passive smoking etc.), oral tobacco use, occupational history, past history of radiotherapy, use of hormone replacement therapy, alcohol intake, physical activity etc. Smoking is associated with around 13 types of cancer and so is obesity/lack of physical activity.
- Family history: It is crucial, especially in cancers of breast, ovary, uterus, pancreas, prostate, colorectal etc. The relative risk of an individual is very high above the normal population if there is one first-degree relative or more than one second-degree relatives with breast, colon, ovarian cancer etc. Mutations of *BRCA*, *p53*, *MMR* genes etc., cause familial cancer syndromes. Pedigree charts help to assess the risk. Different clinical criteria such as the Amsterdam criteria for hereditary non polyposis coli (HNPCC) are used to offer genetic counseling to high-risk individuals along with cancer-screening measures.

TABLE 3 Eastern Co-operative Oncology Group (ECOG) Performance Status.

Grade	Description of patient
0	Fully active, able to carry out all predisease performance without restriction
1	Restricted in physically strenuous activity but ambulatory and able to carry out work of a light and sedentary nature, e.g., house work, office work
2	Ambulatory and capable of all self-care but unable to carry out any work activities; up and about more than 50% of waking hours
3	Capable of only limited self-care; confined to bed or chair more than 50% of waking hours
4	Completely disabled; cannot do any self-care; totally confined to bed or chair
5	Dead

At the end of history, we must be able to summarize them with salient points and to develop differential diagnosis including the benign causes such as tuberculosis (pulmonary, nodal, and other extrapulmonary) in our country.

CLINICAL EXAMINATION

After deriving a differential diagnosis, physical examination helps in localizing the symptoms as due to a particular cancer. Always remember that it is important to assess whether, the patient is in distress due to his/her symptoms, especially due to pain. It is highly recommended that patients are made comfortable if they are in pain before the examiner proceeds with complete physical examination.

Few clinical pearls regarding the clinical examination in oncology are given below. Detailed accounts of physical examination can be obtained in standard clinical (medical/surgical) textbooks mentioned in recommended readings at the end of the chapter.

- General examination: Focus on nutritional status (including anthropometric measurements), pallor, icterus, clubbing, cyanosis, lymphadenopathy, edema, skin/spine (PICCLES). Please make a note of any surgical scars of past surgeries which can give clue to the current symptoms due to metastatic disease. Cancer patients have high risk to develop deep vein thrombosis and hence should be specifically looked for, especially if the patient is having restricted mobility. Pressure sores in dependent positions are also common in bedridden patients.
- Local examination: It depends on the symptoms such as swelling/ulcer and should be examined as per standard protocols. Always remember to assess the regional lymph nodes draining the specific site. Also, assess the functional disability due to disease such as mobility in bone tumors, vocal cord function/feeding status in head and neck cancers.
- System examination: The most common sites of metastases are lung, liver, bone, and brain. Hence, watch out for signs of pleural effusion/lung mass, hepatosplenomegaly, spine tenderness, neurological deficits etc., for all patients, especially in breast and lung cancers. Testicular examination in males is important, especially in cancer of unknown primary. Per rectal and per vaginal examination should be included as per the symptoms of the patient.

Being gentle and empathetic during clinical examination cannot be overemphasized in a cancer patient. The patient–doctor relationship in oncology has multiple dimensions of which meticulous yet considerate physical examination is a vital one.

EVALUATION ASSESSMENT AND PLANNING OF TREATMENT

In cancer, diagnosis, staging, treatment, and follow-up constitute the salient features of an optimal management plan. MDT-based approach is the standard of care, irrespective of the type and stage of cancer. **Figure 1** shows the various components of MDT. Advancements in oncopathology and cancer imaging have helped in accurate histopathological including molecular diagnosis and radiological staging. The close coordination between medical, surgical, and radiation oncology teams ensure best results without treatment delays and with least toxicity. The integration of palliative care, rehabilitation, and psycho-oncology help in improving quality of life of patients. The support of medical specialties (internal medicine/cardiology/gastroenterology/nephrology etc.,) helps both during the treatment phase and later in survivorship issues during follow-up. Medical social workers contribute in providing financial and logistics support with help of government schemes and nongovernment organizations (NGOs).

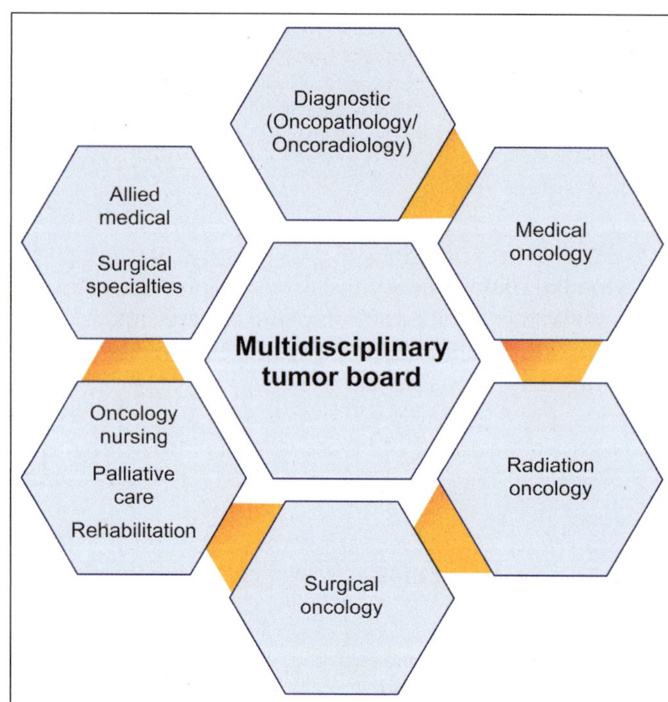

FIGURE 1: Multidisciplinary team approach in cancer.

ROLE OF ONCOPATHOLOGY IN SOLID TUMORS

Histopathological examination is the gold standard of cancer diagnosis. The first step usually involves tissue biopsy from the involved organ or from metastases. Core biopsy (breast), needle biopsy (mostly image guided from internal organs such as lung/kidney), punch biopsy (oral cavity/cervix), excision biopsy (lymph node/small tumors), wedge biopsy (large tumors/skin cancer) etc., are used to provide adequate tissue for examination. Frozen biopsy are used during surgery to give rapid assessment of tumor margins to ensure adequate clearance. Fine-needle aspiration and fluid cytology also helps in making the diagnosis but further tests are not feasible. Cell blocks prepared from body fluids such as pleural effusion and ascites can replace the need for biopsy if adequate. Liquid biopsy are next-generation sequencing (NGS)-based platforms where the circulating tumor DNAs in blood are isolated. Their presence in blood has a prognostic role and subsequent analysis for targetable mutations help in planning treatment, especially in nonsmall-cell lung cancer. This is useful when a repeat tissue biopsy is not possible.

Microscopic examination is followed by immunohistochemistry (IHC) analysis for confirmation. IHC is based on the differential expression of various proteins in and around the tumor which has a distinct pattern for each type of tumor. They also have a role as predictive biomarkers for targeted therapy and immunotherapy in many cancers such as breast. **Table 4** gives the details of morphology and IHC of common solid tumors.

MOLECULAR PATHOLOGY

Molecular pathology has revolutionized the field of oncopathology and has important clinical applications as various genetic mutations such as point mutation, deletion, and translocations form the basis for most cancers. The various technologies in use are fluorescent in situ hybridization (FISH) for cytogenetics, karyotyping (conventional cytogenetics), real-time polymerase chain reaction (RT-PCR), NGS etc. The detailed discussion on these techniques are not within the scope of the chapter. **Table 5** enlists major molecular tests and their implications in solid tumors.

CANCER IMAGING

Once diagnosis is suspected, imaging helps in assessment of the local tumor and the involvement of distant sites due to cancer. Often, CT or USG-guided procedures help to assess the site for tissue biopsy for confirmation in case of lung cancer/renal cancers etc. In the current era, oncoradiology involves both diagnostic and interventional roles.

Diagnostic role: Staging of solid tumors is based on both clinical examination and radiological assessment. The various imaging modalities in oncology are X-rays, ultrasonogram, mammogram, CT, MRI, bone scan, positron emission tomography (PET) etc. In case of CT/MRI, if renal parameters are within limits, use of contrast causes differential enhancement of tumors and helps in delineating the anatomical/vascular relations of the tumor. Diffusion-weighted and perfusion-weighted MRI imaging are very useful in characterizing brain tumors. PET-CT

TABLE 4 Common histology and IHC of solid tumors.

Solid tumors	Histomorphology	Immunohistochemistry
Breast	• Infiltrating ductal adenocarcinoma • Infiltrating lobular carcinoma	AE1/AE3+, Cam5.2+, CK7+, ER+/-, CK20-, GATA3+, mammaglobin+, HER2+/-
Lung	• Small-cell carcinoma • Nonsmall-cell carcinoma (NSCLC): ◦ Adenocarcinoma ◦ Squamous cell Carcinoma	• AE1/AE3+, Cam5.2+, chromogranin+, CK7+/-, CK20-, synaptophysin+, NSE+ • AE1/AE3+, Cam5.2+, CK7+, CK20-, Napsin A+, TTF1+ • AE1/AE3+, Cam5.2+, CK5/6+, CK7+/-, GATA3+, p40+, p63+
Prostate	Adenocarcinoma	AE1/AE3+, Cam5.2+, NKX3-1, PAP+, PSA+
Bladder	Urothelial adenocarcinoma	AE1/AE3+, Cam5.2+, CK7+, CK20+, GATA3+, p40+, p63+
Colorectal	Adenocarcinoma	AE1/AE3+, Cam5.2+, CDX2, CK7-, CK20+, SATB2+, Vilin+
Stomach	Adenocarcinoma	AE1/AE3+, Cam5.2+, CDX2+, CK7+/-, CK20+/-
Pancreas	Adenocarcinoma	AE1/AE3+, Cam5.2+, CDX2+/-, CK7+, CK20-
Ovary	Epithelial adenocarcinoma: • Papillary serous • Endometroid • Mucinous • Clear	AE1/AE3+, Cam5.2+, CK7+/-,CK20-,ER+, Napsin+/-, PAX8+
Germ-cell tumors	Seminoma (M), Dysgerminoma (F) Nonseminomatous germ-cell tumor (NSGCT): • Yolk sac • Embryonal	• AE1/AE3+, Cam5.2+, PLAP, SALL4, Oct4+, CD117+,(D2-40) + • AE1/AE3+, Cam5.2+, PLAP, SALL4, AFP, glypican-3 • AE1/AE3+, Cam5.2+, PLAP, SALL4, Oct4, CD30, SOX2
Head and neck	Squamous cell carcinoma	• AE1/AE3+, Cam5.2+, CK5/6+, CK7+/-, p40+, p63+ • P16 (HPV-positive)
Kidney cancer	Renal cell carcinoma: • Clear cell • Nonclear cell	• AE1/AE3+, Cam5.2+, CD10/RCC, CK7+, CK20-, PAX8+ • AE1/AE3+, Cam5.2+, CD10/RCC, CK7-, CK20-, PAX8+
Liver	Hepatocellular carcinoma	• AE1/AE3+, Cam5.2+, arginase+/HepPar1+, CK7-, CK20-
Thyroid	• Papillary carcinoma • Follicular carcinoma • Anaplastic carcinoma	• AE1/AE3+, Cam5.2+, CK7-, CK20+, Napsin-, TTF1+, thyroglobulin+, PAX8+

(AFP: alpha fetoprotein; CD: cluster of differentiation; CDX2: caudal type homeobox 2; CK: cytokeratin; ER: estrogen receptor; GATA3: GATA-binding protein 3; GCDFP-15: gross cystic disease fluid protein-15; HepPar1: hepatocyte paraffin 1; NSE: neuron-specific enolase; OCT4: octamer-binding transcription factor 4; p40 /p63: protein/tumor protein 40/63; PAP: prostatic acid phosphatase; PAX: paired box gene; PLAP: placental alkaline phosphatase; PSA: prostate-specific antigen; RCC: renal-cell carcinoma; SALL4: spalt-like transcription factor 4; SATB2: special AT-rich sequence-binding protein 2; TTF1: thyroid transcription factor 1)

TABLE 5 Molecular tests in solid tumors.

Solid tumors	Molecular/Cytogenetic tests	Indication
Breast	• Cytogenetics by fluorescent in situ hybridization (FISH) for *HER2* (only done if IHC is indeterminate, 2+)	• Human epidermal growth factor receptor-2 (HER2) is a prognostic and predictive marker. Anti-HER2-directed therapy if positive (trastuzumab, lapatinib, pertuzumab)
Breast, ovary	• *BRCA* gene analysis by next-generation sequencing (NGS)	• For detection of *BRCA* gene mutation, which increases breast and ovarian cancer risk • If mutation positive, PARP inhibitors such as olaparib can be used which provide clinical benefit
Lung	• Real-time polymerase chain reaction (RT-PCR) for epidermal growth factor receptor (EGFR) • Anaplastic lymphoma kinase (*ALK*) or ROS-1 rearrangement by IHC. *ALK* gene rearrangement can be confirmed by FISH • NGS can be used as single test to detect and confirm the above targetable mutations/translocations	• *EGFR* mutations: *Exon 19, L858R* are very sensitive to tyrosine kinase inhibitors (TKI): Gefitinib, erlotinib, osimertinib etc. • Crizotinib, lorlatinib, alectinib etc., are TKI used in ALK or ROS-1 rearrangement-positive adenocarcinoma lung
Gliomas (brain tumors)	• MGMT promoter methylation testing by gene sequencing	• Prognostic marker for glioblastoma as positive patients has better prognosis and predictive marker for better response to temozolamide
Colon cancers	• Microsatellite Instability (MSI) testing by *Mismatch Repair* (*MMR*) gene sequencing by NGS (can also be done by IHC for the MMR proteins: mMSH6, hMLH1, hMSH2, hPMS2) • *KRAS, NRAS, BRAF* mutation testing by sequencing	• If MSI high or deficient MMR (dMMR) in nonmetastatic colon cancer, then they have poor sensitivity to fluorouracil and better prognosis • If mutant, anti-EGFR therapy is not indicated
Sarcoma	• FISH for translocation: ◦ Translocation t(X;18) ◦ der(17)t(X;17)(p11;25) ◦ t(2;13)(q35;q14) or t(1;13)(p36;q14)	• Diagnostic test for: ◦ Synovial sarcoma ◦ Alveolar soft-part sarcoma ◦ Alveolar rhabdomyosarcoma
All solid tumors	• Microsatellite instability (MSI) testing by *MMR* gene sequencing by NGS (can also be done by IHC for the MMR proteins: mMSH6, hMLH1, hMSH2, hPMS2)	• If MSI high or dMMR, then irrespective of cell of origin, cancers are sensitive to immunotherapy (pembrolizumab). This is called tumor agnostic therapy

[IHC: immunohistochemistry; MGMT: O6-methylguanine-DNA methyltransferase; PARP: Poly (ADP-ribose) polymerase]

is functional imaging which captures the high metabolic activity seen in tumors using radioisotope labeled dyes such as F18-fluorodeoxyglucose (F18-FDG).

For metastatic workup in locally advanced breast cancers, either contrast-enhanced CT of neck/thorax/abdomen with bone scan or whole-body PET-CT is done whereas in lung/esophageal/renal cancers and lymphomas, PET-CT is usually preferred. PET-CT has shown to cause stage migration to higher stages when compared to CT and thus causing a change in treatment plan in 10–15% patients. Imaging also is essential for response assessment after treatment such as radiotherapy or systemic therapy. Response Evaluation in Solid Tumors (RECIST) criteria help in defining response as complete response, partial response, stable disease and progressive disease (PD) based on measurements of tumors and lymph nodes. PET-CT responses are defined based on differences between pre-and post-therapy metabolic activity of tumor which is calculated in terms of standard uptake value (SUV). SUV is a mathematically derived ratio of tissue radioactivity concentration at a point in time C(t) and the injected dose of radioactivity per kilogram of the patient's body weight. iRECIST criteria are used for response after immunotherapy.

Therapeutic role: The various therapeutic indications of interventional radiology include palliative (vertebroplasty for bone metastases, angioembolization for bleeding GI ulcers, celiac and other nerve plexus blocks for pain relief etc.) and curative [transarterial chemoembolization (TACE) or transarterial radioembolization (TARE) in hepatocellular carcinoma]. Theranostics is the systematic integration of targeted diagnostics and therapeutics and is commonly used in neuroendocrine tumors (Gallium68-DOTATATE to identify somatostatin receptor expression followed by Lutetium Lu177 DOTATATE-based treatment), prostate cancers etc. The use of radionuclide or radioisotope in molecular-targeted therapy of cancers is known as Particle Radionuclide Radiation therapy (PRRT).

STAGING OF CANCER

Staging of Cancer based on standard universally accepted classification is necessary for understanding cancer burden, planning treatment, assessing response, scientific research and most importantly, communication between oncologists working in different areas of the world. The most commonly used system is TNM staging system, an anatomical system based on extent of Tumor (T), involvement of Node (N), and presence of distant Metastases (M). This system was developed by the American Joint Committee on Cancer (AJCC) and has been adopted by the Union for International Cancer Control (UICC). Recently, the incorporation of biological factors have been done for breast cancer and prognostic stages have been defined apart from anatomic stages. The pathologic staging also follows TNM classification and is denoted with the prefix "p." If the patient has recurrent disease, then "r" is mentioned as a prefix. More details on staging of different cancers are available in the recommended readings.

TREATMENT PLAN

The detailed history with clinical examination, histopathological evaluation, and cancer imaging helps to determine the patient's fitness in terms of PS, comorbidity status, stage of cancer, and burden of disease. The next most important step is a Multidisciplinary Board meeting. Evidence-based medicine is the essence of multidisciplinary tumor board. The medical, radiation, surgical oncologists, palliative-care physicians with input from physicians, radiologists, and pathologists discuss the various aspects of the individual's cancer and decide on the treatment plan. The intent of treatment is decided as curative or palliative (in case of most advanced cancers). The final treatment is planned after discussion with the patient and family depending on physical fitness, social, economic, and logistic issues as per the individual and the treating institution. Breaking bad news is a very important communication skill and various methods have been described, most common is "SPIKES" (S—setting, P—perception, I—invitation or information, K—knowledge, E—empathy, and S—summarize or strategize).

ONCOLOGICAL EMERGENCIES

The clinical behavior of many solid tumors is often insidious until they become symptomatic due to local progression or metastatic disease. Thus, it is clinically challenging to identify cancers early and treat them in initial stages. Due to disease per se or due to cancer treatment, oncologic emergencies can present during the insidious clinical course. It is important to promptly act upon as they have high risk of mortality or morbidity depending on the burden of disease and the treatment received. Involvement of other medical and surgical specialties is often necessary apart from oncologists in their management (**Table 6**).

TABLE 6 Oncological emergencies.

Oncologic emergencies	Salient features	Clinical features	Treatment
Tumor lysis syndrome (TLS)	Due to excessive tumor cell kill either spontaneous or due to treatment. *Common cancers* include solid tumors (small-cell carcinoma lung, germ-cell tumor), high-grade lymphoma, and leukemia. Baseline impaired renal function, dehydration, high tumor burden etc., are risk factors	Diarrhea, nausea, vomiting, decreased urine output, acute renal failure, seizures, altered sensorium etc. Classified by Cairo-Bishop system: • Lab TLS: ≥2 factors below (within 3 days before or 7 day after start of cytotoxic therapy): Uric acid > 8 mg/dL, K^+ > 6 meq/L, PO_4^+ > 4.5 mg/dL, Ca < 8 mg/dL) • Clinical TLS: ≥1 lab + ≥1 clinical Seizure, increased serum creatinine (≥ 1.5 times upper limit of normal), cardiac dysrhythmia	• **Prophylaxis**: Adequate hydration is the key, 2–3 L/m² as per BSA, diuretics, allopurinol, rasburicase IV in high-risk patients • **Treatment**: Management of hyperkalemia, hyperphosphatemia, hypokalemia, and hyperuricemia: ○ Periodic 6–8 hourly monitoring of electrolytes is important. Usually, it improves over first 3–5 days unless patient develops oliguria and needs hemodialysis
Superior vena (SVC) syndrome	Obstruction due to extrinsic compression of SVC by mediastinal mass or lymph nodes. Common cancers include NSCLC, SCLC, lymphoma, metastatic carcinoma, germ-cell tumor etc.	Facial edema, distended neck veins, pleural effusion, dyspnea, cough, arm edema, facial plethora, syncope etc. • Diagnosis: ○ If symptoms moderate or severe, imaging with contrast-enhanced CT or MRI without contrast if high creatinine ○ If the symptoms are mild, Doppler ultrasound of the neck veins should be done to rule out thrombosis	If there is stridor or altered sensorium, emergency endovenous stenting is recommended and also in patients where cancer is not proven • *Intravascular anticoagulation* is preferred if thrombus is present. If not feasible for stenting or in known cancer patient, external beam radiotherapy is preferred. *Chemotherapy* is given in very chemosensitive tumors such as germ cell tumors, small-cell carcinoma etc. Steroids (dexamethasone 4 mg q6 hourly, loop diuretics, elevate head end of bed are supportive measures

Continued...

Continued...

Oncologic emergencies	Salient features	Clinical features	Treatment
Spinal cord compression	Epidural spinal cord compression (ESCC) happens when vertebral metastases invade the thecal sac and the epidural space and causes spinal cord infarction and irreversible loss of neurological function. Most common cancers causing ESCC are lung, breast, prostate, renal cell carcinoma etc.	Thoracic spine most commonly involved followed by lumbar and cervical. Most common symptom is backache. Other symptoms depend on the site: autonomic dysfunction such as bladder retention/ incontinence, anal sphincter incontinence, LMN type paralysis, sensory loss etc. ESCC is graded into Grade 0: only bone, Grade 1A: Epidural sac extension with intact dura,1B: Dural sac deformation, intact cord 1C: Dural sac deformation with cord abutment but no compression, Grade 2: Cord compression with CSF around visible around cord, Grade 3: Cord compression with CSF space obliterated	*Urgent MRI* Whole spine with contrast preferable without waiting for neurological signs to develop. Pretreatment neurologic status is most important prognostic factor for regaining neurological function. *Dexamethasone* 10 mg IV stat followed by 4 mg IV 8th hourly (can increase dose depending on the neurological deficit) is started along with pain medications. *Surgical decompression* is preferred over external beam radiotherapy as neurological recovery is faster, also helps in providing mechanical stability by pedicle fixation and in solid tumors. In case of metastatic disease with multiple levels of cord compression or in advanced disease with high disease burden and expected survival less than 3 months, external beam radiotherapy is the preferred option

(LMN: low motor neuron; NSCLC: nonsmall cell lung cancer; SCLC: small-cell lung cancer)

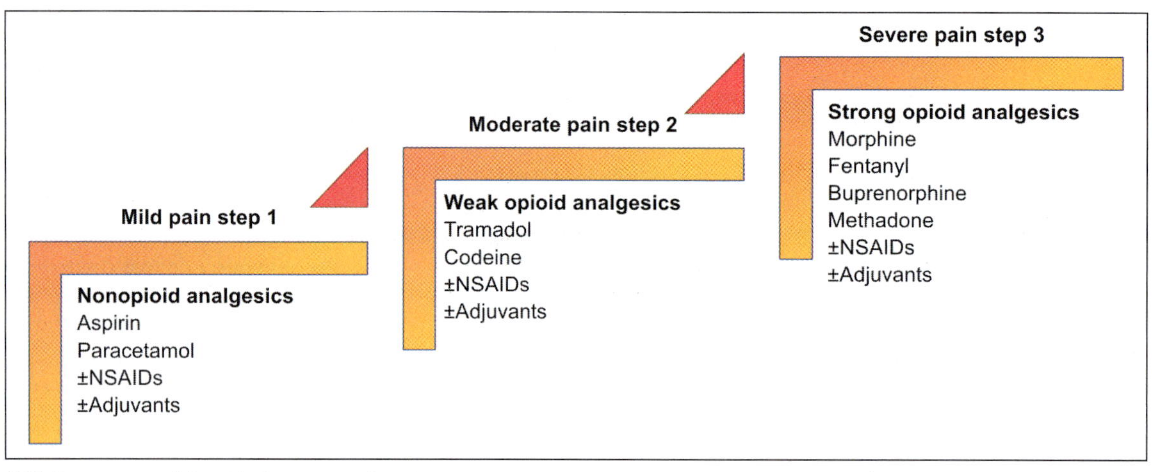

(NSAIDs: nonsteroidal anti-inflammatory drugs)

FIGURE 2: The World Health Organization (WHO) three-step analgesic ladder.

PALLIATIVE CARE IN ONCOLOGY

As a part of multimodality treatment, palliative care assumes a vital place in providing comfort to the patient. The various cancer symptoms that mandate palliative care are pain (often the most distressing symptom), breathlessness, nonhealing ulcers, intestinal obstruction etc. They may be present both in early and late stages of cancer. Pain management follows the World Health Organization (WHO) three-step ladder for pain (**Fig. 2**). In early cancers, the inclusion of palliative care initially itself helps patients to go through their curative treatment with ease. In advanced cancer patients, often palliative care is provided after they progress on multiple lines of treatment. Early palliative care is preferred where the patients get palliative care at the time of diagnosis itself. Palliative care early in the treatment course of advanced cancer patients has been shown to improve the quality of life and even prolong the overall survival of lung and esophageal cancer patients.

Treatment of common solid tumors: Multimodality treatment of solid cancers include surgery, systemic therapy (chemotherapy, targeted therapy, and immunotherapy), radiation therapy, palliative care, and rehabilitation. Care for comorbidities, if present, such as diabetes, cardiac and renal disease is also continued during cancer treatment. **Tables 7** and **8** below summarizes the main treatment schema for the common solid tumors in India. Detailed discussion on each aspect of the different solid tumors are beyond the scope of this chapter and please refer to recommended readings which also has pivotal trials from India enlisted. Also, in the references, pivotal trials from India in management of solid tumors are mentioned.

TABLE 7	Multimodality treatment in solid tumors-I.			
Solid tumor	**Stage**	**Surgery**	**Systemic therapy**	**Radiotherapy**
Breast	• Early breast cancer (EBC) • Locally advanced breast cancer (LABC) • Metastatic breast cancer (MBC)	*Upfront in EBC*: • Breast conservation surgery (BCS) or simple mastectomy with axillary clearance (SMAC) • In LABC, neoadjuvant chemotherapy followed by BCS/SMAC • No role for surgery in MBC except in advanced bleeding/ ulcerated mass for palliation	• Adjuvant/neoadjuvant therapy: 4–6 cycles • Chemotherapy regimen: AC → P or FAC or DC etc. If ER/PR +, addition of endocrine therapy for 5 years (tamoxifen in premenopausal / letrozole or anastrozole in postmenopausal). If HER2 positive, add trastuzumab with chemotherapy as neoadjuvant and also 1 year total as adjuvant therapy **MBC:** • *If ER/PR positive/Her 2-negative* and not in visceral crisis (altered organ function tests /very symptomatic patient), endocrine therapy along with CDK4/6 inhibitors such as palbociclib and ribociclib. If in visceral crisis, chemotherapy followed by endocrine therapy maintenance • *In HER2-positive cancers*, chemotherapy with anti-HER2-directed therapy (trastuzumab) for 6–8 cycles followed by continuation of trastuzumab and endocrine therapy, if ER/PR positive • On progression, second-line endocrine/ chemotherapy/anti-HER2 therapy will be needed	• *Radiotherapy (RT) to involved whole breast* is an essential component of breast conservation surgery, irrespective of the stage. It improves locoregional control and overall survival also • Dose: 50 Gray/25 fractions/5 weeks followed by Boost RT to tumor bed • In LABC, RT is indicated in post mastectomy cases if T3/T4, N2 or above, post NACT, occasionally N1 disease • RT is given to the chest wall and to the supraclavicular nodal area in node-positive cancers and triple-negative breast cancers
Ovary	• Stage I, II (Surgical staging) • Stage III/IV	• *Cytoreductive surgery*: Total abdominal hysterectomy with bilateral salpingo-oophorectomy, peritoneal wash and cytology, peritoneal biopsies and infracolic omentectomy • Interval cytoreductive surgery after 3–4 cycles of chemotherapy to achieve optimal cytoreduction (<1 cm of residual disease)	• *For all stages* postsurgery except, stage Ia and Ib, there is role for adjuvant chemotherapy. Usually paclitaxel/ carboplatin (PC) chemotherapy is given for 6 cycles • *In patients who present in advanced stages* with multiple omental/ peritoneal disease, ascites, pleural effusion etc., initial administration of 3–4 cycles of chemotherapy with PC helps in tumor debulking and enables optimal cytoreductive surgery. Postsurgery, 3–4 cycles of chemotherapy is given to complete the treatment. and then patient is kept on follow-up • In advanced ovarian cancers with liver /bone/lung metastases, the intent of treatment is palliative and PC chemotherapy is given for 6 cycles. On disease progression, second-line chemotherapy (liposomal doxorubicin, gemcitabine) etc., is given • *In BRCA mutation-positive patients*, addition of PARP inhibitors as maintenance after completion of chemotherapy helps in improving the progression-free survival	*No role for RT* in ovarian cancers, except as palliative therapy for metastases to bone/brain etc.

Continued...

Continued...

Solid tumor	Stage	Surgery	Systemic therapy	Radiotherapy
Cervix	• Stage I-IVA • Metastatic (IVB)	• *In stages IA, IB, and IIA; Wertheim hysterectomy* is treatment of choice and includes extrafascial hysterectomy with resection of medial half of uterosacral ligaments, cardinal ligaments, upper 1–2 cm of vagina along with pelvic and para-aortic lymphadenectomy • Minimally invasive hysterectomy is proven inferior to open radical abdominal hysterectomy in cervical cancer patients • No role for surgery in stage IV	• Role of chemotherapy in stage I-IV is as radiosensitizer given weekly with RT. Cisplatin is the preferred drug. Use of cisplatin with radiotherapy in shown to improve disease-free survival and overall survival when compared to RT alone • Also, concurrent chemoradiation was confirmed superior to neoadjuvant chemotherapy followed by surgery in carcinoma cervix, Ib-IIB • In metastatic cervical cancer, paclitaxel carboplatin with or without bevacizumab is considered as first-line therapy	• *External beam RT along with weekly cisplatin as* radiosensitizer followed by brachytherapy is the treatment of choice in cervical cancer, stage IIB-IVA. In stage IB-IIA, also radiotherapy is an option • Dose: 50 Gray/25 fractions to pelvis followed by 3–4 sessions of intracavitary brachytherapy • In metastatic cervical cancer, short-course RT is useful in palliation of symptoms

(AC: doxorubicin/cyclophosphamide; DC: docetaxel, carboplatin; ER: estrogen receptor; FAC: 5 fluorouracil, doxorubicin, cyclophosphamide; MBC: metastatic breast cancer; NACT: neoadjuvant chemotherapy; P: paclitaxel; PR: progesterone receptor; PARP: poly (ADP-ribose) polymerase)

TABLE 8 Multimodality treatment of solid tumors-2.

Solid tumor	Stage	Surgery	Systemic therapy	Radiotherapy
Lung cancer (nonsmall cell lung cancer)	• Stage I, II, IIIA T1/T2, N0/N1(single station, nonbulky node) • IIIA-IIIB (bulky N1, N2) • Metastatic lung cancer	• *Lobectomy* is the preferred surgery for primary along with mediastinal nodal clearance. Video-assisted minimally invasive surgery can reduce postoperative stay and complications but has higher learning curve • In selected cases, neoadjuvant chemotherapy followed by surgery can be considered • *Chemoradiation* is the preferred treatment in most cases • No role for surgery	• *Adjuvant/neoadjuvant therapy*: 4 cycles of vinorelbine cisplatin or pemetrexed cisplatin is given pre- or postsurgery and improves overall survival • *In concurrent chemoradiation*, weekly chemotherapy regimen such as paclitaxel/carboplatin for 5–6 cycles is preferable. The other options include single-agent cisplatin • *Metastatic disease*: In adenocarcinoma, depends on presence of targetable mutations such as EGFR, ALK translocation, ROS-1 rearrangement etc., where the oral TKIs (gefitinib, erlotinib, osimertinib) (anti-EGFR); crizotinib, alectinib (ALK) etc., are the drug of choice • If no target identified, PDL1 by IHC if >50%, immunotherapy (pembrolizumab) is indicated as single agent. If PDL1 < 50%, then chemotherapy with or without immunotherapy is used. Common chemotherapy regimen are paclitaxel/carboplatin, pemetrexed/carboplatin etc.	• Postsurgery, the indications of RT are positive margins, N2 disease • In case of radical chemoradiation in IIIA-IIIB disease, concurrent chemoradiation is preferred over radiation alone • Doses used are 60 Gray/30 fractions/6 weeks • As lung tumors move with respiration, there is need for advanced technology such as image-guided radiotherapy (IGRT) • In case of medically inoperable, early lung cancers, T1/T2, N0/N1: Stereotactic ablative radiotherapy (SART) where high doses per fraction are given in less number of fraction

Continued...

Solid tumor	Stage	Surgery	Systemic therapy	Radiotherapy
Colorectal	• Nonmetastatic (Stage I–III) • Metastatic	• Complete mesocolic excision with central vascular ligation (in case of rectum, total mesorectal excision) is the surgery of choice. The extent of surgery depends on the location of tumor etc., in ascending colon, right hemicolectomy etc. • In oligometastases (<5 metastases), curative surgery is still considered, especially if only liver metastases are there. They are operated upfront along with primary or after completion of 3–4 cycles of chemotherapy • In unresectable, multiple metastases, primary surgery alone is done if there is obstruction or bleeding due to primary colon tumor	• *Adjuvant chemotherapy* is indicated in stage III and in high risk stage II. The most common regimen used are FOLFOX and CAPEOX. The duration of treatment is 3 months or 6 months based on high risk factors such as nodal positivity • *In metastatic colorectal cancer*, the optimum treatment depends on the biological profile. Molecular tests for mutations in *KRAS, NRAS BRAF, HER2* etc., are checked and if not present, anti-EGFR antibodies such as cetuximab and panitumumab are added to the chemotherapy regimen and gives better overall survival and response rates. If the above mutations (*KRAS/NRAS/BRAF*) are present, then anti-VEGF antibody, bevacizumab is added. In case of BRAF mutation, targeted therapy with dabrafenib/trametinib also is an option. In HER2-positive, trastuzumab is added with chemotherapy. Usually, chemotherapy with biological therapy is continued till progression or intolerable side effects • Usual regimens are FOLFOX, CapeOx, FOLFIRI • Immunotherapy for MSI-high tumors also is approved and pembrolizumab is the drug used	• RT has an *important role in rectal cancers.* In T3/T4 or node-positive cancers (Stage III), neoadjuvant radiotherapy with concurrent oral capecitabine is given before surgery to improve chances of TME and downsize the disease. It improves the overall survival and anal sphincter preservation rates. Dose: 50 Gray/25 fractions/5 weeks with oral capecitabine is used • In some patients, short-course radiotherapy (25 Gray/5 fractions/1 week) also is used followed by surgery either immediately or after 4–6 weeks • *Palliative RT* is offered in metastatic colorectal cancers, when there is local bleeding or bone metastases

(ALK: anaplastic lymphoma kinase; CapeOX: capecitabine, oxaliplatin; EGFR: epidermal growth factor receptor; FOLFIRI: 5FU, leucovorin, irinotecan; FOLFOX: 5FU, leucovorin, oxaliplatin; IHC: immunohistochemistry; MSI: microsatellite instability; PDL1: programmed death ligand 1; TKI: tyrosine kinase inhibitor; TME: total mesorectal excision)

FOLLOW-UP AND SURVIVORSHIP ISSUES

Due to advancements in cancer diagnosis and treatment, a majority of cancer patients get cured and survive for many years. Once the treatment is completed, they are advised for regular follow-up as per the standard guidelines. The need for structured follow-up with clinical examination and imaging as and when required cannot be overemphasized in oncology. Follow-up helps to detect any recurrence and more importantly, to identify any posttreatment late-term side effects which can cause morbidity to the patient and impair their physical, psychological, emotional, social, and economic rehabilitation.

Like in pediatric patients, adult patients also have late-term side effects such as cardiac failure (anthracyclines, anti-HER2 therapy, chest radiation), endocrine insufficiency (antiestrogens, androgen blockade, cranial and neck radiation), infertility (chemotherapy, stem cell transplant, radiation), cognitive impairment (brain tumor surgery, radiation, chemotherapy), psychosocial (self-image in mastectomy, head and neck surgery), and sexual (lack of libido— hormonal therapy, vaginal dryness—radiation to reproductive organs). General physicians also play a significant role in detecting them and in treating them. Social and economic rehabilitation needs support from governmental and NGOs.

CONCLUSION

Oncology is a challenging yet fascinating branch of clinical medicine. Its spectrum extends from basic translational research to survivorship issues and exists firmly on evidence-based medicine along with compassionate care. The basic concepts of solid tumors discussed in this chapter should provide a solid platform for the students of medicine to know more about them and take up the responsibility to advance the clinical care and cancer research in our country.

RECOMMENDED READINGS

1. International Agency for Research on Cancer; World Health Organization. Global Cancer Observatory. [Online] Available from https://gco.iarc.fr/.
2. Mathur P, Sathishkumar K, Chaturvedi M, Das P, Sudarshan KL, Santhappan S, et al. Cancer Statistics, 2020: Report From National Cancer Registry Programme, India. JCO Glob Oncol. 2020;6:1063-75.
3. Tomasetti C, Li L, Vogelstein B. Stem cell divisions, somatic mutations, cancer etiology, and cancer prevention. Science. 2017;355(6331):1330-34.
4. Chaturvedi P, Singh A, Chien CY, Warnakulasuriya S. Tobacco related oral cancer. BMJ. 2019;365:l2142.
5. Scott JM, Stene G, Edvardsen E, Jones LW. Performance status in cancer: Not broken, but time for an upgrade? JCO. 2020;38(25):2824-9.
6. Taberna M, Moncayo FG, Jané-Salas E, Antonio M, Arribas L, Vilajosana E, et al. The multidisciplinary team (MDT) approach and quality of care. Front Oncol. 2020;10:85.
7. Schwartz LH, Litière S, de Vries E, Ford R, Gwyther S, Mandrekar S, et al. RECIST 1.1-update and clarification: From the RECIST committee. Eur J Cancer. 2016;62:132-7.
8. Jadvar H, Chen X, Cai W, Mahmood U. Radiotheranostics in cancer diagnosis and management. Radiology. 2018;286(2):388-400.
9. Bousquet G, Orri M, Winterman S, Brugière C, Verneuil L, Revah-Levy A. Breaking bad news in oncology: A metasynthesis. J Clin Oncol. 2015;33(22):2437-43.
10. Temel JS, Greer JA, Muzikansky A, Gallagher ER, Admane S, Jackson VA, et al. Early palliative care for patients with metastatic non-small-cell lung cancer. NEJM. 2010;363:733-42.
11. Drilon A, Postow M, Vasan N, Carlo MI. Pocket Oncology, 2nd edition. USA: Lippincott Williams & Wilkins; 2018.
12. DeVita VT, Lawrence TS, Rosenberg SA. DeVita, Hellman, and Rosenberg's Cancer: Principles & Practice of Oncology, 10th edition. USA: Lippincott Williams & Wilkins; 2018.
13. D'Cruz AK, Vaish R, Kapre N, Dandekar M, Gupta S, Hawalda R, et al. Elective versus therapeutic neck dissection in node-negative oral cancer. NEJM. 2015;373:521-29.
14. Badwe R, Hawaldar R, Nair N, Kaushik R, Parmar V, Siddique S, et al. Locoregional treatment versus no treatment of the primary tumour in metastatic breast cancer: an open-label randomised controlled trial. Lancet Oncol. 2015;16(13):1380-8.
15. Murthy V, Maitre P, Kannan S, Panigrahi G, Krishnatry R, Bakshi G, et al. Prostate-only versus whole-pelvic radiation therapy in high-risk and very high-risk prostate cancer (POP-RT): Outcomes from phase III randomized controlled trial. J Clin Oncol. 2021;39(11):1234-42.
16. Shastri SS, Mittra I, Mishra GA, Gupta S, Dikshit R, Singh S, et al. Effect of VIA screening by primary health workers: randomized controlled study in Mumbai, India. J Natl Cancer Inst. 2014;106(3):dju009.
17. Gupta S, Maheshwari A, Parab P, Mahantshetty U, Hawaldar R, Sastri Chopra S, et al. Neoadjuvant chemotherapy followed by radical surgery versus concomitant chemotherapy and radiotherapy in patients with stage IB2, IIA, or IIB Squamous Cervical Cancer: A randomized controlled trial. J Clin Oncol. 2018;36(16):1548-55.
18. Chopra SJ, Mathew A, Maheshwari A, Bhatla N, Singh S, Rai B, et al. National Cancer Grid of India Consensus Guidelines on the Management of Cervical Cancer. J Glob Oncol. 2018;4:1-15.

CHAPTER 161

Chemotherapy: Principles, Classification, and Toxicity

Manjinder Singh

ABSTRACT

Chemotherapy is systemic therapy for cancer which can be used for curative or palliative intent. Furthermore, based on sequence with local therapy (like surgery) it can be referred as neoadjuvant, concurrent, or adjuvant when given before, along, or after the local therapy, respectively. It is important to note that because only a fraction of the cells in a tumor dies with each treatment (fractional kill), repeated doses must be administered to continue to reduce the size of the tumor.

Based on mode of action chemotherapy are classified as alkylating agents [alkylate proteins and deoxyribonucleic acid (DNA)], antimetabolites [impede DNA and ribonucleic acid (RNA) synthesis], antimicrotubule agents (block cell division by preventing microtubule function), topoisomerase inhibitors (inhibitor of topoisomerase I or II interferes), and cytotoxic antibiotics (interrupt cell division). All these drugs finally lead to apoptosis and cell death. Most chemotherapy drugs are delivered intravenously, as day care procedure through vascular access devices like chemo port or peripherally inserted central catheter (PICC) line.

Chemotherapy drugs mainly affect the fast dividing cells of the body, which is the cause of adverse effects related to chemotherapy. To give an illustration, immunosuppression and myelosuppression occur due to damage of blood cells lead to anemia and neutropenia. Similarly, damage of cells lining the mouth, stomach, and intestines in turn causes mucositis, nausea, vomiting, anorexia, diarrhea, abdominal cramps, and enterocolitis. Likewise, alopecia and infertility are due to damage of hair follicle and gonads. In addition, some chemotherapy agents are cardiotoxic, nephrotoxic, hepatotoxic and ototoxic. To conclude, chemotherapy is one of the important component of oncology treatment provided firstly, it is planned as per performance status of patients secondly, be aware of its toxicity.

"The human spirit is stronger than anything that can happen to it"

—CC Scott

INTRODUCTION

Chemotherapy (often abbreviated to chemo) utilizes drugs that cause selective damage to fast dividing cells by inducing DNA damage leading to programmed cell death known as apoptosis. Systematic therapy is approach to introduce these drugs into blood stream thus is able kill any cancer cells at any anatomic location in body. Systemic therapy is often used in conjunction with local therapy (i.e., surgery or radiotherapy).

TREATMENT STRATEGIES

When cancer is curable then the intent of treatment with chemotherapy is curative. On the other hand, in metastatic disease the aim is palliative to relief the symptoms.

- *Upfront chemotherapy*: This strategy is used for a goal of curative intend.
- *Combined modality chemotherapy* is the use of drugs with other cancer treatment, such as surgery or radiotherapy.
- *Consolidation chemotherapy* is given after remission. In addition, same drug regimen is used as was used in to achieve remission.
- *Intensification chemo strategy* is identical to consolidate chemotherapy with different drug which is used for upfront chemotherapy.
- *Chemotherapy in combination*: Here different combination of drug is used which have different mechanism and side effects. It is important to note that its major advantage is to deal with drug resistance. Furthermore, dose reduction of drugs minimizes toxicity.
- *Neoadjuvant chemotherapy* is given before the local treatment such as surgery, with the aim to downstage/shrink the primary tumor. Furthermore, in tumors with high risk of micrometastasis this strategy is useful.
- *Adjuvant chemotherapy*: This strategy is used for curative tumors after a primary treatment (radiotherapy or surgery) to minimize risk of recurrence, specifically to treat micrometastases thus reducing relapse rate.
- *Maintenance strategy*: These used low-dose chemotherapy protocols to prolong the achieved remission.
- *Salvage or palliative chemotherapy*: This strategy is used in palliative setting when disease has widespread, to decrease tumor burden and to give good quality of expected life.

Dosage of chemotherapy is based on *performance status*. Chemotherapy kill of tumor follows bell-shaped distribution, i.e., cause fractionated kill. Due to this, repeated doses must be administered to continue to reduce the size of the tumor. To minimize toxicity repeated cycles of chemotherapy are given at fixed interval.

The overall effectiveness of chemotherapy depends on chemosensitivity of tumor. It ranges from being curative for some cancers like leukemia, partially effective for tumors like brain tumors and ineffective for tumors nonmelanoma skin.

DOSAGE

Dose response relationship of cell killing by chemotherapeutic drugs on normal and cancer cells is shown in **Figure 1**. Cancer cells follow a Gompertzian model of growth (**Fig. 2**). The ratio of proliferating cancer cells to total cells continues to decrease with increasing tumor size. Consequently, the tumor growth curve has

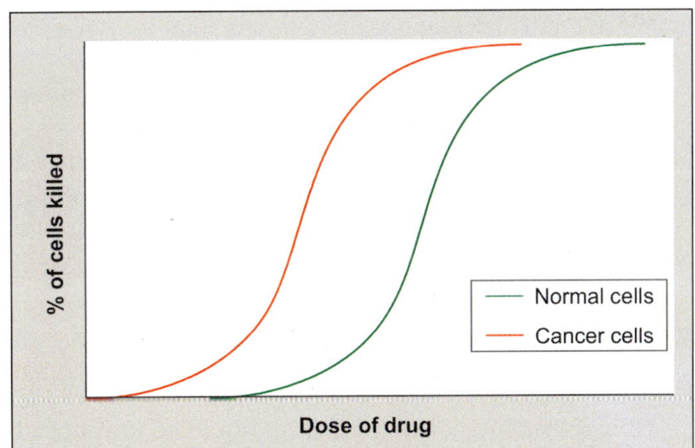

FIGURE 1: Dose response relationship of cell killing by chemotherapeutic drugs on normal and cancer cells. At high doses the percentage of normal and cancer cells killed is very similar. For this reason, doses are chosen where antitumor activity exceeds normal cell death.

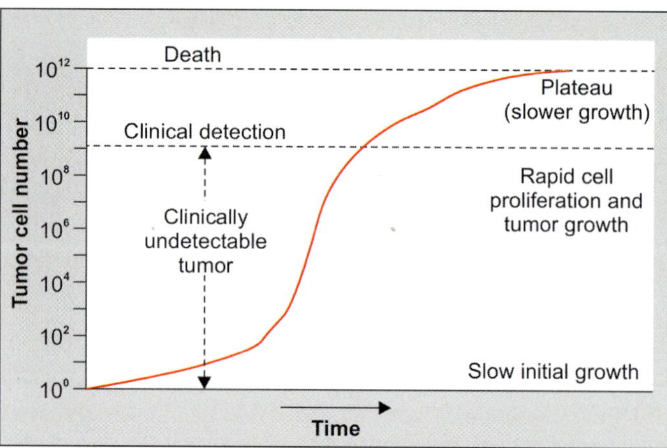

FIGURE 2: Gompertzian model of tumor growth.

N7 interstrand crosslinked DNA

FIGURE 3: Two deoxyribonucleic acid (DNA) bases that are crosslinked by a nitrogen mustard. Different nitrogen mustards will have different chemical groups (R). The nitrogen mustards most commonly alkylate the N7 nitrogen of guanine (as shown here) but other atoms can be alkylated.

TABLE 1 Subtypes and examples of alkylating agents.

Subtypes	Examples
Nitrogen mustards	Mechlorethamine, cyclophosphamide, melphalan, chlorambucil, ifosfamide, and busulfan
Nitrosoureas	N-Nitroso-N-methylurea (MNU), carmustine (BCNU), lomustine (CCNU), semustine (MeCCNU), fotemustine, and streptozotocin
Tetrazines	Dacarbazine, mitozolomide, and temozolomide
Aziridines	Thiotepa, mitomycin, and diaziquone (AZQ)
Cisplatin and derivatives	Cisplatin, carboplatin, and oxaliplatin
Nonclassical alkylating agents	Procarbazine and hexamethylmelamine

three distinct parts: A slow initial phase, a middle phase characterized by rapid growth, and a slow plateau phase. Chemotherapy drugs which target only rapidly proliferating cells, consequently kills only a small fraction of cells when the cancer is advanced and the tumor is large, but kills a higher fraction of cells when the tumor is small or when the cancer is clinically undetectable.

Dosage of chemotherapy has to be such that it should not be too low, neither too high which can lead to toxicity. Method for determining chemotherapy dosage is based on calculated body surface area (BSA). The BSA is usually calculated with a mathematical formula, using the recipient's weight and height.

VARIOUS GROUPS OF CHEMOTHERAPY

ALKYLATING AGENTS

One of first chemotherapeutics group to be introduced was alkylating agents (**Table 1**). These were first originally derived from mustard gas used in World War I, there are now many types of alkylating agents in use. They are named so because of their ability to alkylate many molecules, including proteins, RNA, and DNA. The alkylating agents block covalently to DNA via their alkyl group (**Fig. 3**). This is main mode of action and primary cause for their anticancer effects. These molecules crosslink with DNA chain either by binding twice to one of DNA strand which is called intrastrand crosslink or by binding once to both DNA strand which is called interstrand crosslinks. If the cell tries to replicate crosslinked DNA during cell division, or tries to repair it, the DNA strands can break leading to apoptosis. Alkylating agents are cell cycle independent group of chemotherapy drugs because they can work at any point on cell cycle.

ANTIMETABOLITE AGENTS

Antimetabolites group has chemotherapy agents which have structure similar to building blocks of DNA and RNA thus impede DNA and RNA synthesis. These building blocks of DNA and RNA are called nucleotides (**Fig. 4**). These chemotherapy drugs resemble nucleotides, but have altered chemical groups and exert their effect by either blocking the enzymes required for DNA synthesis or becoming incorporated into DNA or RNA thus prevent mitosis. In addition, misincorporation of these molecules into DNA causes DNA damage leading to apoptosis. Unlike alkylating agents, antimetabolites are cell cycle dependent as they work only in S-phase (the DNA synthesis phase) of cell cycle (**Table 2**).

ANTIMICROTUBULE GROUP OF DRUGS

These agents are derived from plant and they block cell division by preventing microtubule function. More specifically, the two proteins which are building block of microtubules, α-tubulin and β-tubulin. These tubulins are hollow rod-shaped structures that are required for cell division and for cellular functions. Vinca alkaloids and taxanes are the two main groups of antimicrotubule agents which causes microtubule dysfunction (**Table 3**). Vinca alkaloids prevent the assembly of microtubules, whereas taxanes prevent their disassembly. By doing so, they inhibit mitosis leading to apoptosis. In addition, these drugs can also affect blood vessel growth (**Fig. 5**).

Deoxycytidine | Gemcitabine | Decitabine

FIGURE 4: Deoxycytidine (left) and two antimetabolite drugs (centre and right); gemcitabine and decitabine. The drugs are very similar but they have subtle differences in their chemical structure.

TABLE 2 Subtypes and examples of antimetabolites.

Subtypes	Examples
Antifolates	Methotrexate and pemetrexed
Fluoropyrimidines	Fluorouracil and capecitabine
Deoxynucleoside analogs	Cytarabine, gemcitabine, decitabine, azacitidine, fludarabine, nelarabine, cladribine, clofarabine, and pentostatin
Thiopurines	Thioguanine and mercaptopurine

The source of vinca alkaloids is *Catharanthus roseus*, formally called *Vinca rosea*.

Taxanes can be produced naturally like the first drug of this class called paclitaxel, which was originally extracted from *Taxus brevifolia*. Now this drug and other drugs of this class like docetaxel are produced semisynthetically from a chemical found in the bark of another tree called *Taxus baccata*.

Podophyllotoxin is also obtained from plant source primarily from *Podophyllum peltatum* and *Sinopodophyllum hexandrum*. Mode of action of it is microtubule inhibition, action similar to vinca alkaloids. The two drugs in this class are etoposide and teniposide.

TOPOISOMERASE INHIBITORS

Topoisomerase inhibitors inhibit topoisomerase I and topoisomerase II enzyme causing mismatch of unwinding of DNA. Irinotecan and topotecan are two topoisomerase inhibitors which are derived semisynthetically form Chinese tree called *Camptotheca acuminata*. Drugs which act on topoisomerase II are further divided into two major groups. First group mode of action is to increase levels of enzymes bound to DNA, thus preventing DNA replication and transcription leading to programmed cell kill. Drugs under this group are etoposide, teniposide, mitoxantrone, and doxorubicin. The second group includes novobiocin, merbarone, and aclarubicin. These are catalytic inhibitors, which block activity of topoisomerase II thus prevents DNA synthesis, translation, and thus inhibiting unwinding of DNA leading to apoptosis (**Fig. 6**).

CYTOTOXIC ANTIBIOTICS

The cytotoxic antibiotics in common interrupt cell division. Some prominent examples include anthracyclines, bleomycins, mitomycin C, and actinomycin.

Among cytotoxic antibiotics, first to be discovered were doxorubicin and daunorubicin from a bacterium named *Streptomyces peucetius*. Further derivative of these

TABLE 3 Subtypes and examples of antimicrotubule.

Subtypes	Examples
Vinca alkaloids	Vincristine, vinblastine, vinorelbine, vindesine, and vinflunine
Taxanes	Paclitaxel and docetaxel

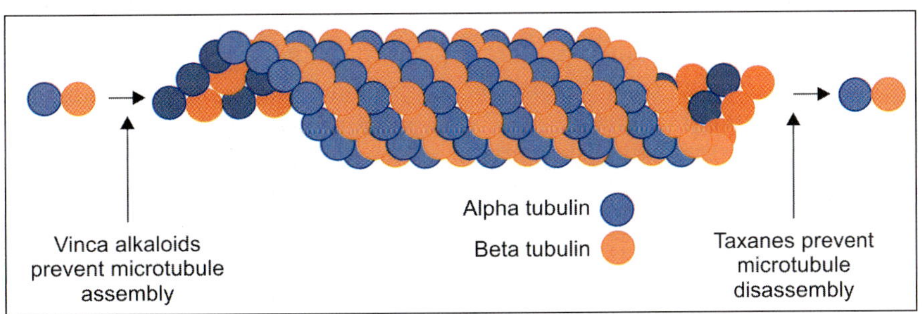

FIGURE 5: Vinca alkaloids prevent the assembly of microtubules, whereas taxanes prevent their disassembly. Both mechanisms cause defective mitosis.

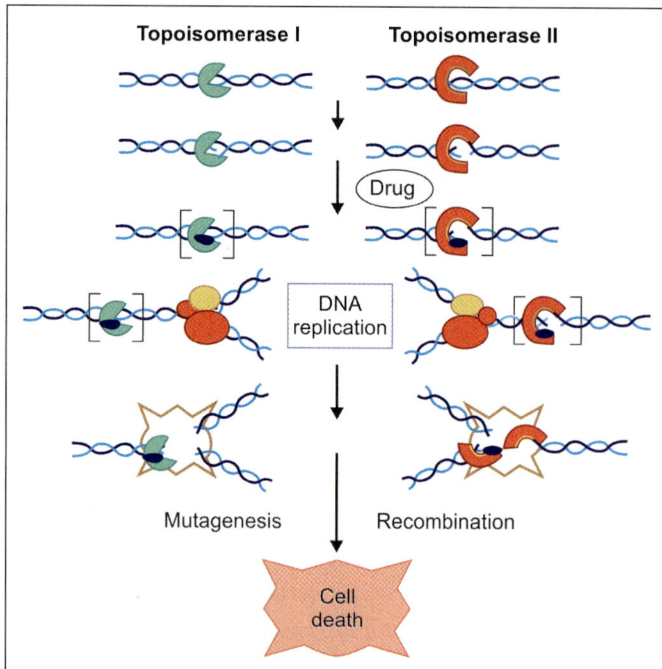

(DNA: deoxyribonucleic acid)

FIGURE 6: Topoisomerase inhibitors.

compounds lead to discovery of pirarubicin and epirubicin. Other important clinically used drugs in chemotherapy regimens of anthracycline group are mitoxantrone, aclarubicin, and pirarubicin. The three main mode of action of these drugs is that these agents insert between the two strands of DNA, process known as intercalation, generation of free radicals which damage intercellular molecules, and topoisomerase inhibition.

Actinomycin drug intercalate DNA and thus prevent RNA synthesis.

Bleomycin is isolated form bacterium named *Streptomyces verticillus*. It is a glycopeptide which damages the DNA firstly by intercalating with it and secondly by generation of free radicals which occur once bleomycin binds to a metal ion, hence become chemically reduced and reacts with oxygen.

Cytotoxic antibiotic which acts by alkylating DNA is Mitomycin.

DELIVERY

Majority of chemotherapy drugs are given intravenously, although some of agents can be administered orally like melphalan, busulfan, and capecitabine. According to a recent (2016) systematic review, oral therapies present additional challenges for patients and care teams to maintain and support adherence to treatment plans.

There are many intravenous methods of drug delivery, known as vascular access devices, which includes:

- Winged infusion device
- Peripheral venous catheter
- Midline catheter
- PICC
- Central venous catheter, and
- Implantable port

The devices have different applications regarding duration of chemotherapy treatment, method of delivery, and types of chemotherapeutic agent.

Chemotherapy regimens may be given on either an inpatient or an outpatient basis as per stage and type of regimen used. For continuous infusion regimens, such as over 24–48 hours infusion, various systems may be surgically inserted into vasculature to maintain access. Commonly used systems are the Hickman line, the port-a-cath, and the PICC line. Main advantages of these are low risk of contamination, much less prone to extravasation, and they eliminate the need of repeated peripheral cannulation.

Another approach is known as isolated limb perfusion. It is used to administer chemotherapy in cases of melanoma or lung tumors. Goal of this approach is to deliver a very high tumoricidal dose of chemotherapy to the tumor site without causing much systemic side effects. This approach is mainly used to treat oligometastatic disease (two to five sites of metastasis), and not wide spread metastatic or micrometastasis disease, hence are not defined as systematic.

Topical application of some chemotherapy drugs which are available as emulsions like 5-flurocils are mainly used for nonmelanoma skin cancers.

When chemotherapy agents are injected in cerebrospinal fluid (CSF) fluid this is as intrathecal therapy and is mainly indicated for widespread central nervous system or meningeal spread metastasis.

ADVERSE EFFECTS

In addition to cancer cells chemotherapeutic medications affect mainly the fast dividing cells of the body, such as blood forming cells and cells lining the gastrointestinal (GI) tract, i.e., cell lining mouth, stomach, and intestines. Common chemotherapy-related side effects are enumerated in **Figure 7**. Chemotherapy-related toxicities can be acute or chronic.

IMMUNOSUPPRESSION AND MYELOSUPPRESSION

Chemotherapeutic regimens weakens the immune system of body, often by paralyzing the bone marrow and leading to a decrease of white blood cells, red blood cells, and platelets. Anemia and thrombocytopenia may require blood transfusion. Neutropenia (a decrease of the neutrophil granulocyte count below 0.5×10^9/L) needs colony stimulating factors like filgrastim.

Patients undergoing chemotherapy are advised to take precautions such as to wash their hands regularly, avoid contact with sick peoples, and to take other infection-reducing steps. It is important to note that about 85% of infections which occur in immunocompromised patients are due to commensals which are naturally occurring microorganisms in the person's own GI tract and skin. Myelosuppression may manifest as systematic infection

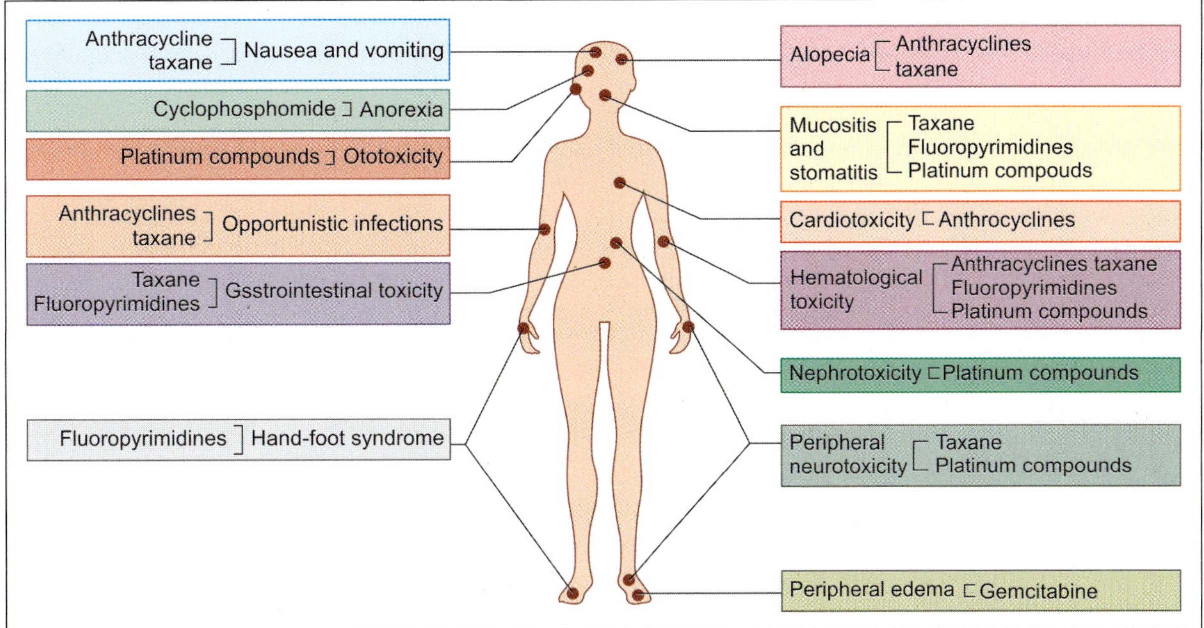

FIGURE 7: Common chemotherapy-related side effects.

leading to sepsis or can manifest as localized infection like herpes simples or shingles.

NEUTROPENIC ENTEROCOLITIS

In neutropenic patients, neutropenic enterocolitis (typhlitis) is a "life-threatening GI complication of chemotherapy". These patients usually manifest with symptoms of vomiting, diarrhea, abdomen distension, fever, chills, or abdomen tenderness.

Typhlitis being a medical emergency with poor prognosis and needs prompt treatment.

GASTROINTESTINAL DISTRESS

Among patient undergoing chemotherapy most commonly and most feared side effect reported are nausea and vomiting. Moreover, this was also addressed by Coates et al. in 1983. CINV is term used for chemotherapy-induced nausea and vomiting. These are common with many chemotherapeutic regimens. Presently there are many new antiemetics such as aprepitant and palonosetron which are used along with emeset and dexamethasone to take care of acute and delayed onset nausea and vomiting due to various chemotherapy regimens.

ANEMIA

Anemia can be due to direct damage of red blood cells by myelosuppressive chemotherapy regimens or due to indirect related to cancer such as bleeding or hemolysis, addition anemia also results due to underlying hereditary disease, kidney disorder, nutritional deficiencies, or due to anemia of chronic disease. Various treatment options to treat anemia include iron supplements, erythropoietin, or blood transfusions. Fatigue occurs due to cancer or its treatment. Aerobic exercise has been found to reduce fatigue.

HAIR LOSS

Alopecia is caused by chemotherapy as hair follicles are also rapidly dividing cells. Hair loss is not permanent side effect of cancer chemotherapy. Sometimes when hair regrow, they become curly which is referred as "chemo curls". Common drugs causing alopecia are doxorubicin, daunorubicin, paclitaxel, docetaxel, cyclophosphamide, ifosfamide, and etoposide.

Chemotherapy induced hair loss are more in women than men.

Scalp cooling offers a means of preventing temporary hair loss; however, concerns about this method have been raised.

SECONDARY NEOPLASM

Development of secondary neoplasia after successful chemotherapy treatment can occur. The most common secondary neoplasm is secondary acute myeloid leukemia, which develops primarily after treatment with alkylating agents or topoisomerase inhibitors.

INFERTILITY

Some types of chemotherapy are gonadotoxic and may cause infertility. High-risk group include alkylating agents, busulfan, chlorambucil, and chlormethine. Medium risk includes platinum agents such as cisplatin and carboplatin and doxorubicin. Low-risk agents include plant derivatives, e.g., vincristine, vinblastine, antibiotics such as dactinomycin and bleomycin, and antimetabolites such as methotrexate (MTX), 5- fluorouracil, and 6-mercaptopurine (6-MP).

Premature ovarian failure is cause of female infertility induced by chemotherapy.

Young patients can opt for fertility preservation prior to chemotherapy by cryopreservation of semen, ovarian tissue, oocytes, or embryos.

TERATOGENICITY

Chemotherapy is teratogenic during pregnancy, especially during the trimester. Teratogenic and risk to cognitive development is not increased during second and third trimester exposure to chemotherapy agents, however it may increase risk of other complications and myelosuppression associated with pregnancy.

In males and females who previously have undergone chemotherapy, there appears to be no increase in genetic defects in their children conceived after therapy. However, possibility of genetic mutations in oocytes exists, especially if in vitro fertilization, and cryopreservations are practiced between or shortly after chemotherapy.

PERIPHERAL NEUROPATHY

Around 30% of patients undergoing chemotherapy experience chemotherapy-induced peripheral neuropathy (CIPN), a progressive, enduring, and often irreversible condition, causing pain, tingling, numbness and sensitivity to cold, beginning in the hands and feet. CINP is mainly observed in regimens which include vinca alkaloids, taxanes, platinum drugs, thalidomide, and epothilone. Usually patient present with sensory symptoms, but is some cases presentation may be motor or autonomic. CIPN usually manifest after first cycle of chemotherapy dosage and usually progress with further cycles, but this progression usually levels off at completion of treatment.

COGNITIVE IMPAIRMENT

Post-chemotherapy cognitive impairment, referred to as "chemo brain". This category includes nonspecific neurocognitive issues such as fatigue, lack of sleep, or lack of concentration.

TUMOR LYSIS SYNDROME

This syndrome is mainly seen in bulky tumors and tumors with high white cell counts, such as lymphomas, teratomas, and some leukemia. Tumor lysis syndrome is consequence of rapid breakdown of cancer cells which causes the release of chemicals. This leads to accumulation of high levels of uric acid, potassium, chloride, and phosphate in the blood. Secondary hypoparathyroidism, resulting in low levels of calcium in the blood occur due to high levels of phosphate. This results in kidney damage and cardiac arrhythmia due to high potassium levels. In cancers suspected to have tumor lysis syndrome after treatment, prophylaxis is started by adequate hydration before chemotherapy to minimize the risk, however this is a dangerous side effect that can lead to death if left untreated.

ORGAN DAMAGE

Cardiotoxicity (heart damage) is especially prominent with the use of anthracycline drugs (doxorubicin, epirubicin, idarubicin, and liposomal doxorubicin). Mechanism of action of cardia toxicity is the production of free radicals.

Many cytotoxic drugs cause hepatotoxicity (liver damage). This hepatotoxicity of chemotherapy has a direct effect by damage to liver cells or cause indirect damage by inducing hepatic sinusoidal syndrome, cholestasis, or liver fibrosis.

Nephrotoxicity (kidney damage) can be caused by tumor lysis syndrome and also due direct effects of drug clearance by the kidneys.

Ototoxicity mainly by damage to the inner ear is main side effect of platinum-based drugs. This damage to inner ear cells produces symptoms such as dizziness and vertigo.

OTHER SIDE EFFECTS

Some drugs can cause erythematous skin, dry skin, xerostomia, fluid retention, and sexual dysfunction.

RECOMMENDED READINGS

1. Rachel A. Cancer chemotherapy: Basic Science to the Clinic. Chichester: Wiley-Blackwell; 2009.
2. Wood M, Brighton D. The Royal Marsden Hospital Handbook of Cancer Chemotherapy: A Guide for the Multidisciplinary Team. St. Louis, Mo: Elsevier Churchill Livingstone; 2005.
3. Perry MJ. The Chemotherapy Source Book. Philadelphia: Wolters Kluwer Health/Lippincott Williams & Wilkins; 2008.
4. Skeel RT. Handbook of Cancer Chemotherapy (paperback), 6th edition. Philadelphia: Lippincott Williams & Wilkins; 2003.
5. Chabner B, Longo DL. Cancer Chemotherapy and Biotherapy: Principles and Practice, 4th edition. Philadelphia: Lippincott Willians & Wilkins; 2005.
6. Lind MJ, Principles of cytotoxic chemotherapy. Medicine. 2008;36(1):19-23.
7. Greer JA, Amoyal N, Nisotel L, Fishbein JN, MacDonald J, Stagl J, et al. A Systematic Review of Adherence to Oral Antineoplastic Therapies. Oncologist. 2016;21(3): 354-76.
8. Huang ES, Wilson Tang WH, Lee DS, Thomson CC, Fischer MA. Internal Medicine: Handbook for Clinicians, Resident Survival Guide. Arlington VA, ISBN 0964546752 (1.9.2000).

CHAPTER

162

Radiotherapy: Principles, Methods, and Application

Subhadeep Bose, Davinder Paul

ABSTRACT

Last two decades have seen unpresented advancements in understanding the basic hallmarks of cancer development, which has resulted in innumerable new treatment options for cancer treatment. Despite this, in view of increasing global burden of cancer, the clinical management of cancer still continues to be a major global health care challenge. Cancer treatment modalities comprises radiation therapy, surgery, chemotherapy, immunotherapy, and hormonal therapy. Radiation therapy continues to remain an important component of cancer treatment with approximately 50% of all cancer patients requiring radiation therapy during the course of their treatment. At most of the sites, radiotherapy is given with a curative intent.

The basic concept of radiotherapy is to cause direct tumor kill and to deprive cancer cells of their multiplying capability. Over the last 100 years, continued advancements in the type of radiotherapy delivery systems and widening indications, supported by the progress in understanding the biology of cancer response to radiotherapy, has led to improved survival and simultaneously reduced radiotherapy side-effects, especially long-term side-effects. Recognizing the role of radiotherapy in cancer alleviation over last 100 years, since Marie Curie won her second Noble prize for her research on radium, year 2011 was designated as year of radiation therapy. In this chapter, we will be discussing the principles, various methods, and applications of radiotherapy in the clinical practice.

"Be patient and tough; some day this pain will be useful to you"

—Ovid

INTRODUCTION

Radiation therapy represents an essential modality in the treatment of patients with many different types of malignancy and differs significantly from other commonly used modalities such as surgery and systemic therapy in its delivery and mechanism of action. Role of radiotherapy, as a means of cancer treatment came into picture after the discovery of X-rays by Wilhelm Conrad Rontgen in 1895. In 1911, Marie Curie won her second Nobel Prize for her research into radium, establishing her as a pioneer in the field of radiation therapy. Along with surgery and medical oncology, radiation therapy remains an important and integral modality in cancer treatment worldwide. About approximately 50% of all cancer patients will receive radiation therapy during their course of anticancer treatment.

Rapid progress in this field continues to be boosted by advances in imaging techniques, computerized treatment planning systems, radiation treatment machines (with improved X-ray production and treatment delivery) as well as improved understanding of the radiobiology of radiation therapy. The purpose of this chapter is to provide a review of the basics of radiation oncology, including an introduction to radiation biology and radiation physics, a summary of patient workflow and treatment delivery and finally, an evaluation of alternative radiation techniques beyond conventional external beam radiation therapy.

RADIATION BIOLOGY AND PHYSICS

Radiation therapy is primarily delivered using external beam radiation therapy via a linear accelerator with the predominant treatment mode being high-energy photons or X-rays, which are nonparticulate form of radiation. These photons represent ionizing radiation and are part of the electromagnetic spectrum. Alternatives to photons are the particulate form of radiation including electrons (available on linear accelerators) and to a lesser degree protons and neutrons (separate devices). **Table 1** documents the various types of radiation. Photon-based radiation therapy is considered indirectly ionizing, in that it does not produce damage directly for the most part but instead has its energy transferred to secondary particles (usually electrons), which produce deoxyribonucleic acid (DNA) damage. This primarily occurs through the Compton process for photons. Heavy charged particles, though less frequently used, are directly ionizing and can cause damage without secondary particles.

Radiation therapy causes biologic effects through DNA damage, in particular double stranded DNA breaks. DNA damage occurs through interactions between particles and DNA, which can occur directly or indirectly, as shown in **Figure 1**. Direct action occurs when the photon transfers energy to an electron, which subsequently interacts with the DNA. Indirect action occurs when the secondary electron interacts to produce free radicals, which can then damage

TABLE 1 Various types of radiation.

Name	Description
Alpha particles	(High energy) helium nuclei consisting of two protons and two neutrons
Beta particles	(High energy) electrons
Positron	Particles with same mass as an electron but with 1 unit of positive charge
Proton	Nuclei of hydrogen atoms
Neutron	Particles with a mass approximately equal to that of a proton but with no charge
Gamma ray	Very high energy electromagnetic radiation

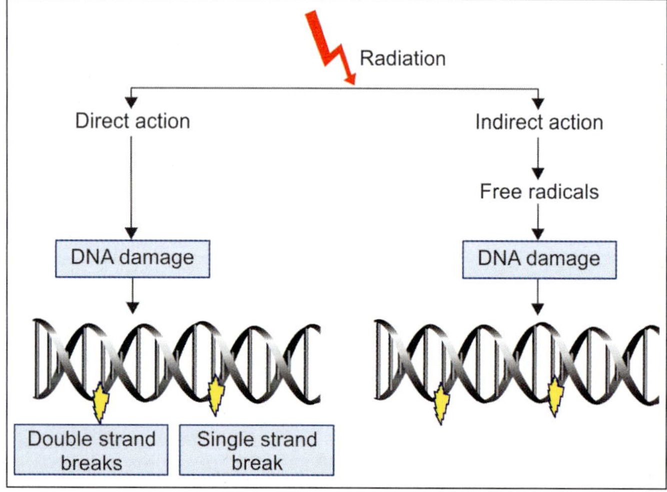

(DNA: deoxyribonucleic acid)

FIGURE 1: Direct and indirect methods of DNA damage by radiotherapy.

DNA. Photon-based radiation therapy works primarily through indirect action while heavy charged particles work primarily through direct action.

Radiation therapy is typically delivered via fractionation, with multiple small radiation doses delivered, allowing for a higher total dose to be delivered, and increasing tumor control probability while reducing the risk of normal tissue toxicity. It should be noted that with improvements in treatment planning, treatment delivery, and image guidance, there is a renewed interest in hypofractionation (larger doses per fraction); further the development of stereotactic body radiotherapy (SBRT) allows for the delivery of radiation therapy in five fractions or less using large doses per fraction.

The four fundamental radiobiologic principles guiding standard fractionation and clinical radiation oncology are: (1) Repair, (2) Reassortment, (3) Repopulation, and (4) Reoxygenation.

Repair: It is essential and one of the key reasons for fractionation. After receiving photon-based radiation therapy, normal tissue cells are able to repair sublethal damage, limiting toxicity while cancer cells are limited in their abilities to repair sublethal damage, and allowing for an improvement in the therapeutic ratio with fractionation.

Reassortment: It is important because cancer cells have varying degrees of radiosensitivity based on the stage of the cell cycle they are in, with the G2-M phase being the most radiosensitive and the S phase being the least sensitive. As such, fractionation allows for reassortment of cells into more radiosensitive phases of the cell cycle, enhancing cell kill.

Repopulation: It is important for two reasons; repopulation with fractionation allows for normal tissues to recover if an adequate time interval is introduced. More importantly, some malignancies have been shown to clinically demonstrate repopulation (e.g., head and neck cancer, cervical cancer) during treatment requiring clinicians to complete treatment within a certain duration of time or risk suboptimal local control and outcomes.

Reoxygenation: It represents a key principle of radiation sensitivity and damage. As most radiation is delivered with photons, the primary mechanism of DNA damage is indirect action via free radicals. The presence of oxygen allows "fixation" of the DNA damage caused by free radicals enhancing the impact of the radiation. Fractionation enhances reoxygenation, and increasing radiation sensitivity of tumors.

TREATMENT WORKFLOW AND DELIVERY

Regardless of treatment location, radiation oncology workflows are fairly consistent. Patients are initially seen in consultation to discuss the role of radiation therapy and inform patients regarding the potential benefits of treatment as well as acute, subacute, and chronic toxicities associated with treatment to allow for informed decision-making.

Planning: This is followed by radiation therapy planning, which begins with a simulation or planning scan. The simulation typically consists of some form of imaging; traditionally, this was done with 2-D films or fluoroscopy but this has been replaced primarily with a computed tomography (CT) simulator. At the time of simulation, immobilization is created to achieve reproducible patient positioning, depending on location [e.g., mask for central nervous system (CNS) and head and neck cases]. Immobilization can also be dependent on the type of treatment; for example, more rigid immobilization may be used when high dose treatments (e.g., SBRT) are performed. At the time of simulation, contrast can be used to enhance assessment of vasculature and lymph nodes, and 4-D scans are performed to assess the impact of respiratory motion on target and organ at risk volumes. The patient is scanned and an isocenter is placed; additionally, tattoos are commonly placed to facilitate patient setup daily.

Once simulation is complete, the images obtained are transferred to a treatment planning computer. The physician will then draw in contours or volumes for the target including the gross tumor volume (GTV), the clinical target volume (CTV), and the planning target volume (PTV) based on physical examination, imaging, and any other procedures [e.g., colonoscopy, esophagogastroduodenoscopy (EGD), and nasopharyngoscopy]. Additionally, if a 4-D scan is performed, an internal target volume (ITV) can be created to account for organ motion. Contours are also made for all critical normal tissue structures in the treatment field. A radiation plan is then created by a dosimetrist and reviewed by the physician. Once approved by the physician, a medical physicist reviews the treatment plan and it undergoes quality assurance checks which are dependent on the technique utilized.

Delivery: Modern radiation therapy is typically delivered with *a linear accelerator*. A linear accelerator working at 50–120 kV, generates high-energy photons by accelerating electrons and having them approach a target, as shown in **Figure 2**. The X-rays/photons are primarily produced when the electrons are deflected (Bremsstrahlung radiation); additionally, electrons can be used as the therapeutic particle when the target is removed. Inside the head of the linear accelerator several structures are designed to allow for safe and efficient treatment delivery. In patients treated with photons, beyond the X-ray target is a flattening filter, which creates a more uniform radiation field as well as ion chambers, which measure radiation dose, and subsequently jaws, which can shape the beam. There is a light field to visualize the treatment field as well as an optical distance indicator to measure the source to surface distance. Modern linear accelerators also include a multileaf collimator, which can be used to shape the beam. A similar set of structures is used for electron treatments with the exception of the target being removed and the use of scattering foils rather than flattening filter. Radiation therapists perform treatment delivery; treatment plans created in the treatment planning system are sent to information systems that communicate with the linear accelerator while also serving as an electronic medical record to document daily treatment.

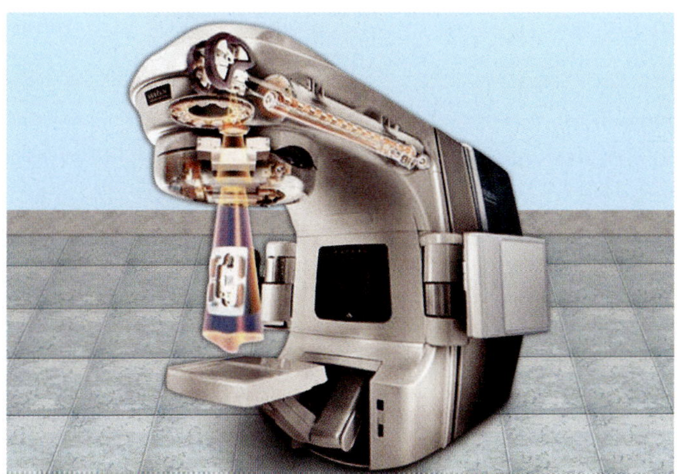

FIGURE 2: Shadow view of linear accelerator. Electron beam (originating at upper right) is accelerated through a linear accelerator wave guide, selected for correct energy in a bending magnet, and then impinges on an X-ray production target. The X-ray beam (originating at target upper left) is flattened and collimated before leaving the treatment head.

Techniques: Multiple treatment techniques can be utilized to deliver external beam radiation therapy. Modern radiation therapy primarily utilizes a *CT simulator* for treatment planning and therefore a three-dimensional approach. Beams can then be shaped using the jaws in the linear accelerator or with leaves within a multileaf collimator. Such approaches are known as three-dimensional conformal radiotherapy (3D-CRT). Over the past two decades, an alternative technique to 3D-CRT has emerged known as *intensity modulated radiation therapy (IMRT)*. IMRT allows for the modulation of the intensity of the beam, providing clinicians the ability to preferentially give dose to one area while sparing another. This is accomplished primarily through inverse treatment planning algorithms where the treatment planning system is provided dose constraints for the target and normal tissue structures (with weighting for each objective provided), as well as beam angles. IMRT is routinely performed in the treatment of many different malignancies including CNS malignancies, head and neck cancers, cancers of the thorax and abdomen, sarcomas, and genitourinary as well as gynecologic malignancies.

External beam radiation therapy can be utilized in many different scenarios. Definitive radiation therapy can be utilized in the management of some CNS tumors, lymphomas, and prostate cancers. Definitive radiation in conjunction with chemotherapy can also be utilized in the treatment of some CNS malignancies, head and neck cancers, inoperable lung cancers, esophageal cancers, pancreas cancers, gynecologic malignancies, and bladder cancers allowing for organ preservation and the potential for improved toxicity and quality of life.

Radiation therapy can also be delivered postoperatively for patients at high risk for recurrence or residual microscopic disease following surgery; this is most commonly seen in breast cancers but is also used in CNS malignancies, head and neck cancers, pancreatic cancer, sarcomas, genitourinary, and gynecologic malignancies. Finally, radiation therapy can be utilized for palliation, most commonly for bone metastases, brain metastases, lung masses, and bleeding. Common oncologic emergencies where radiation therapy is utilized include spinal cord compression, airway compromise, superior vena cava syndrome, and symptomatic brain metastases not amenable to surgery.

Radiosensitizers can be used with radiation therapy to increase the response to treatment. Clinically, this is most commonly done with the addition of concurrent chemotherapy. However, alternatives have been studied including halogenated pyrimidines and hypoxic radio-sensitizers, though both are used sparingly in the clinic at this time. Radioprotectors, compounds that protect the body from radiation, have also been explored. At this time, the only clinically utilized radioprotector is amifostine, which is utilized to prevent xerostomia with data demonstrating no difference in clinical oncologic outcomes when using amifostine in head and neck cancers.

Toxicity: Radiation therapy can be associated with acute, subacute, and chronic toxicities. The most common toxicities noted during treatment are fatigue and skin erythema/irritation. Additional acute toxicities are typically dependent on the area of the body being irradiated. Common acute and subacute side-effects are listed based on treatment site: CNS (headache, nausea, alopecia, and tinnitus), head and neck (mucositis, xerostomia, altered taste, and dysphagia), thorax (esophagitis, and pneumonitis), gastrointestinal (nausea, vomiting, and diarrhea), and genitourinary/gynecologic (urinary frequency/urgency, dysuria, diarrhea, and vaginal irritation). Acute and subacute side-effects tend to resolve within weeks to months of the completion of treatment. Chronic toxicities can be long-lasting; however, use of normal tissue toxicity constraints can limit the risk of chronic toxicities based on treatment site.

ADDITIONAL TECHNIQUES

Stereotactic radiation therapy: As noted above, stereotactic radiation therapy is a technique that allows for the delivery of highly conformal radiation treatments, allowing for large doses per fraction. With respect to terminology, stereotactic radiosurgery (SRS) is usually associated with a single fraction while SBRT typically is more than one fraction and usually up to five fractions. SRS is best known for its use in the CNS and can be performed with a linear accelerator or more specialized treatment machines (e.g., *Gamma Knife*). While most commonly associated with the treatment of brain metastases, SRS can also be used for pituitary adenomas, trigeminal neuralgia, acoustic neuromas, meningiomas, and arteriovenous malformations as well. More recently, SRS has been incorporated into the management of spine metastases as well, replacing standard radiation therapy in some cases and offering the potential for improved local control and pain control.

Stereotactic body radiation therapy (SBRT) is most commonly associated with the treatment of inoperable early stage nonsmall cell lung cancers. Promising initial data from Indiana University led to a multi-institutional study, which confirmed excellent rates of local control and an acceptable toxicity profile. Moving forward, current trials are evaluating optimal dose and fractionation schemes for peripheral and central tumors as well as comparing SBRT to surgery in operable patients. SBRT is also being utilized in the management of prostate cancer with trials evaluating five fraction regimens with promising results leading to comparisons to standard and hypofractionated radiation therapy. More recently, SBRT has been utilized to treat liver metastases and hepatocellular carcinoma (HCCs) with encouraging preliminary outcomes with respect to local control and liver toxicity as well as pancreatic cancers. Additionally, SBRT is being evaluated in a number of treatment sites including soft tissue sarcoma and head and neck cancers.

Brachytherapy is a radiation therapy technique where radioactive sources are implanted on or inside a patient. Brachytherapy can be performed with *low dose rate (LDR) implants* typically associated with prostate seed implants, or *high dose rate (HDR) implants* typically associated with temporary gynecologic or breast implants. Brachytherapy is a commonly utilized treatment in the *management of prostate cancer*. As noted above, many are familiar with LDR brachytherapy for prostate cancer with excellent clinical outcomes and toxicity profiles reported. Additionally, increasing data are available supporting HDR brachytherapy in prostate cancer, which, unlike LDR, allows for modulation of dose once catheters are in place and the potential for improved toxicity profiles. While treatment with brachytherapy in prostate cancer is primarily monotherapy, recent data are available on the use brachytherapy boost in patients with higher-risk prostate cancer.

Brachytherapy (placing radioactive material inside or on the surface of the body) has also emerged as a standard of care treatment option in appropriately selected women with *early stage breast cancer via accelerated partial breast irradiation (APBI)*, which treats the lumpectomy cavity with a margin. Initial studies evaluated APBI using multi-catheter interstitial HDR; however, more recent studies have evaluated single entry applicators, increasing the ability for patients to receive this treatment. At this time, multiple randomized trials comparing brachytherapy with standard whole breast irradiation have been performed, with no difference in local recurrence noted.

Intraoperative radiation therapy (IORT) represents a form of partial breast irradiation different from APBI and can be delivered with multiple techniques at the time of surgery; however, two randomized trials evaluating the technique have demonstrated increased rates of local recurrence compared with whole breast irradiation and as such this technique should not be considered off-protocol at this time. Brachytherapy remains an essential component in the management of gynecologic cancers; in patients with endometrial cancer, postoperative vaginal cylinder brachytherapy is routinely used based on clinical and pathologic factors while brachytherapy remains essential in the management of cervical cancers. Brachytherapy can also be utilized in head and neck cancers, as well as soft tissue sarcomas. **Figure 3** shows the various forms of radiation delivery methods in clinical use.

Proton therapy: Traditionally, radiation therapy was delivered with photons (high energy X-rays) or electrons for superficial treatments. Photons, which are the most commonly utilized form of radiation therapy, are uncharged and are known for characteristics including the need for a build-up region and dose deposition over several centimeters. Protons, on the other hand, are different than photons in that the majority of dose is deposited within a small range (few millimeters) known as the Bragg peak, which can be modulated by changing the energy of the protons. It should be noted however, this range is typically too small for clinical utilization and as such, a spread-out Bragg peak is used. The biology of protons is considered

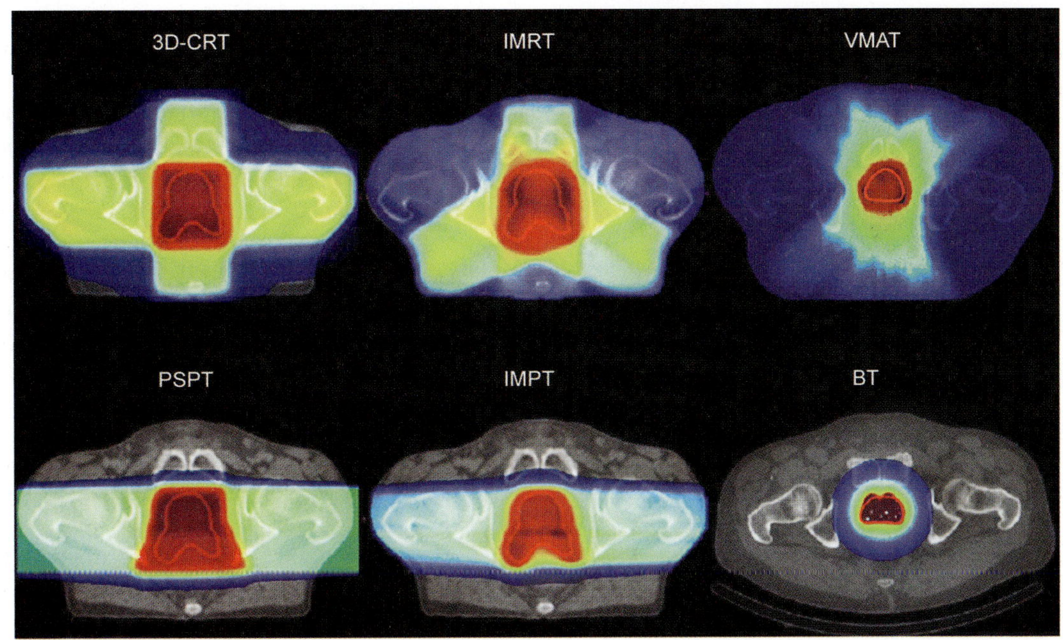

(BT: brachytherapy; 3D-CRT: 3-dimensional conformal radiotherapy; IMPT: intensity modulated proton therapy; IMRT: intensity modulated radiotherapy; PSPT: passively scattered proton therapy; VMAT: volumetric modulated arc therapy)

FIGURE 3: Examples of dose distribution of a 3D-CRT, IMRT-5, VMAT, PSPT, IMPT, and a BT treatment plan calculated on the same carcinoma prostate patient. The red surface represents the high-dose regions, the yellow surface the intermediate-high-dose regions, the dark blue surface the low dose regions, and the azure blue surface the intermediate-dose regions.

similar to photons with the advantage being primarily improved dose distribution rather than greater biologic effect as seen with neutrons for example.

While previously limited to a few centers throughout the United States, the past two decades has seen a significant expansion in the number of proton centers. One of the challenges associated with proton therapy is the amount of resources required to deliver treatment and therefore, the cost of treatment. However, proton therapy is particularly attractive for pediatric malignancies with data available supporting the utilization of protons in pediatric cancers, particularly CNS malignancies. With respect to other malignancies, much has been made of the role of protons in the management of prostate cancer. However, at this time, the data does not consistently support the utilization of protons in the management of prostate cancer and should be only performed on-protocol. Similarly, there is limited data supporting the role of protons in breast cancer; while recent data suggests protons can be used for APBI and may be cost-effective, the limited number of patients treated with this technique mandates further study before patients are routinely treated off-protocol.

Moving forward, further technological advances including intensity modulated proton therapy and advanced image guidance may allow for further improvement in outcomes with proton therapy; in the interim, in light of the limited data suggesting comparable or improved outcomes and the lack of data demonstrating cost-effectiveness, outside of accepted indications (e.g., pediatric cancers), proton therapy should be limited to use on-protocol primarily.

CONCLUSION

Radiation remains an absolutely important modality for anticancer treatment. The ongoing efforts toward designing new radiation treatment modalities and techniques are continuously improving the survival and quality of life of patients. Along with improved radiation therapy efficacy and delivery systems, minimizing radiation therapy related toxicities has also become a priority. The improvements in radiation technology have improved the sparing of normal cells/tissues through dose fractionation and conformal radiation techniques. Radiotherapy is also delivered in combination with molecular targeted therapy with the aim of further improving the therapeutic ratio of the radiation treatment.

RECOMMENDED READINGS

1. Hanahan D, Weinberg R. The hallmarks of cancer. Cell. 2000;100(1):57-70.
2. Delaney G, Jacob S, Featherstone C, Barton M. The role of radiotherapy in cancer treatment: estimating optimal utilization from a review of evidence-based clinical guidelines. Cancer. 2005;104(6):1129-37.
3. Bernier J, Hall EJ, Giaccia A. Radiation oncology: a century of achievements. Nat Rev Cancer. 2004:4(9): 737-47.
4. Eriksson D, Stigbrand T. Radiation-induced cell death mechanisms. Tumour Biol. 2010;31(4):363-72.
5. Jonathan EC, Bernhard EJ, McKenna WG. How does radiation kill cells? Curr Opin Chem Biol. 1999;3(1):77-83.

6. Atun R, Jaffray DA, Barton MB, Bray F, Baumann M, Vikram B, et al. Expanding global access to radiotherapy. Lancet Oncol. 2015;16(10):1153-86.
7. Constine LS, Milano MT, Friedman D, et al. Late effects of cancer treatment on normal tissues. In: Halperin EC, Perez CA, Brady LW (Eds). Perez, Brady's. Principles and practice of radiation oncology, 5th edition. Philedelphia: Lippincott, Williams & Wilkins; 2008. pp. 320-55.
8. Brown JM. Therapeutic targets in radiotherapy. Int J Radiat Oncol Biol Phys. 2001;49(2):319-26.
9. Tofilon PJ, Saxman S, Coleman CN. Molecular targets for radiation therapy: bringing preclinical data into clinical trials. Clin Cancer Res. 2003;9:3518-20.

MULTIPLE CHOICE QUESTIONS

To access the multiple choice questions of this Section online, kindly scan the QR code.